Cardiac Pacing, Defibrillation and Resynchronization

Dedications

To the memory of Henry Hayes (Dad) – DLH

To Mr. Satyanarayan Raju for the encouragement, insight, and willingness to look deeper even when he didn't need to . . . – SJA

To Vicki, Lindsay, Hannah, and Madeline – for your love and encouragement – PAF

Cardiac Pacing, Defibrillation and Resynchronization

A Clinical Approach

THIRD EDITION

David L. Hayes, MD
Consultant, Division of Cardiovascular Diseases
Mayo Clinic;
Professor of Medicine
College of Medicine
Mayo Clinic
Rochester, MN, USA

Samuel J. Asirvatham, MD
Consultant, Division of Cardiovascular Diseases
Mayo Clinic;
Professor of Medicine and of Pediatrics
College of Medicine
Mayo Clinic
Rochester, MN, USA

Paul A. Friedman, MD
Consultant, Division of Cardiovascular Diseases
Director, Implantable Device Lab
Mayo Clinic;
Professor of Medicine
College of Medicine
Mayo Clinic
Rochester, MN, USA

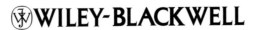

WILEY-BLACKWELL
A John Wiley & Sons, Ltd., Publication

This edition first published 2013 © 2013 by Mayo Foundation for Medical Education and Research

Wiley-Blackwell is an imprint of John Wiley & Sons, formed by the merger of Wiley's global Scientific, Technical and Medical business with Blackwell Publishing.

Registered office: John Wiley & Sons, Ltd, The Atrium, Southern Gate, Chichester, West Sussex, PO19 8SQ, UK

Editorial offices: 9600 Garsington Road, Oxford, OX4 2DQ, UK
   The Atrium, Southern Gate, Chichester, West Sussex, PO19 8SQ, UK
   111 River Street, Hoboken, NJ 07030-5774, USA

For details of our global editorial offices, for customer services and for information about how to apply for permission to reuse the copyright material in this book please see our website at www.wiley.com/wiley-blackwell

Library of Congress Cataloging-in-Publication Data
Cardiac pacing, defibrillation and resynchronization : a clinical approach / edited by David L. Hayes, Samuel J. Asirvatham, Paul A. Friedman. – 3rd ed.
    p. ; cm.
  Includes bibliographical references and index.
  ISBN 978-0-470-65833-8 (hardback : alk. paper)
  I. Hayes, David L.   II. Asirvatham, Samuel J.   III. Friedman, Paul A.   IV. Mayo Foundation for Medical Education and Research.
  [DNLM: 1. Cardiac Pacing, Artificial.   2. Cardiac Resynchronization Therapy Devices.   3. Defibrillators, Implantable.
4. Pacemaker, Artificial. WG 168]
  617.4'120645–dc23
2012021657

A catalogue record for this book is available from the British Library.

Wiley also publishes its books in a variety of electronic formats. Some content that appears in print may not be available in electronic books.

Cover image: with permission from the editors Fig. 11.43
Cover design by OptaDesign.co.uk

Set in 8.75/11 pt Minion by Toppan Best-set Premedia Limited
Printed and bound in Singapore by Markono Print Media Pte Ltd

1 2013

Contents

Contributors, vii

Preface, ix

1 Pacing and Defibrillation: Clinically Relevant Basics for Practice, 1

 T. Jared Bunch, David L. Hayes, Charles D. Swerdlow, Samuel J. Asirvatham, Paul A. Friedman

2 Hemodynamics of Cardiac Pacing: Optimization and Programming to Enhance Cardiac Function, 41

 Faisal F. Syed, David L. Hayes, Paul A. Friedman, Samuel J. Asirvatham

3 Indications for Pacemakers, ICDs and CRT: Identifying Patients Who Benefit from Cardiac Rhythm Devices, 93

 Apoor S. Gami, David L. Hayes, Samuel J. Asirvatham, Paul A. Friedman

4 Choosing the Device Generator and Leads: Matching the Device with the Patient, 133

 Malini Madhavan, David L. Hayes, Paul A. Friedman, Samuel J. Asirvatham

5 Implanting and Extracting Cardiac Devices: Technique and Avoiding Complications, 157

 Malini Madhavan, Samuel J. Asirvatham, Matthew J. Swale, David L. Hayes, Paul A. Friedman

6 Implant-Related Complications: Relevant Anatomy and an Approach for Prevention, 219

 Seth H. Sheldon, David L. Hayes, Paul A. Friedman, Samuel J. Asirvatham

7 Timing Cycles, 255

 David L. Hayes, Paul J. Wang, Samuel J. Asirvatham, Paul A. Friedman

8 Programming: Maximizing Benefit and Minimizing Morbidity Programming, 319

 Paul A. Friedman, Charles D. Swerdlow, Samuel J. Asirvatham, David L. Hayes

9 Sensor Technology for Rate-Adaptive Pacing and Hemodynamic Optimization, 407

 David L. Hayes, Samuel J. Asirvatham, Paul A. Friedman

10 Troubleshooting: Interpreting Diagnostic Information to Ensure Appropriate Function, 427

 Charles D. Swerdlow, Paul A. Friedman, Samuel J. Asirvatham, David L. Hayes

11 Radiography of Implantable Devices, 553

 David L. Hayes, Paul A. Friedman, Samuel J. Asirvatham

12 Electromagnetic Interference: Sources, Recognition, and Management, 591

 David L. Hayes, Paul A. Friedman, Samuel J. Asirvatham

13 Follow-up, 613

 David L. Hayes, Niloufar Tabatabaei, Michael Glikson, Samuel J. Asirvatham, Paul A. Friedman

Index, 651

Contributors

Samuel J. Asirvatham, MD
Consultant, Division of Cardiovascular Diseases
Mayo Clinic;
Professor of Medicine and of Pediatrics
College of Medicine
Mayo Clinic
Rochester, MN, USA

T. Jared Bunch, MD
Heart Rhythm Specialist
Intermountain Medical Group
Logan, UT, USA

Paul A. Friedman, MD
Consultant, Division of Cardiovascular Diseases
Director, Implantable Device Lab
Mayo Clinic;
Professor of Medicine
College of Medicine
Mayo Clinic
Rochester, MN, USA

Apoor S. Gami, MD
Research Collaborator in Cardiovascular Diseases
Mayo School of Graduate Medical Education
College of Medicine
Mayo Clinic
Rochester, MN, USA

Michael Glikson, MD
Director, Davidai Arrhythmia Center
Sheba Medical Center and Tel Aviv University
Tel Hashomer, Israel

David L. Hayes, MD
Consultant, Division of Cardiovascular Diseases
Mayo Clinic;
Professor of Medicine
College of Medicine
Mayo Clinic
Rochester, MN, USA

Malini Madhavan, MBBS
Fellow in Cardiovascular Diseases
Mayo School of Graduate Medical Education
College of Medicine
Mayo Clinic
Rochester, MN, USA

Seth H. Sheldon, MD
Fellow in Cardiovascular Diseases
Mayo School of Graduate Medical Education
College of Medicine
Mayo Clinic
Rochester, MN, USA

Matthew J. Swale, MBBS
Resident in Cardiovascular Diseases
Mayo School of Graduate Medical Education
College of Medicine
Mayo Clinic
Rochester, MN, USA

Charles D. Swerdlow, MD
Cedars-Sinai Heart Center
at Cedars-Sinai Medical Center
Los Angeles, CA;
Clinical Professor of Medicine
David Geffen School of Medicine
University of California, Los Angeles
Los Angeles, CA, USA

Faisal F. Syed, MB, ChB
Fellow in Cardiovascular Diseases
Mayo School of Graduate Medical Education
College of Medicine
Mayo Clinic
Rochester, MN, USA

Niloufar Tabatabaei, MD
Consultant, Cardiovascular Diseases
Olmsted Medical Center
Rochester, MN, USA

Paul J. Wang, MD
Director of Cardiac Arrhythmia Service
and Cardiac Electrophysiology
Professor of Medicine
Stanford School of Medicine
Stanford University
Stanford, CA, USA

Preface

I'm often asked how many editions of this pacing text have been done. The answer is not entirely straightforward. The original version of this text was written by Drs. Sy Furman, David Hayes and David Holmes. After a number of editions for this original text, we mutually agreed that the original authors would not proceed with the next edition and instead the next edition would be written with Drs. Paul Friedman and Margaret Lloyd. This was officially the first "Mayo only" edition. Subsequently, Paul and I published a revised text in 2008 and this 2013 text represents the third edition. This edition adds Dr. Samuel Asirvatham as an editor. Sam made significant contributions to the second edition and is now a part of the entire text.

The goal of the current text is the same as that of the original text by Furman/Hayes/Holmes: to provide a practical approach to clinical understanding and management of issues related to pacemakers, implantable cardioverter-defibrillators (ICDs) and cardiac resynchronization therapy (CRT) devices. There have been two principles that we have adhered to from the beginning and apply to this edition as well. Although we have a number of contributors to this edition, Paul, Sam, and I are all involved in each chapter to maintain a uniformity of style and level of detail. Although there are number of outstanding multiauthored texts available on implantable cardiac devices, we have always believed there was a distinct advantage in limiting the number of editors and involving them in the writing of the entire text in an effort to have a consistent style and message. The second principle has to do with the level of detail. This text is *not* meant to be an encyclopedic approach to implantable cardiac device therapy. Excellent sources exist that do provide a much greater level of detail, and these sources may be needed to find detailed or perhaps a more obscure issue related to implantable cardiac device therapy. For the purpose of finding a practical approach to everyday issues that arise with pacemakers, ICDs and CRT devices, our goal is to provide those answers within this text. We're also frequently told by individuals who have studied for one or more of the available board examinations that include questions on implantable cardiac devices that they felt that previous editions of this text served them well in their endeavors.

As with previous editions we owe a great debt of thanks to all of the contributors. In addition to the contributors who are included as authors on various chapters, we have others to thank. The nursing staff in our heart rhythm group at Mayo Clinic Rochester is a great resource. They not only provide outstanding patient care, they often provide us with great teaching cases and are often the ones to be credited with the troubleshooting examples that we use. We also have great support from the various device manufacturers. All of them have provided examples and information for this text. There are too many names to list individually but we do appreciate all of the assistance from Biotronik, Boston Scientific, Medtronic, Sorin Medical and St. Jude Medical.

This is a field that has changed tremendously over the years, and it will continue to evolve given continued advances in technology. As a result, textbooks, examinations, and, most importantly, patient care will also continue to evolve. Although our (DLH, PAF, SJA) ultimate goal is to see you succeed in any and all efforts related to implantable cardiac devices, we definitely hope that this text will assist you in the day-in and day-out management of patients with implantable devices that we are all so very privileged to serve.

David L. Hayes
Samuel J. Asirvatham
Paul A. Friedman

1 Pacing and Defibrillation: Clinically Relevant Basics for Practice

T. Jared Bunch[1], David L. Hayes[2], Charles D. Swerdlow[3], Samuel J. Asirvatham[2], Paul A. Friedman[2]

[1]Intermountain Heart Institute, Intermountain Medical Center, Murray, Utah, USA

[2]Mayo Clinic, Rochester, MN, USA

[3]Cedars-Sinai Heart Center at Cedars-Sinai Medical Center; David Geffen School of Medicine, University of California, Los Angeles, CA, USA

Anatomy and physiology of the cardiac conduction system 2
Electrophysiology of myocardial stimulation 2
Pacing basics 4
Stimulation threshold 4
Variations in stimulation threshold 6
Sensing 7
Lead design 9
Bipolar and unipolar pacing and sensing 13
Left ventricular leads 13
Pulse generators 14
Pacemaker nomenclature 16
Defibrillation basics 16
Critical mass 18
Upper limit of vulnerability 18
Progressive depolarization 19
Virtual electrode depolarization 19
Defibrillation theory summary 21
The importance of waveform 21
Biphasic waveforms 22
Phase duration and tilt 23

Polarity and biphasic waveforms 24
Mechanism of improved efficacy with biphasic waveforms 24
Measuring shock dose 24
Measuring the efficacy of defibrillation 25
Threshold and dose–response curve 25
Relationship between defibrillation threshold and dose–response curve 25
Patient-specific defibrillation threshold and safety margin testing 26
Clinical role of defibrillation testing at implantation 27
Management of the patient who fails defibrillation testing 29
Upper limit of vulnerability to assess safety margin 33
Drugs and defibrillators 33
Antitachycardia pacing 34
References 35

Cardiac Pacing, Defibrillation and Resynchronization: A Clinical Approach, Third Edition.
David L. Hayes, Samuel J. Asirvatham, and Paul A. Friedman.
© 2013 Mayo Foundation for Medical Education and Research. Published 2013 by John Wiley & Sons, Ltd.

Anatomy and physiology of the cardiac conduction system

The cardiac conduction system consists of specialized tissue involved in the generation and conduction of electrical impulses throughout the heart. In this book, we review how device therapy can be optimally utilized for various forms of conduction system disturbances, tachyarrhythmias, and for heart failure. Knowledge of the normal anatomy and physiology of the cardiac conduction system is critical to understanding appropriate utilization of device therapy.

The sinoatrial (SA) node, located at the junction of the right atrium and the superior vena cava, is normally the site of impulse generation (Fig. 1.1). The SA node is composed of a dense collagen matrix containing a variety of cells. The large, centrally located P cells are thought to be the origin of electrical impulses in the SA node, which is surrounded by transitional cells and fiber tracts extending through the perinodal area into the right atrium proper. The SA node is richly innervated by the autonomic nervous system, which has a key function in heart rate regulation. Specialized fibers, such as Bachmann's bundle, conduct the impulse throughout the right and left atria. The SA node has the highest rate of spontaneous depolarization and under normal circumstances is responsible for generating most impulses. Atrial depolarization is seen as the P wave on the surface ECG (Fig. 1.1).

Atrial conduction fibers converge, forming multiple inputs into the atrioventricular (AV) node, a small subendocardial structure located within the interatrial septum (Fig. 1.1). The AV node likewise receives abundant autonomic innervation, and it is histologically similar to the SA node because it is composed of a loose collagen matrix in which P cells and transitional cells are located. Additionally, Purkinje cells and myocardial contractile fibers may be found. The AV node allows for physiologic delay between atrial and ventricular contraction, resulting in optimal cardiac hemodynamic function. It can also function as a subsidiary "pacemaker" should the SA node fail. Finally, the AV node functions (albeit typically suboptimally) to regulate the number of impulses eventually reaching the ventricle in instances of atrial tachyarrhythmia. On the surface ECG, the majority of the PR interval is represented by propagation through the AV node and through the His–Purkinje fibers (Fig. 1.1).

Purkinje fibers emerge from the distal AV node to form the bundle of His, which runs through the membranous septum to the crest of the muscular septum, where it divides into the various bundle branches. The bundle branch system exhibits significant individual variation and is invariably complex. The right bundle is typically a discrete structure running along the right side of the interventricular septum to the anterior papillary muscle, where it divides. The left bundle is usually a large band of fibers fanning out over the left ventricle, sometimes forming functional fascicles. Both bundles eventually terminate in individual Purkinje fibers interdigitating with myocardial contractile fibers. The His–Purkinje system has little in the way of autonomic innervation.

Because of their key function and location, the SA and AV nodes are the most common sites of conduction system failure; it is therefore understandable that the most common indications for pacemaker implantation are SA node dysfunction and high-grade AV block. It should be noted, however, that conduction system disease is frequently diffuse and may involve the specialized conduction system at multiple sites.

Electrophysiology of myocardial stimulation

Stimulation of the myocardium requires the initiation of a propagating wave of depolarization from the site of initial activation, whether from a native "pacemaker" or from an artificial stimulus. Myocardium exhibits "excitability," which is a response to a stimulus out of proportion to the strength of that stimulus.[1] Excitability is maintained by separation of chemical charge, which results in an electrical transmembrane potential. In cardiac myocytes, this electrochemical gradient is created by differing intracellular and extracellular concentrations of sodium (Na^+) and potassium (K^+) ions; Na^+ ions predominate extracellularly and K^+ ions predominate intracellularly. Although this transmembrane gradient is maintained by the high chemical resistance intrinsic to the lipid bilayer of the cellular membrane, passive leakage of these ions occurs across the cellular membrane through ion channels. Passive leakage is offset by two active transport mechanisms, each transporting three positive charges out of the myocyte in exchange for two positive charges that are moved into the myocyte, producing cellular polarization.[2,3] These active transport mechanisms require energy and are susceptible to disruption when energy-generating processes are interrupted.

The chemical gradient has a key role in the generation of the transmembrane action potential (Fig. 1.2). The membrane potential of approximately −90 mV drifts upward to the threshold potential of approximately −70 to −60 mV. At this point, specialized membrane-bound channels modify their conformation from an inactive to an active state, which allows the abrupt influx of extracellular Na^+ ions into the myocyte,[4,5] creating phase 0 of the action potential and rapidly raising the transmembrane potential to approximately +20 mV.[6,7] This rapid upstroke creates a short period of overshoot potential

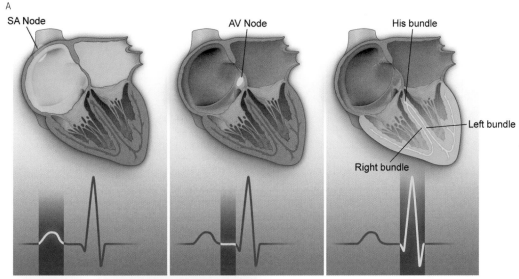

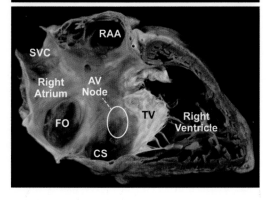

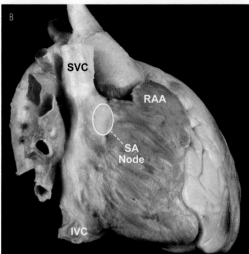

Fig. 1.1 (A) The cardiac conduction system. AV, atrioventricular; SA, sinoatrial. Conduction begins with impulse generation in the SA node (left panel). Impulse propagation through the atria gives rise to the P wave on the surface ECG (bottom of left panel). The impulse is then delayed in the AV node to allow blood to flow to the ventricles; wavefront travel through the AV node is not seen on the surface ECG. The wavefronts then pass through the His–Purkinje system, to rapidly activate the ventricular myocardium. The larger mass of the ventricles give rise to the large amplitude QRS complex. Further details in text. (B) An anatomic specimen showing the location of key conduction system elements. The top panel shows an external view of the heart with the region of the SA node in the epicardium at the juncture of the superior vena cava (SVC) and right atrium (RA) indicated. The structure itself is not visible to the naked eye. IVC, inferior vena cava. In the bottom panel the right atrial and ventricular free wall has been removed to reveal the position of the AV node anterior to the coronary sinus (CS) and atrial to the tricuspid valve (TV), situated in Koch's triangle (bounded by the TV, CS, and tendon of Todaro, not shown). FO, fossa ovalis.

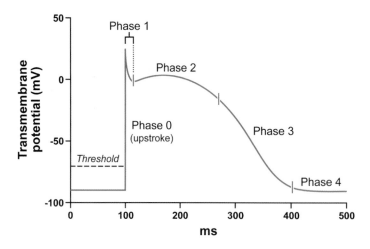

Fig. 1.2 Action potential of a typical Purkinje fiber, with the various phases of depolarization and repolarization (described in the text). (From Stokes KB, Kay GN. Artificial electric cardiac stimulation. In: Ellenbogen KA, Kay GN, Wilkoff BL, eds. Clinical Cardiac Pacing. Philadelphia: WB Saunders Co., 1995: 3–37, by permission of the publisher.)

(phase 1), which is followed by a plateau period (phase 2) created by the inward calcium (Ca^{2+}) and Na^+ currents balanced against outward K^+ currents.[8–10] During phase 3 of the action potential, the transmembrane potential returns to normal, and during phase 4 the gradual upward drift in transmembrane potential repeats. The shape of the transmembrane potential and the relative distribution of the various membrane-bound ion channels differ between the components of the specialized cardiac conduction system and working myocytes.

Depolarization of neighboring cells occurs as a result of passive conduction via low-resistance intercellular connections called "gap junctions," with active regeneration along cellular membranes.[11,12] The velocity of depolarization throughout the myocardium depends on the speed of depolarization of the various cellular components of the myocardium and on the geometric arrangement and orientation of the myocytes. Factors such as myocardial ischemia, electrolyte imbalance, metabolic abnormalities, myocardial scar, diseased tissue, and drugs affect the depolarization and depolarization velocity.

Pacing basics
Stimulation threshold
Artificial pacing involves delivery of an electrical impulse from an electrode of sufficient strength to cause depolarization of the myocardium in contact with that electrode and propagation of that depolarization to the rest of the myocardium. The minimal amount of energy required to produce this depolarization is called the stimulation threshold. The components of the stimulus include the pulse amplitude (measured in volts) and the pulse duration (measured

in milliseconds). An exponential relationship exists between the stimulus amplitude and the duration, resulting in a hyperbolic strength–duration curve. At short pulse durations, a small change in the pulse duration is associated with a significant change in the pulse amplitude required to achieve myocardial depolarization; conversely, at long pulse durations, a small change in pulse duration has relatively little effect on threshold amplitude (Fig. 1.3). Two points on the strength–duration curve should be noted (Fig. 1.4). The *rheobase* is defined as the smallest amplitude (voltage) that stimulates the myocardium at an infinitely long pulse duration (milliseconds). The *chronaxie* is the threshold pulse duration at twice the rheobase voltage. The chronaxie is important in the clinical practice of pacing because it approximates the point of minimum threshold energy (microjoules) required for myocardial depolarization.

The relationship of voltage, current, and pulse duration to stimulus energy is described by the formula

$$E = V^2/R \times t$$

in which E is the stimulus energy, V is the voltage, R is the total pacing impedance, and t is the pulse duration. This formula demonstrates the relative increase in energy with longer pulse durations. The energy increase due to duration is offset by a decrement in the needed voltage. The strength–duration curve discussed thus far has been that of a constant voltage system, which is used in all current pacemakers and defibrillators. Constant current devices are no longer used.

Impedance is the term applied to the resistance to current flow in the pacing system. Ohm's law describes

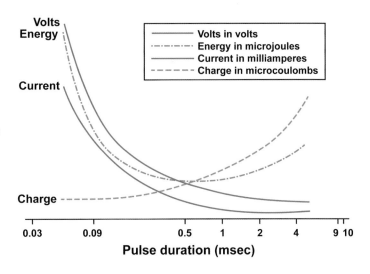

Fig. 1.3 Relationship of charge, energy, voltage, and current to pulse duration at stimulation threshold. As the pulse duration is shortened, voltage and current requirements increase. Charge decreases as pulse duration shortens. At threshold, energy is lowest at a pulse duration of 0.5–1.0 ms and increases at pulse widths of shorter and longer duration. (Modified from Furman S. Basic concepts. In: Furman S, Hayes DL, Holmes DR Jr, eds. A Practice of Cardiac Pacing. Mount Kisco, NY: Futura Publishing Co., by permission of the publisher.)

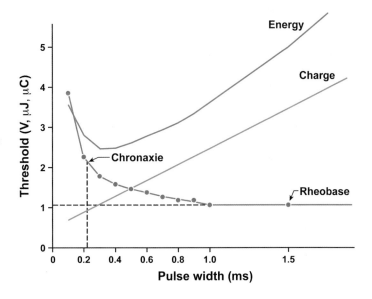

Fig. 1.4 Relationships among chronic ventricular strength–duration curves from a canine, expressed as potential (V), charge (μC), and energy (μJ). Rheobase is the threshold at infinitely long pulse duration. Chronaxie is the pulse duration at twice rheobase. (From Stokes K, Bornzin G. The electrode–biointerface stimulation. In: Barold SS, ed. Modern Cardiac Pacing. Mount Kisco, NY: Futura Publishing Co., 1985: 33–77, by permission of the publisher.)

the relationship among voltage, current, and resistance as

$$V = IR$$

in which V is the voltage, I is the current, and R is the resistance. Although Ohm's law is used for determining impedance, technically impedance and resistance are not interchangeable terms. Impedance implies inclusion of all factors that contribute to current flow impediment, including lead conductor resistance, elec-

trode resistance, resistance due to electrode polarization, capacitance, and inductance. Technically, the term "resistance" does not include the effects of capacitance (storage of charge) or inductance (storage of current flow) to impede current flow. Nevertheless, Ohm's law (substituting impedance for R) is commonly used for calculating impedance. In constant voltage systems, the lower the pacing impedance, the greater the current flow; conversely, the higher the pacing impedance, the lower the current flow. Lead conductors are designed to have a low resistance to minimize the generation of energy-wasting heat as current flows along the lead, and electrodes are designed to have a high resistance to minimize current flow and to have negligible electrode polarization. Decreasing the electrode radius minimizes current flow by providing greater electrode resistance and increased current density, resulting in greater battery longevity and lower stimulation thresholds.[13]

"Polarization" refers to layers of oppositely charged ions that surround the electrode during the pulse stimulus. It is related to the movement of positively charged ions (Na^+ and H_3O^+) to the cathode; the layer of positively charged ions is then surrounded by a layer of negatively charged ions (Cl^-, HPO_4^{2-}, and OH^-). These layers of charge develop during the pulse stimulus, reaching peak formation at the termination of the pulse stimulus, after which they gradually dissipate. Polarization impedes the movement of charge from the electrode to the myocardium, resulting in a need for increased voltage for stimulation. As polarization develops with increasing pulse duration, one way to combat formation of polarization is to shorten the pulse duration. Electrode design has incorporated the use of materials that minimize polarization, such as platinum black, iridium oxide, titanium nitride, and activated carbon.[14] Finally, polarization is inversely related to the surface area of the electrode. To maximize the surface area (to reduce polarization) but minimize the radius (to increase electrode impedance), electrode design incorporates a small radius but a porous, irregular surface construction.[15] Fractal coatings on the lead tip increase the surface area 1000-fold without the need to increase the axial diameter. Leads designed to maximize these principles are considered "high-impedance" leads.

Variations in stimulation threshold

Myocardial thresholds typically fluctuate, occasionally dramatically, during the first weeks after implantation. After implantation of earlier generations of endocardial leads, the stimulation threshold would typically rise rapidly in the first 24 h and then gradually increase to a peak at approximately 1 week (Fig. 1.5). Over the ensuing 6–8 weeks, the stimulation threshold would usually decline to a level somewhat higher than that at implantation, but less than the peak threshold, known as the "chronic threshold."[16,17] The magnitude and duration of this early increase in threshold was highly dependent on lead design, the interface between the electrode and the myocardium, and individual patient variation, but chronic thresholds would typically be reached by 3 months. The single most important lead design change to alter pacing threshold evolution was the incorporation of steroid elution at the lead tip, to blunt the local inflammatory response (Fig. 1.6). With steroid elution there may be a slight increase in thresholds post-implantation, with subsequent reduction to almost that of acute thresholds.[18,19]

Transvenous pacing leads have used passive or active fixation mechanisms to provide a stable electrode–myocardium interface. Active fixation leads may have higher initial pacing thresholds acutely at implantation, but thresholds frequently decline significantly within the first 5–30 min after placement.[16] This effect has been attributed to hyperacute injury due to advancement of the screw into the myocardium. On a cellular level,

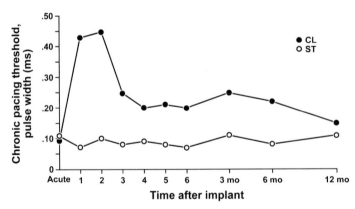

Fig. 1.5 Long-term pacing thresholds from a conventional lead (no steroid elution) (CL; *closed circles*) and a steroid-eluting lead (ST; *open circles*). With the conventional lead, an early increase in threshold decreases to a plateau at approximately 4 weeks. The threshold for the steroid-eluting lead remains relatively flat, with no significant change from short-term threshold measurements. (From Furman S. Basic concepts. In: Furman S, Hayes DL, Holmes DR Jr, eds. A Practice of Cardiac Pacing, 2nd edn. Mount Kisco, NY: Futura Publishing Co., 1989: 23–78, by permission of Mayo Foundation.)

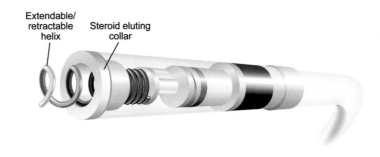

Extendable/
retractable
helix

Steroid eluting
collar

Fig. 1.6 Diagram of a steroid-eluting active fixation lead. The electrode has a porous, platinized tip. A silicone rubber collar is impregnated with 1 mg of dexamethasone sodium.

implantation of a transvenous pacing lead results in acute injury to cellular membranes, which is followed by the development of myocardial edema and coating of the electrode surface with platelets and fibrin. Subsequently, various chemotactic factors are released, and an acute inflammatory reaction develops, consisting of mononuclear cells and polymorphonuclear leukocytes. After the acute response, release of proteolytic enzymes and oxygen free radicals by invading macrophages accelerates cellular injury. Finally, fibroblasts in the myocardium begin producing collagen, leading to production of the fibrotic capsule surrounding the electrode. This fibrous capsule ultimately increases the effective radius of the electrode, with a smaller increase in surface area.[20,21] Steroid-eluting leads are believed to minimize fibrous capsule formation. In both atrial and ventricular active fixation leads, steroid elution results in long-term reduction in energy consumption with maintenance of stimulation thresholds, lead impedance values, and sensing thresholds.[22,23]

The stimulation threshold may vary slightly with a circadian pattern, generally increasing during sleep and decreasing during the day, probably reflecting changes in autonomic tone. The stimulation threshold may also rise after eating; during hyperglycemia, hypoxemia, or acute viral illnesses; or as a result of electrolyte fluctuations. In general, these threshold changes are minimal. However, in the setting of severe hypoxemia or electrolyte abnormalties they can lead to loss of capture. Certain drugs used in patients with cardiac disease may also increase pacing thresholds (see Chapter 8: Programming).

The inflammatory reaction and subsequent fibrosis that occur after lead implantation may act as an insulating shield around the electrode. These processes effectively increase the distance between the electrode and the excitable tissue, allowing the stimulus to disperse partially before reaching the excitable cells. These changes result in an increased threshold for stimulation and attenuate the amplitude and slew rate of the endo-

cardial signal being sensed. This is a process termed "lead maturation." Improvements in electrode design and materials have reduced the severity of the inflammatory reaction and thus improved lead maturation rates.[18,24] When the capture threshold exceeds the programmed output of the pacemaker, exit block will occur; loss of capture will result if the capture threshold exceeds the programmed output of the pacemaker.[16,25] Exit block, a consequence of lead maturation, results from the progressive rise in thresholds over time.[16,25] This phenomenon occurs despite initial satisfactory lead placement and implantation thresholds, often but not always occurs in parallel in the atrium and ventricle, and usually recurs with placement of subsequent leads. Steroid-eluting leads prevent exit block in most, but not all patients (Fig. 1.6).

Sensing

The first pacemakers functioned as fixed-rate, VOO devices. All contemporary devices offer demand-mode pacing, which pace only when the intrinsic rate is below the programmed rate. For such devices to function as programmed, accurate and consistent sensing of the native rhythm is essential.

Intrinsic cardiac electrical signals are produced by the wave of electrical current through the myocardium (Fig. 1.7). As the wavefront of electrical energy approaches an endocardial unipolar electrode, the intracardiac electrogram records a positive deflection. As the wavefront passes directly under the electrode, a sharp negative deflection is recorded, referred to as the intrinsic deflection.[26] The intrinsic deflection is inscribed as the advancing wavefront passes directly underneath a unipolar electrode. Smaller positive and negative deflections preceding and following the intrinsic deflection represent activation of surrounding myocardium. The analog on the surface ECG is the peak of the R wave, referred to as the intrinsicoid deflection, because the electrical depolarization is measured at a distance (from the surface), rather than directly on the myocardium. However, the

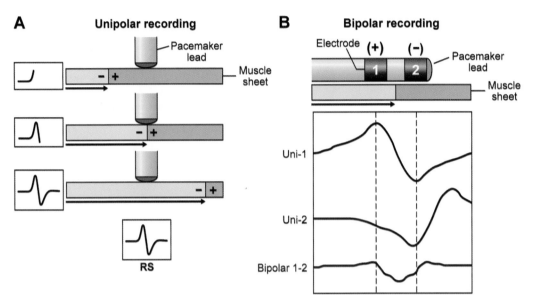

Fig. 1.7 Schema of the relationship of the pacing lead to the recorded electrogram with unipolar (left) and bipolar (right) sensing. Top left: as the electrical impulse moves toward the cathode (lead tip), a positive deflection is created in the electrogram. Middle left: as the electrical impulse passes the cathode, the deflection suddenly moves downward, at the intrinsic deflection. Bottom left: as the impulse moves away from the cathode, a negative deflection occurs. The right panel shows the same phenomena occur for each electrode of a bipolar lead when considered independently (uni-1 and uni-2). When these are put together as a bipolar signal, the resultant tracing is seen at bottom (bipolar 1–2). (Adapted from Stevenson WG, Soejima K. Recording techniques for clinical electrophysiology. J Cardiovasc Electrophysiol 2005; 16:1–6.)

intrinsic deflection is a local endocardial event; it does not necessarily time with the intrinsicoid deflection in any ECG lead. Bipolar electrograms (Fig. 1.7) represent the difference in potential recorded between two closely spaced intracardiac electrodes. Due to the close spacing of two typically small electrodes, far-field signals (i.e., signals not generated by the tissue the lead electrode is in contact with) are smaller and thus more easily rejected by pacemakers and defibrillators. Ventricular electrograms typically are much larger than atrial electrograms because ventricular mass is greater. Typical amplitude ranges for ventricular electrograms are 5–25 mV, and for atrial electrograms 1.5–5 mV (Fig. 1.8). The maximum frequency densities of electrograms in sinus rhythm are in the range of 80–100 Hz in the atrium and 10–30 Hz in the ventricle (these frequencies may differ slightly depending on leads and/or technologies). Pulse generator filtering systems are designed to attenuate signals outside of these ranges. Filtering and use of blanking and refractory periods (discussed later) have markedly reduced unwanted sensing, although myopotential frequencies (ranging from 10 to 200 Hz) considerably overlap with those generated by atrial and ventricular depolarization and are difficult to filter out, especially during sensing in a unipolar configuration.[27–29] Shorten-

ing of the tip-to-ring spacing has also improved atrial sensing and rejection of far-field R waves.

A second important metric of the intracardiac electrogram in addition to amplitude is the slew rate, i.e., the peak slope of the developing electrogram[30] (Fig. 1.8). The slew rate represents the maximal rate of change of the electrical potential between the sensing electrodes and is the first derivative of the electrogram (dV/dt). An acceptable slew rate should be at least 0.5 V/s in both the atrium and the ventricle. In general, the higher the slew rate, the higher the frequency content and the more likely the signal will be sensed. Slow, broad signals, such as those generated by the T wave, are less likely to be sensed because of a low slew rate and lower frequency density.

Polarization also affects sensing function. After termination of the pulse stimulus, an excess of positive charge surrounds the cathode, which then decays until the cathode is electrically neutral. Afterpotentials can be sensed, resulting in inappropriate inhibition or delay of the subsequent pacing pulse (Fig. 1.9). The amplitude of afterpotentials is directly related to both the amplitude and the duration of the pacing pulse; thus, they are most likely to be sensed when the pacemaker is programmed to high voltage and long pulse duration in combination with maximal sensitivity.[30] The use of programmable sensing refractory and blanking periods has helped to prevent the pacemaker from reacting to afterpotentials, although in dual-chamber systems, atrial afterpotentials of sufficient strength and duration to be sensed by the ventricular channel may result in inappropriate ventricular inhibition (crosstalk), especially in unipolar systems.[31,32] Afterpotentials may be a source of problems in devices with automatic threshold measurement and capture detection; the use of leads designed to minimize afterpotentials may increase the effectiveness of such algorithms.[33]

"Source impedance" is the impedance from the heart to the proximal portion of the lead, and it results in a voltage drop from the site of the origin of the intracardiac electrogram to the proximal portion of the lead.[34] Components include the resistance between the electrode and the myocardium, the resistance of the lead conductor material, and the effects of polarization. The resistance between the electrode and the myocardium, as well as polarization, is inversely related to the surface area of the electrode; thus, the effects of both can be minimized by a large electrode surface area. The electrogram actually seen by the pulse generator is determined by the ratio between the sensing amplifier (input) impedance and the lead (source) impedance. Less attenuation of the signal from the myocardium occurs when there is a greater ratio of input impedance to source impedance. Clinically, impedance mismatch is seen with insulation or conductor failure, which results in sensing abnormalities or failure.

Lead design

Pacing lead components include the electrode and fixation device, the conductor, the insulation, and the connector pin (Figs 1.10 and 1.11). Leads function in the harsh environment of the human body, and are subject to biologic, chemical, and mechanical repetitive stress. They must be constructed of materials that provide mechanical longevity, stability, and flexibility; they must satisfy electrical conductive and resistive requirements; they must be insulated with material that is durable and that has a low friction coefficient to facilitate implantation; and they must include an electrode that provides good mechanical and electrical

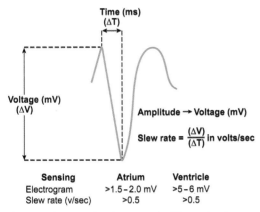

Amplitude → Voltage (mV)

$$\text{Slew rate} = \frac{(\Delta V)}{(\Delta T)} \text{ in volts/sec}$$

	Sensing	Atrium	Ventricle
Electrogram		>1.5–2.0 mV	>5–6 mV
Slew rate (v/sec)		>0.5	>0.5

Fig. 1.8 In the intracardiac electrogram, the difference in voltage recorded between two electrodes is the amplitude, which is measured in millivolts. The slew rate is volts per second and should be at least 0.5.

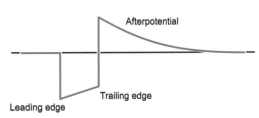

Fig. 1.9 Diagram of a pacing pulse, constant voltage, with leading edge and trailing edge voltage and an afterpotential with opposite polarity. As described in the text, afterpotentials may result in sensing abnormalities.

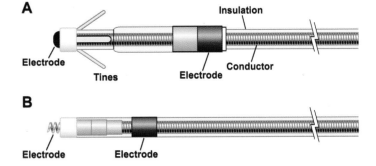

Fig. 1.10 (A) Basic components of a passive fixation pacing lead with tines. (B) Active fixation lead in which the helix serves as the distal electrode.

contact with the myocardium. Industry continues to improve lead design to achieve these goals.

Optimal stimulation and sensing thresholds favor an electrode with a small radius and a large surface area. Electrode shape and surface composition have evolved over time. Early models utilized a round, spherical shape with a smooth metal surface. Electrodes with an irregular, textured surface allow for increased surface area without an increase in electrode radius.[15,33,35] To achieve increased electrode surface area, manufacturers have used a variety of designs, including microscopic pores, coatings of microspheres, and wire filament mesh.

Unfortunately, relatively few conductive materials have proven to be satisfactory for use in pacing electrodes. Ideally, electrodes are biologically inert, resist degradation over time, and do not elicit a marked tissue reaction at the myocardium–electrode interface. Certain metals, such as zinc, copper, mercury, nickel, lead, and silver, are associated with toxic reactions with

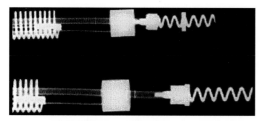

Fig. 1.11 Radiographic example of an active fixation screw-in lead with a retractable screw rather than a screw that is always extended. The screw is extended in the lower image.

the myocardium. Stainless steel alloys are susceptible to corrosion. Titanium, tantalum, platinum, and iridium oxide acquire a surface coating of oxides that impedes current transfer. Materials currently in use are platinum–iridium, platinized titanium-coated platinum, iridium oxide, and platinum (Fig. 1.12). Carbon electrodes seem to be least susceptible to corrosion. Also, they are improved by activation, which roughens the surface to increase the surface area and allow for tissue ingrowth.[36]

Lead fixation may be active or passive. Passive fixation endocardial leads usually incorporate tines at the tip that become ensnared in trabeculated tissue in the right atrium or ventricle, providing lead stability. Leads designed for coronary venous placement usually incorporate a design that wedges the lead against the wall of the coronary vein. Active fixation leads deploy an electrically active screw into the myocardium to provide lead stability. There are advantages and disadvantages to active and passive designs. Passive fixation leads are simple to deploy. However, considerable myocardial and fibrous tissue enveloping the tip typically develops with passive fixation leads. The encasement of the tines of a passive fixation lead by fibrous tissue often makes the extraction of passive fixation leads more difficult than that of active fixation leads. Active fixation leads are often preferable in patients with distorted anatomy, such as those with congenital cardiac defects or those with surgically amputated atrial appendages. Active fixation leads are also preferable in patients with high right-sided pressures. As alternative site pacing has evolved, i.e., the placements of leads outside the right atrial appendage and right ventricular apex, screw-in leads have become more popular because

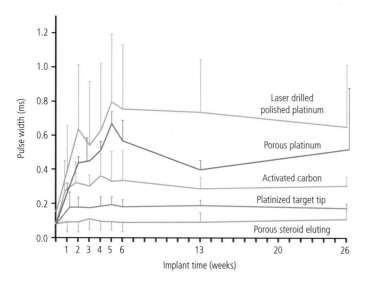

Fig. 1.12 Capture thresholds from implantation to 26 weeks from a variety of unipolar leads with similar geometric surface area electrodes. From top to bottom, the curves represent laser drilled polished platinum; porous surface platinum; activated carbon; platinized target tip; and porous steroid eluting leads. (From Stokes KB, Kay GN. Artificial electric cardiac stimulation. In: Ellenbogen KA, Kay GN, Wilkoff BL, eds. Clinical Cardiac Pacing. Philadelphia: WB Saunders Co., 1995: 3–37, by permission of the publisher.)

of the ability to stabilize them mechanically in non-traditional locations.

In active fixation leads, various mechanism are used to keep the screw unexposed (to avoid tissue injury) until it is in position for fixation. In many leads, the helix is extendable and retractable by rotation of the proximal connector using a simple tool (Bisping screwdriver). This allows the operator to control the precise time and location of helix deployment. Another approach entails covering a fixed helix with a material such as mannitol which dissolves in the blood stream

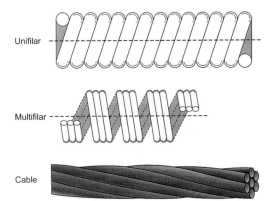

Fig. 1.13 Conductor coils may be of unifilar, multifilar, or cable design. The multifilar and cable designs allow the conductor to be more flexible and more resistant to fracture.

after approximately 5 minutes. This permits placement of the lead atraumatically at the desired location. Fixation is accomplished by rotating the entire lead body.

Conductors are commonly of a multifilament design to provide tensile strength and reduce resistance to metal fatigue (Fig. 1.13). Alloys such as MP35N (cobalt, nickel, chromium, and molybdenum) and nickel silver are typically used in modern pacing leads. Bipolar leads may be of coaxial design, with an inner coil extending to the distal electrode and an outer coil terminating at the proximal electrode (Fig. 1.14). This design requires that the conductor coils be separated by a layer of inner insulation. Coaxial designs remain commonly used in the treatment of bradyarrhythmias. Some bipolar leads are coradial, or "parallel-wound"; that is, two insulated coils are wound next to each other. Leads may also be constructed with the conductor coils parallel to each other (multiluminal), again separated by insulating material (Fig. 1.14). This type of design is typically used for tachyarrhythmia leads. Additionally, leads may use a combination of coils and cables. The coil facilitates the passage of a stylet for lead implantation, and the cable allows a smaller lead body.

Two materials have predominated in lead insulation: silicone and polyurethane. Each has its respective advantages and disadvantages, but the overall performances of both materials have been excellent.[37] Table 4.2 in Chapter 4 compares the advantages and disadvantages of these two insulating materials.

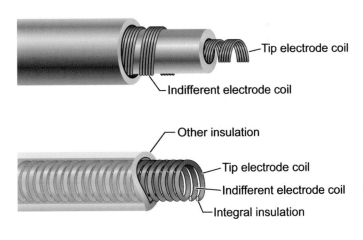

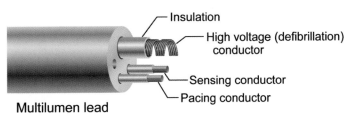

Fig. 1.14 Varieties of conductor construction. Top: bipolar coaxial design with an inner multifilar coil surrounded by insulation (inner), an outer multifilar coil, and outer insulation. Middle: individually insulated wires wound together in a single multifilar coil for bipolar pacing. Bottom: multilumen lead body design in which each conductor has its own lumen.

The two grades of polyurethane that have had the widest use are Pellathane 80A (P80A) and Pellathane 55D. Early after the introduction of polyurethane as an insulating material, it became clear that clinical failure rates with specific leads were higher than acceptable; further investigation revealed that the failures were occurring primarily in leads insulated with the P80A polymer.[35,38] Microscopic cracks developed in the P80A polymer, initially occurring as the heated polymer cooled during manufacture; with additional environmental stress, these cracks propagated deeper into the insulation, resulting in failure of the lead insulation.

Polyurethane may also undergo oxidative stress in contact with conductors containing cobalt and silver chloride, resulting in degradation of the lead from the inside and subsequent lead failure. Some current leads use silicone with a polyurethane coating, incorporating the strength and durability of silicone with the ease of handling of polyurethane while maintaining a satisfactory external lead diameter. Silicone rubber is well known to be susceptible to abrasion wear, cold flow due to cyclic compression, and wear from lead-to-lead and lead-to-can contact. Current silicone leads have surface modifications that improve lubricity and reduce friction in blood. Preliminary studies have suggested that a hybrid coating of silicone and polyurethane may offer improved wear.[39] Despite lead improvements, laboratory testing, and premarketing, clinical trials have been inadequate to predict the long-term performance of leads, so that clinicians implanting the devices or performing follow-up in patients with pacing systems must vigilantly monitor lead status. Increasingly, the use of internet-enabled remote monitoring and pulse generator based algorithms permits automatic alert generation in the event of impending lead fracture.

Contemporary leads and connectors are standardized to conform to international guidelines (IS-1 standard), which mandate that leads have a 3.2-mm diameter inline bipolar connector pin.[40] These standards were established many years ago because some leads and connector blocks were incompatible, requiring the development of multiple adaptors. The use of the IS-1 standard permits using one manufacturer's leads with another manufactuer's pulse generator. Similarly, the DF-1 standard insures a common site for high-voltage connections in defibrillators. The newer IS-4 standard permits a single inline connection of four low-voltage electrodes, permitting coronary sinus leads to include four (rather than two) pacing sites, increasing the likelihood of a lead having an acceptable threshold and/or pacing site. The DF-4 connectors (Fig. 1.15A) contain

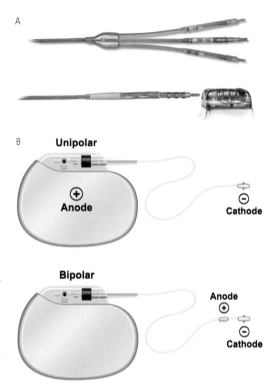

Fig. 1.15 Lead connectors and configurations. (A) Connector types in defibrillator leads. The top panel shows the proximal end of a defibrillation lead with a three connectors. Top and bottom pins are DF-1 connectors used for high voltage shock delivery for defibrillation, while the middle pin is an IS-1 connector used for pacing and sensing. Bottom images shows a DF-4 connector, in which all four conductors (two for defibrillation and two for pace/sense) are mounted on a single pin. (B) Unipolar vs. bipolar leads pacing leads. In a unipolar configuration, the pacemaker case serves as the anode, or (+), and the electrode lead tip as the cathode, or (−). In a bipolar configuration, the anode is located on the ring, often referred to as the "ring electrode," proximal to the tip, or cathode. The distance between tip and ring electrode varies among manufacturers and models.

two high-voltage and two low-voltage connections so that a single connector (with single screw) can provide pace-sense and dual coil defibrillation support, significantly decreasing pocket bulk. The limitation introduced by the DF-4 connector is the inability to use a separate lead and connect it to the proximal coil port in the header. While not commonly required, this is useful when the defibrillation threshold (DFT) is high and a strategy of placing a defibrillation coil in the coronary sinus, azygous vein, or subcutaneous tissues is planned.

Bipolar and unipolar pacing and sensing

In unipolar pacing systems, the lead tip functions as the cathode and the pulse generator as the anode (unipolar vs. bipolar leads; Fig. 1.15B). In bipolar systems, the lead tip serves as the cathode and a lead ring acts as the anode (Fig. 1.15B). Unipolar leads are of simpler design (only one conductor) and have a smaller external diameter. Unipolar leads have historically demonstrated greater durability than bipolar leads. In recent years the difference in durability has been less distinct. Unipolar leads do not offer the option of bipolar function. Although unipolar and bipolar leads are readily available, present usage of transvenous leads is almost exclusively bipolar in the USA. Bipolar leads may function in the unipolar mode if the pacemaker is so programmed. They are available in several designs, generally coaxial or multiluminal. Regardless of design, the external diameter of a bipolar lead is usually greater than that of unipolar leads because each coil must be electrically separated by insulating material. Bipolar pacing is generally preferred over unipolar pacing because it cannot cause extracardiac stimulation at the pulse generator (pectoralist muscle stimulation), which may occasionally occur with unipolar pacing due to current returning to the generator. Also, because closely spaced electrodes result in a smaller "antenna," bipolar sensing is less susceptible to myopotential and far-field oversensing and to electromagnetic interference.[41] All implantable defibrillators utilize bipolar sensing to minimize the risk of inappropriate shock caused by oversensing.

There are historical controversies regarding unipolar versus bipolar pacing and sensing configurations and which, if either, is superior.[41] Nonetheless, the majority of leads implanted are bipolar. There are certain advantages with unipolar leads. They employ a simpler design and smaller size. Smaller, more compliant and flexible unipolar leads can be placed in difficult coronary sinus venous tributaries. Traditionally, they have very low failure rates.[42] Unipolar leads are less prone to short

circuit when there are insulation breaches (due the absence of an adjacent conductor), although this benefit may be outweighed by their susceptibility to oversensing. Importantly, a lead that is malfunctioning in the bipolar mode may function satisfactorily when programmed to the unipolar configuration (see Chapter 8: Programming).

All pulse generators offer independently programmable pacing and sensing in each channel; however, bipolar programming of a device attached to a unipolar lead results in no output. Bipolar leads can function in the unipolar mode; the converse is not true.

Left ventricular leads

Cardiac resynchronization therapy with biventricular pacing is an established treatment for patients with chronic moderate–severe congestive heart failure, low left ventricular ejection fraction, and New York Heart Association class III or IV heart failure.[43] In order to pace the left ventricle, a pacing lead is implanted transvenously through the coronary sinus and one of its venous tributaries to stimulate the left ventricular free wall. Resynchronization is obtained by stimulating both ventricles to contract with minimal intraventricular delay, thereby improving the left ventricular performance.[44]

New technologies have emerged to assist in the placement of leads to targeted anatomic sites. Catheter-delivered systems use a deflectable sheath that is braided to allow the simultaneous ability to torque and advance the catheter. A second, smaller lumen sheath can be used within the first sheath to enhance access to the coronary sinus and its venous tributaries, as well as serve as a conduit for contrast injections and lead delivery. A second technology developed to reach difficult anatomic targets is to use an over-the-wire lead delivery system (Fig. 1.16). With this system the lead can be advanced to a stable position over a guidewire used initially to navigate tortuous regions of the coronary veins similar to techniques used extensively for

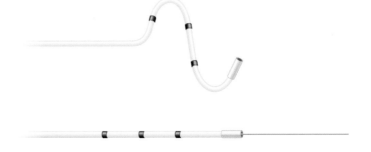

Fig. 1.16 Over the wire leads to facilitate placement in coronary vein branches. Top: lead with wire advanced beyond the distal end. The wire acts as a track over which the lead is advanced to provide stability. Bottom: lead with wire removed for final deployment.

coronary angiography. Using stiffer wires like a stylette that do not exit the left ventricular lead, the leads can be pushed into position as well as have their relative geometries changed by the constraints of the stiff wire. Tip geometry changes allow the operator to change the early contour of the lead system dynamically to allow passage through tortuous veins. Flexibility in tool selection improves access to target sites across a broad range of anatomies and decreases injury to coronary venous structures. Through availability and/or combining of these multiple technologies, access to target sites has improved greatly, in particular, coronary vein subselection for left ventricular lead placement.

Modifications of tip geometries as well as a family of left ventricular leads to choose from have improved the stability of these passive leads. Furthermore, newer multipolar left ventricular leads provide a broad array of pacing configurations to facilitate favorable pacing thresholds and avoid phrenic nerve stimulation.[45] Establishing a well-positioned left ventricular lead position, and avoiding apical pacing, favorably influence long-term outcomes with cardiac resynchronization.[46]

Pulse generators

All pulse generators include a power source, an output circuit, a sensing circuit, a timing circuit, and a header with a standardized connector (or connectors) to attach a lead (or leads) to the pulse generator.[47] Essentially, all devices are capable of storing some degree of diagnostic information that can be retrieved at a later time. Most pacemakers incorporate a rate-adaptive sensor. Despite increasing complexity, device size has continued to decrease. This has led to a variable effect on the potential longevity.

Many power sources have been used for pulse generators over the years. Lithium iodine cells have been the energy source for almost all contemporary pacemaker pulse generators. Newer pacemakers and implantable cardioverter-defibrillators (ICDs) that can support higher current drains for capacitor charging and high-rate antitachycardia pacing use lithium–silver oxide–vanadium chemistries. Lithium is the anodal element and provides the supply of electrons; iodine is the cathodal element and accepts the electrons. The cathodal and anodal elements are separated by an electrolyte, which serves as a conductor of ionic movement but a barrier to the transfer of electrons. The circuit is completed by the external load, i.e., the leads and myocardium. The battery voltage of the cell depends on the chemical composition of the cell; at the beginning of life for the lithium iodine battery, the cell generates approximately 2.8V, which decreases to 2.4V when approximately 90% of the battery life has been used.

The voltage then exponentially declines to 1.8V as the battery reaches end-of-life. However, the voltage at which the cell reaches a specific degree of discharge is load dependent. The elective replacement voltages were chosen based on the shape of the discharge curves under expected operating conditions. When the battery is at end-of-service, most devices lose telemetry and programming capabilities, frequently reverting to a fixed high-output pacing mode to maintain patient safety. This predictable depletion characteristic has made lithium-based power cells common in current devices. Nickel–cadmium technology is being used once again in at least one investigational implantable device.

The battery voltage can be telemetered from the pulse generator. In addition, most devices provide battery impedance (which increases with battery depletion) for additional information about battery life. The battery life can also be estimated by the magnet rate of the device, which changes with a decline in battery voltage. Unfortunately, the magnet rates are not standardized, and rate change characteristics vary tremendously among manufacturers and even among devices produced by the same manufacturer. Therefore, it is important to know the magnet rate characteristics of a given device before using this feature to determine battery status.

The longevity of any battery is determined by several factors, including chemical composition of the battery, size of the battery, external load (pulse duration and amplitude, stimulation frequency, total pacing lead impedance, and amount of current required to operate device circuitry and store diagnostic information), amount of internal discharge, and voltage decay characteristics of the cell. The basic formula for longevity determination is $114 \times$ [battery capacity (A-HR)/current drain (μA)] = longevity in years. However, this formula is subject to how the power cell's ampere-hours is specified by the manufacturer; thus, the longevity will vary somewhat by company. High-performance leads, automatic capture algorithms, and programming options that minimize pacing may further enhance device longevity if not offset by energy consumption from running the software.[48,49]

The pacing pulse is generated first by charging an output capacitor with subsequent discharge of the capacitor to the pacing cathode and anode. Because the voltage of a lithium iodine cell is fixed, obtaining multiple selectable pulse amplitudes requires the use of a voltage amplifier between the battery and the output capacitor. Contemporary pulse generators are constant-voltage (rather than constant-current) devices, implying delivery of a constant-voltage pulse throughout the pulse duration. In reality, some voltage drop occurs between the leading and the trailing edges of the impulse; the size of this decrease depends on the pacing impedance and pulse duration. The lower the impedance, the greater the current flow from the fixed quantity of charge on the capacitor and the greater the voltage drop throughout the pulse duration.[50] The voltage drop is also dependent on the capacitance value of the capacitor and the pulse duration.

The output waveform is followed by a low-amplitude wave of opposite polarity, the afterpotential. The afterpotential is determined by the polarization of the electrode at the electrode–tissue interface; formation is due to electrode characteristics as well as to pulse amplitude and duration. The sensing circuit may sense afterpotentials of sufficient amplitude, especially if the sensitivity threshold is low. Newer pacemakers use the output circuit to discharge the afterpotential quickly, thus lowering the incidence of afterpotential sensing. The afterpotential also helps to prevent electrode corrosion.

The intracardiac electrogram results from current conducted from the myocardium to the sensing circuit via the pacing leads, where it is then amplified and filtered. The input impedance must be significantly larger than the sensing impedance to minimize attenuation of the electrogram. A bandpass filter attenuates signals on either side of a center frequency, which varies between manufacturers (generally ranging from 20 to 40 Hz).[51,52] After filtering, the electrogram signal is compared with a reference voltage, the sensitivity setting; signals with an amplitude of this reference voltage or higher are sensed as true intracardiac events and are forwarded to the timing circuitry, whereas signals with an amplitude below the reference amplitude are categorized as noise, extracardiac or other cardiac signal, such as T waves.

Sensing circuitry also incorporates noise reversion that cause the pacemaker to revert to a noise reversion mode (asynchronous pacing) whenever the rate of signal received by the sensing circuit exceeds the noise reversion rate. This feature is incorporated to prevent inhibition of pacing when the device is exposed to electromagnetic interference. Pulse generators also use Zener diodes designed to protect the circuitry from high external voltages, which may occur, for example, with defibrillation. When the input voltage presented to the pacemaker exceeds the Zener voltage, the excess voltage is shunted back through the leads to the myocardium.

The timing circuit of the pacemaker is an electronic clock that regulates the pacing cycle length, refractory periods, blanking periods, and AV intervals with extreme accuracy. The output from the clock (as well as signals from the sensing circuitry) is sent to a timing and logic control board that operates the internal clocks, which in turn regulate all the various timing cycles of the pulse generator. The timing and logic control circuitry also contains an absolute maximal upper rate cut-off to prevent "runaway pacing" in the event of random component failure.[53,54]

Each new generation of pacemakers contains more microprocessor capability. The circuitry contains a combination of read-only memory (ROM) and random-access memory (RAM). ROM is used to operate the sensing and output functions of the device, and RAM is used in diagnostic functions. Larger RAM capability has allowed devices to store increased amounts of retrievable diagnostic information and patient-specific longitudinal data, with the potential to allow downloading of new features externally into an implanted device.

External telemetry is supported in all implantable devices and in some pacemakers. The pulse generator can receive information from the programmer and send information back by radiofrequency signals. Each manufacturer's programmer and pulse generator operate on an exclusive radiofrequency, preventing the use of one manufacturer's programmer with a pacemaker from another manufacturer. Through telemetry, the programmer can retrieve both diagnostic information and real-time information about battery status, lead impedance, current, pulse amplitude, and pulse duration. Real-time electrograms and marker channels can also be obtained with most devices. The device can also be directed to operate within certain limits and to store specific types of diagnostic information via the programmer.

The most recent change in telemetry is that of "remote" capability. Information exchange has traditionally occurred by placing and leaving the programming "head" of the programmer over the pulse generator for the duration of the interrogation and programming changes. New telemetry designs allow the programming "head" or "wand" to be placed briefly over the pulse generator, or in the near vicinity of the device, to establish identity of the specific model and pulse generator and then complete the bidirectional informational exchange at a distance, i.e., the "wand" does not need to be kept in a position directly over the pulse generator. Finally, even the use of a wand for certain pulse generators is not required for remote programming. These technology advances have allowed remote monitoring of all implantable devices and in some pacemakers using home telemetry systems that upload patient and device-specific data to a central, secure database. With home monitoring, devices can be routinely monitored, patient alerts transmitted in real time, and patient cardiac status updates communicated on a programmable criteria basis. Remote monitoring of patients with ICDs improves survival and readily identifies risk markers of mortality.[55]

Table 1.1 The North American Society of Pacing and Electrophysiology and the British Pacing and Electrophysiology Group (NBG) code.

I	II	III	IV	V
Chamber(s) paced	**Chamber(s) sensed**	**Response to sensing**	**Programmability, rate modulation**	**Multisite pacing**
O = None	O =None	O = None	O = None	O = None
A = Atrium	A = Atrium	T = Triggered	P = Simple programmable	A = Atrium
V = Ventricle	V = Ventricle	I = Inhibited	M = Multiprogrammable	V = Ventricle
D = Dual (A + V)	D = Dual (A + V)	D = dual (T + I)	C = Communicating	D = Dual (A + V)

Source: modified from Bernstein AD, Daubert JC, Fletcher RD, *et al*. The revised NASPE/BPEG generic code for antibradycardia, adaptive-rate, and multisite pacing. North American Society of Pacing and Electrophysiology/British Pacing and Electrophysiology Group. Pacing Clin Electrophysiol 2002; 25:260–4, by permission of Futura Publishing Company.

Pacemaker nomenclature

A lettered code to describe the basic function of pacing devices, initially developed by the American Heart Association and the American College of Cardiology, has since been modified and updated by the members of the North American Society of Pacing and Electrophysiology and the British Pacing and Electrophysiology Group (currently the Heart Rhythm Society).[56] This code has five positions to describe basic pacemaker function, although it obviously cannot incorporate all of the various special features available on modern devices (Table 1.1).

The first position describes the chamber or chambers in which electrical stimulation occurs. **A** reflects pacing in the atrium, **V** implies pacing in the ventricle, **D** signifies pacing in both the atrium and the ventricle, and **O** is used when the device has antitachycardia pacing (ATP) or cardioversion-defibrillation capability but no bradycardia pacing capability.

The second position describes the chamber or chambers in which sensing occurs. The letter code is the same as that in the first position, except that an **O** in this position represents lack of sensing in any chamber, i.e., fixed-rate pacing. (Manufacturers may use an **S** in both the first and the second positions to indicate single-chamber capability that can be used in either the atrium or the ventricle.)

The third position designates the mode of sensing, i.e., how the device responds to a sensed event. **I** indicates that the device inhibits output when an intrinsic event is sensed and starts a new timing interval. **T** implies that an output pulse is triggered in response to a sensed event. **D** indicates that the device is capable of dual modes of response (applicable only in dual-chamber systems).

The fourth position reflects both programmability and rate modulation. **O** indicates that none of the pacemaker settings can be changed by noninvasive programming, **P** suggests "simple" programmability (i.e.,

one or two variables can be modified), **M** indicates multiprogrammability (three or more variables can be modified), and **C** indicates that the device has telemetry capability and can communicate noninvasively with the programmer (which also implies multiprogrammability). Finally, an **R** in the fourth position designates rate-responsive capability. This means that the pacemaker has some type of sensor to modulate the heart rate independent of the intrinsic heart rate. All modern devices are multiprogrammable and have telemetry capability; therefore, the **R** to designate rate-responsive capability is the most commonly used currently.

The fifth position was originally used to identify antitachycardia treatment functions. However, this has been changed, and antitachycardia options are no longer included in the nomenclature. The fifth position now indicates whether multisite pacing is not present (O), or present in the atrium (A), ventricle (V), or both (D). Multisite pacing is defined for this purpose as stimulation sites in both atria, both ventricles, more than one stimulation site in any single chamber, or any combination of these.

All pacemaker functions (whether single, dual or multi-chamber) are based on timing cycles. Even the function of the most complex devices can be readily understood by applying the principles of pacemaker timing intervals. This understanding is critical for accurate interpretation of pacemaker electrocardiograms, especially during troubleshooting. Pacemaker timing cycles are described in detail in Chapter 7: Timing Cycles.

Defibrillation basics

In 1899, Prevost and Battelli[57] noted that the "fibrillatory tremulations produced in the dog" could be arrested with the re-establishment of the normal heartbeat if one submitted the animal "to passages of current of high voltage." Despite these early observa-

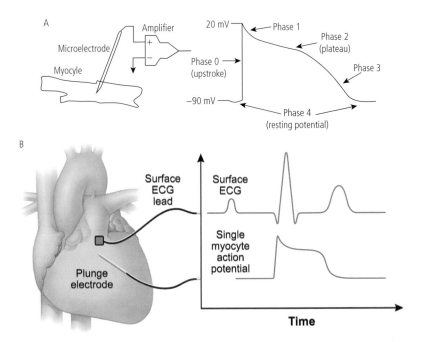

Fig. 1.17 (A) The cardiac action potential. Left: impalement of a single myocyte by a microelectrode. This permits recording of the change in voltage potential over time in a single cell. Right: on the graph, voltage (in millivolts) is on the ordinate, time on the abscissa. The action potential in ventricular myocytes begins with a rapid upstroke (phase 0), which is followed by transient early repolarization (phase 1), a plateau (phase 2), and terminal repolarization (phase 3), which returns the membrane potential back to the resting value. (B) Correlation of cellular and clinical electrical activity. The QRS complex of the surface ECG is generated by the action potential upstroke (phase 0) of ventricular myocytes and the propagation of the upstroke through the ventricular myocardium. Similarly, the T wave is the result of ventricular repolarization (phase 3).

tions, decades elapsed before broad clinical applicability fueled interest in more widespread investigation of the mechanism underlying defibrillation. With the development of internal defibrillators in the late 1970s came a greater need to quantify defibrillation effectiveness, to understand the factors governing waveform and lead design, and to determine the effect of pharmacologic agents on defibrillation. Remarkably, much of this work was carried out without a complete understanding of the fundamental mechanism of defibrillation.

This section reviews the emerging insights to the electrophysiologic effects of shocks and how they are related to defibrillation. It also reviews the means of assessing the efficacy of defibrillation and the important effects of waveform, lead design and placement, and pharmacologic agents on defibrillation, with an emphasis on those principles pertaining to clinical practice.

Despite great strides made in understanding the technology required for defibrillation (e.g., lead design and position, waveform selection), the basic underlying mechanisms have not been definitively determined. A few hypotheses have been proposed to explain how an electric shock terminates fibrillation: critical mass, upper limit of vulnerability, progressive depolarization, and virtual electrode depolarization. These hypotheses, which are not entirely mutually exclusive, are summarized below.

In its resting state, the myocardium is excitable, and a pacing stimulus, or current injected by the depolarization of a neighboring myocyte, can bring the membrane potential to a threshold value, above which a new action potential ensues (Fig. 1.17). The ability of the action potential of a myocyte to depolarize adjacent myocardium results in propagation of electrical activity through cardiac tissue. Importantly, immediately after depolarization, the myocardium is refractory and cannot be stimulated to produce another action potential until it has recovered excitability (Fig. 1.18). The interval immediately after an action potential, during which another action potential cannot be elicited by a pacing stimulus, is referred to as the "refractory period."

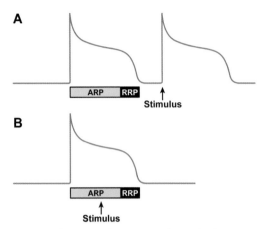

Fig. 1.18 Refractory periods. Myocytes can be stimulated to generate new action potentials, except in their absolute refractory period (ARP). In (A), a stimulus occurs after the myocyte has fully recovered from the preceding action potential, and a new action potential ensues. In contrast, in (B), the same stimulus is delivered earlier, the myocyte remains in its absolute refractory period because of the preceding action potential, and no new action potential is elicited. RRP, relative refractory period.

Ventricular fibrillation (VF) results when an electrical wavebreak induces re-entry and results in a cascade of new wavebreaks. In patients with a structurally abnormal or diseased heart, the underlying tissue heterogeneity results in a predisposition to wavebreak, then re-entry, and finally fibrillation.[58] These wandering wavelets are self-sustaining once initiated. In the 1940s, Gurvich and Yuniev[59] predicted that electric shocks led to premature tissue stimulation in advance of propagating wavefronts, preventing continued progression of the wavefront. This concept of defibrillation as a large-scale stimulation remains a central tenet of many of the currently held theories of defibrillation.

Critical mass

The critical mass theory proposed that shocks need only eliminate fibrillatory wavelets in a critical amount of myocardium to extinguish the arrhythmia. Experiments in canine models found that injection of potassium chloride (which depolarizes myocardium, rendering it unavailable for fibrillation) into the right coronary artery or the left circumflex artery failed to terminate VF as often as injection into both the left circumflex and the left anterior descending arteries together. Similarly, electrical shocks of equal magnitude terminated fibrillation most frequently when the electrodes were positioned at the right ventricular apex and the posterior left ventricle, as opposed to two right ventricular electrodes. Thus, it was concluded that if a "critical mass" of myocardium

was rendered unavailable for VF either by potassium injection or by defibrillatory shock, the remaining excitable tissue was insufficient to support the wandering wavelets, and the arrhythmia terminated.[60] However, it was not critical to depolarize every ventricular cell to terminate fibrillation.

Upper limit of vulnerability

Studies mapping electrical activation after failed shocks led to several observations not accounted for by the critical mass hypothesis, giving rise to the upper limit of vulnerability theory. First, an isoelectric interval (an electrical pause) was seen after failed shocks before resumption of fibrillation. The relatively long pause suggested that VF was terminated by the shock and then secondarily regenerated by it.[61] The concept that failed shocks are unsuccessful because they reinitiate fibrillation rather than because they fail to halt continuing wavelets was further buttressed by a second observation – that post-shock conduction patterns were not the continuation of preshock wavefronts.[62] If a failed shock resulted from the inability to halt continuing fibrillation, the assumption was that the post-shock wavefronts should be a continuation of the propagating wavefronts present before shock delivery and that new wavefronts at sites remote from the preshock wavefronts would not be expected. Furthermore, VF was frequently reinitiated in the regions of lowest shock intensity, suggesting that these low-intensity regions were responsible for reinitiating fibrillation. Shocks that fall into the vulnerable period (which overlaps the T wave during normal rhythm) with an energy above the lower limit of vulnerability and below the upper limit of vulnerability induce VF. Shocks with energies above the upper limit of vulnerability never induce VF, and thus defibrillate (Fig. 1.19).

Elegant mapping studies demonstrated that shocks with potential gradients less than a minimum critical value – termed the upper limit of vulnerability (ULV) (6 V/cm for monophasic shocks, 4 V/cm for biphasic shocks) – could induce fibrillation when applied to myocardium during its vulnerable period. Low-energy shocks did so by creating regions of functional block in vulnerable myocardium at "critical points" that initiated re-entry and subsequent fibrillation.[63] Importantly, this theory permits linking of defibrillation and fibrillation. In sinus rhythm, low-energy shocks delivered during the vulnerable period (the T wave) induce VF; higher energy shocks – with energy above the ULV – do not (Fig. 1.19). Because at any given time during fibrillation a number of myocardial regions are repolarizing and thus vulnerable, a shock with a potential gradient below the ULV may create a critical point and reinitiate fibrillation. Conversely, a shock with a

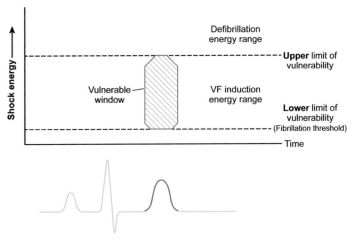

Fig. 1.19 Window of vulnerability during sinus rhythm. During sinus rhythm, the ventricles are vulnerable to ventricular fibrillation (VF) when a shock is delivered on the T wave, in the vulnerable window. To induce fibrillation, the shock energy must be greater than the lower limit of vulnerability (the fibrillation threshold) and below the upper limit of vulnerability (ULV). Shocks with energy above the upper limit of vulnerability do not induce fibrillation. Because during VF there is dyssynchrony of activation, at any given instant a number of regions are repolarizing (equivalent to the T wave in sinus rhythm), so that a shock with a gradient that is less than the ULV can reinduce fibrillation in these regions. In contrast, shocks with energy above the ULV throughout the myocardium cannot reinitiate VF and are successful. The ULV is correlated with the defibrillation threshold. Further details appear in the text.

gradient above the ULV across the entire myocardium does not reinduce VF and should therefore succeed. During defibrillator testing, shocks are intentionally delivered in the vulnerable zone to induce fibrillation (Fig. 1.20); the zone of vulnerability has been defined in humans.[64] The fact that the vulnerable zone exists and that the ULV has been correlated with the DFT supports the ULV hypothesis as a mechanism of defibrillation, and permits its use at implant testing (see later).[65]

Progressive depolarization

A third theory of defibrillation, the progressive depolarization theory (also referred to as the "refractory period extension theory") incorporates some elements of both critical mass and ULV theories. Using voltage-sensitive optical dyes, Dillon and Kwaku[66] have demonstrated that shocks of sufficient strength were able to elicit responses, even from supposedly refractory myocardium. Thus, as seen in Fig. 1.21, the duration of an action potential can be prolonged (and the refractory period extended) despite refractory myocardium when a sufficiently strong shock is applied.[67] This phenomenon may result from sodium channel reactivation by the shock. The degree of additional depolarization time is a function of both shock intensity and shock timing.[68] Because the shock stimulates new action potentials in myocardium that is late in repolarization and produces additional depolarization

time when the myocardium is already depolarized, myocardial resynchronization occurs. This is manifested by myocardial repolarization at a constant time after the shock (second dashed line in Fig. 1.21, labeled "constant repolarization time"). Thus, the shock that defibrillates extends overall ventricular refractoriness, limiting the excitable tissue available for fibrillation. Thus, it extinguishes continuing wavelets and resynchronizes repolarization, so that distant regions of myocardium become excitable simultaneously, preventing dispersion of refractoriness and renewed re-entry. Experimental evidence has demonstrated that shocks with a potential gradient above the ULV result in time-dependent extension of the refractory period. In contrast, lower energy shocks may result in a graded response that could create transient block and a critical point, thereby reinducing fibrillation.[68] Note that while progressive depolarization and virtual electrode depolarization (discussed below) address cellular mechanisms of shock induced re-entry, the ULV and critical mass hypotheses do not postulate a specific mechanism, but only that shock-induced re-entry is an important mechanism of failed subthreshold shocks.

Virtual electrode depolarization

More recently, optical signal measurements of transmembrane potentials have demonstrated the concept of the "virtual electrode."[69] The virtual electrode effect

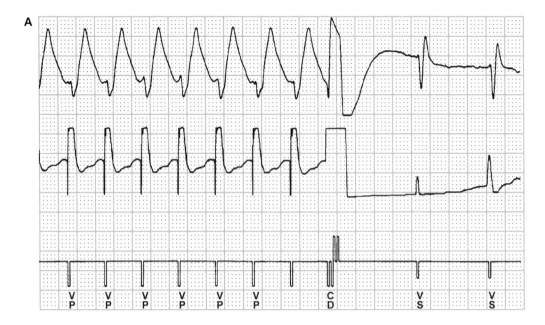

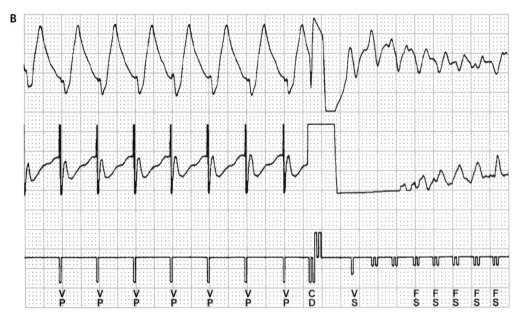

Fig. 1.20 Induction of ventricular fibrillation by a T-wave shock during testing of an implantable defibrillator. In (A), a 1-J shock is delivered 380 ms after the last paced beat. Fibrillation is not induced, because this shock is delivered outside the window of vulnerability. In (B), the timing of the shock is adjusted to 300 ms after the last paced complex, so that it is delivered more squarely on the T wave, in the window of vulnerability, and fibrillation is induced. The window of vulnerability is defined by both shock energy and timing. CD, charge delivered; FS, fibrillation sense; VP, ventricular pacing; VS, ventricular sensing.

refers to stimulation of tissue far from site and implanted electrode. This effect makes the defibrillation electrode effectively much larger than the physical electrode. In the virtual electrode, the anode cells are brought close to their resting potential, increasing their responsiveness to stimulation. More importantly, the region of depolarization or hyperpolarization near the physical electrode is surrounded by regions with opposite polarity. Anodal shocking produces a wavefront of depolarization that begins at the boundary of positively

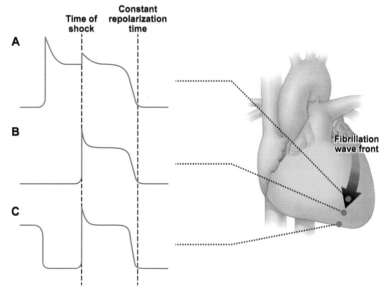

Fig. 1.21 Progressive depolarization. A fibrillatory wavefront is depicted by the arrow, and the action potential response to a defibrillatory shock is demonstrated at several points surrounding the wavefront. The fibrillatory wavefront has just passed through a myocyte at point A when the shock is delivered. The myocyte is in its plateau (phase 2), when it would ordinarily be refractory to additional stimulation. However, when a sufficiently strong shock is delivered, the myocyte can generate an active response with prolongation of the action potential and of the refractory period. The response is referred to as "additional depolarization time." The tissue at point B is at the leading edge of the fibrillatory wavefront. The shock strikes this myocardium at the time of the upstroke (phase 0) and has little effect on the action potential. The tissue at point C is excitable (it is the excitable gap that the fibrillatory wave front was about to enter) when the shock is delivered. The shock elicits a new action potential in this excitable tissue. Despite the different temporal and anatomical locations of the three action potentials depicted, after the shock there is resynchronization by the "constant repolarization time." This resynchronization helps prevent continuation of fibrillation.

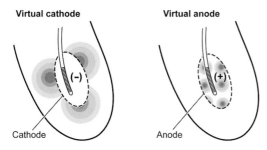

Fig. 1.22 The cathodal shocks (left) produce wavefronts that expand and propagate away from the right ventricular coil. In comparison, anodal shocks (right) produced wavefronts that collapse and propagate towards the right ventricular coil (Adapted from Figure 4, Kroll MW, Efimov IR, Tchou PJ. Present understanding of shock polarity for internal defibrillation: the obvious and non-obvious clinical implications. Pacing Clin Electrophysiol 2006; 29:885–91, with permission.)

charged regions and then spreads toward the negatively charged region of the physical anode.[70] This produces "collapsing" wavefronts which frequently collide and neutralize one another and thereby are less likely to result in a sustained arrhythmia (Fig. 1.22).[71]

Defibrillation theory summary

To summarize and to put defibrillation theory into clinical perspective, the effects of the application of a voltage gradient across myocardium are a function of field strength and timing. Although the biologic effects of shocks may overlap, this concept is summarized in Fig. 1.23, extremely low energy pulses may have no effect on the myocardium. Stronger pulses (in the microjoule range), such as those used for cardiac pacing, result in action potential generation in nonrefractory myocardium, which leads to a propagating impulse. With increasing electric field strength (to the 1-J area), VF can be induced with shocks delivered during the vulnerable period in normal rhythm. Increasing the shock strength above the ULV (and above the DFT) puts the shock in the defibrillation zone. Very high-energy shocks can lead to toxic effects, including disruption of cell membranes, post-shock block, mechanical dysfunction, and new tachyarrhythmias.[68]

The importance of waveform

The shape of a defibrillating waveform can dramatically affect its defibrillation efficacy. As in pacing, the battery

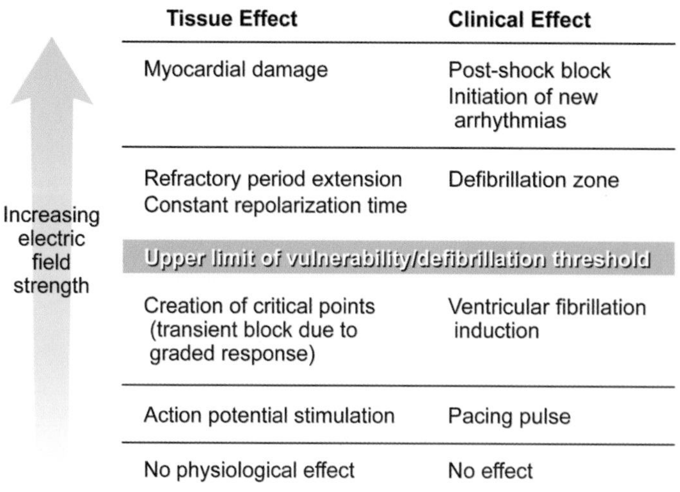

Tissue Effect	Clinical Effect
Myocardial damage	Post-shock block Initiation of new arrhythmias
Refractory period extension Constant repolarization time	Defibrillation zone
Upper limit of vulnerability/defibrillation threshold	
Creation of critical points (transient block due to graded response)	Ventricular fibrillation induction
Action potential stimulation	Pacing pulse
No physiological effect	No effect

Increasing electric field strength →

Fig. 1.23 Effects of increasing shock (electrical field) strength on myocardial tissue.

serves as the source of electrical charge for cardiac stimulation in defibrillation. Before a high-energy shock can be delivered, the electrical charge must be accumulated in a capacitor, because a battery cannot deliver the amount of required charge in the short time of a defibrillation shock. A capacitor stores charge by means of two large surface area conductors separated by a dielectric (poorly conducting) material, and capacitor size is an important determinant of implantable defibrillator volume, typically accounting for approximately 30% of device size. If fluid analogies are used for electricity – voltage as water pressure and current as water flow) – the capacitor is analogous to a water balloon, which has a compliance defined by the ratio of volume to pressure. To increase the amount of water put into the balloon, one can increase the pressure or, alternatively, use a balloon with a greater compliance (more stretch for a given amount of pressure). Similarly, the charge stored can be increased by increasing capacitance or by applying greater voltage. The trend in implantable devices has been toward smaller capacitors to create smaller devices.

The charge stored by a capacitor is defined by

$$\text{Charge} = \text{capacitance} \times \text{voltage}.$$

The voltage waveform of a capacitor discharged into a fixed-resistance load (Fig. 1.24) is determined by

$$V(t) = Vi \cdot e^{-t/RC}$$

and the energy associated with the waveform is given by

$$\text{Energy} = 0.5\, CV^2.$$

Because the "tail" of the waveform in longer pulses (≥10 ms) refibrillates the ventricle, truncated waveforms have been used clinically. The classic monophasic truncated waveform is shown in Fig. 1.24b. The waveform is characterized by the initial voltage (Vi), the final voltage (Vf), and the pulse width or tilt. Tilt is an expression of the percentage decay of the initial voltage. The tilt of a waveform is a function of the size of the capacitor used, the resistance of the leads and tissues through which current passes, and the duration of the pulse. Tilt is defined by the percentage decrease of the initial voltage:

$$\text{Tilt} = (Vi - Vf)/Vi \times 100\%.$$

Tilt can have an important effect on defibrillation efficacy, with progressive improvement in defibrillation efficacy with decreasing tilt, for a trapezoidal waveform of constant duration. For monophasic waveforms formerly used clinically, the optimal tilt was 50–80%.

Biphasic waveforms
Appropriately characterized biphasic shocks can result in significant improvement in defibrillation efficacy, with reductions in defibrillation thresholds (DFTs, a measure of defibrillation energy requirements, discussed below) of 30–50%.[72] All currently available commercial defibrillators use biphasic waveforms; a typical biphasic waveform is shown in Fig. 1.24c. Biphasic waveforms have numerous clinical advantages, all stemming from their improved defibrillation efficacy.

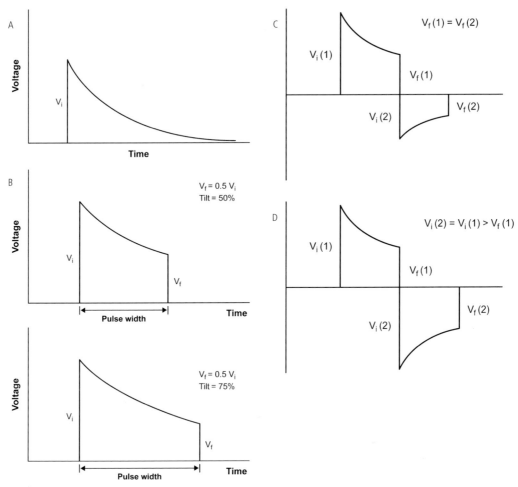

Fig. 1.24 Defibrillation waveforms. (A) Standard capacitor discharge. (B) Monophasic truncated waveform with initial voltage (V_i), final voltage (V_f) and pulse width labeled. Top waveform has 50% tilt, and bottom waveform has 75% tilt. (C) Biphasic waveform with leading edge of the first pulse ($V_{i(1)}$), trailing edge of the first pulse ($V_{f(1)}$), leading edge of the second pulse ($V_{i(2)}$), and trailing edge of the second pulse ($V_{f(2)}$) labeled. As $V_{i(2)}$ equals $V_{f(1)}$, this waveform can be generated by reversing the polarity of a single capacitor after the first pulse is completed. (D) In contrast, $V_{i(2)}$ is greater than $V_{f(1)}$, so that a second capacitor is needed to create this waveform.

Biphasic waveforms have been shown to result in higher implantation success rates because of their lower DFTs, and thereby higher safety margins.[73] Because safety margins are increased, most patients do not require high-energy shocks, and smaller devices can be designed.[74] The improved efficacy of biphasic waveforms permits a greater tolerance in electrode positioning than that required for monophasic waveforms, facilitating the implanting procedure. Additionally, biphasic shocks have been shown to result in faster post-shock recurrence of sinus rhythm and to have greater efficacy than monophasic shocks in terminating VF of long duration.[75,76]

With the development of biphasic defibrillation waveforms the energy required for defibrillation has been reduced.[77–79] Simultaneously, advances in capacitor and battery technology have allowed for a reduction in pulse generator size. Further advances that will reduce the generator size will occur when the energy required for defibrillation is reduced.[77]

Phase duration and tilt

In most commercially available ICDs, pulse duration and tilt are preset to values found to be optimal based on experimental evidence (Fig. 1.25). Some devices permit individualization of the pulse widths, based on

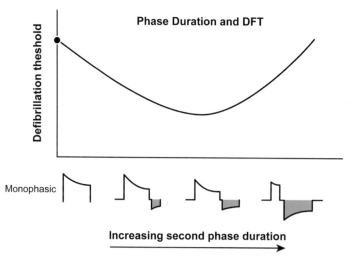

Fig. 1.25 Idealized curve demonstrating the relationship between second phase duration and defibrillation threshold (DFT). Details are in the text. (From Wessale JL, Bourland JD, Tacker WA, Geddes LA. Bipolar catheter defibrillation in dogs using trapezoidal waveforms of various tilts. J Electrocardiol 1980; 13:359–65, by permission of Churchill Livingstone.)

the concept that individual variations in cellular time constants result in varying optimal pulse durations. Anecdotal observations and small studies support pulse width optimization in high DFT patients.[80,81] Waveform optimization is used infrequently in clinical practice, but may be useful in some high DFT patients (discussed further below).

Polarity and biphasic waveforms

Polarity is an important determinant of monophasic defibrillation, with lower DFTs found for transvenous systems when the right ventricular electrode is the anode (+).[82,83] The results of studies of biphasic polarity are less uniform, with some reports showing an effect of biphasic polarity but others indicating no effect.[84,85] However, all studies demonstrating a polarity effect have found that waveforms with a first phase in which the right ventricular electrode is the anode (+) are more effective. Additionally, biphasic polarity has the greatest effect on patients with elevated DFTs. In a study of 60 patients, use of biphasic waveforms with a right ventricular anodal first phase resulted in a 31% reduction in DFT in patients with DFT ≥15 J, whereas polarity made no difference in patients with DFTs <15 J.[86] Despite the fairly uniform population improvement in DFT with a ventricular anodal first phase polarity among studies in which an effect was seen, there is clearly individual variability, so that if an adequate safety margin cannot be found in a patient, a trial of the opposite polarity is reasonable, particularly if the

initial polarity tested was not anodal in the right ventricle for the first phase.

Mechanism of improved efficacy with biphasic waveforms

Several theories have been proposed to explain the observed superiority of biphasic over monophasic waveforms. None provide a complete explanation for the benefits seen, and the fundamental mechanism remains to be determined. However, the clinical superiority of biphasic shocks has been a consistent and reproducible finding. All ICDs today use biphasic defibrillation.

Measuring shock dose

The shape of the waveform is a function of the initial voltage, the size of the capacitor, and the resistance of the load. If a smaller capacitor is used to diminish device size, a larger initial voltage may be needed to deliver an equivalent amount of charge into the fibrillating tissue. Thus, two waveforms may have different leading edge voltages, but the same energy if there are differences in capacitance (Fig. 1.26). Therefore, the question of how to determine the "dose" of a shock arises. The "dose" of defibrillation is usually given in units of energy (joules) on the basis of tradition and ease of measurement. Physiologically, however, energy has little bearing on defibrillation; the voltage gradient is the factor that affects membrane channel conductance, and at the tissue level several decades of animal

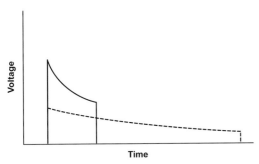

Fig. 1.26 Two waveforms with different voltages but the same energy. The solid waveform has a higher initial voltage but a smaller capacitance and, consequently, a shorter pulse width. The dashed waveform starts with a lower voltage but has a greater capacitance and pulse width, resulting in the same energy delivery despite the marked differences in the voltages. Further details in the text.

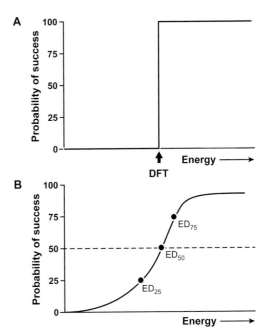

Fig. 1.27 Defibrillation "threshold" (DFT). (A) The expected response to shock if a true threshold value existed. In reality, the likelihood of success is a sigmoidal dose–response curve, as shown in (B). The ED_{50} is the energy dose with a 50% likelihood of success, and so on.

and human research have shown current to be the most important factor for generating action potentials and for defibrillation.[68] To add to the complexity, energy can be described as the stored energy – the amount of energy stored in the capacitor before shock delivery – or the energy delivered. Because the waveforms are truncated, usually around 10% of the stored energy is not delivered. Additionally, although the term is used clinically, "delivered energy" is highly variable, depending on where the delivery is recorded; energy delivered at the lead surface is not the same as energy delivered only a few millimeters into the tissue. Some device manufacturers, in fact, simply report an arbitrary percentage of the stored energy as the delivered energy. Stored energy, although not a direct indicator of the factors responsible for biologic defibrillation, indicates the size of the device necessary to generate a given energy shock. Over the range of clinically utilized capacitor size and biologic tissue resistance in a given system, a change in energy up or down is reflected by a similar change in voltage and current. In practice, "energy" is the most commonly used term to indicate shock dose.

Measuring the efficacy of defibrillation
Threshold and dose–response curve
A measure frequently used to assess the ability of a system to terminate VF is the DFT. The term "threshold" suggests that there is a threshold energy above which defibrillation is uniformly successful and below which shocks fail (Fig. 1.27A). The multitude of factors that affect whether a shock will succeed – patient characteristics, fibrillation duration, degree of ischemia and potassium accumulation, distribution of electrical activation at the time of the shock, circulating pharmacologic agents, and others – result in defibrillation behavior

that is best modeled as a random variable, with a calculable probability of success for any given shock strength. Thus, defibrillation is more accurately described by a dose–response curve, with an increasing probability of success as the defibrillation energy increases (Fig. 1.27B). The curve can be characterized by its slope and intercept, and specific points on the curve can be identified, such as ED_{50}, the energy dose with a 50% likelihood of success. Factors adversely affecting defibrillation shift the curve to the right, so that a higher dose of energy is required to achieve a 50% likelihood of success, and improvements in defibrillation (such as superior lead position and improved waveforms or lead design) shift the curve to the left (Fig. 1.28). Because of the large number of fibrillation episodes required to define a curve (30–40 inductions), the dose–response curve is not determined in clinical practice, but it remains a useful research tool and conceptual framework. However, because the term "defibrillation threshold" (DFT) is widely used in the literature, it is adopted in this chapter.

Relationship between defibrillation threshold and dose–response curve
The probability of successful defibrillation at the DFT energy depends on the steps taken to define the

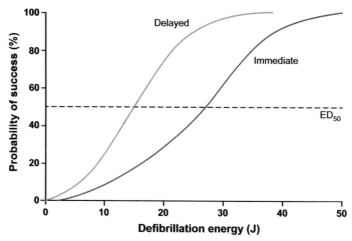

Fig. 1.28 Use of dose–response curve to measure effects of an intervention on defibrillation efficacy. The graph shows the effect of thoracotomy on defibrillation in a canine model. The "immediate" group had defibrillation threshold testing performed immediately after thoracotomy. Note that the curve is shifted to the right and that the energy with a 50% probability of success is 27 J, compared with 15 J for the "delayed" group, which was allowed 48–72 h recovery before defibrillation testing. Defibrillation is more effective in the "delayed" group because the probability of success at a given energy is higher in this group. Thus, the curves graphically display diminished defibrillation efficacy immediately after thoracotomy. (From Friedman PA, Stanton MS. Thoracotomy elevates the defibrillation threshold and modifies the defibrillation dose–response curve. J Cardiovasc Electrophysiol 1997; 8:68–73, by permission of Futura Publishing Company.)

threshold. Consider a step-down to failure DFT, in which shocks are delivered beginning at a relatively high energy (e.g., energy with a 99% success rate) and decremented by several joules with each VF induction until a shock fails (at which point a rescue shock is delivered). The DFT in this protocol is defined as the lowest energy shock that succeeds (Fig. 1.29). Because the initial energies tested are at the upper end of the dose–response curve, successive shocks may have a 98%, 95%, 88%, 85% (and so on) likelihood of success, depending on the starting energy and size of the steps taken. Despite the fairly high likelihood of success for each shock individually, the sheer number of shocks delivered in this range on average result in a shock failing (thus defining the DFT) at a relatively high point on the curve. If this process is repeated many times, a population of DFTs is created, with a mean and expected range. In humans, step-down to failure algorithms have a mean DFT with likelihood of success near 70%, but with a standard deviation near 25%.[87,88] Thus, the likelihood of success of a shock delivered at the energy defined as the DFT at a single determination ranges from 25% to 88%, with an average of 71%.[88] In other words, if a defibrillator is programmed to the step-down to failure DFT energy for its first shock, the likelihood that the first shock will succeed can range from 25% to 88%, but on average will be 71%.

In contrast to the step-down to failure DFT, in a step-up to success DFT, low-energy shocks are delivered during VF with incremental doses of energy until a first success occurs, which defines the DFT. In this case, despite the fairly low likelihood of success at each low-energy shock, if enough shocks are delivered, one is likely to succeed, defining the DFT. With this protocol, the mean DFT has a likelihood of success near 30%. Iterative increment–decrement DFT or binary search algorithms that begin in the middle zone of the curve have been shown to approximate the ED_{50}. In this type of protocol, if the first shock defibrillates the heart, the first shock of the next fibrillation episode uses a lower energy. If the first shock does not defibrillate the heart, a second shock at a higher energy is delivered. Regardless of the DFT protocol, a DFT determination is best conceptualized as a means of approximating a point on the dose–response curve, with the specific point estimated being a function of the DFT algorithm chosen.

Patient-specific defibrillation threshold and safety margin testing

Patient-specific DFT testing determines the lowest energy that reliably defibrillates an individual patient. This permits programming a low first shock strength. The rationale for adopting this strategy is that the lower shock strength will result in the shortest charge time and consequent battery preservation, and diminished risk of syncopy, post-shock AV block, myocardial damage, and impaired sensing.[89,90] The disadvantage of patient-specific DFT termination is that a greater

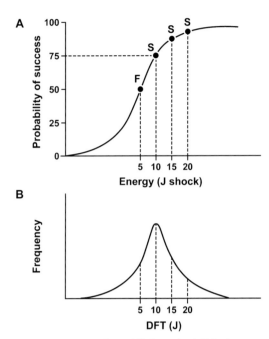

Fig. 1.29 Step-down to failure defibrillation threshold (DFT) testing. In this hypothetical example (A), four shocks are required to define the DFT. The first shock is delivered at 20 J and is successful (S). The next shock, delivered at 15 J, also succeeds. A 10-J shock succeeds, and a 5-J shock fails (F), defining the DFT as 10 J (the lowest successful energy). Note from the curve that the likelihood of success at the DFT energy (10 J) is 70%. Now, if the DFT process were repeated, it is possible that the second shock might fail on one occasion (defining the DFT as 20 J) or that all four shocks might succeed on another occasion (and that a lower energy shock would fail to define the DFT), and so on. Thus, repeating the DFT determinations may result in different values for the DFT with each determination. However, if enough repetitions were performed, a population of DFTs, as shown in (B), would be created. The most commonly observed DFT in this example would be 10 J, which has a 70% likelihood of success. Further details in text.

number of shocks (and often VF inductions) are required. As with current biphasic technology, charge times are short, and syncope due to shock delay and shock-related block are uncommon, safety margin testing is often performed instead of patient-specific defibrillation assessment. With safety margin testing, the goal is to deliver the minimum number of shocks or induce the fewest possible VF episodes to determine whether a sufficient safety margin exists between the maximum ICD shock strength and reliable defibrillation. Following a safety margin test, the first shock is typically programmed to maximum output.

Clinical role of defibrillation testing at implantation

Defibrillation testing also confirms integrity of the shock system, appropriate sensing of ventricular fibrillation, and establishes an adequate safety margin for defibrillation. DFT testing was an integral part of ICD implantation with early monophasic systems, when initial shock failure was not uncommon at implantation, system optimization was frequently required, and patients received devices for secondary prevention, and thus had a higher incidence of spontaneous clinical arrhythmias. With biphasic high output devices available from all device manufacturers, the necessity of defibrillation assessment during implantation has been questioned.[91-93] A biphasic active pulse generator device placed in the left pectoral position has a 95% probability of passing a 10-J safety margin test, and most patients who fail an implant test do so because of a false negative result.[94] The sensitivity of passing an implant test with a low DFT and the specificity of failing with a high DFT depends on the defibrillation test performed (Table 1.2). Despite its limitations, defibrillation efficacy is commonly assessed at implant for several reasons. Defibrillation testing was performed in nearly

Table 1.2 Predicted performance of different implant criteria.

Protocol	Criterion	Passing (%)	Sensitivity (%)	Specificity (%)
2 inductions	2/2 successes at 24 J	93	96	53
1 induction	1/1 success at 15 J	91	94	52
1 induction	1/1 success at 12 J	87	90	61
Step-down	DFT ≤ 24 J	96	98	32
Step-down	DFT ≤ 18 J	87	91	74
Binary search	DFT ≤ 24 J	99	100	11
Binary search	DFT ≤ 12 J	87	90	61

DFT, defibrillation threshold.

Source: Swerdlow CD, Russo AM, Degroot PJ. The dilemma of ICD implant testing. Pacing Clin Electrophysiol 2007; 30:675–700.

all patients enrolled in the clinical trials that demonstrated a mortality benefit with ICD therapy. Assessing defibrillation efficacy is the legal standard of practice in the USA, and the labeling of US manufactured ICDs recommends defibrillation assessment and programming the first VF shock with a 10-J safety margin.[94] The role of testing is in evolution, with a recent survey from Europe indicating that 19% of centers perform no testing at the time of implantation.[95] Patient factors that tend to favor testing include implantation in children and young adults, presence of congenital heart disease, and a secondary prevention indication; testing was avoided in patients with long-standing atrial fibrillation with inadequate anticoagulation.[95]

In deciding whether to perform DFT testing, the risks and benefits of the procedure must be considered. Risks of testing include the risks attributable to anesthesia, to VF itself, and to shock delivery in patients with significant cardiovascular disease and comorbidities. In a recent study from Canada, in 19,067 ICD implantations, eight serious DFT testing-related complications occurred (three deaths and five strokes).[96] These data suggest that when the testing is performed by experienced practitioners the risks are low, even in high-risk patients. A risk of not performing testing includes failure to identify a patient who will not be adequately defibrillated. Clinical variables, including baseline ejection fraction, do not accurately identify patients who may have a high DFT.[97] In general, the likelihood of a high DFT is low, although in one contemporary observation study >6% of patients required modification of their ICD system because of an inadequate safety margin.[91] DFT testing can identify lead dysfunction, demonstrate appropriate sensing and charging of the device, and test complete system integrity.[98] In our practice, most patients undergo implant DFT testing. Testing is favored by the presence of a nonstandard shock vector (i.e., right-sided or abdominal pulse generator, congenital heart disease, unusual superior vena cava [SVC] coil position, or extreme left ventricular [LV] enlargement), clinical conditions that might have an increased risk of an elevated DFT or for which the overall ICD experience is relatively limited (hypertrophic cardiomyopathy, channelopathies, arrhythmogenic right ventricular dysplasia), and a secondary prevention indication. Testing is not performed in patients with absolute contraindications (Table 1.3),[94] and is less commonly performed in primary prevention cardiac resynchronization recipients, in whom the role of testing has been questioned, and the perceived risks higher.[99]

Given the improved efficacy of modern ICDs, there has been a trend towards safety margin testing in order to minimize shocks and VF inductions.

Table 1.3 Contraindications to implantable cardioverter-defibrillator implant testing.

Absolute contraindication
Risk of thromboembolism
Left atrial thrombus
Left ventricular thrombus, not organized
Atrial fibrillation in the absence of anticoagulation
Inadequate anesthesia or anesthesia support
Known inadequate external defibrillation
Severe aortic stenosis
Critical, nonrevascularized coronary artery disease with jeopardized myocardium
Hemodynamic instability requiring inotropic support
Relative contraindication
Left ventricular mural thrombus with adequate systemic anticoagulation
Questionable external defibrillation (e.g., massive obesity)
Severe unrevascularized coronary artery disease
Recent coronary stent
Hemodynamic instability
Recent stroke or transient ischemic attack
Questionable stability of coronary venous lead

Source: Swerdlow CD, Russo AM, Degroot PJ. The dilemma of ICD implant testing. Pacing Clin Electrophysiol 2007; 30:675–700, by permission of Blackwell Publishing.

One common technique utilizes two VF inductions. The first shock is set to 10 J less than the maximum device output. If successful, rather than stepping down by 5–6 J, for the second induction the first shock is programmed to 14 or 15 J, and the second shock is programmed to the same as the first shock. If the first shock succeeded, the approximate "DFT" is said to be ≤15 J, and if the second shock succeeds, the DFT is defined as that energy (typically 25 J). In our experience, patients with an active can, pectoral, biphasic DFT <15 J have a very low risk of subsequent inadequate defibrillation, and no additional testing is performed until the time of pulse generator change out.[100] In patients in whom the DFT approximation is higher, additional testing may be performed at implant or, more commonly, annually until a chronically stable DFT is confirmed. Two successes at an energy 10 J less than the maximum device output confirm a 10-J safety margin. If not achieved, system modification is performed, as discussed below.

A second and increasingly common strategy is based on the results of the Low Energy Safety Study (LESS) trial.[101] In a substudy, Higgins et al.[102] reported that a single conversion success at 14 J with the first ventricular induction yielded a similar positive predictive accuracy (91%) as two successes at 17 or 21 J in determining a successful outcome with a device that provided 31 J.

The results were durable, in that those patients in whom a single VF induction was successfully terminated with a 14-J shock at implantation, regardless of additional induction tests, had similar long-term VF conversion success rates as all ICD recipients when the device was programmed to provide 31 J.

Management of the patient who fails defibrillation testing

Before taking steps to manage defibrillation testing failure the diagnosis should be confirmed, because a

Table 1.4 Options in a patient with high energy requirements or an inadequate safety margin at defibrillation threshold testing.

Check for metabolic abnormalities or pneumothorax

Assess vector (insure RV lead is apical, exclude SVC coil if it is low in the RA or move it proximally, exclude the pulse generator with right-sided implants)

Reverse polarity (particularly if initial shock was not RV anode for the first phase) or modify the waveform (if available)

Exchange the generator to a "high-output" device (if not already in use)

Add a subcutaneous array or patch, or add an azygous lead or coronary sinus coil to include more of the left ventricule in the defibrillation field

Move the generator to a left pectoral position if located on the right

RA, right atrium; RV, right ventricle; SVC, superior vena cava.

single failed shock may occur by chance alone. If a test shock fails, but a maximum output rescue shock from the device succeeds, it is reasonable to repeat the test shock. If the maximum output shock also fails, or if the test shock fails twice, reliable defibrillation with a 10-J safety margin is likely absent and system modification is warranted.

Defibrillation efficacy is modified by changing the waveform, altering the vector, or (at times) substituting the pulse generator for one with a higher output (Table 1.4). In general, the following steps are performed. First, if the implant procedure was prolonged, metabolic abnormalities may be present; if so, it may be reasonable to defer testing if they are not readily corrected. Screening for a pneumothorax also may also identify a treatable cause of an elevated DFT.

Second, it is important to insure an adequate vector, by assessing the position of the leads and can relative to the heart, and in particular the left ventricle. An anterior chest wall can to a right ventricular (RV) lead coil may fail because both electrodes are relatively anterior. Insuring the RV lead is apical and that the SVC coil is in the high SVC or inominate vein optimizes vectors (Fig. 1.30). If the coil is low, it should be excluded (performed electronically in many devices). With a right-sided pulse generator, removing the can from the circuit may improve defibrillation. If the maximum output shock succeeded but the safety margin failed,

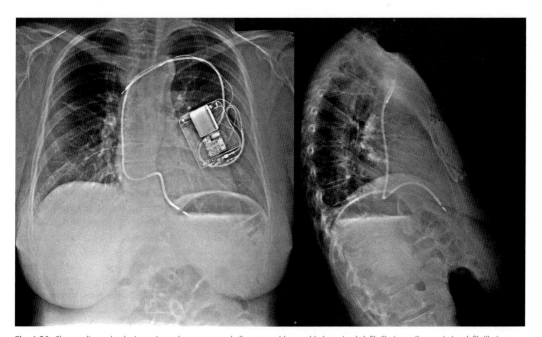

Fig. 1.30 Chest radiographs depict active pulse generator shell system with an added proximal defibrillation coil to optimize defibrillation threshold.

reversing polarity (if the default polarity is not RV anodal for the first phase) or reprogramming shock pulse width (if an option for the pulse generator in use) may help.

If these approaches fail to result in adequate defibrillation, a subcutaneous lead is added (see Chapter 5 for implantation technique). With current biphasic waveform systems, subcutaneous leads are required in only 3.7% of devices implanted.[103] Alternatives to placing a subcutaneous lead (which may be associated with patient discomfort and increased fracture risk) is the addition of a defibrillation coil in the azygous vein (which lies directly behind the left ventricle), or in the branches of the coronary sinus (Fig. 1.31A). The authors often favor this approach over subcutaneous arrays.

In a single-center observational study of three types of subcutaneous leads (single-element subcutaneous array electrode, three-finger electrodes, subcutaneous patch electrodes), all types performed well.[104] Although there was no significant difference in complications, 7.3–9.5% of patients developed a major complication (predominantly lead fracture). Therefore, with use of a subcutaneous ICD lead, patients require close follow-up.

Because the pulse generator shell serves as an electrode, its position can also affect defibrillation efficacy. Implantable defibrillators are most commonly placed in the left pectoral region, typically in the prepectoral (subcutaneous) plane. However, the site of pulse generator placement and vascular access is influenced by multiple factors, including patient and physician preference, anatomic anomalies, previous operations, integrity of the vascular system, and whether a pre-existing permanent pacing system is present. In addition to factors specific to the patient, choice of the implantation site can affect ease of technical insertion, defibrillation effectiveness, and long-term rates of lead failure.

Right pectoral implantation may be considered in left-handed persons, hunters who place the rifle butt on the left shoulder, and patients with previous mastectomy, other surgical procedures, or anatomy that precludes left-sided insertion. In systems with both distal and proximal defibrillation coils, the proximal coil is either shifted toward the right hemithorax (if both coils are on the same lead) or, often, advanced to a lower SVC position for greater cardiac proximity (in two-lead systems) with right-sided placement. With active can pulse generators, the largest defibrillation lead surface, the device shell, is shifted away from the ventricular myocardium (Fig. 1.32). This unfavorable position decreases defibrillation effectiveness.[105,106] With biphasic waveforms, right-sided implantation results in a 6-J

increase in DFT compared with left-sided placement (11.3 ± 5.3 J, left-sided; 17.0 ± 4.9 J, right-sided; $P <$ 0.0001).[105] Even with the increase, right-sided devices were successfully placed in 19 of 20 patients; in one patient, an acceptable right-sided threshold could not be achieved and that approach was abandoned. Despite the concern that a right-sided active can might be detrimental by diverting a significant portion of the electrical field away from the ventricles, the large surface area of the shell compensates for this, so that when right-sided implantation is required, active can devices are preferable (Fig. 1.33).[105] In general, however, left-sided insertion is superior to right-sided placement and is used if there are no compelling factors against it. Placement of a defibrillation coil in the azygous vein or coronary sinus branch is infrequently required, but may result in a favorable vector and improved DFT (Fig. 1.31).

An alternative site for device placement is the abdomen, but this site is only rarely used. Although not as effective for defibrillation as the left pectoral position, the abdomen appears superior to the right pectoral location for active can placement.[107] However, abdominal insertion is technically more challenging, requiring two incisions, lead tunneling, abdominal dissection (often necessitating surgical assistance), and general anesthesia. Additionally, because of the greater risk of infection, threat of peritoneal erosion, and increased risk of lead fracture, even with totally transvenous systems this position is used only in rare circumstances.[108]

There are many factors that may result in elevated DFT: drug therapy; underlying cardiac disease; the size, configuration, and number of defibrillating leads; the time that VF persists before shock delivery; ischemia; hypoxia; amplitude of the VF waveform; temperature; heart weight; body weight; direction of the delivered shock and waveform; and chronicity of lead implantation.[109] In patients with inherited channelopathies, such as Brugada syndrome, high DFTs may be prevalent and problematic.[110] In one series of patients who received a high-output generator for an elevated DFT, the majority had underlying coronary artery disease, with reduced left ventricular function, and were on amiodarone.[109] An important finding in this study was that in patients with high DFTs who receive an ICD, arrhythmia death remained a significant long-term risk (42% of the deaths were arrhythmia related).

An interesting observation is that there is a circadian variation in the DFT. The DFT has a morning peak that is 16% higher than that measured after noon.[111] In addition, the first failed shock rate is more likely to occur in the morning compared with other times during the day. This variability in DFT is clinically

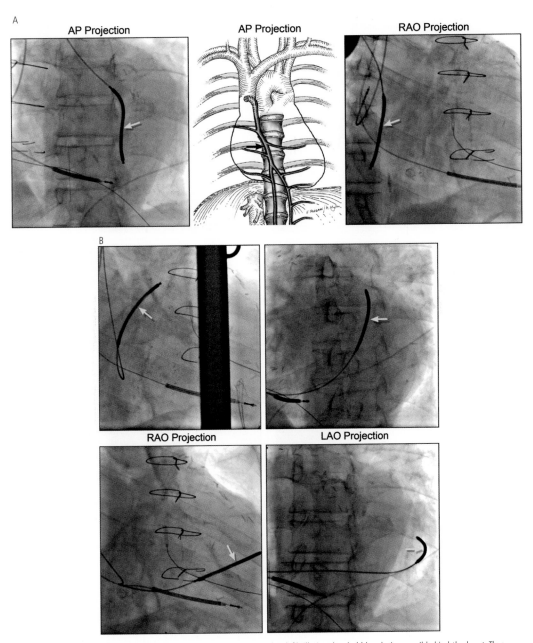

Fig. 1.31 (A) Placement of defibrillation coil in azygous vein to lower the defibrillation threshold by placing a coil behind the heart. Thus, current flows from behind the heart (azygous vein) to the anterior chest (pulse generator). The left panel shows a fluoroscopic AP projection; the middle panel shows a cartoon of the relevant anatomy (adapted from Cooper JA, Smith TW. How to implant a defibrillation coil in the azygous vein. Heart Rhythm J 2009; 6:1677–80); the right panel shows the right anterior oblique (RAO) projection. The arrow in each case points to the coil in the azygous vein. (B) Placement of a coil in the coronary sinus (CS). Top two panels: coil in main body of the CS. Bottom two panels: coil in the posterolateral branch of the CS in the same patient. This position resulted in effective defibrillation. Note that the in the left anterior oblique (LAO) view the coil clearly encompasses the lateral aspects of the cardiac silhouette, suggesting the defibrillation vector effectively surrounds the heart.

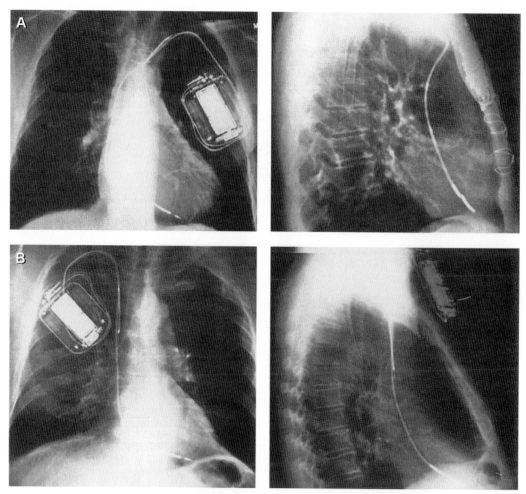

Fig. 1.32 (A) Posteroanterior and lateral chest radiographs from a patient with a left-sided defibrillator. Note that the proximal defibrillation lead is in the left subclavian vein. (B) Posteroanterior and lateral chest radiographs from a patient with right-sided defibrillator placement. Note that the proximal defibrillation lead is in the superior vena cava.

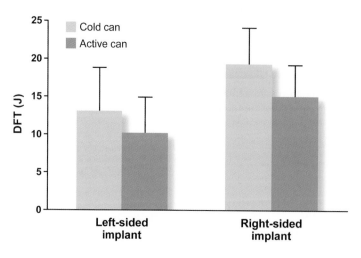

Fig. 1.33 Defibrillation thresholds with right-sided and left-sided cardioverter-defibrillator implantation of active can and cold can devices. Defibrillation threshold (DFT) is on ordinate, and side of placement and can type are on abscissa. (From Friedman PA, Rasmussen MJ, Grice S, Trusty J, Glikson M, Stanton MS. Defibrillation thresholds are increased by right-sided implantation of totally transvenous implantable cardioverter defibrillators. Pacing Clin Electrophysiol 1999; 22:1186–92, by permission of Futura Publishing Company.)

important in patients with high thresholds, in whom a 10-J safety margin becomes more difficult to achieve.

Upper limit of vulnerability to assess safety margin

The ULV is the lowest energy above which shocks delivered during the vulnerable period do not induce fibrillation. Numerous studies have demonstrated that the DFT and ULV are strongly linked, with the ULV approximating the E90 (shock with 90% likelihood of success).[112–117] Because the DFT and ULV are correlated, delivery of a shock during the vulnerable period (T wave) that fails to induce VF indicates that the shock is of sufficient strength to terminate VF.[112] During sinus rhythm, test shocks are delivered at and around the peak of the T wave at a single energy (margin testing) or at progressively lower energies until VF is induced (patient-specific testing). Because the ULV may be dependent on the coupling interval, shocks are delivered at various intervals before the T-wave peak to "scan" repolarization. Shocks programmed 5 J above the ULV terminate spontaneous VF as reliably as shocks programmed using the DFT with a 10-J safety margin.[116,117] Because ULV margin testing assesses defibrillation efficacy with no VF induction in 75–90% of patients (its major advantage), sensing of VF is not directly tested.[118,119] Therefore, the R wave should be ≥7 mV to insure adequate sensing of VF has been proposed, although the correlation between the normal rhythm R wave and VF electrogram amplitude is poor. In the small subset of patients with ULV > 20 J, some experts advocate performing DFT testing at implant.[120] Because of the need to record 6–12 surface leads to insure proper shock timing, the lack of experience by many implanters with determining the timing of the test shocks, and the modest increase in time required to deliver 3–4 sinus rhythm shocks as opposed to a single VF induction, ULV testing has only been adopted as routine clinical practice in a few centers. However, automatic algorithms in which the ICD identifies the vulnerable window using the intracardiac electrogram and scans the T wave with shocks automatically have recently been developed and tested. If commercially released, ULV testing may become more widespread because of its ability to assess defibrillation efficacy without VF inductions in most patients and the possibility of automated testing by the ICD.

Drugs and defibrillators

Antiarrhythmic drugs are frequently used in patients with ICDs to treat supraventricular arrhythmias (particularly atrial fibrillation), suppress ventricular tachyarrhythmias, and slow ventricular tachycardia (VT) to increase the responsiveness of antitachycardia pacing.

In the implantable defibrillator trials, concomitant use of membrane-active agents (Vaughan-Williams class I or III drugs) has ranged from 11% to 31%.[121–124] Several important device–drug interactions must be considered.[125]

1. **Detection:** Most drugs slow VT. If slowed below the detection cut-off rate, VT is not detected by the device and remains untreated. Initiation of antiarrhythmic drugs in patients with VT is usually followed by device testing to assess detection of VT. This is the most important device–drug interaction with modern ICDs.

2. **Pacing thresholds:** Bradycardia and antitachycardia pacing thresholds may be affected by pharmacologic agents, as discussed in Chapter 13: Follow-up.

3. **Pacing requirements:** Drugs may exacerbate conduction defects or slow the sinus rate, necessitating pacing for bradycardia.

4. **Drug-induced proarrhythmia.**

5. **Changes in DFT:** Although it is well known that pharmacologic agents can modulate defibrillation effectiveness, drug–defibrillation interactions are complex. Moreover, assessment of the influence of drugs on defibrillation is confounded by the effects of anesthetic agents, variability in lead systems and waveforms across studies, and heterogeneity in study subjects (i.e., human, canine, and porcine). In general, however, agents that impede the fast inward sodium current (such as lidocaine) or calcium channel function (such as verapamil) increase the DFT, whereas agents that block repolarizing potassium currents (such as sotalol) lower the DFT. The effects of amiodarone are legion; clinically, long-term administration of amiodarone increases DFTs, whereas intravenous administration has little immediate effect. In addition to antiarrhythmic agents, other drugs have been shown to increase the DFT, such as sildenafil,[126] venlafaxine,[127] and alcohol.[128]

Importantly, with current generation biphasic ICDs, the clinical effect of most drugs, including amiodarone, is modest.[129] In general, then, ICD evaluation should be performed when administration of membrane active drugs that can increase the threshold (especially amiodarone) is initiated, particularly in patients with borderline DFTs. Drug effects on defibrillation are summarized in Table 1.5. In patients with a low DFT, testing for slow VTs or, less commonly, empirically lengthening the detection interval (to allow for VT slowing) is most important. As a general rule, ICD evaluation should be considered whenever administration of Vaughan-Williams class I or III drugs is initiated or their dosage significantly increased. These drugs are listed in Table 1.6. Drug and defibrillator interactions are also discussed in Chapter 13: Follow-up.

It is equally important to remember that use of cardiovascular medications outside of membrane active

Table 1.5 Effects of drugs on defibrillation.

Drug	Class*	Effect on defibrillation threshold†
Quinidine	IA	Increase
Procainamide	IA	No change
N-acetyl-procainamide	IA	Decrease
Disopyramide	IA	No change
Mexiletine	IB	Increase
Flecainide	IC	Increase
Moricizine	IC	Increase
Propafenone	IC	No change
Propranolol	II	Increase
Atenolol	II	No change
Isoproterenol		Decrease
Sotalol	III	Decrease
Ibutilide	III	Decrease
Dofetilide	III	Decrease
Amiodarone	III	
Oral		Increase
Intravenous		No change or decrease
Dronedarone	III	No change
Diltiazem	IV	Increase
Verapamil	IV	Increase

*Vaughan-Williams classification.
†If study results conflict, the most frequently reported effect is noted.
Source: modified from Carnes CA, Mehdirad AA, Nelson SD. Drug and defibrillator interactions. Pharmacotherapy 1998; 18:516–25, by permission of Pharmacotherapy Publications.

drugs (i.e., use of angiotensin-converting enzyme (ACE) inhibitors, angiotensin receptor blockers, β-blockers, statins, aspirin, warfarin, and other evidence-based medications) have been shown to reduce mortality in various clinical situations and do not interact with ICD function in any clinically significant way, and should therefore be encouraged.

Antitachycardia pacing

In monomorphic VT, a re-entrant circuit utilizing abnormal tissue (adjacent to an infarct in the post-myocardial infarction patient) is responsible for the arrhythmia (Fig. 1.34). For the re-entrant circuit to perpetuate itself, the tissue immediately in front of the

Table 1.6 Membrane-active drugs. These agents may significantly affect defibrillator function, often mandating device testing on initiation.

Vaughan-Williams classification	Medication
IA	Quinidine, procainamide, disopyramide
IB	Lidocaine, tocainide, phenytoin
IC	Flecainide, propafenone, encainide, moricizine
III	Sotalol, ibutilide, dofetilide, amiodarone, dronedarone

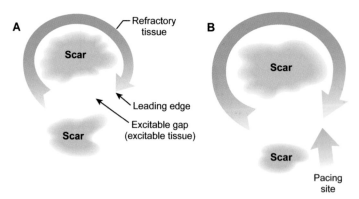

Fig. 1.34 Re-entrant ventricular tachycardia circuit. In (A), a circuit around a fixed scar is depicted by the arrow. The head of the arrow depicts the leading edge of the wavefront, and the body of the arrow back to the tail consists of tissue that is still refractory (because the wavefront has just propagated through it). The tissue between the tip and the tail of the arrow is excitable and is called the "excitable gap." For the arrow head to continue its course around the scar, an excitable gap must be present; if the wavefront encounters refractory tissue, it cannot proceed. In (B), a wavefront generated by an antitachycardia pacing impulse enters the excitable gap and terminates tachycardia. Tachycardias with a small excitable gap (i.e., the head of the arrow follows the tail very closely, so that only a small "moving rim" of excitable tissue is in the circuit) are more difficult to terminate with antitachycardia pacing.

leading edge of the wavefront must have recovered excitability so that it can be depolarized (Fig. 1.34). Thus, an excitable gap of tissue must be present in advance of the leading tachycardia wavefront or the arrhythmia will terminate. ATP – delivered as a short burst of pacing impulses at a rate slightly greater than the tachycardia rate – can terminate VT by depolarizing the tissue in the excitable gap, so that the tissue in front of the advancing VT wavefront becomes refractory, preventing further arrhythmia propagation (Fig. 1.34B). The ability of a train of impulses to travel to the site of the re-entrant circuit and interrupt VT depends on several factors, including the site of pacing (the closer to the circuit entrance, the greater the likelihood of circuit penetration and termination), the length of the tachycardia cycle, and the size of the excitable gap. With delivery of ATP, faster and more remote circuits with smaller excitable gaps are generally more difficult to terminate and have a greater risk of degeneration to less organized tachyarrhythmias, including fibrillation.

ATP has been applied successfully to treat slow VT (<188–200 bpm, success rate 78–91%),[130] and recently fast VT (200–250 bpm, success rate 50–81%).[131,132] These therapy success rates are reinforced by the observation that ATP did not result in an increased risk of acceleration of the arrhythmia, syncope, or mortality in comparison with patients who receive defibrillation shocks only.[131] Patients with ATP, rather than those programmed to defibrillation shocks only, also report statistically higher quality of life of scores. If ATP fails, or if the frequency of the VT is too high to apply ATP, the device diverts immediately to deliver a defibrillation shock. The use of ATP in the ventricle is important in limiting shocks, and is further discussed in Chapter 8: Programming. Most defibrillators offer ATP immediately before or during charging, because many tachyarrhythmias with cycle lengths in the VF zone are actually fast monomorphic VT. ATP is also available in the atrium in some dual-chamber ICDs, although its efficacy and role in clinical practice is far more limited.

References

1 Hodgkin AL, Huxley AF. A quantitative description of membrane current and its application to conduction and excitation in nerve. J Physiol 1952; 117:500–44.

2 Gadsby DC. The Na/K pump of cardiac cells. Annu Rev Biophys Bioeng 1984; 13:373–98.

3 Glitsch HG. Electrogenic Na pumping in the heart. Annu Rev Physiol 1982; 44:389–400.

4 Balser JR. Structure and function of the cardiac sodium channels. Cardiovasc Res 1999; 42:327–38.

5 Makielski JC, Sheets MF, Hanck DA, January CT, Fozzard HA. Sodium current in voltage clamped internally perfused canine cardiac Purkinje cells. Biophys J 1987; 52:1–11.

6 Kunze DL, Lacerda AE, Wilson DL, Brown AM. Cardiac Na currents and the inactivating, reopening, and waiting properties of single cardiac Na channels. J Gen Physiol 1985; 86:691–719.

7 Cohen CJ, Bean BP, Tsien RW. Maximal upstroke velocity as an index of available sodium conductance: comparison of maximal upstroke velocity and voltage clamp measurements of sodium current in rabbit Purkinje fibers. Circ Res 1984; 54:636–51.

8 Hume JR, Giles W. Ionic currents in single isolated bullfrog atrial cells. J Gen Physiol 1983; 81:153–94.

9 Reuter H. Divalent cations as charge carriers in excitable membranes. Prog Biophys Mol Biol 1973; 26:1–43.

10 Hume JR, Giles W, Robinson K, et al. A time- and voltage-dependent K+ current in single cardiac cells from bullfrog atrium. J Gen Physiol 1986; 88:777–98.

11 Barr L, Dewey MM, Berger W. Propagation of action potentials and the structure of the nexus in cardiac muscle. J Gen Physiol 1965; 48:797–823.

12 De Mello WC. Intercellular communication in cardiac muscle. Circ Res 1982; 51:1–9.

13 Lindemans FW, Denier Van der Gon JJ. Current thresholds and liminal size in excitation of heart muscle. Cardiovasc Res 1978; 12:477–85.

14 de Voogt WG. Pacemaker leads: performance and progress. Am J Cardiol 1999; 83:187D–91D.

15 Timmis G, Helland J, Westveer D. The evolution of low threshold leads. Clin Prog Pacing Electrophysiol 1983; 1:313–34.

16 Kay GN, Anderson K, Epstein AE, Plumb VJ. Active fixation atrial leads: randomized comparison of two lead designs. Pacing Clin Electrophysiol 1989; 12:1355–61.

17 de Buitleir M, Kou WH, Schmaltz S, Morady F. Acute changes in pacing threshold and R- or P-wave amplitude during permanent pacemaker implantation. Am J Cardiol 1990; 65:999–1003.

18 Kruse IM, Terpstra B. Acute and long-term atrial and ventricular stimulation thresholds with a steroid-eluting electrode. Pacing Clin Electrophysiol 1985; 8:45–9.

19 Mond H, Stokes K, Helland J, et al. The porous titanium steroid eluting electrode: a double blind study assessing the stimulation threshold effects of steroid. Pacing Clin Electrophysiol 1988; 11:214–9.

20 Guarda F, Galloni M, Assone F, Pasteris V, Luboz MP. Histological reactions of porous tip endocardial electrodes implanted in sheep. Int J Artif Organs 1982; 5:267–73.

21 Beyersdorf F, Schneider M, Kreuzer J, Falk S, Zegelman M, Satter P. Studies of the tissue reaction induced by transvenous pacemaker electrodes. I. Microscopic examination of the extent of connective tissue around the electrode tip in the human right ventricle. Pacing Clin Electrophysiol 1988; 11:1753–9.

22 Schwaab B, Frohlig G, Berg M, Schwerdt H, Schieffer H. Five-year follow-up of a bipolar steroid-eluting ventricular pacing lead. Pacing Clin Electrophysiol 1999; 22:1226–8.

23 Wiegand UK, Potratz J, Bonnemeier H, et al. Long-term superiority of steroid elution in atrial active fixation platinum leads. Pacing Clin Electrophysiol 2000; 23:1003–9.

24 Klein HH, Steinberger J, Knake W. Stimulation characteristics of a steroid-eluting electrode compared with three conventional electrodes. Pacing Clin Electrophysiol 1990; 13:134–7.

25 King DH, Gillette PC, Shannon C, Cuddy TE. Steroid-eluting endocardial pacing lead for treatment of exit block. Am Heart J 1983; 106:1438–40.

26 Furman S, Hurzeler P, DeCaprio V. The ventricular endocardial electrogram and pacemaker sensing. J Thorac Cardiovasc Surg 1977; 73:258–66.

27 Kleinert M, Elmqvist H, Strandberg H. Spectral properties of atrial and ventricular endocardial signals. Pacing Clin Electrophysiol 1979; 2:11–9.

28 Watson W. Myopotential sensing in cardiac pacemakers. In: Barold SS, ed. Modern Cardiac Pacing. Mount Kisco, NY: Futura Publishing Co., 1985: 813–37.

29 Parsonnet V, Myers GH, Kresh YM. Characteristics of intracardiac electrograms. II: Atrial endocardial electrograms. Pacing Clin Electrophysiol 1980; 3:406–17.

30 Hurzeler P, De Caprio V, Furman S. Endocardial electrograms and pacemaker sensing. Med Instrum 1976; 10: 178–82.

31 Sweesy MW, Batey RL, Forney RC. Crosstalk during bipolar pacing. Pacing Clin Electrophysiol 1988; 11: 1512–6.

32 Janosik DL, Redd RM, Kennedy HL. Crosstalk inhibition of a dual-chamber pacemaker diagnosed by ambulatory electrocardiography. Am Heart J 1990; 120:435–8.

33 Clarke M, Liu B, Schuller H, et al. Automatic adjustment of pacemaker stimulation output correlated with continuously monitored capture thresholds: a multicenter study. European Microny Study Group. Pacing Clin Electrophysiol 1998; 21:1567–75.

34 Kay GN. Basic aspects of cardiac pacing. In: Ellenbogen K, ed. Cardiac Pacing. Boston: Blackwell Scientific Publications, 1992: 32–119.

35 Raymond RD, Nanian KB. Insulation failure with bipolar polyurethane pacing leads. Pacing Clin Electrophysiol 1984; 7:378–80.

36 Bornzin GA, Stokes KB, Wiebusch WA. A low threshold, low polarization platinized endocardial electrode (abstract). Pacing Clin Electrophysiol 1983; 6:A-70.

37 Kertes P, Mond H, Sloman G, Vohra J, Hunt D. Comparison of lead complications with polyurethane tined, silicone rubber tined, and wedge tip leads: clinical experience with 822 ventricular endocardial lads. Pacing Clin Electrophysiol 1983; 6:957–62.

38 Hanson JS. Sixteen failures in a single model of bipolar polyurethane-insulated ventricular pacing lead: a 44-month experience. Pacing Clin Electrophysiol 1984; 7:389–94.

39 Mond HG, Grenz D. Implantable transvenous pacing leads: the shape of things to come. Pacing Clin Electrophysiol 2004; 27:887–93.

40 Calfee RV, Saulson SH. A voluntary standard for 3.2 mm unipolar and bipolar pacemaker leads and connectors. Pacing Clin Electrophysiol 1986; 9:1181–5.

41 Mond HG. Unipolar versus bipolar pacing: poles apart. Pacing Clin Electrophysiol 1991; 14:1411–24.

42 Gregoratos G, Abrams J, Epstein AE, et al. ACC/AHA/NASPE 2002 guideline update for implantation of cardiac pacemakers and antiarrhythmia devices: summary article. A report of the American College of Cardiology/American Heart Association Task Force on Practice Guidelines (ACC/AHA/NASPE Committee to Update the 1998 Pacemaker Guidelines). J Cardiovasc Electrophysiol 2002; 13:1183–99.

43 Abraham WT, Hayes DL. Cardiac resynchronization therapy for heart failure. Circulation 2003; 108: 2596–603.

44 Sogaard P, Egeblad H, Kim WY, et al. Tissue Doppler imaging predicts improved systolic performance and reversed left ventricular remodeling during long-term cardiac resynchronization therapy. J Am Coll Cardiol 2002; 40:723–30.

45 Shetty AK, Duckett SG, Bostock J, Rosenthal E, Rinaldi CA. Use of a quadripolar left ventricular lead to achieve successful implantation in patients with previous failed attempts at cardiac resynchronization therapy. Europace 2011; 13:992–6.

46 Singh JP, Klein HU, Huang DT, et al. Left ventricular lead position and clinical outcome in the multicenter automatic defibrillator implantation trial: cardiac resynchronization therapy (MADIT-CRT) trial. Circulation 2011; 123:1159–66.

47 Furman S. Basic concepts. In: Furman S, Hayes DL, Holmes DR Jr, eds. A Practice of Cardiac Pacing, 3rd edn. Armonk, NY: Futura Publishing Co., 1993: 29–88.

48 Schoenfeld MH. Contemporary pacemaker and defibrillator device therapy: challenges confronting the general cardiologist. Circulation 2007; 115:638–53.

49 Ribeiro AL, Rincon LG, Oliveira BG, et al. Automatic adjustment of pacing output in the clinical setting. Am Heart J 2004; 147:127–31.

50 Tyers GF, Brownlee RR. Power pulse generators, electrodes, and longevity. Prog Cardiovasc Dis 1981; 23: 421–34.

51 Irnich W. Muscle noise and interference behavior in pacemakers: a comparative study. Pacing Clin Electrophysiol 1987; 10:125–32.

52 Bicik V, Kristan L. Sine2/triangle/square wave generator for pacemaker testing. Pacing Clin Electrophysiol 1985; 8:484–93.

53 Hauser RG, Kallinen L. Deaths associated with implantable cardioverter defibrillator failure and deactivation reported in the United States Food and Drug Administration Manufacturer and User Facility Device Experience Database. Heart Rhythm 2004; 1:399–405.

54 Zaim S, Sunthorn H, Adatte JJ, Kursteiner K, Burgener D, Huehn C. Inappropriate high-rate ventricular pacing in a patient with a defibrillator. Europace 2002; 4:427–30.

55 Saxon LA, Hayes DL, Gilliam FR, et al. Long-term outcome after ICD and CRT implantation and influence of remote device follow-up: the ALTITUDE survival study. Circulation 2010; 122:2359–67.

56 Bernstein AD, Daubert JC, Fletcher RD, et al. The revised NASPE/BPEG generic code for antibradycardia, adaptive-rate, and multisite pacing. North American Society of

Pacing and Electrophysiology/British Pacing and Electrophysiology Group. Pacing Clin Electrophysiol 2002; 25: 260–4.

57 Prevost J, Battelli F. Some effects of electrical discharge on the hearts of mammals. Comptes Rendus Acad Sci 1899; 129:1267–8.

58 Weiss JN, Qu Z, Chen PS, et al. The dynamics of cardiac fibrillation. Circulation 2005; 112:1232–40.

59 Gurvich NL, Yuniev GS. Restoration of regular rhythm in the mammalian fibrillating heart. Am Rev Sov Med 1946; 3:236–9.

60 Zipes DP, Fischer J, King RM, Nicoll AD, Jolly WW. Termination of ventricular fibrillation in dogs by depolarizing a critical amount of myocardium. Am J Cardiol 1975; 36:37–44.

61 Chen PS, Shibata N, Dixon EG, et al. Activation during ventricular defibrillation in open-chest dogs: evidence of complete cessation and regeneration of ventricular fibrillation after unsuccessful shocks. J Clin Invest 1986; 77:810–23.

62 Chen PS, Wolf PD, Melnick SD, Danieley ND, Smith WM, Ideker RE. Comparison of activation during ventricular fibrillation and following unsuccessful defibrillation shocks in open-chest dogs. Circ Res 1990; 66:1544–60.

63 Frazier DW, Wolf PD, Wharton JM, Tang AS, Smith WM, Ideker RE. Stimulus-induced critical point: mechanism for electrical initiation of reentry in normal canine myocardium. J Clin Invest 1989; 83:1039–52.

64 Swerdlow CD, Martin DJ, Kass RM, et al. The zone of vulnerability to T wave shocks in humans. J Cardiovasc Electrophysiol 1997; 8:145–54.

65 Chen PS, Feld GK, Kriett JM, et al. Relation between upper limit of vulnerability and defibrillation threshold in humans. Circulation 1993; 88:186–92.

66 Dillon SM, Kwaku KF. Progressive depolarization: a unified hypothesis for defibrillation and fibrillation induction by shocks. J Cardiovasc Electrophysiol 1998; 9:529–52.

67 Sweeney RJ, Gill RM, Steinberg MI, Reid PR. Ventricular refractory period extension caused by defibrillation shocks. Circulation 1990; 82:965–72.

68 Dillon SM. The electrophysiological effects of defibrillation shocks. In: Kroll MW, Lehmann MH, eds. Implantable Cardioverter Defibrillator Therapy: The Engineerin–Clinical Interface. Norwell, MA: Kluwer Academic Publishers, 1996: 31–61.

69 Kroll MW, Efimov IR, Tchou PJ. Present understanding of shock polarity for internal defibrillation: the obvious and non-obvious clinical implications. Pacing Clin Electrophysiol 2006; 29:885–91.

70 Yamanouchi Y, Cheng Y, Tchou PJ, Efimov IR. The mechanisms of the vulnerable window: the role of virtual electrodes and shock polarity. Can J Physiol Pharmacol 2001; 79:25–33.

71 Efimov IR, Cheng Y, Yamanouchi Y, Tchou PJ. Direct evidence of the role of virtual electrode-induced phase singularity in success and failure of defibrillation. J Cardiovasc Electrophysiol 2000; 11:861–8.

72 Olsovsky MR, Hodgson DM, Shorofsky SR, Kavesh NG, Gold MR. Effect of biphasic waveforms on transvenous

defibrillation thresholds in patients with coronary artery disease. Am J Cardiol 1997; 80:1098–100.

73 Wyse DG, Kavanagh KM, Gillis AM, et al. Comparison of biphasic and monophasic shocks for defibrillation using a nonthoracotomy system. Am J Cardiol 1993; 71: 197–202.

74 Bardy GH, Ivey TD, Allen MD, Johnson G, Mehra R, Greene HL. A prospective randomized evaluation of biphasic versus monophasic waveform pulses on defibrillation efficacy in humans. J Am Coll Cardiol 1989; 14:728–33.

75 Jones JL, Swartz JF, Jones RE, Fletcher R. Increasing fibrillation duration enhances relative asymmetrical biphasic versus monophasic defibrillator waveform efficacy. Circ Res. 1990; 67:376–84.

76 Schuder JC, McDaniel WC, Stoeckle H. Defibrillation of 100 kg calves with asymmetrical, bidirectional, rectangular pulses. Cardiovasc Res 1984; 18:419–26.

77 Shorofsky SR, Rashba E, Havel W, et al. Improved defibrillation efficacy with an ascending ramp waveform in humans. Heart Rhythm 2005; 2:388–94.

78 Kavanagh KM, Tang AS, Rollins DL, Smith WM, Ideker RE. Comparison of the internal defibrillation thresholds for monophasic and double and single capacitor biphasic waveforms. J Am Coll Cardiol 1989; 14:1343–9.

79 Fain ES, Sweeney MB, Franz MR. Improved internal defibrillation efficacy with a biphasic waveform. Am Heart J 1989; 117:358–64.

80 Denman RA, Umesan C, Martin PT, et al. Benefit of millisecond waveform durations for patients with high defibrillation thresholds. Heart Rhythm 2006; 3:536–41.

81 Natarajan S, Henthorn R, Burroughs J, et al. "Tuned" defibrillation waveforms outperform 50/50% tilt defibrillation waveforms: a randomized multi-center study. Pacing Clin Electrophysiol 2007; 30(Suppl 1):S139–42.

82 Strickberger SA, Hummel JD, Horwood LE, et al. Effect of shock polarity on ventricular defibrillation threshold using a transvenous lead system. J Am Coll Cardiol 1994; 24:1069–72.

83 Bardy GH, Ivey TD, Allen MD, Johnson G, Greene HL. Evaluation of electrode polarity on defibrillation efficacy. Am J Cardiol 1989; 63:433–7.

84 Natale A, Sra J, Dhala A, et al. Effects of initial polarity on defibrillation threshold with biphasic pulses. Pacing Clin Electrophysiol 1995; 18:1889–93.

85 Strickberger SA, Man KC, Daoud E, et al. Effect of first-phase polarity of biphasic shocks on defibrillation threshold with a single transvenous lead system. J Am Coll Cardiol 1995; 25:1605–8.

86 Olsovsky MR, Shorofsky SR, Gold MR. Effect of shock polarity on biphasic defibrillation thresholds using an active pectoral lead system. J Cardiovasc Electrophysiol 1998; 9:350–4.

87 Strickberger SA, Daoud EG, Davidson T, et al. Probability of successful defibrillation at multiples of the defibrillation energy requirement in patients with an implantable defibrillator. Circulation 1997; 96:1217–23.

88 Davy JM, Fain ES, Dorian P, Winkle RA. The relationship between successful defibrillation and delivered energy in

open-chest dogs: reappraisal of the "defibrillation thresh-old" concept. Am Heart J 1987; 113:77–84.

89 Brady PA, Friedman PA, Stanton MS. Effect of failed defibrillation shocks on electrogram amplitude in a noninte-grated transvenous defibrillation lead system. Am J Cardiol 1995; 76:580–4.

90 Ideker RE, Hillsley RE, Wharton JM. Shock strength for the implantable defibrillator: can you have too much of a good thing? Pacing Clin Electrophysiol 1992; 15:841–4.

91 Russo AM, Sauer W, Gerstenfeld EP, et al. Defibrillation threshold testing: is it really necessary at the time of implantable cardioverter-defibrillator insertion? Heart Rhythm. 2005; 2:456–61.

92 Strickberger SA, Klein GJ. Is defibrillation testing required for defibrillator implantation? J Am Coll Cardiol 2004; 44:88–91.

93 Gula LJ, Massel D, Krahn AD, Yee R, Skanes AC, Klein GJ. Is defibrillation testing still necessary? A decision analysis and Markov model. J Cardiovasc Electrophysiol 2008; 19:400–5.

94 Swerdlow CD, Russo AM, Degroot PJ. The dilemma of ICD implant testing. Pacing Clin Electrophysiol 2007; 30:675–700.

95 Morgan JM, Marinskis G. Defibrillation testing at the time of implantable cardioverter defibrillator implanta-tion: results of the European Heart Rhythm Association survey. Europace 2011; 13:581–2.

96 Birnie D, Tung S, Simpson C, et al. Complications associ-ated with defibrillation threshold testing: the Canadian experience. Heart Rhythm 2008; 5:387–90.

97 Val-Mejias JE, Oza A. Does defibrillation threshold increase as left ventricular ejection fraction decreases? Europace 2010; 12:385–8.

98 Ideker RE, Epstein AE, Plumb VJ. Should shocks still be administered during implantable cardioverter-defibrillator insertion? Heart Rhythm 2005; 2:462–3.

99 Michowitz Y, Lellouche N, Contractor T, et al. Defibrilla-tion threshold testing fails to show clinical benefit during long-term follow-up of patients undergoing cardiac resynchronization therapy defibrillator implantation. Europace 2011; 13:683–8.

100 Luria D, Glikson M, Brady PA, et al. Predictors and mode of detection of transvenous lead malfunction in implant-able defibrillators. Am J Cardiol 2001; 87:901–4.

101 Gold MR, Higgins S, Klein R, et al. Efficacy and temporal stability of reduced safety margins for ventricular defi-brillation: primary results from the Low Energy Safety Study (LESS). Circulation 2002; 105:2043–8.

102 Higgins S, Mann D, Calkins H, et al. One conversion of ventricular fibrillation is adequate for implantable cardioverter-defibrillator implant: an analysis from the Low Energy Safety Study (LESS). Heart Rhythm 2005; 2:117–22.

103 Trusty JM, Hayes DL, Stanton MS, Friedman PA. Factors affecting the frequency of subcutaneous lead usage in implantable defibrillators. Pacing Clin Electrophysiol 2000; 23:842–6.

104 Kettering K, Mewis C, Dornberger V, et al. Long-term experience with subcutaneous ICD leads: a comparison among three different types of subcutaneous leads. Pacing Clin Electrophysiol 2004; 27:1355–61.

105 Friedman PA, Rasmussen MJ, Grice S, Trusty J, Glikson M, Stanton MS. Defibrillation thresholds are increased by right-sided implantation of totally transvenous implant-able cardioverter defibrillators. Pacing Clin Electrophysiol 1999; 22:1186–92.

106 Epstein AE, Kay GN, Plumb VJ, Voshage-Stahl L, Hull ML. Elevated defibrillation threshold when right-sided venous access is used for nonthoracotomy implantable defibrilla-tor lead implantation. The Endotak Investigators. J Car-diovasc Electrophysiol 1995; 6:979–86.

107 Heil JE, Lin Y, Derfus DL, Lang DJ. Impact of ICD elec-trode position on transvenous defibrillation thresholds (abstract). Pacing Clin Electrophysiol 1995; 18:873.

108 Brady PA, Friedman PA, Trusty JM, Grice S, Hammill SC, Stanton MS. High failure rate for an epicardial implant-able cardioverter-defibrillator lead: implications for long-term follow-up of patients with an implantable cardioverter-defibrillator. J Am Coll Cardiol 1998; 31:616–22.

109 Epstein AE, Ellenbogen KA, Kirk KA, Kay GN, Dailey SM, Plumb VJ. Clinical characteristics and outcome of patients with high defibrillation thresholds: a multicenter study. Circulation 1992; 86:1206–16.

110 Watanabe H, Chinushi M, Sugiura H, et al. Unsuccessful internal defibrillation in Brugada syndrome: focus on refractoriness and ventricular fibrillation cycle length. J Cardiovasc Electrophysiol 2005; 16:262–6.

111 Venditti FJ Jr, John RM, Hull M, Tofler GH, Shahian DM, Martin DT. Circadian variation in defibrillation energy requirements. Circulation 1996; 94:1607–12.

112 Glikson M, Gurevitz OT, Trusty JM, et al. Upper limit of vulnerability determination during implantable cardioverter-defibrillator placement to minimize ven-tricular fibrillation inductions. Am J Cardiol 2004; 94: 1445–9.

113 Hwang C, Swerdlow CD, Kass RM, et al. Upper limit of vulnerability reliably predicts the defibrillation threshold in humans. Circulation 1994; 90:2308–14.

114 Chen PS, Shibata N, Dixon EG, Martin RO, Ideker RE. Comparison of the defibrillation threshold and the upper limit of ventricular vulnerability. Circulation 1986; 73:1022–8.

115 Behrens S, Li C, Franz MR. Effects of myocardial ischemia on ventricular fibrillation inducibility and defibrillation efficacy. J Am Coll Cardiol 1997; 29:817–24.

116 Swerdlow CD, Peter CT, Kass RM, et al. Programming of implantable cardioverter-defibrillators on the basis of the upper limit of vulnerability. Circulation 1997; 95:1497–504.

117 Swerdlow CD, Ahern T, Kass RM, Davie S, Mandel WJ, Chen PS. Upper limit of vulnerability is a good estimator of shock strength associated with 90% probability of suc-cessful defibrillation in humans with transvenous implantable cardioverter-defibrillators. J Am Coll Cardiol 1996; 27:1112–8.

118 Swerdlow C, Shivkumar K, Zhang J. Determination of the upper limit of vulnerability using implantable

cardioverter-defibrillator electrograms. Circulation 2003; 107:3028–33.

119 Swerdlow CD. Implantation of cardioverter defibrillators without induction of ventricular fibrillation. Circulation 2001; 103:2159–64.

120 Gurevitz OT, Friedman PA, Glikson M, *et al.* Discrepancies between the upper limit of vulnerability and defibrillation threshold: prevalence and clinical predictors. J Cardiovasc Electrophysiol 2003; 14:728–32.

121 Buxton AE, Lee KL, DiCarlo L, *et al.* Electrophysiologic testing to identify patients with coronary artery disease who are at risk for sudden death. Multicenter Unsustained Tachycardia Trial Investigators. N Engl J Med 2000; 342:1937–45.

122 Bardy GH, Lee KL, Mark DB, *et al.* Amiodarone or an implantable cardioverter-defibrillator for congestive heart failure. N Engl J Med 2005; 352:225–37.

123 123 Antiarrhythmics Versus Implantable Defibrillators (AVID) Investigators. A comparison of antiarrhythmic-drug therapy with implantable defibrillators in patients resuscitated from near-fatal ventricular arrhythmias. N Engl J Med 1997; 337:1576–83.

124 Moss AJ, Zareba W, Hall WJ, *et al.* Prophylactic implantation of a defibrillator in patients with myocardial infarction and reduced ejection fraction. N Engl J Med 2002; 346:877–83.

125 Carnes CA, Mehdirad AA, Nelson SD. Drug and defibrillator interactions. Pharmacotherapy 1998; 18:516–25.

126 Shinlapawittayatorn K, Sungnoon R, Chattipakorn S, Chattipakorn N. Effects of sildenafil citrate on defibrillation efficacy. J Cardiovasc Electrophysiol 2006; 17:292–5.

127 Carnes CA, Pickworth KK, Votolato NA, Raman SV. Elevated defibrillation threshold with venlafaxine therapy. Pharmacotherapy 2004; 24:1095–8.

128 Papaioannou GI, Kluger J. Ineffective ICD therapy due to excessive alcohol and exercise. Pacing Clin Electrophysiol 2002; 25:1144–5.

129 Hohnloser SH, Dorian P, Roberts R, *et al.* Effect of amiodarone and sotalol on ventricular defibrillation threshold: the optimal pharmacological therapy in cardioverter defibrillator patients (OPTIC) trial. Circulation 2006; 114:104–9.

130 Luceri RM, Habal SM, David IB, Puchferran RL, Muratore C, Rabinovich R. Changing trends in therapy delivery with a third generation noncommitted implantable defibrillator: results of a large single center clinical trial. Pacing Clin Electrophysiol 1993; 16:159–64.

131 Wathen MS, DeGroot PJ, Sweeney MO, *et al.* Prospective randomized multicenter trial of empirical antitachycardia pacing versus shocks for spontaneous rapid ventricular tachycardia in patients with implantable cardioverter-defibrillators: Pacing Fast Ventricular Tachycardia Reduces Shock Therapies (PainFREE Rx II) trial results. Circulation 2004; 110:2591–6.

132 Swerdlow CD, Shehata M. Antitachycardia pacing in primary-prevention ICDs. J Cardiovasc Electrophysiol 2010; 21:1355–7.

2 Hemodynamics of Cardiac Pacing: Optimization and Programming to Enhance Cardiac Function

Faisal F. Syed, David L. Hayes, Paul A. Friedman, Samuel J. Asirvatham

Mayo Clinic, Rochester, MN, USA

Cardiovascular physiology 42
Abnormal physiology 43
Basics of hemodynamic pacing 43
Chronotropic response 43
Atrioventricular dissociation and ventriculoatrial
conduction 43
Atrioventricular synchrony 45
Atrioventricular optimization 49
Principles of echocardiographic atrioventricular
optimization 52
Atrial mechanical function 56
**Effect of pacing mode on morbidity and
mortality 56**
Optimal ventricular pacing sites 61
Pacing in heart failure 66
Influence of pacing site 66
Mechanisms underlying the benefits of left
ventricular and biventricular pacing 67
Left ventricular diastolic function 70
**AV optimization in cardiac resynchronization
therapy 70**
**Ventricular timing optimization (V-V
optimization) 71**
Optimizing site of pacing (LV and/or RV) 71
Varying the pacing vector 72

Impact of diseased myocardium proximate to the
pacing electrodes 72
Electrical parameters for V-V optimization 72
QRS vector fusion 72
Echocardiography for ventricular timing
optimization 75
Clinical approaches to V-V optimization 75
Other end-points for optimization 77
Mitral regurgitation 77
Arrhythmogenesis 77
Left atrial pacing 77
Right ventricular function 77
Cardiac contractility modulation pacing 78
Ventricular rate regulation 78
**Less common indications for pacing for
hemodynamic improvement 78**
Pacing in hypertrophic obstructive cardiomyopathy 78
Hemodynamic benefits of pacing in neurocardiogenic
syndromes 79
Hemodynamic benefits of pacing in first-degree
atrioventricular block 80
Conclusions 80
Addendum 80
References 80

Our understanding of the hemodynamic consequences of cardiac pacing has evolved dramatically over past decades. Dual-chamber pacing, rate-responsive pacing, rate-adaptive and differential atrioventricular (AV) intervals, alternative-site pacing, ventricular pacing avoidance algorithms, ventricular rate regularization and cardiac resynchronization therapy are all attempts to mimic and/or restore normal cardiac conduction and physiology.

Application of the appropriate pacing therapy first requires understanding of normal physiology, the various interrelated components contributing to the normally functioning cardiovascular system, and the effects of cardiac and noncardiac diseases on these individual components as well as on function of the whole. Given that our understanding of cardiac function in normal and abnormal conditions is incomplete and that current technology is imperfect, the goal to mimic the normal cardiovascular system perfectly under all conditions has yet to be met. Nevertheless, hemodynamically optimized pacing continues to attract intense interest as technologic advances bring us closer to that goal.

Cardiovascular physiology

Challenge to the cardiovascular system, such as exercise or emotion, usually results in an increase in cardiac output, which is determined by heart rate and stroke volume. The relative contribution of each is variable and in part determined by age, the type and intensity of activity, baseline cardiovascular conditioning, and whether there is underlying disease (Fig. 2.1).

The cardiovascular demands incurred with exercise are usually met primarily by an increase in heart rate and secondarily by increases in stroke volume. Aerobically trained athletes can increase stroke volume proportionally more, thus enabling them to reach the same cardiac output with a smaller increase in heart rate. Stroke volume is defined as the amount of blood ejected with each ventricular contraction, i.e., end-diastolic volume minus end-systolic volume. In the normal heart, end-diastolic volume depends on diastolic filling pressure, total blood volume, distribution of that blood volume, and atrial systole (preload). End-systolic volume depends on myocardial contractility and afterload. The Frank–Starling law relates the degree of left ventricular (LV) filling pressure to cardiac output at various degrees of contractility (Fig. 2.2).

All of these relationships are modulated by metabolic alterations, autonomic tone, pharmacologic agents, and the cardiac rhythm. For example, the increase in sympathetic tone associated with an increase in heart rate decreases the AV interval. Antiarrhythmic drugs can

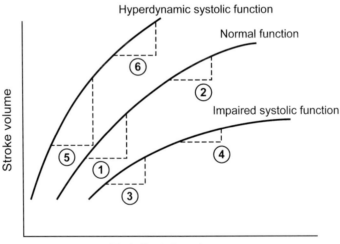

Fig. 2.1 Left ventricular (LV) function curve indicating the relationship between LV end-diastolic volume and stroke volume. Normal LV function is represented by the middle curve. If LV systolic function is on the ascending limb of the curve, an increase in end-diastolic volume results in a significant increase in stroke volume (1). This increase is even greater for patients with hyperdynamic systolic function (5) and less for patients with impaired systolic function (3). At greater end-diastolic volumes, i.e., higher LV filling pressures, further increasing the end-diastolic volume results in smaller increments in stroke volume. Even though patients with normal (2) or hyperdynamic (6) LV function may have a greater absolute increase in stroke volume, any increase in stroke volume for patients with LV dysfunction may be critically important (4). (Modified from Greenberg B, Chatterjee K, Parmley WW, Werner JA, Holly AN. The influence of left ventricular filling pressure on atrial contribution to cardiac output. Am Heart J 1979; 98:742–51, by permission of Mosby.)

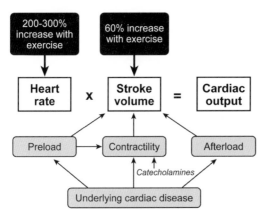

Fig. 2.2 Determinants of cardiac output during exercise. (Modified from Janosik DL, Labovitz AJ. Basic physiology of cardiac pacing. In: Ellenbogen KA, Kay GN, Wilkoff BL, eds. Clinical Cardiac Pacing. Philadelphia: WB Saunders Co., 1995:367–98, by permission of WB Saunders Co.)

increase or decrease the heart rate at rest and in response to exercise, either by a direct effect on the sinus node or by effects on the autonomic nervous system.

Abnormal physiology

A large segment of the pacing population has cardiac disease or other comorbidities that affect cardiac performance. These conditions can be characterized as those affecting heart rate, stroke volume, or both.

Chronotropic incompetence (an inadequate heart rate increase with exercise or stress) may be caused by isolated sinus node dysfunction, autonomic dysfunction, or drugs. Individuals with normal LV function may be asymptomatic at rest but experience symptoms with activity, depending on activity level, comorbid conditions (such as pulmonary disease), and the severity of chronotropic incompetence. Patients with significant LV dysfunction may be less tolerant of chronotropic incompetence because their impaired stroke volume makes them more dependent on heart rate to maintain cardiac output. Patients may be unaware of how symptomatic they are unless objectively evaluated.

Myocardial contractility may be impaired by coronary artery disease, myocardial infarction, nonischemic cardiomyopathy, valvular disease, or pericardial disease. Patients with LV dysfunction regardless of cause are more dependent on preload and afterload to maintain optimal stroke volume. Many of these patients have associated conduction system disease, such as sinus node dysfunction, AV nodal disease, or His–Purkinje disease. AV dissociation and interventricular and

intraventricular dyssynchrony can worsen already impaired myocardial performance. Interventricular dyssynchrony refers to activation of the right (RV) and left ventricles (LV) at different times; intraventricular dyssynchrony refers to temporal delay in mechanical contraction of different LVr segments (Fig. 2.3). It has been the focus of extensive study, as it adversely impacts clinical heart failure. Metabolic abnormalities, such as chronic acidosis, hypoxia, and hypercarbia, may depress cardiac performance. Patients with severe LV dysfunction may also have autonomic dysfunction that further limits the ability of the heart to increase heart rate and stroke volume with physiologic stress.

Many individuals with LV dysfunction have a number of associated comorbidities, e.g., concomitant renal failure, diabetes mellitus, coronary artery disease, hypertension, chronic obstructive pulmonary disease, and many others, all of which may affect indices of preload, afterload, and autonomic function as well as directly impair myocardial contractility (Fig. 2.4).[1] Drugs used in the treatment of these conditions, atrial fibrillation, and coronary artery disease may further affect these functions and directly suppress intrinsic conduction. Understandably, determining which patients will benefit from hemodynamic pacing techniques and which pacing technique will most benefit any individual patient is complex and incompletely understood.

Basics of hemodynamic pacing
Chronotropic response

Appropriate heart rate response during exercise, i.e., chronotropic competence, is the most important contributor to cardiac output, especially at moderate or extreme degrees of exercise (Fig. 2.5).[2-4] At rest and at lower levels of activity, AV synchrony contributes significantly to achieving an appropriate cardiac output (Fig. 2.6). Because many paced patients are at the lower end of the activity curve most of the time and a significant proportion of these patients are also dependent on adequate preload because of decreased ventricular compliance, AV synchrony is perhaps just as important as rate responsiveness for achieving optimal cardiovascular hemodynamics in the typical patient. Restoration of both rate responsiveness and AV synchrony should be the goal of physiologic pacing and should be viewed as complementary.

Atrioventricular dissociation and ventriculoatrial conduction

The earliest indication for pacing was complete heart block, and ventricular-only pacing was the only mode available. Establishing a stable ventricular rhythm was lifesaving and overshadowed the fact that normal

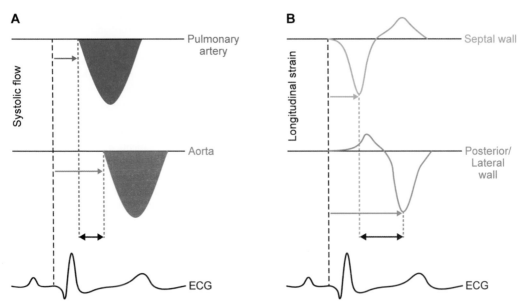

Fig. 2.3 Echocardiographic assessment of interventricular (A) and intraventricular (B) dyssynchrony. In (A), the flow of blood across the pulmonary valve (top) and aortic valve (middle) is charted as velocity (vertical axis) against time (horizontal axis). The difference in pre-ejection time (i.e., time delay from onset of the QRS [bottom] to onset of pulmonary or aortic flow), is a measure of *inter*ventricular dyssynchrony. In (B), the degree of myocardial tissue deformation ("strain", in this case measured in the longitudinal plane) of the septal (top) and posterior/lateral (middle) walls is charted vertically. The difference in time to peak strain between the two opposing walls, as calibrated by the ECG (bottom), is a measure of intraventricular dyssynchrony.

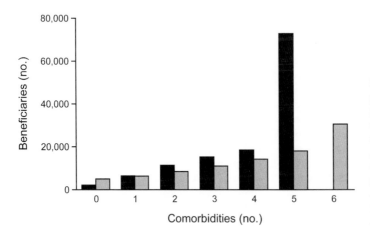

Fig. 2.4 Number of comorbidities per patient in congestive heart failure population (dark bars). Cost per additional comorbidity: total Medicare expenditures (light bars). Reproduced from Braunstein JB, Anderson GF, Gerstenblith G, *et al.* Noncardiac comorbidity increases preventable hospitalizations and mortality among Medicare beneficiaries with chronic heart failure. J Am Coll Cardiol 2003; 42:1226–33, by permission of Elsevier.)

cardiac function was not re-established. However, some patients experienced hemodynamic decline with this mode of pacing. Later it was established that hemodynamic impairment could be caused by ventriculoatrial conduction and atrial contraction against a closed AV valve, which could result in pacemaker syndrome.[5] Ventriculoatrial conduction can activate mechanical stretch receptors in the walls of the atria and pulmonary veins (Fig. 2.7). Vagal afferents transmit these impulses centrally, and reflex peripheral vasodilatation results. In addition, various neurohormonal agents, such as atrial natriuretic peptide, are activated. Pacemaker syndrome may be manifested by a variety of symptoms and physical signs (Table 2.1; Fig. 2.8). Pacemaker syndrome was

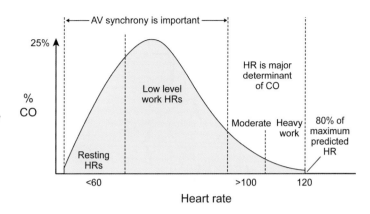

Fig. 2.5 Schematic representation of the contribution of atrioventricular synchrony and rate response to cardiac output (CO) at various levels of activity. At rest and low levels of activity, maintenance of atrioventricular synchrony makes a proportionately greater contribution to cardiac output. At higher exercise levels, cardiac rate (HR) clearly contributes more to cardiac output.

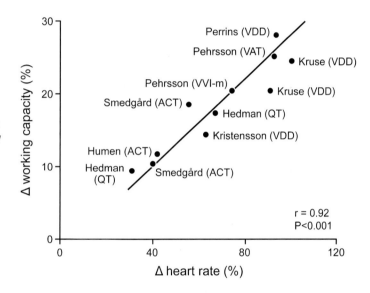

Fig. 2.6 Representation of multiple studies comparing the relative contribution of heart rate and atrioventricular synchrony to work capacity. All studies agree that heart rate is the greatest contributor during exercise. ACT, VVIR activity sensor; QT, VVIR QT sensor; VVI-m, rate-matched ventricular pacing. (From Nordlander R, Hedman A, Pehrsson SK. Rate responsive pacing and exercise capacity: a comment. Pacing Clin Electrophysiol 1989; 12:749–51, by permission of Futura Publishing Co.)

initially identified as a complication of VVI pacing; however, it may occur with any pacing mode when there is AV dissociation. It may also occur in persons with a markedly prolonged AV delay, with atrial systole effectively occurring concurrently with or after ventricular systole (Fig. 2.9).

The prevalence of pacemaker syndrome is difficult to determine and depends in part on how it is identified. Older studies evaluating objective clinical impairment with pacing in a nontracking mode suggest that the incidence may be in the range of 7–10%.[6] In a substudy of the Mode Selection Trial (MOST) trial, investigators noted the development of "severe" pacemaker syndrome in approximately 20% of patients paced in the VVIR mode. Improvement was noted with reprogram-

ming to a dual-chamber pacing mode.[7] However, in an older crossover study[8] of patients with pacing in each of the DDD and VVI modes for 1 week in randomized order, 83% of subjects experienced some degree of pacemaker syndrome with pacing in the VVI mode. This finding suggests that when patients have a basis for comparison, they are more aware of symptoms of pacemaker syndrome (Fig. 2.10).

Atrioventricular synchrony

The contribution of AV synchrony to maintaining physiologic cardiac performance is well established. AV synchrony is estimated to increase stroke volume by as much as 50% and in normal hearts may decrease left atrial pressure and increase cardiac index by as

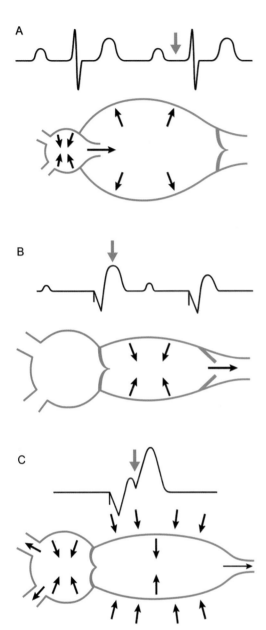

Table 2.1 Pacemaker syndrome.

Potential symptoms
Weakness
Chest pain
Syncope or near-syncope
Dyspnea
Cough
Neck pulsations
Apprehension
Abdominal pulsations
Potential physical findings
Hypotension
Congestive heart failure
Cannon "a" waves
Blood pressure decline during ventricular pacing
Decrease in cardiac output and arterial pressure
Increase in peripheral vascular resistance during monitoring

Fig. 2.7 (A) Optimal cardiac filling with atrioventricular (AV) synchrony. (B) With VVI pacing, the ventricle is not optimally filled and there is contraction against a closed AV valve. (C) As a result of the loss of AV synchrony, venous pressure is increased, and multiple symptoms may ensue. (From Levine PA, Mace RC. Pacing Therapy: A Guide to Cardiac Pacing for Optimum Hemodynamic Benefit. Mount Kisco, NY: Futura Publishing Co., 1983: 29, 36, by permission of the publisher.)

much as 25–30%. Although patients with normal ventricular function may have the greatest absolute degree of improvement with restoration of AV synchrony, a greater degree of relative improvement is typical in patients with severe LV systolic dysfunction. In these patients, any improvement derived from appropriately timed atrial systole may be beneficial.

Mitral valve closure and diastolic filling are influenced by the timing of atrial and ventricular contraction. Identifying the optimal AV interval for a given patient can be difficult. Regardless of whether the AV interval is programmed too long or too short, optimal AV interval timing leads to premature mitral closure. If the AV interval is too long, ventricular contraction does not immediately follow atrial emptying. Thus, the AV valves "float" back towards the atria, resulting in near closure of these valves prior to the onset of ventricular systole. This results in a soft first heart sound and, when extreme, regurgitation of blood through the AV valves during diastole (diastolic AV regurgitation). If the AV interval is unduly short, ventricular contraction and closure of the AV valves occurs before completion of atrial emptying. Because in patients with cardiomyopathy and heart failure there can be considerable differences in the timing of RV and LV contraction and relaxation, optimal AV closure for one side of the circulation may not be ideal for the other. Patients with severe diastolic dysfunction benefit even more from appropriately timed atrial systole because dependence on optimal preload is even greater to maintain satisfactory cardiac output.

The influence of pacing mode on factors indirectly but importantly related to cardiovascular performance

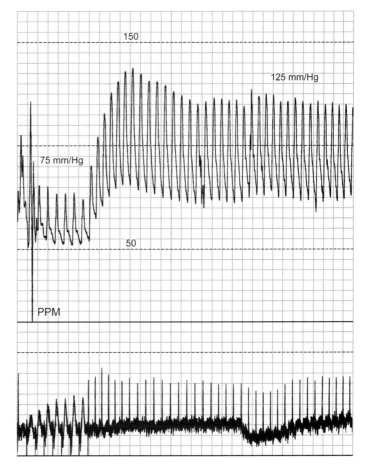

Fig. 2.8 Hemodynamic tracing from a patient with a VVI pacemaker. The arterial blood pressure increases with the transition from VVI pacing to normal sinus rhythm. (From Hayes DL, Holmes DR Jr. Hemodynamics of cardiac pacing. In: Furman S, Hayes DL, Holmes DR Jr, eds. A Practice of Cardiac Pacing, 3rd edn. Mount Kisco, NY: Futura Publishing Co., 1993: 195–218, by permission of Mayo Foundation.)

has also been studied. P-synchronous pacing has been shown to result not only in significantly higher cardiac outputs than VVI pacing, but also in lower systemic vascular resistance, lower serum lactate levels, smaller AV oxygen gradients, and lower levels of circulating vasoactive peptides and norepinephrine.

Mechanical AV delay varies between paced and sensed atrial beats because of the intrinsic delay in atrial activation after atrial pacing, i.e., intra-atrial conduction. The absolute intra-atrial conduction delay varies significantly among patients and also depends on underlying conduction or myocardial disease (Fig. 2.11). The right intra-atrial conduction time is measured from the beginning of the P wave, or the intracardiac signal recorded in the upper right atrium, to the onset of atrial depolarization in the para-Hisian bundle region. The normal right intra-atrial conduction time is usually between 30 and 60 ms. Interatrial conduction time, measured from the beginning of the P wave or depolarization in the upper right atrium to the onset of left

atrial depolarization, is recorded at the level of the distal coronary sinus. The interatrial conduction time is generally between 60 and 85 ms.[9] Taking the interatrial and intra-atrial delay into consideration and programming the differential AV interval accordingly will result in improved hemodynamics.[10]

Because intra-atrial conduction delay varies from patient to patient and the relative timing of left and right atrial contraction depends on the actual site in the atrium of earliest activation, it can be very difficult to predict consistently when atrial systole will actually be complete for both atria (Fig. 2.12). Added to this, the extent of intra-atrial conduction delay is dependent on the site of activation (pacing site within diseased/ scarred area, etc.) during atrially paced complexes, further complicating the issue. Clues on the ECG that suggest echocardiographic AV optimization may be particularly helpful include a P-wave duration >120 ms, an absent or negative PR segment, and notching and/ or isoelectric periods during the inscription of the P

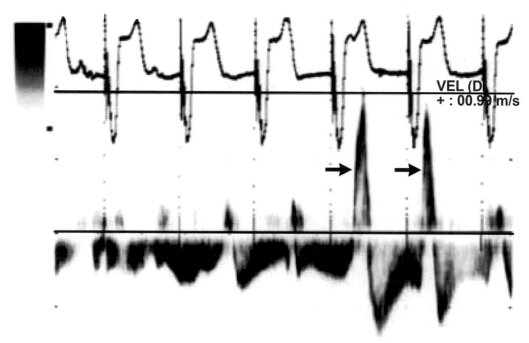

Fig. 2.9 Right-sided pacemaker syndrome. Pulsed wave hepatic vein Doppler from an 81-year-old man with heart failure and a history of atrioventricular conduction block treated with a VVI pacemaker. Transthoracic echocardiography indicated normal ventricular systolic function, elevated right ventricular systolic pressures, and a dilated inferior vena cava. Arrows point to hepatic vein flow reversals in timing with atrial systole, consistent with canon-waves. After upgrading to a DDD pacemaker was accompanied by resolution of clinical signs of heart failures and normalization of right ventricular systolic pressures as well as the above flow reversals. (From de Zuttere D, Galey A, Jolly G, Rocha P. Diagnosis of pacemaker syndrome by suprahepatic vein pulsed Doppler echocardiography. Eur J Echocardiogr 2011; 12:E25, with permission of the publisher.)

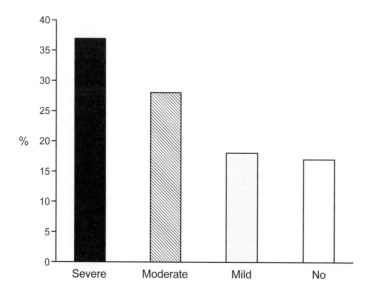

Fig. 2.10 Degree of symptoms detected in patients randomized to DDD and VVI pacing modes. Overall, 83% of patients had some symptoms consistent with pacemaker syndrome. (Modified from Heldman D, Mulvihill D, Nguyen H, *et al.* True incidence of pacemaker syndrome. Pacing Clin Electrophysiol 1990; 13:1742–50, by permission of Futura Publishing Co.)

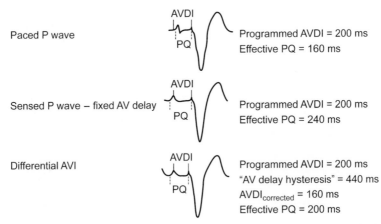

Fig. 2.11 A differential atrioventricular interval (AVDI) attempts to correct for the timing differences between a paced and a sensed atrial event. When the atrium is paced, the atrioventricular interval (AVI) begins with delivery of the pacing artifact. However, there is latency between delivery of the pacing artifact and actual depolarization. Depending on interatrial conduction time, the pacedsensed difference can be great. In this diagram, the AVI is programmed to 200 ms for each event, but the effective AVI is 160 ms after the sensed atrial event and 240 ms after the paced atrial event. (From Janosik DL, Pearson AC, Buckingham TA, Labovitz AJ, Redd RM. The hemodynamic benefit of differential atrioventricular delay intervals for sensed and paced atrial events during physiologic pacing. J Am Coll Cardiol 1989; 14:499–507, by permission of the American College of Cardiology.)

wave. In practice, with the exception of cardiac resynchronization devices, echocardiographic optimization is rarely performed. Programming the AV interval is discussed further below.

In addition to independently programmable paced and sensed AV intervals, dual-chamber pacemakers provide rate-adaptive AV intervals. Conduction time through the AV node normally decreases because of sympathetic nervous system activity with physiologic increases in heart rate, resulting in shorter AV intervals at higher heart rates. Any variation in heart rate has been demonstrated to result in an immediate, precise, and inversely proportional variation in the AV interval in normal hearts.[11] A linear relationship exists between heart rate and the AV interval, independent of age or baseline PR interval (Fig. 2.13).[12] In patients with conduction system disease or autonomic dysfunction, the AV delay may not shorten with heart rate increase. Rate-adaptive AV interval attempts to mirror normal physiology and allow a higher maximal tracking rate, and has been shown to improve hemodynamic indices during exercise compared with those with a fixed AV interval.[11,13]

Optimization of the AV interval has been a source of frustration for many years. When dual-chamber pacemakers were first introduced and only a fixed AV interval was possible, very simple programming guidelines were followed. In general, if the patient had intact AV conduction, the AV interval was programmed long enough to allow intrinsic conduction. If the patient had

AV block, the AV interval was programmed to mimic what was considered to be a normal PR interval, i.e., 150–200 ms. However, this outdated approach fails to account for the previously described mechanical intra-atrial delay from atrial pacing to atrial depolarization, the effect of any interatrial conduction delay, and the deleterious effects of RV apical pacing that may be avoided if a significantly longer AV interval allows intrinsic conduction to occur. In addition, optimization of the AV interval becomes a significantly more important hemodynamic issue with the introduction of cardiac resynchronization therapy.

Atrioventricular optimization

Optimizing the AV interval serves to optimize LV preload. Selection of the best AV interval often depends on echocardiographic or invasive hemodynamic measurement. Patients who require biventricular systems typically have abnormal and variable intra-atrial and intraventricular conduction. This makes the prediction of left-sided atrial ventricular mechanical delay difficult using right atrial pacing. Thus, a given AV interval will result in markedly different left-sided AV mechanical delays in different patients based on their individual intra-atrial and intraventricular conduction delay. The site of both ventricular and atrial leads also impacts optimization of AV timing. For example, an atrial lead placed on the intra-atrial septum with an LV lead placed near the base of the LV will give rise to a completely different AV mechanical interval than a right

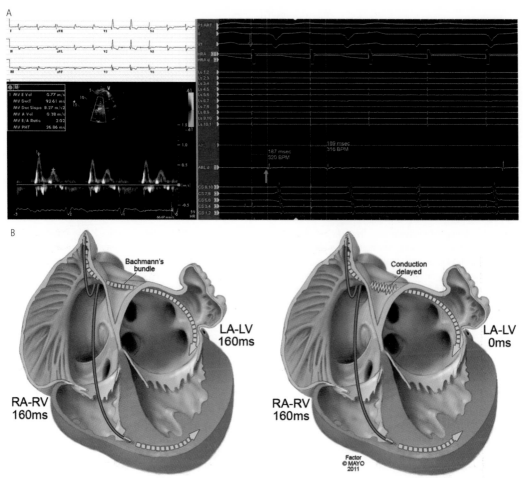

Fig. 2.12 Interatrial conduction delay. The PR interval or the paced AV interval does not always correlate with LA–LV timing. In (A), despite a markedly prolonged PR interval (380 ms, top left), the timing of the mitral valve Doppler inflow (bottom left) is normal on account of a delay of 187 ms (right) between the right (hollow arrow, paced signal) and left (filled arrow, sensed signal) atria as determined by intracardiac electrograms. (Courtesy of Dr. Brian Powell, Mayo Clinic, Rochester, MN). (B) With normal conduction (A), an adequate delay in the paced RA–RV interval results in an adequate LA–LV interval. In B, interatrial delay results in a delayed LA activation, such that the effective LA–LV interval results in simultaneous LA and LV contraction, or the equivalent of a left-sided pacemaker syndrome.

atrial appendage position used with LV apical pacing, even though the AV interval is set similarly.

The rationale for cardiac resynchronization therapy is primarily to normalize the ventricular activation sequence and coordinate septal and free wall contraction, thereby improving cardiac efficiency.[14] Although this primary utility of ventricular resynchronization is independent of AV conduction and mechanical AV delays, an incremental benefit above that achieved with ventricular resynchronization has been demonstrated with a range of ideal AV delays,[15] and others have demonstrated the effects of suboptimal AV delays in heart failure.[16] With long AV delays, there is a suboptimal contribution of atrial systole. This gives rise to diastolic mitral regurgitation and limits the diastolic filling that occurs as a result of active atrial systole. Shortening the AV delay decreases the amount of diastolic mitral regurgitation and dilated cardiomyopathy, thereby decreasing pulmonary capillary wedge pressures, etc. Conversely, an AV delay that is too short gives rise to a suboptimally shortened filling period for the LV and thus decreased preload and cardiac output.

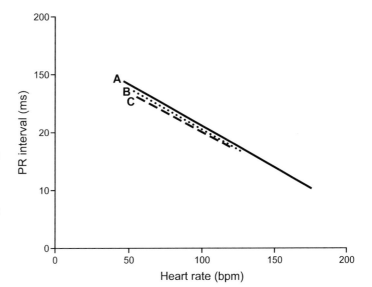

Fig. 2.13 Linear regression of PR interval (ms) and heart rate (bpm) from electrocardiograms of young healthy subjects (A), older healthy subjects (B), and patients after myocardial infarction (C). Linear shortening of the interval occurs as exercise intensity increases. (From Rees M, Haennel RG, Black WR, Kappagoda T. Effect of rate-adapting atrioventricular delay on stroke volume and cardiac output during atrial synchronous pacing. Can J Cardiol 1990; 6:445–52, by permission of Pulsus Group.)

The degree and extent of intra-atrial conduction delay in patients with heart failure and abnormal heart is highly variable. In the normal state, sinus impulses from the right atrial–superior vena caval junction reach the left atrium primarily through the roof of the atrium (Bachmann's bundle) and secondarily through the fossa ovalis and the musculature of the coronary sinus.[17] Once the impulse reaches the atria, a distinct sequence of activations involving predictable differences in activation of the posterior atrium, left atrial appendages, and pulmonary vein are observed. While this intra-atrial conduction is occurring, conduction via the AV node to the ventricle is also occurring. In patients without bundle branch block there is near-simultaneous activation of the right and left mid endo-cardial surfaces of the intraventricular septum. With AV pacing using a right atrial appendage lead and a RV apical lead configuration, increased intra-atrial conduction delay may give rise to near-simultaneous left atrial and LV activation, producing the equivalent of a left-sided pacemaker syndrome (Fig. 2.12). On the other hand, placement of the atrial lead in the Bach-mann's bundle region in a patient with insignificant intra-atrial conduction delay, but with significant conduction delay from the RV pacing site to the LV, will cause marked prolongation of the left-sided mechanical AV interval. Intra-atrial conduction delay also affects the AV interval during atrial sensing. During atrial tracking, right atrial events are sensed after the onset of atrial depolarization. In some patients, sinus activation occurs first on the septal side of the right

atrial superior vena caval junction. There may be marked intra-atrial delay from this site to the right atrial appendage where the pacing lead is required. In these patients, by the time the atrial event is sensed, left atrial activation may be ongoing or even completed, giving rise to a very long left atrium to LV mechanical delay with usual AV timing.

Thus, the location of the atrial, the RV and the LV leads, the magnitude and difference between intra-atrial conduction and intraventricular conduction delay and the lead function at any given time (atrial pacing vs. sensing) all impact LA–LV mechanical intervals in a manner that is difficult to predict.[18]

LV end-diastolic pressures may change significantly based on the actual AV delay, and this change is largely independent of the site of ventricular pacing.[18] LV contractility as measured as dP/dt is also affected by the AV delay, and this effect is incremental to the benefit seen with LV-based pacing over RV pacing.[19] In the PATH-CHF trial, a hemodynamic benefit as seen with increased LV maximal dP/dt and increased impulse pressure was demonstrated with either LV or biventricular pacing in comparison with RV-based pacing. The effect, however, was seen best at AV delays between 25% and 75% of the intrinsic PR interval.[15] A benefit of LV free-wall pacing when compared with an anterior site in the LV when measuring a percent increase in dP/dt has also been demonstrated. This effect was also optimal at AV delays between 50 and 100 ms and prolongation of the AV delay showed a decrease in this beneficial effect on contractility irrespective of the site of pacing.[20]

Principles of echocardiographic atrioventricular optimization

The AV or PR interval is usually simply measured from either the atrial pacemaker artifact or from the start of the P wave to the beginning of the QRS complex. The mechanically relevant AV interval is the time between mechanical atrial contraction and ventricular contraction. The echocardiographic parameter most useful in studying the filling characteristics of the LV is the mitral valve inflow Doppler velocity. The mitral valve inflow pattern in sinus rhythm is biphasic. Distinct filling waves can be recognized (Fig. 2.14). The first is the early filling wave (E wave). This represents blood flow into the LV during diastole. The velocity and magnitude of this flow are dependent primarily on the relaxation characteristics of the LV. The second distinct wave is the A wave, which occurs only in sinus rhythm and is from active atrial contraction. Because of electromechanical delays in the atrium and the ventricle there is a distinct interval between the start of the P wave and the start of the A wave measured by mitral Doppler inflow. In fact, the QRS complex itself is usually inscribed typically before the start of the A wave. When the PR–AV interval is short, the QRS is inscribed early and this results in aortic ejection and mitral valve closure occurring (forced by ventricular contraction) prior to complete

inscription of the atrial Doppler inflow (truncation of the A wave) (Fig. 2.15). Thus, with short AV delays, diastolic flow is limited and the full benefit of atrial contraction is not obtained. This is important in all patients with heart failure, but extremely important in patients with significant diastolic dysfunction/ relaxation abnormality. In these patients, because of problems with ventricular relaxation, the E wave is limited and a greater portion of diastolic filling is from atrial systole and the A wave. Conversely, with a long AV interval (PR interval) the A wave is completed. However, a significant gap between the end of atrial filling (A wave) and the beginning of ventricular contraction and aortic ejection occurs. During this delay the mitral valve has passively closed (soft first heart sound) and diastolic mitral regurgitation may occur. Thus, in an optimal AV interval the atrial filling wave has completed and there is no excessive delay between this completion and the beginning of aortic ejection. Most methods of echocardiographic AV optimization use this principle. In one technique the mitral inflow Doppler velocity and aortic outflow are continuously monitored echocardiographically. During this monitoring the AV interval is first set at or about the patient's intrinsic PR interval (long AV interval). The AV interval is then progressively shortened until truncation of the A wave is just seen. This AV interval with or without a small positive offset is taken as the optimized AV interval. Using the principle that optimal AV delay results when spontaneous mitral valve closure occurs at about the same time as forced closure (ventricular contraction) and therefore aortic ejection, Ritter et al.[21] have described the following method. Initially, a short AV

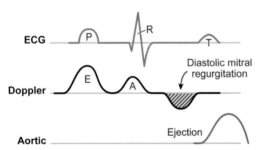

Fig. 2.14 There exists a significant delay between electrical and mechanical events that need to be understood to provide optimal atrioventricular programming in resynchronization devices. This figure shows the situation where the PR interval is too long following the electrical event (P waves). Diastolic mechanical flow from atrium to ventricle (the A wave) as a result of atrial contraction occurs slightly later. Similarly, following the QRS complex aortic ejection occurs after a definite and significant electromechanical delay interval. Because atrial filling has been completed and the ventricle has not yet started contracting, blood flows back into the atrium during diastole (diastolic mitral regurgitation). Programming a shorter PR interval (AV interval) will prevent this from occurring. (From Hayes DL, Wang P, Sackner-Bernstein J, Asirvatham S. Resynchronization and Defibrillation for Heart Failure: A Practical Approach. Blackwell-Futura, 2004: 145. Copyrighted and used with permission of Mayo Foundation for Medical Education and Research.)

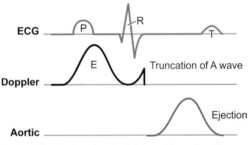

Fig. 2.15 The situation when the P–R interval is too short. Now ventricular systole (mechanical contraction of the ventricle) occurs even before complete emptying of the atrium (truncation of the A wave). Thus, in a mechanical sense the patient is the equivalent of atrial fibrillation (no effective hemodynamic contribution of the atrium). (From Hayes DL, Wang P, Sackner-Bernstein J, Asirvatham S. Resynchronization and Defibrillation for Heart Failure: A Practical Approach. Blackwell-Futura, 2004: 145.)

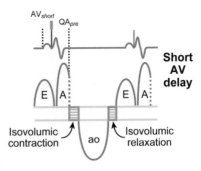

- Program short AV delay (AV$_{short}$), forcing closure of mitral valve

- Note premature shortening of A-wave, reducing diastolic filling prior to aortic out-flow (ao); QA is time for QRS onset to the premature end of the A-wave

- Program long AV delay (AV$_{long}$), maintaining ventricular pre-excitation but allowing spontaneous MV closure

- Note delay between MV closure and start of systole marked by beginning of isovolumic contraction period; QA$_{spont}$ is the time from QRS onset to the spontaneous end of the A-wave

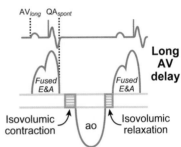

Fig. 2.16 Echocardiographic example for atrioventricular (AV) delay optimization. With the short AV delay, truncation of the A wave is seen. Gradually lengthening the AV delay takes away the truncation while further lengthening (long AV delay) allows diastolic mitral regurgitation (see text). (Data from Ritter P, Dib JC, Mahaux V, *et al*. PACE 1995; 18:855 (abstract). Reproduced with permission from Blackwell Publishing.)

- Optimized AV delay (AV$_{opt}$) is calculated from the formula below

- End of diastolic filling coincides with beginning of systole

- Results in
  - R-wave and A-wave separation
  - Maximized LV diastolic filling time

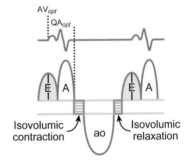

$$AV_{opt} = AV_{short} + d$$
where
$$d = (AV_{long} - AV_{short}) - (QA_{pre} - QA_{spont})$$

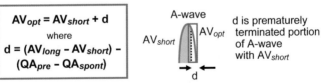

Fig. 2.17 Calculation of the optimal atrioventricular (AV) interval using the Ritter formula. (Data from Ritter P, Dib JC, Mahaux V, *et al*. PACE 1995; 18:855 (abstract). Reproduced with permission from Blackwell Publishing.)

delay (AV1) is programmed and the interval between the onset of the QRS to the end of the truncated A wave (QA1) is measured (Fig. 2.16). Next there is a long AV delay (AV2) that maintains ventricular capture (prior to spontaneous AV conduction), but allowing mitral valve closure before aortic ejection is measured (Fig. 2.16). The interval between the start of the QRS to the end of the nontruncated A wave is noted (QA2). The optimal AV interval according to the Ritter calculation is AV1 + [(AV2 − AV1) − (QA1 − QA2)] (Fig. 2.17).

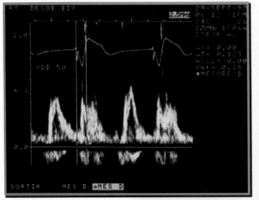 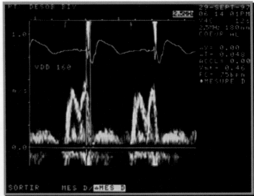

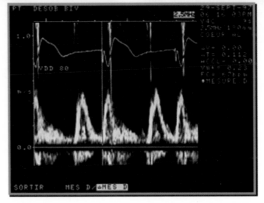

Fig. 2.18 Echocardiographic images demonstrating the Ritter method for atrioventricular (AV) interval optimization. The upper left panel obtained with a short AV interval; upper right panel obtained with a long AV interval; lower panel demonstrates optimal separation of E and A waves.

Thus, the greater the difference in the AV interval that allows complete inscription of the A wave and the short AV interval the larger the optimal AV interval will be. On the other hand, a large difference between the start of the QRS and the end of the A wave when allowing for complete AV inscription (long atrial filling) will result in the optimal AV interval being short. Echocardiographic images demonstrating use of the Ritter method are demonstrated in Fig. 2.18.

An alternative method for AV optimization was also proposed many years ago (Fig. 2.19).[22] In this somewhat simpler method, a slightly prolonged AV delay is set. From this number is subtracted the interval between the end of the A wave and complete closure of the mitral valve. This interval from the end of the A wave to the beginning of aortic ejection or complete closure of the mitral valve is the duration of diastolic mitral regurgitation. Thus, from a single long AV interval the optimal AV interval can be calculated. The steps for using the Ishikawa method would be to set a long AV interval and measure the mitral Doppler inflow. The interval between the end of the complete A wave and the beginning of aortic ejection can be measured. This measurement is subtracted from the long AV interval.

Several observations with regard to AV optimization in the PATH-CHF study also allow for relatively simpler AV interval optimization. Patients with a wide QRS complex demonstrated shorter optimal AV delay sensations with a narrow QRS complex. This is likely to be because intraventricular conduction delay is more prominent than interatrial conduction delay. The optimal average AV interval for patients with a QRS >150 ms was 43% of the intrinsic AV interval. On the other hand, for patients with a normal or narrower QRS, optimal AV intervals were about 80% of the intrinsic AV interval. This, of course, will be affected by the position of the LV lead. For example, if the LV lead is located at a site causing early aortic ejection, then a longer AV interval despite the wider QRS will be required.

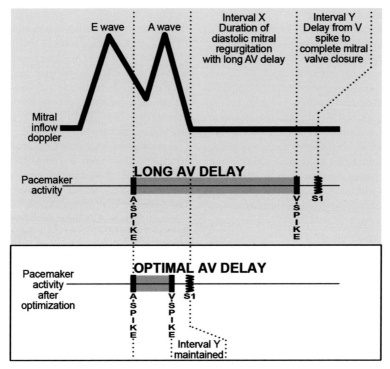

Fig. 2.19 Ishikawa method for atrioventricular (AV) optimization (see text). (Modified from Ishikawa T, Sumita S, Kimura K, *et al.* Critical PQ interval for the appearance of diastolic mitral regurgitation and optimal PQ interval in patients implanted with DDD pacemakers. Pacing Clin Electrophysiol 1994; 17:1989–94.)

Acute hemodynamic studies suggest that optimal ventricular contractility is further enhanced in individual patients when a patient's specific AV interval is programmed. It has been shown that there is a close correlation between impedance-measured AV interval and echo Doppler-derived AV interval and externally applied impedance signals are a relatively straightforward bedside method to adjust the AV interval.[23–25]

A major weakness that remains is the inability to optimize the AV interval during exercise. Optimization of the AV interval at rest does not reflect the optimal AV interval during exercise, which can be longer, shorter, or the same as that at rest.[26] Programming the AV delay during exercise results in superior exercise hemodynamics than derivations from the resting AV delay.[26] Techniques have been hypothesized for AV interval optimization during stress in cardiac resynchronization systems.[27] While adaptive algorithms to optimize the AV interval during exercise would be a step forward, several problems remain. The actual optimal AV interval during exercise may vary with loading conditions on the heart, e.g., when over-

diuresis or incipient heart failure occurs. Even with real-time physiologic parameter monitoring as part of a feedback system, the optimal AV interval may be difficult to determine, as no single parameter may be representative of all factors that need to be considered. The optimal AV interval for diastolic function is difficult to determine; only measuring mitral inflow Doppler measurements and making sure that all of atrial contraction has contributed to diastole is probably too simplistic. Ventricular stretch, efficiency of ventricular relaxation, and optimization of early filling may involve different AV interval optimizing algorithms from systolic function optimization. Even if the AV interval has been carefully optimized, if radiofrequency ablation is performed in the atrium, antiarrhythmic drugs are used, or myocardial infarctions have occurred, a completely different relative atrial and ventricular timing may result. Another confounding variable is optimal RA–RV timing. The operator may perfectly optimize LA–LV timing, only to find that there is significant diastolic tricuspid regurgitation giving rise to hepatic engorgement and right-sided heart failure.

Atrial mechanical function

Enhanced atrial contraction should follow optimal atrial conduction. In a study of cardiac resynchronization therapy recipients, atrial sensed beats (allowing for intrinsic intra-atrial and interatrial conduction), compared with right atrial paced beats, resulted in improved LV output and filling as well as improved tissue Doppler strain indices of right and left atrial function and interatrial mechanical synchrony.[28] Similarly, compared with those with interatrial delay, whether intrinsic or pacing-induced, atrial contraction and mechanical synchrony improved with pacing the right atrial septum, Bachman's bundle, or with biatrial pacing.[29–33] Whether these observations translate into clinically significant outcomes, such as long-term benefits with atrial remodeling and cardiac output, is currently unknown.

Effect of pacing mode on morbidity and mortality

An early study of the effect of pacing mode on morbidity and mortality[34] paved the way for intense clinical interest in and subsequent clinical trials on the effect of pacing mode on morbidity and mortality and on the potential adverse effects of VVI pacing (Figs 2.20 and 2.21). In this early study, at 4 years of follow-up, atrial fibrillation had occurred in 47% of the patients receiving VVI pacing, but in only 7% of those receiving AAI pacing ($P < 0.0005$); heart failure occurred in 37% of the VVI group and in 15% of the AAI group ($P < 0.005$); and mortality was 23% in the VVI group and 8% in the AAI group ($P < 0.025$).

Many other investigators have performed retrospective reviews to assess the effect of pacing mode on mortality. Despite the inherent weaknesses of retrospective analyses, it is difficult to dismiss the similar finding

among all the studies of significantly lower mortality with DDD or AAI pacing than with VVI pacing and significantly lower incidences of atrial fibrillation.[35]

Survival was assessed in a large population of patients (20,948) with sinus node dysfunction.[36] This random sample was from the complete US cohort of Medicare patients receiving pacing for sinus node dysfunction in 1988 through 1990. The DDD/DDDR pacing mode was an independent correlate of survival.

A number of prospective trials have assessed the effect of pacing mode on morbidity and mortality. Andersen et al.[37] published the first prospective data on pacing mode and survival. (This trial is referred to as the Andersen Trial or the Danish Pacemaker Trial.) Among 225 patients (mean age 76 years) with sinus

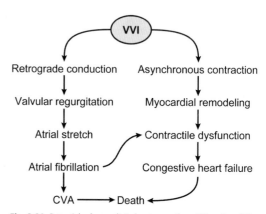

Fig. 2.20 Potential adverse clinical outcomes from VVI pacing. CVA, cerebrovascular accident. (Modified from Gillis AM. Pacing to prevent atrial fibrillation. Cardiol Clin 2000; 18:25–36, by permission of WB Saunders Co.)

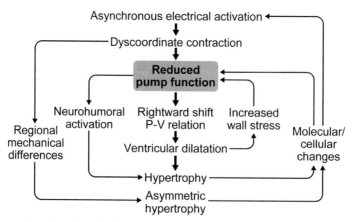

Fig. 2.21 Elegant representation of the adverse hemodynamic consequences of ventricular pacing. (Reprinted with permission from Sweeney MO, Prinzen FW. A new paradigm for physiologic ventricular pacing. J Am Coll Cardiol 2006; 47:282.)

node dysfunction randomized to AAI or VVI pacing, the incidence of atrial fibrillation was higher in the VVI group (AAI group 14%; VVI group 23%; $P = 0.12$) and the incidence of thromboembolism was also higher in the VVI group than in the AAI group ($P = 0.0083$). Although no difference in mortality could be detected at the initial analysis at 3.3 years, subsequent analysis at 5.5 years showed improved survival and less heart failure in the AAI group.[38] In addition, there was a persistent reduction in the incidence of atrial fibrillation and thromboembolic events. This trial stands alone in demonstrating lower mortality with physiologic pacing. This may be explained by the fact that the physiologic pacing mode implemented was AAI mode. With AAI pacing, the patient maintains intrinsic AV conduction; perhaps more important, this avoids the abnormal depolarization pattern of RV pacing that would occur with VVI or DDD pacing.

In a smaller trial,[39] paroxysmal atrial fibrillation occurred more frequently with VVI pacing than with DDD pacing. However, the Pac-A-Tach trial[40] found no significant difference in recurrence of atrial tachyarrhythmias by intention to treat at 1 year—48% in DDDR and 43% in VVI.

The Pacemaker Selection in the Elderly (PASE) trial, a prospective, randomized, single-blind trial, compared DDDR with VVIR pacing modes.[41] There was no statistically significant difference in quality of life between DDDR and VVIR pacing modes, but there was a trend toward improved quality of life in patients with sinus node dysfunction randomized to dual-chamber pacing. Perhaps more significant was a crossover of 26% of patients from ventricular pacing to dual-chamber pacing because of pacemaker syndrome.

The Canadian Trial of Physiologic Pacing (CTOPP)[42] compared VVIR with DDDR or AAIR and had primary end-points of overall mortality and cerebrovascular accidents and secondary end-points of atrial fibrillation, hospitalizations for CHF, and death from a cardiac cause. CTOPP demonstrated that physiologic pacing (DDD/AAI) was associated with a reduced rate in the development of chronic atrial fibrillation, from 3.78% to 2.87% per year, at the 3-year analysis. No significant improvement in quality of life or mortality was demonstrated with dual-chamber pacing. However, there was a slight divergence of the mortality curves favoring dual-chamber pacing. In addition, quality of life was improved in subsets of patients. These included patients who were pacemaker-dependent and patients with severe diastolic or systolic dysfunction.[43]

The UK Pacing and Cardiovascular Events (UKPACE) trial compared DDD with VVI pacing modes in patients ≥70 years old who required permanent pacing for second- or third-degree AV block.[43] UKPACE demon-

strated no significant difference between pacing modes in the primary end-point of all-cause mortality or in the composite secondary end-point of cardiovascular deaths, atrial fibrillation, heart failure hospitalizations, cerebrovascular accidents or thromboembolic events, and reoperation.

Of the major trials assessing the effect of pacing mode on morbidity and mortality, the Mode Selection Trial (MOST) and subsequent substudies have probably had the most profound effect on the practice of pacing.[44] MOST randomized 2010 patients with sinus node dysfunction to either VVI or DDD pacing. The primary end-points were all causes of mortality and cerebrovascular accidents. This trial failed to demonstrate any difference in mortality, but did demonstrate a lower incidence of atrial fibrillation with physiologic pacing and reduced the signs and symptoms of heart failure. Quality of life was slightly improved. The rates of hospitalization for heart failure and of death, stroke, or hospitalization for heart failure were not significant in unadjusted analyses, but with adjusted analyses became marginally significant. The study concluded that, overall, dual-chamber pacing offers significant improvement compared with ventricular pacing.

Substudies of the MOST trial,[45] DAVID (Dual Chamber and VVI Implantable Defibrillator),[46] and MADIT-II (Multicenter Automatic Defibrillator Trial II)[47] have demonstrated the adverse effects of RV apical pacing when no ventricular pacing was required, i.e., the patient had intact AV conduction at some AR interval.

The DAVID trial was designed to assess the effect of dual-chamber pacing vs. backup ventricular pacing in patients with an implantable cardioverter-defibrillator (ICD) indication but no indication for antibradycardia pacing, no history of recurrent atrial arrhythmias and an LV ejection fraction of ≤40%.[46] Patients were randomized to effectively no pacing, VVI backup pacing at 40 bpm, or DDDR pacing with a lower rate of 70 bpm. Dual-chamber pacing offered no advantage and actually increased the combined end-point of death or hospitalization for heart failure (Fig. 2.22).

Given these findings, DAVID II[48] tested the hypothesis that atrial pacing is as safe as VVI backup pacing. Six hundred patients with LV ejection fraction of 40% or less and meeting criteria for ICD placement were randomized to AAI (at 70 bpm) or VVI (at 40 bpm). No difference in mortality, heart failure, atrial fibrillation, or quality of life was seen between the groups.

Investigators from the MOST trial demonstrated that in patients with a normal baseline QRS duration, cumulative percent of ventricular pacing is a strong predictor of hospitalization for heart failure, and the risk of atrial fibrillation also increased linearly with

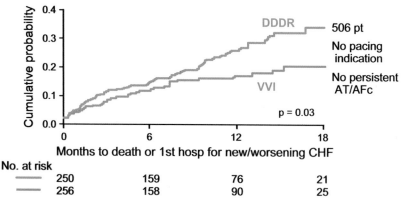

Fig. 2.22 Survival in the DAVID trial. Survival was significantly improved in patients in whom ventricular pacing was avoided. DDDR mode vs. VVI mode an composite end-point of death or new/worsening heart failure hospitalization. In DDDR group, patients who survived to 3 months' follow-up had worse 12-month event-free rates when percentage of RV pacing was >40% (*P* = 0.09). (Reprinted with permission from Wilkoff BL, Cook JR, Epstein AE, *et al.* Dual-chamber pacing or ventricular backup pacing in patients with an implantable defibrillator: the Dual Chamber and VVI Implantable Defibrillator (DAVID) Trial. JAMA 2002; 288:3115–23. Copyrighted and used with permission of Mayo Foundation for Medical Education and Research.)

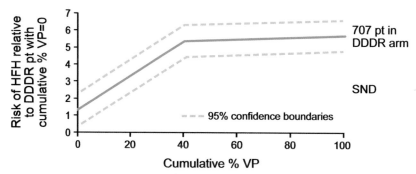

Fig. 2.23 Sweeney and colleagues demonstrated a relationship between percentage ventricular pacing (VP) and subsequent hospitalization for heart failure and the occurrence of atrial fibrillation. DDDR mode, cumulative percentage VP and risk of first heart failure hospitalization (HFH). Risk of HFH increased between 0 and 40% with VP, but RR was level above 40% VP. Risk is reduced to about 2% if VP is minimized. (Reprinted with permission from Sweeney MO, Hellkamp AS, Ellenbogen KA, *et al.* MOde Selection Trial Investigators. Adverse effect of ventricular pacing on heart failure and atrial fi brillation among patients with normal baseline QRS duration in a clinical trial of pacemaker therapy for sinus node dysfunction. Circulation 2003; 107:2932–7, by permission of American Heart Association.)

cumulative percent of ventricular pacing. This occurs even when AV synchrony is preserved (Figs 2.23 and 2.24).

In the MADIT-II trial, patients with myocardial infarction and LV ejection fraction ≤30% were randomized to receive an ICD or conventional therapy. Those in the ICD group had a significant lower mortality. However, in those in whom the RV was paced more than 50% of the time, this mortality benefit was attenuated such that after 4 years there was no significant difference in mortality than in control subjects, whereas in those with <50% RV pacing the benefit in mortality was maintained (Fig. 2.25).[49]

These findings led to the development and widespread use of pacing algorithms that avoid ventricular pacing. Rather than placing a pacemaker capable only of atrial pacing and therefore not providing backup ventricular pacing in the event of AV block, ventricular pacing avoidance algorithms may dynamically alter the AV interval to allow intrinsic ventricular depolarization, and other algorithms may allow one or more P waves to occur without a subsequent pacemaker output in an effort to promote intrinsic ventricular depolarization (Figs 2.26 and 2.27). Three prospective trials (INTRINSIC RV, SAVE-PACe, and DANPACE) have investigated whether pacing modes and device algorithms that mini-

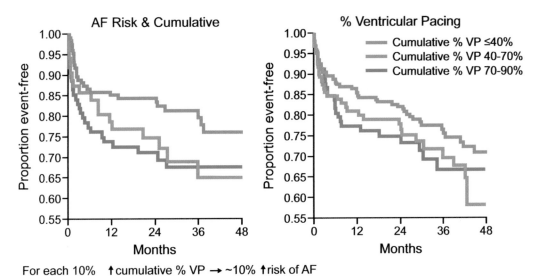

For each 10% ↑cumulative % VP → ~10% ↑risk of AF

Fig. 2.24 From Sweeney and colleagues, a representation of the relationship between cumulative percentage ventricular pacing and the incidence of atrial fibrillation (AF). (Reprinted with permission from Sweeney MO, Hellkamp AS, Ellenbogen KA, *et al*. Mode Selection Trial Investigators. Adverse effect of ventricular pacing on heart failure and atrial fibrillation among patients with normal baseline QRS duration in a clinical trial of pacemaker therapy for sinus node dysfunction. Circulation 2003; 107:2932–7, by permission of American Heart Association.)

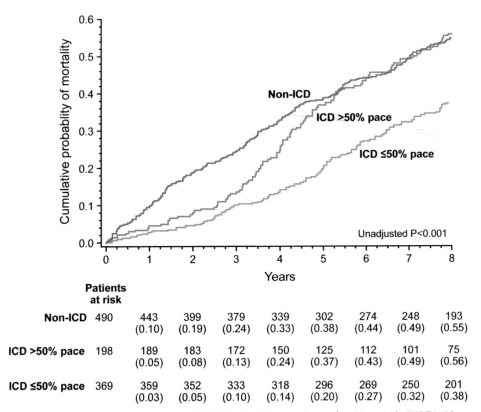

Patients at risk									
Non-ICD	490	443 (0.10)	399 (0.19)	379 (0.24)	339 (0.33)	302 (0.38)	274 (0.44)	248 (0.49)	193 (0.55)
ICD >50% pace	198	189 (0.05)	183 (0.08)	172 (0.13)	150 (0.24)	125 (0.37)	112 (0.43)	101 (0.49)	75 (0.56)
ICD ≤50% pace	369	359 (0.03)	352 (0.05)	333 (0.10)	318 (0.14)	296 (0.20)	269 (0.27)	250 (0.32)	201 (0.38)

Fig. 2.25 Outcome with right ventricular apical pacing in MADIT-II. Kaplan–Meier survival curve of participants in the MADIT-II trial, comparing implantable cardioverter-defibrillator (ICD) recipients with RV pacing >50% with ≤50%. Those with frequent RV pacing had a similar mortality to those stratified to the non-ICD arm of the trial. See main text. (From Barsheshet A, Moss AJ, McNitt S, *et al*. Long-term implications of cumulative right ventricular pacing among patients with an implantable cardioverter-defibrillator. Heart Rhythm 2011; 8:212–8.)

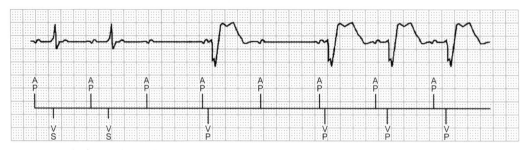

Fig. 2.26 Example of managed ventricular pacing. One QRS complex is allowed to "drop" in an effort to maintain intrinsic atrioventricular (AV) conduction and intrinsic ventricular determination.

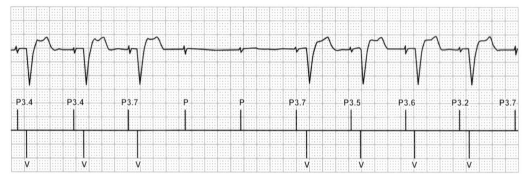

Fig. 2.27 Example of AAIR Safe Pace. Again, in an attempt to maintain intrinsic ventricular conduction, this algorithm will allow up to two P waves to occur without pacing.

mize RV pacing influence outcome. The INTRINSIC RV (Inhibition of Unnecessary RV Pacing With AVSH in ICDs)[50] study tested the hypothesis that minimizing RV pacing using a device algorithm called AVSH (AV search hysteresis) was noninferior to VVI backup pacing. No difference in mortality or heart failure was seen at 1 year. The SAVE-PACe (Search AV Extension and Managed Ventricular Pacing for Promoting Atrioventricular Conduction)[51] trial randomized 1065 patients with sinus node disease requiring dual pacemaker implantation to conventional dual-chamber pacing or dual chamber with features designed to permit automatic lengthening or elimination of the pacemaker's AV interval in order to withhold ventricular pacing. There was no difference in mortality or heart failure between the two allocation groups, though there was an increase in atrial fibrillation with minimized ventricular pacing. In DANPACE (Danish Multicenter Randomized Trial on Single Lead Atrial Pacing versus Dual Chamber Pacing in Sick Sinus Syndrome),[52] patients with sick sinus syndrome requiring pacemaker implantation were randomized to AAIR or DDDR. The

two groups were similar with respect to mortality and heart failure occurrence. A surprising finding was a greater incidence of paroxysmal atrial fibrillation in the AAIR group. Reasons are unclear, but may relate to paradoxical effects in patients with pro-longed AV conduction. The findings are similar to the MVP (Managed Ventricular Pacing) trial[53] assessing the equivalence of atrial pacing plus ventricular backup at 60 bpm versus ventricular backup at 40 bpm in a randomized study of 1030 ICD recipients. Patients were in sinus rhythm without bradycardia at baseline. The study was terminated prematurely because those with a PR interval of $\geq$230 ms had increased mortality and heart failure occurrence.

Information emerging, but not yet published, from large cohorts of patients followed on remote-monitoring networks is concordant with the trials discussed above demonstrating lower mortality when unnecessary RV stimulation is avoided.

The potential advantage of extending RV pacing avoidance to cardiac resynchronization therapy (CRT) has also been studied. In one investigation, synchro-

Table 2.2 Clinical studies of the adverse effects of right ventricular (RV) apical pacing.

Trial	No. of patients	Mean age (years)	Mean FU (years)	LA diameter	LV function	CHF	AF
Tantengco et al.[202]	24	19.5	9.5	NA	↓	2 patients	NA
Karpawich et al.[203]	14	15.5	5.5	NA	Altered histology	NA	NA
Thambo et al.[204]	23	24	10	NA	↓/DS	NA	NA
Tse et al.[56]	12	72	1.5	NA	↓/MPD	NA	NA
Hamdan et al.[205]	13	66	NA*	NA	↓/↑SNA	NA	NA
DAVID[206]	506	64	1	NA	NA	↑	NA
MADIT II[207,208] Substudy	567	64	1.7	NA	NA	↑	NA
Wonisch et al.[209]	17	59	0.25	NA	NA	†	NA
Thackray et al.[210]	307	72	5.2	NA	NA	↑	↑
MOST[45]	1339	74	6	NA	NA	↑	↑
Nielsen et al.[211]	177	74	2.9	↑	↓	NA	↑
O'Keefe et al.[212]	59	69	1.5	NA	↓	NA	NA
Ichiki et al.[213]	76	64	3.6	↓/↑	↓	NA	NA
Tops et al.[214]	58	61	3.8	NA	↓/DS	↑	NA
Shimano et al.[215]	18	63	6.8	↑	↓	↑	NA
Pastore et al.[216]	153	73	NA*	NA	↓DS	NA	NA
Albertsen et al.[217]	50	72	1	NA	↓DS	↓/↑	NA
Zhang et al.[218]	304	68	7.8	NA	↓/↑	↑	↑
Wolber et al.[219]	26	58	NA*	NA	↓,↓DS	NA	NA

AF, atrial fibrillation; CHF, congestive heart failure; DS, dyssynchrony; FU, follow-up; LA, left atrium; LBBB, left bundle branch block; LV, left ventricular; MPD, myocardial perfusion defects; NA, not available/not assessed; SNA, sympathetic nerve activity.

*Acute study.

†Permanent RV pacing significantly reduced exercise capacity and submaximal cardiorespiratory parameters.

Source: Manolis AS. The deleterious consequences of right ventricular apical pacing: time to seek alternate site pacing. Pacing Clin Electrophysiol 2006; 29:298–315, by permission of Blackwell Publishing.

nized LV pacing, i.e., eliminating RV stimulation produced acute LV and systemic hemodynamic benefits similar to biventricular pacing. This pacing configuration provided superior RV hemodynamics compared with biventricular pacing.[54]

Optimal ventricular pacing sites

Given the potential adverse effects of RV apical pacing, significant attention has been given to other RV pacing sites that may avoid these adverse effects (Table 2.2). Although there is no definitive answer regarding optimal RV pacing site(s), there have been multiple studies assessing different pacing configurations and their impact on hemodynamics (Fig. 2.28). Tables 2.3 and 2.4 summarize some of the studies to date. Although a number of studies have now been published, many of the series are small, some involving long-term pacing and others short-term observation only, and overall there is no trend or concordance of the results. A series of trials are underway that may better address the issue.[55]

In a study of 24 patients randomized to RV apical or RV outflow tract (RVOT) pacing, the mean QRS duration was significantly longer with apical pacing than during outflow tract pacing (151 ± 6 vs. 134 ± 4 ms; $P = 0.03$). At 18 months, the incidence of myocardial perfusion defects (83% vs. 33%) and regional wall motion abnormalities (75% vs. 33%) were higher and LV ejection fraction (47 ± 3 vs. 56 ± 1%) was lower in those patients paced apically than in those patients with outflow tract pacing (all $P < 0.05$). Investigators concluded that preserving synchronous ventricular activation with RVOT pacing prevented the long-term deleterious effects of RV apical pacing on LV function and perfusion (Fig. 2.29).[56] Inadvertently placing the lead onto the RV anterior or free wall instead of the septum results in a longer QRS duration (158.1 ± 4.7 ms vs. 140.7 ± 3.9 ms).[57] The mid-RV septum and RVOT septum yield similar paced QRS duration.[58,59] Reviews of procedural outcomes from large volume centers performing RVOT lead placement report it to be safe and durable.[60,61]

In addition to investigations of alternate RV pacing sites, there have been multiple additional studies that have investigated the hemodynamics of LV pacing, multisite RV pacing, and pacing the ventricles in three

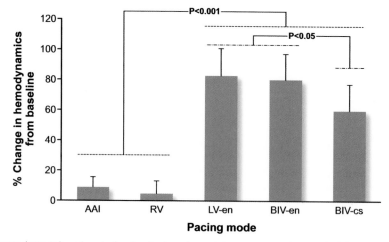

Fig. 2.28 Percentage change in hemodynamics from baseline by pacing mode in response to pacing at optimal site. AAI, atrial pacing only; BIV-cs, conventional CRT; BIV-en, DDD biventricular endocardial; LV-en, DDD LV endocardial; RV, DDD right ventricular. (From Ginks MR, Lambiase PD, Duckett SG, *et al*. A simultaneous X-Ray/MRI and noncontact mapping study of the acute hemodynamic effect of left ventricular endocardial and epicardial cardiac resynchronization therapy in humans. Circ Heart Fail 2011; 4:170–9.)

Table 2.3 Studies comparing hemodynamic and/or clinical effects of right ventricular (RV) apical pacing and alternate site pacing in the RV outflow tract (RVOT), RV septal (RVS), the His bundle (His), left ventricular (LV) or biventricular (Biv) site.

Study	No. of patients	Mean age (years)	Hemodynamic/clinical variables	Improved results	
				Acute	**Chronic**
Cowell *et al.*[220]	15	59	CO (Cath)	RVS	NA
Giudici *et al.*[221]	89	68	CO (Echo)	RVOT	NA*
Buckingham *et al.*[222]	11	48	CO (Echo)	RVOT	NA
Karpawich and Mital[223]	22	10	LVEDP (Cath)	RVS	NA
Blanc *et al.*[104]	23	66	PWP (Cath)	LV/BiV	NA
De Cock *et al.*[224]	17	58	CO (Echo)	RVOT	NA
Mera *et al.*[225]	12	68	FS/EF (Echo/RNV)	NA	RVS
Buckingham *et al.*[226]	14	55	12 (Echo/Cath)	RVOT/BF	NA
Victor *et al.*[227]	16	69	4 (Echo/RNV)	NA	None
Schwaab *et al.*[228]	14	71	EF (RNV)	RVS	NA
Kolettis *et al.*[229]	20	62	CO (Echo)	RVOT	NA
Bourke *et al.*[230]	20	64	8 (RNV)	NA	RVOT
Tse *et al.*[56]	24	75	WMA/EF (RNS/RNV)	NA	RVOT
Hamdan *et al.*[205]	13	66	BP/CVP/SNA	LV/Biv	NA
Kass *et al.*[14]	18	66	10 (Cath)	LV/Biv	NA
Yu *et al.*[231]	33	66	14 (Echo)	Biv	NA
Leclercq *et al.*[232]	37	63	6 (Clinical)	NA	Biv
Leon *et al.*[233]	20	70	6 (Echo/Clinical)	NA	Biv
Leclercq *et al.*[234]	56	73	5 (Clinical)	NA	Biv
ROVA[235]†	103	69.5	6 (Clinical/Echo)	ND	ND
OPSITE[236]†	56	70	QOL/Exercise capacity	Biv/LV	NA
PAVE[237]†	252	NA	4 (Clinical)	NA	Biv
Catanzariti *et al.*[238]	23	75	3 (Echo)	His	NA
Lieberman *et al.*[239]	31	61	12 (Cath)	BiV/LV	NA
Occhetta *et al.*[240]†	18	71	8 (Echo/Clinical)	His	NA
Hoijer *et al.*[241]†	10	68	11 (Clinical, NP, Echo)	BiV	NA
Victor *et al.*[242]†	28	63	4 (Clinical/Echo)	RVS	NA

Table 2.3 (Continued)

Study	No. of patients	Mean age (years)	Hemodynamic/clinical variables	Improved results	
				Acute	Chronic
Leclercq et al.[234]†	56	73	8 (Echo/ECG/Clinical)	BiV	NA
Albertsen et al.[243]†	50	76	5 (EF/Strain/NP/Clinical)	RAA	NA
Fornwalt et al.[244]	14	13	DS	RAA	NA
Kypta et al.[245]†	98	72	EF, NP, Clinical	No change	NA
Zanon et al.[246]	12	74	8 (Echo/DS/SPECT/Clinical/NP)	His	NA
Leclercq et al.[92]†	44	73	11 (Clinical, Echo)	BiV	NA
Vanerio et al.[247]	150	72	Mortality	NA	RVOT
ten Cate et al.[248]	14	69	4 (Echo)	RVOT	NA
Tse et al.[249]†	24	71	6MHW, EF	RVS=RVA	RVS
Tse et al.[250]	12	73	3 (Clinical, Nuclear)	RVS	NA
Yu et al.[251]†	177	69	5 (Echo, Clinical)	BiV	NA
Flevari et al.[252]†	36	73	5 (Echo)	RVS	RVS
Gong et al.[253]†	96	70	6 (Echo, DS)	RVOT	NA
Wang et al.[254]	25	72	4 (Echo)	BiV	NA
Yoon et al.[255]	30	49	DS	RVOT/RVS	NA
van Gendorp et al.[256]†	36	65	6 (Echo, Clinical)	BiV	NA
Cano et al.[257]†	93	72	14 (Clinical, NP, Echo)	RVS	NA
Ji et al.[258]	31	40	Strain, twist	RVOT and RVA equal reduction in function	NA
Leong et al.[259]†	58	75	4 (Echo)	RVOT	NA
Liu et al.[260]	36	76	4 (Echo, DS)	RVOT reduction in function c/w no pacing	NA
Orlov et al.[261]†	108	72	6 (Echo, Clinica)	BiV	NA
Martinelli Filho et al.[262]†	60	58	4 (Echo, Clinical)	BiV	NA
Inoue et al.[263]	46	73	DS, torsion, twist	RVS	NA
Pastore et al.[264]	142	78	DS	His (>RVS)	NA
Sanagala et al.[265]	31	62	LA volume, ejection fraction, LV diastolic function	BiV	NA
Rubaj et al.[266]	73	71	Impedance cardiography (CO)	RVOT+RVA dual site	NA
Yamano et al.[267]	20	54	3 (Echo, DS, Coronary flow)	RVOT	NA
Hara et al.[268]	31	73	Twist	NA	RVOT

BF, bifocal; BP, arterial blood pressure; Cath, cardiac catheterization; CO, cardiac output; CVP, central venous pressure; DS, dyssynchrony; ECG, electrocardiographic; Echo, echocardiography; EF, (left ventricular) ejection fraction; FS, (left ventricular) fractional shortening; LVEDP, left ventricular end-diastolic pressure; 6MHW, 6-minute hall walk test; NA, not available/not assessed; ND, no difference; NP, natriuretic peptide; PWP, pulmonary wedge pressure; RAA, right atrial appendage; RNS, radionuclide scintigraphy; RNV, radionuclide ventriculography; SNA, sympathetic neural activity (measured by microneurography); WMA, wall motion abnormalities.

*Only five patients were evaluated at 6 months and demonstrated a similar improvement in cardiac output with RV outflow tract pacing compared with RV apical pacing.

†Randomized studies; ROVA compared quality of life between RV apical and RV outflow tract pacing only after 3 months of pacing in patients with heart failure and chronic atrial fibrillation; OPSITE: randomized, single-blind, 3-month crossover comparison between RV and LV pacing and between RV and BiV pacing in patients with atrial fibrillation and heart failure undergoing AV node ablation; PAVE: randomized study evaluating BiV vs. RV pacing in atrial fibrillation patients receiving ablate and pace therapy.

Source: Modified from Manolis AS. The deleterious consequences of right ventricular apical pacing: time to seek alternate site pacing. Pacing Clin Electrophysiol 2006; 29:298–315, by permission of Blackwell Publishing.

Table 2.4 Other studies of alternate site pacing.

Study	No. of patients	Target population	Pacing site	Studied variables	Improvement
Turner et al.[269]	10	HF	LV	Hemodynamic	Yes
Vanagt et al.[270]	8	Children during cardiac surgery	LV apex	Hemodynamic	Yes*
Gebauer et al.[271]	32	Children with AV block	Epicardial LV apex, RV apex, RV free wall	Clinical/Echo	LV apex preserves LV synchrony best
Touiza et al.[272]	18	HF/LBBB	LV	Clinical/Echo	Yes
Blanc et al.[273]	22	HF/LBBB	LV	Clinical/Echo	Yes
Auricchio et al.[274]	57	HF/LBBB	LV	Clinical	Yes
Garrigue et al.[275]	13	HF/AF/LBBB	LV/BiV	Clinical/Pm sensor	Yes
Vlay[276]	22	HF/LBBB	Bifocal RV (RVA+RVOT)	Clinical/Echo	Yes
Pachon et al.[277]	39	HF/LBBB	Bifocal RV (RVA+RVS)	Clinical/Echo/Nuclear	Yes†
O'Donnell et al.[94]	6	HF/LBBB	Bifocal RV (RVA+RVOT)	Clinical/Echo	Yes‡
ROVA[235]	50	HF/AF	Bifocal RV (RVA+RVOT)	Clinical/Echo	NS§
Deshmukh and Romanyshyn[278]	39	HF/AF	HB	Clinical/Echo	Yes
Zamparelli and Martiniello[279]	25	HF/LBBB	Bifocal RV (RVA+RVS)	Clinical/Echo	Yes
Aonuma et al.[280]	13	HF	Trifocal (RVA+LV+RVOT)	(Acute) hemodynamic/ clinical	Yes
Valzania et al.[281]	22	HF/LBBB	BiV vs. LV	Clinical/Echo	Yes, with no difference
Sirker et al.[82]	18	HF/LBBB	BiV vs. LV	Clinical/Echo	Yes, with no difference between groups

BF, bifocal; BP, arterial blood pressure; Cath, cardiac catheterization; CO, cardiac output; CVP, central venous pressure; Echo, echocardiography; EF, (left ventricular) ejection fraction; FS, (left ventricular) fractional shortening; HB, His bundle; HF, heart failure; LBBB, left bundle branch block; LV, left ventricle; NS, no significant (differences); pm, pacemaker; RV, right ventricle; RVA, right ventricular apex; RVOT, right ventricular outflow tract; RVS, right ventricular septum.

*Comparison made with RV apical pacing (parameters were maintained at sinus rhythm level with left ventricular apex pacing).

†Comparison made with RV apical and RV septal pacing.

‡Comparison made with biventricular pacing.

§Comparison was made with RV apical and RVOT pacing; at 3 months, physical functioning score was worse than during RV apical pacing and mental health scores were worse than during RVOT pacing. New York Heart Association (NYHA) class during dual-site RV pacing was slightly better than during RVOT ($P = 0.03$), but not different than RV apical pacing; there were no other significant differences in other studied parameters.

Source: Manolis AS. The deleterious consequences of right ventricular apical pacing: time to seek alternate site pacing. Pacing Clin Electrophysiol 2006; 29:298–315, by permission of Blackwell Publishing.

sites (Table 2.4). However, a definitive answer regarding the optimal ventricular pacing site(s) is still not available. Also, the literature is confusing because of the anatomic terms used to describe alternative RV pacing sites. The difficulty in comparing different ventricular pacing sites has led to proposed nomenclature to describe alternative RV pacing sites, i.e., other than the apical pacing site.[60,62] The RVOT, once defined fluoroscopically as the area between the pulmonary valve above (the exact border of which can be discerned by the change in the local QRS signal as it is traversed) and an imaginary straight line extending from the apex of

the tricuspid valve to the RV border, can be subdivided into high and low halves midway between these boundaries. Thus, the four recognized pacing sites in the RVOT are the high and low septum and the high and low free wall (Fig. 2.30). With RV septal pacing, the QRS in lead I is negative, whereas in RV free wall pacing it is positive. Pacing in the higher RVOT will result in a more positive QRS in a VF, and vice versa. The exact site of RVOT pacing is critical to the pattern of LV activation. For example, cephalad to the crista supraventricularis on the free wall, the wavefront of activation will spread to the RV significantly ahead of the intra-

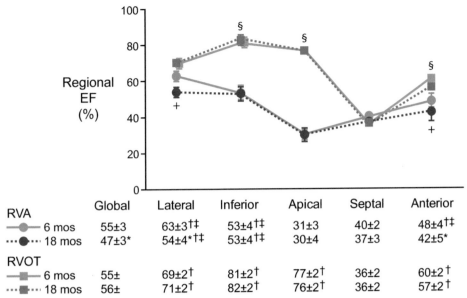

	Global	Lateral	Inferior	Apical	Septal	Anterior
RVA						
——⬤—— 6 mos	55±3	63±3†‡	53±4†‡	31±3	40±2	48±4†‡
····⬤···· 18 mos	47±3*	54±4*†‡	53±4†‡	30±4	37±3	42±5*
RVOT						
——◼—— 6 mos	55±	69±2†	81±2†	77±2†	36±2	60±2†
····◼···· 18 mos	56±	71±2†	82±2†	76±2†	36±2	57±2†

Fig. 2.29 Changes in regional ejection fraction comparing right ventricular apical (RVA) and RV outflow tract (RVOT) pacing groups studied by Tse. $+P < 0.05$ RVA 18 months vs. RVA 6 months; $§P < 0.05$ RVOT vs. RVA at 6 months and 18 months; $*P < 0.05$ compared with RVA pacing at 6 months; $†P < 0.05$ compared with septal region; $‡P < 0.05$ compared with apical region; data are expressed as mean value ± SEM. (From Tse HF, Yu C, Wong KK, et al. Functional abnormalities in patients with permanent right ventricular pacing: the effect of sites of electrical stimulation. J Am Coll Cardiol 2002; 40:1451–8, by permission of the American College of Cardiology.)

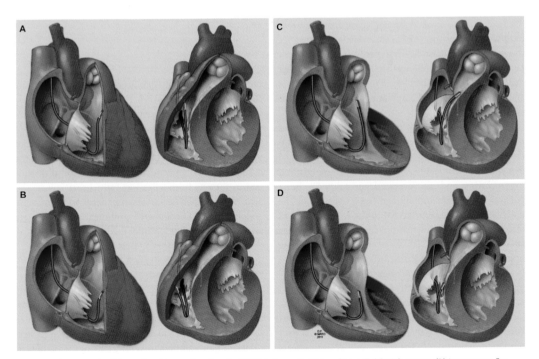

Fig. 2.30 Alternative site RV septal and free wall pacing site. (A) High free wall. (B) Low free wall. (C) High septum. (D) Low septum. For each, the left image depicts orientation in the right anterior oblique fluoroscopic projection and the right depicts the left anterior oblique projection. See text for details. (Adapted from the information in Vlay SC. Right ventricular outflow tract pacing: practical and beneficial: a 9-year experience of 460 consecutive implants. Pacing Clin Electrophysiol 2006; 29:1055–62.)

ventricular septum and LV. On the other hand, a posterior pacing site above the crista supraventricularis may pre-excite the LV free wall because of the myocardial architecture and direction of spiral lamination of the myocardium in this location. Further, the remnants of an extensive embryologic infra-Hisian conduction system (right superior fascicles) if present in a patient will result in more rapid and early conduction via the His–Purkinje system than in patients who do not have such remnants and thus rely entirely on intraventricular conduction for wave propagation.

Pacing in heart failure

Heart failure affects approximately 1% of the over-65-year-old population in the USA.[63] Over 1 million hospitalizations with a primary diagnosis of heart failure occur each year[64] and approximately 1 in 9 death certificates lists heart failure as a cause.[63] The rationale for pacing as therapy for heart failure was first proposed in the 1990s. Improvement by dual-chamber pacing was shown to be related to optimal synchronization of atrial and ventricular contractions.[16] However, only patients with heart failure who have prolonged PR intervals, in which atrial contraction occurs so prematurely that the atrial "kick" to ventricular contraction is lost, appear to derive benefit from dual-chamber pacing. Conversely, in patients with normal or short AV conduction, the diastolic filling period does not change and cardiac output decreases by 23%, most likely because of the systolic and diastolic dyssynergy induced by RV pacing.[16] Overall, the clinical trials demonstrated that dual-chamber pacing had limited long-term efficacy as an adjunct to medical therapy in relieving heart failure symptoms.[65,66]

Progressive QRS widening frequently accompanies heart failure, in particular when associated with LV remodeling and reduced ejection fraction. The electrical dyssynchrony that results is associated with mechanical dyssynchrony and an increased mortality in heart failure.[67–69] Understanding and intervening on the underlying mechanisms has led to the well-established discipline of cardiac resynchronization therapy. Similar to the hemodynamic effects of isolated left bundle branch block (LBBB), LBBB in cardiomyopathy increases isovolumic contraction and relaxation times, thereby increasing the duration of mitral regurgitation and shortening LV filling time, with the net effect of decreasing preload (Fig. 2.31). The duration of mitral regurgitation is more sensitive to heart rate in patients with LBBB than in those without.[70] The magnitude of these effects is proportional to the QRS duration. Regionally diminished myocardial function or disturbed temporal sequence of contraction secondary to abnormal electrical activation disproportionately worsens systolic dys-

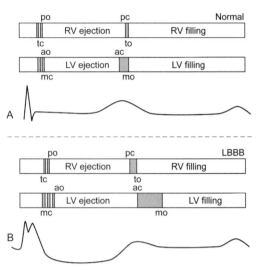

Fig. 2.31 Relationship between right ventricular (RV) and left ventricular (LV) events in normal subjects (A) and in patients with left bundle branch block (LBBB) (B). In the normal group, LV events either precede or occur simultaneously with RV events. In LBBB, the sequence is reversed, with RV events preceding those of the left ventricle. po, to, ao, mo: time of pulmonic, tricuspid, aortic and mitral valve openings; pc, tc, ac, mc: time of respective valve closures. (Modified from Grines CL, Bashore TM, Boudoulas H, Olson S, Shafer P, Wooley CF. Functional abnormalities in isolated left bundle branch block: the effect of interventricular asynchrony. Circulation 1989; 79:845–53, by permission of the American Heart Association.)

function in cardiomyopathy, because the remaining myocardium cannot provide the compensatory increase in fiber shortening necessary to maintain stroke volume.[71]

On the above premise, a number of randomized trials have now prospectively evaluated biventricular pacing (usually with a LV epicardial lead placed via the coronary sinus) in reducing all-cause mortality, outcomes such as hospitalization from heart failure and symptoms in specific subsets of patients with severe LV systolic dysfunction and QRS prolongation who remain symptomatic despite optimal medical therapy.[72,73]

Influence of pacing site

The site of latest LV activation during RV apical pacing is the posterior or posteroinferior base.[74] Because the electrical activation sequence in LBBB is very similar to that in RV pacing, LV pacing at the posterior or posteroinferior base should have a normalizing effect on ventricular activation. Consequently, monoventricular LV pacing in patients with severe LV dysfunction and LBBB yields a hemodynamic response similar to that of biventricular pacing (and may even be higher than biventricular pacing, providing that LV pacing is associated with ventricular complex fusion from intrinsic activation)[75] and significantly higher than that of RV pacing.[76–79] Studies have since prospectively compared the effects of LV pacing to biventricular pacing on clinical status and LV function in patients with LV systolic dysfunction and wide QRS. The BELIEVE trial randomized 74 patients with heart failure undergoing CRT therapy to biventricular or LV pacing and found similar response rates between the two modalities at 2 months.[80] The DECREASE-HF trial randomized 306 patients with heart failure undergoing CRT therapy to sequential biventricular, simultaneous biventricular or isolated LV pacing.[81] At 6 months, the simultaneous biventricular pacing group had the greatest reduction in LV end-systolic dimension, while stroke volume and LV ejection fraction improved in all groups with no difference across groups. The LOLA ROSE study, a small crossover trial of 18 patients, also reported similar functional performance measures and quality of life after 8 weeks of biventricular pacing compared with LV pacing.[82] The B-LEFT HF was a double-blind, noninferiority trial which randomized 176 patients with CRT-D to programming of biventricular or isolated LV pacing.[83] At 6 months, no difference in New York Heart Association (NYHA) functional status or LV volumes was present between the groups. In contrast to these relatively larger studies, a smaller randomized study of 40 heart failure patients undergoing CRT found increased reverse LV remodeling with biventricular when compared with LV pacing after 12 months.[84]

Pacing of the midlateral area or posterior area of the LV in this situation leads to greater improvement in pulse pressure and dP/dt than pacing of anterior or apical LV sites[15,20] and greater improvement in LV size at 6 months,[85] while an apical lead position is associated with an increased risk of heart failure or death.[86,87] When an optimal site cannot be reached via the coronary sinus, direct epicardial placement has been demonstrated to be a viable alternative.[88–90] Hemodynamic improvement following multifocal LV pacing in CRT has also been reported from small clinical studies[91,92] and a randomized trial is underway to assess the effect on clinical end-points.[93] Several small clinical studies have compared the utility of bifocal RV pacing, which utilizes conjunctive septal pacing, as an alternative means to achieve resynchronization.[94–99] Initial results in functional and echocardiographic improvement are favorable but larger studies comparing longer term procedural and clinical outcomes with biventricular pacing are not available.

With the above considerations in mind, in practice, the functional status of the myocardium in the paced segment affects the hemodynamic results. Dekker et al.[100] have demonstrated that the position of the LV lead determines the acute hemodynamic response to biventricular pacing, and the most and least optimal positions vary between patients. Pacing of ischemic or scarred myocardium is not as effective as pacing of myocardium with normal regional function[101] and adversely affects the relationship of LV dP/dt to end-diastolic volume.

When comparing patterns of LV activation during intrinsic rhythm and RV pacing, two factors are important. First, the location of the RV pacing site relative to the normal exit of the right bundle branch. When pacing exactly at the exit site of the right bundle branch, one would expect that LV activation would be identical to that seen with LBBB. With varying the RV pacing site, however, intrinsic conduction with LBBB may have either less or more disorganized activation when compared with RV pacing. Second, when considering LV pacing simultaneous with the RV pacing site and comparing this with intrinsic conduction, one must keep in mind that the normal left bundle exit (if it was conducting normally) would be on the left side of the intraventricular septum and not on the free wall.

Mechanisms underlying the benefits of left ventricular and biventricular pacing

The mechanisms by which LV and biventricular pacing improve mechanical LV function in patients with heart failure and LBBB are not entirely understood. Up to four levels of dyssynchrony have been described (Fig. 2.32): AV dyssynchrony (discussed above); interventricular dyssynchrony (between the RV and LV); intraventricular dyssynchrony (within segment of the LV); and intramural dyssynchrony within the walls of the LV (least well established).[102] Intraventricular dyssynchrony is probably the most significant clinically. Electrical resynchronization between the RV and LV should eliminate the adverse effects of LBBB-induced mechanical ventricular dyssynchrony on regional LV systolic function. However, biventricular pacing in the absence of conduction system disease is hemodynamically superior to RV pacing, despite similarly paced QRS duration.[103] Also, hemodynamic improvement with LV pacing in LBBB is equivalent to, if not better than biventricular pacing even though it does not shorten the QRS complex.[14,79,104] The improvement in systolic dP/dt by LV pacing in LBBB is proportional to the reduction of the electromechanical delay within the LV.[105] It follows that positioning the coronary sinus lead to obtain the optimal dP/dt during LV pacing results in the highest degree of LV reverse remodeling following biventricular CRT,[106,107] which is important because the prognostic benefits from CRT are associated with improvement in LV geometry and systolic function.[108]

A

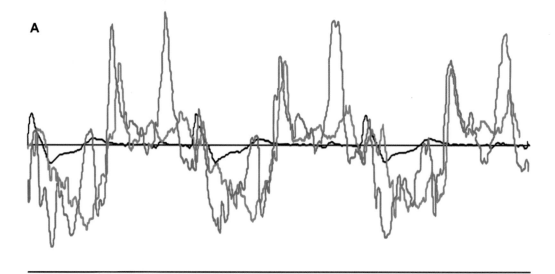

B

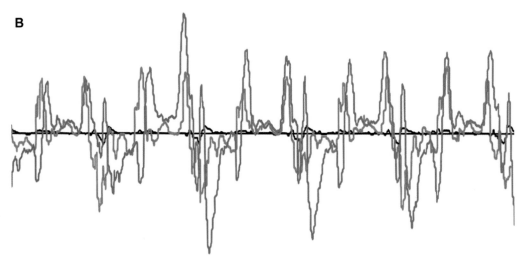

Fig. 2.32 Electromechanical dyssynchrony may be due to atrioventricular, interventricular, intraventricular, and intramural delays. This figure demonstrates intraventricular dyssynchrony. Strain rate profiles of septal (blue line) and lateral (red line) basal segments (arrows, peak systolic strain rate). Note the reduction in time delay between the septal and lateral walls post-cardiac resynchronization therapy (CRT) (lower panel, B) compared with pre-CRT (upper panel, A). (From Hayes DL, Wang P, Sackner-Bernstein J, Asirvatham S. Resynchronization and Defibrillation for Heart Failure: A Practical Approach. Blackwell-Futura, 2004: 167.)

In practice, the lead configuration resulting in the optimal acute hemodynamic effect is highly variable between patients.[109] Pacing at the site of latest LV activation, identified from speckle-track myocardial strain imaging, has also been shown to correlate with LV reverse remodeling and outcome after CRT.[69,110] These findings imply that synchronization of LV wall motion is important in the improvement of systolic function. Furthermore, in an experimental model, the magnitude of mechanical dyssynchrony exceeded that of electrical dyssynchrony, because the time interval between electrical activation and onset of fiber shortening is larger the later a particular region is activated.[111] Therefore, for achieving benefit from pacing therapy, electrical resynchronization evidenced by QRS narrowing may be less important than the LV pacing site and the associated change in LV contraction efficiency. The hemodynamic improvements in systolic LV function with pacing may not be a result of mechanical factors alone. Systemic or intramyocardial release of catecholamines, reflex-mediated baroreceptor and autonomic nervous system activation, and release of vasodilatory substances, such as natriuretic peptides, have all been demonstrated for dual-chamber pacing and may well have a role in biventricular and LV pacing.

Approximately 30% of patients with severe LV systolic dysfunction and electrical dyssynchrony, as identified by prolonged QRS duration, do not respond to CRT and in many this is in spite of device setting optimization.[72] Reasons for failure, as with those of success, are not completely clear. The lack of prediction of response from mechanical dyssynchrony assessment,[112,113] despite its ability to predict mortality from heart failure,[68,69] suggests that procedural factors may be responsible, such as suboptimal placement of the LV lead which, as discussed earlier in the chapter, importantly determines the hemodynamic response to this therapy. The observation that dyssynchrony, or rather its echocardiographic assessment, is dependent on the loading conditions of the ventricle[114] suggests that dyssynchrony may be a temporally dynamic entity which would confound prediction. Another possible explanation may be that electrical dyssynchrony and pacing each has a variable effect on myocardial mechanical function, depending on the sequence of activation and the condition of myocardial tissue. Thus, even though greater improvements in myocardial function are seen after CRT in those with longer QRS duration,[115] benefit is more fre-

quent in those with LBBB,[115–118] which has a greater association with LV intraventricular mechanical dyssynchrony than right bundle branch block.[119] Another example is ischemic cardiomyopathy, which is associated with more frequent treatment failure with CRT than nonischemic cardiomyopathy.[115,117,120,121] In addition to comparatively less mechanical dyssynchrony in the context of QRS prolongation,[122] there are more areas of scar which are associated with slowed conduction and ineffective pacing,[123–125] while avoiding these results in an improved hemodynamic response.[124,125] However, others[126,127] have not found a significant role for scar in determining response to CRT and difference between studies may relate to methodologic techniques in ascertainment of scar and dyssynchrony.

Measures of dyssynchrony may themselves be subject to error. For example, low-voltage conduction within diseased myocardium may not be evident as surface ECG changes such as QRS prolongation, yet these patients may still have significant mechanical dyssynchrony, though mechanical dyssynchrony is reported less frequently in those with normal QRS duration heart failure than when the QRS is prolonged.[128] Measurable improvement in mechanical synchrony is associated with significant survival benefit, such that for patients in the MADIT-CRT trial, every 20 ms improvement in intraventricular synchrony (measured in this study using radial speckle-track strain) was associated with a 7% reduction in death or heart failure at 1 year (Fig. 2.33).[115] Similarly, persistence of QRS prolongation after CRT therapy was an adverse prognostic factor in

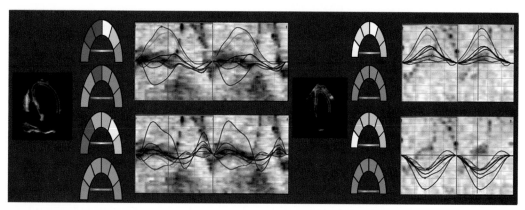

Fig. 2.33 Improvement in intraventricular mechanical dyssynchrony with cardiac resynchronization therapy. Two-dimensional speckle-tracking imaging in the apical four-chamber view in a patient before (left panel) and after cardiac resynchronization therapy defibrillator implantation (right panel). Upper curves represent transverse strain curves, which were used to measure left ventricular dyssynchrony and lower curves represent longitudinal strain that were used to measure contractile function. Improvement in left ventricular dyssynchrony and left ventricular contractile function was shown at follow-up. (From Pouleur AC, Knappe D, Shah AM, *et al.* Relationship between improvement in left ventricular dyssynchrony and contractile function and clinical outcome with cardiac resynchronization therapy: the MADIT-CRT trial. Eur Heart J 2011; 32:1720–9, by permission of European Heart Journal.)

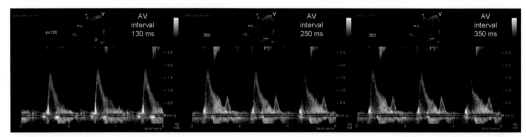

Fig. 2.34 AV optimization in cardiac resynchronization therapy. Mitral inflow pulsed Doppler echocardiography demonstrating increasing atrial emptying with sequentially longer programmed AV intervals of 130 ms (left), 250 ms (middle) and 350 ms (right). Given that the patient's intrinsic PR interval was 360 ms, a shorter AV interval of 250 ms was programmed to allow for ventricular synchronous pacing, whereas 130 ms was deemed overly short on account of compromising atrial emptying. (Courtesy of Dr. Brian Powell, Mayo Clinic, Rochester, MN.)

the CARE-HF trial.[116] Even though mechanical dyssynchrony may exist in patients with narrow QRS, and with some evidence that it responds to CRT,[129] trials of CRT in this setting have reported on functional end-points and have yielded conflicting results on benefit,[130,131] while larger studies (CRT-Narrow [NCT00821938] and EchoCRT [NCT00683696]) designed to assess the impact on clinical events are currently underway.

Delgado *et al.*[69] measured radial speckle-track strain on 397 patients with ischemic cardiomyopathy treated with CRT to identify radial intraventricular dyssynchrony, sites of latest mechanical activation of the LV, and regions of scar. At 3-year follow-up, independent predictors of mortality on a multivariate hazards analysis were age (hazard ratio [HR] 1.027 [1.003–1.051]), plasma creatinine levels (HR 1.004 [1.002–1.007]), LV dyssynchrony (HR per 1 ms 0.995 [0.992–0.998], LV lead placement discordant to the site of latest activation (HR 2.086 [1.336–3.258]), and myocardial scar in the targeted segment (HR 2.913 [1.740–4.877]).

Both electrical and mechanical parameters therefore appear to be important and outcomes are worst when both QRS duration is short and mechanical dyssynchrony is absent and best when both are present.[68] The QRS duration therefore remains an important tool for identifying those who stand to benefit from CRT; this is intuitive in part because CRT is itself an electrical therapy.

Left ventricular diastolic function
Measures of impaired ventricular relaxation and increased filling pressures at baseline (i.e., prior to resynchronization) also have prognostic significance for the period that follows resynchronization.[132] Dyssynchronous relaxation appears to be common in heart failure.[133] Resynchronization has varying reported effects on LV diastolic function, with some reporting

Table 2.5 Arteriovenous (AV) delay programming methods in cardiac resynchronization therapy (CRT).

Fixed, preprogrammed AV delay
Invasive hemodynamic assessment of left ventricular (LV) dP/dT or pulse pressure
Determination of cardiac output using thermodilution[282]
Doppler echocardiography (Ritter's method, iterative method, Ishikawa method, LV outflow tract velocity–time integral optimization, mitral inflow velocity–time integral optimization,[140] mitral regurgitation derived dP/dT estimation[283])
Electrogram-based calculation of AV delay[142]
Intracardiac impedence[147,162,284]
Prediction using intrinsic AV conduction time[285]
Acoustic cardiography[286]
Impedance cardiography[23,287]

no change[134] and others reporting improvement only with improvement in systolic function.[133,135–138] Possible reasons for the variation include interindividual differences in acute responses to pacing,[139] variation in programmed diastolic emptying,[140] and etiology of cardiomyopathy (ischemic vs. non-ischemic).[115,117,120–122]

AV optimization in cardiac resynchronization therapy
There are similar considerations for AV optimization in CRT as in conventional pacing, such as attention to atrial conduction times.[141] Allowing for complete atrial emptying through an adequately long programmed AV delay must be balanced with activating the ventricles in a synchronous fashion before intrinsic dyssynchronous depolarization occurs (Fig. 2.34).

A number of methods for programming the AV delay have been proposed (Table 2.5). Most of these methods result in similar LV dP/dt when in direct comparison.[142] The SMART-AV trial compared three of these methods, randomizing 1014 patients undergoing CRT implantation to a fixed AV delay of 120 ms, echocardiographically optimized AV delay, or electrocardiographically optimized AV delay (via a device-automated protocol based on the intrinsic AV interval and QRS width [SmartDe-lay™]).[143] After 6 months, there were no differences in LV end-diastolic volume or ejection fraction, 6-minute walk, quality of life measures, or NYHA classification between the three groups.

Ventricular timing optimization (V-V optimization)

Once it was recognized that not all LV pacing sites were equivalent in a given patient in terms of providing symptomatic benefits, methods to optimize biventricular pacing began to be developed. Table 2.6 summarizes currently available techniques to assess V-V optimiza-

Table 2.6 V-V optimization methods in cardiac resynchronization therapy (CRT).

Optimization modality	Measurements
Surface ECG[148,150,288,289]	QRS duration LV–RV difference in time from pacing stimulus to first fast deflection on precordial leads[288]
Invasive hemodynamic assessment[106,107,290]	dP/dt_{max}
Echocardiographic hemodynamic assessment[109,152,291,292]	LV outflow tract velocity–time integral to calculate stroke volume
Echocardiographic dyssynchrony assessment[288,293]	Interventricular dyssynchrony (difference between aortic and pulmonary pre-ejection times) Tissue Doppler (difference in time to peak velocity) Speckle-track imaging (difference in time to peak strain) Real-time 3-D (systolic dyssynchrony index)
Device-based algorithms[81]	Expert Ease for Heart Failure™
Others	Blood pressure[294] Acoustic cardiography[286,295] Impedance cardiography[147,287,296] Radionuclide ventriculography[297] Intracardiac ECGs (QuickOpt™)[298,299] stimulation to sense timing intervals between LV and RV leads[300] Finger photo-plethysmography[294] Inert gas breathing (noninvasive cardiac output measurement)[127,301]

tion, of which surface ECG and transthoracic echocardiography are used routinely. Optimal V-V settings are individual specific and have not been shown to be predictable through clinical parameters[144] and vary (as with optimal A-V settings) with time during follow-up,[145] characterizing the challenge in V-V optimization, particularly in understanding its effect on longer term outcome. Optimization may take the form of attempting various pacing sites in the coronary venous system at implant, placing the RV pacing lead at varying sites, varying the vector of pacing (bipolar vs. LV tip to RV ring, etc.), varying the timing of LV and RV pacing, and utilizing or avoiding anodal stimulation.

Optimizing site of pacing (LV and/or RV)

It is generally recognized that the ideal LV pacing site is on the midportion of the free wall of the LV placed as far away as possible from the RV pacing lead when observed in the left anterior oblique (or lateral X-ray) image. There are obvious difficulties with this simplification, because some patients will have a lateral wall infarction or have an inordinate amount of exit delay related to the lateral pacing site, and the least dyssynchrony-producing LV site may depend on the location of the RV pacing lead, etc. An optimal lead position is associated not only with immediate optimization of cardiac output, but also longer term outcome from CRT.[69,106–108,110,146] Techniques generally involve either optimizing cardiac output and function at the time of implantation with invasive pressure monitoring or echocardiography, or identifying sites of ventricular contraction that are delayed and occurring once aortic ejection is underway. The latter was initially through M-mode analysis but has been superseded with tissue Doppler techniques. One construct for predicting the ideal location to place the LV pacing lead is to aim for early stimulation at a location where, without pacing, the latest activation occurs. Using the QRS duration or morphology to identify this location is difficult. For example, if the latest sites of activation are within a diseased peri-infarct ventricular region, the fragmented local electrograms that result from the wavefront propagating to this region may not contribute (and hence be invisible in) the surface QRS. On the other hand, if the abnormally slow area of conduction is just proximal to the last site to be activated, a discernible deflection at the terminal portion of the QRS (as the wavefront exits the diseased region), possibly separated from the initial QRS by an isoelectric period (reflecting conduction through the diseased tissue), may result. Despite these ECG differences, the optimal pacing location, assuming it is the last site activated, would be very similar. Auricchio and Abraham[102] found marked differences in endocardial activation despite a near-identical LBBB morphology on the QRS complex. Endocardial activation depended on the site of intraventricular conduction delay as identified with electroanatomic and noncontact mapping. Because of these issues, mechanical parameters have been more frequently used to find the last site of ventricular activation. The important problem that remains even when an echocardiographic parameter (tissue velocity/M-mode contractility latest from the onset of the QRS, etc.) is used is that LV pacing at that location may not necessarily produce the maximal benefit. This is because one may simply change the pattern of dyssynchrony with another location now being the latest to activate. Which pattern of dyssynchrony is *in toto* least conducive to normal hemodynamic is difficult to predict. One elegant study demonstrated that the effectiveness of V-V optimization, as determined by cardiac output estimation using impedance cardiography, was limited to those whose LV lead was positioned in a segment adjacent to, but not at nor remote from, the most delayed segment.[147] Algorithms that either simulate or predict resultant total LV dyssynchrony following LV stimulation prior to placing the lead are being investigated.

Varying the pacing vector

With bipolar stimulation using closely spaced electrodes, the pacing site coincides with the location of the electrodes. The situation is more complex when pacing occurs between widely spaced electrodes on the LV pacing lead or between a LV electrode and a RV ring or coil electrode. The QRS morphology, activation pattern, and actual site of stimulation (cathode vs. anode) can vary quite markedly. There are no clear data in the literature in terms of impact on symptom improvement and long-term outcomes when the pacing vectors are changed.

Impact of diseased myocardium proximate to the pacing electrodes

At times, the LV pacing lead may be optimally located; however, because of prominent exit delay, only a small region of LV is captured by the LV electrode, so that effectively, the LV is predominantly activated via the RV pacing lead. During threshold testing at high outputs, because of recruitment of larger areas of myocardium, there is less capture latency and more rapid intraventricular conduction, with true LV stimulation during biventricular pacing. On the other hand, at lower output, despite LV capture, capture latency is prolonged and conduction slowed with effective loss of LV lead contribution to LV depolarization during simultaneous biventricular stimulation. In this situation, providing an offset (pacing the LV earlier than the RV) can remedy the situation by allow greater time for LV depolarization via the LV lead-initiated wavefront, prior to RV stimulation. Although increasing the LV pacing output is an alternative solution, the obvious limitation is shortened battery longevity.

Electrical parameters for V-V optimization

When optimizing the pacing site at implantation, the parameter used to identify the optimal site or pacing configuration must be determined. The QRS duration is the most easily obtained electrical parameter to use during implant procedures, as well as in follow-up to optimize ventricle to ventricle timing. Lecoq *et al.*[148] studied whether ECG parameters can predict response from CRT. They found that of all the variables studied in predicting response to CRT, the amount of QRS shortening associated with biventricular stimulation was the only independent predictor. Notably, in this study, the RV implantation site was specifically manipulated to obtain the shortest possible QRS duration. However, contrary conclusions were drawn in other studies.[149] Tamborero *et al.*[150] randomized 156 patients with LBBB meeting criteria for CRT to V-V optimization defined by optimal intraventricular mechanical synchrony assessed tissue Doppler imaging versus optimal electrical synchrony determined by the narrowest obtainable QRS duration. Echocardiographic response, as determined by >10% LV end-systolic volume reduction, was higher in the ECG optimized group (68% vs. 50%; $P = 0.023$) at 6 months' follow-up, with no difference in 6-minute walk test.

There are clear limitations to the use of the QRS duration alone for optimization. First, isoelectric periods during QRS inscription may occur when the activation wavefront proceeds through areas of extremely slow conduction involving diseased myocardium. The location of the slow zones and/or abnormal tissue will determine whether the QRS appears wide or not. If a slow zone of myocardial conduction is the first or last site to be activated following stimulation, the QRS may appear normal (if normal portions not seen in the routine 12-lead ECG). On the other hand, if the slow zone is mid-LV and the pacing site is RV or intrinsic rhythm with LBBB is present, a wide QRS results. Similarly, when optimizing the V-V timing or LV lead pacing site, a narrow QRS may result from true synchronous electrical activation of the ventricles or from activation of a slow zone at the beginning or end of the QRS inscription.

QRS vector fusion

The premise for this method to optimize biventricular devices is that the QRS morphology (vector) is specific for a given pacing site (Fig. 2.35). Thus, LV pacing from the lateral wall typically results in a QS complex in lead

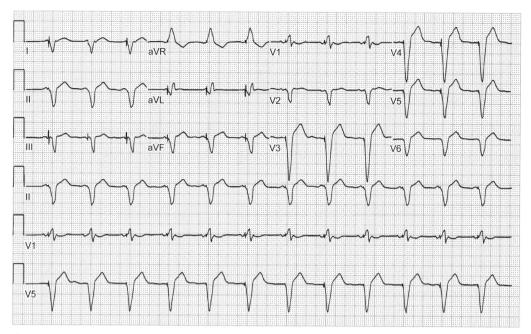

Fig. 2.35 Twelve-lead electrocardiogram obtained from a patient with a biventricular pacing system. The QRS demonstrates a right bundle branch block morphology suggesting left ventricular simulation. To further localize the site of the left ventricular pacing lead we note that leads II, III, and aVF are all negative, suggesting a posterior and/or inferiorly located pacing lead. However, we note further that lead I is negative, suggesting a lateral left ventricular location for the left ventricular pacing lead. An additional finding is that the degree of negativity (depth of QF complex) is deeper in lead II (left-sided lead) than in lead III (a right-sided lead). Each left ventricular lead pacing site has a specific signature electrocardiogram and this example is consistent with a left ventricular lead located in a posterolateral site.

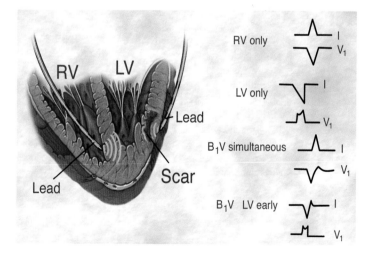

Fig. 2.36 EKG vector fusion. (By permission of Mayo Foundation.)

I, right bundle branch block patterns, and negative or isoelectric complexes in leads II, III and aVF; and RV apical pacing results in a tall R wave in lead I and a LBBB pattern. With biventricular stimulation, a fused vector, in which the QRS morphology is a hybrid between lone-RV and lone-LV pacing, is expected (Fig. 2.36) If, the biventricular paced QRS morphology matches the lone-RV pacing morphology despite a good LV threshold, then either prolonged capture latency or significant conduction delay from the LV

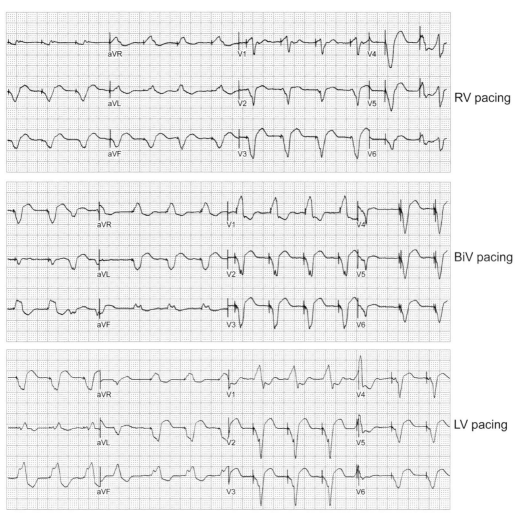

Fig. 2.37 The top panel shows the characteristic 12-lead electrocardiogram when pacing from a right ventricular (RV) apex. Note, in lead V1 the predominant morphology is that of left bundle branch block, but as is commonly observed in patients with enlarged left ventricles, a small R wave is noted in lead V1. The bottom panel shows the 12-lead electrocardiogram when pacing from a left free wall anterolateral location. Note, the deep negative QS complex in lead I, right bundle branch block configuration and the positive QRS complexes in leads II, III and aVF. The middle panel shows biventricular (BiV) pacing with simultaneous left and right ventricular stimulation. Most of the leads depicted are more akin to left ventricular (LV) pacing (bottom panel). This suggests that the patient may have a septal infarction such that the RV pacing wavefront does not effectively depolarize a significant portion of the myocardium. An improvement in ventricular synchrony may be obtained by programming an offset for RV simulation to occur prior to LV stimulation. This situation is exceptional, with most cases requiring an offset with LV pre-excitation.

pacing site is present. By progressively pacing the LV lead earlier than the RV lead while monitoring the QRS for fusion (hybrid QRS complexes) during biventricular stimulation, the V-V can be optimized (Fig. 2.37). In certain situations (septal infarcts) an offset may need to be programmed whereby the RV lead is paced earlier than the LV lead. Some studies have indicated that electromechanical delay as well as possible tethering of the infarct region to nearby myocardium may be more prominent in ischemic cardiomyopathy than in idiopathic dilated cardiomyopathy.[151]

Therefore, when using the ECG to optimize V-V timing, the QRS duration and QRS vector fusion are analyzed, which may compensate for some the vagaries of capture latency and intraventricular conduction heterogeneity. Attention should also be paid to abrupt changes in QRS morphology which result from anodal stimulation or change in the pacing vector configuration. Anodal stimulation is discussed in detail in Chapter 10: Troubleshooting. Although QRS-based optimization is straightforward for use during implant, by definition it optimizes the surface ECG. As noted above, important electromechanical delay may be present despite optimization of the QRS. Thus, electrical synchronization, although feasible and usually quite straightforward, lacks the appeal of mechanical optimization of ventricular lead placement.

Echocardiography for ventricular timing optimization

The most common echocardiographic methods currently in practice for optimizing the V-V interval are estimation of cardiac output from measuring the LV outflow tract velocity–time integral (LVOT VTI) on blood pool, with the largest LVOT VTI defining the optimal V-V interval, or assessing mechanical dyssynchrony, either by comparing pre-ejection RV with LV times using blood pool Doppler, which identifies blood flow, or the variation in timing of regional ventricular contraction using tissue Doppler, which identifies tissue motion (interventricular vs. intraventricular synchrony; Fig. 2.3).

The use of 2-D and standard Doppler echocardiography, including cardiac output measurement using LVOT-VTI and interventricular dyssynchrony assessment to optimize V-V delays, has been prospectively studied in 121 patients randomized 1:3 to standard simultaneous biventricular pacing (RHYTHM II study).[152] Those randomized to optimized V-V intervals had significantly better exercise capacity and quality of life at baseline, but at 6 months there was no difference between the groups. Changes in AV and VV delays were seen over the 6-month follow-up period, which may be partly why the groups had similar outcomes over time.

The advent of strain imaging has allowed for analysis of myocardial deformation (i.e., strain), which involves assessing myocardial motion in relation to itself (using two samples within a small area of myocardium) and is therefore independent of the artifactual effects of translation or tethering. With speckle-track imaging, which utilizes spaciotemporal tracking of the unique echocardiographic speckling pattern of tissue during the cardiac cycle, planes of motion are no longer required to be tangential to the sampling volume as the technology is independent of measuring the Doppler effect. Radial (in addition to longitudinal) strain can be quantified, a reproducible method for identifying mechanical dyssynchrony which is more sensitive at identifying dys-

synchrony than tissue-velocity derived indices[153] and correlates with response to CRT and mortality.[68,69,115,154] A dispersion of strain from peak to end-systole has also been correlated with response to CRT,[155,156] as has the absence of low amplitude of strain (indicating reduced myocardial contraction) at the pacing site present prior to lead placement.[157] Given that speckle-track imaging is able to measure strain in rotational planes, it allows for measurement of myocardial twist, which is the gradient of radial rotation during the cardiac cycle from apex to base (degrees/cm). Myocardial twist reflects global LV function and is sensitive to dyssynchrony.[158,159] An immediate improvement in LV twist following CRT has been shown to predict symptomatic improvement and LV reverse remodeling with incremental value over other established measures of dyssynchrony.[158–160]

Though promising, these imaging modalities have not been tested prospectively in optimizing V-V function.

Clinical approaches to V-V optimization

With the option to program an offset between RV and LV stimulation, methods have been sought to optimize the V-V stimulus interval. Thus, QRS duration and QRS vector summation decreasing the site of maximal mechanical delay, delayed tissue Doppler-derived contraction sites and global indices improvement of tissue contraction have been studied with varying the V-V interval. The frame rate or firing rate in case of echocardiographic imaging is of paramount importance when dealing with electrical and electromechanical phenomena. The frame rate has to be sufficiently high to track electrical conduction. Electrical conduction velocities, even in diseased myocardium, are sufficiently rapid that ideal frame rates are required in the range of 700–1200 frames/s. With echocardiographic 2-D imaging, the usual rate is 30–50 frames/s, while the temporal resolution of "pulsed" tissue Doppler is 250–300 frames/s.[161] Thus, what is actually perceived as dyssynchrony between two segments is quite different when imaged with frame rates of 10/s or 1000/s. With the lower frame rates, two sites may be thought to activate simultaneously when in fact this is an artifact of the slow change in frame rate. One of the challenges of echocardiographic assessment of hemodynamics is distinguishing physiologic effects from measurement variability, which if implemented may result in no improvement and even a paradoxical deterioration.[162]

Several early investigations were performed to demonstrate the hemodynamic advantage of optimizing the V-V interval in patients with severe heart failure and LBBB.[163,164] In one study, 3-D echocardiography and Doppler tissue imaging were performed before and after implant and re-examination at 3 months. Although

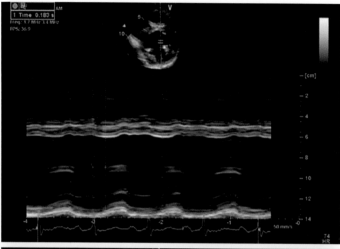

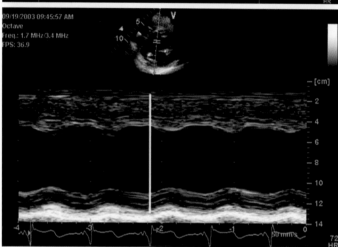

Fig. 2.38 M-mode echocardiogram obtained through a short axis view visualizing the septum and free wall of the left ventricle. In the upper panel, peak systolic contraction occurs on the free wall late after the QRS and is significantly preceded by peak contraction on the septum. In the lower panel, simultaneous peak contraction of both the septum and free wall occur soon after the QRS complex following biventricular pacing stimulation and signifies likely synchronous left ventricular contraction.

simultaneous cardiac resynchronization did reduce the extent of myocardium displaying delayed longitudinal contraction (DLC, a Doppler measure of local mechanical activation) and improved the LV ejection fraction, there was an incremental benefit with sequential cardiac resynchronization. In this study, patients with idiopathic dilated cardiomyopathy had delayed longitudinal contraction in the lateral and posterior walls of the LV. In contrast, DLC was more frequent in the septum and inferior walls in patients with ischemic cardiomyopathy. Preactivation of the LV lead was helpful in nine patients, whereas preactivation of the RV lead was superior in the remaining 11 patients. LV preactivation tended to be more beneficial in patients with delayed lateral wall contraction, i.e., patients with dilated cardiomyopathy. The degree of preactivation was surprisingly modest at about 20 ms. It is important to note that the actual area of mechanical asynchrony

is not reflected by the LBBB pattern alone but is specific based on the nature of the cardiomyopathy and location of ischemia and infarction. Also noted in this study was significant improvement in the 6-minute hall walk test, where the walking distance doubled.

Pitzalis *et al.*[165] assessed the role of septal-to-posterior wall motion delay (SPWMD) on the echocardiogram as a predictor of CRT response (Fig. 2.38). In a study of 60 patients followed over a 14-month period, multivariate analysis determined that a long SPWMD was significantly associated with a decreased risk of heart failure progression (HR 0.91; 95% confidence interval 0.83, 0.99; $P < 0.05$). In 79% of patients with a baseline SPWMD of ≥130 ms there was improvement in the LV ejection fraction, but in only 9% of those with an SPWMD of <130 ms ($P < 0.0001$). They concluded that the baseline SPWMD is a strong predictor of CRT response in patients with LBBB and severe heart failure.[165] However, when data from patients from the CONTAK-CD trial were analyzed, the SPWMD did not correlate with clinical parameters of improvement.[166]

On this premise, one could ask whether the presence of mechanical dyssynchrony can be used to predict response to CRT. This was investigated by the PROS-PECT study (Predictors of Response to CRT),[112] a multicenter, blinded study which analyzed 12 echocardiographic dyssynchrony assessments (derived from M-mode, conventional Doppler, tissue Doppler, and tissue Doppler strain imaging) in 498 unselected patients with standard indications for CRT. No echocardiographic measure of dyssynchrony at baseline predicted response to CRT. Similar findings were reported from a single-center study of 184 patients.[113] Therefore, despite the close association between improvement in mechanical dyssynchrony and outcome after CRT, the demonstration of mechanical dyssynchrony at baseline has not been shown to identify those who benefit.

In summary, in the light of currently available evidence, identification of mechanical dyssynchrony using techniques such as echocardiography does not predict outcome from CRT. The prospective randomized clinical trials that provide the evidence base for CRT nearly universally used surface ECG criteria for patient selection. Echocardiography has an important role in device optimization, is used to address the issue of nonresponders and, in conjunction with other imaging modalities such as magnetic resonance imaging (MRI), provides insight into reasons for nonresponse and optimal lead placement.

Other end-points for optimization

Although both AV and ventricle-to-ventricle optimization has primarily targeted improvements in mechanical function and, in some instances, its translation to effort tolerance,[167] other end-points also need to be considered.

Mitral regurgitation

Disruption to normal mitral valve function results from LV dilatation and reduced contractility. Papillary muscle dyssynchrony has also been implicated.[168,169] The extent of mitral regurgitation has been shown to decrease with LV stimulation. Improvement in the short term has been shown to be related to reduction in valve coaptation height and LV dyssynchrony, while longer term improvement requires remodeling and restoration of normal papillary muscle geometry.[170]

Arrhythmogenesis

Certain pacing sites may be associated with an increased propensity for re-entrant ventricular arrhythmia, whereas other sites may actually serve to decrease the likelihood of a re-entrant circuit developing. Currently, it is not possible to predict which pacing site will be beneficial and which will be arrhythmogenic, as methods to reliably locate the arrhythmogenic slow zones necessary for re-entry are lacking. Coronary sinus lead placement pre-excites the epicardium relative to the endocardium, whereas the RV lead pre-excites the endocardium. Wedge preparations suggest epicardial pacing may be arrhythmogenic relative to endocardial pacing.[171] Finally, the actual location of the RV pacing leads, even if nonarrhythmogenic, would need to be located at a site likely to terminate ventricular tachycardia should it occur as part of defibrillator function (antitachycardia pacing).

Reverse LV remodeling with CRT is associated with a reduction in ventricular arrhythmia.[47,172]

Left atrial pacing

At times, it is impossible to provide optimal LA–LV synchrony while maintaining RA–RV synchrony. This is because a single atrial site with variable intra-atrial conduction is present, yet with two different intraventricular sites. Additionally, when the V timing is varied, reoptimization of AV timing for both sides of the circulation may be required. In such cases, it becomes necessary to have the ability to pre-excite the left atrium if needed. Although this may be partially accomplished with Bachmann's bundle pacing or coronary sinus pacing, ideally, a separate left atrial pacing lead should be placed. This is typically done via the coronary sinus and utilizing a patent vein of Marshall (oblique vein of the left atrium). Although theoretically attractive, the clinical benefit of using a fourth (dedicated left atrial) pacing lead has not been established, and it is not routinely performed in practice.

Right ventricular function

Biventricular pacing results in improved parameters of RV contractile function in the short term, compared with intrinsic dyssynchronous activation or RV apical pacing.[173,174] Longer term recovery in RV function, including improvement in RV dyssynchrony,[175] is associated with overall clinical improvement after CRT. However, this appears to be mediated through improvements in LV function, rather than a direct effect.[176,177] Severe RV dysfunction at baseline is associated with a reduced likelihood of LV functional improvement after CRT.[120,177] The strategy of targeting RV function and synchrony, for example using protocols avoiding RV pacing,[54] to improve outcomes from CRT is currently untested.

Cardiac contractility modulation pacing

Cardiac contractility modulation (CCM) involves increasing myocardial contractility by applying a biphasic square-wave electrical impulse to the ventricle during its refractory period. An internal right atrial sense lead can be used to time delivery of the ventricular impulse onto the septum. Underlying mechanisms have not been fully elucidated but studies of both myocardial cellular preparations and *in vivo* models demonstrate that the effects are mediated through local autonomic neural modulation with resultant normalization of the abnormal gene and protein expression involved in aberrant calcium handling. Echocardiographic studies in humans have demonstrated improved systolic indices, even in walls remote to the stimulation site, with reverse remodeling and reduction in mitral regurgitation.[178] Randomized clinical trials have been conducted in patients with normal QRS duration with severe LV systolic dysfunction (ejection fraction [EF] ≤35%) and NYHA class III and IV dyspnea. The FIX-HF4 trial randomized 164 patients in a double-blind fashion to 3 months of CCM followed by 3 months of a sham device setting, and vice versa.[179] Although there was no change in LV ejection fraction, exercise tolerance (measured using peak oxygen uptake) and quality of life was improved with CCM. This study was followed by the multicenter, non-blinded FIX-HF5 trial which randomized 428 patients in a 1:1 fashion to CCM, demonstrating an improvement in peak oxygen uptake (but not anaerobic threshold, the trial's primary end-point) and quality of life at 6 months.[180] Interestingly, this trial demonstrated a greater effect in those with less severe symptoms (NYHA class III) and less severe LV systolic dysfunction (EF > 25%) at baseline. At present, though promising, this pacing modality requires further investigation into mechanism of action, optimal delivery of the CCM signal, long-term safety, and effectiveness. It is currently not implemented into routine clinical practice.

Ventricular rate regulation

Ventricular rate regulation (VRR) or ventricular rate stabilization algorithms are intended to minimize ventricular cycle length variation in patients with atrial fibrillation. In some patients the use of a VRR algorithm will result in better tolerance of atrial fibrillation. It has been shown to stabilize the ventricular rate effectively without significantly increasing the pacing rate and may result in a more favorable autonomic balance and lead to improved rate recovery after exercise.[181]

In a multicenter trial, assessing the potential benefits of a ventricular pacing response algorithm did decrease the severity of atrial fibrillation-related symptoms. However, it did not improve the general quality of life assessed by the SF-36, functional capacity by 6-minute hall walk, or performance of routine activities as assessed by the Duke Activity Status Index.[182]

Although the overall impact of VRR on hemodynamic status will vary from patient to patient, it appears that this type of algorithm has potential hemodynamic advantage in patients with atrial fibrillation requiring permanent pacing.

Algorithms are also available to limit irregularities caused by pauses after premature ventricular contractions. It had been hoped that these might prevent arrhythmias by mitigating arrhythmogenic short–long–short intervals that introduce variable repolarization and arrhythmogenesis. Although these might be attractive in subsets of patients (e.g., long QT syndrome), in a heterogeneous representative population of ICD recipients, these algorithms did not appear to prevent arrhythmias. Notably, the devices tested were standard ICDs, capable of pacing the ventricles only from the RV.[183]

Less common indications for pacing for hemodynamic improvement

Pacing in hypertrophic obstructive cardiomyopathy

Pacing in hypertrophic obstructive cardiomyopathy (HCM) has been the subject of several randomized single-center and multicenter trials. A single-center, randomized, crossover trial demonstrated symptomatic improvement in 63% of patients with pacing in the DDD mode.[184] However, 42% of patients had improvement with programming to a low pacing rate in the AAI mode, i.e., effectively no pacing, suggesting a significant placebo effect.

In the PIC (Pacing in Cardiomyopathy) study, a multicenter, randomized, crossover study,[185] dual-chamber pacing resulted in a 50% reduction of the LV outflow tract gradient, a 21% increase in exercise duration, and improvement in NYHA functional class compared with baseline status. When clinical features, including chest pain, dyspnea, and subjective health status, were compared between DDD and backup AAI pacing, there was no significant difference, again suggesting a significant placebo effect.

In a double-blind, crossover study, the M-PATHY (Multicenter Study of Pacing Therapy for Hypertrophic Cardiomyopathy) trial, patients were randomized to 3 months each of DDD or AAI pacing (rate, 30) in a crossover design. No significant differences were evident between pacing and no pacing, either subjectively or objectively, when exercise capacity, quality of life score, treadmill exercise time, and peak oxygen consumption were compared.[186] Patients reported symptomatic improvement with pacing, a result suggesting a substantial placebo effect, and a small subset of patients >65 years old had significant objective improvement, a suggestion that DDD pacing might be a viable option in these patients. The investigators concluded that pacing should not be considered a primary treatment for HCM and that subjective benefit without objective evidence of improvement should be interpreted cautiously.

As a result of these trials, pacing is almost never used for the HCM patient unless the patient has a symptomatic bradycardia or ICD implantation is indicated for those HCM patients felt to be at significant risk for sudden cardiac death.

Hemodynamic benefits of pacing in neurocardiogenic syndromes

Hemodynamic considerations are important during pacing for neurocardiogenic syncope.[187–190] Understanding the physiology involved is crucial to understanding the hemodynamics.[191] The carotid sinus reflex is the physiologic response to pressure exerted on the carotid sinus. Stimulation results in activation of baroreceptors within the wall of the carotid sinus, and they initiate an afferent response. Discharge from vagal efferents then results in cardiac slowing. Although this reflex is physiologic, some persons have an exaggerated or even pathologic response. This reflex has two components: cardio-inhibitory and vasodepressor. A cardio-inhibitory response results from increased parasympathetic tone and may be manifested by sinus arrest, sinus bradycardia, PR prolongation, or advanced AV block. The vasodepressor response is caused by sympathetic withdrawal and secondary hypotension. Although a pure cardio-inhibitory or pure vasodepressor response can occur, a mixed response is most common.

Tilt-table testing can provide the physiologic environment to reproduce vasovagal syncope (Fig. 2.39). With head-up tilt, susceptible patients have decreased venous return and subsequent decrease in LV filling. This response triggers stimulation of baroreceptors and adrenergic discharge, which can result in efferent vagal discharge and sympathetic withdrawal. Vasodilatation and hypotension as well as cardiac slowing may result. It is important to document whether the predominant cause of symptoms is cardio-inhibitory or vasodepressor, because therapy differs. Tilt-table testing is often helpful in determining the predominant cause.

A number of mechanical interventions, such as orthostatic training and support stockings, and medications including β-adrenergic blockers, serotonin uptake inhibitors, and α-receptor antagonists are used

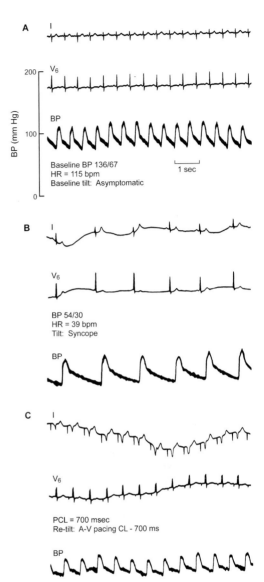

Fig. 2.39 Electrocardiographic and arterial blood pressure recordings obtained during tilt testing. (A) Tilt with the patient asymptomatic demonstrates normal sinus rhythm at a heart rate (HR) of 115 bpm and baseline blood pressure (BP) of 136/67 mmHg. (B) Tilt during syncope; the heart rate is 39 bpm and the blood pressure 54/30 mmHg. (C) Subsequent tilt with atrioventricular (A-V) sequential pacing at a cycle length (PCL) of 700 ms (86 bpm). Significant vasodepression remains, but with the heart rate maintained, the patient experienced only presyncope. (Courtesy of Dr. W-K. Shen, Mayo Clinic.)

in treatment. For refractory cases, although significant controversy persists, vasovagal syncope can be aborted or blunted by dual-chamber pacing, and even if syncope does occur, pacing can prolong consciousness to avoid injury.[187]

VVI pacing usually fails to ameliorate symptoms even if a bradycardic response prevails,[192] because the absence of AV synchrony aggravates the peripheral vasodilatation that generally accompanies this condition. However, existing data suggest that dual-chamber pacing may provide a beneficial effect. The results of randomized clinical trials have been inconsistent. In two trials of highly symptomatic patients with bradycardia, permanent pacing increased the time to first syncopal event. In one study the pacemaker was programmed to DDI at 80 bpm with hysteresis at 45 bpm vs. no pacing.[193] In the other trial the pacemaker was programmed to β-blocker therapy or dual-chamber pacemaker with a sudden rate drop algorithm.[194] In this study, pacemakers were more effective than β-blocker therapy in the prevention of recurrent syncope.

In the initial Vasovagal Pacemaker Study (VPS-1), the rate of recurrent syncope was 18.5% for pacemaker patients and 59.7% for control patients at 1 year.[195]

The same group of investigators subsequently performed VPS-2.[196] In this double-blind, randomized trial, in which all patients received a pacemaker and were randomized to pacing vs. no pacing, pacing therapy did not reduce the risk of recurrent syncopal events. This contrasts with VPS-1, in which patients were randomized to pacemaker implant vs. no pacemaker.

The pacemakers used in these trials depended on sensing heart rate changes whereas a number of patients with neurocardiogenic syndromes may have significant blood pressure reductions without an appreciable change in pulse rate. Closed loop pacemakers may be better suited to detect such hemodynamic alterations as they are able to detect changes in myocardial contractility, with observational data suggesting some benefit in preventing syncope.[197,198]

Pacing therapy is not considered first-line therapy for many patients with neurocardiogenic syncope. However, permanent pacing does have a role for some patients. In those patients who have little or no warning prior to their syncopal event, those with profound bradycardia or asystole during a documented event, and those in whom other therapies have failed, a permanent pacemaker should be considered and may be effective in reducing symptoms if a significant cardio-inhibitory component is felt to be contributing to the cause of the patient's symptoms.

Hemodynamic benefits of pacing in first-degree atrioventricular block

Hemodynamic compromise due to marked first-degree AV block is well documented.[199,200] It is unfortunate that the symptoms have been described as those of pacemaker syndrome.[200] The hemodynamic compromise and symptoms in these patients are caused by loss of optimal AV relationships (Fig. 2.32). Although loss of AV synchrony is a factor in pacemaker syndrome, as previously discussed, other adverse hemodynamic conditions, such as atrial stretch, contribute as well. Pacing therapy should not be limited to first-degree AV block. Patients with type I second-degree AV block, traditionally not an indication for pacing, who have hemodynamic compromise brought about by AV dyssynchrony and not necessarily bradycardia, should also probably be considered for permanent pacing.[201]

Conclusions

The goal of physiologic pacing should be to restore normal physiology to the greatest extent possible. This includes restoration of rate responsiveness in all patients and restoration of AV synchrony in all patients with the exception of those with chronic atrial fibrillation. In CRT it also includes restoration of interatrial and intraventricular synchrony.

The hemodynamic importance of optimizing the AV interval is well established, and differential AV intervals and rate-adaptive AV intervals are important considerations. Data from DAVID and MOST studies have also established the importance of avoiding ventricular pacing whenever possible.

Hemodynamic superiority of different pacing sites or multiple pacing sites has yet to be definitively proven.

Addendum

Two important trials of pacing have been published since the initial writing of this chapter—TARGET (Khan FZ, et al, J Am Coll Cardiol 2012; 59:1590–18) and ISSUE-3 (Brignole M et al, Circulation 2012; 125: 2566–71). The TARGET (Targeted Left Ventricular Lead Placement to Guide Cardiac Resynchronization Therapy) study randomized 220 patients eligible for CRT to the use of speckle-tracking radial strain imaging to guide LV lead placement at the most delayed viable segment, versus no echocardiographic guidance. Compared to unguided LV lead placement, strain imaging guidance resulted in improvement in LV volumes, functional class, quality of life, and reduced heart-failure related hospitalizations. ISSUE-3 (Third International Study on Syncope of Uncertain Etiology) randomized 77 patients with neurally mediated syncope and documented asystole to dual-chamber pacing, versus no pacing. By 2 years, 57% without pacing had syncope versus 25% with pacing.

References

1 Braunstein JB, Anderson GF, Gerstenblith G, et al. Noncardiac comorbidity increases preventable hospitalizations and mortality among Medicare beneficiaries with

chronic heart failure. J Am Coll Cardiol 2003; 42:1226–33.

2 Nordlander R, Hedman A, Pehrsson SK. Rate responsive pacing and exercise capacity: a comment. Pacing Clin Electrophysiol 1989; 12:749–51.

3 Fananapazir L, Srinivas V, Bennett DH. Comparison of resting hemodynamic indices and exercise performance during atrial synchronized and asynchronous ventricular pacing. Pacing Clin Electrophysiol 1983; 6:202–9.

4 Kruse I, Arnman K, Conradson TB, Ryden L. A comparison of the acute and long-term hemodynamic effects of ventricular inhibited and atrial synchronous ventricular inhibited pacing. Circulation 1982; 65:846–55.

5 Ausubel K, Furman S. The pacemaker syndrome. Ann Intern Med 1985; 103:420–9.

6 Ausubel K, Boal BH, Furman S. Pacemaker syndrome: definition and evaluation. Cardiol Clin 1985; 3:587–94.

7 Link MS, Hellkamp AS, Estes NA 3rd, et al. High incidence of pacemaker syndrome in patients with sinus node dysfunction treated with ventricular-based pacing in the Mode Selection Trial (MOST). J Am Coll Cardiol 2004; 43:2066–71.

8 Heldman D, Mulvihill D, Nguyen H, et al. True incidence of pacemaker syndrome. Pacing Clin Electrophysiol 1990; 13:1742–50.

9 Daubert JC, Pavin D, Jauvert G, Mabo P. Intra- and interatrial conduction delay: implications for cardiac pacing. Pacing Clin Electrophysiol 2004; 27:507–25.

10 Janosik DL, Pearson AC, Buckingham TA, Labovitz AJ, Redd RM. The hemodynamic benefit of differential atrioventricular delay intervals for sensed and paced atrial events during physiologic pacing. J Am Coll Cardiol 1989; 14:499–507.

11 Khairy P, Talajic M, Dominguez M, et al. Atrioventricular interval optimization and exercise tolerance. Pacing Clin Electrophysiol 2001; 24:1534–40.

12 Rees M, Haennel RG, Black WR, Kappagoda T. Effect of rate-adapting atrioventricular delay on stroke volume and cardiac output during atrial synchronous pacing. Can J Cardiol 1990; 6:445–52.

13 Sheppard RC, Ren JF, Ross J, McAllister M, Chandrasekaran K, Kutalek SP. Doppler echocardiographic assessment of the hemodynamic benefits of rate adaptive AV delay during exercise in paced patients with complete heart block. Pacing Clin Electrophysiol 1993; 16: 2157–67.

14 Kass DA, Chen CH, Curry C, et al. Improved left ventricular mechanics from acute VDD pacing in patients with dilated cardiomyopathy and ventricular conduction delay. Circulation 1999; 99:1567–73.

15 Auricchio A, Stellbrink C, Block M, et al. Effect of pacing chamber and atrioventricular delay on acute systolic function of paced patients with congestive heart failure. The Pacing Therapies for Congestive Heart Failure Study Group. The Guidant Congestive Heart Failure Research Group. Circulation 1999; 99:2993–001.

16 Nishimura RA, Hayes DL, Holmes DR Jr, Tajik AJ. Mechanism of hemodynamic improvement by dual-chamber pacing for severe left ventricular dysfunction: an acute Doppler and catheterization hemodynamic study. J Am Coll Cardiol 1995; 25:281–8.

17 Asirvatham S, Packer DL. Longitudinal disassociation of atrial and coronary sinus conduction in man. Circulation 2000; 102:II–441.

18 Cazeau S, Leclercq C, Lavergne T, et al. Effects of multisite biventricular pacing in patients with heart failure and intraventricular conduction delay. N Engl J Med 2001; 344:873–80.

19 Kass DA. Pathophysiology of physiologic cardiac pacing: advantages of leaving well enough alone. JAMA 2002; 288:3159–61.

20 Butter C, Auricchio A, Stellbrink C, et al. Effect of resynchronization therapy stimulation site on the systolic function of heart failure patients. Circulation 2001; 104:3026–9.

21 Ritter P, Padeletti L, Gillio-Meina L, Gaggini G. Determination of the optimal atrioventricular delay in DDD pacing: comparison between echo and peak endocardial acceleration measurements. Europace 1999; 1:126–30.

22 Ishikawa T, Sumita S, Kimura K, et al. Critical PQ interval for the appearance of diastolic mitral regurgitation and optimal PQ interval in patients implanted with DDD pacemakers. Pacing Clin Electrophysiol 1994; 17: 1989–94.

23 Braun MU, Schnabel A, Rauwolf T, Schulze M, Strasser RH. Impedance cardiography as a noninvasive technique for atrioventricular interval optimization in cardiac resynchronization therapy. J Interv Card Electrophysiol 2005; 13:223–9.

24 Santos JF, Parreira L, Madeira J, Fonseca N, Soares LN, Ines L. Non invasive hemodynamic monitorization for AV interval optimization in patients with ventricular resynchronization therapy. Rev Port Cardiol 2003; 22: 1091–8.

25 Tse HF, Yu C, Park E, Lau CP. Impedance cardiography for atrioventricular interval optimization during permanent left ventricular pacing. Pacing Clin Electrophysiol 2003; 26:189–91.

26 Mokrani B, Lafitte S, Deplagne A, et al. Echocardiographic study of the optimal atrioventricular delay at rest and during exercise in recipients of cardiac resynchronization therapy systems. Heart Rhythm 2009; 6:972–7.

27 Rom R, Erel J, Glikson M, Rosenblum K, Ginosar R, Hayes DL. Adaptive cardiac resynchronization therapy device: a simulation report. Pacing Clin Electrophysiol 2005; 28:1168–73.

28 Liang HY, Cheng A, Chang KC, et al. Influence of atrial function and mechanical synchrony on LV hemodynamic status in heart failure patients on resynchronization therapy. JACC Cardiovasc Imaging 2011; 4:691–8.

29 Dabrowska-Kugacka A, Lewicka-Nowak E, Rucinski P, Zagozdzon P, Raczak G, Kutarski A. Atrial electromechanical sequence and contraction synchrony during single- and multisite atrial pacing in patients with bradytachycardia syndrome. Pacing Clin Electrophysiol 2009; 32:591–603.

30 Burri H, Bennani I, Domenichini G, et al. Biatrial pacing improves atrial haemodynamics and atrioventricular

timing compared with pacing from the right atrial appendage. Europace 2011; 13:1262–7.

31 Dabrowska-Kugacka A, Lewicka-Nowak E, Rucinski P, Kozlowski D, Raczak G, Kutarski A. Single-site Bachmann's bundle pacing is beneficial while coronary sinus pacing results in echocardiographic right heart pacemaker syndrome in brady-tachycardia patients. Circ J 2010; 74:1308–15.

32 Wang M, Siu CW, Lee KL, et al. Effects of right low atrial septal vs. right atrial appendage pacing on atrial mechanical function and dyssynchrony in patients with sinus node dysfunction and paroxysmal atrial fibrillation. Europace 2011; 13:1268–74.

33 Yasuoka Y, Abe H, Umekawa S, et al. Interatrial septum pacing decreases atrial dyssynchrony on strain rate imaging compared with right atrial appendage pacing. Pacing Clin Electrophysiol 2011; 34:370–6.

34 Rosenqvist M, Brandt J, Schuller H. Long-term pacing in sinus node disease: effects of stimulation mode on cardiovascular morbidity and mortality. Am Heart J 1988; 116:16–22.

35 Barold SS, Santini M. Natural history of sick sinus syndrome after pacemaker implantation. In Barold SS, Mugica J, eds: New Perspectives in Cardiac Pacing. Mount Kisco, NY: Futura Publishing, 1993: 169–211.

36 Lamas GA, Pashos CL, Normand SL, McNeil B. Permanent pacemaker selection and subsequent survival in elderly Medicare pacemaker recipients. Circulation 1995; 91:1063–9.

37 Andersen HR, Thuesen L, Bagger JP, Vesterlund T, Thomsen PE. Prospective randomised trial of atrial versus ventricular pacing in sick-sinus syndrome. Lancet 1994; 344:1523–8.

38 Andersen HR, Nielsen JC, Thomsen PE, et al. Long-term follow-up of patients from a randomised trial of atrial versus ventricular pacing for sick-sinus syndrome. Lancet 1997; 350:1210–6.

39 Schrepf R, Koller B, Pache J, Hofmann M, Goedel-Meinen L, Schoemig A. Results of the randomized prospective DDD vs. VVI trial in patients with paroxysmal atrial fibrillation (abstract). Pacing Clin Electrophysiol 1997; 20:1152.

40 Wharton JM, Sorrentino RA, Campbell P, Investigators atPA-T. Effect of pacing modality on atrial tachyarrhythmia recurrence in the tachycardia-bradycardia syndrome: preliminary results of the Pacemaker Atrial Tachycardia trial (abstract). Circulation 1998; 98(Suppl. I):494.

41 Lamas GA, Orav EJ, Stambler BS, et al. Quality of life and clinical outcomes in elderly patients treated with ventricular pacing as compared with dual-chamber pacing. Pacemaker Selection in the Elderly Investigators. N Engl J Med 1998; 338:1097–104.

42 Connolly SJ, Kerr CR, Gent M, et al. Effects of physiologic pacing versus ventricular pacing on the risk of stroke and death due to cardiovascular causes. Canadian Trial of Physiologic Pacing Investigators. N Engl J Med 2000; 342:1385–91.

43 Tang AS, Roberts RS, Kerr C, et al. Relationship between pacemaker dependency and the effect of pacing mode on cardiovascular outcomes. Circulation 2001; 103:3081–5.

44 Lamas GA, Lee KL, Sweeney MO, et al. Ventricular pacing or dual-chamber pacing for sinus-node dysfunction. N Engl J Med 2002; 346:1854–62.

45 Sweeney MO, Hellkamp AS, Ellenbogen KA, et al. Adverse effect of ventricular pacing on heart failure and atrial fibrillation among patients with normal baseline QRS duration in a clinical trial of pacemaker therapy for sinus node dysfunction. Circulation 2003; 107:2932–7.

46 Wilkoff BL, Cook JR, Epstein AE, et al. Dual-chamber pacing or ventricular backup pacing in patients with an implantable defibrillator: the Dual Chamber and VVI Implantable Defibrillator (DAVID) Trial. JAMA 2002; 288:3115–23.

47 Barsheshet A, Wang PJ, Moss AJ, et al. Reverse remodeling and the risk of ventricular tachyarrhythmias in the MADIT-CRT (Multicenter Automatic Defibrillator Implantation Trial-Cardiac Resynchronization Therapy). J Am Coll Cardiol 2011; 57:2416–23.

48 Wilkoff BL, Kudenchuk PJ, Buxton AE, et al. The DAVID (Dual Chamber and VVI Implantable Defibrillator) II trial. J Am Coll Cardiol 2009; 53:872–80.

49 Barsheshet A, Moss AJ, McNitt S, et al. Long-term implications of cumulative right ventricular pacing among patients with an implantable cardioverter-defibrillator. Heart Rhythm 2011; 8:212–8.

50 Olshansky B, Day JD, Moore S, et al. Is dual-chamber programming inferior to single-chamber programming in an implantable cardioverter-defibrillator? Results of the INTRINSIC RV (Inhibition of Unnecessary RV Pacing With AVSH in ICDs) study. Circulation 2007; 115:9–16.

51 Sweeney MO, Bank AJ, Nsah E, et al. Minimizing ventricular pacing to reduce atrial fibrillation in sinus-node disease. N Engl J Med 2007; 357:1000–8.

52 Nielsen JC, Thomsen PE, Hojberg S, et al. A comparison of single-lead atrial pacing with dual-chamber pacing in sick sinus syndrome. Eur Heart J 2011; 32:686–96.

53 Sweeney MO, Ellenbogen KA, Tang AS, et al. Atrial pacing or ventricular backup-only pacing in implantable cardioverter-defibrillator patients. Heart Rhythm 2010; 7:1552–60.

54 Lee KL, Burnes JE, Mullen TJ, Hettrick DA, Tse HF, Lau CP. Avoidance of right ventricular pacing in cardiac resynchronization therapy improves right ventricular hemodynamics in heart failure patients. J Cardiovasc Electrophysiol 2007; 18:497–504.

55 Kaye G, Stambler BS, Yee R. Search for the optimal right ventricular pacing site: design and implementation of three randomized multicenter clinical trials. Pacing Clin Electrophysiol 2009; 32:426–33.

56 Tse HF, Yu C, Wong KK, et al. Functional abnormalities in patients with permanent right ventricular pacing: the effect of sites of electrical stimulation. J Am Coll Cardiol 2002; 40:1451–8.

57 Hillock RJ, Stevenson IH, Mond HG. The right ventricular outflow tract: a comparative study of septal, anterior wall, and free wall pacing. Pacing Clin Electrophysiol 2007; 30:942–7.

58 Rosso R, Teh AW, Medi C, Hung TT, Balasubramaniam R, Mond HG. Right ventricular septal pacing: the success of stylet-driven active-fixation leads. Pacing Clin Electrophysiol 2010; 33:49–53.

59 Rosso R, Medi C, Teh AW, et al. Right ventricular septal pacing: a comparative study of outflow tract and mid ventricular sites. Pacing Clin Electrophysiol 2010; 33:1169–73.

60 Vlay SC. Right ventricular outflow tract pacing: practical and beneficial: a 9-year experience of 460 consecutive implants. Pacing Clin Electrophysiol 2006; 29:1055–62.

61 Medi C, Mond HG. Right ventricular outflow tract septal pacing: long-term follow-up of ventricular lead performance. Pacing Clin Electrophysiol 2009; 32:172–6.

62 Lieberman R, Grenz D, Mond HG, Gammage MD. Selective site pacing: defining and reaching the selected site. Pacing Clin Electrophysiol 2004; 27:883–6.

63 Roger VL, Go AS, Lloyd-Jones DM, et al. Heart disease and stroke statistics – 2011 update: a report from the American Heart Association. Circulation 2011; 123: e18–e209.

64 Gheorghiade M, Pang PS. Acute heart failure syndromes. J Am Coll Cardiol 2009; 53:557–73.

65 Gold MR, Feliciano Z, Gottlieb SS, Fisher ML. Dual-chamber pacing with a short atrioventricular delay in congestive heart failure: a randomized study. J Am Coll Cardiol 1995; 26:967–73.

66 Linde C, Gadler F, Edner M, Nordlander R, Rosenqvist M, Ryden L. Results of atrioventricular synchronous pacing with optimized delay in patients with severe congestive heart failure. Am J Cardiol 1995; 75:919–23.

67 Iuliano S, Fisher SG, Karasik PE, Fletcher RD, Singh SN. QRS duration and mortality in patients with congestive heart failure. Am Heart J 2002; 143:1085–91.

68 Gorcsan J 3rd, Oyenuga O, Habib PJ, et al. Relationship of echocardiographic dyssynchrony to long-term survival after cardiac resynchronization therapy. Circulation 2010; 122:1910–8.

69 Delgado V, van Bommel RJ, Bertini M, et al. Relative merits of left ventricular dyssynchrony, left ventricular lead position, and myocardial scar to predict long-term survival of ischemic heart failure patients undergoing cardiac resynchronization therapy. Circulation 2011; 123:70–8.

70 Xiao HB, Lee CH, Gibson DG. Effect of left bundle branch block on diastolic function in dilated cardiomyopathy. Br Heart J 1991; 66:443–7.

71 Herman MV, Heinle RA, Klein MD, Gorlin R. Localized disorders in myocardial contraction: asynergy and its role in congestive heart failure. N Engl J Med 1967; 277:222–32.

72 Holzmeister J, Leclercq C. Implantable cardioverter defibrillators and cardiac resynchronisation therapy. Lancet 2011; 378:722–30.

73 Jessup M, Abraham WT, Casey DE, et al. 2009 focused update: ACCF/AHA Guidelines for the Diagnosis and Management of Heart Failure in Adults: a report of the American College of Cardiology Foundation/American Heart Association Task Force on Practice Guidelines: developed in collaboration with the International Society for Heart and Lung Transplantation. Circulation 2009; 119:1977–2016.

74 Vassallo JA, Cassidy DM, Miller JM, Buxton AE, Marchlinski FE, Josephson ME. Left ventricular endocardial activation during right ventricular pacing: effect of underlying heart disease. J Am Coll Cardiol 1986; 7:1228–33.

75 van Gelder BM, Bracke FA, Meijer A, Pijls NH. The hemodynamic effect of intrinsic conduction during left ventricular pacing as compared to biventricular pacing. J Am Coll Cardiol 2005; 46:2305–10.

76 Bordachar P, Lafitte S, Reuter S, et al. Biventricular pacing and left ventricular pacing in heart failure: similar hemodynamic improvement despite marked electromechanical differences. J Cardiovasc Electrophysiol 2004; 15:1342–7.

77 Kurzidim K, Reinke H, Sperzel J, et al. Invasive optimization of cardiac resynchronization therapy: role of sequential biventricular and left ventricular pacing. Pacing Clin Electrophysiol 2005; 28:754–61.

78 Riedlbauchova L, Fridl P, Kautzner J, Peichl P. Performance of left ventricular versus biventricular pacing in chronic heart failure assessed by stress echocardiography. Pacing Clin Electrophysiol 2004; 27:626–31.

79 Delnoy PP, Ottervanger JP, Luttikhuis HO, et al. Pressure–volume loop analysis during implantation of biventricular pacemaker/cardiac resynchronization therapy device to optimize right and left ventricular pacing sites. Eur Heart J 2009; 30:797–804.

80 Gasparini M, Bocchiardo M, Lunati M, et al. Comparison of 1-year effects of left ventricular and biventricular pacing in patients with heart failure who have ventricular arrhythmias and left bundle-branch block: the Bi vs Left Ventricular Pacing: an International Pilot Evaluation on Heart Failure Patients with Ventricular Arrhythmias (BELIEVE) multicenter prospective randomized pilot study. Am Heart J 2006; 152:155 e15–7.

81 Rao RK, Kumar UN, Schafer J, Viloria E, De Lurgio D, Foster E. Reduced ventricular volumes and improved systolic function with cardiac resynchronization therapy: a randomized trial comparing simultaneous biventricular pacing, sequential biventricular pacing, and left ventricular pacing. Circulation 2007; 115:2136–44.

82 Sirker A, Thomas M, Baker S, et al. Cardiac resynchronization therapy: left or left-and-right for optimal symptomatic effect – the LOLA ROSE study. Europace 2007; 9:862–8.

83 Boriani G, Kranig W, Donal E, et al. A randomized double-blind comparison of biventricular versus left ventricular stimulation for cardiac resynchronization therapy: the Biventricular versus Left Univentricular Pacing with ICD Back-up in Heart Failure Patients (B-LEFT HF) trial. Am Heart J 2010; 159:1052–8.

84 Sedlacek K, Burianova L, Mlcochova H, Peichl P, Marek T, Kautzner J. Isolated left ventricular pacing results in worse long-term clinical outcome when compared with biventricular pacing: a single-centre randomized study. Europace 2010; 12:1762–8.

85 Buck S, Maass AH, Nieuwland W, Anthonio RL, Van Veldhuisen DJ, Van Gelder IC. Impact of interventricular lead distance and the decrease in septal-to-lateral delay on response to cardiac resynchronization therapy. Europace 2008; 10:1313–9.

86 Singh JP, Klein HU, Huang DT, et al. Left ventricular lead position and clinical outcome in the multicenter automatic defibrillator implantation trial-cardiac resynchronization therapy (MADIT-CRT) trial. Circulation 2011; 123:1159–66.

87 Mortensen PT, Herre JM, Chung ES, et al. The effect of left ventricular pacing site on cardiac resynchronization therapy outcome and mortality: the results of a PROSPECT substudy. Europace 2010; 12:1750–6.

88 Doll N, Piorkowski C, Czesla M, et al. Epicardial versus transvenous left ventricular lead placement in patients receiving cardiac resynchronization therapy: results from a randomized prospective study. Thorac Cardiovasc Surg 2008; 56:256–61.

89 Patwala A, Woods P, Clements R, et al. A prospective longitudinal evaluation of the benefits of epicardial lead placement for cardiac resynchronization therapy. Europace 2009; 11:1323–9.

90 Goscinska-Bis K, Bis J, Krejca M, et al. Totally epicardial cardiac resynchronization therapy system implantation in patients with heart failure undergoing CABG. Eur J Heart Fail 2008; 10:498–506.

91 Padeletti L, Colella A, Michelucci A, et al. Dual-site left ventricular cardiac resynchronization therapy. Am J Cardiol 2008; 102:1687–92.

92 Leclercq C, Gadler F, Kranig W, et al. A randomized comparison of triple-site versus dual-site ventricular stimulation in patients with congestive heart failure. J Am Coll Cardiol 2008; 51:1455–62.

93 Bordachar P, Alonso C, Anselme F, et al. Addition of a second LV pacing site in CRT nonresponders rationale and design of the multicenter randomized V(3) trial. J Card Fail 2010; 16:709–13.

94 O'Donnell D, Nadurata V, Hamer A, Kertes P, Mohamed U. Bifocal right ventricular cardiac resynchronization therapies in patients with unsuccessful percutaneous lateral left ventricular venous access. Pacing Clin Electrophysiol 2005; 28(Suppl 1):S27–30.

95 Res JC, Bokern MJ, de Cock CC, van Loenhout T, Bronzwaer PN, Spierenburg HA. The BRIGHT study: bifocal right ventricular resynchronization therapy: a randomized study. Europace 2007; 9:857–61.

96 Rocha EA, Gondim TP, Abreu S, et al. Ventricular resynchronization: comparing biventricular and bifocal right ventricular pacemakers. Arq Bras Cardiol 2007; 88:674–82.

97 Lane RE, Mayet J, Peters NS, Davies DW, Chow AW. Comparison of temporary bifocal right ventricular pacing and biventricular pacing for heart failure: evaluation by tissue Doppler imaging. Heart 2008; 94:53–8.

98 Bulava A, Lukl J. Similar long-term benefits conferred by apical versus mid-septal implantation of the right ventricular lead in recipients of cardiac resynchronization therapy systems. Pacing Clin Electrophysiol 2009; 32 (Suppl 1):S32–7.

99 Malecka B, Zabek A, Lelakowski J. Shortening of paced QRS complex and clinical improvement following upgrading from apical right ventricular pacing to bifocal right ventricular or biventricular pacing in patients with permanent atrial fibrillation. Kardiol Pol 2010; 68: 1234–41.

100 Dekker AL, Phelps B, Dijkman B, et al. Epicardial left ventricular lead placement for cardiac resynchronization therapy: optimal pace site selection with pressure-volume loops. J Thorac Cardiovasc Surg 2004; 127: 1641–7.

101 Raichlen JS, Campbell FW, Edie RN, Josephson ME, Harken AH. The effect of the site of placement of temporary epicardial pacemakers on ventricular function in patients undergoing cardiac surgery. Circulation 1984; 70:I118–23.

102 Auricchio A, Abraham WT. Cardiac resynchronization therapy: current state of the art: cost versus benefit. Circulation 2004; 109:300–7.

103 Auricchio A, Salo RW. Acute hemodynamic improvement by pacing in patients with severe congestive heart failure. Pacing Clin Electrophysiol 1997; 20:313–24.

104 Blanc JJ, Etienne Y, Gilard M, et al. Evaluation of different ventricular pacing sites in patients with severe heart failure: results of an acute hemodynamic study. Circulation 1997; 96:3273–7.

105 Gras D, Mabo P, Tang T, et al. Multisite pacing as a supplemental treatment of congestive heart failure: preliminary results of the Medtronic Inc. InSync Study. Pacing Clin Electrophysiol 1998; 21:2249–55.

106 Duckett SG, Ginks M, Shetty AK, et al. Invasive acute hemodynamic response to guide left ventricular lead implantation predicts chronic remodeling in patients undergoing cardiac resynchronization therapy. J Ame Coll Cardiol 2011; 58:1128–36.

107 Butter C, Wellnhofer E, Seifert M, et al. Time course of left ventricular volumes in severe congestive heart failure patients treated by optimized AV sequential left ventricular pacing alone: a 3-dimensional echocardiographic study. Am Heart J 2006; 151:115–23.

108 Solomon SD, Foster E, Bourgoun M, et al. Effect of cardiac resynchronization therapy on reverse remodeling and relation to outcome: multicenter automatic defibrillator implantation trial – cardiac resynchronization therapy. Circulation 2010; 122:985–92.

109 van Campen CM, Visser FC, de Cock CC, Vos HS, Kamp O, Visser CA. Comparison of the haemodynamics of different pacing sites in patients undergoing resynchronisation treatment: need for individualisation of lead localisation. Heart 2006; 92:1795–800.

110 Ypenburg C, van Bommel RJ, Delgado V, et al. Optimal left ventricular lead position predicts reverse remodeling and survival after cardiac resynchronization therapy. J Am Coll Cardiol 2008; 52:1402–9.

111 Prinzen FW, Augustijn CH, Allessie MA, Arts T, Delhaas T, Reneman RS. The time sequence of electrical and mechanical activation during spontaneous beating and ectopic stimulation. Eur Heart J 1992; 13:535–43.

112 Chung ES, Leon AR, Tavazzi L, et al. Results of the Predictors of Response to CRT (PROSPECT) trial. Circulation 2008; 117:2608–16.

113 Miyazaki C, Redfield MM, Powell BD, et al. Dyssynchrony indices to predict response to cardiac resynchronization therapy: a comprehensive prospective single-center study. Circ Heart Fail 2010; 3:565–73.

114 Park HE, Chang SA, Kim HK, et al. Impact of loading condition on the 2D speckle tracking-derived left ventricular dyssynchrony index in nonischemic dilated cardiomyopathy. Circ Cardiovasc Imaging 2010; 3:272–81.

115 Pouleur AC, Knappe D, Shah AM, et al. Relationship between improvement in left ventricular dyssynchrony and contractile function and clinical outcome with cardiac resynchronization therapy: the MADIT-CRT trial. Eur Heart J 2011; 32:1720–9.

116 Gervais R, Leclercq C, Shankar A, et al. Surface electrocardiogram to predict outcome in candidates for cardiac resynchronization therapy: a sub-analysis of the CARE-HF trial. Eur J Heart Fail 2009; 11:699–705.

117 Linde C, Abraham WT, Gold MR, Daubert C. Cardiac resynchronization therapy in asymptomatic or mildly symptomatic heart failure patients in relation to etiology: results from the REVERSE (REsynchronization reVErses Remodeling in Systolic Left vEntricular Dysfunction) study. J Am Coll Cardiol 2010; 56:1826–31.

118 Zareba W, Klein H, Cygankiewicz I, et al. Effectiveness of Cardiac Resynchronization Therapy by QRS Morphology in the Multicenter Automatic Defibrillator Implantation Trial-Cardiac Resynchronization Therapy (MADIT-CRT). Circulation 2011; 123:1061–72.

119 Haghjoo M, Bagherzadeh A, Farahani MM, Haghighi ZO, Sadr-Ameli MA. Significance of QRS morphology in determining the prevalence of mechanical dyssynchrony in heart failure patients eligible for cardiac resynchronization: particular focus on patients with right bundle branch block with and without coexistent left-sided conduction defects. Europace 2008; 10:566–71.

120 Ghio S, Freemantle N, Scelsi L, et al. Long-term left ventricular reverse remodelling with cardiac resynchronization therapy: results from the CARE-HF trial. Eur J Heart Fail 2009; 11:480–8.

121 Sutton MG, Plappert T, Hilpisch KE, Abraham WT, Hayes DL, Chinchoy E. Sustained reverse left ventricular structural remodeling with cardiac resynchronization at one year is a function of etiology: quantitative Doppler echocardiographic evidence from the Multicenter InSync Randomized Clinical Evaluation (MIRACLE). Circulation 2006; 113:266–72.

122 Tournoux F, Donal E, Leclercq C, et al. Concordance between mechanical and electrical dyssynchrony in heart failure patients: a function of the underlying cardiomyopathy? J Cardiovasc Electrophysiol 2007; 18:1022–7.

123 Bleeker GB, Kaandorp TA, Lamb HJ, et al. Effect of posterolateral scar tissue on clinical and echocardiographic improvement after cardiac resynchronization therapy. Circulation 2006; 113:969–76.

124 Ypenburg C, Schalij MJ, Bleeker GB, et al. Impact of viability and scar tissue on response to cardiac resynchronization therapy in ischaemic heart failure patients. Eur Heart J 2007; 28:33–41.

125 Ginks MR, Lambiase PD, Duckett SG, et al. A simultaneous X-Ray/MRI and noncontact mapping study of the acute hemodynamic effect of left ventricular endocardial and epicardial cardiac resynchronization therapy in humans. Circ Heart Fail 2011; 4:170–9.

126 Jansen AH, Bracke F, van Dantzig JM, et al. The influence of myocardial scar and dyssynchrony on reverse remodeling in cardiac resynchronization therapy. Eur J Echocardiogr 2008; 9:483–8.

127 Riedlbauchova L, Brunken R, Jaber WA, et al. The impact of myocardial viability on the clinical outcome of cardiac resynchronization therapy. J Cardiovasc Electrophysiol 2009; 20:50–7.

128 Tatsumi K, Tanaka H, Matsumoto K, et al. Mechanical left ventricular dyssynchrony in heart failure patients with narrow QRS duration as assessed by three-dimensional speckle area tracking strain. Am J Cardiol 2011; 108:867–72.

129 van Bommel RJ, Tanaka H, Delgado V, et al. Association of intraventricular mechanical dyssynchrony with response to cardiac resynchronization therapy in heart failure patients with a narrow QRS complex. Eur Heart J 2010; 31:3054–62.

130 Beshai JF, Grimm RA, Nagueh SF, et al. Cardiac-resynchronization therapy in heart failure with narrow QRS complexes. N Engl J Med 2007; 357:2461–71.

131 Foley PW, Patel K, Irwin N, et al. Cardiac resynchronisation therapy in patients with heart failure and a normal QRS duration: the RESPOND study. Heart 2011; 97:1041–7.

132 Gradaus R, Stuckenborg V, Loher A, et al. Diastolic filling pattern and left ventricular diameter predict response and prognosis after cardiac resynchronisation therapy. Heart 2008; 94:1026–31.

133 Shanks M, Bertini M, Delgado V, et al. Effect of biventricular pacing on diastolic dyssynchrony. J Am Coll Cardiol 2010; 56:1567–75.

134 Fung JW, Zhang Q, Yip GW, Chan JY, Chan HC, Yu CM. Effect of cardiac resynchronization therapy in patients with moderate left ventricular systolic dysfunction and wide QRS complex: a prospective study. J Cardiovasc Electrophysiol 2006; 17:1288–92.

135 Waggoner AD, Faddis MN, Gleva MJ, de las Fuentes L, Davila-Roman VG. Improvements in left ventricular diastolic function after cardiac resynchronization therapy are coupled to response in systolic performance. J Am Coll Cardiol 2005; 46:2244–9.

136 Jansen AH, van Dantzig J, Bracke F, et al. Improvement in diastolic function and left ventricular filling pressure induced by cardiac resynchronization therapy. Am Heart J 2007; 153:843–9.

137 Aksoy H, Okutucu S, Kaya EB, et al. Clinical and echocardiographic correlates of improvement in left ventricular

diastolic function after cardiac resynchronization therapy. Europace 2010; 12:1256–61.

138 Shanks M, Antoni ML, Hoke U, et al. The effect of cardiac resynchronization therapy on left ventricular diastolic function assessed with speckle-tracking echocardiography. Eur J Heart Fail 2011; 13:1133–9.

139 de Cock CC, Vos DH, Jessurun E, Allaart CP, Visser CA. Effects of stimulation site on diastolic function in cardiac resynchronization therapy. Pacing Clin Electrophysiol 2007; 30(Suppl 1):S40–2.

140 Jansen AH, Bracke FA, van Dantzig JM, et al. Correlation of echo-Doppler optimization of atrioventricular delay in cardiac resynchronization therapy with invasive hemodynamics in patients with heart failure secondary to ischemic or idiopathic dilated cardiomyopathy. Am J Cardiol 2006; 97:552–7.

141 Levin V, Nemeth M, Colombowala I, et al. Interatrial conduction measured during biventricular pacemaker implantation accurately predicts optimal paced atrioventricular intervals. J Cardiovasc Electrophysiol 2007; 18:290–5.

142 Gold MR, Niazi I, Giudici M, et al. A prospective comparison of AV delay programming methods for hemodynamic optimization during cardiac resynchronization therapy. J Cardiovasc Electrophysiol 2007; 18:490–6.

143 Ellenbogen KA, Gold MR, Meyer TE, et al. Primary results from the SmartDelay determined AV optimization: a comparison to other AV delay methods used in cardiac resynchronization therapy (SMART-AV) trial: a randomized trial comparing empirical, echocardiography-guided, and algorithmic atrioventricular delay programming in cardiac resynchronization therapy. Circulation 2010; 122:2660–8.

144 Fischer A, Hansalia R, Buckley S, et al. Lack of clinical predictors of optimal V-V delay in patients with cardiac resynchronization devices. J Interv Card Electrophysiol 2009; 25:153–8.

145 Boriani G, Biffi M, Muller CP, et al. A prospective randomized evaluation of VV delay optimization in CRT-D recipients: echocardiographic observations from the RHYTHM II ICD study. Pacing Clin Electrophysiol 2009; 32(Suppl 1):S120–5.

146 Ansalone G, Giannantoni P, Ricci R, Trambaiolo P, Fedele F, Santini M. Doppler myocardial imaging to evaluate the effectiveness of pacing sites in patients receiving biventricular pacing. J Am Coll Cardiol 2002; 39:489–99.

147 Khan FZ, Virdee MS, Read PA, et al. Impact of VV optimization in relation to left ventricular lead position: an acute haemodynamic study. Europace 2011; 13:845–52.

148 Lecoq G, Leclercq C, Leray E, et al. Clinical and electrocardiographic predictors of a positive response to cardiac resynchronization therapy in advanced heart failure. Eur Heart J 2005; 26:1094–100.

149 Reuter S, Garrigue S, Barold SS, et al. Comparison of characteristics in responders versus nonresponders with biventricular pacing for drug-resistant congestive heart failure. Am J Cardiol 2002; 89:346–50.

150 Tamborero D, Vidal B, Tolosana JM, et al. Electrocardiographic versus echocardiographic optimization of the

interventricular pacing delay in patients undergoing cardiac resynchronization therapy. J Cardiovasc Electrophysiol 2011; 22:1129–34.

151 Ashikaga H, Mickelsen SR, Ennis DB, et al. Electromechanical analysis of infarct border zone in chronic myocardial infarction. Am J Physiol Heart Circ Physiol 2005; 289:H1099–105.

152 Boriani G, Muller CP, Seidl KH, et al. Randomized comparison of simultaneous biventricular stimulation versus optimized interventricular delay in cardiac resynchronization therapy. The Resynchronization for the HemodYnamic Treatment for Heart Failure Management II implantable cardioverter defibrillator (RHYTHM II ICD) study. Am Heart J 2006; 151:1050–8.

153 Faletra FF, Conca C, Klersy C, et al. Comparison of eight echocardiographic methods for determining the prevalence of mechanical dyssynchrony and site of latest mechanical contraction in patients scheduled for cardiac resynchronization therapy. Am J Cardiol 2009; 103: 1746–52.

154 Tanaka H, Nesser HJ, Buck T, et al. Dyssynchrony by speckle-tracking echocardiography and response to cardiac resynchronization therapy: results of the Speckle Tracking and Resynchronization (STAR) study. Eur Heart J 2010; 31:1690–700.

155 Lim P, Buakhamsri A, Popovic ZB, et al. Longitudinal strain delay index by speckle tracking imaging: a new marker of response to cardiac resynchronization therapy. Circulation 2008; 118:1130–7.

156 Lim P, Donal E, Lafitte S, et al. Multicentre study using strain delay index for predicting response to cardiac resynchronization therapy (MUSIC study). Eur J Heart Fail 2011; 13:984–91.

157 Khan FZ, Virdee MS, Read PA, et al. Effect of low-amplitude two-dimensional radial strain at left ventricular pacing sites on response to cardiac resynchronization therapy. J Am Soc Echocardiogr 2010; 23:1168–76.

158 Bertini M, Marsan NA, Delgado V, et al. Effects of cardiac resynchronization therapy on left ventricular twist. J Am Coll Cardiol 2009; 54:1317–25.

159 Sade LE, Demir O, Atar I, Muderrisoglu H, Ozin B. Effect of mechanical dyssynchrony and cardiac resynchronization therapy on left ventricular rotational mechanics. Am J Cardiol 2008; 101:1163–9.

160 Bertini M, Delgado V, Nucifora G, et al. Effect of cardiac resynchronization therapy on subendo- and subepicardial left ventricular twist mechanics and relation to favorable outcome. Am J Cardiol 2010; 106:682–7.

161 Powell BD, Espinosa RE, Yu C, Oh JK. Tissue Doppler imaging, strain imaging and dyssynchrony assessment. In Oh JK, Seward JB, Tajik AJ, eds. The Echo Manual. Rochester: Lippincott Williams & Wilkins, 2007; 80–98.

162 Turcott RG, Witteles RM, Wang PJ, Vagelos RH, Fowler MB, Ashley EA. Measurement precision in the optimization of cardiac resynchronization therapy. Circ Heart Fail 2010; 3:395–404.

163 Sogaard P, Egeblad H, Pedersen AK, et al. Sequential versus simultaneous biventricular resynchronization for

severe heart failure: evaluation by tissue Doppler imaging. Circulation 2002; 106:2078–84.

164 Sogaard P, Egeblad H, Kim WY, et al. Tissue Doppler imaging predicts improved systolic performance and reversed left ventricular remodeling during long-term cardiac resynchronization therapy. J Am Coll Cardiol 2002; 40:723–30.

165 Pitzalis MV, Iacoviello M, Romito R, Luzzi G, Anaclerio M, Forleo C. Role of septal to posterior wall motion delay in cardiac resynchronization therapy. J Am Coll Cardiol 2006; 48:596–7.

166 Marcus GM, Rose E, Viloria EM, et al. Septal to posterior wall motion delay fails to predict reverse remodeling or clinical improvement in patients undergoing cardiac resynchronization therapy. J Am Coll Cardiol 2005; 46:2208–14.

167 Alboni P, Scarfo S, Fuca G, Mele D, Dinelli M, Paparella N. Short-term hemodynamic effects of DDD pacing from ventricular apex, right ventricular outflow tract and proximal septum. G Ital Cardiol 1998; 28:237–41.

168 Kanzaki H, Bazaz R, Schwartzman D, Dohi K, Sade LE, Gorcsan J. 3rd A mechanism for immediate reduction in mitral regurgitation after cardiac resynchronization therapy: insights from mechanical activation strain mapping. J Am Coll Cardiol 2004; 44:1619–25.

169 Ypenburg C, Lancellotti P, Tops LF, et al. Acute effects of initiation and withdrawal of cardiac resynchronization therapy on papillary muscle dyssynchrony and mitral regurgitation. J Am Coll Cardiol 2007; 50:2071–7.

170 Matsumoto K, Tanaka H, Okajima K, et al. Relation between left ventricular morphology and reduction in functional mitral regurgitation by cardiac resynchronization therapy in patients with idiopathic dilated cardiomyopathy. Am J Cardiol 2011; 108:1327–34.

171 Medina-Ravell VA, Lankipalli RS, Yan GX, et al. Effect of epicardial or biventricular pacing to prolong QT interval and increase transmural dispersion of repolarization: does resynchronization therapy pose a risk for patients predisposed to long QT or torsade de pointes? Circulation 2003; 107:740–6.

172 Gold MR, Linde C, Abraham WT, Gardiwal A, Daubert JC. The impact of cardiac resynchronization therapy on the incidence of ventricular arrhythmias in mild heart failure. Heart Rhythm 2011; 8:679–84.

173 Donal E, Vignat N, De Place C, et al. Acute effects of biventricular pacing on right ventricular function assessed by tissue Doppler imaging. Europace 2007; 9:108–12.

174 Rajagopalan N, Suffoletto MS, Tanabe M, et al. Right ventricular function following cardiac resynchronization therapy. Am J Cardiol 2007; 100:1434–6.

175 Vitarelli A, Franciosa P, Nguyen BL, et al. Additive value of right ventricular dyssynchrony indexes in predicting the success of cardiac resynchronization therapy: a speckle-tracking imaging study. J Card Fail 2011; 17:392–402.

176 Burri H, Domenichini G, Sunthorn H, et al. Right ventricular systolic function and cardiac resynchronization therapy. Europace 2010; 12:389–94.

177 Kjaergaard J, Ghio S, St John Sutton M, Hassager C. Tricuspid annular plane systolic excursion and response to

cardiac resynchronization therapy: results from the REVERSE trial. J Card Fail 2011; 17:100–7.

178 Yu CM, Chan JY, Zhang Q, et al. Impact of cardiac contractility modulation on left ventricular global and regional function and remodeling. JACC Cardiovasc Imaging 2009; 2:1341–9.

179 Borggrefe MM, Lawo T, Butter C, et al. Randomized, double blind study of non-excitatory, cardiac contractility modulation electrical impulses for symptomatic heart failure. Eur Heart J 2008; 29:1019–28.

180 Kadish A, Nademanee K, Volosin K, et al. A randomized controlled trial evaluating the safety and efficacy of cardiac contractility modulation in advanced heart failure. Am Heart J 2011; 161:329–37.

181 Ciaramitaro G, Sgarito G, Solimene F, et al. Role of rate control and regularization through pacing in patients with chronic atrial fibrillation and preserved ventricular function: the VRR study. Pacing Clin Electrophysiol 2006; 29:866–74.

182 Tse HF, Newman D, Ellenbogen KA, Buhr T, Markowitz T, Lau CP. Effects of ventricular rate regularization pacing on quality of life and symptoms in patients with atrial fibrillation (Atrial fibrillation symptoms mediated by pacing to mean rates [AF SYMPTOMS study]). Am J Cardiol 2004; 94:938–41.

183 Friedman PA, Jalal S, Kaufman S, et al. Effects of a rate smoothing algorithm for prevention of ventricular arrhythmias: results of the Ventricular Arrhythmia Suppression Trial (VAST). Heart Rhythm 2006; 3:573–80.

184 Nishimura RA, Hayes DL, Ilstrup DM, Holmes DR Jr, Tajik AJ. Effect of dual-chamber pacing on systolic and diastolic function in patients with hypertrophic cardiomyopathy. Acute Doppler echocardiographic and catheterization hemodynamic study. J Am Coll Cardiol 1996; 27:421–30.

185 Kappenberger L, Linde C, Daubert C, et al. Pacing in hypertrophic obstructive cardiomyopathy: a randomized crossover study. PIC Study Group. Eur Heart J 1997; 18:1249–56.

186 Maron BJ, Nishimura RA, McKenna WJ, Rakowski H, Josephson ME, Kieval RS. Assessment of permanent dual-chamber pacing as a treatment for drug-refractory symptomatic patients with obstructive hypertrophic cardiomyopathy: a randomized, double-blind, crossover study (M-PATHY). Circulation 1999; 99:2927–33.

187 Fitzpatrick A, Theodorakis G, Ahmed R, Williams T, Sutton R. Dual chamber pacing aborts vasovagal syncope induced by head-up 60 degrees tilt. Pacing Clin Electrophysiol 1991; 14:13–9.

188 Fitzpatrick A, Sutton R. Tilting towards a diagnosis in recurrent unexplained syncope. Lancet 1989; 1:658–60.

189 Morgan JM, Amer AS, Ingram A, Fitzpatrick A, Sutton R. Diagnosis and management of vasovagal syndrome (abstract). Pacing Clin Electrophysiol 1991; 14:667.

190 Sutton R. Vasovagal syncope: clinical presentation, classification and management. In Aubert AE, Ector H, Stroobandt R, eds. Cardiac Pacing and Electrophysiology: a Bridge to the 21st Century. The Netherlands: Kluwer Academic Publishers, 1994; 15–22.

191 Maloney JD, Jaeger FJ, Rizo-Patron C, Zhu DW. The role of pacing for the management of neurally mediated syncope: carotid sinus syndrome and vasovagal syncope. Am Heart J 1994; 127:1030–7.

192 Sra JS, Jazayeri MR, Avitall B, et al. Comparison of cardiac pacing with drug therapy in the treatment of neurocardiogenic (vasovagal) syncope with bradycardia or asystole. N Engl J Med 1993; 328:1085–90.

193 Sutton R, Brignole M, Menozzi C, et al. Dual-chamber pacing in the treatment of neurally mediated tilt-positive cardioinhibitory syncope: pacemaker versus no therapy: a multicenter randomized study. The Vasovagal Syncope International Study (VASIS) Investigators. Circulation 2000; 102:294–9.

194 Ammirati F, Colivicchi F, Santini M. Permanent cardiac pacing versus medical treatment for the prevention of recurrent vasovagal syncope: a multicenter, randomized, controlled trial. Circulation 2001; 104:52–7.

195 Connolly SJ, Sheldon R, Roberts RS, Gent M. The North American Vasovagal Pacemaker Study (VPS). A randomized trial of permanent cardiac pacing for the prevention of vasovagal syncope. J Am Coll Cardiol 1999; 33:16–20.

196 Connolly SJ, Sheldon R, Thorpe KE, et al. Pacemaker therapy for prevention of syncope in patients with recurrent severe vasovagal syncope: Second Vasovagal Pacemaker Study (VPS II): a randomized trial. JAMA 2003; 289:2224–9.

197 Occhetta E, Bortnik M, Audoglio R, Vassanelli C. Closed loop stimulation in prevention of vasovagal syncope. Inotropy Controlled Pacing in Vasovagal Syncope (INVASY): a multicentre randomized, single blind, controlled study. Europace 2004; 6:538–47.

198 Kanjwal K, Karabin B, Kanjwal Y, Grubb BP. Preliminary observations on the use of closed-loop cardiac pacing in patients with refractory neurocardiogenic syncope. J Interv Card Electrophysiol 2010; 27:69–73.

199 Barold SS, Ilercil A, Leonelli F, Herweg B. First-degree atrioventricular block: clinical manifestations, indications for pacing, pacemaker management and consequences during cardiac resynchronization. J Interv Card Electrophysiol 2006; 17:139–52.

200 Barold SS. Optimal pacing in first-degree AV block. Pacing Clin Electrophysiol 1999; 22:1423–4.

201 Shaw DB, Gowers JI, Kekwick CA, New KH, Whistance AW. Is Mobitz type I atrioventricular block benign in adults? Heart 2004; 90:169–74.

202 Tantengco MV, Thomas RL, Karpawich PP. Left ventricular dysfunction after long-term right ventricular apical pacing in the young. J Am Coll Cardiol 2001; 37:2093–100.

203 Karpawich PP, Rabah R, Haas JE. Altered cardiac histology following apical right ventricular pacing in patients with congenital atrioventricular block. Pacing Clin Electrophysiol 1999; 22:1372–7.

204 Thambo JB, Bordachar P, Garrigue S, et al. Detrimental ventricular remodeling in patients with congenital complete heart block and chronic right ventricular apical pacing. Circulation 2004; 110:3766–72.

205 Hamdan MH, Zagrodzky JD, Joglar JA, et al. Biventricular pacing decreases sympathetic activity compared with right ventricular pacing in patients with depressed ejection fraction. Circulation 2000; 102:1027–32.

206 Wilkoff BL. The Dual Chamber and VVI Implantable Defibrillator (DAVID) Trial: rationale, design, results, clinical implications and lessons for future trials. Card Electrophysiol Rev 2003; 7:468–72.

207 Moss AJ. MADIT-II: substudies and their implications. Card Electrophysiol Rev 2003; 7:430–3.

208 Steinberg JS, Fischer A, Wang P, et al. The clinical implications of cumulative right ventricular pacing in the multicenter automatic defibrillator trial II. J Cardiovasc Electrophysiol 2005; 16:359–65.

209 Wonisch M, Lercher P, Scherr D, et al. Influence of permanent right ventricular pacing on cardiorespiratory exercise parameters in chronic heart failure patients with implanted cardioverter defibrillators. Chest 2005; 127:787–93.

210 Thackray SD, Witte KK, Nikitin NP, Clark AL, Kaye GC, Cleland JG. The prevalence of heart failure and asymptomatic left ventricular systolic dysfunction in a typical regional pacemaker population. Eur Heart J 2003; 24:1143–52.

211 Nielsen JC, Kristensen L, Andersen HR, Mortensen PT, Pedersen OL, Pedersen AK. A randomized comparison of atrial and dual-chamber pacing in 177 consecutive patients with sick sinus syndrome: echocardiographic and clinical outcome. J Am Coll Cardiol 2003; 42:614–23.

212 O'Keefe JH Jr, Abuissa H, Jones PG, et al. Effect of chronic right ventricular apical pacing on left ventricular function. Am J Cardiol 2005; 95:771–3.

213 Ichiki H, Oketani N, Hamasaki S, et al. Effect of right ventricular apex pacing on the Tei index and brain natriuretic peptide in patients with a dual-chamber pacemaker. Pacing Clin Electrophysiol 2006; 29:985–90.

214 Tops LF, Suffoletto MS, Bleeker GB, et al. Speckle-tracking radial strain reveals left ventricular dyssynchrony in patients with permanent right ventricular pacing. J Am Coll Cardiol 2007; 50:1180–8.

215 Shimano M, Tsuji Y, Yoshida Y, et al. Acute and chronic effects of cardiac resynchronization in patients developing heart failure with long-term pacemaker therapy for acquired complete atrioventricular block. Europace 2007; 9:869–74.

216 Pastore G, Noventa F, Piovesana P, et al. Left ventricular dyssynchrony resulting from right ventricular apical pacing: relevance of baseline assessment. Pacing Clin Electrophysiol 2008; 31:1456–62.

217 Albertsen AE, Nielsen JC, Poulsen SH, et al. DDD(R)-pacing, but not AAI(R)-pacing induces left ventricular desynchronization in patients with sick sinus syndrome: tissue-Doppler and 3D echocardiographic evaluation in a randomized controlled comparison. Europace 2008; 10:127–33.

218 Zhang XH, Chen H, Siu CW, et al. New-onset heart failure after permanent right ventricular apical pacing in patients with acquired high-grade atrioventricular block and

normal left ventricular function. J Cardiovasc Electrophysiol 2008; 19:136–41.

219 Wolber T, Haegeli L, Huerlimann D, Brunckhorst C, Luscher TF, Duru F. Altered left ventricular contraction pattern during right ventricular pacing: assessment using real-time three-dimensional echocardiography. Pacing Clin Electrophysiol 2011; 34:76–81.

220 Cowell R, Morris-Thurgood J, Ilsley C, Paul V. Septal short atrioventricular delay pacing: additional hemodynamic improvements in heart failure. Pacing Clin Electrophysiol 1994; 17:1980–3.

221 Giudici MC, Thornburg GA, Buck DL, et al. Comparison of right ventricular outflow tract and apical lead permanent pacing on cardiac output. Am J Cardiol 1997; 79:209–12.

222 Buckingham TA, Candinas R, Schlapfer J, et al. Acute hemodynamic effects of atrioventricular pacing at differing sites in the right ventricle individually and simultaneously. Pacing Clin Electrophysiol 1997; 20:909–15.

223 Karpawich PP, Mital S. Comparative left ventricular function following atrial, septal, and apical single chamber heart pacing in the young. Pacing Clin Electrophysiol 1997; 20:1983–8.

224 de Cock CC, Meyer A, Kamp O, Visser CA. Hemodynamic benefits of right ventricular outflow tract pacing: comparison with right ventricular apex pacing. Pacing Clin Electrophysiol 1998; 21:536–41.

225 Mera F, DeLurgio DB, Patterson RE, Merlino JD, Wade ME, Leon AR. A comparison of ventricular function during high right ventricular septal and apical pacing after his-bundle ablation for refractory atrial fibrillation. Pacing Clin Electrophysiol 1999; 22:1234–9.

226 Buckingham TA, Candinas R, Attenhofer C, et al. Systolic and diastolic function with alternate and combined site pacing in the right ventricle. Pacing Clin Electrophysiol 1998; 21:1077–84.

227 Victor F, Leclercq C, Mabo P, et al. Optimal right ventricular pacing site in chronically implanted patients: a prospective randomized crossover comparison of apical and outflow tract pacing. J Am Coll Cardiol 1999; 33:311–6.

228 Schwaab B, Frohlig G, Alexander C, et al. Influence of right ventricular stimulation site on left ventricular function in atrial synchronous ventricular pacing. J Am Coll Cardiol 1999; 33:317–23.

229 Kolettis TM, Kyriakides ZS, Tsiapras D, Popov T, Paraskevaides IA, Kremastinos DT. Improved left ventricular relaxation during short-term right ventricular outflow tract compared to apical pacing. Chest 2000; 117:60–4.

230 Bourke JP, Hawkins T, Keavey P, et al. Evolution of ventricular function during permanent pacing from either right ventricular apex or outflow tract following AV-junctional ablation for atrial fibrillation. Europace 2002; 4:219–28.

231 Yu CM, Lin H, Fung WH, Zhang Q, Kong SL, Sanderson JE. Comparison of acute changes in left ventricular volume, systolic and diastolic functions, and intraventricular synchronicity after biventricular and right

ventricular pacing for heart failure. Am Heart J 2003; 145: E18.

232 Leclercq C, Victor F, Alonso C, et al. Comparative effects of permanent biventricular pacing for refractory heart failure in patients with stable sinus rhythm or chronic atrial fibrillation. Am J Cardiolo 2000; 85:1154–6, A1159.

233 Leon AR, Greenberg JM, Kanuru N, et al. Cardiac resynchronization in patients with congestive heart failure and chronic atrial fibrillation: effect of upgrading to biventricular pacing after chronic right ventricular pacing. J Am Coll Cardiol 2002; 39:1258–63.

234 Leclercq C, Cazeau S, Lellouche D, et al. Upgrading from single chamber right ventricular to biventricular pacing in permanently paced patients with worsening heart failure: The RD-CHF Study. Pacing Clin Electrophysiol 2007; 30(Suppl 1):S23–30.

235 Stambler BS, Ellenbogen K, Zhang X, et al. Right ventricular outflow versus apical pacing in pacemaker patients with congestive heart failure and atrial fibrillation. J Cardiovasc Electrophysiol 2003; 14:1180–6.

236 Brignole M, Gammage M, Puggioni E, et al. Comparative assessment of right, left, and biventricular pacing in patients with permanent atrial fibrillation. Eur Heart J 2005; 26:712–22.

237 Doshi RN, Daoud EG, Fellows C, et al. Left ventricular-based cardiac stimulation post AV nodal ablation evaluation (the PAVE study). Cardiovasc Electrophysiol 2005; 16:1160–5.

238 Catanzariti D, Maines M, Cemin C, Broso G, Marotta T, Vergara G. Permanent direct his bundle pacing does not induce ventricular dyssynchrony unlike conventional right ventricular apical pacing: an intrapatient acute comparison study. J Intervent Card Electrophysiol 2006; 16:81–92.

239 Lieberman R, Padeletti L, Schreuder J, et al. Ventricular pacing lead location alters systemic hemodynamics and left ventricular function in patients with and without reduced ejection fraction. J Am Coll Cardiol 2006; 48:1634–41.

240 Occhetta E, Bortnik M, Magnani A, et al. Prevention of ventricular desynchronization by permanent para-Hisian pacing after atrioventricular node ablation in chronic atrial fibrillation: a crossover, blinded, randomized study versus apical right ventricular pacing. J Am Coll Cardiol 2006; 47:1938–45.

241 Hoijer CJ, Meurling C, Brandt J. Upgrade to biventricular pacing in patients with conventional pacemakers and heart failure: a double-blind, randomized crossover study. Europace 2006; 8:51–5.

242 Victor F, Mabo P, Mansour H, et al. A randomized comparison of permanent septal versus apical right ventricular pacing: short-term results. J Cardiovasc Electrophysiol 2006; 17:238–42.

243 Albertsen AE, Nielsen JC, Poulsen SH, et al. Biventricular pacing preserves left ventricular performance in patients with high-grade atrio-ventricular block: a randomized comparison with DDD(R) pacing in 50 consecutive patients. Europace 2008; 10:314–20.

244 Fornwalt BK, Cummings RM, Arita T, *et al.* Acute pacing-induced dyssynchronous activation of the left ventricle creates systolic dyssynchrony with preserved diastolic synchrony. J Cardiovasc Electrophysiol 2008; 19:483–8.

245 Kypta A, Steinwender C, Kammler J, Leisch F, Hofmann R. Long-term outcomes in patients with atrioventricular block undergoing septal ventricular lead implantation compared with standard apical pacing. Europace 2008; 10:574–9.

246 Zanon F, Bacchiega E, Rampin L, *et al.* Direct His bundle pacing preserves coronary perfusion compared with right ventricular apical pacing: a prospective, cross-over mid-term study. Europace 2008; 10:580–7.

247 Vanerio G, Vidal JL, Fernandez Banizi P, Banina Aguerre D, Viana P, Tejada J. Medium- and long-term survival after pacemaker implant: improved survival with right ventricular outflow tract pacing. J Intervent Card Electrophysiol 2008; 21:195–201.

248 ten Cate TJ, Scheffer MG, Sutherland GR, Verzijlbergen JF, van Hemel NM. Right ventricular outflow and apical pacing comparably worsen the echocardiographic normal left ventricle. Eur J Echocard 2008; 9:672–7.

249 Tse HF, Wong KK, Siu CW, *et al.* Impacts of ventricular rate regularization pacing at right ventricular apical vs. septal sites on left ventricular function and exercise capacity in patients with permanent atrial fibrillation. Europace 2009; 11:594–600.

250 Tse HF, Wong KK, Siu CW, Zhang XH, Ho WY, Lau CP. Upgrading pacemaker patients with right ventricular apical pacing to right ventricular septal pacing improves left ventricular performance and functional capacity. J Cardiovasc Electrophysiol 2009; 20:901–5.

251 Yu CM, Chan JY, Zhang Q, *et al.* Biventricular pacing in patients with bradycardia and normal ejection fraction. N Engl J Med 2009; 361:2123–34.

252 Flevari P, Leftheriotis D, Fountoulaki K, *et al.* Long-term nonoutflow septal versus apical right ventricular pacing: relation to left ventricular dyssynchrony. Pacing Clin Electrophysiol 2009; 32:354–62.

253 Gong X, Su Y, Pan W, Cui J, Liu S, Shu X. Is right ventricular outflow tract pacing superior to right ventricular apex pacing in patients with normal cardiac function? Clin Cardiol 2009; 32:695–9.

254 Wang YC, Lin YH, Liu YB, *et al.* The immediate effects of pacemaker-related electric remodelling on left ventricular function in patients with sick sinus syndrome. Europace 2009; 11:1660–5.

255 Yoon HJ, Jin SW, Her SH, *et al.* Acute changes in cardiac synchrony and output according to RV pacing sites in Koreans with normal cardiac function. Echocardiography 2009; 26:665–74.

256 van Geldorp IE, Vernooy K, Delhaas T, *et al.* Beneficial effects of biventricular pacing in chronically right ventricular paced patients with mild cardiomyopathy. Europace 2010; 12:223–9.

257 Cano O, Osca J, Sancho-Tello MJ, *et al.* Comparison of effectiveness of right ventricular septal pacing versus right ventricular apical pacing. Am J Cardiol 2010; 105: 1426–32.

258 Ji L, Hu W, Yao J, *et al.* Acute mechanical effect of right ventricular pacing at different sites using velocity vector imaging. Echocardiography 2010; 27:1219–27.

259 Leong DP, Mitchell AM, Salna I, *et al.* Long-term mechanical consequences of permanent right ventricular pacing: effect of pacing site. J Cardiovasc Electrophysiol 2010; 21:1120–6.

260 Liu WH, Guo BF, Chen YL, *et al.* Right ventricular outflow tract pacing causes intraventricular dyssynchrony in patients with sick sinus syndrome: a real-time three-dimensional echocardiographic study. J Am Soc Echocardiogr 2010; 23:599–607.

261 Orlov MV, Gardin JM, Slawsky M, *et al.* Biventricular pacing improves cardiac function and prevents further left atrial remodeling in patients with symptomatic atrial fibrillation after atrioventricular node ablation. Am Heart J 2010; 159:264–70.

262 Martinelli Filho M, de Siqueira SF, Costa R, *et al.* Conventional versus biventricular pacing in heart failure and bradyarrhythmia: the COMBAT study. J Card Fail 2010; 16:293–300.

263 Inoue K, Okayama H, Nishimura K, *et al.* Right ventricular pacing from the septum avoids the acute exacerbation in left ventricular dyssynchrony and torsional behavior seen with pacing from the apex. J Am Soc Echocardiogr 2010; 23:195–200.

264 Pastore G, Zanon F, Noventa F, *et al.* Variability of left ventricular electromechanical activation during right ventricular pacing: implications for the selection of the optimal pacing site. Pacing Clin Electrophysiol 2010; 33:566–74.

265 Sanagala T, Johnston SL, Groot GD, Rhine DK, Varma N. Left atrial mechanical responses to right ventricular pacing in heart failure patients: implications for atrial fibrillation. J Cardiovasc Electrophysiol 2011; 22:866–74.

266 Rubaj A, Rucinski P, Sodolski T, *et al.* Comparison of the acute hemodynamic effect of right ventricular apex, outflow tract, and dual-site right ventricular pacing. Ann Noninvasive Electrocardiol 2010; 15:353–9.

267 Yamano T, Kubo T, Takarada S, *et al.* Advantage of right ventricular outflow tract pacing on cardiac function and coronary circulation in comparison with right ventricular apex pacing. J Am Soc Echocardiogr 2010; 23:1177–82.

268 Hara M, Nishino M, Taniike M, *et al.* Chronic effect of right ventricular pacing on left ventricular rotational synchrony in patients with complete atrioventricular block. Echocardiography 2011; 28:69–75.

269 Turner MS, Bleasdale RA, Mumford CE, Frenneaux MP, Morris-Thurgood JA. Left ventricular pacing improves haemodynamic variables in patients with heart failure with a normal QRS duration. Heart 2004; 90:502–5.

270 Vanagt WY, Verbeek XA, Delhaas T, Mertens L, Daenen WJ, Prinzen FW. The left ventricular apex is the optimal site for pediatric pacing: correlation with animal experience. Pacing Clin Electrophysiol 2004; 27:837–43.

271 Gebauer RA, Tomek V, Kubus P, *et al.* Differential effects of the site of permanent epicardial pacing on left ventricular synchrony and function in the young: implications for lead placement. Europace 2009; 11:1654–9.

272 Touiza A, Etienne Y, Gilard M, Fatemi M, Mansourati J, Blanc JJ. Long-term left ventricular pacing: assessment and comparison with biventricular pacing in patients with severe congestive heart failure. J Am Coll Cardiol 2001; 38:1966–70.

273 Blanc JJ, Bertault-Valls V, Fatemi M, Gilard M, Pennec PY, Etienne Y. Midterm benefits of left univentricular pacing in patients with congestive heart failure. Circulation 2004; 109:1741–4.

274 Auricchio A, Stellbrink C, Butter C, et al. Clinical efficacy of cardiac resynchronization therapy using left ventricular pacing in heart failure patients stratified by severity of ventricular conduction delay. J Am Coll Cardiol 2003; 42:2109–16.

275 Garrigue S, Bordachar P, Reuter S, et al. Comparison of permanent left ventricular and biventricular pacing in patients with heart failure and chronic atrial fibrillation: prospective haemodynamic study. Heart 2002; 87: 529–34.

276 Vlay SC: Alternate site biventricular pacing: Bi-V in the RV – is there a role? Pacing Clin Electrophysiol 2004; 27:567–9.

277 Pachon JC, Pachon EI, Albornoz RN, et al. Ventricular endocardial right bifocal stimulation in the treatment of severe dilated cardiomyopathy heart failure with wide QRS. Pacing Clin Electrophysiol 2001; 24:1369–76.

278 Deshmukh PM, Romanyshyn M. Direct His-bundle pacing: present and future. Pacing Clin Electrophysiol 2004; 27:862–70.

279 Zamparelli L, Martiniello AR. Right ventricular bifocal DDD pacing as primary choice for cardiac resynchronization in heart failure patients with severe mitral regurgitation (abstract). Heart Rhythm 2005; 2(Suppl.): S250.

280 Aonuma K, Yokoyama Y, Seo Y, et al. Tri-ventricular pacing: a novel concept of resynchronization therapy for better left ventricular performance in end-stage heart failure (abstract). Heart Rhythm 2005; 2(Suppl.): S131.

281 Valzania C, Rocchi G, Biffi M, et al. Left ventricular versus biventricular pacing: a randomized comparative study evaluating mid-term electromechanical and clinical effects. Echocardiography 2008; 25:141–8.

282 Kara T, Novak M, Nykodym J, et al. Short-term effects of cardiac resynchronization therapy on sleep-disordered breathing in patients with systolic heart failure. Chest 2008; 134:87–93.

283 Morales MA, Startari U, Panchetti L, Rossi A, Piacenti M. Atrioventricular delay optimization by doppler-derived left ventricular dP/dt improves 6-month outcome of resynchronized patients. Pacing Clin Electrophysiol 2006; 29:564–8.

284 Bocchiardo M, Meyer zu Vilsendorf D, Militello C, et al. Resynchronization therapy optimization by intracardiac impedance. Europace 2010; 12:1589–95.

285 Khaykin Y, Exner D, Birnie D, Sapp J, Aggarwal S, Sambelashvili A. Adjusting the timing of left-ventricular pacing using electrocardiogram and device electrograms. Europace 2011; 13:1464–70.

286 Zuber M, Toggweiler S, Quinn-Tate L, Brown L, Amkieh A, Erne P. A comparison of acoustic cardiography and echocardiography for optimizing pacemaker settings in cardiac resynchronization therapy. Pacing Clin Electrophysiol 2008; 31:802–11.

287 Heinroth KM, Elster M, Nuding S, et al. Impedance cardiography: a useful and reliable tool in optimization of cardiac resynchronization devices. Europace 2007; 9:744–50.

288 Vidal B, Tamborero D, Mont L, et al. Electrocardiographic optimization of interventricular delay in cardiac resynchronization therapy: a simple method to optimize the device. J Cardiovasc Electrophysiol 2007; 18:1252–7.

289 Bertini M, Ziacchi M, Biffi M, et al. Interventricular delay interval optimization in cardiac resynchronization therapy guided by echocardiography versus guided by electrocardiographic QRS interval width. Am J Cardiol 2008; 102:1373–7.

290 van Gelder BM, Meijer A, Bracke FA. The optimized V-V interval determined by interventricular conduction times versus invasive measurement by LVdP/dtMAX. J Cardiovasc Electrophysiol 2008; 19:939–44.

291 Leon AR, Abraham WT, Brozena S, et al. Cardiac resynchronization with sequential biventricular pacing for the treatment of moderate-to-severe heart failure. J Am Coll Cardiol 2005; 46:2298–304.

292 Bordachar P, Lafitte S, Reuter S, et al. Echocardiographic parameters of ventricular dyssynchrony validation in patients with heart failure using sequential biventricular pacing. J Am Coll Cardiol 2004; 44:2157–65.

293 van Gelder BM, Bracke FA, Meijer A, Lakerveld LJ, Pijls NH. Effect of optimizing the VV interval on left ventricular contractility in cardiac resynchronization therapy. Am J Cardiol 2004; 93:1500–3.

294 Whinnett ZI, Davies JE, Willson K, et al. Haemodynamic effects of changes in atrioventricular and interventricular delay in cardiac resynchronisation therapy show a consistent pattern: analysis of shape, magnitude and relative importance of atrioventricular and interventricular delay. Heart 2006; 92:1628–34.

295 Taha N, Zhang J, Ranjan R, et al. Biventricular pacemaker optimization guided by comprehensive echocardiography-preliminary observations regarding the effects on systolic and diastolic ventricular function and third heart sound. J Am Soc Echocardiogr 2010; 23:857–66.

296 Sciaraffia E, Malmborg H, Lonnerholm S, Blomstrom P, Blomstrom Lundqvist C. The use of impedance cardiography for optimizing the interventricular stimulation interval in cardiac resynchronization therapy: a comparison with left ventricular contractility. J Interv Card Electrophysiol 2009; 25:223–8.

297 Burri H, Sunthorn H, Somsen A, et al. Optimizing sequential biventricular pacing using radionuclide ventriculography. Heart Rhythm 2005; 2:960–5.

298 Baker JH 2nd, McKenzie J 3rd, Beau S, et al. Acute evaluation of programmer-guided AV/PV and VV delay optimization comparing an IEGM method and echocardiogram for cardiac resynchronization therapy in heart

failure patients and dual-chamber ICD implants. J Cardiovasc Electrophysiol 2007; 18:185–91.

299 Porciani MC, Rao CM, Mochi M, *et al*. A real-time three-
dimensional echocardiographic validation of an intracardiac electrogram-based method for optimizing cardiac
resynchronization therapy. Pacing Clin Electrophysiol
2008; 31:56–63.

300 Sassone B, Gabrieli L, Sacca S, *et al*. Value of right ventricular-
left ventricular interlead electrical delay to predict reverse

remodelling in cardiac resynchronization therapy: the
INTER-V pilot study. Europace 2010; 12:78–83.

301 Reinsch N, Konorza T, Woydowski D, *et al*. Iterative
cardiac output measurement for optimizing cardiac
resynchronization therapy: a randomized, blinded,
crossover study. Pacing Clin Electrophysiol 2010; 33:
1188–94.

3 Indications for Pacemakers, ICDs and CRT: Identifying Patients Who Benefit from Cardiac Rhythm Devices

Apoor S. Gami[1], David L. Hayes[2], Samuel J. Asirvatham[2], Paul A. Friedman[2]

[1]Midwest Heart Specialists, Elmhurst, IL, USA.

[2]Mayo Clinic, Rochester, MN, USA

Indications for permanent pacing 94
Atrioventricular block 94
Acute myocardial infarction 100
Chronic bifascicular and trifascicular block 101
Sinus node dysfunction 101
Neurally mediated reflex syncope 104
Tachyarrhythmias 106
Hypertrophic cardiomyopathy 107
Congestive heart failure 107
 QRS duration 111
 Right bundle branch block 111
 Atrial fibrillation 112
 Nonresponders 112
Pacing after cardiac transplantation 112
Indications for the implantable cardioverter-defibrillator 112
Secondary prevention 113
Primary prevention 113

Coronary artery disease 114
Dilated cardiomyopathy 116
Long QT syndrome 117
Brugada syndrome and sudden unexplained death syndrome 120
Other channelopathies 121
Arrhythmogenic right ventricular dysplasia 121
Hypertrophic cardiomyopathy 122
Congenital heart disease 125
Contraindications to implantable cardioverter-defibrillator therapy 126
Acknowledgement 127
References 127

Cardiac Pacing, Defibrillation and Resynchronization: A Clinical Approach, Third Edition.
David L. Hayes, Samuel J. Asirvatham, and Paul A. Friedman.
© 2013 Mayo Foundation for Medical Education and Research. Published 2013 by John Wiley & Sons, Ltd.

Guidelines for the use of cardiac pacemakers and the internal cardioverter-defibrillator (ICD) were first established in 1984 by a task force formed jointly by the American College of Cardiology (ACC) and the American Heart Association (AHA). These were most recently updated in 2008 in conjunction with the North American Society of Pacing and Electrophysiology, now named the Heart Rhythm Society (HRS).[1] In 2006, the ACC, AHA, and European Society of Cardiology (ESC) published guidelines for prevention of sudden cardiac death, which included updated guidelines for ICD implantation.[2] Based on the strength of available data and expert opinion, the indications have been divided into the following three classes:

Class I: there is evidence and/or general agreement that device implantation is beneficial, useful, and effective.

Class IIa: there is conflicting evidence and/or a divergence of opinion, and the weight of the evidence or opinion is in favor of the usefulness or efficacy of device implantation.

Class IIb: there is conflicting evidence and/or a divergence of opinion, and the usefulness or efficacy of device implantation is less established.

Class III: there is evidence and/or general agreement that device implantation is not useful or effective and in some cases may be harmful. Device implantation is contraindicated.

Indications for permanent pacing

As the guidelines classification implies, some conduction disturbances are accepted as definite indications for permanent pacing, but for others there is general agreement that permanent pacing is not required. However, expert clinicians disagree about criteria for pacemaker use and whether to use single- or dual-chamber devices for many clinical scenarios, and in a number of conduction disturbances the need for permanent pacing depends on the unique circumstances of the patient. Because of changes in diagnosis and therapy, the absolute indications for permanent pacing are constantly evolving.

Before concluding that permanent pacing is indicated, the physician must carefully assess whether it is in the best interest of the patient. This assessment should include the specifics of the cardiac rhythm disturbance, the patient's general medical status, and the patient's concerns and preferences. As a rule of thumb, bradycardias caused by nontemporary conditions that are associated with symptoms warrant pacing. These are discussed in more detail below.

Indications for permanent pacing are categorized by the underlying conduction system disorder or disease process, including:

- Atrioventricular (AV) block
- Acute myocardial infarction
- Chronic bifascicular and trifascicular block
- Sinus node dysfunction
- Neurally mediated syncope
- Tachyarrhythmias
- Hypertrophic cardiomyopathy
- Congestive heart failure
- Cardiac transplantation

The ACC/AHA/HRS guidelines also include a section on pacing indications for pediatric patients. In this chapter, specific pediatric considerations are included within the broader categories; e.g., congenital AV block is included in the section on AV block.

Atrioventricular block

AV block is the impairment of conduction of a cardiac impulse from the atrium to the ventricles. It can occur at different levels: proximal to the AV node, in the AV node, or in the His–Purkinje system. Indications for permanent pacing in patients with AV block are summarized in Table 3.1.

Electrocardiographically, AV block is divided into first-degree, second-degree, and third-degree (complete) heart block. First-degree heart block is reflected by a prolonged PR interval with conduction to the ventricle. The normal PR interval is defined electrocardiographically as a range of 120–200 ms. First-degree AV block is usually secondary to a delay of impulse conduction through the atrium or AV node (Fig. 3.1).

Second-degree AV block occurs when an atrial impulse that should be conducted to the ventricle is not conducted. The blocked impulses may be intermittent or frequent, at regular or irregular intervals, and preceded by fixed or lengthening PR intervals. A distinguishing feature of second-degree heart block is that impulse conduction occurs in a recurrent pattern rather than randomly (i.e., there is a recognizable pattern in the relationship between P waves and QRS complexes). Second-degree AV block is further classified as Mobitz type I (also called Wenckebach block), Mobitz type II block, or advanced second-degree AV block. Typical type I second-degree AV block is characterized by progressive PR interval prolongation that culminates with a nonconducted P wave (Fig. 3.2). In type II second-degree AV block, the PR interval remains constant before the nonconducted P wave (Fig. 3.3), and a P wave abruptly fails to conduct to the ventricles. The AV block is intermittent and generally repetitive. Advanced second-degree AV block is characterized by more than one nonconducted P wave in a row, with the presence of some conducted beats. Type II second-degree AV block often precedes the development of higher grades of AV block, whereas type I second-

Table 3.1 Indications for pacing in atrioventricular (AV) block.

Class I	
1	Third-degree or advanced second-degree AV block at any anatomic level associated with any one of the following conditions:
a	Symptoms (including heart failure) attributable to AV block
b	Arrhythmias and other medical conditions that require drugs that result in symptomatic bradycardia
c	Documented periods of asystole >3.0 s, any escape rate ≤40 bpm, or any esacpe rhythm below the AV junction (e.g., a wide QRS morphology) in awake, asymptomatic patients in sinus rhythm
d	A documented period of asystole >5 s in awake, asymptomatic patients in atrial fibrillation
e	After catheter ablation of the AV junction
f	Postoperative AV block that is not expected to resolve after cardiac surgery
g	Neuromuscular diseases, such as myotonic muscular dystrophy, Kearns–Sayre syndrome, Erb's (limb-girdle) dystrophy, and peroneal muscular atrophy, with or without symptoms of bradycardia
2	Asymptomatic third-degree AV block at any anatomic site with an average awake ventricular rate >40 bpm in patients with cardiomegaly or left ventricular dysfunction
3	Second-degree or third-degree AV block during exercise in the absence of myocardial ischemia
4	Symptomatic second-degree AV block regardless of type or site of block
5	Congenital third-degree AV block with a wide QRS escape rhythm, complex ventricular ectopy, or ventricular dysfunction
6	Congenital third-degree AV block in an infant with a ventricular rate <50–55 bpm or with congenital heart disease and a ventricular rate <70 bpm
Class IIa	
1	Advanced second-degree or third-degree AV block at any anatomic site with an average ventricular rate >40 bpm in the absence of cardiomegaly or hypertrophy
2	Asymptomatic type I second-degree AV block at intra- or infra-His levels found at electrophysiologic study
3	First-degree or second-degree AV block with symptoms similar to those of pacemaker syndrome
4	Congenital third-degree AV block after the first year of life with an average ventricular rate <50 bpm or abrupt pauses in ventricular rate that are two to three times the basic cycle length
5	Long QT syndrome with third-degree or advanced second-degree AV block
6	Congenital heart disease and loss of AV synchrony with impaired hemodynamics
Class IIb	
1	Severe first-degree AV block (>0.30 s) in patients with ventricular dysfunction and symptoms of heart failure in whom a shorter AV interval results in hemodynamic improvement
2	AV block due to drug use or toxicity when the block is expected to recur even after withdrawal of the drug
3	Neuromuscular diseases, such as myotonic muscular dystrophy, Kearns–Sayre syndrome, Erb's (limb-girdle) dystrophy, and peroneal muscular atrophy with any degree of AV block (including first-degree AV block), with or without symptoms of bradycardia
4	Pediatric patient with transient postoperative third-degree AV block that reverts to sinus rhythm with residual bifascicular block
5	Infant, child, adolescent, or young adult with asymptomatic congenital third-degree AV block, an acceptable rate, narrow QRS complex, and normal ventricular function
Class III	
1	Asymptomatic first-degree AV block
2	Asymptomatic type I second-degree AV block at a site above the His (i.e., the AV node) or not known to be intra- or infra-Hisian by electrophysiology study
3	AV block expected to resolve and unlikely to recur (e.g., drug toxicity, Lyme disease, nocturnally in sleep apnea, early postoperative status, transient increases in vagal time)

degree AV block is usually a less severe conduction disturbance that does not consistently progress to more advanced AV block.

Anatomically, type I second-degree AV block with a normal QRS complex usually occurs at the level of the AV node, proximal to the bundle of His. AV block that is 2 : 1 may be type I or II second-degree AV block. If the QRS complex is narrow, the block is more likely to be type I and one should search for transition of the 2 : 1 block to 3 : 2 block, during which the PR interval lengthens in the second cardiac cycle (Fig. 3.4). If the QRS complex is wide, the level of block is more

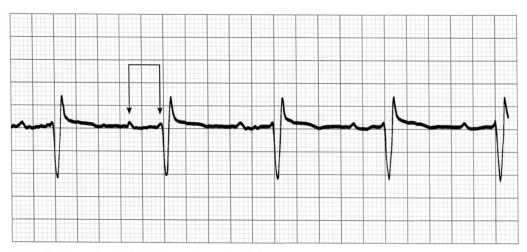

Fig. 3.1 First-degree atrioventricular block. Here, with a PR interval of 300 ms.

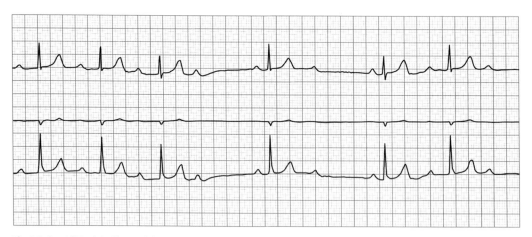

Fig. 3.2 Type I (Wenckebach) second-degree atrioventricular block.

likely to be distal to the His bundle and the escape focus is usually less reliable (Figs 3.5 and 3.6). If pre-existing bundle branch block is present, it is difficult to distinguish whether the block is located in the AV node or the His–Purkinje system. An attempt to alter the AV conduction ratio, either by exercise or by pharmacologic means (e.g., with atropine) may allow localization of the conduction abnormality and assist with diagnosis. AV block that develops or worsens during exercise reflects conduction disease in the His–Purkinje system, which warrants implantation of a permanent pacemaker. During exercise, increased adrenergic drive facilitates AV nodal conduction; a diseased distal conduction system is unable to accom-modate the increased rate and block occurs. In contrast, block in the AV node is more often physiologic, due to increased vagal tone. Exercise changes the autonomic balance, leading to diminished vagal tone and improved conduction. Pacing is generally not needed in this situation.

Third-degree AV block (complete heart block) is defined by lack of conduction of atrial impulses to the ventricle (Fig. 3.7). It is important to distinguish this from AV dissociation due to a subsidiary pacemaker, usually junctional, that discharges more rapidly than the underlying sinus rate. In contrast, in third-degree AV block, the atrial rate is faster than the ventricular escape and there is no AV nodal conduction.

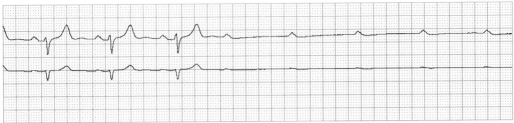

00:07:41-2

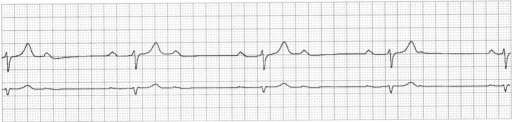

00:11:32-2

Fig. 3.3 Advanced atrioventricular block, in which there is sporadic failure to conduct from the atrium to the ventricle. Here, the first and last P waves result in ventricular depolarization, with a PR interval of 220 ms. However, nine P waves are not conducted through the AV node, and the result is a 7.4-s period of ventricular asystole.

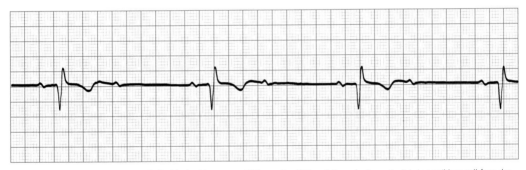

Fig. 3.4 Second-degree 2:1 atrioventricular block with a narrow QRS complex. With a 2:1 conduction ratio, it is impossible to tell from the electrocardiogram exactly where in the atrioventricular junction the conduction disturbance occurs. A narrow QRS complex suggests that the conduction defect is "supra-His" (at the level of the atrioventricular node or His bundle) rather than "infra-His," which would result more commonly in a wide QRS complex.

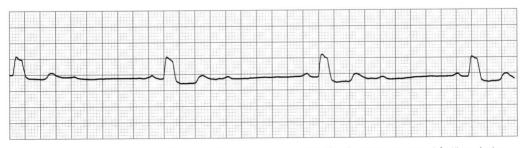

Fig. 3.5 Second-degree 2:1 atrioventricular block with left intraventricular conduction delay. This pattern suggests an infra-His conduction defect.

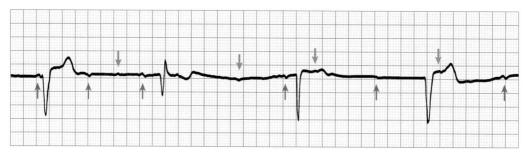

Fig. 3.6 Subsequent electrocardiogram from the patient whose recording is shown in Fig. 3.5. Here, there is intermittent third-degree atrioventricular block with junctional escape beats (arrows indicate P waves).

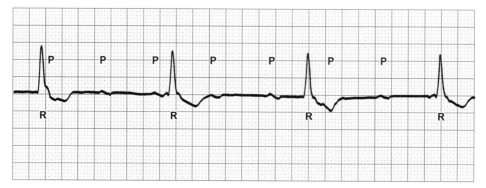

Fig. 3.7 Third-degree atrioventricular block (complete heart block) is characterized by complete lack of conduction from atrium to ventricle and dissociation of atrial and ventricular activity. Here, the atrial activity (identified by P's on the tracing) occur at approximately 100 bpm, whereas the ventricular complexes (R's) occur at just under 40 bpm.

Third-degree AV block may be congenital or acquired. In the congenital form, there is anatomic discontinuity in the conduction pathway. Pacing for this disorder was controversial for many years, because many patients with congenital complete heart block consider themselves asymptomatic, and there was conflicting information on the risk of sudden death associated with the condition. However, subjective improvement is usually noted once chronotropic competency is restored with permanent pacing. In addition, data support improved survival with permanent pacing.[3,4] Indications for pacing in patients with congenital complete heart block are the presence of a wide QRS escape rhythm, complex ventricular ectopy, or ventricular dysfunction; or, in an infant, a ventricular rate of <50–55 bpm, or a ventricular rate <70 bpm if congenital heart disease is also present. In addition, a class IIa indication is congenital complete heart block after the first year of life with an average ventricular rate <50 bpm or abrupt pauses in ventricular rate that are

two or three times the basic cycle length. Finally, congenital complete heart block in an asymptomatic infant, child, adolescent, or young adult with an acceptable rate, narrow QRS, and normal ventricular function is considered a class IIb indication.[1] In summary, pacing can be justified in any patient with congenital complete heart block, although the strength of evidence varies depending on the clinical circumstance.

Acquired third-degree AV block is due most commonly to aging, with or without calcification of the conduction system, or ischemic disease (e.g., myocardial infarction with damage involving the conduction system). Complete heart block has been associated with a number of systemic illnesses, many of which have been described in case reports (Table 3.2). Iatrogenic complete heart block can occur with open heart surgery or with inadvertent AV node ablation during treatment of supraventricular tachyarrhythmias. Acquired complete heart block can be either intermittent or fixed. Patients may be asymptomatic or experience severe

Table 3.2 Causes of acquired atrioventricular (AV) block.

Idiopathic (senescent) AV block
Coronary artery disease
Calcific valvular disease
Postoperative or traumatic
AV node ablation
Therapeutic radiation to the chest

Infections:
• Syphilis
• Diphtheria
• Chagas' disease
• Tuberculosis
• Toxoplasmosis
• Lyme disease
• Viral myocarditis
• Infective endocarditis

Collagen-vascular diseases:
• Rheumatoid arthritis
• Scleroderma
• Dermatomyositis
• Ankylosing spondylitis
• Polyarteritis nodosa
• Systemic lupus erythematosus
• Marfan's syndrome

Infiltrative diseases:
• Sarcoidosis
• Amyloidosis
• Hemochromatosis
• Malignant disease (lymphomatous or solid tumor)

Neuromuscular diseases:
• Progressive external ophthalmoplegia, Kearns–Sayre syndrome
• Myotonic muscular dystrophy
• Peroneal muscular atrophy, Charcot–Marie–Tooth disease
• Scapuloperoneal syndrome
• Erb's (limb-girdle) dystrophy

Drug effects:
• Digoxin
• β-Blockers
• Calcium-blocking agents
• Amiodarone
• Procainamide
• Class 1C agents: propafenone, encainide, flecainide

symptoms related to profound bradycardia, AV dissociation, or ventricular arrhythmias. It has been well documented that patients with complete heart block have improved survival with permanent pacing.[5]

The most important factor in the decision to implant a pacemaker in a patient with AV block is whether or not the patient has symptoms that may be directly attributed to the arrhythmia. These symptoms include overt or near syncope, lightheadedness, fatigue, activity intolerance, dyspnea, confusion or other cognitive changes, or symptoms of heart failure. Another important factor in the decision to implant a pacemaker for AV block is the expected irreversibility of the conduction disturbance. Potentially reversible causes of AV block include electrolyte abnormalities, Lyme disease, perioperative hypothermia or inflammation, sleep apnea, and vagally mediated bradyarrhythmias related to medical illness or physiologic changes in autonomic tone (e.g., bradycardia during emesis).

Atrial fibrillation with a slow ventricular response reflects the presence of AV block, although it is often categorized as sinus node dysfunction. Patients with this condition should receive a pacemaker if the bradycardia is causing symptoms (Fig. 3.8).

Areas of controversy exist in the indications for permanent pacing for AV block, and there are situations in which deviations from the ACC/AHA/HRS guidelines may be appropriate. Although the guidelines designate asymptomatic complete heart block with ventricular escape rates >40 bpm as a class IIa indication for pacing, we believe it should be a class I indication. The rate cut-off of 40 bpm is arbitrary, and it is not the escape rate per se that is critical to stability, but rather the site of origin of the escape rhythm (i.e., the AV node, His bundle, His–Purkinje system, or the ventricle). No definitive evidence exists regarding the conduction system localization or long-term stability of an escape rate of 40 bpm. Unfortunately, rate stability is not obvious or predictable. Clinically, one must grapple with whether the patient is truly asymptomatic and whether any diagnostic procedures, such as ambulatory monitoring or exercise testing, should be performed. No clinical trials or observational studies provide

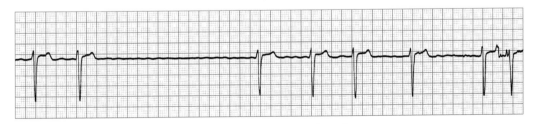

Fig. 3.8 Atrial fibrillation with a variable ventricular response and a 3.5-s episode of asystole.

answers to these questions. From a practical and safety standpoint, we believe that permanent pacing is warranted for irreversible, acquired, complete heart block.

Some asymptomatic patients with type I second-degree AV block have as poor a prognosis as patients with type II second-degree AV block, and permanent pacing improves survival in those patients >45 years old.[6,7] Asymptomatic type I second-degree AV block not known to be at intra- or infra-Hisian levels is a class III indication (a contraindication) for pacing. Generally, an electrophysiology study to obtain His bundle recordings is not recommended. However, if an electrophysiology study is performed for other reasons and asymptomatic type I second-degree AV block with a narrow QRS is found to be infranodal, then pacemaker implantation is a class IIa indication according to the current guidelines. In this setting, a patient is likely to have diffuse conduction system disease, and we believe permanent pacing is warranted.

In patients with specific neuromuscular diseases, pacing is advocated as a class I indication in third-degree AV block and as a class IIb indication in first-degree or second-degree AV block. The potential for sudden death in this group of patients is well documented.[8–11] Because of the unpredictable progression to symptomatic bradycardia in patients with first-degree or second-degree AV block, the safest and most rational approach may be to offer pacing once any conduction abnormality is noted and subsequent follow-up reveals any progression. As discussed later, ICD therapy may also need to be considered for these patients.[12]

Acute myocardial infarction

Conduction disturbances associated with acute myocardial infarction are largely related to the site of the infarction and the extent of myocardial injury.[13,14] Given a greater awareness of the symptoms of acute myocardial infarction, the seeking of healthcare earlier, and more aggressive acute intervention, there are fewer extensive infarcts and permanent pacing is becoming less frequently required in this situation. Inferior myocardial infarctions are accompanied by a variety of conduction disturbances, including sinus bradycardia, sinus arrest, atrial fibrillation, atrial flutter, and all grades of AV block.[15] Anterior myocardial infarctions are more likely to be accompanied by AV block or intraventricular conduction defects (or both).[16]

The indications for permanent pacemaker implantation after an acute myocardial infarction are based on the persistence of AV block and the presence of concomitant intraventricular conduction disturbances (Table 3.3). A general rule is that a permanent pace-

Table 3.3 Indications for permanent pacing after acute myocardial infarction (MI).

Class I	
1	Third-degree atrioventricular (AV) block within or below the His–Purkinje system after ST-segment elevation MI or persistent second-degree AV block in the His–Purkinje system with alternating bundle branch block
2	Transient second- or third-degree infranodal AV block and associated bundle branch block. If the site of block is uncertain, an electrophysiologic study may be necessary
3	Persistent and symptomatic second- or third-degree AV block
Class IIa	
	None
Class IIb	
	Persistent second- or third-degree transient AV block at the AV node level, with or without symptoms
Class III	
1	Transient AV block without intraventricular conduction defects
2	Transient AV block with isolated left anterior fascicular block
3	Acquired left anterior fascicular block without AV block
4	Asymptomatic first-degree AV block with bundle branch or fasicular block

maker is not indicated in a patient with an acute myocardial infarction if AV block is expected to resolve and if the conduction disturbance is not associated with a poor long-term prognosis.[15,16] The indications are less dependent on the presence or absence of symptoms, unlike pacing indications in other clinical settings. Clear class I indications are persistent, severe conduction disturbances (second-degree AV block in the His–Purkinje system with bilateral bundle branch block, or third-degree AV block at or below the His–Purkinje system). Also considered a class I indication is transient advanced (second-degree or third-degree) infranodal AV block and associated bundle branch block. A reasonable rule of thumb is useful in the patient with transient second-degree or third-degree AV block and associated bundle branch block: after an anterior wall myocardial infarction, a pacemaker is indicated if vagal block is excluded, because the block is almost certainly infranodal; after an inferior wall myocardial infarction no pacemaker is needed, because the prognosis is good and is not adversely affected by the AV block. Also, it is important to note that a requirement for temporary pacing in a patient with acute myocardial infarction

Table 3.4 Indications for pacing in chronic bifascicular and trifascicular block.

Class I
1   Intermittent third-degree or advanced second-degree atrioventricular (AV) block
2   Type II second-degree AV block
3   Alternating bundle branch block.
Class IIa
1   Syncope not demonstrated to be due to AV block when other likely causes, specifically ventricular tachycardia, have been excluded
2   Incidental finding at electrophysiologic study of markedly prolonged HV interval (≥100 ms) in asymptomatic patients
3   Incidental finding at electrophysiologic study of pacing-induced infra-His block that is not physiologic
Class IIb
Neuromuscular diseases, such as myotonic muscular dystrophy, Kearns–Sayre syndrome, Erb's (limb-girdle) dystrophy, and peroneal muscular atrophy with any degree of fascicular block, with or without symptoms of bradycardia
Class III
1   Fascicular block without AV block or symptoms
2   Fascicular block with first-degree AV block without symptoms

does not constitute an indication for permanent pacing for that patient.

Chronic bifascicular and trifascicular block

Bifascicular block is defined as a conduction disturbance of two fascicles of the ventricular conduction system (e.g., isolated left bundle branch block, right bundle branch block [RBBB] and left anterior fascicular block, or RBBB and left posterior fascicular block). Trifascicular block is defined as a conduction disturbance in all three fascicles (either simultaneously or in successive ECGs) or the presence of first-degree AV block and bifascicular block. A special example of trifascicular block is alternating bundle branch block (also referred to as bilateral bundle branch block).

Indications for permanent pacing in patients with bifascicular or trifascicular block depend on the risk of development of transient or permanent advanced AV block (Table 3.4).[17] This is because patients with bifascicular or trifascicular block and advanced AV block have higher rates of sudden death and all-cause death. Syncope is common in patients with bifascicular block, but it is not associated with an increased risk of sudden

death. Thus, defining the cause of syncope in patients with bifascicular and trifascicular block is important, and a permanent pacemaker should be implanted if transient or persistent, advanced AV block is documented. If, after investigation, the cause of syncope is undetermined, then implantation of a permanent pacemaker is reasonable (class IIa indication), because the syncope may be due to intermittent advanced AV block. However, it is notable that the incidence of progression of bifascicular block to complete heart block is low, and that there are no reliable predictors of death from progression of the conduction disease. Patients with RBBB and left anterior hemiblock are at higher risk of cardiovascular death, but this is not specifically due to bradycardia or conduction disease, and permanent pacing is not recommended in these patients in the absence of symptoms or advanced AV block.

Although the incidence of progression to advanced AV block is relatively low in patients with bifascicular or trifascicular block, measurement of the HV interval (a measure of conduction of the His–Purkinje system) may rarely help in identifying patients at higher risk of developing symptomatic advanced AV block. The degree of HV interval lengthening necessary to justify prophylactic pacemaker placement is controversial. Some have advocated pacing for an HV interval of >100 ms, and others have considered pacing for an HV interval of >70 ms, especially if the patient is to receive cardioactive drugs that have the potential for further impairment of the conduction system. The development of nonphysiologic infra-His block with increasingly rapid atrial pacing during an electrophysiology study may reflect increased risk of progression to advanced AV block or symptomatic bradycardias (and thus has a class IIa indication for permanent pacing); however, failure to develop infra-His block is not a reliable indicator that advanced AV block will not develop in the future. Electrophysiologic studies to measure HV intervals are not routinely performed in patients with bifascular or trifascular block in the absence of symptoms or other findings.

Sinus node dysfunction

Sinus node dysfunction (sick sinus syndrome) includes a variety of cardiac arrhythmias, including sinus bradycardia (Fig. 3.9), sinus arrest (Fig. 3.10), and sinoatrial block. It also includes the tachycardia-bradycardia syndrome, in which paroxysmal supraventricular tachycardias alternate with periods of bradycardia or asystole (Fig. 3.11). Indications for permanent pacing in patients with sinus node dysfunction are summarized in Table 3.5.

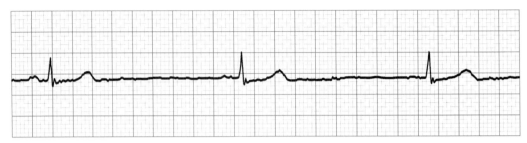

Fig. 3.9 Sinus bradycardia with a rate of 39 bpm. The patient had symptoms that resolved after DDD pacing.

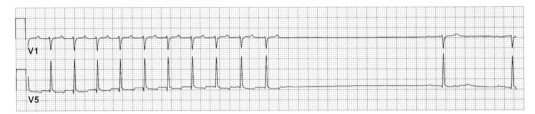

Fig. 3.10 Continuous electrocardiographic tracing from a patient with tachycardia-bradycardia syndrome (sinus node dysfunction). Here, sinus rhythm alternates with atrial flutter, and an episode of sinus arrest with a 4.5-s pause occurs.

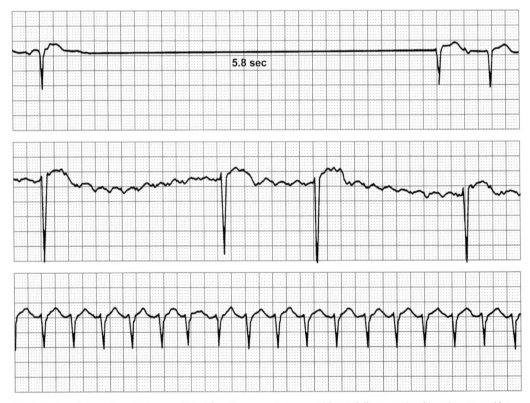

Fig. 3.11 Three electrocardiographic tracings obtained from the same patient over a 12-h period. The top tracing shows sinus arrest with a 5.8-s pause terminated by a junctional escape beat. The middle tracing shows atrial flutter with a slow ventricular response. The bottom tracing shows supraventricular tachycardia.

Table 3.5 Indications for pacing in sinus node dysfunction.

Class I
1   Sinus node dysfunction with symptomatic bradycardia or frequent symptomatic sinus pauses. In some patients, bradycardia is iatrogenic and occurs as a consequence of essential long-term drug therapy for which there is no acceptable alternative. The definition of bradycardia varies with the patient's age and expected heart rate
2   Symptomatic chronotropic incompetence

Class IIa
1   Sinus node dysfunction occurring spontaneously or as a result of necessary drug therapy, with heart rate <40 bpm, when a clear association between significant symptoms consistent with bradycardia and the actual presence of bradycardia has not been documented
2   Syncope of unknown etiology when sinus node dysfunction is provoked or discovered during electrophysiologic testing that is felt to be clinically significant

Class IIb
    In minimally symptomatic patients, chronic heart rate <40 bpm while awake

Class III
1   Sinus node dysfunction in asymptomatic patients
2   Sinus node dysfunction in patients with symptoms that are clearly documented in the absence of bradycardia
3   Sinus node dysfunction with symptomatic bradycardia due to nonessential drug therapy

Table 3.6 Indications for pacing in neurally mediated reflex syncope.

Class I
    Recurrent syncope caused by carotid sinus hypersensitivity, defined as minimal carotid sinus pressure inducing ventricular asystole of ≥3 s in patients not receiving medication that depress the sinus node or AV conduction

Class IIa
    Syncope in the absence of definite provocative event with a pause of ≥3 s with carotid massage

Class IIb
    Recurrent symptomatic neurocardiogenic syncope with a cardioinhibitory response during tilt-table testing

Class III
1   A cardioinhibitory response during carotid sinus stimulation without symptoms or vague symptoms
2   Situational vasovagal syncope in which avoidance behavior is effective

The definition of clinically significant bradycardia varies, but it is generally agreed to denote rates of <40 bpm during waking hours. Sinus pauses of ≥3 s or symptomatic sinus rates <40 bpm in the awake patient are indications for permanent pacing. However, it should be recognized that there is disagreement about the absolute cycle length of an asystolic period that requires pacing. The patient's entire clinical condition should be considered, including age, associated diseases, medications, and symptoms. For example, sleeping endurance athletes have sinus rates as low as 30 bpm, but are asymptomatic and do not require pacing. Sinus bradycardia during sleep in an asymptomatic patient is not an indication for pacing. Sleep apnea is a potential cause of nocturnal bradycardias that should be treated if considered clinically significant.[18,19] This is particularly true if atrial fibrillation is also present, because approximately half of patients with atrial fibrillation also have obstructive sleep apnea.[20]

In sinus node dysfunction, correlation of symptoms with the specific arrhythmia is essential. The use of ambulatory ECG monitors and event loop recorders is helpful to document patients' rhythms during specific symptoms. Patients who develop symptomatic bradycardias due to required pharmacologic therapy for other conditions require permanent pacing, but pacing is unnecessary if the bradycardias are asymptomatic. Chronotropic incompetence may be demonstrated by the absence of an appropriate physiologic increase in sinus rate with exercise, and it is a class I indication for implantation of a rate-responsive permanent pacemaker.

When permanent pacing is indicated for patients with sinus node dysfunction, special thought should be given to selection of the appropriate device and programming. Single-chamber ventricular pacemakers are not appropriate for patients with sinus node dysfunction. Single-chamber atrial pacemakers with rate-responsive capability are attractive because of their relative simplicity and lower cost compared with dual-chamber pacemakers. In patients without coexisting AV block, AAIR pacing may be appropriate. The major concern is that AV block develops in patients with sinus node dysfunction after atrial pacemaker implantation at an annual rate of 0.6–5%, with a higher risk in patients with pre-existing bundle branch block.[21,22] Although this risk is relatively low, there is some benefit to provide ventricular pacing in the event it is needed. Conversely, pacing the ventricle unnecessarily can result in a higher incidence of atrial fibrillation and congestive heart failure.[23–26] Avoidance of ventricular pacing can be accomplished by programming a very

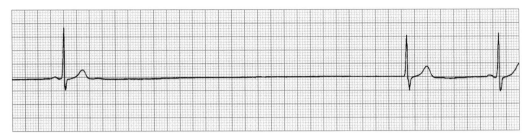

Fig. 3.12 Carotid sinus massage may demonstrate carotid sinus hypersensitivity, which may be a cause of syncope. Here, carotid sinus massage produced prolonged sinus arrest with a junctional escape.

long AV interval, or by use of an algorithm that effectively avoids ventricular pacing except when absolutely required by predefined criteria (discussed further in Chapter 8: Programming). Thus, the best options for sinus node dysfunction are either a single-chamber atrial pacemaker or a dual-chamber pacemaker that is programmed either manually or via an algorithm to avoid ventricular pacing. The decision must be made on an individual basis, with consideration of the extent of conduction disease, severity of its clinical manifestations, comorbidities, risk of future revision to a dual-chamber system, and the patient's own preferences. In the USA, dual-chamber pacemakers are most commonly used.

Neurally mediated reflex syncope

Permanent pacing is indicated in the proper clinical setting for some types of neurally mediated reflex syncope, which includes carotid sinus syndrome and neurocardiogenic (vasovagal) syncope (Table 3.6). Understanding the physiology involved in these different types of syncope is crucial to understanding their clinical manifestations and the appropriateness of permanent pacing.[27]

The carotid sinus reflex is the physiologic bradycardic response to stimulation of the carotid sinus baroreceptors. Although this reflex is normal, some individuals have an exaggerated response that may be pathologic. This reflex has two components. The first, a cardio-inhibitory response, results from increased parasympathetic tone and may be manifested by any or all of the following: sinus bradycardia, sinus arrest (Fig. 3.12), PR prolongation, and advanced AV block. The second component, a vasodepressor response, is due to decreased sympathetic activity and results in peripheral vasodilatation and hypotension (independently of changes in heart rate). Pure cardio-inhibitory or pure vasodepressor responses may occur, but a mixed response is most common.

The definitions of normal and abnormal responses to carotid sinus stimulation are somewhat arbitrary. Generally, an abnormal response is defined as development of ventricular asystole of $\geq 3\,$s and/or a decrease in blood pressure of 30–50 mmHg. As many as 40% of patients ≥ 65 years old have carotid sinus hypersensitivity;[28] thus, the causal relationship between carotid sinus hypersensitivity and symptoms is critical to decisions regarding therapy. Patients with syncope may have a typical history related to a tight collar or neck extension, but more commonly definite provocative maneuvers cannot be identified. If carotid sinus massage reproduces the patient's symptoms and is associated with significant cardio-inhibition or vasodepression, a diagnosis of carotid sinus syndrome can be made and treatment should be initiated. If carotid sinus massage yields a positive result but does not reproduce the patient's symptoms, a hypersensitive carotid reflex has been demonstrated, but it may not be of clinical significance, and other causes for syncope should be investigated. Situations exist where it is difficult to correlate symptoms. If the result of carotid sinus massage is negative, tilt testing may be indicated to identify other mechanisms of neurally mediated reflex syncope.

Neurocardiogenic (vasovagal) syncope may be benign or malignant. The exact pathophysiology of these syndromes is unclear, but important mechanisms include prolonged orthostatic stress, venous pooling, activation of cardiac mechanoreceptors, and an abnormal decrease in sympathetic activity. These processes result in bradycardia, peripheral vasodilatation, and syncope.[27] The episodes can be triggered by various stimuli, such as pain, warm environments, visceral sensations, and acute psychologic stress. Manifestations include a prodrome of nausea, diaphoresis, and light-headedness followed by a brief episode of unconsciousness, after which there is quick and complete cognitive recovery. In the elderly, prodromal symptoms

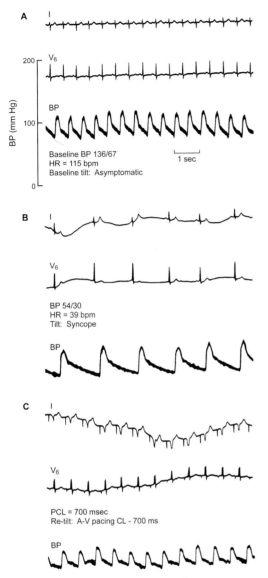

Fig. 3.13 Electrocardiographic and arterial blood pressure recordings obtained during head-up tilt-table testing. (A) Recordings made during tilt with the patient asymptomatic demonstrate normal sinus rhythm at a heart rate (HR) of 115 bpm and baseline blood pressure (BP) of 136/67 mmHg. (B) Recordings during syncope, at which time the HR was 39 bpm and the BP was 54/30 mmHg. (C) After atrioventricular sequential pacing at a cycle length of 700 ms (86 ppm), a subsequent tilt-table test produced significant vasodepression, but the patient experienced only presyncope. (Courtesy of Dr. W.K. Shen, Mayo Clinic, Rochester, MN.)

are often absent and loss of consciousness may occur suddenly, mimicking other causes of syncope.[29]

Head-up tilt-table testing can reproduce neurocardiogenic syncope in susceptible patients. Passive head-up tilt creates an exaggerated orthostatic state by stressing the autonomic system in the absence of the usual compensatory skeletal muscle tone. This triggers the cascade of mechanisms described above. Tilt-table testing can help identify whether the predominant cause of symptoms is vasodepressor or cardio-inhibitory in origin (Fig. 3.13), which is important because therapy may differ for each situation.

Benign vasovagal syncope, or a "simple faint," usually does not require therapy. Associated rhythms are usually prolonged sinus arrest without a junctional or ventricular escape rhythm (Fig. 3.14). Situational syncope, which occurs stereotypically with swallowing, cough, micturition, or defecation, does not significantly increase mortality and usually does not require permanent pacing. However, recurrent events may be disabling to some patients, and the situations during which the events occur, such as operation of a motor vehicle or heavy machinery, may predispose the patient or bystanders to danger. In these cases, permanent pacemaker implantation may be an effective means of preventing syncope; however, this is unproven and controversial.

In patients with significant cardio-inhibition, permanent pacing is a seemingly intuitive intervention. Despite early promise,[30–32] randomized trials have shown that permanent pacing does not improve outcomes in patients with neurocardiogenic syncope.[33,34] The data suggested a benefit with permanent pacing only in patients with severe cardio-inhibition (i.e., asystole) compared with those with less severe bradycardias during tilt-table testing. The indications for permanent pacing in patients with neurocardiogenic syncope include: (i) a significant cardio-inhibitory component with severe bradycardia or asystole during syncope; (ii) lack of a prodrome; and (iii) recurrent syncope despite maximally tolerated medical therapy.[35] Pacemakers with the capability of triggering a faster pacing rate for a defined period of time in response to a specified sudden drop in heart rate have been developed specifically for this syndrome. For all patients with neurocardiogenic syncope, principal therapy includes diet and lifestyle modification, compression stockings, and pharmacologic agents. Most patients have a mixed cardio-inhibitory and vasodepressor response, and it is most common for hypotension to precede bradycardia during an episode, so the medical therapies must continue even after pacemaker implantation, when pacing is offered.

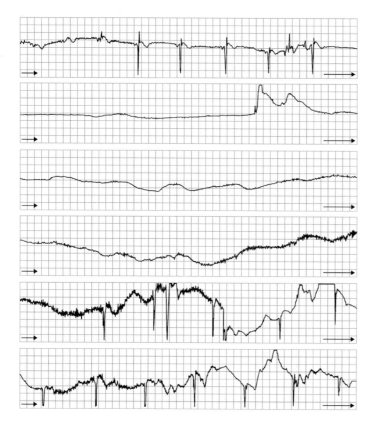

Fig. 3.14 Continuous electrocardiographic recording in a 55-year-old man who has hypervagotonia, with an asystolic period >30 s. Recovery with sinus bradycardia occurs in the fifth panel.

Tachyarrhythmias

Previously, national guidelines recognized a number of class I indications for implantation of permanent pacemakers that detect and pace to terminate tachyarrhythmias. These devices initiate programmed stimulation or bursts of rapid pacing to terminate re-entrant arrhythmias after their automatic detection or after user activation (by magnet application). However, because of the wide availability and success of treatment by catheter ablation, there are currently no class I indications for permanent pacemakers to treat supraventricular tachyarrhythmias (Tables 3.7 and 3.8). Indications for device implantation in the treatment of ventricular tachyarrhythmias is discussed in a subsequent section (see Indications for the implantable cardioverter-defibrillator).

The implantation of a permanent pacemaker to prevent or treat tachyarrhythmias is still indicated in rare situations. A class I indication is for patients with or without a long QT interval who experience recurrent pause-dependent ventricular tachycardia (VT). The device of choice in these individuals is an implanted cardioverter-defibrillator with a bradycardia pacing function. The use of pacemakers to terminate supraventricular tachycardias or to prevent AV node re-entrant or AV re-entrant tachycardias when drugs or catheter ablation fail are class IIa indications. The success rate typically exceeds 95% with catheter ablation for these arrhythmias, so pacing is rarely used. Atrial fibrillation, atrial flutter, and atrial tachycardia are common in patients with sinus node dysfunction and an implanted pacemaker. Some devices have atrial fibrillation-prevention algorithms, including rate-adaptive atrial overdrive pacing, pacing to suppress premature atrial complexes, and rate response to limit the rate of decrease in heart rate after exercise. Some devices also provide atrial antitachycardia pacing therapy, which is about 50% effective in terminating organized atrial arrhythmias. These algorithms have been shown to reduce the overall burden of atrial arrhythmias in some patient populations.[36–40] However, important improvements in clinical outcomes have not been shown, limiting the role of pacing for prevention or termination of atrial arrhythmias to patients who

Table 3.7 Indications for pacemakers to terminate tachycardia.

Class I
None
Class IIa
Symptomatic recurrent supraventricular tachycardia that is reproducibly terminated by pacing in the unlikely event that catheter ablation and/or drugs fail to control the arrhythmia or produce intolerable side effects
Class III
The presence of accessory pathways with the capacity for rapid anterograde conduction

Table 3.8 Indications for pacemakers to prevent tachycardia.

Class I
Pause-dependent sustained ventricular tachycardia with or without prolonged QT
Class IIa
Pacing is reasonable for patients with congenital long-QT syndrome considered to be high-risk
Class IIb
Prevention of symptomatic, drug-refractory recurrent atrial fibrillation in patients with coexisting sinus node dysfunction
Class III
1 Frequent or complex ventricular ectopic activity without sustained ventricular tachycardia in patients without long QT syndrome
2 Torsades de pointes ventricular tachycardia due to reversible causes

also have another device indication. Implantation of a pacemaker for prevention, reduction, or treatment of atrial arrhythmias is a class IIb indication. In patients with an implanted pacemaker and recurrent symptomatic atrial arrhythmias, consideration could be given to the use of a device with atrial antitachycardia pacing capabilities. However, in patients with atrial tachyarrhythmias and no bradycardia pacing indication, atrial ablation is offered for patients who are candidates, whereas AV nodal ablation and pacing controls symptoms when atrial ablation is not appropriate.

Hypertrophic cardiomyopathy

Standard indications for permanent pacing related to sinus node dysfunction or AV block, discussed above, apply equally to patients with hypertrophic cardiomyopathy (HCM). Patients who undergo transcatheter septal ablation to alleviate an outflow gradient have an estimated 11% chance of developing subacute complete heart block, and they are treated with dual-chamber permanent pacing.[41] Although an additional class IIb indication exists for the use of dual-chamber pacing in patients with HCM who have a demonstrable significant left ventricular outflow gradient and continue to have symptoms despite medical and/or surgical treatment, randomized trials have not demonstrated that this intervention significantly improves symptoms or outcomes.[42–44] Indications for ICD therapy in patients with HCM are discussed in a subsequent section (see Indications for the implantable cardioverter-defibrillator).

Congestive heart failure

One-quarter to one-third of patients with congestive heart failure have left bundle branch block,[45] which has been associated with increased mortality.[45,46] With left bundle branch block, the left ventricle is initially activated at the anteroseptum, with delayed activation and contraction of the left ventricular lateral wall (Fig. 3.15). This dyssynchrony of ventricular activation leads to impaired pumping efficiency. In selected patients with refractory heart failure, pacing both ventricles (referred to as biventricular pacing or cardiac resynchronization therapy [CRT]) restores synchrony and improves exercise tolerance, clinical and biochemical markers of heart failure, ejection fraction, quality of life, and survival.[47–52] The left ventricle is most commonly paced by placing an electrode in a coronary sinus tributary (Fig. 3.16). The implant technique is discussed in detail in Chapter 5. Most patients with depressed ventricular function and heart failure are also at risk for sudden cardiac arrest due to ventricular tachyarrhythmias, and they commonly receive a device capable of both resynchronization and defibrillation (CRT-D, as opposed to a device solely for resynchronization pacing [CRT-P]). The indications for CRT-D are discussed in a subsequent section (see Indications for the implantable cardioverter-defibrillator).

The 2012 ACCF/AHA/HSR Focused Update of the guidelines provide recommendation for CRT in specific populations based on the current data (summarized in Table 3.9). It is helpful to consider the indications for CRT in two broad categories:

1 Patients with left ventricular dysfunction and conventional indications for antibradycardia pacing

Standard indications for permanent pacing related to sinus node dysfunction or AV block, discussed earlier, apply equally to patients with heart failure. However, there are special considerations when pacing patients

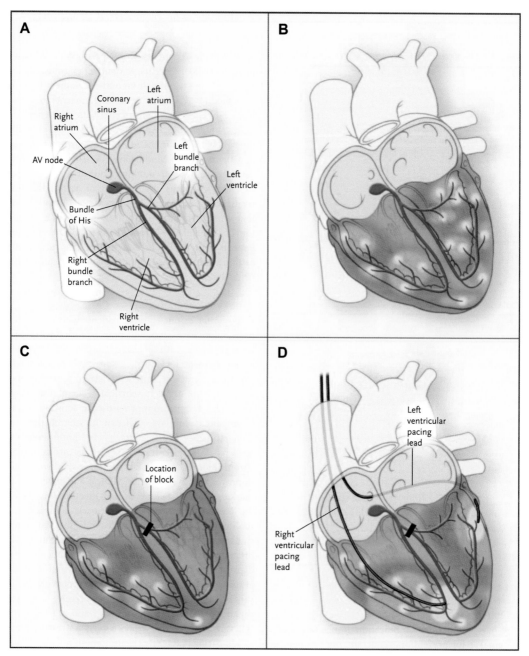

Fig. 3.15 Sequence of left ventricular activation in patients with left bundle branch block. The left ventricular lateral wall is depolarized last and leads to dyssynchronous global ventricular function that impairs hemodynamics. (Reproduced from Jarcho J. Biventricular pacing. N Engl J Med 2006; 355:288–94, by permission of Massachusetts Medical Society.)

Fig. 3.16 (A) Chest X-ray showing typical biventricular pacemaker lead placement. Three pacemaker leads are implanted via the extrathoracic veins and superior vena cava. One lead is placed in the right atrium, a second lead is placed across the tricuspid valve into the right ventricle, and a third lead is placed via the coronary sinus into a venous tributary on the lateral wall of the left ventricle. Ideally, the left and right ventricular pacing leads are spatially separated as shown on the posteroanterior and lateral chest radiographs. This provides nearly simultaneous activation of the ventricles and produces a narrow QRS complex on the electrocardiogram. (B) left panel: view of ventricles with atrial removed. The coronary sinus (CS) drains into the right atrium, near the tricuspid valve (TV). Advancement of a lead into the CS, which wraps around the mitral valve (MV), permits advancement to a lateral left ventricular position. Right panel: left lateral view of the epicardial surface of the heart. Arrow indicates a lateral epicardial vein, an ideal target for a left ventricular lead. AV, aortic valve; LAD, left anterior descending artery; LCX, left circumflex artery; PV, pulmonic valve.

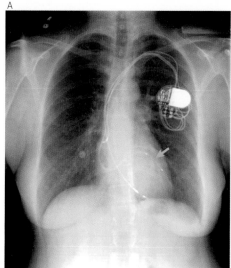

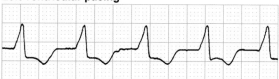

Left ventricular pacing

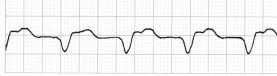

Right ventricular pacing

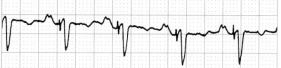

Biventricular pacing

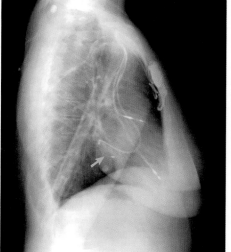

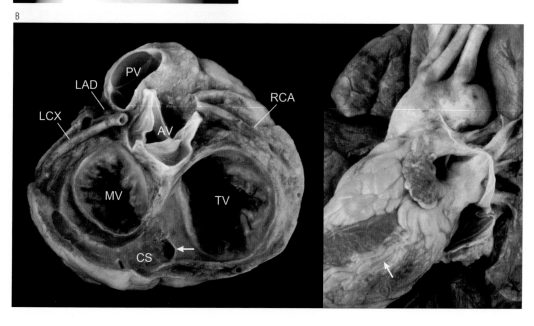

Table 3.9 Recommendations for CRT in patients with systolic heart failure.*

Class I	
1	LVEF ≤35%, sinus rhythm, LBBB with QRS ≥150 ms, NYHA class II, III, or ambulatory IV symptoms on GDMT
Class IIa	
1	LVEF ≤35%, sinus rhythm (level of evidence A) or atrial fibrillation (level of evidence B), LBBB with QRS 120–149 ms, NYHA class II, III, or ambulatory IV symptoms on GDMT
2	LVEF ≤35%, sinus rhythm (level of evidence A) or atrial fibrillation (level of evidence B), non-LBBB with QRS ≥150 ms, NYHA class III, or ambulatory IV symptoms on GDMT
3	LVEF ≤35%, atrial fibrillation, and expected near 100% ventricular pacing, on GDMT (Level of evidence B)
4	LVEF ≤35%, expected >40% frequency of ventricular pacing, on GDMT. (Level of evidence C)
Class IIb	
1	LVEF ≤35%, ischemic cardiomyopathy, sinus rhythm, LBBB with QRS ≥150 ms, NYHA class I on GDMT
2	LVEF ≤35%, sinus rhythm, non-LBBB with QRS 120–149 ms, NYHA class III or ambulatory IV symptoms on GDMT
3	LVEF ≤35%, sinus rhythm, non-LBBB with QRS ≥150 ms, NYHA class II symptoms on GDMT
Class III	
1	NYHA class I or II symptoms, non-LBBB pattern with QRS <150 ms.
2	Expected survival <1 year

CRT, cardiac resynchronization therapy; GDMT, guideline-directed medical therapy; LBBB, left bundle branch block; LVEF, left ventricular ejection fraction; NYHA, New York Heart Association.
*Adapted from 2012 ACCF/AHA/HRS Focused Update of the 2008 Guidelines for Device-Based Therapy of Cardiac Rhythm Abnormalities: A Report of the American College of Cardiology Foundation/American Heart Association Task Force on Practice Guidelines. Tracy CM, Epstein AE, Darbar D, Dimarco JP, Dunbar SB, Estes NA 3rd, Ferguson TB Jr, Hammill SC, Karasik PE, Link MS, Marine JE, Schoenfeld MH, Shanker AJ, Silka MJ, Stevenson LW, Stevenson WG, Varosy PD. *J Am Coll Cardiol* 2012 Aug 31 [Epub ahead of print]. PMID: 22975230.

with depressed ventricular function. Right ventricular apex (RVA) pacing results in a left bundle branch block morphology on the surface ECG. As with naturally occurring left bundle branch block, RVA pacing causes dyssynchrony due to earlier depolarization of the left ventricular septum relative to the lateral wall. In patients with ejection fraction under 40%, a prospective, randomized trial has found that the DDD mode incurs a greater risk for the development of atrial fibrillation, progression of heart failure, heart failure hospitalizations, and death than backup VVI pacing.[24,26] *Post hoc* analysis of several trials has shown this risk results from RVA pacing.[23,26] This concept is further supported by the observation that upgrading patients with refractory congestive heart failure and chronic RVA pacing leads improves New York Heart Association (NYHA) functional class, ejection fraction, and other clinical parameters.[53] The risk of adverse clinical outcomes as a consequence of RVA pacing is a function of a patient's substrate and the severity of dyssynchrony. Patient risk factors for RVA pacing-induced heart failure include a low ejection fraction, history of heart failure, and wide baseline QRS. The severity of dyssynchrony is a function of the

paced QRS duration and the RVA pacing frequency; AV dyssynchrony also has a role. These findings explain the clinical observation that most patients with preserved ventricular function and no history of heart failure tolerate pacing systems incorporating an RVA lead well, whereas patients with a history of heart failure and low ejection fraction are prone to RVA pacing-associated heart failure exacerbation. In practice, in patients with existing pacemakers who have a low ejection fraction (<40%) and persistent heart failure, strong consideration is given to revising (upgrading) the system to a biventricular pacemaker.[53–55] For *de novo* implants for bradycardia in patients with clinical heart failure and ejection fraction ≤40%, we usually offer CRT, particularly when the ventricular pacing frequency is anticipated to exceed 40%. This necessarily includes patients undergoing AV nodal ablation. The exception to the rule are patients in whom tachycardia-induced cardiomyopathy is implicated. One-third of such patients will experience improved ventricular function following AV node ablation with RVA pacing alone due to improved rate control and ventricular regularity.[56] At this time CRT is not indicated in patients with only mildly depressed ventricular function (ejection fraction 40–55%). In such patients cardiac function is periodically assessed and the pacing system upgraded to CRT if function declines. Recent randomized trials support extending this strategy to patients with dyssynchrony who have minimal heart failure symptoms, because CRT has been shown to prevent heart failure and improve survival in these patients.[50–52] In the MADIT CRT study, patients with an ejection fraction of ≤30%, QRS duration of ≥150 ms, and NYHA class I or II symptoms (ischemic cardiomyopathy), or NYHA class II symptoms (nonischemic) had a 41% reduction in the risk of heart failure events, a significant reduction in left ventricular volumes, and improvement in ejection fraction.[51]

2 Patients with left ventricular dysfunction and no indications for antibradycardia pacing

Prospective, randomized, clinical trials have demonstrated that CRT improves left ventricular systolic function, heart failure symptoms, exercise tolerance, quality of life, and survival.[48] Patient selection for CRT is based on the inclusion criteria used in these trials and extrapolating based on these data (Table 3.9).[47–52,57–60] Traditional criteria include nonischemic or ischemic cardiomyopathy, systolic dysfunction with left ventricular ejection fraction ≤35%, stable NYHA class III or IV heart failure symptoms, sinus rhythm, a QRS duration >120 ms, and maximally tolerated medical therapy (including dietary management, β-blockers, angiotensin-converting enzyme inhibitors or angiotensin receptor blockers, aldosterone antagonists, and diuretics).[61] As noted above, recent prospective, randomized, clinical trials have demonstrated the ben-

efits of extending CRT to patients with NYHA class I and II heart failure symptoms, in whom CRT was shown to improve left ventricular systolic function, prevent development or progression of heart failure symptoms, and in one trial improve survival (Table 3.10).[50–52] The latest guidelines provide a class IIb indication for biventricular pacing in these patients but, based on more recent data, we believe biventricular pacing should have a class I indication in patients with NYHA class I and II heart failure who meet all other criteria. Lastly, patients' symptoms and therapy should be stable for 3 months prior to consideration of biventricular pacing.

QRS duration

The presumed mechanism by which patients improve with CRT is restoration of synchrony. The QRS duration has been used as a surrogate for electrical and mechanical dyssynchrony in nearly all large, randomized, clinical trials. Limitations to use of the QRS duration as a marker for dyssynchrony exist, and indeed may partially explain the nonresponse rate to CRT of approximately 30% in most trials. Efforts to use imaging to identify dyssynchrony and CRT response have been disappointing.[62] Because the large, prospective, randomized trials enrolled patients predominantly based on the presence of a wide QRS, and because of the unreliability of imaging modalities to predict clinical response, patients with NYHA class III or ambulatory class IV heart failure and ejection fraction <35% with a QRS >120 ms are offered CRT if they are otherwise appropriate candidates. For patients with ejection fraction ≤35% and ischemic NYHA class I heart failure or class II heart failure of any etiology, CRT is offered if the QRS is >150 ms. Given that a meta-analysis of the major CRT trials has suggested that resynchronization is most effective when the QRS is >150 ms,[63] irrespective of NYHA class, for patients with QRS >120 and <150 it may be preferable that other characteristics that suggest a favorable outcome such as a left bundle branch block ECG pattern, dilated left ventricle, nonischemic etiology, or female gender be present.

Right bundle branch block

Resynchronization advances left ventricular free wall activation to coordinate electrical and mechanical activity to improve cardiac output and alleviate heart failure. In the absence of left ventricular free wall activation delay, it is not clear that CRT has a beneficial role. Patients with RBBB may have delay in both the right and left bundles, with greater delay in the right bundle leading to the RBBB pattern on the surface ECG. While inclusion in the randomized trials of CRT

Table 3.10 Clinical trials of biventricular pacing in patients with New York Heart Association (NYHA) class I and II heart failure (HF) symptoms.

Trial	REVERSE[50]	MADIT-CRT[51]	RAFT[52]
Patients	610	1820	1798
NYHA class I	18%	15%	0%
NYHA class II	82%	85%	80%
NYHA class III	0%	0%	20%
LVEF criteria	≤40%	≤30%	≤30%
QRS criteria	>120 ms	>130 ms	>120 ms
Outcome: HF hospitalization	HR = 0.47; $P = 0.03$	HR = 0.59; $P < 0.001$	HR = 0.68; $P < 0.001$
Outcome: death	HR = NA; $P = 0.63$	HR = 1.00; $P = 0.99$	HR = 0.75; $P = 0.003$

HR, heart rate; LVEF, left ventricular ejection fraction.

was based on a prolonged QRS duration irrespective of morphology, only 5–13% of patients had RBBB. Small studies have had mixed results, and a systematic review of the five large randomized studies that reported data for patients with RBBB (total 485 patients) demonstrated no benefits with CRT.[64] However, the data were not granular enough to permit a meta-analysis. Until better data are available, current indications are predicated on the original trial inclusion criteria, i.e., the QRS duration regardless of its morphology, and thus it is reasonable to offer CRT to patients with RBBB who meet the other criteria, in the absence of significant comorbidities or elevated procedural risk.. Nonetheless, the emerging data that suggest the presence of a RBBB may limit CRT response should be considered in weighing the risk–benefit ratio for an individual patient.

Atrial fibrillation

Patients with atrial fibrillation thus far have been excluded from all but a few observational studies and three small controlled trials assessing CRT.[52,65] MUSTIC-AF was a crossover trial of 59 patients (of whom only 58% completed the trial) with NYHA class III heart failure, chronic atrial fibrillation, right ventricular pacemakers, and wide-paced QRS complexes (>200 ms). Those with effective CRT therapy had improved exercise tolerance and decreased hospitalizations compared with right ventricular pacing alone.[52] The PAVE trial was a randomized trial of 184 patients with atrial fibrillation undergoing AV node ablation for control of rapid ventricular rates. Those who received CRT, particularly those with decreased left ventricular systolic function and NYHA class II or III heart failure, had improved exercise tolerance and increased left ventricular ejection fraction compared with those who received a conventional right ventricular lead.[65] A meta-analysis has demonstrated a trend toward reduced all-cause mortality in patients with congestive heart failure and atrial fibrillation treated with CRT.[66] While awaiting larger trials in broader groups of patients, we recommend that patients with atrial fibrillation receive CRT if they meet all other criteria (class IIa indication). In this population, care is taken to insure a high frequency of ventricular pacing (>90%) following device implantation. We found an improved response to CRT and a survival benefit in patients with atrial fibrillation who received AV node ablation compared with those with CRT alone, and thus have a low threshold for offering AV node ablation to this population.[67]

Nonresponders

Up to 25% of patients in clinical trials did not respond to CRT. Reasons for nonresponse to CRT include poor patient selection (absence of electrical or mechanical dyssynchrony), poor lead location, or insufficient pacing frequency. Management of nonresponders is covered in Chapter 10: Troubleshooting.

Pacing after cardiac transplantation

The incidence of bradyarrhythmias after cardiac transplantation is 8–23%.[68] Sinus node dysfunction is the usual cause of bradyarrhythmias in these patients, but risk factors for its development are unknown. Most bradyarrhythmias are transient, and half will resolve 6–12 months after transplantation.[69] Pacing is indicated (class I) for symptomatic, persistent, inappropriate bradyarrhythmias or chronotropic incompetence are not expected to resolve, and also indicated for sinus node dysfunction or AV block, as discussed above for the general population.[1] Pacing may be considered (class IIb) when relative bradycardia is recurrent or prolonged, thus preventing rehabilitation on discharge after transplantation, and when syncope occurs after cardiac transplantation even if a bradyarrhythmia has not been documented.

Indications for the implantable cardioverter-defibrillator

Development of the ICD was pioneered by Dr. Michel Mirowski in the late 1960s after the death of a close friend and mentor, who had been hospitalized with recurrent ventricular tachyarrhythmias. His frustration with the limitations of available therapies for high-risk patients led to the concept of an implantable device that continuously monitors cardiac rhythm and delivers defibrillating shocks for ventricular tachyarrhythmias when they occur. During the 1970s, experimental models were built and refined, leading to the first implantation of an ICD in 1980 in a patient with two previous cardiac arrests.[70] By the next decade, the indications had broadened to include patients with drug-refractory ventricular fibrillation (VF) or VT, patients with VT or VF in whom arrhythmias could not be induced (so that electrophysiologic study could not assess drug effectiveness), and patients who did not tolerate antiarrhythmic drugs.[71] With additional significant refinements in ICD technology, disillusionment with effectiveness of drug therapy, and the publication of prospective clinical data demonstrating effectiveness, the ICD has become the gold standard therapy for patients at high risk for lethal arrhythmias.[1,2]

It is useful to consider ICD indications in terms of secondary or primary prevention. Secondary prevention refers to ICD use in patients who have previously experienced an out-of-hospital cardiac arrest or life-threatening arrhythmia. Primary prevention refers to

Table 3.11 Indications for the implantable cardioverter-defibrillator for secondary prevention of sudden cardiac death.

1	Cardiac arrest due to VF or VT not within 24–48h of acute myocardial infarction and not due to a transient or reversible cause. *Class I*
2	Cardiac arrest when clear evidence of acute myocardial ischemia is documented to immediately precede the onset of VF, but when coronary revascularization cannot be carried out. *Class I*
3	Spontaneous sustained VT or VF in patients with structural heart disease. *Class I*
4	Unexplained syncope with clinically relevant, significant VT or VF induced at electrophysiology study. *Class I*
5	Sustained ventricular arrhythmias in patients with ischemic or nonischemic cardiomyopathy but normal or near-normal left ventricular function. *Class IIa*
6	Unexplained syncope in patients with significant left ventricular dysfunction who are receiving chronic optimal medical therapy. *Class IIa*

VF, ventricular fibrillation; VT, ventricular tachycardia.

ICD use in patients who may have significant cardiovascular disease, but who have never experienced a life-threatening arrhythmia. Current indications for the ICD for primary and secondary prevention of sudden cardiac death are detailed below.

Secondary prevention

Indications for an ICD for secondary prevention of sudden cardiac death are summarized in Table 3.11. The ICD has a well-established survival benefit in patients with prior out-of-hospital cardiac arrest, documented VF or VT, or syncope in association with structural heart disease and inducible ventricular arrhythmias.[2] Patients who have a cardiac arrest due to VF or VT without acute myocardial infarction or a clearly reversible cause are at high risk for recurrent cardiac arrest (30–50% recurrence within 2 years). Randomized controlled trials have shown more than a 50% relative risk reduction of death in patients with prior events who receive an ICD compared with patients treated empirically with amiodarone or treated with sotalol guided by electrophysiologic testing.[72] Furthermore, they showed that the ICD was effective regardless of the presence or absence of structural heart disease, revascularization, or type of dysrhythmia (VT or VF).[72] Electrophysiologic study is not required, as it does not alter the decision to implant an ICD in a patient with a fatal or near-fatal arrhythmic event. However, the study may guide ICD programming, inform device selection (by assessing concomitant need for pacing

modalities), and detect VT that is amenable to ablation.

In patients with ventricular dysfunction and hemodynamically stable VT, catheter-based ablation is palliative, and an ICD remains indicated because of the risk of subsequent unstable VT.[2,73] In patients with stable VT and preserved left ventricular function (i.e., ejection fraction >40%), antiarrhythmic drugs or catheter-based treatments are often helpful; however, the decision not to implant an ICD after the occurrence of sustained VT is controversial. Exceptions to this rule include the well-characterized idiopathic VTs in the setting of a structurally normal heart, for which catheter ablation is accepted primary therapy (discussed further below).

Syncope of undetermined etiology in patients with either ventricular dysfunction or normal ventricular function but hemodynamically significant sustained VT or VF induced at electrophysiology study is an indication for an ICD, regardless of adjunctive drug therapy.[2]

Lastly, for patients at high risk of recurrent VT or VF, but in whom comorbidities preclude immediate ICD implantation or for whom the risk is transient (i.e., awaiting cardiac transplantation), a reasonable option is a wearable cardioverter defibrillator.[2,74–76]

Primary prevention

Given that the majority of sudden cardiac death occurs in people without a prior event, identification of individuals at high risk of a first potentially fatal arrhythmia who would benefit from prophylactic implantation of an ICD is paramount. A large proportion of these events occur in asymptomatic community-dwelling individuals without recognized cardiac disease. A smaller proportion of these events occur in asymptomatic or symptomatic patients with established cardiac disease, and it is in this population that major strides have been made in primary prevention of sudden cardiac death. Importantly, if a strategy of implanting ICDs only in patients with an antecedent life-threatening event were adopted, 60–90% of individuals who might benefit from the device would not receive therapy, as they would have succumbed to the initial event. As shown in Fig. 3.17, a strategy that focuses only on the highest risk patients will provide benefit to those individuals, with little impact on sudden death rates for society as a whole; conversely, implanting ICDs in excessively broad populations results in exposing individuals at low risk to device implantation. Strategies focusing on patients with depressed ventricular function and heart failure lead to device placement in patients who benefit and whose conditions are sufficiently common for a societal benefit to be seen. Thus,

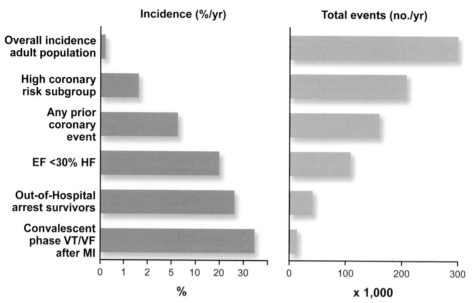

Fig. 3.17 The incidence of sudden cardiac death and the absolute number of sudden cardiac deaths in different populations. Despite the fact that the risk is lowest (about 0.1% per year) for the general adult population, it is in this group that the most sudden cardiac deaths occur. Conversely, those at highest risk of sudden cardiac death comprise the smallest number of patients at risk. A strategy that targets patients in the middle group (patients with reduced ventricular function and heart failure) results in implantation of a defibrillator in individuals who benefit from therapy and may impact the general population's risk. However, the challenge of broadly applying preventive therapy to the general population is apparent in this graph. EF, ejection fraction; HF, heart failure; MI, myocardial infarction. (Figure adapted from Myerburg RJ, Kessler KM, Castellanos A. Sudden cardiac death: structure, function, and time-dependence of risk. Circulation 1992; 85 [Suppl. I]:I2–I10, by permission of the American Heart Association.)

it has become increasingly clear that the severity of underlying organic heart disease is an important prognostic factor and influences the decision to implant an ICD. The greatest information regarding future sudden death risk is available for patients with coronary artery disease, dilated cardiomyopathy, or congestive heart failure. A disease-specific approach to selecting candidates for prophylactic ICD follows, and indications are summarized in Table 3.12. Lastly, for many of the clinical scenarios below in which a "waiting period" exists for ICD candidacy, the wearable cardioverter-defibrillator is an excellent option to prevent sudden cardiac arrest until either the patient's risk diminishes or an ICD is implanted.[2,74–76]

Coronary artery disease

Patients with a history of myocardial infarction and reduced left ventricular function are at increased risk of sudden cardiac death. This occurs most commonly as a result of VT due to re-entry around infarct scars or electrically heterogeneous areas in infarct border zones. Other arrhythmia mechanisms are contributory.

In the past, patients with prior myocardial infarction, ventricular dysfunction, and nonsustained VT were further risk stratified by assessing the inducibility of VT or VF during an electrophysiology study.[77] Randomized trial data from the MADIT study[78] and observational data from a subanalysis of the MUSTT study[79] showed that patients with inducible VT or VF survived longer when treated with an ICD compared with medical therapy. However, this approach had important limitations. First, those patients with ventricular dysfunction who had negative electrophysiologic studies and were not treated with an ICD still had a high risk of death.[80] Additionally, a strategy to determine ICD utility that required an invasive electrophysiology study in all potential candidates had inherent practical limitations.

Consequently, the pivotal MADIT II trial assessed the benefit of the ICD in patients with prior myocardial infarction and significant left ventricular dysfunction (ejection fraction ≤30%) without requiring an electrophysiology study.[81] It showed that ICD implantation led to a 31% relative risk reduction (a 6% absolute risk

Table 3.12 Indications for the implantable cardioverter-defibrillator for primary prevention of sudden cardiac death in patients with ischemic or nonischemic cardiomyopathy.

1	LVEF <35% and NYHA functional class II–III symptoms in patients with a myocardial infarction ≥40 days prior and no coronary revascularization in the last 3 months who are receiving optimal medical therapy. *Class I*
2	LVEF <35% and NYHA functional class II–III symptoms in patients with nonischemic heart disease who are receiving optimal medical therapy. *Class I*
3	LVEF <30% and NYHA functional class I symptoms in patients with a myocardial infarction ≥40 days prior and no coronary revascularization in the last 3 months who are receiving optimal medical therapy. *Class I*
4	LVEF <40%, prior MI, nonsustained VT, and inducible sustained VT or VF at electrophysiologic study. *Class I*
5	LVEF ≤35% and NYHA functional class I symptoms in patients with nonischemic heart disease who are receiving optimal medical therapy. *Class IIb*
6	In combination with CRT in patients with LVEF ≤35% and NYHA functional class III–IV symptoms who meet all other criteria for CRT

CRT, cardiac resynchronization therapy; LVEF, left ventricular ejection fraction; MI, myocardial infarction; NYHA, New York Heart Association.

Table 3.13 Patient characteristics to consider when assessing indications for a prophylactic implantable cardioverter-defibrillator.

1	Left ventricular ejection fraction
2	New York Heart Association functional class
3	Use of optimal medical therapy for heart failure
4	Timing relative to myocardial infarction or coronary revascularization
5	Comorbidities
6	Patient life expectancy

reduction) in death. These findings were extended by the SCD-HeFT trial, which assessed the benefits of the ICD in patients with ischemic or nonischemic heart disease, significant left ventricular dysfunction (ejection fraction ≤35%), and NYHA functional class II or III.[82] The SCD-HeFT study found that therapy with an ICD compared with amiodarone or standard medical treatment yielded a 23% relative risk reduction (7% absolute risk reduction) in death. Subsequent to these trials, routine invasive electrophysiology has been abandoned.

Currently, the main determinant of candidacy for an ICD for the primary prevention of sudden cardiac death is the severity of left ventricular dysfunction.[2] In general, patients with an ejection fraction ≤35% are likely to benefit from a prophylactic ICD. Although incompletely supported by randomized trials, recent guidelines promote the use of NYHA functional class to determine which patients with less severely depressed ventricular function (i.e., ejection fraction 35–40%) may benefit from an ICD. Implantation has been recommended if NYHA functional class II or III is present in this setting.[2] Current ICD indications for primary prevention are summarized in Table 3.12.[2] In addition to the left ventricular ejection fraction, other important factors that should be considered when determining

whether to place a prophylactic ICD are listed in Table 3.13. Of these, the timing of implantation relative to myocardial infarction and revascularization is discussed in greater detail below.

For patients with ischemic cardiomyopathy, trial data provide guidance regarding the timing of ICD implantation. Most ICD trials excluded patients with recent myocardial infarction (usually within 1 month). Despite the fact that the risk of sudden cardiac death is high immediately after acute myocardial infarction, the DINAMIT trial, which prospectively randomized patients to ICD or medical therapy 6–40 days after acute infarction, did not show a survival benefit with the ICD.[83] As a result, routine prophylactic ICD implantation should be delayed at least 40 days after an acute myocardial infarction. Additionally, as over half of patients with left ventricular dysfunction during acute myocardial infarction will experience an increase in systolic function within 3 months of the acute infarct, left ventricular ejection fraction should be reassessed after that time period to determine long-term risk and ICD candidacy.[84] An exception to this approach are patients with chronic left ventricular dysfunction (and ICD candidacy) who experience a recent troponin rise.[85]

Also excluded from most prophylactic ICD trials were patients with recent (within 3 months) coronary artery bypass graft (CABG) surgery. The CABG-Patch trial randomized patients with left ventricular dysfunction undergoing CABG surgery to ICD or medical therapy, and found that an ICD placed at the time of surgery did not improve survival.[86] As a result of this study and the exclusion from the primary prevention ICD trials of patients who had CABG in the prior 3 months, implantation of a prophylactic ICD is deferred for 3 months after CABG surgery or percutaneous coronary intervention. A subanalysis of the MADIT II trial showed no ICD survival benefit in patients who had coronary revascularization 3–6 months before implantation of the ICD, suggesting that the ICD can be further deferred up to 6 months after coronary revascularization.[87] Taken together, these trials highlight the importance of revascularization and biologic healing following a cardiac insult. Because left ventricular function may improve after revascularization,[88] left ventricular ejection fraction and ICD candidacy should be reassessed after a 3–6-month time period. Importantly, these findings apply only to prophylactic ICD placement, and not to patients with significant clinical dysrhythmias.

The other common clinical scenario is management of the patient with reduced left ventricular function due to a remote infarction who is clinically stable and has no arrhythmic symptoms. Available evidence suggests these patients do benefit from a prophylactic ICD, and that the benefit of ICD implantation increases as the time from infarction increases (Fig. 3.18).[89]

In patients with coronary artery disease, ejection fraction <35%, and QRS ≥120 ms with NYHA class III or IV heart failure, or QRS ≥150 with NYHA class I or II heart failure, an ICD with cardiac resynchronization pacing is indicated for the treatment of heart failure. This is discussed in detail above (see Congestive heart failure).

Dilated cardiomyopathy

Patients with left ventricular dysfunction that is not attributable to coronary artery disease (i.e., nonischemic cardiomyopathy) are also at increased risk of arrhythmic death and all-cause death.[90–92] The cause of sudden cardiac death in nonischemic cardiomyopathy is usually VT due to re-entry around areas of myocardial fibrosis that result from the underlying pathophysiology of the cardiomyopathy. In contrast to ischemic heart disease, in which there are usually discrete areas of scar, fibrosis in nonischemic cardiomyopathy may be diffusely scattered throughout the myocardium. The extent of this fibrosis, which is the substrate for ventricular arrhythmias, is demonstrable with recent advances in cardiac imaging and correlates with the risk of ventricular arrhythmias and sudden cardiac death.[93,94]

Invasive electrophysiology study is insensitive in predicting significant ventricular arrhythmias and sudden cardiac death in nonischemic cardiomyopathy.[95–100] Other risk stratification tools have been studied in this population, including signal-averaged ECG, baroreflex sensitivity, heart rate variability, and T wave alternans; however, none has been as robust a risk marker for sudden cardiac death as left ventricular ejection fraction.[101]

Several randomized controlled trials have assessed the role of the ICD for primary prevention of sudden cardiac death in patients with nonischemic cardiomyopathy. The first two trials, CAT and AMIOVIRT, did not show a survival benefit with the ICD, but their study samples were small.[102,103] CAT randomized 104 patients with an ejection fraction ≤30% and within 9 months of their diagnosis of cardiomyopathy to receive either an ICD or no device, and survival was not different between the two groups after 4 years of follow-up.[102] AMIOVIRT randomized 103 patients with an ejection

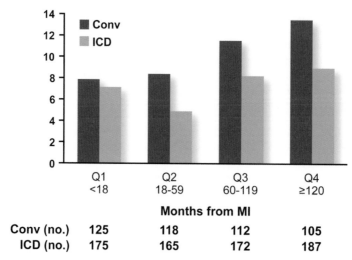

Fig. 3.18 Relationship between the time after myocardial infarction (MI) and benefit from the implantable cardioverter-defibrillator (ICD) for primary prevention of sudden cardiac death. (Modified from Wilber DJ, Zareba W, Hall WJ, *et al*. Time dependence of mortality risk and defibrillator benefit after myocardial infarction. Circulation 2004; 109:1082–4, by permission of the American Heart Association.)

fraction ≤35% and nonsustained VT to receive either an ICD or amiodarone, and survival was not different between the two groups after 3 years of follow-up.[103] The first larger trial, DEFINITE, randomized 458 patients with nonischemic cardiomyopathy, ejection fraction <36%, a history of heart failure symptoms, and nonsustained ventricular arrhythmias to receive either an ICD or no device in the setting of optimal medical therapy.[104] After an average of 29 months' follow-up, the risk of death was 35% less and the risk of sudden arrhythmic death was 80% less in the patients who had received an ICD. The most recent and definitive data come from SCD-HeFT, which randomized 2521 patients with an ejection fraction ≤35% and NYHA class II or III heart failure to either an ICD, amiodarone, or placebo (all in addition to conventional medical therapy).[82] Compared with placebo, patients who received an ICD had a 23% relative reduction and a 7% absolute reduction in the risk of death after an average follow-up of 46 months. The overall results were similar regardless of the etiology of heart failure (48% of the study population had nonischemic cardiomyopathy).

Based on these data, current indications for a prophylactic ICD in patients with nonischemic cardiomyopathy are NYHA class II or III symptoms, an ejection fraction <35%, and chronic medical therapy (Tables 3.12 and 3.13). Also, despite the relative lack of data for patients with NYHA class I symptoms, current guidelines provide a class IIb indication for the ICD in these patients.

For patients diagnosed with nonischemic cardiomyopathy, the optimal time to implant an ICD is controversial. The COMPANION trial excluded patients within 9 months of the diagnosis of cardiomyopathy, and the SCD-HeFT and DEFINITE trials did not specify a specific time interval, but excluded patients if they had a reversible cause of cardiomyopathy.[48,82,104] The uncertainty regarding the appropriate timing of ICD implantation centers on our limited ability to identify the causes of nonischemic cardiomyopathy and to predict the occurrence and magnitude of improvements in cardiac function after diagnosis. Currently, Medicare and Medicaid reimburse ICD implantations performed 9 months after the diagnosis of nonischemic cardiomyopathy. They also reimburse ICD implants performed 3–9 months after the diagnosis of nonischemic cardiomyopathy for patients enrolled in a national registry, which was created to clarify the benefits of the ICD during this early time period.[105] A recent analysis from this registry at one institution[106] and a *post hoc* subgroup analysis of the DEFINITE trial[104] have shown that the ICD was beneficial immediately after the diagnosis of nonischemic cardiomyopathy when a reversible cause was excluded. Because

unrecognized persistent tachycardia may result in reduced ventricular systolic function, it is important to recognize the potential impact of both atrial fibrillation and frequent premature ventricular contractions on the etiology of cardiomyopathy. Recovery from tachycardia-induced cardiomyopathy may be evident months after adequate control of ventricular rates is achieved.[56,107] While current practice is to implant the ICD 3 months after diagnosis of nonischemic cardiomyopathy, the optimal patient selection for earlier ICD implantation will be honed by future research regarding clinical and laboratory-based predictors of irreversible ventricular dysfunction.[108]

The ICD is also indicated for primary prevention of sudden cardiac death as part of a CRT-D system in selected subgroups of patients who meet all other criteria for conventional CRT (as discussed above, see Congestive heart failure). Patients with NYHA class III heart failure with an ejection fraction ≤35%, sinus rhythm, and QRS interval >120 ms, as well as some patients with NYHA class II heart failure meeting these criteria, benefit from CRT-D as opposed to CRT-P.[2] In the COMPANION trial, 1520 patients with ischemic or nonischemic cardiomyopathy, NYHA functional class III or IV, and a QRS ≥120 ms were randomized to CRT-P, CRT-D, or no device therapy (all combined with optimal medical therapy).[48] CRT-D reduced the risk of all-cause mortality by 36% (which was similar to the risk reduction with CRT-P and significantly greater than that with no device therapy). The indications for each therapy (CRT and ICD) can be considered independently of one another for a given patient and then prescribed accordingly as CRT-P, ICD, or CRT-D. Lastly, while the ICD is generally contraindicated in NYHA class IV heart failure (due to the limited prognosis in these patients), it has a proven survival benefit and is indicated as part of a CRT-D system when CRT is otherwise indicated in patients with NYHA class IV symptoms.[97]

Long QT syndrome

Long QT syndrome (LQTS) comprises a group of uncommon inherited disorders of cardiac ion channels, which result in abnormal repolarization and usually manifest on the surface ECG with a long corrected QT interval and abnormal T-wave morphology (Fig. 3.19; Table 3.14).[109] Patients with LQTS have a propensity for syncope, seizures, and/or sudden cardiac death secondary to polymorphic VT (torsades de pointes).[110] For the highest risk subset, the untreated mortality is approximately 5–10% per year.[110] Because this is primarily an electrical disorder typically seen in patients without significant cardiac structural or functional abnormalities, arrhythmia control results in an excellent prognosis.

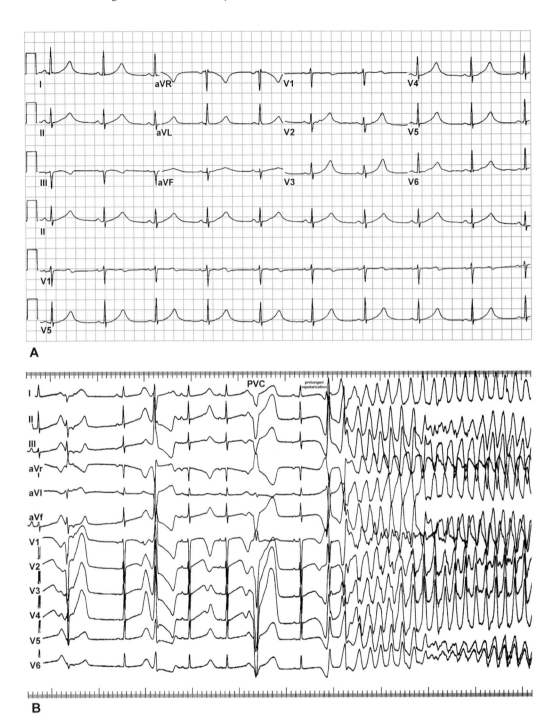

Fig. 3.19 Long QT syndrome. (A) ECG shows a QTc of 575 ms, suggesting increased risk of an arrhythmic event. This patient had a confirmed mutation affecting the cardiac potassium channel KVLQT1. (B) In a rhythm strip from a different patient, torsades de pointes is initiated during a dobutamine challenge. A short interval is terminated by a premature ventricular contraction (PVC), which in turn is followed by a long interval. The short–long sequence results in prolongation of repolarization, and a second PVC initiates the dysrhythmia.

Table 3.14 Electrocardiographic findings in long QT syndrome (LQTS) 1, 2, and 3.

LQTS Type	ECG (lead V5)	Mutation
LQTS 1		KCNQ1
LQTS 2		KCNH2
LQTS 3		SCN5A

LQTS 1 is usually associated with broad-based T waves, LQTS 2 is usually associated with low-amplitude T waves, and LQTS 3 is usually associated with a long ST segment and peaked T waves; however, much variability exists.

Images reproduced from Moss AJ, Zareba W, Benhorin J, *et al*. ECG T-wave patterns in genetically distinct forms of the hereditary long QT syndrome. Circulation 1995; 92:2929–34, by permission of the American Heart Association.

β-Blockers are first-line therapy, and they improve symptoms and reduce significantly (but do not eliminate) the risk of death, especially for patients with type 1 LQTS (LQTS 1), in whom the response is quite effective.[111] Unfortunately, about 30% of patients remain symptomatic despite high-dose β-blocker therapy, and 9% of sudden deaths among patients with LQTS occur in those taking β-blockers.[109] Both antibradycardia pacing (to prevent proarrhythmic pauses and to shorten depolarization) and left cardiac sympathetic denervation also reduce the risk of sudden death in these patients.[110] Avoidance of QT-prolonging drugs is essentially component to sudden death prevention.

ICD therapy is recommended for patients with LQTS and previous aborted sudden death (class I indication) and those with sustained ventricular arrhythmias or recurrent syncope despite β-blocker therapy (class IIa indications).[2] Observational data from a series of patients with LQTS and aborted sudden death or recurrent syncope demonstrated 1.3% mortality during an average 3 years' follow-up in the 73 patients with an ICD, compared with 16% mortality during an average 8 years' follow-up in the 161 patients without an ICD.[112]

At present, it is unclear whether a positive family history provides relevant information regarding an individual's risk for sudden death and the potential benefit from ICD implantation. Patients with LQTS and a strong family history of sudden death are often offered an ICD (class IIb indication), particularly if other risk factors are present (deafness, syncope, female sex, or corrected QT interval >500 ms). However, it is possible that family history provides an emotional impetus for more aggressive therapy rather than an evidence-based one. In persons with a strong family history and a normal corrected QT interval, familial genetic evaluation can be helpful. Family members found to have a putative mutation but who do not have symptoms or a prolonged corrected QT interval are generally observed or treated with β-blockers, whereas those with significant risk factors may be offered an ICD.

ICD therapy should be strongly considered in patients who are noncompliant or cannot tolerate β-blocker therapy, because β-blocker noncompliance can be fatal. Indications for the ICD in patients with LQTS are individualized as risk stratification continues to evolve. Table 3.15 lists patient groups at high risk for sudden cardiac death in patients with LQTS.[2,113] Genetic analysis is increasingly having a role in risk stratification, and genetic testing is now commercially available. The unique issues to programming ICDs in patients with LQTS are discussed in Chapter 8:: Programming.

Brugada syndrome and sudden unexplained death syndrome

Individuals with the Brugada syndrome, now recognized also to include the sudden unexplained death syndrome (SUDS) which predominantly afflicts young South East Asian men, have an increased risk of sudden cardiac death despite a structurally normal heart. It is an inherited condition with autosomal dominant

Table 3.15 High-risk long QT patients in whom an ICD should be considered.

1	Prior cardiac arrest
2	Therapy intolerance or breakthrough
3	QTc >550 ms (especially if not LQTS 1)
4	Female gender, LQTS 2, QTc >500 ms
5	Infants with 2 : 1 AV block

QTc, corrected QT interval.

transmission and increased manifestation in men. Various mutations in the gene encoding the α subunit of the cardiac sodium channel SCN5A have been identified, but <20% of familial cases of Brugada syndrome are associated with recognized mutations of this gene.[114] Diagnosis depends on the demonstration of an ECG with incomplete RBBB and coved ST-segment elevation in leads V_1–V_3 (which sometimes is evident only after administration of a sodium-channel blocker, such as procainamide or ajmaline) (Fig. 3.20). Other precipitants of the typical electrocardiographic pattern are vagotonic agents, α-adrenergic receptor agonists, β-adrenergic receptor blockers, tricyclic or tetracyclic antidepressants, alcohol, cocaine, hyperthermia, or hypokalemia.

The risk of sudden cardiac death in the Brugada syndrome has been found to be 0.35–4% per year, depending on the population being studied.[115] A meta-analysis of over 30 prospective studies estimated that sudden death, syncope, or ICD therapy occurred in 10% of patients during an average 32 months' follow-up.[116] Pharmacologic therapy to prevent sudden death is relatively ineffective. Patients at highest risk of sudden death for whom the ICD is recommended have the typical ECG findings and either prior cardiac arrest (class I indication) or prior syncope or VT (class IIa indications).[2] A randomized trial of ICD therapy has not been performed in the broader Brugada syndrome population, but one randomized controlled trial in 86

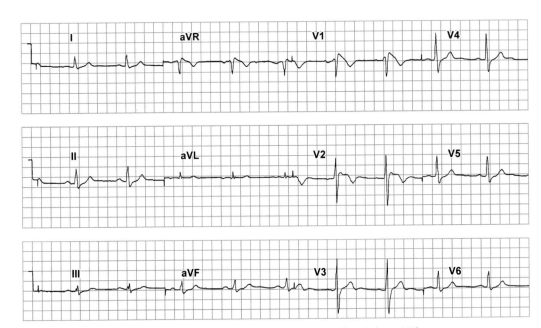

Fig. 3.20 Characteristic ECG of Brugada syndrome. (Courtesy of Dr. M. Ackerman, Mayo Clinic, Rochester, MN.)

Table 3.16 Risk factors for sudden cardiac death in the Brugada and sudden unexplained death syndromes.

1	Prior cardiac arrest
2	Male sex
3	Spontaneous electrocardiographic Brugada pattern
4	Prior syncope and a spontaneous electrocardiographic Brugada pattern
5	Inducible ventricular tachycardia or fibrillation (controversial)
6	Fever

South East Asian patients with SUDS with prior confirmed or suspected cardiac arrest showed a clear benefit of the ICD for preventing recurrent sudden cardiac death in this specific subgroup.[117] Patients at an intermediate risk of sudden death have the typical ECG findings, but no history of syncope. Previously, the decision to implant an ICD was aided by electrophysiology study;[118] however, this strategy is controversial.[115,116] Finally, those at lowest risk of sudden death are asymptomatic individuals who either have the typical ECG findings only with pharmacologic challenge or are known from screening to be silent carriers of the gene mutation.[118] The best approach to risk stratification and treatment of these different presentations of the Brugada syndrome and SUDS is unknown. Significant risk factors for sudden cardiac death in these syndromes are listed in Table 3.16.[2,119]

Other channelopathies

The short QT syndrome is a condition characterized by a structurally normal heart with a short QT interval (<300–320 ms) and narrow, peaked T waves. Published case reports in very few individuals with these findings have suggested that it is associated with a markedly increased risk of sudden cardiac death.[120] To date, mutations in three genes encoding different cardiac potassium channels that result in abnormally short ventricular repolarization have been identified.[2] However, selection bias and the lack of a controlled study limit the inferences regarding risk that can be made from these series of cases. Recent controlled studies in large populations have shown that a short QT interval is exceedingly rare (no QT interval ≤300 ms was identified among 118,444 people in these studies) and that individuals with QT intervals in the shortest half centile of the normal distribution did not experience increased mortality after an average of 8 years' follow-up.[121,122] The duration of the QT interval that might be associated with an increased risk of sudden death, other clinical characteristics associated with an increased risk of sudden death, the role of electrophysi-

ology study, pharmacologic management, and the role of the ICD in these patients are currently unknown.

Catecholaminergic polymorphic ventricular tachycardia (CPVT) is a condition characterized by sustained ventricular arrhythmias that occur during acute emotional or physical stress. These arrhythmias can include sustained monomorphic VT, bidirectional VT (i.e., alternating QRS axis), polymorphic VT, and VF.[123] It is an inherited condition with autosomal dominant and autosomal recessive modes of transmission, and it usually manifests during childhood. Associated mutations have been identified in the genes encoding the cardiac ryanodine receptor and calsequestrin, both responsible for intracellular handling of calcium. Implantation of an ICD is generally indicated for all patients with CPVT who have had a prior cardiac arrest (class I) or syncope or sustained VT while receiving β-blocker therapy (class IIa). Currently, other clinical characteristics and the results of genetic testing do not add to risk stratification and the decision to implant an ICD.[2]

Arrhythmogenic right ventricular dysplasia

Arrhythmogenic right ventricular dysplasia (ARVD) is characterized by fibrous and fatty replacement of right ventricular myocardium, although both ventricles can be involved.[124] Over half of recognized patients have a family history, and mutations in genes encoding specific cell adhesion proteins have been identified.[125] Patients present with asymptomatic premature ventricular contractions, palpitations, syncope due to fast monomorphic VT, or sudden death. Up to 10% of unexplained sudden deaths in young patients are thought to be due to ARVD in some geographic regions.[124] The ECG manifestations of ARVD include inverted T waves in leads V_1–V_3, RBBB, and epsilon waves (Fig. 3.21). The premature ventricular contractions and VT usually have a left bundle branch block pattern due to their origin in the right ventricle (Fig. 3.22). The diagnosis is sometimes challenging and requires cardiac imaging to identify the presence and extent of fibrous or fatty tissue within the ventricular myocardium. Endomyocardial biopsy is insensitive because of the apical location and patchy nature of the involved tissue, but it may be performed to distinguish ARVD from other cardiomyopathies.[126] The diagnostic criteria for ARVD are listed in Table 3.17.

Indications for the ICD in patients with ARVD are based on emerging data regarding the risk factors for sudden death. Aborted sudden death defines an individual as high risk with a clear secondary prevention indication. In patients without prior cardiac arrest, a history of syncope or sustained VT or VF are class I indications for the ICD.[2] Other factors associated with

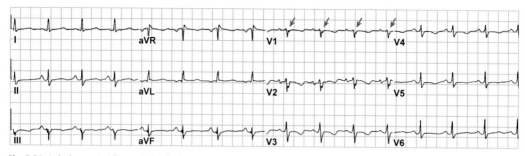

Fig. 3.21 Arrhythmogenic right ventricular dysplasia. ECG shows right precordial T wave inversions and epsilon waves (arrows).

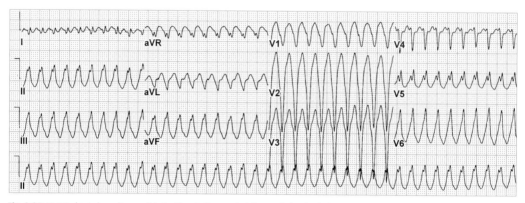

Fig. 3.22 Ventricular tachycardia associated with arrhythmogenic right ventricular dysplasia.

death or ICD firings include severe right ventricular dilatation, inducible VT during electrophysiology study, early onset of symptoms, male gender, increased QT dispersion, and left ventricular involvement.[126–128] Class IIa indications for the ICD include "extensive disease," involvement of the left ventricle, family members with ARVD and sudden death, and undiagnosed syncope when VT and VF have not been excluded as its cause.[2] The frequency of ventricular arrhythmias in patients with ARVD may be high, necessitating other therapies to prevent excessive shocks while maintaining ICD therapy as a life-saving backup measure.[129] In these cases, alternative or adjuvant treatment approaches include medications, catheter ablation, and surgical ventriculotomy or disarticulation of the involved myocardium.

Hypertrophic cardiomyopathy

HCM is a heterogeneous disease, associated with various mutations of the genes encoding myocardial contractile proteins, as well as variable cardiac structural abnormalities and clinical presentations.[130] The natural history of HCM is characterized by slow progression of symptoms such as dyspnea and angina, but also by sudden cardiac death. The characteristic myocardial disarray and interstitial fibrosis provide the substrate for re-entrant ventricular arrhythmias, which are probably the cause of sudden death in most patients and may be triggered or modulated by autonomic dysfunction, subendocardial ischemia, or conduction abnormalities.[130] The annual risk of sudden death is 5% in patients without prior cardiac arrest and 11% for patients with a history of resuscitated arrest.[131] About 50% of sudden deaths in young athletes are due to HCM, and about 50% of deaths in patients with HCM occur suddenly.[130–132]

The 2008 ACC/AHA/ESC guidelines assign a class IIa indication for an ICD for the primary prevention of sudden cardiac death in patients with HCM who have one or more major risk factors (Table 3.18).[2,133] The ICD is undoubtedly a necessary and proven therapy in these patients,[131] but identifying the patients most likely to benefit is challenging. About 50% of patients with HCM who have sudden death do not have any of the

Table 3.17 Diagnostic criteria for arrhythmogenic right ventricular dysplasia (ARVD).

Original Task Force Criteria	Revised Task Force Criteria
I. Global or regional dysfunction and structural alterations*	
Major	
• Severe dilatation and reduction of RV ejection fraction with no (or only mild) LV impairment • Locafized RV aneurysms (akinetic or dyskinetic areas with diastolic bulging) • Severe segmental dilatation of the RV	**By 2D echo:** • Regional RV akinesia, dyskinesia. or aneurysm • *and* 1 of the following (end diastole): – PLAX RVOT ≥32 mm (corrected lor body size [PLAXIBSA]) ≥19 mm/m^2 – PSAX RVOT ≥36 mm (corrected lor body size [PSAX/BSA]) ≥21 mm/m^2) – Or fractional area change ≤33% **By MRI:** • Regional RV akilesia or dyskinesia or dyssynchronous RV contraction • *and* 1 of the following: – Ratio of RV end-diastolic volume to BSA ≥110 mL/m^2 (male) or ≥100 mL/m^2 (female) – Or RV ejection fraction ≤40% **By RV angiography:** • Regional RV akilesia, dyskinesia. or aneurysm
Minor	
• Mild global RV dilalalion and/or ejection fraction reduction with normal LV • Mild segmental dilatation of the RV • Regional RV hypokinesia	**By 2D echo:** • Regional RV akinesia or dyskinesia • *and* 1 of the following (end diastole): – PLAX RVOT ≥29 to <32 mm (corrected for body size [PIAX/BSA]) ≥16 to <19 mm/m^2 – PSAX RVOT ≥32 to <36 mm (corrected for body size [PSAX/BSA]) ≥18 to <21 mm/m^2 – Or fractional area change >33% to ≤40% **By MRI:** • Regional RV akilesia or dyskinesia or dyssynchronous RV contraction • *and* 1 of the following: – Ratio of RV end-diastolic volume to BSA ≥100 to <110 mL/m^2 (male) or ≥90 to <100 mL/m^2 (female) – Or RV ejection fraction >40% to ≤45%
II. Tissue characterization of wall	
Major	
• Fibrofatty replacement of myocardium on endomyocardial biopsy	• Residual myocytes <60% by morphometric analysis (or <50% if estimated), with fibrous replacement of the RV free wall myocardium in ≥1 sample, with or without fatty replacement of tissue on endomyocardial biopsy
Minor	
	• Residual myocytes 60% to 75% by morphometric analysis (or 50% to 65% if estimated), with fibrous replacement of the RV free wall myocardium in ≥1 sample, with or without fatty replacement of tissue on endomyocardial biopsy
III. Repolarization abnormalities	
Major	
	• Inverted T waves in right precordial leads (V$_1$, V$_2$ and V$_3$) or beyond in individuals >14 years of age (in the absence of complete right bundle-branch block QRS ≥120 ms)
Minor	
• Inverted T waves in right precordial leads (V$_2$ and V$_3$) (people age >12years, in absence of right bundle-branch block)	• Inverted T waves in leads V$_1$ and V$_2$ in individuals >14 years of age (in the absence of complete right bundle-branch block) or in V$_4$, V$_5$, or V$_6$ • Inverted T waves in leads V$_1$, V$_2$, V$_3$ and V$_4$ in individuals >14 years of age in the presence of complete right bundle-blanch block

(Continued)

Table 3.17 *(Continued)*

Original Task Force Criteria	Revised Task Force Criteria
IV. Depolarization/conduction abnormalities	
Major	
• Epsilon waves or localized prolongation(>110 ms) of the QRS complex in right precordial leads (V$_1$ to V$_3$)	• Epsilon wave (reproducible low-amplitude signals between end of QRS complex to onset of the T wave) in the right precordial leads (V$_1$ to V$_2$)
Minor	
• Late polentials (SAECG)	• Late potentials by SAECG in ≥1 of 3 parameters in the absence of a QRS duration of ≥110 ms on the standard ECG
	• Filtered QRS duration (fQRS) ≥114 ms
	• Ouration of terminal QRS <40 μV (low-amplitude signal duration) ≥38 ms
	• Root-mean-square voltage of terminal 40 ms ≤ 20 μV
	• Terminal activation duration of QRS ≥55 ms measured from the nadir of the S wave to the end of the QRS. including R', in V$_1$, V$_2$ or V$_3$ in the absence of comlplete right bundle-branch block
V. Arrhythmias	
Major	
	• Nonsustained or sustained ventricular tachycardia of left bundle-branch morphology with superior axis (negative or indeterminate QRS in leads II, III, and aVf and positive in lead aVL)
Minor	
• Left bundle-branch block-type ventricular tachycardia (sustained and nonsustained) (ECG, Holter, exercise)	• Nonsustained or sustained ventricular tachycardia of RV outflow configuration, left bundle-branch block morphology with inferior axis (positive QRS in leads II, III, and aVF and negative in lead aVL) or of unknown axis
• Frequent ventricular extrasystoles (>1000 per 24 hours) (Holter)	• >500 ventricular extrasystoles per 24 hours (Holter)
VI. Family history	
Major	
• Familial disease confirmed at necropsy or surgery	• ARVC/D confirmed in a first-degree relative who meets current Task Force criteria
	• ARVC/D confirmed pathologically at autopsy or surgery in a first-degree relative
	• Identification of a pathogenic mutation[†] categorized as associated or probably associated with ARVC/D in the patient under evaluation
Minor	
• Family history of premature sudden death (<35 years of age) due 10 suspected ARVC/D	• History of ARVC/D in a first-degree relative in whom it is not possible or practical to determine whether the family member meets current Task Force criteria
• Familial history (clinical diagnosis based on present criteria)	• Premature sudden death(<35 years of age) due to suspected ARVC/D in a first-degree relative
	• ARVC/D confirmed pathologically or by current Task Force Criteria in second-degree relative

PLAX indicates parasternal long-axis view; RVOT, RV outflow tract; BSA, body surface area; PSAX, parasternal short-axis view; aVF, augmented voltage unipolar left toot lead; and aVL, augmented voltage unipolar left arm lead.

Diagnostic terminology for original criteria: This diagnosis is fulfilled by the presence of 2 major, or 1 major plus 2 minor criteria or 4 minor criteria from different groups. Diagnostic terminology for revised criteria: definite diagnosis: 2 major or 1 major and 2 minor criteria or 4 minor from different categories; borderline: 1 major and 1 minor or 3 minor criteria from different categories; possible: 1 major or 2 minor criteria from different categories.

*Hypokinesis is not included in this or subsequent definitions of RV regional wall motion abnormalities for the proposed modified criteria.

†A pathogenic mutation is a DNA alteration associated with ARVC/D that alters or is expected to alter the encoded protein, is unobserved or rare in a large non-ARVC/D control population, and either alters or is predicted to alter the structure or function of the protein or has demonstrated linkage to the disease phenotype in a conclusive pedigree.

Source: Table 1 from Marcus FI, McKenna WJ, Sherrill D, *et al.* Diagnosis of arrhythmogenic right ventricular cardiomyopathy/dysplasia. Circulation 2010; 121:1533–41. Reproduced with permission.

Table 3.18 Risk factors for sudden cardiac death in hypertrophic cardiomyopathy.

Prior aborted sudden cardiac death
Spontaneous sustained ventricular tachycardia
History of sudden cardiac death in multiple first-degree relatives
Recurrent or exertional syncope
Nonsustained ventricular tachycardia
Failure to increase blood pressure >20 mmHg with exercise testing in patients <50 years old
Interventricular septal wall thickness >30 mm
Possible risk factors:
- Specific genetic mutations of the myosin heavy chain, troponin T, or α-tropomyosin
- Atrial fibrillation
- Myocardial ischemia
- LV outflow obstruction
- Intense (competitive) physical exertion

Source: Adapted from Epstein AE, DiMarco JP, Ellenbogen KA, et al. American College of Cardiology/American Heart Association Task Force on Practice Guidelines (Writing Committee to Revise the ACC/AHA/NASPE 2002 Guideline Update for Implantation of Cardiac Pacemakers and Antiarrhythmia Devices); American Association for Thoracic Surgery; Society of Thoracic Surgeons. ACC/AHA/HRS 2008 Guidelines for Device-Based Therapy of Cardiac Rhythm Abnormalities: a report of the American College of Cardiology/American Heart Association Task Force on Practice Guidelines (Writing Committee to Revise the ACC/AHA/NASPE 2002 Guideline Update for Implantation of Cardiac Pacemakers and Antiarrhythmia Devices) developed in collaboration with the American Association for Thoracic Surgery and Society of Thoracic Surgeons. J Am Coll Cardiol 2008; 51:e1–62. Errata in: J Am Coll Cardiol 2009; 53:1473; J Am Coll Cardiol 2009; 53:147.

recognized major risk factors.[134] Despite these challenges, there are several areas of broad consensus. Patients who survived cardiac arrest or who have spontaneous sustained ventricular tachyarrhythmias clearly should receive an ICD (class I indication). Strong consideration should be given to ICD implantation in patients with multiple risk factors, particularly the following: young age (<35 years old); sudden death related to HCM in multiple family members; unexplained syncope, especially if recurrent or occurring during exertion; a hypotensive response to exercise, especially in patients <50 years old; a left ventricular wall thickness ≥30 mm, especially in younger patients; significant left ventricular outflow tract obstruction; and a high-risk mutation.[2,130] The presence of even one risk factor, when considered significant for that individual (such as a malignant family history), is sufficient to warrant ICD implantation.[2,130,133] Because of low implant morbidity and the uncertain effectiveness of antiarrhythmic drugs for this disease, we often offer ICD therapy to these

patients with a highly individualized approach. Each patient's preferences must be understood regarding the commitment to lifelong device implantation, the long-term need for system revisions, and the possibility of inappropriate shocks and associated anxiety.

Therapies such as β-blockers, alcohol septal ablation, and septal myectomy are successful in treating the symptoms of HCM related to left ventricular outflow tract obstruction and heart failure but, of these, only septal myectomy may provide survival benefit and reduce the rate of sudden death.[135] However, septal myectomy is performed in only about 5% of patients with HCM, and it does not eliminate the risk of sudden cardiac death.[135] Further risk stratification is required in patients who have undergone septal myectomy, and ICD therapy should continue to be offered to these patients based on their risk factor profile.

Congenital heart disease

Success in palliating many congenital heart defects during infancy and childhood has resulted in a growing population of adult patients with post-surgical congenital heart disease. These patients often have altered hemodynamics, abnormal cardiac chamber sizes, and reduced ventricular function. Specific conditions that have been associated with an increased risk of sudden cardiac death in adulthood are the tetralogy of Fallot, transposition of the great arteries, and the univentricular heart. Most available data regarding risk stratification have been derived in patients with corrected tetralogy of Fallot due to its higher prevalence. Characteristics associated with sudden cardiac death are older age at surgery, ventricular dysfunction, wide QRS (>180 ms) and hemodynamic abnormality due to pulmonary regurgitation.[136] The role of invasive electrophysiology study has been controversial.[137,138] A recent, large, multicenter study that included more than 250 tetralogy of Fallot patients found that inducible monomorphic or polymorphic VT predicted ventricular arrhythmias and sudden cardiac death.[139] In tetralogy of Fallot patients with clinical symptoms or documented arrhythmias, the negative predictive value of electrophysiology study was 86% and the positive predictive value was 67%. These data suggest that invasive electrophysiology study, while imperfect, has a role in conjunction with other clinical characteristics for risk stratification and decision-making regarding ICD therapy. In general, these strategies, which have been demonstrated in patients with tetralogy of Fallot, are often extrapolated to patients with other congenital heart defects due to the paucity of data in these other conditions.

Class I indications for ICD therapy in patients with congenital heart disease include resuscitated cardiac arrest in patients for whom a reversible etiology of the cardiac arrest is excluded and who are receiving optimal medical therapy, or the occurrence of sustained VT that cannot be managed by catheter ablation or cardiac surgery.[2] Class IIa indications for ICD therapy include unexplained syncope in patients with reduced ventricular systolic function after electrophysiology and hemodynamic studies. As discussed above, ICD therapy should be considered in patients at high risk of sudden cardiac death based on clinical characteristics and the results of electrophysiology study.

Contraindications to implantable cardioverter-defibrillator therapy

Contraindications to ICD therapy are summarized in Table 3.19. Patients who have incessant arrhythmias that cannot be controlled by adjuvant medical, catheter-based, or surgical therapy are not candidates for the ICD.

Table 3.19 Contraindications to the implantable cardioverter-defibrillator.

1	Syncope of undetermined cause in a patient without inducible ventricular tachyarrhythmias and without structural heart disease
2	Incessant VT or ventricular fibrillation
3	Ventricular fibrillation or VT resulting from arrhythmias amenable to surgical or catheter ablation; e.g., atrial arrhythmias associated with the Wolff–Parkinson–White syndrome, right ventricular outflow tract VT, idiopathic left VT, or fascicular VT
4	Ventricular tachyarrhythmias due to a transient or reversible disorder (e.g., acute myocardial infarction, electrolyte imbalance, drugs, trauma)
5	Significant psychiatric illnesses that may be aggravated by device implantation or may preclude systematic follow-up
6	Expected survival with acceptable functional status <1 year
7	Patients with coronary artery disease who have left ventricular dysfunction and prolonged QRS duration without spontaneous or inducible sustained or nonsustained VT and who are undergoing coronary bypass surgery
8	New York Heart Association class IV drug-refractory congestive heart failure in patients who are not candidates for biventricular pacing or cardiac transplantation

VT, ventricular tachycardia.

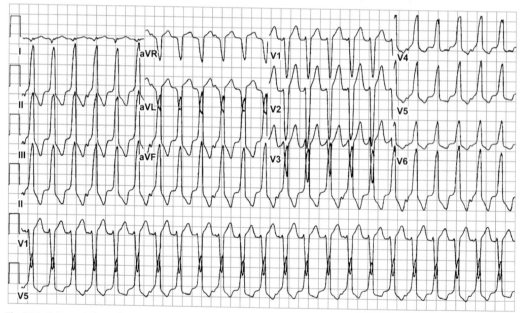

Fig. 3.23 Right ventricular outflow tract ventricular tachycardia (VT). Because of the origin of the tachycardia in the high outflow tract, the ECG pattern is that of left bundle branch block with positive QRS complexes in II, III, and aVF (inferior axis). This tracing also demonstrates atrioventricular dissociation (best seen in lead II). Because of the rapid rate of the tachycardia, only every third VT complex can conduct retrogradely to the AV node, resulting in 3:1 ventriculoatrial conduction. AV dissociation in this situation is not indicative of AV block; in fact, this patient has normal AV nodal conduction during sinus rhythm. Right ventricular outflow tract VT is best treated with catheter ablation, and defibrillator therapy is not indicated.

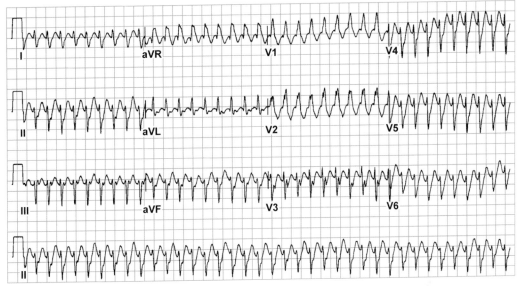

Fig. 3.24 ECG showing fascicular ventricular tachycardia. Note the right bundle branch block pattern with far-left axis deviation, consistent with an arrhythmia focus in the left posterior fascicle. Ablation success rates exceed 90% for this arrhythmia, so defibrillator therapy is not typically indicated.

Patients whose arrhythmias are clearly due to a transient or reversible disorder, such as acute myocardial infarction, significant electrolyte imbalance, drug ingestion, or trauma, do not have a greatly increased risk of recurrent arrhythmia and should not receive an ICD. Patients with significant psychiatric illnesses that may be aggravated by device shocks and patients with terminal illness and unacceptable functional status should not receive an ICD. This includes patients with NYHA class IV drug-refractory congestive heart failure who are not candidates for transplantation (except when ICD therapy is offered as part of an appropriately indicated CRT device). Also, in general, patients should not undergo ICD therapy for arrhythmias amenable to surgical or catheter ablation, such as right ventricular outflow tract VT, idiopathic left ventricular VT, fascicular VT, or Wolff–Parkinson–White syndrome with ventricular tachyarrhythmias secondary to rapid anterograde conduction of atrial fibrillation (Figs 3.23 and 3.24).

Acknowledgement

The authors thank Dr. Michael Ackerman for his review of the LQTS section of this chapter.

References

1 Epstein AE, DiMarco JP, Ellenbogen KA, et al. ACC/AHA/HRS 2008 Guidelines for Device-Based Therapy of Cardiac Rhythm Abnormalities: a report of the American College of Cardiology/American Heart Association Task Force on Practice Guidelines (Writing Committee to Revise the ACC/AHA/NASPE 2002 Guideline Update for Implantation of Cardiac Pacemakers and Antiarrhythmia Devices) developed in collaboration with the American Association for Thoracic Surgery and Society of Thoracic Surgeons. J Am Coll Cardiol 2008; 51:e1–62.

2 Zipes DP, Camm AJ, Borggrefe M, et al. ACC/AHA/ESC 2006 guidelines for management of patients with ventricular arrhythmias and the prevention of sudden cardiac death: a report of the American College of Cardiology/American Heart Association Task Force and the European Society of Cardiology Committee for Practice Guidelines (Writing Committee to Develop Guidelines for Management of Patients With Ventricular Arrhythmias and the Prevention of Sudden Cardiac Death). J Am Coll Cardiol 2006; 48:e247–346.

3 Dewey RC, Capeless MA, Levy AM. Use of ambulatory electrocardiographic monitoring to identify high-risk patients with congenital complete heart block. N Engl J Med 1987; 316:835–9.

4 Balmer C, Fasnacht M, Rahn M, Molinari L, Bauersfeld U. Long-term follow up of children with congenital complete atrioventricular block and the impact of pacemaker therapy. Europace 2002; 4:345–9.

5 Shen WK, Hammill SC, Hayes DL, et al. Long-term survival after pacemaker implantation for heart block in patients > or = 65 years. Am J Cardiol 1994; 74:560–4.

6 Shaw DB, Kekwick CA, Veale D, Gowers J, Whistance T. Survival in second degree atrioventricular block. Br Heart J 1985; 53:587–93.

7 Shaw DB, Gowers JI, Kekwick CA, New KH, Whistance AW. Is Mobitz type I atrioventricular block benign in adults? Heart 2004; 90:169–74.

8 Bialer MG, McDaniel NL, Kelly TE. Progression of cardiac disease in Emery–Dreifuss muscular dystrophy. Clin Cardiol 1991; 14:411–6.

9 Young TJ, Shah AK, Lee MH, Hayes DL. Kearns–Sayre syndrome: a case report and review of cardiovascular complications. Pacing Clin Electrophysiol 2005; 28: 454–7.

10 Komajda M, Frank R, Vedel J, Fontaine G, Petitot JC, Grosgogeat Y. Intracardiac conduction defects in dystrophia myotonica: electrophysiological study of 12 cases. Br Heart J 1980; 43:315–20.

11 Fragola PV, Autore C, Magni G, Antonini G, Picelli A, Cannata D. The natural course of cardiac conduction disturbances in myotonic dystrophy. Cardiology 1991; 79:93–8.

12 Subbiah RN, Kuchar D, Baron D. Torsades de pointes in a patient with Kearns–Sayre syndrome: a fortunate finding. Pacing Clin Electrophysiol 2007; 30:137–9.

13 Aplin M, Engstrom T, Vejlstrup NG, Clemmensen P, Torp-Pedersen C, Kober L. Prognostic importance of complete atrioventricular block complicating acute myocardial infarction. Am J Cardiol 2003; 92:853–6.

14 Opolski G, Kraska T, Ostrzycki A, Zielinski T, Korewicki J. The effect of infarct size on atrioventricular and intraventricular conduction disturbances in acute myocardial infarction. Int J Cardiol 1986; 10:141–7.

15 Berger PB, Ruocco NA Jr, Ryan TJ, Frederick MM, Jacobs AK, Faxon DP. Incidence and prognostic implications of heart block complicating inferior myocardial infarction treated with thrombolytic therapy: results from TIMI II. J Am Coll Cardiol 1992; 20:533–40.

16 Meine TJ, Al-Khatib SM, Alexander JH, et al. Incidence, predictors, and outcomes of high-degree atrioventricular block complicating acute myocardial infarction treated with thrombolytic therapy. Am Heart J 2005; 149:670–4.

17 Englund A, Bergfeldt L, Rehnqvist N, Astrom H, Rosenqvist M. Diagnostic value of programmed ventricular stimulation in patients with bifascicular block: a prospective study of patients with and without syncope. J Am Coll Cardiol 1995; 26:1508–15.

18 Simantirakis EN, Schiza SE, Chrysostomakis SI, et al. Atrial overdrive pacing for the obstructive sleep apnea-hypopnea syndrome. N Engl J Med 2005; 353:2568–77.

19 Krahn AD, Yee R, Erickson MK, et al. Physiologic pacing in patients with obstructive sleep apnea: a prospective, randomized crossover trial. J Am Coll Cardiol 2006; 47:379–83.

20 Gami AS, Pressman G, Caples SM, et al. Association of atrial fibrillation and obstructive sleep apnea. Circulation 2004; 110:364–7.

21 Brandt J, Anderson H, Fahraeus T, Schuller H. Natural history of sinus node disease treated with atrial pacing in 213 patients: implications for selection of stimulation mode. J Am Coll Cardiol 1992; 20:633–9.

22 Sutton R, Kenny RA. The natural history of sick sinus syndrome. Pacing Clin Electrophysiol 1986; 9:1110–4.

23 Sharma AD, Rizo-Patron C, Hallstrom AP, et al. Percent right ventricular pacing predicts outcomes in the DAVID trial. Heart Rhythm 2005; 2:830–4.

24 Wilkoff BL, Cook JR, Epstein AE, et al. Dual-chamber pacing or ventricular backup pacing in patients with an implantable defibrillator: the Dual Chamber and VVI Implantable Defibrillator (DAVID) Trial. JAMA 2002; 288:3115–23.

25 Lamas GA, Lee KL, Sweeney MO, et al. Ventricular pacing or dual-chamber pacing for sinus-node dysfunction. N Engl J Med 2002; 346:1854–62.

26 Sweeney MO, Hellkamp AS, Ellenbogen KA, et al. Adverse effect of ventricular pacing on heart failure and atrial fibrillation among patients with normal baseline QRS duration in a clinical trial of pacemaker therapy for sinus node dysfunction. Circulation 2003; 107:2932–7.

27 Grubb BP. Neurocardiogenic syncope and related disorders of orthostatic intolerance. Circulation 2005; 111: 2997–3006.

28 Kerr SR, Pearce MS, Brayne C, Davis RJ, Kenny RA. Carotid sinus hypersensitivity in asymptomatic older persons: implications for diagnosis of syncope and falls. Arch Intern Med 2006; 166:515–20.

29 Del Rosso A, Alboni P, Brignole M, Menozzi C, Raviele A. Relation of clinical presentation of syncope to the age of patients. Am J Cardiol 2005; 96:1431–5.

30 Ammirati F, Colivicchi F, Santini M. Permanent cardiac pacing versus medical treatment for the prevention of recurrent vasovagal syncope: a multicenter, randomized, controlled trial. Circulation 2001; 104:52–7.

31 Connolly SJ, Sheldon R, Roberts RS, Gent M. The North American Vasovagal Pacemaker Study (VPS). A randomized trial of permanent cardiac pacing for the prevention of vasovagal syncope. J Am Coll Cardiol 1999; 33:16–20.

32 Sutton R, Brignole M, Menozzi C, et al. Dual-chamber pacing in the treatment of neurally mediated tilt-positive cardioinhibitory syncope: pacemaker versus no therapy – a multicenter randomized study. The Vasovagal Syncope International Study (VASIS) Investigators. Circulation 2000; 102:294–9.

33 Connolly SJ, Sheldon R, Thorpe KE, et al. Pacemaker therapy for prevention of syncope in patients with recurrent severe vasovagal syncope: Second Vasovagal Pacemaker Study (VPS II): a randomized trial. JAMA 2003; 289:2224–9.

34 Raviele A, Giada F, Menozzi C, et al. A randomized, double-blind, placebo-controlled study of permanent cardiac pacing for the treatment of recurrent tilt-induced vasovagal syncope. The vasovagal syncope and pacing trial (SYNPACE). Eur Heart J 2004; 25:1741–8.

35 Sutton R. Has cardiac pacing a role in vasovagal syncope? J Interv Card Electrophysiol 2003; 9:145–9.

36 Friedman PA, Dijkman B, Warman EN, et al. Atrial therapies reduce atrial arrhythmia burden in defibrillator patients. Circulation 2001; 104:1023–8.

37 Israel CW, Hugl B, Unterberg C, et al. Pace-termination and pacing for prevention of atrial tachyarrhythmias: results from a multicenter study with an implantable device for atrial therapy. J Cardiovasc Electrophysiol 2001; 12:1121–8.

38 Lee MA, Weachter R, Pollak S, et al. The effect of atrial pacing therapies on atrial tachyarrhythmia burden and

frequency: results of a randomized trial in patients with bradycardia and atrial tachyarrhythmias. J Am Coll Cardiol 2003; 41:1926–32.

39 Gillis AM, Koehler J, Morck M, Mehra R, Hettrick DA. High atrial antitachycardia pacing therapy efficacy is associated with a reduction in atrial tachyarrhythmia burden in a subset of patients with sinus node dysfunction and paroxysmal atrial fibrillation. Heart Rhythm 2005; 2:791–6.

40 Carlson MD, Ip J, Messenger J, et al. A new pacemaker algorithm for the treatment of atrial fibrillation: results of the Atrial Dynamic Overdrive Pacing Trial (ADOPT). J Am Coll Cardiol 2003; 42:627–33.

41 Alam M, Dokainish H, Lakkis N. Alcohol septal ablation for hypertrophic obstructive cardiomyopathy: a systematic review of published studies. J Interv Cardiol 2006; 19:319–27.

42 Nishimura RA, Trusty JM, Hayes DL, et al. Dual-chamber pacing for hypertrophic cardiomyopathy: a randomized, double-blind, crossover trial. J Am Coll Cardiol 1997; 29:435–41.

43 Kappenberger L, Linde C, Daubert C, et al. Pacing in hypertrophic obstructive cardiomyopathy: a randomized crossover study. PIC Study Group. Eur Heart J 1997; 18:1249–56.

44 Maron BJ, Nishimura RA, McKenna WJ, Rakowski H, Josephson ME, Kieval RS. Assessment of permanent dual-chamber pacing as a treatment for drug-refractory symptomatic patients with obstructive hypertrophic cardiomyopathy: a randomized, double-blind, crossover study (M-PATHY). Circulation 1999; 99:2927–33.

45 Hawkins NM, Wang D, McMurray JJ, et al. Prevalence and prognostic impact of bundle branch block in patients with heart failure: evidence from the CHARM programme. Eur J Heart Fail 2007; 9:510–7.

46 Baldasseroni S, Opasich C, Gorini M, et al. Left bundle-branch block is associated with increased 1-year sudden and total mortality rate in 5517 outpatients with congestive heart failure: a report from the Italian network on congestive heart failure. Am Heart J 2002; 143:398–405.

47 Abraham WT, Fisher WG, Smith AL, et al. Cardiac resynchronization in chronic heart failure. N Engl J Med 2002; 346:1845–53.

48 Bristow MR, Saxon LA, Boehmer J, et al. Cardiac-resynchronization therapy with or without an implantable defibrillator in advanced chronic heart failure. N Engl J Med 2004; 350:2140–50.

49 Cleland JG, Daubert JC, Erdmann E, et al. The effect of cardiac resynchronization on morbidity and mortality in heart failure. N Engl J Med 2005; 352:1539–49.

50 Linde C, Abraham WT, Gold MR, St. John Sutton M, Ghio S, Daubert C. Randomized trial of cardiac resynchronization in mildly symptomatic heart failure patients and in asymptomatic patients with left ventricular dysfunction and previous heart failure symptoms. J Am Coll Cardiol 2008; 52:1834–43.

51 Moss AJ, Hall WJ, Cannom DS, et al. Cardiac-resynchronization therapy for the prevention of heart-failure events. N Engl J Med 2009; 361:1329–38.

52 Tang AS, Wells GA, Talajic M, et al. Cardiac-resynchronization therapy for mild-to-moderate heart failure. N Engl J Med 2010; 363:2385–95.

53 Hoijer CJ, Meurling C, Brandt J. Upgrade to biventricular pacing in patients with conventional pacemakers and heart failure: a double-blind, randomized crossover study. Europace 2006; 8:51–5.

54 Eldadah ZA, Rosen B, Hay I, et al. The benefit of upgrading chronically right ventricle-paced heart failure patients to resynchronization therapy demonstrated by strain rate imaging. Heart Rhythm 2006; 3:435–42.

55 Witte KK, Pipes RR, Nanthakumar K, Parker JD. Biventricular pacemaker upgrade in previously paced heart failure patients: improvements in ventricular dyssynchrony. J Card Fail 2006; 12:199–204.

56 Ozcan C, Jahangir A, Friedman PA, et al. Significant effects of atrioventricular node ablation and pacemaker implantation on left ventricular function and long-term survival in patients with atrial fibrillation and left ventricular dysfunction. Am J Cardiol 2003; 92: 33–7.

57 Cazeau S, Leclercq C, Lavergne T, et al. Effects of multisite biventricular pacing in patients with heart failure and intraventricular conduction delay. N Engl J Med 2001; 344:873–80.

58 Auricchio A, Stellbrink C, Sack S, et al. Long-term clinical effect of hemodynamically optimized cardiac resynchronization therapy in patients with heart failure and ventricular conduction delay. J Am Coll Cardiol 2002; 39:2026–33.

59 Young JB, Abraham WT, Smith AL, et al. Combined cardiac resynchronization and implantable cardioversion defibrillation in advanced chronic heart failure: the MIRACLE ICD Trial. JAMA 2003; 289:2685–94.

60 Higgins SL, Hummel JD, Niazi IK, et al. Cardiac resynchronization therapy for the treatment of heart failure in patients with intraventricular conduction delay and malignant ventricular tachyarrhythmias. J Am Coll Cardiol 2003; 42:1454–9.

61 Strickberger SA, Conti J, Daoud EG, et al. Patient selection for cardiac resynchronization therapy: from the Council on Clinical Cardiology Subcommittee on Electrocardiography and Arrhythmias and the Quality of Care and Outcomes Research Interdisciplinary Working Group, in collaboration with the Heart Rhythm Society. Circulation 2005; 111:2146–50.

62 Miyazaki C, Redfield MM, Powell BD, et al. Dyssynchrony indices to predict response to cardiac resynchronization therapy: a comprehensive prospective single-center study. Circ Heart Fail 2010; 3:565–73.

63 Sipahi I, Carrigan TP, Rowland DY, Stambler BS, Fang JC. Impact of QRS duration on clinical event reduction with cardiac resynchronization therapy: meta-analysis of randomized controlled trials. Arch Intern Med 2011; 171:1454–62.

64 Nery PB, Ha AC, Keren A, Birnie DH. Cardiac resynchronization therapy in patients with left ventricular systolic dysfunction and right bundle branch block: a systematic review. Heart Rhythm 2011; 8:1083–7.

65 Doshi RN, Daoud EG, Fellows C, *et al.* Left ventricular-based cardiac stimulation post AV nodal ablation evaluation (the PAVE study). J Cardiovasc Electrophysiol 2005; 16:1160–5.

66 Bradley DJ, Shen WK. Atrioventricular junction ablation combined with either right ventricular pacing or cardiac resynchronization therapy for atrial fibrillation: the need for large-scale randomized trials. Heart Rhythm 2007; 4:224–32.

67 Dong K, Shen WK, Powell BD, *et al.* Atrioventricular nodal ablation predicts survival benefit in patients with atrial fibrillation receiving cardiac resynchronization therapy. Heart Rhythm 2010; 7:1240–5.

68 DiBiase A, Tse TM, Schnittger I, Wexler L, Stinson EB, Valantine HA. Frequency and mechanism of bradycardia in cardiac transplant recipients and need for pacemakers. Am J Cardiol 1991; 67:1385–9.

69 Payne ME, Murray KD, Watson KM, *et al.* Permanent pacing in heart transplant recipients: underlying causes and long-term results. J Heart Lung Transplant 1991; 10:738–42.

70 Mirowski M, Reid PR, Mower MM, *et al.* Termination of malignant ventricular arrhythmias with an implanted automatic defibrillator in human beings. N Engl J Med 1980; 303:322–4.

71 Dreifus LS, Fisch C, Griffin JC, Gillette PC, Mason JW, Parsonnet V. Guidelines for implantation of cardiac pacemakers and antiarrhythmia devices. A report of the American College of Cardiology/American Heart Association Task Force on Assessment of Diagnostic and Therapeutic Cardiovascular Procedures (Committee on Pacemaker Implantation). J Am Coll Cardiol 1991; 18:1–13.

72 Connolly SJ, Hallstrom AP, Cappato R, *et al.* Meta-analysis of the implantable cardioverter defibrillator secondary prevention trials. AVID, CASH and CIDS studies. Antiarrhythmics vs. Implantable Defibrillator study. Cardiac Arrest Study Hamburg. Canadian Implantable Defibrillator Study. Eur Heart J 2000; 21:2071–8.

73 Glikson M, Lipchenca I, Viskin S, *et al.* Long-term outcome of patients who received implantable cardioverter defibrillators for stable ventricular tachycardia. J Cardiovasc Electrophysiol 2004; 15:658–64.

74 Auricchio A, Klein H, Geller CJ, Reek S, Heilman MS, Szymkiewicz SJ. Clinical efficacy of the wearable cardioverter-defibrillator in acutely terminating episodes of ventricular fibrillation. Am J Cardiol 1998; 81: 1253–6.

75 Feldman AM, Klein H, Tchou P, *et al.* Use of a wearable defibrillator in terminating tachyarrhythmias in patients at high risk for sudden death: results of the WEARIT/BIROAD. Pacing Clin Electrophysiol 2004; 27:4–9.

76 Chung MK, Szymkiewicz SJ, Shao M, *et al.* Aggregate national experience with the wearable cardioverter-defibrillator: event rates, compliance, and survival. J Am Coll Cardiol 2010; 56;194–203.

77 Wilber DJ, Olshansky B, Moran JF, Scanlon PJ. Electrophysiological testing and nonsustained ventricular tachycardia: use and limitations in patients with coronary artery disease and impaired ventricular function. Circulation 1990; 82:350–8.

78 Moss AJ, Hall WJ, Cannom DS, *et al.* Improved survival with an implanted defibrillator in patients with coronary disease at high risk for ventricular arrhythmia. Multicenter Automatic Defibrillator Implantation Trial Investigators. N Engl J Med 1996; 335:1933–40.

79 Buxton AE, Lee KL, Fisher JD, Josephson ME, Prystowsky EN, Hafley G. A randomized study of the prevention of sudden death in patients with coronary artery disease. Multicenter Unsustained Tachycardia Trial Investigators. N Engl J Med 1999; 341:1882–90.

80 Buxton AE, Lee KL, Hafley GE, *et al.* Relation of ejection fraction and inducible ventricular tachycardia to mode of death in patients with coronary artery disease: an analysis of patients enrolled in the multicenter unsustained tachycardia trial. Circulation 2002; 106:2466–72.

81 Moss AJ, Zareba W, Hall WJ, *et al.* Prophylactic implantation of a defibrillator in patients with myocardial infarction and reduced ejection fraction. N Engl J Med 2002; 346:877–83.

82 Bardy GH, Lee KL, Mark DB, *et al.* Amiodarone or an implantable cardioverter-defibrillator for congestive heart failure. N Engl J Med 2005; 352:225–37.

83 Hohnloser SH, Kuck KH, Dorian P, *et al.* Prophylactic use of an implantable cardioverter-defibrillator after acute myocardial infarction. N Engl J Med 2004; 351:2481–8.

84 Solomon SD, Glynn RJ, Greaves S, *et al.* Recovery of ventricular function after myocardial infarction in the reperfusion era: the healing and early afterload reducing therapy study. Ann Intern Med 2001; 134:451–8.

85 Packer DL, Gillis AM, Calkins H, Deering TF, Fogel RI, Wilkoff BL. ICDs: evidence, guidelines and glitches. Heart Rhythm 2011; 8:800–3.

86 Bigger JT Jr. Prophylactic use of implanted cardiac defibrillators in patients at high risk for ventricular arrhythmias after coronary-artery bypass graft surgery. Coronary Artery Bypass Graft (CABG) Patch Trial Investigators. N Engl J Med 1997; 337:1569–75.

87 Goldenberg I, Moss AJ, McNitt S, *et al.* Time dependence of defibrillator benefit after coronary revascularization in the Multicenter Automatic Defibrillator Implantation Trial (MADIT)-II. J Am Coll Cardiol 2006; 47:1811–7.

88 Bax JJ, Visser FC, Poldermans D, *et al.* Time course of functional recovery of stunned and hibernating segments after surgical revascularization. Circulation 2001; 104 (Suppl 1):314–8.

89 Wilber DJ, Zareba W, Hall WJ, *et al.* Time dependence of mortality risk and defibrillator benefit after myocardial infarction. Circulation 2004; 109:1082–4.

90 Grzybowski J, Bilinska ZT, Ruzyllo W, *et al.* Determinants of prognosis in nonischemic dilated cardiomyopathy. J Card Fail 1996; 2:77–85.

91 Bart BA, Shaw LK, McCants CB Jr, *et al.* Clinical determinants of mortality in patients with angiographically diagnosed ischemic or nonischemic cardiomyopathy. J Am Coll Cardiol 1997; 30:1002–8.

92 Felker GM, Thompson RE, Hare JM, *et al.* Underlying causes and long-term survival in patients with initially

unexplained cardiomyopathy. N Engl J Med 2000; 342:1077–84.

93 Nazarian S, Bluemke DA, Lardo AC, *et al.* Magnetic resonance assessment of the substrate for inducible ventricular tachycardia in nonischemic cardiomyopathy. Circulation 2005; 112:2821–5.

94 Assomull RG, Prasad SK, Lyne J, *et al.* Cardiovascular magnetic resonance, fibrosis, and prognosis in dilated cardiomyopathy. J Am Coll Cardiol 2006; 48:1977–85.

95 Poll DS, Marchlinski FE, Buxton AE, Josephson ME. Usefulness of programmed stimulation in idiopathic dilated cardiomyopathy. Am J Cardiol 1986; 58:992–7.

96 Das SK, Morady F, DiCarlo L Jr, *et al.* Prognostic usefulness of programmed ventricular stimulation in idiopathic dilated cardiomyopathy without symptomatic ventricular arrhythmias. Am J Cardiol 1986; 58:998–1000.

97 Constantin L, Martins JB, Kienzle MG, Brownstein SL, McCue ML, Hopson RC. Induced sustained ventricular tachycardia in nonischemic dilated cardiomyopathy: dependence on clinical presentation and response to antiarrhythmic agents. Pacing Clin Electrophysiol 1989; 12:776–83.

98 Chen X, Shenasa M, Borggrefe M, *et al.* Role of programmed ventricular stimulation in patients with idiopathic dilated cardiomyopathy and documented sustained ventricular tachyarrhythmias: inducibility and prognostic value in 102 patients. Eur Heart J 1994; 15:76–82.

99 Turitto G, Ahuja RK, Caref EB, Elsherif N. Risk stratification for arrhythmic events in patients with nonischemic dilated cardiomyopathy and nonsustained ventricular-tachycardia: role of programmed ventricular stimulation and the signal-averaged electrocardiogram. J Am Coll Cardiol 1994; 24:1523–28.

100 Grimm W, Hoffmann J, Menz V, Luck K, Maisch B. Programmed ventricular stimulation for arrhythmia risk prediction in patients with idiopathic dilated cardiomyopathy and nonsustained ventricular tachycardia. J Am Coll Cardiol 1998; 32:739–45.

101 Grimm W, Christ M, Bach J, Muller HH, Maisch B. Noninvasive arrhythmia risk stratification in idiopathic dilated cardiomyopathy: results of the Marburg cardiomyopathy study. Circulation 2003; 108:2883–91.

102 Bansch D, Antz M, Boczor S, *et al.* Primary prevention of sudden cardiac death in idiopathic dilated cardiomyopathy: the cardiomyopathy trial (CAT). Circulation 2002; 105:1453–58.

103 Strickberger SA, Hummel JD, Bartlett TG, *et al.* Amiodarone versus implantable cardioverter-defibrillator: randomized trial in patients with nonischemic dilated cardiomyopathy and asymptomatic nonsustained ventricular tachycardia (AMIOVIRT). J Am Coll Cardiol 2003; 41:1707–12.

104 Kadish A, Dyer A, Daubert JP, *et al.* Prophylactic defibrillator implantation in patients with nonischemic dilated cardiomyopathy. N Engl J Med 2004; 350:2151–8.

105 McClellan MB, Tunis SR. Medicare coverage of ICDs. N Engl J Med 2005; 352:222–4.

106 Makati KJ, Fish AE, England HH, Tighiouart H, Estes NA 3rd, Link MS. Equivalent arrhythmic risk in patients recently diagnosed with dilated cardiomyopathy compared with patients diagnosed for 9 months or more. Heart Rhythm 2006; 3:397–403.

107 Chugh SS, Shen WK, Luria DM, Smith HC. First evidence of premature ventricular complex-induced cardiomyopathy: a potentially reversible cause of heart failure. J Cardiovasc Electrophysiol 2000; 11:328–9.

108 Marchlinski FE, Jessup M. Timing the implantation of implantable cardioverter-defibrillators in patients with nonischemic cardiomyopathy. J Am Coll Cardiol 2006; 47:2483–5.

109 Schwartz PJ, Priori SG, Spazzolini C, *et al.* Genotype-phenotype correlation in the long-QT syndrome: gene-specific triggers for life-threatening arrhythmias. Circulation 2001; 103:89–95.

110 Schwartz PJ. The congenital long QT syndromes from genotype to phenotype: clinical implications. J Intern Med 2006; 259:39–47.

111 Vincent GM, Schwartz PJ, Denjoy I, *et al.* High efficacy of beta-blockers in long-QT syndrome type 1: contribution of noncompliance and QT-prolonging drugs to the occurrence of beta-blocker treatment "failures". Circulation 2009; 119:215–21.

112 Zareba W, Moss AJ, Daubert JP, Hall WJ, Robinson JL, Andrews M. Implantable cardioverter defibrillator in high-risk long QT syndrome patients. J Cardiovasc Electrophysiol 2003; 14:337–41.

113 Sauer AJ, Moss AJ, McNitt S, *et al.* Long QT syndrome in adults. J Am Coll Cardiol 2007; 49:329–37.

114 Priori SG, Napolitano C, Gasparini M, *et al.* Clinical and genetic heterogeneity of right bundle branch block and ST-segment elevation syndrome: a prospective evaluation of 52 families. Circulation 2000; 102:2509–15.

115 Priori SG, Napolitano C. Should patients with an asymptomatic Brugada electrocardiogram undergo pharmacological and electrophysiological testing? Circulation 2005; 112:279–92.

116 Gehi AK, Duong TD, Metz LD, Gomes JA, Mehta D. Risk stratification of individuals with the Brugada electrocardiogram: a meta-analysis. J Cardiovasc Electrophysiol 2006; 17:577–83.

117 Nademanee K, Veerakul G, Mower M, *et al.* Defibrillator Versus beta-Blockers for Unexplained Death in Thailand (DEBUT): a randomized clinical trial. Circulation 2003; 107:2221–6.

118 Priori SG, Napolitano C, Gasparini M, *et al.* Natural history of Brugada syndrome: insights for risk stratification and management. Circulation 2002; 105:1342–7.

119 Antzelevitch C, Brugada P, Borggrefe M, *et al.* Brugada syndrome: report of the second consensus conference: endorsed by the Heart Rhythm Society and the European Heart Rhythm Association. Circulation 2005; 111:659–70.

120 Gussak I, Brugada P, Brugada J, *et al.* Idiopathic short QT interval: a new clinical syndrome? Cardiology 2000; 94:99–102.

121 Reinig MG, Engel TR. The shortage of short QT intervals. Chest 2007; 132:246–9.

122 Gallagher MM, Magliano G, Yap YG, *et al.* Distribution and prognostic significance of QT intervals in the lowest

half centile in 12,012 apparently healthy persons. Am J Cardiol 2006; 98:933–5.

123 Priori SG, Napolitano C, Memmi M, et al. Clinical and molecular characterization of patients with catecholaminergic polymorphic ventricular tachycardia. Circulation 2002; 106:69–74.

124 Thiene G, Nava A, Corrado D, Rossi L, Pennelli N. Right ventricular cardiomyopathy and sudden death in young people. N Engl J Med 1988; 318:129–33.

125 McKoy G, Protonotarios N, Crosby A, et al. Identification of a deletion in plakoglobin in arrhythmogenic right ventricular cardiomyopathy with palmoplantar keratoderma and woolly hair (Naxos disease). Lancet 2000; 355:2119–24.

126 Sen-Chowdhry S, Lowe MD, Sporton SC, McKenna WJ. Arrhythmogenic right ventricular cardiomyopathy: clinical presentation, diagnosis, and management. Am J Med 2004; 117:685–95.

127 Roguin A, Bomma CS, Nasir K, et al. Implantable cardioverter-defibrillators in patients with arrhythmogenic right ventricular dysplasia/cardiomyopathy. J Am Coll Cardiol 2004; 43:1843–52.

128 Corrado D, Leoni L, Link MS, et al. Implantable cardioverter-defibrillator therapy for prevention of sudden death in patients with arrhythmogenic right ventricular cardiomyopathy/dysplasia. Circulation 2003; 108:3084–91.

129 Fontaine G. The use of ICDs for the treatment of patients with Arrhythmogenic Right Ventricular Dysplasia (ARVD). J Interv Card Electrophysiol 1997; 1:329–30.

130 Maron BJ. Hypertrophic cardiomyopathy: a systematic review. JAMA 2002; 287:1308–20.

131 Maron BJ, Shen WK, Link MS, et al. Efficacy of implantable cardioverter-defibrillators for the prevention of sudden death in patients with hypertrophic cardiomyopathy. N Engl J Med 2000; 342:365–73.

132 Firoozi S, Sharma S, McKenna WJ. Risk of competitive sport in young athletes with heart disease. Heart 2003; 89:710–4.

133 Maron BJ, McKenna WJ, Danielson GK, et al. American College of Cardiology/European Society of Cardiology clinical expert consensus document on hypertrophic cardiomyopathy. A report of the American College of Cardiology Foundation Task Force on Clinical Expert Consensus Documents and the European Society of Cardiology Committee for Practice Guidelines. J Am Coll Cardiol 2003; 42:1687–713.

134 Elliott PM, Poloniecki J, Dickie S, et al. Sudden death in hypertrophic cardiomyopathy: identification of high risk patients. J Am Coll Cardiol 2000; 36:2212–8.

135 Ommen SR, Maron BJ, Olivotto I, et al. Long-term effects of surgical septal myectomy on survival in patients with obstructive hypertrophic cardiomyopathy. J Am Coll Cardiol 2005; 46:470–6.

136 Gatzoulis MA, Balaji S, Webber SA, et al. Risk factors for arrhythmia and sudden cardiac death late after repair of tetralogy of Fallot: a multicentre study. Lancet 2000; 356:975–81.

137 Chandar JS, Wolff GS, Garson A Jr, et al. Ventricular arrhythmias in postoperative tetralogy of Fallot. Am J Cardiol 1990; 65:655–61.

138 Alexander ME, Walsh EP, Saul JP, Epstein MR, Triedman JK. Value of programmed ventricular stimulation in patients with congenital heart disease. J Cardiovasc Electrophysiol 1999; 10:1033–44.

139 Khairy P, Landzberg MJ, Gatzoulis MA, et al. Value of programmed ventricular stimulation after tetralogy of fallot repair: a multicenter study. Circulation 2004; 109:1994–2000.

4 Choosing the Device Generator and Leads: Matching the Device with the Patient

Malini Madhavan, David L. Hayes, Paul A. Friedman, Samuel J. Asirvatham

Mayo Clinic, Rochester, MN, USA

Pacemaker selection 134
  Symptomatic bradycardia 135
  Pure sinus node dysfunction 136
  Pure atrioventricular block 136
  Neurocardiogenic syncope and carotid sinus hypersensitivity 136
Choosing specific programmable options 136
Choosing the rate-adaptive sensor 136
Choosing the lead or leads 136
  Threshold reduction 137
  Lead polarity 137
  Electrode design 139
  Lead conductor 139
  Lead insulation 139
  Lead diameter 140
  Compatibility of lead and pulse generator 141
  Epicardial leads 141
  Resources for lead performance and survival data 142
Generator and lead selection in defibrillators 144
  Lead design considerations for ICD leads 144
    Coaxial and multilumen leads 144

ICD lead conductor 145
ICD lead defibrillation coil 145
ICD lead insulation material 145
Integrated and bipolar sensing 146
ICD lead connector 147
Size and longevity 148
Programmable waveforms 149
Dual-chamber or single-chamber ICD? 149
  Factors favoring single-chamber defibrillators 149
  Factors favoring dual-chamber defibrillators 149
  Specific device and lead features influencing selection 150
  Avoiding adverse effects from the lead or from frequent and unnecessary pacing 150
  Cardiac resynchronization therapy 151
  Promoting continuous biventricular pacing 151
  Leads for resynchronization devices 151
  RV–LV pacing offset and vector of pacing 153
Conclusions 154
References 154

Cardiac Pacing, Defibrillation and Resynchronization: A Clinical Approach, Third Edition.
David L. Hayes, Samuel J. Asirvatham, and Paul A. Friedman.
© 2013 Mayo Foundation for Medical Education and Research. Published 2013 by John Wiley & Sons, Ltd.

The purpose of this chapter is to provide direction in choosing the most appropriate pulse generator – pacemaker, internal cardioverter-defibrillator (ICD) or cardiac resynchronization therapy (CRT) – and leads for a given patient. It is not possible to provide guidelines that meet the needs of every patient; indeed, pulse generator selection, whether pacemaker, ICD, or CRT, must be individualized. Our goal is to provide practical considerations and a generic approach to determine the type of hardware most appropriate for the patient who is receiving an implantable cardiac device.

Pacemaker selection

Pacemaker selection today involves a decision as to whether cardiac resynchronization is required. A significant proportion of patients receiving devices have combined abnormalities that may include chronotropic incompetence, atrioventricular (AV) nodal dysfunction, intraventricular conduction delay (electrical ventricular dyssynchrony), and the propensity for ventricular arrhythmia. Thus, decisions for patients requiring pacemakers may involve consideration and exclusion of the need for a defibrillator lead or a left ventricular (LV) pacing lead. The data supporting the hemodynamic benefits of cardiac resynchronization and the present indications are discussed in Chapters 2 and 3. In this chapter, after a brief summary of the generally used algorithm for deciding which pulse generator, mode selection, and leads are to be used, we point out specific issues relevant to cardiac resynchronization devices.

While substantive algorithms have been described for pacemaker mode selection (Figs 4.1 and 4.2)[1], a simplified approach is presented here. For patients with chronic atrial fibrillation who require pacing, a single-chamber device with VVIR mode selection is preferred. For all other patients, a dual-chamber device with DDDR pacing and automatic mode switch to a non-tracking mode during paroxysms of atrial fibrillation is done. Occasionally, patients with limited longevity or highly limited activity levels may do best with a single lead and VVI or VVIR modes.[2]

Even for a patient with another irreversible and possibly progressive medical illness and marked limitations in activity in whom a decision is made to implant a pacemaker, if VVI pacing results in pacemaker syndrome, the patient may actually feel worse. Although such an outcome may be impossible to predict, it should at least be considered and, at a minimum, blood pressures should be compared in the native underlying rhythm vs. ventricular pacing.

At one time there were significant cost differences between simpler devices (VVI) and those that had rate-adaptive pacing, etc. Today, these differences are largely negligible in most parts of the world, and the main decision that needs to be made is whether a single-

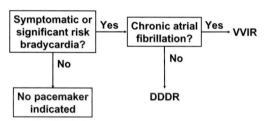

Fig. 4.2 Algorithm for pacing mode selection that includes only DDDR and VVIR pacing modes.

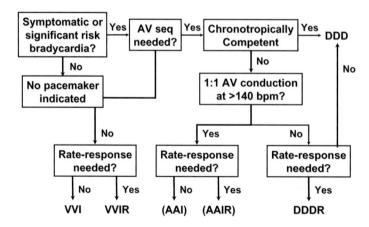

Fig. 4.1 Algorithm for pacing mode selection that includes most available pacing modes. AV, atrioventricular; seq, sequential.

chamber device will suffice (chronic atrial fibrillation). Internationally, however, the simplest device (single-chamber non-rate-adaptive) may be necessary to save lives amidst more significant economic constraints. In most practices, however, devices retaining options for more complex pacing requirements are placed and programmed "on" when required (Table 4.1).

Symptomatic bradycardia

For most patients with bradyarrhythmias requiring pacing who do not have chronic atrial fibrillation, a dual-chamber pacemaker is indicated. Using a dual-chamber pacemaker with rate-adaptive capabilities (DDDR) in all patients provides the greatest long-term flexibility, and most patients with symptomatic

Table 4.1 Indications for various pacing modes.

Mode	Generally agreed-upon indications	Controversial indications	Contraindications
VVI		Symptomatic bradycardia in the patient with associated terminal illness or other medical conditions from which recovery is not anticipated and pacing is life-sustaining only	Patients with known PM syndrome or hemodynamic deterioration with ventricular pacing at the time of implantation CI patient who will benefit from rate response Patients with hemodynamic need for dual-chamber pacing
VVIR	Fixed atrial arrhythmias (AF or atrial flutter) with symptomatic bradycardia	Same as for VVI	Patients with known PM syndrome or hemodynamic deterioration with ventricular pacing at the time of implantation Patients with hemodynamic need for dual-chamber pacing
AAI	Symptomatic bradycardia as a result of SND in the otherwise CC patient when AV conduction can be proven normal		SND with associated AV block demonstrated either spontaneously or during preimplantation testing In the unlikely event that atrial sensing is inadequate
AAIR	Symptomatic bradycardia as a result of SND in the CI patient when AV conduction can be proven normal		Same as for AAI
VDD	Congenital AV block AV block when sinus node function can be proven normal	AV block when sinus node function can be proven normal	SND AV block accompanied by SND When adequate atrial sensing cannot be attained AV block accompanied by paroxysmal supraventricular tachycardias
VDDR	Same as for VDD, but when a potential need for ventricular rate-adaptive pacing also exists		Same as for VDD
DDD*	AV block and SND in the CC patient Need for AV synchrony, e.g., to maximize cardiac output, inactive patients Previous PM syndrome with VVI(R) pacemaker	For any rhythm disturbance when atrial sensing and capture are possible, with the exception of AF or atrial flutter, potentially to minimize future AF, reduce morbidity, and improve survival For the suppression of tachyarrhythmias by overdrive suppression	Chronic AF, atrial flutter, giant inexcitable atrium, or other frequent paroxysmal supraventricular tachyarrhythmias When adequate atrial sensing cannot be attained
DDDR	AV block and SND in the CI patient	Same as for DDD	Same as for DDD

AF, atrial fibrillation; AV, atrioventricular; CC, chronotropically competent; CI, chronotropically incompetent; PM, pacemaker; SND, sinus node dysfunction.

*DDI and DDIR are not included as separate modes in this table because they are not commonly used as the preimplantation modes of choice.

bradycardia often have associated chronotropic incompetence or at least the potential for this to occur. In some situations, however, rate-adaptive pacing is essential, including dual-chamber devices placed specifically for patients with sick sinus syndrome and fatigue from documented chronotropic incompetence and patients with chronic atrial fibrillation with slow ventricular rates. Because rate responsiveness in patients with chronic atrial fibrillation depends on autonomic regulation of the AV node (poorly regulated), these patients necessarily require sensor-driven pacing. For example, if chronic atrial fibrillation with a slow ventricular response develops at a later date, the DDDR pacemaker could be reprogrammed to VVIR. A DDD pacemaker, which has no rate-adaptive capability, could be programmed only to VVI, potentially a suboptimal option.

Pure sinus node dysfunction

For the patient with pure sinus node disease, i.e., no documented or provocable abnormalities in AV nodal conduction, AAIR pacing may be appropriate. (Preimplantation criteria for AAI/AAIR pacing are described in Chapter 3.) If preimplantation testing has established normal AV nodal conduction, the annual risk of AV block developing is 1–2%.[3,4] If AV block develops, another procedure is required to implant a ventricular lead and upgrade the pacemaker. This additional procedure is obviated if a DDDR pacemaker is used initially.

Although DDDR pacing gives the most flexibility of options, some disadvantages of placing a ventricular lead and pacing the right ventricle require consideration. The adverse effects of right ventricular pacing are discussed in Chapter 2: Hemodynamics, and ventricular avoidance pacing algorithms are discussed in Chapter 7: Timing Cycles and Chapter 8: Programming.

Pure atrioventricular block

For the patient with pure AV node disease, i.e., no documented abnormalities in sinus node behavior, VDD or VDDR pacing may be appropriate. Specifically, the patient with congenital complete heart block may do well with VDD(R) pacing.[5,6] As before, a problem arises if sinus node dysfunction develops in the future, resulting in a suboptimal pacing mode without reasonable programming options. However, from a "hardware" perspective, use of a single-lead VDD or VDDR pacing system helps to minimize the amount of hardware needed. This can be especially important for pediatric patients.

Single-pass VDD(R) systems are occasionally favored in pediatric patients, but otherwise this pacing mode is not commonly used. Single-pass VDD leads, i.e., atrial sensing occurs via "floating" electrodes in the atrialized portion of the lead, have generally been passive fixation leads, and for pediatric patients many implanters, including our institution, would prefer active-fixation leads.

It should be mentioned that single-pass leads have also been used for DDD pacing, i.e., the floating atrial electrodes are capable of pacing and sensing.[7] This approach to DDD pacing has never been widely embraced. Concerns have been the requirement for high atrial outputs in order to achieve capture and phrenic nerve stimulation. Placing a single-pass DDD lead in the coronary sinus has also been attempted for left atrial and left ventricular stimulation.[8]

Neurocardiogenic syncope and carotid sinus hypersensitivity

If a patient requires pacing for neurocardiogenic syncope, whether the vasovagal variety or carotid sinus hypersensitivity, dual-chamber pacing is necessary for several reasons.[9–11] In a patient with vasovagal syncope that most likely has some component of vasodepression together with the cardio-inhibition that requires pacing, ventricular pacing alone could result in pacemaker syndrome and further aggravate symptoms caused by hypotension. The bradycardia that occurs in patients with carotid sinus hypersensitivity may be due to either AV block or sinus arrest. Therefore, ventricular pacing support is required, and dual-chamber pacing is superior for the reasons already noted. For specific programmable options that are desirable when pacing patients with these disorders see Chapter 8: Programming and Chapter 7: Timing Cycles.

Choosing specific programmable options

Programming and the wide variety of programmable options available in current devices are covered in Chapter 8: Programming.

Choosing the rate-adaptive sensor

When choosing hardware for a specific patient, there may be advantages of one rate-adaptive sensor over another. This is discussed in Chapter 9: Rate-Adaptive Pacing.

Choosing the lead or leads

A detailed discussion of the merits of various lead types is beyond the scope of this chapter, as is a thorough discussion of the evolution of pacing leads. Rather, the purpose of the chapter is to provide the reader with an understanding of the types of leads that are available and future trends that are likely to be seen.

With the exception of a few specific circumstances, choice of the pacing lead or leads becomes one of personal preference and personal bias. Choice of pacing

4A Active;

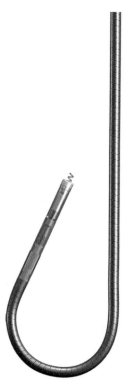

4B Passive

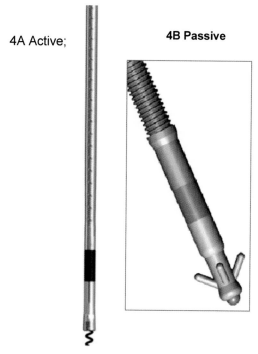

Fig. 4.3 Active fixation atrial "J" lead.

Fig. 4.4 (A) Active fixation lead which could be used in either chamber; active fixation leads may be straight or preformed J, unipolar or bipolar. Preformed J leads are used only in the atrium, and straight active fixation leads may be used in either chamber. The fixation mechanism varies, that is, the screw may be retractable or nonretractable. In some, the nonretractable screw is coated with a material that dissolves once in the bloodstream. This allows the lead to be passed into the heart without an exposed screw catching on the vascular tree. (B) Passive fixation lead which is typically used for right ventricular pacing. Passive fixation leads may also be unipolar or bipolar. Tines represent the nearly exclusive passive fixation mechanism used in contemporary passive fixation leads.

leads should also be based on performance data of the specific model. Options that must be considered for all leads are as follow:

- Type of insulation: silicone or polyurethane or a "hybrid" combination (such as in a bipolar coaxial lead where the inner and outer insulations are different materials)
- Mechanism of fixation: active or passive
- Polarity: unipolar or bipolar
- Compatibility of lead and pulse generator connection system.

Choice of an atrial pacing lead must take into account insulation, fixation, polarity, and whether the lead is straight or preformed J type (Fig. 4.3). The same decisions must be made for choice of the ventricular lead, except that right ventricular leads are straight (Fig. 4.4). Specific issues related to LV pacing are discussed below.

Threshold reduction

Although multiple mechanisms have been used to achieve lower thresholds, steroid elution has been the most successful and most widely used method for threshold reduction.[12,13] Steroid elution has been accomplished in several ways, such as from a steroid-saturated silicone plug within the lead's tip electrode or from a steroid-eluting collar adjacent to the tip

electrode (Fig. 4.5). Steroid elution significantly minimizes the post-implant pacing threshold increases and peaking that typically occurs with nonsteroid-eluting electrodes. The steroid-eluting plug or collar contains a very small amount of steroid, e.g., <1 mg dexamethasone sodium phosphate or dexamethasone acetate, which does not have any systemic effect. Steroid elution is available on atrial and ventricular leads with both active and passive fixation means, and is also available in coronary venous and epicardial leads. In nearly all institutions, steroid-eluting leads are used routinely.

Fractal coating (Fig. 4.6) and other techniques have also been used to lower pacing thresholds.

Lead polarity

Unipolar leads have an electrode at the tip that functions as the cathode and the pulse generator serves as

Steroid-lead

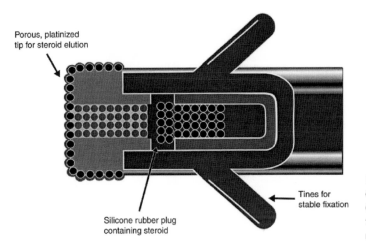

Porous, platinized
tip for steroid elution

Tines for
stable fixation

Silicone rubber plug
containing steroid

Fig. 4.5 Diagrammatic representation of a steroid-eluting lead. Steroid (dexamethasone) is slowly eluted through the porous, platinized tip of a silicone rubber plug.

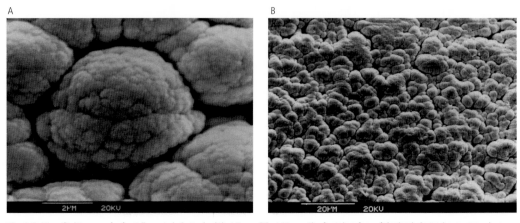

A

B

Fig. 4.6 Magnified images of a fractally coated electrode: (A) at 2 μm; (B) at 20 μm. The fractal surface of the lead electrodes creates a larger effective surface area, and as a result maximizes the myocardial interface, which is a major factor in determining a lead's sensing characteristics.

the anode. Bipolar leads have a both electrodes within the heart – the tip electrode functions as the cathode and a ring electrode proximal to the tip functions as the anode. Because the unipolar lead has a large interelectrode distance or a "big antenna," they are more susceptible to sensing of intracardiac and extracardiac far-field signals than bipolar leads.

Bipolar leads are used more frequently in the USA. This preference exists largely because of a lower susceptibility to electromagnetic interference and other far-field signals when pacemakers are in a bipolar sensing configuration.[14–16] If examined over decades of use, bipolar leads have had an overall higher incidence of failure than unipolar leads, largely because of the specific bipolar leads which utilized the 80A version of

polyurethane that failed in high numbers in the 1980s. If these leads were excluded from the analysis, the survival difference between unipolar and bipolar leads would be minimal.

The interelectrode distance of a bipolar lead also deserves consideration. This distance may not only affect the duration of the intracardiac electrogram signals, but it also usually has an effect on the amplitude and slew rate of the electrogram's signals, depending on the low- and high-frequency band pass filters in the input amplifiers of the device. A lead with a greater distance between electrodes will generally have larger amplitude far-field signals (i.e., R-waves sensed on an atrial lead). This characteristic may affect the reliability of mode switching. In pacing systems with more than one ventricular sensing lead, i.e., pacemaker and ICD in the same patient or ICD with biventricular pacing, minimizing far-field signals may also be of increased importance.

Electrode design

The choice of electrode material is guided by the metal–tissue impedance properties, tissue fibrotic reaction, long-term function, and susceptibility to corrosion. Platinum, platinum-iridium and Elgiloy (an alloy of cobalt, chromium, molybdenum, manganese, nickel, and iron) are commonly used. However, these metals are prone to corrosion in the body. Vitreous carbon electrodes are inert and have been shown to have lower chronic thresholds than platinum electrodes.

The impedance of the electrode–tissue interface is determined by electrode material, tissue characteristics, and electrode surface area in contact with tissue. Older leads had a large electrode surface area which resulted in low lead impedance resulting in high current drain and high pacing threshold. Contemporary electrode tips employ very a small surface area (e.g., the Medtronic CapSure 5054 lead has a 1.2-mm^2 electrode tip) which results in a high current density at the tip, higher lead impedance, lower pacing threshold, and improved generator longevity. Contemporary tip electrodes are made porous by using sintered or laser drilled tips. Porous electrodes have lower pacing threshold and dislodgement rates than smooth-tipped electrodes.

Lead conductor

The conductor is made of a high strength material such as MP35N (alloy of nickel, cobalt, chromium and molybdenum) made into a coil or drawn into a cable. Unipolar leads have one and bipolar leads have two conductors. Bipolar lead conductors can be arranged in parallel or coaxially. Coaxial leads have a central lumen that allows passage of a stylet for ease of lead placement. Traditionally, the two conductors in a coaxial bipolar lead were arranged concentrically and each surrounded by insulation material which resulted in bulkier and stiffer lead bodies. Current coaxial leads employ thin ETFE (ethylene tetrafluoroethylene) insulation on each conductor wire, such that both wires can be coiled into a single coil to reduce lead diameter and increase flexibility.

Lead insulation

With few exceptions, the materials that have been used for most pacing leads for almost five decades are silicone rubber and polyurethane. Historically, both have generally had excellent performance records. Table 4.2 compares the basic characteristics of silicone rubber and polyurethane. When first introduced, polyurethane insulated leads were widely used by many implanters because they could be designed to have a smaller lead body diameter than many of the contemporary silicone rubber insulated leads and were said to handle better when two leads were implanted due to their greater lubricity in the body. Improvements in silicone insulation and use of lubricious coatings have made these differences less significant.

Manufacturers often make the same lead available with either silicone or polyurethane outer insulation. Implanters base their choice on past experience, ideally taking into account product surveillance reports that detail the survival of specific leads. Not all agree on what is advantageous or disadvantageous about the characteristics of the insulating material.

For silicone rubber, being "very flexible" may or may not be an advantage. This quality means that something else in the design, such as the conductor coil, must increase the stiffness of the lead to the optimal value. A lead that is too flexible can damage the heart with excessive movement and may cause lead dislodgment or deterioration of the lead's electrical parameters. A lead that is too stiff may cause perforation or dislodgment. A stiff conductor coil can be more prone to fracture. Some currently available bipolar coaxial leads utilize both silicone (inner insulation) and polyurethane (outer insulation) to benefit maximally from both their properties. A new insulation material, created specifically for cardiac leads, is available and used in various types of leads, which is a silicone rubber–polyurethane copolymer (Optim®; St Jude Medical, Inc.).

"Smaller diameter possible" is not included in Table 4.2 because it is neither an advantage nor a disadvantage. It is the result of the polymer's mechanical properties such as high tear strength and higher stiffness. That is, even if silicone rubber had the same tear strength as polyurethane, smaller diameter insulation could make a lead like a whipsaw. Higher stiffness allows a thinner tube to maintain high torque strength for implantability, but the thinner tube makes the structure more flexible in bending. Therefore, an advantage of polyurethane in certain designs is "higher stiffness" combined with "higher tear strength."

Polyurethane has vastly superior compressive properties, specifically low creep or "cold-flow." It is also much less prone to abrasion from physical rubbing contact with other leads or the device. In addition, some believe that polyurethane is inherently less thrombogenic than silicone rubber. Although silicone rubber has been available longer, polyurethane has been used in humans as lead insulation for >30 years.

Polyurethane has been available in a softer, more flexible version known as "80A" and a harder, less flexible version known as "55D." Early leads made with the 80A polyurethane exhibited higher levels of

Table 4.2 Lead insulation: comparison of silicone rubber and polyurethane.

Silicone rubbe	Polyurethane
Advantages	
Performance record >30 years	High tear strength
Excellent biostability	High cut resistance
Flexibility	Low friction in blood
	High abrasion resistance
	Inherently less thrombogenic
	Superior compressive properties
Disadvantages	
Tears easily	Relatively stiff (55D)
Abrades easily	Potential for environmental
Cuts easily	stress cracking (true for
Higher friction in blood	Pellethane 80A)
Subject to cold flow failure	Potential for metal ion
More thrombogenic	oxidation (true for
	Pellethane 80A and 55D)
	More susceptible to cautery
	heat damage

degradation of the polyurethane insulation. Most current polyurethane leads utilize the 55D version insulation, which is much less prone to the degradation.

Silicone rubber is sometimes criticized for "absorbing lipids (calcifications)." Although lipid absorption is reported in the literature for ball and cage heart valves, it has not been proven to be clinically significant in pacing leads and does not appear to result in failures. Lipid absorption and calcification are two different phenomena. Even though mineralization of encapsulating sheaths (extrinsic mineralization) is common, there is no evidence that it causes lead insulation failure (although it greatly hinders removal of old leads). Mineralization of the silicone rubber per se (intrinsic mineralization) has also been rarely observed, but lead failures from this mechanism have been very rare.

Polyurethane, being "relatively stiffer," is often used advantageously, especially in a portion or certain segment of a lead, and allows manufacturers to make smaller, tough leads that can have greater torquability, resulting in easier implantability.

At one time, not being "repairable" was a disadvantage for polyurethane insulated leads vs. silicone leads. In the earlier years of cardiac pacing, experienced individuals would at times attempt outer insulation repair of silicone rubber insulated leads with medical adhesive and silicone film. This worked relatively well if done correctly. Also, terminal pin replacement on unipolar leads could be performed, if necessary, with specific repair "kits" from the manufacturers. At this time, repair of any portion of the lead should not be attempted. If a lead is malfunctioning or grossly damaged, it should be abandoned and capped, or extracted and replaced.

Although no longer a significant issue, "sensitivity to manufacturing process" can also be a disadvantage for both materials. Knowledge is required to work with either one. The potential for environmental surface cracking remains true for the 80A polyurethane, but is not a significant mechanism of clinical failure in contemporary 55D polyurethane leads. The potential for metal ion oxidation remains an issue for contemporary 55D polyurethane insulated leads. Despite a blemish on polyurethane leads due to a high failure rate in the 1980s of the 80A version of polyurethane, the overall survival rate for other, newer polyurethane leads utilizing the 55D version has been excellent.[17,18]

What is an acceptable rate of lead failure? Ideally, leads would never fail, but this level of reliability will never be reached. The acceptable failure rate for permanent pacing and defibrillation leads (and pulse generators for that matter) is a matter of continued debate.[19] During the preparation of this text there were a number of leads and pulse generators that were placed on advisory status, which has significantly fueled this debate. Some experts have suggested that no worse than 5% cumulative failure rate at 10 or 20 years should be goals for ICD and pacing leads, respectively. However, at this time, no specific acceptable failure rate can be quoted for any component of a pacing, defibrillation, or CRT system.

Lead diameter

Over the years the diameter of pacing leads has decreased. In general, lead diameters have decreased over the years, and while this is of benefit for ease of vascular access and preventing tricuspid regurgitation, SVT stenosis, etc., lead failure and lack of pain with manipulating with very small leads are potential disadvantages. There is still significant variation in the lead body size. Contemporary stylet-driven leads are commonly in the range of 4.5–7 Fr in size. Lead selection may be driven by "size" in some patients. It may be advantageous to use preferentially a small-diameter lead in children and in patients with existing transvenous leads in whom the vessel lumen is compromised.

More recently, a lumenless pacemaker lead (Select-Secure lead model 3830, Medtronic, Inc.) (Fig. 4.7) has become available which replaces the coil cathode with a cable conductor (Fig. 4.8). The lead is delivered using a deflectable catheter (deflectable model 10600 catheter, Medtronic, Inc.) without the use of a stylet. This allows for further reduction in lead diameter (4.1 Fr), increased lead body tensile strength, site-specific lead placement, and lead extraction without locking stylet. Implantation of this lead was shown to be feasible, but preliminary data suggest higher implantation complications including lead dislodgement and cardiac perforation as well as higher, but acceptable, pacing thresholds at 18 months' follow-up. Long-term experience with the lead is limited at this time.[20]

Compatibility of lead and pulse generator

The pacemaker lead or leads and pulse generator selected do not need to be from the same manufacturer. It is generally acceptable to "mix and match" leads from company X with a pulse generator from company Y, assuming similar functionality. What is mandatory is that the lead connector be compatible with the connector cavity of the pulse generator.

Historically, unipolar leads were 5 or 6 mm in diameter and bipolar leads were of the bifurcated design with similar 5 or 6-mm sizes. Most leads currently used are of "inline" bipolar design with a 3.2-mm diameter (Fig. 4.9). In 1986, a voluntary standard for lead connectors and connector cavities was established. This voluntary standard for leads and connectors incorporated sealing rings on a 3.2-mm lead connector and is referred to as VS-1.[21] Subsequently, an industry-wide, international standard configuration known as IS-1

(International Standard 1) was developed and accepted. Figure 4.10 shows the types of lead connectors available, and Fig. 4.11 demonstrates varieties of inline bipolar pulse generator headers. "Unipolar" leads comply with the same design features, but the ring electrode on a dedicated unipolar lead is electrically inactive. Currently, virtually all pacing leads comply with the IS-1 connector standard configuration.

Epicardial leads

Epicardial pacing may still be necessary in patients with congenital cardiac anomalies that prevent the access needed for transvenous leads, with a prosthetic tricuspid valve, or with other tricuspid valve abnormalities that preclude lead placement across the valve. Figure 4.12 demonstrates available types of epicardial fixation mechanisms. Epicardial leads have historically had higher pacing thresholds and less mechanical reliability than transvenous leads. Platinized and steroid-eluting epicardial leads are used in an attempt to keep epicardial pacing thresholds lower.[22,23]

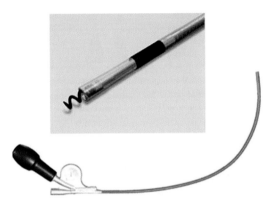

Fig. 4.7 An example of a lumenless lead, SelectSecure™, Medtronic, Inc., that is not stylet driven. Instead, the lead is advanced through a deflectable sheath that is maneuvered to the specific site of interest. The lead is then passed through the sheath and the helix advanced into the myocardium at that site. (Used with permission from Medtronic, Inc.)

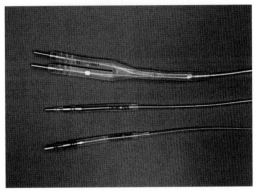

Fig. 4.9 Three pacemaker lead connectors. Top, Bifurcated bipolar lead – these leads are no longer manufactured, but there are still some in service. Middle, VS-1 in-line bipolar lead. Bottom, VS-1 unipolar lead; the ring electrode is inactive.

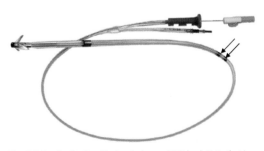

Fig. 4.8 Passive fixation bipolar single-pass VDD lead. Note that in the portion of the lead that will be positioned within the atrium, there are two ring electrodes (arrows). Sensing occurs via these "floating" atrial electrodes and allows P-synchronous pacing with a single lead.

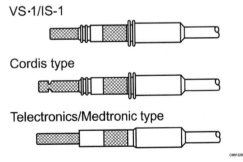

Fig. 4.10 Varieties of VS-1 leads. Top diagram, IS-1, VS-1 lead type. Middle diagram, 3.2-mm connector with sealing rings, referred to as the Cordis type. Bottom diagram, 3.2-mm connector pin without sealing rings, referred to as the Medtronics or Telectronics type.

Resources for lead performance and survival data

Lead choice is often determined by the implanter's personal experience. As new leads become available, it is important to be aware of resources of lead survival and performance. Resources include the following:
• Manufacturers' data (e.g., active lead registries, returned lead analysis)
• Published information from individual centers or consortium of larger medical centers
• Public databases.

Manufacturers are required by law to collect post-market surveillance data on hardware performance.

Various manufacturers use different approaches for collection and analysis of this information, but performance data should be available from any manufacturer on request. Figure 4.13 is an example of lead performance and survival data from one manufacturer in a report that is regularly updated.

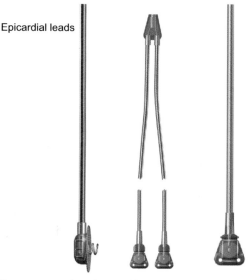
Fig. 4.12 Commonly used epicardial fixation mechanisms. From left to right: Medtronic 5071 screw-in lead; Medtronic 4968 steroid-eluting suture on bipolar epicardial lead; Metronic 4965 steroid-eluting suture-on unipolar epicardial lead.

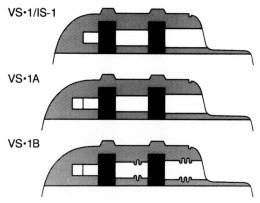
Fig. 4.11 Available types of in-line pulse generator headers. Few VS-1B pulse generators remain in service.

A
7274 Marquis DR

Product Characteristics

US Market Release	Mar-02	NBD Code	VVED
Registered US Implants	48,000	Serial Number Prefix/X-ray ID	PKC
Estimated Active US Implants	24,000	Max Delivered Energy	30 J
Normal Battery Depletions	145	Estimated Longevity	See page 33
Malfunctions	104 (30 related to advisory)		
Therapy Function Not Compromised	49 (2 related to advisory)		
Therapy Function Compromised	55 (28 related to advisory)		
Advisories	1 see page 156 – 2005 Potential Premature Battery Depletion Due to Battery Short		

Device Survival Probability (%)

Years After Implant — **Malfunction-Free Survival** - - - - - All-Cause Survival

		1 yr	2 yr	3 yr	4 yr	at 57 mo
%	——	100.0	99.9	99.7	99.5	99.5
%	- - - -	99.8	99.6	98.6	97.4	97.2
#		42,000	32,000	16,000	5,000	100
Effective Sample Size						

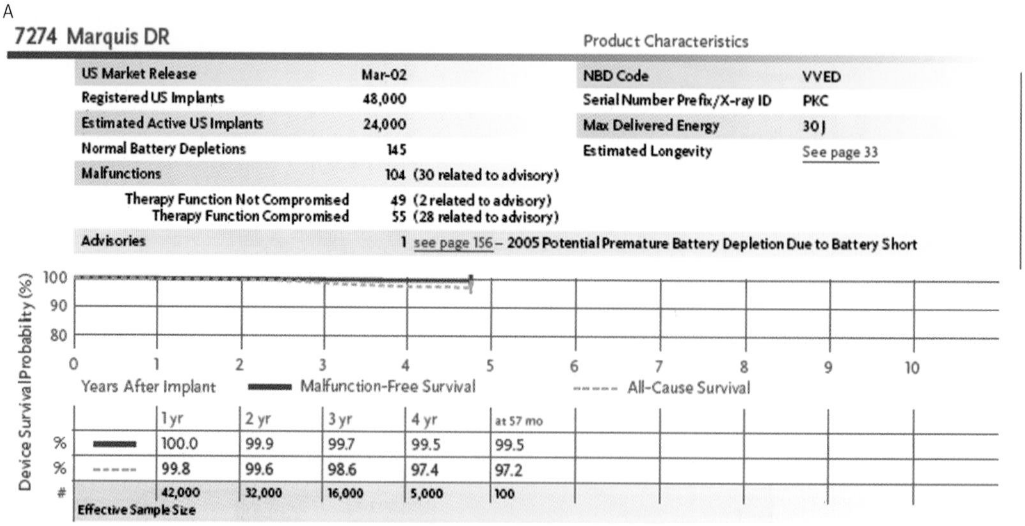

Fig. 4.13 Examples of product performance data from three manufacturers taken from the product performance reports available for use by caregivers. (Information is in the public domain so anyone can access the product performance information.) Post-market surveillance data from product performance report by (A) Medtronic: data regarding a dual-chamber ICD; (B) St. Jude Medical: data regarding a dual-chamber pacemaker; (C) Boston Scientific: data regarding specific "family" of pacing leads.

B

Integrity® AFx DR (Models 5342 & 5346)			
US Market Release	(5342) April 2000	Normal Battery Depletion	4083
	(5346) July 2001	Malfunctions	56
Registered US Implants	47,329	Malfunctions w/ Compromised Therapy	6
Estimated Active US Implants	26,959	Malfunctions w/o Compromised Therapy	50
Estimated Longevity	6.3 Years	Number of Advisories	None

Including Normal Battery Depletion

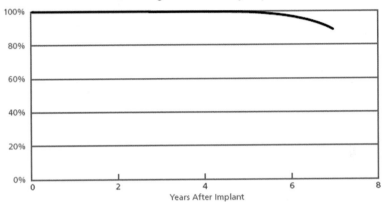

Year	2	4	6	at 84 months
Survival Probability	99.93%	99.80%	97.03%	89.02%
± 1 standard error	0.01%	0.02%	0.07%	0.15%
Sample Size	42100	33500	17400	500

Excluding Normal Battery Depletion

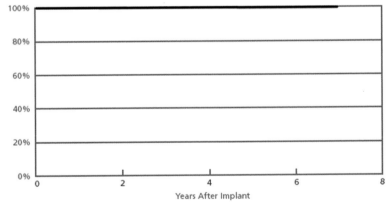

Year	2	4	6	at 84 months
Survival Probability	99.95%	99.89%	99.77%	99.76%
± 1 standard error	0.01%	0.02%	0.03%	0.03%

Fig. 4.13 (*Continued*)

(*Continued*)

C

FINELINE II/FINELINE II Sterox Atrial J (Polyurethane) — Models 4477/4478/4479/4480

U.S. Registered Implants: 33,000	U.S. Unconfirmed Reports of Lead Complications: 174	U.S. Confirmed Malfunctions: 13 Without Compromised Therapy: 12 With Compromised Therapy: 1	99.96% No Confirmed Malfunction
U.S. Approval Date: November 1996			
U.S. Estimated Active Implants: 24,000		U.S Average Device Age: 32.3 mo.	0.04% Confirmed Malfunction

	Registered U.S. Implants	Yr 1 (%)	Yr 2 (%)	Yr 3 (%)	Yr 4 (%)	Yr 5 (%)	Yr 6 (%)	Yr7 (%)	Yr 8 (%)	Yr 9 (%)	Yr 10(%)
Non Advisory Population	33,000	99.68 (-0.1/+0.1)	99.53 (-0.1/+0.1)	99.32 (-0.1/+0.1)	99.18 (-0.1/+0.1)	98.99 (-0.2/+0.2)	98.88 (-0.2/+0.2)	98.58 @ 79 mo. (-0.5/+0.4)	–	–	–

Data are representative of Guidant FINELINE II (poly) and Intermedics THINLINE II (poly) lead performance.

FINELINE II/FINELINE II Sterox Passive Fixation (Silicone) — Models 4454/4455/4458/4459

U.S. Registered Implants: 11,000	U.S. Unconfirmed Reports of Lead Complications: 128	U.S. Confirmed Malfunctions: 5 Without Compromised Therapy: 0 With Compromised Therapy: 5	99.95% No Confirmed Malfunction
U.S. Approval Date: November 1996			
U.S. Estimated Active Implants: 7,000		U.S Average Device Age: 38.2 mo.	0.05% Confirmed Malfunction

	Registered U.S. Implants	Yr 1 (%)	Yr 2 (%)	Yr 3 (%)	Yr 4 (%)	Yr 5 (%)	Yr 6 (%)	Yr7 (%)	Yr 8 (%)	Yr 9 (%)	Yr 10(%)
Non Advisory Population	11,000	99.72 (-0.1/+0.1)	99.34 (-0.2/+0.3)	98.87 (-0.3/+0.2)	98.48 (-0.3/+0.3)	98.14 (-0.4/+0.3)	97.38 (-0.6/+0.5)	96.87 @ 80 mo. (-1.0/+0.7)	–	–	–

Data are representative of Guidant FINELINE II (silicone) and Intermedics THINLINE II (silicone) lead performance.

FINELINE II EZ/FINELINE II Sterox EZ Positive Fixation (Silicone) — Models 4466/4467/4468/4472/4473/4474

U.S. Registered Implants: 33,000	U.S. Unconfirmed Reports of Lead Complications: 291	U.S. Confirmed Malfunctions: 17 Without Compromised Therapy: 1 With Compromised Therapy: 16	99.95% No Confirmed Malfunction
U.S. Approval Date: November 1996			
U.S. Estimated Active Implants: 24,000		U.S Average Device Age: 34.0 mo.	0.05% Confirmed Malfunction

	Registered U.S. Implants	Yr 1 (%)	Yr 2 (%)	Yr 3 (%)	Yr 4 (%)	Yr 5 (%)	Yr 6 (%)	Yr7 (%)	Yr 8 (%)	Yr 9 (%)	Yr 10(%)
Non Advisory Population	33,000	99.70 (-0.1/+0.1)	99.40 (-0.1/+0.1)	99.10 (-0.1/+0.1)	98.75 (-0.2/+0.2)	98.08 (-0.3/+0.3)	97.38 (-0.4/+0.4)	97.25 @ 81 mo. (-0.5/+0.4)	–	–	–

Data are representative of Guidant FINELINE II (silicone) and Intermedics THINLINE II (silicone) lead performance.

Fig. 4.13 (*Continued*)

Follow-up data may be obtained from active registry information[24,25] or from centers that publish survival and performance data on individual leads (see Chapter 10: Troubleshooting). A literature search is likely to yield implanters with information on many of the most widely used leads.[26]

There is no independent comprehensive database of leads or pulse generators in the USA. Although there have been attempts at developing such a database, it has yet to be accomplished.

In 2005 in the USA, the Center for Medicare and Medicaid Services initiated regulations that require implanting centers and hospitals to supply certain follow-up information about ICD patients in order to obtain reimbursement. However, the registry, the National Cardiovascular Device Registry (https://www.ncdr.com/webncdr/ICD/Default.aspx), is run privately with the American College of Cardiology and Heart Rhythm Society jointly involved with ICD data management.[27]

Another database is operational for documenting hardware failures for leads, pacemakers and ICDs. Because only failures are reported, the database does not provide the incidence with which specific failures might occur, but it may alert one to a potential problem or allow a search to see if others have reported a similar problem (www.pacerandicdregistry.com).[24,25]

Generator and lead selection in defibrillators

Many of the considerations in selecting an appropriate pacing system for a patient, e.g., the use of tined or active fixation leads, the need for specific pacing features, are identical in defibrillator selection and are not repeated here. Other issues, however, either are unique to defibrillators or take on added dimensions, including the following:

- Use of integrated or bipolar sensing
- Pulse generator size in relation to longevity
- Maximum shock output
- Upper pacing rate
- Pacing and defibrillation with a dual-chamber or a single-chamber device and arrhythmia discrimination
- Features of a specific device (or lead) to allow solving commonly encountered ICD problems (e.g., inappropriate shocks, far-field oversensing).

Lead design considerations for ICD leads

Coaxial and multilumen leads

Historically, two basic ICD lead designs have been used. The coaxial design has a layered structure in which the electrodes are coiled over each other with layers of insulation in between. Coaxial leads had larger diameter, greater stiffness, and higher failure rates and have been superseded by the multiluminal design. Multilumen leads incorporate all the electrodes and shocking coils in parallel within a single insulation framework.

ICD lead conductor

The conductor is critical to the design of the ICD lead and is made of the alloy MP35N and silver to provide low resistance required for high energy defibrillation. Silver is incorporated into MP35N in one of two different designs: drawn brazed strand has silver around the MP35N and drawn filled tube has a core of silver surrounded by MP35N. Conductors can have either multifilar coil or multifilar cable design. The coil design has a central lumen and allows the passage of a stylet to facilitate lead placement. However, higher conductor fracture rate was observed with coils that led to the development of multifilar braided cables. Cable conductors are more resistant to fracture and allow a smaller lead diameter, but do not have a lumen for insertion of a stylet. Current ICD leads have only one coil conductor, the cathode tip, for stylet insertion and helix deployment and the other conductors can be cabled. However, the coil conductor continues to predispose the lead to fracture and limits the ability to reduce the lead diameter.

ICD lead defibrillation coil

ICD lead pace sense electrode is similar in structure to the pacing leads dicussed above. The defibrillation coil is a unique feature of ICDs and is made of platinum iridium alloy or platinum coated with tantalum or iridium oxide. Bare metal coils cause vigorous fibrous reaction making extraction difficult, even dangerous. Several designs have been developed to overcome this.

Defibrillation coils are "backfilled" with silicone rubber in the spaces between the coil metal. However, in the rounded coils, a bare metal surface area for interface with the tissue is still required for high voltage defibrillation. Hence the risk of fibrous encapsulation is not completely eliminated by backfilling. The isodiametric flat surface coils further reduce the risk of encapsulation by abrading away any excess coil surface to create a flat exposed surface (Fig. 4.14). Another design to prevent fibrosis is the use of extended polytetrafluoroethylene (ePTFE) jacket over the coil. The material is able to conduct electricity because of the expanded porous structure. The ePTFE coated coil has been shown to be easier to extract from the coronary venous system in an animal model.

ICD lead insulation material

Considerations regarding the choice of insulating material are similar to those described for pacemaker leads. Current ICD leads often employ a combination of different insulation materials. One common combination is silicone rubber body with an outer polyurethane coating and PTFE (polytetrafluoroethylene)

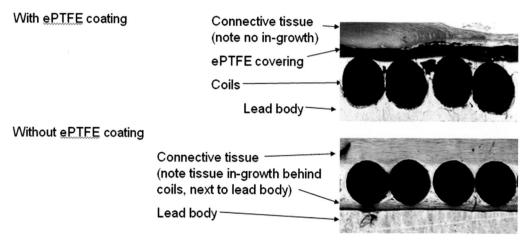

Fig. 4.14 Extended polytetrafluoroethylene (ePTFE) coating on the shock coil in the Boston Scientific Endotak Reliance G ICD lead. The ePTFE covering prevents tissue ingrowth because the pores in the ePTFE do not allow blood and tissue cells to pass through, but can permit electrically conductive plasma to pass through. The figure shows histology from preclinical studies illustrating connective tissue ingrowth behind the defibrillation coils of a lead without ePTFE coating, and the absence of tissue ingrowth in ePTFE covered lead. (Courtesy of Boston Scientific.)

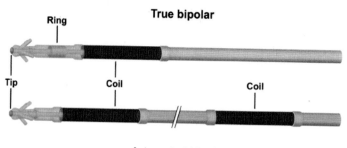

Fig. 4.15 True bipolar (top) and integrated bipolar (bottom) leads. The true bipolar lead senses between the distal tip and the proximal ring, which are dedicated for pacing and sensing. True bipolar leads have a single coil. In contrast, integrated bipolar leads pace and sense between the tip and the distal coil. The distal coil is used for sensing, pacing, and defibrillation. Integrated bipolar leads also contain a second, proximal coil, increasing the lead surface area for defibrillation.

or ETFE (ethylenetetrafluoroethylene) jacket around each conductor.

Integrated and bipolar sensing

The transvenous defibrillator lead, typically placed in the right ventricle, serves to sense signals (local electrogram), pace the heart (antibradycardia and antitachycardia pacing [ATP]), and deliver shocks. ICD leads are tripolar (tip and ring electrodes with one coil, or tip electrode with two coils) or quadripolar (tip and ring with two coils) with variation in the distribution of function across these electrodes. True bipolar sensing occurs between the tip electrode and a closely spaced dedicated ring (Fig. 4.15). Because the spacing between this bipolar pair is small, far-field electrograms for noise related to lead interaction or electromagnetic interference is less likely to be sensed.

Integrated sensing lead systems are constructed with a distal tip electrode for pacing and sensing, a distal coil for both pacing and sensing and for defibrillation, and a proximal coil for defibrillation (Fig. 4.15). This design has the advantage of incorporating two defibrillation coils, which in conjunction with an active can device lowers defibrillation thresholds (DFTs), although this effect has not been uniformly observed.[28,29] In early lead designs, the distance from the tip to the distal coil was small (6 mm) to minimize detection of far-field signals; however, it was found that with a distally placed coil, the amplitude of the recorded electrogram diminished significantly after a shock, an effect that could on rare occasions lead to failure to redetect continuing ventricular fibrillation if an initial shock was unsuccessful (Fig. 4.16).[30] Subsequent to this early experience, integrated leads have been redesigned with a greater distance between the distal coil and the lead tip (12 mm), ameliorating post-shock electrogram diminution, so

that it is no longer a clinical consideration.[31,32] Although the greater distance between the tip and the coil has resolved post-shock sensing problems, the trade-off is an increased risk of oversensing of far-field signals. The cause is the effectively larger antenna created by the greater intrabipole distance. Moreover, to detect the small-amplitude fibrillation signals that may follow a relatively large R wave, defibrillators utilize dynamic sensing or gain. In most defibrillators, the effective sensitivity after a sensed R wave increases with each passing millisecond until the maximum sensitivity is reached (Fig. 4.17).[33] Thus, patients with slow heart rates – which allow more time after a QRS complex for the effective sensitivity to increase – are at increased risk for this type of oversensing. Because sensitivity (or gain) is rapidly maximized after a paced event, patients with slow rates of pacing are the most likely to experience far-field myopotential oversensing, often because phrenic potentials are oversensed (Fig. 4.18). When it occurs, it can result in suppression of bradycardia pacing or inappropriate detection of ventricular tachyarrhythmias.[34] Increasing the lower rate and decreasing sensitivity usually eliminate the problem. In our practice, the predominant situation in which true bipolar sensing is preferred is in the setting of abandoned intravascular leads. In theory, the distal coil in integrated lead systems may make contact with an abandoned lead and generate lead noise. In practice, this is an uncommon occurrence (unpublished observation), and it may be further mitigated with the use of ePTFE-insulated coils.[35]

Although having two coils in the ICD leads offers modest advantages in terms of lowering DFT, disadvantages exist. When lead extraction becomes necessary, the proximal [superior vena cava (SVC)] coil is often densely adherent to the SVC and may be difficult to

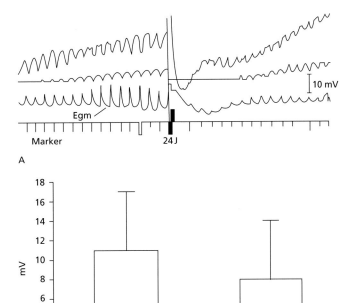

Fig. 4.16 (A) Recording from a failed 24-J shock. The endocardial electrogram (Egm) amplitude is diminished by the 24-J shock, although undersensing does not occur in this example from a true bipolar lead. (B) Mean ventricular fibrillation electrogram amplitude before (Pre) and just after (Post) failed shocks. (Modified from Brady PA, Friedman PA, Stanton MS. Effect of failed defibrillation shocks on electrogram amplitude in a nonintegrated transvenous defibrillation lead system. Am J Cardiol 1995; 76:580–4, by permission of Excerpta Medica.)

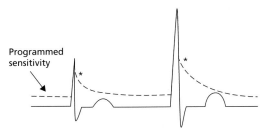

Fig. 4.17 Schematic illustration of dynamic sensing used by many defibrillators. When a QRS event is sensed (*), the sensitivity is decreased to avoid detecting the T wave that follows. The sensitivity progressively increases over time until the next QRS complex is sensed. This progressive sensitivity (or gain adjustment, depending on device) permits defibrillators to detect small fibrillation electrograms and at the same time avoid double counting of QRS complexes and T waves. Because of the progressive increase in gain, the risk of oversensing noncardiac signals is greater with slower heart rates.

remove. In a small minority of patients (<5%), the location of the proximal coil may be ill suited for defibrillation, necessitating excluding it from the shocking circuit or the addition of other defibrillation leads. Because of this, some implanters prefer to use a single coil true bipolar sensing lead and then add an additional lead if DFTs are high. The additional lead may be placed in the SVC or in the coronary sinus and its ventricular tributaries or the inferior vena cava. The additional coil may also be placed in a branch of the SVC such as the azygous vein.

In summary, for most patients dual-coil or single-coil and true or integrated bipolar systems are effective. Single-coil systems are favored in younger patients who have a potential need for future extraction, although ePTFE-coated leads may mitigate the disadvantage of dual coils. True bipolar sensing is preferred in pacemaker-dependent patients, in the setting of abandoned leads, and for patients who may be at increased risk for exposure to electromagnetic interference (e.g., a factory worker). Dual-coil systems may be preferable when higher DFTs are anticipated (hypertrophic cardiomyopathy, antiarrhythmic therapy, some sodium channel defects), although clinical predictors of high DFTs have been limited, and <5% of patients require system revision.[36–38]

ICD lead connector

Modern ICD lead connectors and headers have standardized design allowing the combination of ICD lead

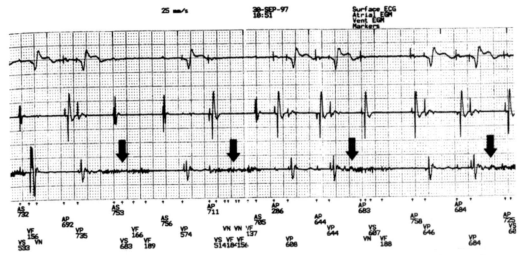

Fig. 4.18 Myopotential oversensing. Real-time recordings are from the surface ECG, atrial electrogram, and ventricular electrogram (top to bottom). During labored breathing with the patient at rest, bursts of diaphragmatic myopotential activity (arrows) result in inhibition of bradycardia pacing with periods of asystole. Note detection of sensed ventricular fibrillation events in association with oversensing. AP, atrial pace; AS, atrial sense; VF, ventricular fibrillation zone sense; VN, ventricular noise during noise response window; VP, ventricular pace; VS, ventricular sense. (From Deshmukh P, Anderson K. Myopotential sensing by a dual chamber implantable cardioverter defibrillator: two case reports. J Cardiovasc Electrophysiol 1998; 9:767–72, by permission of Futura Publishing Co.)

and generator from different manufacturers. The pace-sense component of the lead has an IS-1 lead connector as described above for pacemaker leads. Each shock coil has a standard DF-1 lead connector. Thus, a dual-coil ICD lead has two DF-1 and one IS-1 connector pins, each with its own port in the ICD header which adds considerable bulk to the header. The three lead connectors are connected at a trifurcated yoke, which in turn adds extra length to the lead and bulk to the pocket. The presence of multiple connectors also increases the complexity of lead implantation, creates the potential for DF-1 lead reversal in the header, and lead damage during dissection at generator replacement.

These disadvantages of the current standardized ICD connector design led to the development of a new standard in ICD connector technology – the DF-4 connector. The DF-4 standard was developed in collaboration by the major device manufacturers to simplify ICD lead connection. It incorporates four conductors into a quadrupole connection replacing the defibrillator coil DF-1 and pace-sense coil IS-1 connections with the DF-4 connection (Fig. 4.19). As a result, the three ports previously required for a defibrillation lead are replaced by a single port and connection, the header is smaller, and the lead is 7–10 cm shorter. The sealing rings are moved from the lead to the header reducing the chance of damage during implantation.

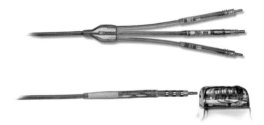

Fig. 4.19 Example of IS-4 connectology (bottom image), St. Jude Medical, SJ-4 header and Durata SJ-4 header compared with a standard DF-4 connector (top image). (Used with permission from St. Jude Medical.)

Size and longevity

In general, larger devices have greater battery capacity and thus greater longevity. Patient size, particularly in smaller patients or children, may rarely constrain the site of device placement, because of either limited pectoral tissue to support the device or cosmetic concerns. In these situations, the options available are smaller devices with shorter longevity, subpectoral placement, and less commonly used sites. When device size becomes a significant factor, technically the simplest solution may be to use the smallest available device and insert it prepectorally, despite potential limits to longevity. Even with selection of the smallest device, alternative insertion sites may be preferable at times. Submuscular placement is discussed in greater detail in Chapter 5: Implantation Techniques. Further technologic advancements will result in progressively smaller devices in the near future.

Programmable waveforms

Elevated DFTs are an uncommon but challenging problem affecting approximately 5–10% of the ICD population, and 5% of current implants. Patients with elevated DFTs and reduced safety margins may have reduced survival compared with other ICD recipients. Most ICDs utilize fixed tilt biphasic waveform. At present, a single manufacturer (St. Jude) manufactures ICDs in which the waveforms are programmable. Small studies suggest that tuning waveforms improves defibrillation and permits most high DFT patients to achieve implant criteria,[39,40] although experts disagree about the benefit of pulse-width-based waveform "tuning."[38,41]

Dual-chamber or single-chamber ICD?

The single most important decision in selecting a defibrillator is determining whether to implant a single-chamber or a dual-chamber system.[42] This decision may be influenced by several considerations:
• The need for dual-chamber bradycardia pacing because of a standard indication, such as sinus node dysfunction or AV block
• Specific conditions (e.g., long QT syndrome or hypertrophic cardiomyopathy) that may respond to dual-chamber pacing
• Congestive heart failure, which occasionally may require traditional dual-chamber or, more commonly, biventricular pacing
• Paroxysmal atrial arrhythmias, for improved specificity, prevention, and therapy.

These are discussed in greater detail below. Table 4.3 summarizes conditions favoring the use of dual-chamber systems. For any given patient, the potential advantages of dual-chamber systems must be weighed against the strengths of single-chamber defibrillator system simplicity, reduced risk of lead dislodgment, reduced cost, and greater longevity per unit size (Table 4.4).

Factors favoring single-chamber defibrillators

Patients with chronic atrial fibrillation or patients who lack the factors favoring dual-chamber devices should receive single-chamber defibrillators. This is particularly true for younger or smaller patients, in whom the greater longevity per unit size and minimal intravascu-

Table 4.3 Factors favoring use of a dual-chamber defibrillator

- Need for dual-chamber bradycardia pacing, particularly sinus node dysfunction (strongest indication for a dual-chamber device)
- Specific conditions that may "respond" to dual-chamber pacing (long QT syndrome, hypertrophic cardiomyopathy)
- Significant left ventricular dysfunction (assumes patient is not a candidate for CRT, in which case a CRT-D would be selected)
- Patients in whom medications that impair chronotropic function are required
- Paroxysmal atrial arrhythmias
- Improved specificity (i.e., differentiate supraventricular from ventricular arrhythmias)
- Known VT <200 ppm (because in this zone dual-chamber detection enhancements are particularly useful)
- Atrial therapies needed (limited to devices that include specific atrial therapies beyond pacing)

Table 4.4 Advantages of single-chamber systems

- Simplified implantation
- Greater longevity per unit size
- Less intravascular hardware
- Reduced risk of lead dislodgment
- Reduced cost

lar hardware requirements of single-chamber systems may be more compelling. In addition to simplicity and longevity, single-chamber benefits include fewer complications. Although previous studies suggested no significant difference in overall complication rates between single-chamber and dual-chamber pacemakers, the preponderance of evidence suggests that atrial leads dislodge more frequently than do ventricular leads.[43,44] Unless dislodged atrial leads are electrically abandoned (thus functionally reducing the implanted system to a single-chamber ICD), this increased rate of dislodgment may result in higher reoperation rates for dual-chamber ICDs. Thus, for patients who have infrequent pacing, who lack episodic atrial arrhythmias, and who do not have specific conditions warranting dual-chamber devices, single-chamber devices are preferred.

Factors favoring dual-chamber defibrillators

Dual-chamber defibrillators are preferred in patients with an accepted indication for dual-chamber pacing. In sinus node dysfunction, atrial pacing (combined with avoidance of ventricular pacing) modestly lowers the risk of atrial fibrillation.[45–47] The addition of β-adrenergic blockers or antiarrhythmic medications may further exacerbate bradycardia and the need for atrial pacing support. In patients with high-grade AV block, a dual-chamber biventricular device is preferred if heart failure is present, given the association of heart failure and chronic right ventricular apical pacing.[47,48] These are discussed further below.

In addition to providing dual-chamber pacing functionality, dual-chamber defibrillators use the information acquired simultaneously from atrial and ventricular leads to enhance arrhythmia diagnosis. Early dual-chamber ICDs were similar or slightly superior to single ICDs in correctly discriminating supraventricular tachycardia (SVT) from ventricular tachycardia (VT). More recently, prospective, randomized trials have found that the odds of inappropriate detection of SVT as VT were decreased by half with the use of dual-chamber detection.[49] As expected, the improved rhythm classification led to a reduction in inappropriate therapy. In this study, more ATP was programmed in the single-chamber arm, and shock rates did not differ, but another study has demonstrated a reduction by one-third in clinically significant adverse events with use of dual-chamber detection enhancements.[50] Although expert opinion is divided, selection of a dual-chamber ICDs to improve SVT-VT rhythm classification is reasonable in patients in whom a VT zone with rates <200 ppm will be programmed who are not in chronic atrial fibrillation and who do not have complete or high-grade AV block (Table 4.4).

Clinical factors that should be considered when making an ICD selection are summarized in Table 4.5.

Specific device and lead features influencing selection

When selecting a particular device or lead for an ICD system, the implanter should briefly consider whether any specific patient characteristic warrants a distinct programmable feature or lead characteristic. In general, today's generators and leads are highly flexible in their programming options and lead characteristics (true bipolar sensing along with dual coil, etc.), so that any choice will work in most situations.[26] However, in certain situations, specific features may be more appropriate on a certain device to offset the likelihood of the most common ICD-related problem, i.e., inappropriate shock for SVTs and sensing-related issues.[51–53]

Avoiding adverse effects from the lead or from frequent and unnecessary pacing

As discussed above (see Pacemaker selection), frequent right ventricular pacing may promote cardiomyopathy. Some ICDs incorporate similar methods to decrease ventricular pacing in addition to enhanced program-

Table 4.5 Clinical factors and defibrillator selection.

Clinical factor	Lead and device considerations
Pacemaker-dependent patient	True bipolar sensing preferable
Need for bradycardia pacing	Confirm that appropriate pacing (sensor, dual-chamber) is made available
Paroxysmal atrial arrhythmias	Dual-chamber devices enhance specificity and lower risk of inappropriate therapy (particularly if VTs with HR <200 are present)
	Atrial pacing modestly reduces paroxysmal atrial fibrillation (in sinus node dysfunction) as long as ventricular pacing minimized
	In patients with atrial flutter, previous heart surgery and incisional atrial flutters, atrial ATP may be useful
	Atrial shocks are infrequently used
Chronic atrial fibrillation	Single-chamber device (VVIR or rarely VVI)
Anticipated elevated defibrillation threshold (previously high defibrillation threshold, hypertrophic cardiomyopathy, marked enlargement)	Higher output device Dual coil lead Consider programmable waveform if fixed tilt waveform has failed
Small body habitus; younger patient; need for limited intravascular hardware	Smaller size, single chamber preferable; consider single coil lead or ePTFE-coated lead
Very slow ventricular tachycardia	Consider relationship of upper rate limit to ventricular tachycardia detection zone

ATP, antitachycardia pacing; ePTFE, expanded polytetrafluoroethylene; HR, heart rate; VT, ventricular tachycardia.

mability of the AV intervals (AV search hysteresis, MVP). When dual-chamber devices are selected for a patient primarily because of possible improved discrimination between SVT and VT, care must be taken to minimize ventricular pacing. This may be done algorithmically, or by utilizing a nontracking pacing mode at sufficiently low rates to minimize pacing.

Tricuspid valve regurgitation as a result of the lead crossing this valve appears more likely to occur with ICD leads than with standard pacing leads.[54,55] The exact incidence of tricuspid regurgitation and relative benefits of choosing a particular lead or lead location are not currently known. In general, smaller profile ICD leads placed with care to avoid perforation and avoiding placement close to the insertion of the papillary muscle on the moderator band are likely to be beneficial.

While a detailed analysis of the differences in programmable features between devices is beyond the scope of this book, the implanter must be familiar with the principles described above in choosing a device and lead.[56–58] When specific patient populations or unique characteristics (pediatrics, right ventricular dysplasia, right bundle aberrancy with high rates) have been noted by the physician, specific enquiries into differences in the options available to deal with these issues should be made prior to selecting the appropriate device and lead.[59,60]

Cardiac resynchronization therapy

There are some specific considerations when selecting a generator, lead, and device function when using cardiac resynchronization devices. In order for the patient to benefit, as close to 100% of QRS complexes should be resynchronized (i.e., paced with capture). CRT pulse generators require particular timing algorithms to maximize biventricular pacing, and LV pacing leads employ special design to maximize stability and minimize extracardiac stimulation.

Promoting continuous biventricular pacing

Unnecessary right ventricular pacing may promote ventricular dysfunction and is possibly disadvantageous; thus, pacing algorithms have evolved to minimize unnecessary right ventricular pacing.

The exact opposite goal is the cornerstone of CRT. The goal when implanting these devices is to have near-continuous biventricular stimulation (perhaps with a programmed RV–LV offset). The main interruptors of resynchronization are atrial fibrillation with rapid intrinsic conduction, an inappropriately long programmed AV interval, and frequent premature ventricular contractions. A variety of programmable variables exist to help manage these specific challenges (see Chapter 10: Troubleshooting and Chapter 8: Programming).

Because continuous biventricular pacing is the goal, in general, generator replacement is required earlier with CRT devices than with standard pacemakers. In addition, LV pacing thresholds are often higher than those obtained from endocardial right ventricular pacing. Specific device features have been developed to try to optimize battery life without compromising biventricular pacing. Algorithms have been developed to determine the minimum amplitude that consistently results in ventricular capture and calculate the new amplitude based on a programmable safety margin and the programmed maximum LV adapted amplitude. In essence, the LV output is kept at a safe margin as determined by these programmed guidelines, yet maintaining capture and optimizing device longevity. Such features should be considered when device selection is made.

Leads for resynchronization devices

As discussed in Chapter 5: Implantation, distinct challenges are present when negotiating the coronary venous tree and create unique requirements for LV pacing leads.

LV pacing leads should be sufficiently flexible in negotiating sharp angulation and tortuosity of the venous system without traumatizing or dissecting these veins. The lead must be large enough to wedge into a venous tributary, yet small enough to negotiate collateral veins, often requiring subcannulation to reach the LV free wall.

Coronary venous leads should be maneuverable to an intramyocardial location to decrease the likelihood of extracardiac stimulation and should be designed to allow multisite or multivector stimulation (see later).

Historically, when LV pacing was first being performed, standard tined right ventricular pacing leads were maneuvered into the coronary sinus and into the ventricular branches with appropriate shaping of the inserted stylet. Shapes were made mimicking standard preformed coronary sinus mapping catheters used in electrophysiology.[61] Later, dedicated LV pacing leads that had a relatively more flexible curved distal segment (Medtronic model 2187) were developed. This lead and another similar lead (Medtronic 2188) were those used in the first large multicenter trial evaluating LV pacing.[62] Despite some designed facilitation of lead delivery, these leads were stylet driven and could not be passed through the then available coronary sinus guiding sheaths. Dislodgment rates were high (8%), and extracardiac stimulation required lead positioning or device reprogramming in 2.5% of patients.

A major advance that simplified LV pacing was the development of over-the-wire LV leads. The lead used in a subsequent large resynchronization study (Medtronic InSync 3), an over-the-wire lead (Medtronic 4193) that allowed an angioplasty wire to be passed through it, was utilized. The smaller profile of this lead along with the over-the-wire technology significantly enhanced successful lead implant rates (95%) and often allowed purposeful manipulation to targeted sites for pacing, often on the LV lateral wall. Although dislodgment rates with these leads were generally lower (3.4%), extracardiac stimulation continued to be a significant

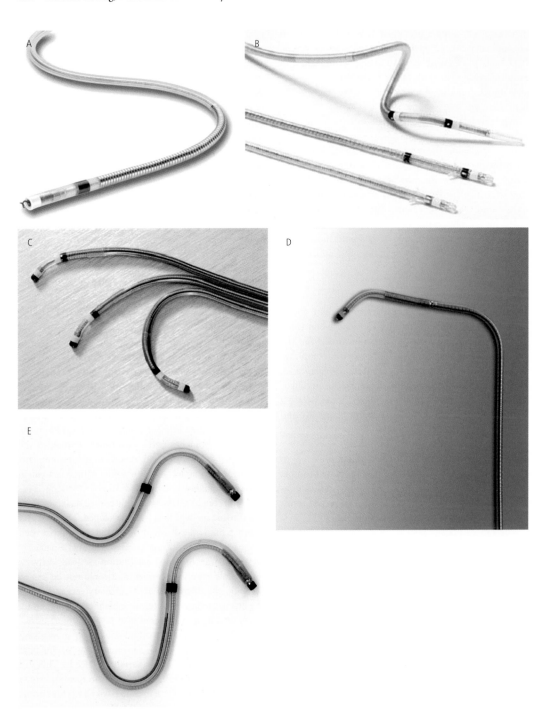

Fig. 4.20 Examples of contemporary coronary venous lead designs. (A) Biotronik, Inc. Linox® lead with S-shaped design. (B) Boston Scientific Easytrak® over-the-wire (OTW) family of leads. From bottom to top, EasyTrak 1,2,3. (C) Boston Scientific Accuity® family of leads. These leads are "steerable," allowing the operator to deflect, push, and torque the lead. (D) Medtronic Attain® OTW lead. (E) St. Jude Medical coronary sinus lead. (F) Sorin Group Situs® left ventricular lead. The orientation curve is intended to orient the electrode toward the epicardium and the contact curve is meant to maintain contact of a half annular electrode with epicardium. (G) Sorin Group Situs® OTW left ventricular lead that is described as having "pseudo-active fixation" mechanism.

F

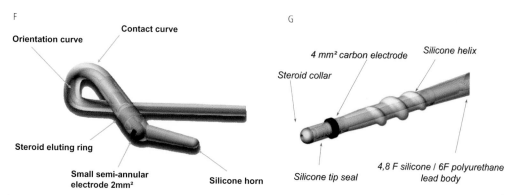

G

Orientation curve

Contact curve

Steroid eluting ring

Small semi-annular
electrode 2mm²

Silicone horn

4 mm² carbon electrode

Silicone helix

Steroid collar

Silicone tip seal

4,8 F silicone / 6F polyurethane
lead body

Fig. 4.20 (*Continued*)

problem, with reprogramming to turn off the LV lead occurring in 8.8% of patients. Further acute hemodynamic studies suggested that the midlateral LV free wall should be the target for pacing,[63] and maximal separation from the right ventricular lead was thought desirable.

As implanters attempted to place leads at specific sites thought to optimize synchrony, stability of these leads at these specific sites became more important. Sometimes the coronary venous system is large (varices) making lead contact with myocardium suboptimal, and at other times excess tortuosity makes judging "slack" on these leads difficult and results in extrusion of the lead from the vein with patient movement or deep respiration. The St. Jude QuickFlex LV lead (5.6 Fr polyurethane body and 5 Fr silicone distal tip) is a lead that promotes stabilization in the coronary vein with an S-shaped tip designed to stabilize itself on opposing walls of a larger vein of interest. Another attempt to optimize stability in relatively larger veins is Boston Scientific's Easy Track 3 lead (6 Fr polyurethane body and 5.7 Fr silicone distal tip). When the stylet or guidewire is removed from this lead, a terminal helix curls and shortens in the coronary vein, promoting stability. Other leads do not have a preformed helix or curve mechanism and are essentially straight (Boston Scientific's Easy Track 2 lead and Medtronic's Attain Ability Straight 4396 lead) to allow ease of maneuverability into the distal coronary venous system. In the Medtronic 4194 lead, the construction of the proximal electrode is essentially a coil rather than an annular electrode with a large (38 mm²) surface area. While leads mentioned above utilize passive fixation, the Medtronic Attain StarFix is the first active fixation LV lead. This lead employs three polyurethane lobes near the lead tip which when deployed fix the lead in place against the venous walls. The lobes can be deployed multiple times

for acute repositioning of the lead to variable diameters up to 24 Fr to fit the size of vein in which the lead is implanted.

Examples of contemporary coronary venous leads are shown in Fig. 4.20. Developing approaches include active fixation mechanism, extrusion of adhesion molecules, and multiple electrodes, all aiming to promote stability or continued capture even if the lead is unstable.

RV–LV pacing offset and vector of pacing

The benefits and technique for sequential biventricular pacing are discussed elsewhere in this book. In observational studies,[64] acute hemodynamic improvement and more optimal Doppler indices of resynchronization are observed when the LV output occurs earlier than that of the right ventricle by approximately 40 ms. Several presently available CRT generators allow programmability of the V-V interval.[65,66] In addition, bipolar or multipolar pacing leads allow noninvasive manipulation of the pacing vector. For example, if a bipolar LV pacing lead is placed, bipolar LV stimulation may be chosen or stimulation between the LV lead tip (or vein) at the cathode and the right ventricular defibrillator coils. This may not only allow adequate pacing thresholds when bipolar capture thresholds are high, but a different pacing vector that may promote better synchrony.[67] Manipulation of the pacing vector may also help in troubleshooting extracardiac stimulation and anodal stimulation (see Chapter 10: Troubleshooting).[66,67]

In addition to the general requirements for optimal pacemaker/ICD generator programmability and lead characteristics, unique requirements thus exist for CRT devices because of the requirements for continuous pacing and the unique lead location in the coronary venous system.

Conclusions

The broad array of devices and lead systems now available has enhanced the opportunity to tailor device therapy to the individual patient.

Pacemaker selection should be made after consideration is given not only to the underlying rhythm disturbance but also to the patient's activity level and need for specific programmable options. For ICD selection, factors such as pacemaker dependency, anticipated defibrillation threshold, need for bradycardia pacing, and paroxysmal or chronic atrial arrhythmias can all affect the choice of system (summarized in Table 4.5). Although most defibrillator systems are suitable for most patients, careful selection of system components can provide the best match between patient and device.

Depending on whether the CRT patient requires CRT-P or CRT-D, multiple factors need to be weighed in choosing a system for this subset of patients. The patient's underlying rhythm also needs to be carefully considered in order to maintain biventricular advantage and take complete advantage of resynchronization.

References

1 Kühne M, Schaer B, Kaufmann C, et al. A randomized trial comparing two different approaches of pacemaker selection. Europace 2007; 9:1185–90.
2 Naegeli B, Kurz DJ, Koller D, et al. Single-chamber ventricular pacing increases markers of left ventricular dysfunction compared with dual-chamber pacing. Europace 2007; 9:194–9.
3 Albertsen AE, Nielsen JC. Selecting the appropriate pacing mode for patients with sick sinus syndrome: evidence from randomized clinical trials. Card Electrophysiol Rev 2003; 7:406–10.
4 Kristensen L, Nielsen JC, Pedersen AK, Mortensen PT, Andersen HR. AV block and changes in pacing mode during long-term follow-up of 399 consecutive patients with sick sinus syndrome treated with an AAI/AAIR pacemaker. Pacing Clin Electrophysiol 2001; 24:358–65.
5 Celiker A, Başpinar O, Karagöz T. Transvenous cardiac pacing in children: problems and complications during follow-up. Anadolu Kardiyol Derg 2007; 7:292–7.
6 Beaufort-Krol GC, Stienstra Y, Bink-Boelkens MT. Sinus node function in children with congenital complete atrioventricular block. Europace 2007; 9:844–7.
7 Izquierdo R, Rodrigo G, Pelegrin J, et al. Single lead DDD pacing using electrodes with longitudinal and diagonal atrial floating dipoles. PACE 2002; 25:1692–8.
8 Merkely B, Vágó H, Bartha E. Permanent left atrial and left ventricular single-lead DDD pacing with a coronary sinus electrode. PACE 2002; 25:992–5.
9 Richardson DA, Bexton RS, Shaw FE, Kenny RA. Prevalence of cardioinhibitory carotid sinus hypersensitivity in patients 50 years or over presenting to the accident and emergency department with "unexplained" or "recurrent" falls. Pacing Clin Electrophysiol 1997; 20:820–3.
10 Connolly SJ, Sheldon R, Roberts RS, Gent M. The North American Vasovagal Pacemaker Study (VPS). A randomized trial of permanent cardiac pacing for the prevention of vasovagal syncope. J Am Coll Cardiol 1999; 33: 16–20.
11 Brignole M, Menozzi C, Lolli G, Bottoni N, Gaggioli G. Long-term outcome of paced and nonpaced patients with severe carotid sinus syndrome. Am J Cardiol 1992; 69: 1039–43.
12 Yeh KH, Wang CC, Wen MS, Chou CC, Yeh SJ, Wu D. Long-term performance of transvenous, steroid-eluting, high impedance, passive-fixation ventricular pacing leads. Pacing Clin Electrophysiol 2004; 27:1399–404.
13 Cornacchia D, Fabbri M, Puglisi A, et al. Latest generation of unipolar and bipolar steroid eluting leads: long-term comparison of electrical performance in atrium and ventricles. Europace 2000; 2:240–4.
14 Toivonen L, Valjus J, Hongisto M, Metso R. The influence of elevated 50 Hz electric and magnetic fields on implanted cardiac pacemakers: the role of the lead configuration and programming of the sensitivity. PACE 1991; 14: 2114–22.
15 Jain P, Kaul U, Wasir HS. Myopotential inhibition of unipolar demand pacemakers: utility of provocative manoeuvres in assessment and management. Int J Cardiol 1992; 34:33–9.
16 Gabry MD, Behrens M, Andrews C, Wanliss M, Klementowicz PT, Furman S. Comparison of myopotential interference in unipolar-bipolar programmable DDD pacemakers. Pacing Clin Electrophysiol 1987; 10:1322–30.
17 Hayes DL, Graham KJ, Irwin M, et al. A multicenter experience with a bipolar tined polyurethane ventricular lead. Pacing Clin Electrophysiol 1992; 15:1033–9.
18 Stokes KB. Polyether polyurethanes: biostable or not? J Biomater Appl 1988; 3:228–59.
19 Maisel WH. Transvenous implantable cardioverter-defibrillator leads: the weakest link. Circulation 2007; 115:2461–3.
20 Gammage MD, Lieberman RA, Yee R, et al.; for the Worldwide Select Secure Clinical Investigators. Multi-center clinical experience with a lumenless, catheter-delivered, bipolar, permanent pacemaker lead: implant safety and electrical performance. Pacing Clin Electrophysiol 2006; 29:858–65.
21 Calfee RV, Saulson SH. A voluntary standard for 3.2 mm unipolar and bipolar pacemaker leads and connectors. Pacing Clin Electrophysiol 1986; 9:1181–5.
22 Horenstein MS, Hakimi M, Walters H 3rd, Karpawich PP. Chronic performance of steroid-eluting epicardial leads in a growing pediatric population: a 10-year comparison. Pacing Clin Electrophysiol 2003; 26:1467–71.
23 Karpawich PP, Stokes KB, Proctor K, Schallhorn R, McVenes R. "In-line" bipolar, steroid-eluting, high impedance, epimyocardial pacing lead. Pacing Clin Electrophysiol 1998; 21:503–8.
24 Hauser RG, Hayes DL, Kallinen LM, et al. Clinical experience with pacemaker pulse generators and transvenous leads: an 8-year prospective multicenter study. Heart Rhythm 2007; 4:154–60.

25 Hauser RG, Hayes DL, Epstein AE, *et al.* Multicenter experience with failed and recalled implantable cardioverter-defibrillator pulse generators. Heart Rhythm 2006; 3:640–4.

26 Ellenbogen K, Wood M, Shepard R. Detection and management of an implantable cardioverter defibrillator lead failure. J Am Coll Cardiol 2003; 41:73–80.

27 Hammill SC, Stevenson LW, Kadish AH, *et al.* Review of the registry's first year, data collected, and future plans. Heart Rhythm 2007; 4:1260–3.

28 Gold MR, Foster AH, Shorofsky SR. Lead system optimization for transvenous defibrillation. Am J Cardiol 1997; 80:1163–7.

29 Bardy GH, Dolack GL, Kudenchuk PJ, Poole JE, Mehra R, Johnson G. Prospective, randomized comparison in humans of a unipolar defibrillation system with that using an additional superior vena cava electrode. Circulation 1994; 89:1090–3.

30 Brady PA, Friedman PA, Stanton MS. Effect of failed defibrillation shocks on electrogram amplitude in a nonintegrated transvenous defibrillation lead system. Am J Cardiol 1995; 76:580–4.

31 Isbruch FM, Block M, Bocker D, *et al.* Improved sensing signals after endocardial defibrillation with a redesigned integrated sense pace defibrillation lead. Pacing Clin Electrophysiol 1996; 19:1211–18.

32 Cooklin M, Tummala RV, Peters RW, Shorofsky SR, Gold MR. Comparison of bipolar and integrated sensing for redetection of ventricular fibrillation. Am Heart J 1999; 138:133–6.

33 Friedman PA, Stanton MS. The pacer-cardioverter-defibrillator: function and clinical experience. J Cardiovasc Electrophysiol 1995; 6:48–68.

34 Deshmukh P, Anderson K. Myopotential sensing by a dual chamber implantable cardioverter defibrillator: two case reports. J Cardiovasc Electrophysiol 1998; 9:767–72.

35 Cooper JM, Sauer WH, Garcia FC, Krautkramer MJ, Verdino RJ. Covering sleeves can shield the high-voltage coils from lead chatter in an integrated bipolar ICD lead. Europace 2007; 9:137–42.

36 Gold MR, Khalighi K, Kavesh NG, Daly B, Peters RW, Shorofsky SR. Clinical predictors of transvenous biphasic defibrillation thresholds. Am J Cardiol 1997; 79:1623–7.

37 Khalighi K, Daly B, Leino EV, *et al.* Clinical predictors of transvenous defibrillation energy requirements. Am J Cardiol 1997; 79:150–3.

38 Swerdlow CD, Russo AM, Degroot PJ. The dilemma of ICD implant testing. PACE 2007; 30:675–700.

39 Natrajan S, Henthorn R, Burroughs J, *et al.* "Tuned" defibrillation waveforms outperform 50/50% tilt defibrillation waveforms: a randomized multi-center study. Pacing Clin Electrophysiol; 30 (Suppl. 1):S139–S142.

40 Keane D, Aweh N, Hynes B, *et al.* Achieving sufficient safety margins with fixed duration waveforms and the use of multiple time constants. PACE 2007; 30:596–602.

41 Irnich W. Tilt or pulse duration: which is the decisive parameter in defibrillation? Pacing Clin Electrophysiol 2007; 30:1181–2.

42 Mehra R, DeGroot P. Where are we, and where are we heading in the device management of ventricular tachycardia/ventricular fibrillation? Heart Rhythm 2007; 4:99–103.

43 Aggarwal RK, Connelly DT, Ray SG, Ball J, Charles RG. Early complications of permanent pacemaker implantation: no difference between dual and single chamber systems. Br Heart J 1995; 73:571–5.

44 Chauhan A, Grace AA, Newell SA, *et al.* Early complications after dual chamber versus single chamber pacemaker implantation. Pacing Clin Electrophysiol 1994; 17:2012–15.

45 Sweeney MO, Bank AJ, Nsah E, *et al.* Search AV Extension and Managed Ventricular Pacing for Promoting Atrioventricular Conduction (SAVE PACe) Trial. Minimizing ventricular pacing to reduce atrial fibrillation in sinus-node disease. N Engl J Med 2007; 357:1000–8.

46 Connolly SJ, Kerr CR, Gent M, *et al.* Effects of physiologic pacing versus ventricular pacing on the risk of stroke and death due to cardiovascular causes. Canadian Trial of Physiologic Pacing Investigators. N Engl J Med 2000; 342:1385–91.

47 Sweeney MO, Hellkamp AS, Ellenbogen KA, *et al.*; MOde Selection Trial Investigators. Adverse effect of ventricular pacing on heart failure and atrial fibrillation among patients with normal baseline QRS duration in a clinical trial of pacemaker therapy for sinus node dysfunction. Circulation 2003; 107:2932–7.

48 Sharma AD, Rizo-Patron C, Hallstrom AP, *et al.*; DAVID Investigators. Percent right ventricular pacing predicts outcomes in the DAVID trial. Heart Rhythm 2005; 2: 830–4.

49 Friedman PA, McClelland RL, Bamlet WR, *et al.* Dual-chamber versus single-chamber detection enhancements for implantable defibrillator rhythm diagnosis: the detect supraventricular tachycardia study. Circulation 2006; 113: 2871–9.

50 Almendral J, Arribas F, Quesada A, *et al.* Are dual chamber ICDs beneficial? The DATAS trial: a randomised trial focused on clinically significant adverse events. Presented at 15th Cardiostim, Nice, 16 June 2006.

51 Friedmann E, Thomas SA, Inguito P, *et al.* Quality of life and psychological status of patients with implantable cardioverter defibrillators. J Interv Card Electrophysiol 2006; 17:65–72.

52 Danik SB, Mansour M, Singh J, *et al.* Increased incidence of subacute lead perforation noted with one implantable cardioverter-defibrillator. Heart Rhythm 2007; 4:439–42.

53 Kroll MW, Swerdlow CD. Optimizing defibrillation waveforms for ICDs. J Interv Card Electrophysiol 2007; 18: 247–63.

54 Lin G, Nishimura RA, Connolly HM, Dearani JA, Sundt TM 3rd, Hayes DL. Severe symptomatic tricuspid valve regurgitation due to permanent pacemaker or implantable cardioverter-defibrillator leads. J Am Coll Cardiol 2005; 45:1672–5.

55 Kucukarslan N, Kirilmaz A, Ulusoy E, *et al.* Tricuspid insufficiency does not increase early after permanent implantation of pacemaker leads. J Card Surg 2006; 21:391–4.

56 Matthews JC, Betley D, Morady F, Pelosi F Jr. Adverse interaction between a left ventricular assist device and an

implantable cardioverter defibrillator. J Cardiovasc Electrophysiol 2007; 18:1107–8.

57 Mehra R, DeGroot P. Where are we, and where are we heading in the device management of ventricular tachycardia/ventricular fibrillation? Heart Rhythm 2007; 4:99–103.

58 Walsh EP. Interventional electrophysiology in patients with congenital heart disease. Circulation 2007; 115:3224–34.

59 Boriani G, Artale P, Biffi M, *et al.* Outcome of cardioverter-defibrillator implant in patients with arrhythmogenic right ventricular cardiomyopathy. Heart Vessels 2007; 22: 184–92.

60 Chun TU, Collins KK, Dubin AM. Implantable cardioverter defibrillators in children. Expert Rev Cardiovasc Ther 2004; 2:561–71.

61 Rea R. New resynchronization lead systems and devices. In: Wang P, ed. New Arrhythmia Technologies. Malden: Blackwell Futura, 2005: 145–53.

62 Abraham WT. Cardiac resynchronization therapy for heart failure: biventricular pacing and beyond. Curr Opin Cardiol 2002; 17: 346–52.

63 Auricchio A, Stellbrink C, Sack S, *et al.* The Pacing Therapies for Congestive Heart Failure (PATH-CHF) study: rationale, design, and endpoints of a prospective randomized multicenter study. Am J Cardiol 1999; 83(5B): 130D–135D.

64 Mortensen PT, Sogaard P, Mansour H, *et al.* Sequential biventricular pacing: evaluation of safety and efficacy. Pacing Clin Electrophysiol 2004; 27: 339–45.

65 Mehra R, DeGroot P. Where are we, and where are we heading in the device management of ventricular tachycardia/ventricular fibrillation? Heart Rhythm 2007; 4:99–103.

66 Sogaard P, Egeblad H, Pedersen AK, *et al.* Sequential versus simultaneous biventricular resynchronization for severe heart failure: evaluation by tissue Doppler imaging. Circulation 2002; 106:2078–84.

67 Pitzalis MV, Iacoviello M, Romito R, *et al.* Cardiac resynchronization therapy tailored by echocardiographic evaluation of ventricular asynchrony. J Am Coll Cardiol 2002; 40:1615–22.

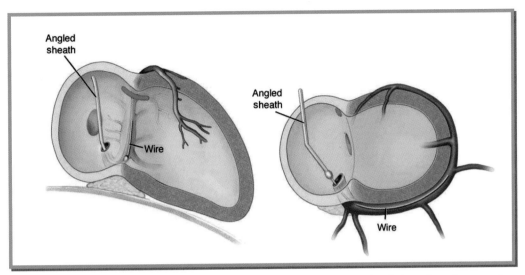

Fig. 5.28 Cannulating the coronary sinus with a guidewire. If a curved or angled sheath is employed, guidewire can be used to engage the coronary sinus and its tributaries. With the sheath rotated counterclockwise so that it points septally in the left anterior oblique projection, the wire is advanced gently, and it is seen to take the typical course of the vein in both the right and left anterior oblique projections. (From Chapter 4, Biventricular device implantation. In: Hayes DL, Wang PJ, Sackner-Bernstein J, Asirvatham SJ, eds. Resynchronisation and Defibrillation for Heart Failure: A Practical Approach. Oxford, UK: Blackwell Futura, 2004.)

been cannulated, pulling back on the catheter slightly while advancing the sheath will allow the sheath to be deployed into the CS (Figs 5.29–5.31).

A third option entails using preformed curved sheaths designed to facilitate CS access, in conjunction with gentle puffs of contrast to confirm cannulation. The sheath may have an obdurator within it to provide mechanical support, or a smaller sheath with a 50–90° bend at the distal end. Most commonly, such a sheath or sheath-within-a-sheath system is positioned in the RV at the septum. Gentle counterclockwise torque and slight retraction of the guiding sheath results in the distal tip approaching the ostium of the CS. Gentle puffs of contrast outline characteristic endocardial contours until the CS itself is seen. The advantage of this technique is that with current preformed guide catheters, CS access is rapid and reproducible. Disadvantages include the need for extra contrast, the risk of injury and/or dissection if contrast is injected too forcefully, and the fact that the large curves used to access the CS often are better suited for subsequently cannulating distal branches, making access to the middle cardiac vein more difficult.

In most cases, any technique – angiographic wires, contrast puffs, or deflectable electrophysiologic catheters – is successful. The advantage of angiographic wires is that their small size and soft tip allow repeated advancements into the appropriate radiographic planes; also, they engage and advance through tortuous, small-

diameter, or partially dissected coronary veins. When the Eustachian ridge is prominent, the guiding sheath has to be placed clearly in the ventricle anterior to the prominent ridge so that counterclockwise torque will place the sheath in the sub-Eustachian isthmus (between the Eustachian ridge and the tricuspid valve). If the guiding sheath is placed on the floor of this structure, gently advancing the wire with slight changes in the torque applied to the sheath will allow cannulation of the CS. This can be a difficult maneuver. Deflectable electrophysiologic catheters have the advantage of recording electrograms, which should show a balanced atrial and ventricular signal to identify annular locations in the patient. Furthermore, catheters with bidirectional curves can be used to negotiate sharp bends over prominent Eustachian ridges and around near circumferential thebesian valves (Fig. 5.32).[25] In choosing between techniques, the operator should make the decision on the basis of his or her experience. For example, an interventionalist may prefer trying various wires or contrast approaches, whereas an electrophysiologist is likely to be more comfortable with deflectable catheters. Regardless, deflectable catheters are larger in diameter and may not allow cannulation in patients with coronary vein stenosis or spasm. It is imperative that minimal force be applied with slow and gentle movements. because CS dissection is more likely with stiff catheters, which should be avoided. This risk is minimized if the

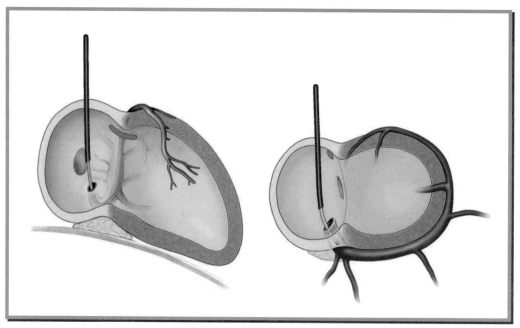

Fig. 5.29 Either straight or curved sheaths can be used with a deflectable catheter to engage the coronary sinus. The catheter is deflected just above the posterior fat pad in an end-on manner in the right anterior oblique projection and points septally and leftward in the left anterior oblique projection. Care should be taken that once the catheter has engaged the coronary sinus, the sheath should be advanced to the ostium of the coronary sinus with gentle pulling back of the catheter (see text). (From Chapter 4, Biventricular device implantation. In: Hayes DL, Wang PJ, Sackner-Bernstein J, Asirvatham SJ, eds. Resynchronisation and Defibrillation for Heart Failure: A Practical Approach. Oxford, UK: Blackwell Futura, 2004.)

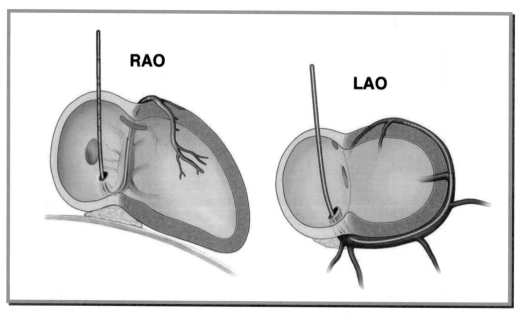

Fig. 5.30 Advancing the guiding sheath into the coronary sinus. After the sheath has been placed in the ostium of the coronary sinus, the deflectable catheter is advanced to the region of the desired vein. While pulling back on the catheter, advance the sheath and then advance the catheter again. Repeat this maneuver until the desired location in the venous system has been obtained. LAO, left anterior oblique; RAO, right anterior oblique. (From Chapter 4, Biventricular device implantation. In: Hayes DL, Wang PJ, Sackner-Bernstein J, Asirvatham SJ, eds. Resynchronisation and Defibrillation for Heart Failure: A Practical Approach. Oxford, UK: Blackwell Futura, 2004.)

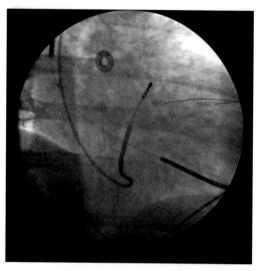
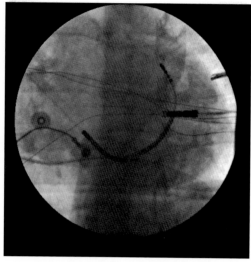

Fig. 5.31 Right anterior oblique (left panel) and left anterior oblique (right panel) projections showing cannulation of the great cardiac vein using a defl ectable catheter. (From Chapter 4, Biventricular device implantation. In: Hayes DL, Wang PJ, Sackner-Bernstein J, Asirvatham SJ [eds] Resynchronisation and Defibrillation for Heart Failure: A Practical Approach. Oxford, UK: Blackwell Futura, 2004.)

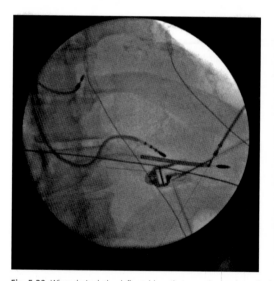
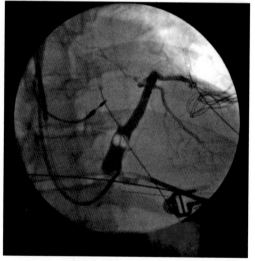

Fig. 5.32 When desired, the defl ectable catheter can be used to subselect the vein of interest and, using the maneuver described above, the sheath can be advanced into the ventricular vein. Note that angiography failed to visualize the branch that was located with gentle probing with the defl ectable catheter. (From Chapter 4, Biventricular device implantation. In: Hayes DL, Wang PJ, Sackner-Bernstein J, Asirvatham SJ, eds. Resynchronisation and Defibrillation for Heart Failure: A Practical Approach. Oxford, UK: Blackwell Futura, 2004.)

operator avoids advancing the sheath when the tip of the catheter is not free, avoids advancing into atrial coronary veins, and matches the French size of the catheter with the sheath.

Depending on operator preference and patient anatomy, one might choose ostial placement of the guiding sheath as opposed to subselection into a ventricular vein. The description of these techniques and advantages and disadvantages of each are beyond the scope of this text. However, multiple resources are available for in-depth description.[26,27]

Coronary sinus venography

After the guiding sheath has been placed at the ostium of the CS, coronary venography may be performed (Fig. 5.33). CS angiography can be performed

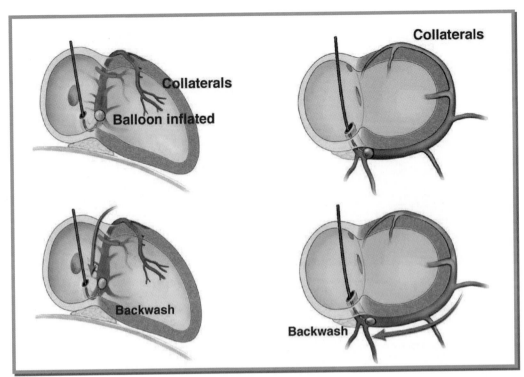

Fig. 5.33 When performing coronary sinus angiography with balloon catheters, the distal coronary sinus, great cardiac vein, and ventricular veins are best visualized with complete inflation of the balloon and occlusion of the coronary sinus. More proximal branches and the middle cardiac vein can be visualized when collaterals reforming these veins are seen or with continuous imaging when the balloon is defl ated and the ostia of the proximal veins are visualized with a backwash of contrast. (From Chapter 4, Biventricular device implantation. In: Hayes DL, Wang PJ, Sackner-Bernstein J, Asirvatham SJ, eds. Resynchronisation and Defibrillation for Heart Failure: A Practical Approach. Oxford, UK: Blackwell Futura, 2004.)

effectively with end-hole, balloon-tipped catheters (with injection of the contrast through the guiding sheath with or without a balloon on the sheath) or with deflectable electrophysiologic catheters that allow the injection of contrast dye. The technique most commonly used is balloon occlusion angiography. Care should be taken to ensure that the tip of the balloon catheter is free; the catheter should be advanced approximately 1 cm beyond the guiding sheath tip. If further advancement is not possible, the catheter should be pulled back to a point where the tip is clearly free before the injection of contrast dye is contemplated. The balloon is then inflated and gently pulled back towards the guiding sheath. Complete deployment of the balloon aids visualization of the distal coronary venous tree (Fig. 5.34). The contrast agent is injected under cine fluoroscopy. The anatomy of the coronary venous tree is visualized in at least two orthogonal planes, usually the RAO and LAO projections. To obtain maximal anatomic information from balloon angiography, it is important that:

(i) complete occlusion is performed; (ii) injection and cine fluoroscopy are continued until more proximal veins are seen to fill through anastomoses; and (iii) fluoroscopy is continued after the balloon has been deflated, because the backwash of contrast dye often demonstrates the ostia of the middle cardiac vein, proximal posterolateral veins, and the small cardiac vein.

Performed in this way, contrast CS venography provides a map for further manipulation of the ventricular lead (Figs 5.35 and 5.36). However, CS angiography is not without limitations. First, if care is not taken to ensure free motion of the tip of the catheter before injection, CS dissection or perforation (or both) may result. Second, in some patients, the contrast may adversely affect renal function or promote pulmonary edema. Third, the sheath may become dislodged during manipulation of the balloon catheter. Although CS angiography is helpful in some cases, effective lead deployment, especially with over-the-wire leads, can be accomplished without CS angiography. It is probably

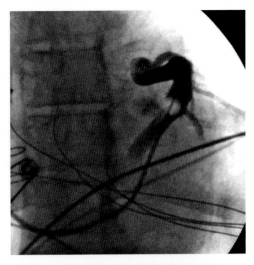

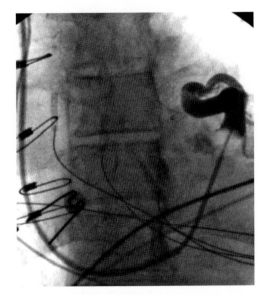

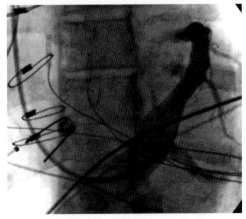

Fig. 5.34 At times during coronary sinus angiography, visualization is best with a graded pull-back technique. Initially, the balloon is placed distally and the distal vessels visualized. The balloon is then deflated more proximally to visualize mid-level branches. Either during the backwash phase or with gradual deflation of the balloon while pulling back the catheter, proximal ventricular as well as atrial branches can be visualized. This technique can be useful with large coronary veins. (From Chapter 4, Biventricular device implantation. In: Hayes DL, Wang PJ, Sackner-Bernstein J, Asirvatham SJ, eds. Resynchronisation and Defibrillation for Heart Failure: A Practical Approach. Oxford, UK: Blackwell Futura, 2004.)

beneficial for an operator to use CS angiography for the first 20–30 implants to become familiar with coronary venous anatomy and to correlate this anatomy with fluoroscopic views and the "feel" of the lead engaging a particular vein. However, some experienced implanters prefer to attempt placing the ventricular lead without performing CS angiography initially; if unsuccessful, a venogram is performed.

Technique for cannulating the coronary sinus

The primary imaging modality used for cannulation of the CS is fluoroscopy. Any projection is potentially useful to effectively engage the ostium of the CS. However, because of the rotation of the heart in the chest cavity, the true orthogonal views along the cardiac axes are the RAO and LAO projections (Fig. 5.37). The LAO projection is along the plane of the interventricular and interatrial septa. Therefore, the left-sided and right-sided cardiac structures are readily distinguished in this view, as are septal and free-wall positions. In the standard presentation, the right atrium and ventricle are seen to the left of the screen, and vice versa. Note that in the LAO projection ventricular and atrial structures cannot be distinguished. In most hearts, an LAO

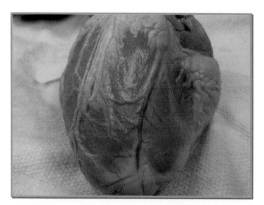

Fig. 5.35 Autopsy specimen showing extensive anastomoses between the primary ventricular veins. (From Chapter 4, Biventricular device implantation. In: Hayes DL, Wang PJ, Sackner-Bernstein J, Asirvatham SJ, eds. Resynchronisation and Defibrillation for Heart Failure: A Practical Approach. Oxford, UK: Blackwell Futura, 2004.)

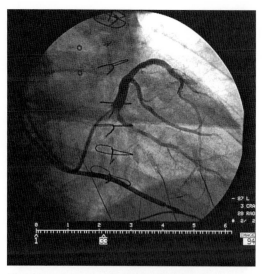

Fig. 5.36 Coronary vein angiogram showing multiple lateral veins with anastomotic branches connecting the lateral and anterolateral veins. (From Chapter 4, Biventricular device implantation. In: Hayes DL, Wang PJ, Sackner-Bernstein J, Asirvatham SJ, eds. Resynchronisation and Defibrillation for Heart Failure: A Practical Approach. Oxford, UK: Blackwell Futura, 2004.)

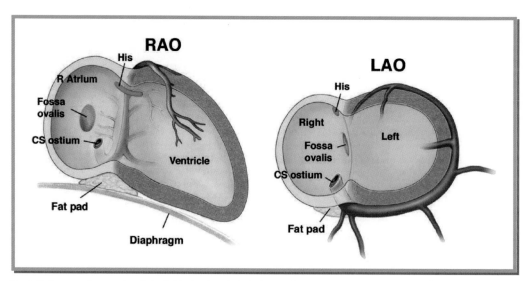

Fig. 5.37 Important fluoroscopic and electrical landmarks include the fat pad of the posteroseptal space and the bundle of His. In the right anterior oblique (RAO) projection, the consistent landmark is the translucency between the hemidiaphragm and the cardiac silhouette caused by the fat pad of the posteroseptal space. Either the guidewire or a deflectable catheter can be aimed at this translucency. The wire or catheter is then advanced leftward from this space in the left anterior oblique (LAO) projection and in an end-on (appearing to come toward the operator) fashion in the RAO projection. In grossly distorted hearts, particularly with a large right (R) atrium, and in congenital anomalies, placing an electrical mapping catheter to locate the His bundle electrogram can help to define the interatrial septum. The catheter can be advanced toward the spine from this electrocardiogram with counterclockwise torque to engage the coronary sinus (CS) ostium. (From Chapter 4, Biventricular device implantation. In: Hayes DL, Wang PJ, Sackner-Bernstein J, Asirvatham SJ, eds. Resynchronisation and Defibrillation for Heart Failure: A Practical Approach. Oxford, UK: Blackwell Futura, 2004.)

projection angle of approximately 30° will align along the interventricular septum. However, implantation of a biventricular device is often required for patients with grossly abnormal hearts, requiring a deviation from the standard approach. To define the septum in an asymmetrically enlarged heart, a catheter can be placed at the location where the His electrogram is recorded, or the RV pacing lead can be placed in the RV apex. After the septum has been defined by one of these techniques, the LAO angle can be adjusted so that this septal catheter (His bundle or RV apex) is viewed end-on. In particularly difficult cases, echocardiography can be used to define the location of the interventricular septum. It is not unusual that an LAO angle >80° is required to achieve the usual septal viewing plane. The natural viewing angle of the RAO projection is through the plane of the AV septum. With this viewing plane, it is easy to differentiate ventricular (i.e., toward the sternum) from atrial (i.e., toward the vertebral column) locations. Either of these viewing planes can easily distinguish superior and inferior positions.

To locate the CS fluoroscopically, the following steps are performed:

1 In the RAO projection (approximately 30°), the epicardial posteroseptal fat pad is visualized. This is usually seen near the angle of the right hemidiaphragm and the cardiac silhouette. If necessary, higher intensity fluoroscopy can be used briefly to visualize the structure. Often, the annulus can be visualized as a relatively radiolucent area. Occasionally, stents and coronary arterial calcifications define the annulus, as does a mechanoprosthetic cardiac AV valve.

2 The angiographic wire, the guide catheter, or deflectable electrophysiologic catheter is moved to a location just posterior and cephalad to the epicardial posteroseptal fat pad.

3 Mild counterclockwise torque is applied to the catheter guide, or sheath with wire, and the wire or catheter is gently advanced.

4 Now, the LAO viewing angle is used to ensure that the catheter or wire is advancing to the left side.

5 After the catheter or wire has advanced for approximately 1–2 cm into the CS (i.e., leftward in the LAO projection and along the AV groove in the RAO projection), the sheath is advanced gently to engage the coronary sinus, as described above.

There are multiple causes for difficulty in engaging the CS. This is again beyond the scope of this text and readers are referred to other sources.[26,27] However, issues to consider include the following:
- The coronary sinus ostium and course of the CS are not in the expected fluoroscopic planes
- Presence of a large right atrium
- Prominent thebesian valve

- Abnormalities of the CS, e.g., CS stenosis, extreme tortuosity of the CS, and congenital anomalies
- Complete occlusion of the CS.

Complications associated with coronary sinus cannulation

Dissection of the CS may occur when engaging the CS or attempting to advance the sheath into the CS.[28] Angiography from the CS will show staining of the CS musculature, the CS wall, or occasionally extensive staining of the entire coronary venous tree. Mild localized dissections of the CS are probably inconsequential, and the procedure can be performed in the usual fashion. More extensive dissections may result in closure of the coronary venous system, precluding placement of the lead (Figs 5.38 and 5.39).[29] The natural history of these occlusions is not known. When a CS dissection is diagnosed, the pericardium should be carefully examined fluoroscopically during injection of dye.[29] If no perforation is seen, certain techniques can be used to continue with the procedure.[26,27]

True CS perforations are recognized by the extravasation of contrast dye injected in the CS. Also, the clinical or echocardiographic features of pericardial effusion are usually seen. Tamponade is unusual because of the low-flow coronary venous system. However, if a sheath is advanced inadvertently through a perforated segment, life-threatening tamponade may occur.

Left ventricular lead deployment

After the CS has been cannulated, the guiding sheath is used to advance the left ventricular pacing lead through the sinus into a ventricular vein. Considerations in choosing the left ventricular pacing site include lead stability and obtaining sufficient separation from the RV lead. Early acute intraoperative epicardial lead data suggest that maximal benefit is achieved with a mid-lateral positioning of the lead.[30] Although a lateral wall position may be ideal for many patients, other issues that need to be considered include: viability of the tissue where the lead is being placed; pattern of mechanical dyssynchrony; and pattern of electrical dyssynchrony and the location of the left phrenic nerve.

General considerations

Both stylet-driven and over-the-wire leads are available for clinical use. Operators are usually familiar with stylet-driven leads. The stylet can be preformed to various curvatures. Also, retracting and inserting the stylet at the tip of the lead can change the angulation at the tip so the lead can be maneuvered into a ventricular venous branch (Fig. 5.40). In many cases, over-the-wire leads are preferable because it is easier to

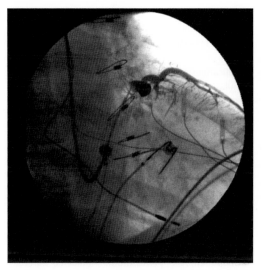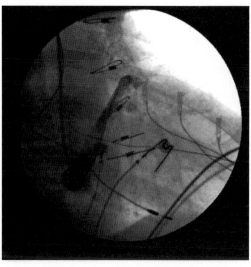

Fig. 5.38 Coronary sinus angiogram in a patient with highly tortuous distal great cardiac vein and ventricular veins. Forceful injection to visualize adequately the distal veins resulted in a pericardial blush (staining), which can result from coronary sinus dissection, pericardial infiltration, or contrast within the thebesian vein network. Cine fluoroscopy will show characteristic annular movement with coronary sinus dissection, but movement with the cardiac silhouette in pericardial and intramyocardial staining. (From Chapter 4, Biventricular device implantation. In: Hayes DL, Wang PJ, Sackner-Bernstein J, Asirvatham SJ, eds. Resynchronisation and Defibrillation for Heart Failure: A Practical Approach. Oxford, UK: Blackwell Futura, 2004.)

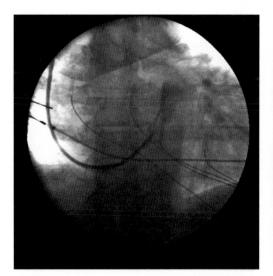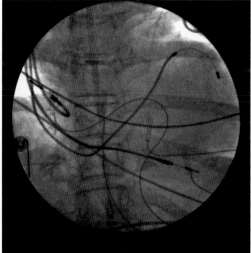

Fig. 5.39 Extravasation of contrast within the coronary veins. (From Chapter 4, Biventricular device implantation. In: Hayes DL, Wang PJ, Sackner-Bernstein J, Asirvatham SJ, eds. Resynchronisation and Defibrillation for Heart Failure: A Practical Approach. Oxford, UK: Blackwell Futura, 2004.)

Fig. 5.40 Fluoroscopy of a stylet-driven pacing lead in a lateral cardiac vein. Stylet-driven leads are more difficult to manipulate than the commonly used over-the-wire pacing leads; however, because of their larger diameter, they can be useful when placing leads in the proximal portion of dilated cardiac veins (see text). (From Chapter 4, Biventricular device implantation. In: Hayes DL, Wang PJ, Sackner-Bernstein J, Asirvatham SJ, eds. Resynchronisation and Defibrillation for Heart Failure: A Practical Approach. Oxford, UK: Blackwell Futura, 2004.)

negotiate more distal locations in the venous system. If the over-the-wire system is used, the wire is first inserted through the sheath and placed in the vein of interest, and then the lead is loaded on the over-the-wire system and advanced into the vein (Fig. 5.41). Typically, small French-size leads are preferred so that the lead tip can be left in a sub-branch or tributary of a major ventricular vein, aiding stability. In some instances, however, the CS and ventricular veins may be grossly dilated and the small French-size lead cannot make adequate contact with the myocardial surface. In this case, larger stylet-driven leads can be used and placed more proximally in the coronary venous system to make better contact. Alternatively, leads with marked preformed bend may be used; withdrawal of the guide-wire results in the development of complex tertiary geometries designed to stabilize the lead in a larger vessel. Similarly, larger stylet-driven leads may be useful when pacing thresholds are poor in the mid and distal portions of the ventricle or when a lead needs to be placed in the proximal venous system, where venous diameter is large and smaller leads may not make adequate contact with the myocardium (Fig. 5.41).

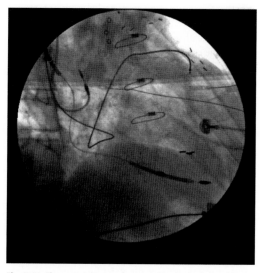

Fig. 5.41 Fluoroscopic image of an over-the-wire lead placed in a lateral branch of the anterior interventricular vein. Collaterals or anastomotic branches exist between the anterior and lateral venous systems. Longer leads may be required to navigate through these collaterals to achieve eventually a location in the mid-lateral left ventricular wall. (From Chapter 4, Biventricular device implantation. In: Hayes DL, Wang PJ, Sackner-Bernstein J, Asirvatham SJ, eds. Resynchronisation and Defibrillation for Heart Failure: A Practical Approach. Oxford, UK: Blackwell Futura, 2004.)

Techniques to ensure lead stability

When the left ventricular lead is advanced, gentle pressure should cause mild buckling in the CS and proximal ventricular vein so that the lead conforms to the curvature of the venous system. Another technique to enhance stability is to advance the lead through a main ventricular venous branch, e.g., the posterolateral vein, and use the wire to subselect a tributary and advance this to a yet secondary tributary that is in parallel with the primary vein. This U-shaped placement is usually highly resistant to dislodgment during removal of the sheath. Care should be taken to prevent excess slack or buckling proximal to the ostium of the CS. After the sheath has been removed, the tricuspid annular region should be inspected carefully. If the lead prolapses beyond the tricuspid valve into the RV, the slack should be removed. Excess slack within a large dilated CS may cause coiling or looping of the lead in the CS. In our experience at Mayo Clinic, this has not affected lead stability and we have elected to leave the loop within the CS. Occasionally, excessive slack causes prolapse of the proximal portion of the lead into the inferior vena cava. It is probably best to pull back on the lead to minimize the slack (Fig. 5.42).

If the coronary venous system is very large (dilated and nearly variceal), obtaining contact and adequate stability is a problem with even larger leads. To overcome this challenge, two techniques may be used: (i) the over-the-wire lead system can be advanced through the large venous system from, for example, the postero-lateral vein all the way to the apex and then advanced through either the anterior interventricular vein or middle cardiac vein to a more proximal location, where the lead can be placed in a smaller venous tributary; (ii) the left ventricular lead is purposely curled on itself and advanced as a loop into the dilated venous system. To do this, the wire is first advanced to engage a venous branch. Thus engaged, the lead is continuously pushed until the body of the lead begins to prolapse as a loop into the great cardiac vein. The wire is then retracted and the lead is advanced as a loop into another venous branch. Advancing the lead with this loop sometimes affords better myocardial contact and adequate thresholds when previous maneuvers were unsuccessful. This same maneuver can also be helpful in avoiding diaphragmatic stimulation when a proximal posterolateral or middle cardiac vein is used. When advanced as a loop, the tip of the lead can be manipulated to be oriented more toward the myocardium than the diaphragm.

Thresholds should be checked before and after the sheath has been removed. High output (at the highest output and pulse width setting) should be performed during both inspiration and expiration to check for phrenic or diaphragmatic stimulation. In our

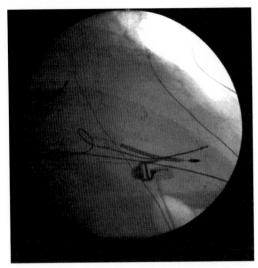 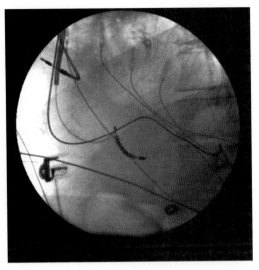

Fig. 5.42 Fluoroscopic images of over-the-wire leads placed in the region of the lateral left ventricle. Various techniques can be used to enhance lead stability. Left, note a loop within the proximal dilated coronary veins. Loops may enhance stability in certain venous locations. Respiratory maneuvers and patient repositioning should be performed before closure. Right, an ideal positioning of the lead tip is shown. The tip has been advanced through a main coronary vein into a subsidiary branch that is parallel to this vein. This type of positioning is particularly useful in very dilated hearts and when dislodgment occurs repeatedly within the main vein. (From Chapter 4, Biventricular device implantation. In: Hayes DL, Wang PJ, Sackner-Bernstein J, Asirvatham SJ, eds. Resynchronisation and Defibrillation for Heart Failure: A Practical Approach. Oxford, UK: Blackwell Futura, 2004.)

experience, if diaphragmatic stimulation occurs, it is preferable to obtain access in a different venous branch than to attempt repositioning the lead in the same vein, because diaphragmatic stimulation may occur subacutely with movement or change in respiration.

Deployment in the middle cardiac vein will be necessary in some patients, and the operator should be familiar with this special technique.[26,27]

Sheath removal

After the lead has been placed satisfactorily and preliminary thresholds have been checked to ensure local ventricular capture and to exclude extracardiac stimulation, the guiding sheath needs to be removed. Several methods are available for removing the sheath, including peel-away type sheaths and cutting-away systems. Also, with certain combinations of lead and sheath, the sheath can be pulled over the lead, although this type of system is rarely used. Regardless of the system used, certain principles need to be followed. A stylet should be reintroduced into the lead before the sheath is removed. Depending on the lead system, the stylet may be introduced all the way to the tip of the lead or into the main body of the CS. Despite these variations, the stylet should be of medium stiffness (in most cases) and placed at least 1 cm into the CS and preferably in the great cardiac vein. If the stylet is placed too close to the CS or in the right atrium, pulling back on the sheath

may cause excessive inferior force and dislodge the lead. Whether the sheath is cut away, peeled away, or removed over the lead, the lead should be held firmly in place while the sheath is removed. In the case of the cut-away system, the cutting blade should be secured to the lead and the blade and lead held firmly onto the patient with one hand. The sheath should be pulled back against the blade and care taken not to change the existing rotational torque on the sheath. In other words, the sheath should be pulled back in the angle in which it lays and not be maneuvered to suit the operator. This is to avoid dislodging the lead as the sheath is cut back. The movement should be smooth and fluid, and the hand that stabilizes the lead should not be moved. Similarly, with peel-away or over-the-lead removal, the hand that stabilizes the lead should not move, and the tendency to push the lead further into the body should be resisted. After the sheath has been removed, the lead is secured to its sleeve and the sleeve to the underlying muscle. Most operators remove the stylet for suturing the lead and introduce the stylet up to the junction of the SVC and right atrium before manipulating other leads. Fluoroscopy should be performed after the stylet has been removed and the lead has been secured to ensure there is no excess slack, specifically slack that causes the body of the lead to prolapse into the RV.

Multiple approaches can be used to cannulate the CS and deploy a left ventricular lead. The choice of a particular approach depends on the training and background of the operator and the resources available. Also, it is desirable to know several solutions to any problem that may develop. No single sheath, curvature, deflectable catheter, wire, or technique is ideally suited for all patients. Although most operators become familiar with a particular set of techniques, they should be willing to try another technique that may be helpful in a difficult case.

Securing permanent leads

If pacing and sensing thresholds are satisfactory and there is no diaphragmatic stimulation measured with pacing at 10V, the silicone rubber sleeve provided on the lead is positioned over the lead at the point of entry into the vein. Synthetic nonabsorbable ligature is used to fix the sleeve to the lead and to the muscle or the vein itself. It is essential to use the sleeve and not affix the lead directly to the adjacent tissue (Fig. 5.43). Ligatures applied directly to the lead may damage the insulation and act as a fulcrum, with eventual lead fracture at the ligature site.

Dual-chamber pulse generator implantation

The introducer technique can be used to place two leads. Three variations of the technique can be selected. Two venepunctures can be made, one for each catheter to be inserted, the ventricular lead generally being placed first (Fig. 5.44). This technique reduces the

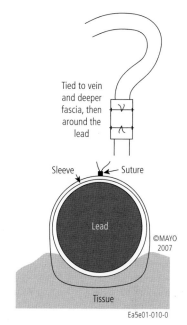

Fig. 5.43 The permanent lead is secured with a ligature placed around the sleeve provided on the lead and then to the underlying tissue. Some implanters prefer to place two ligatures around each sleeve to ensure stability. Copyrighted and used with permission of Mayo Foundation for Medical Education and Research.

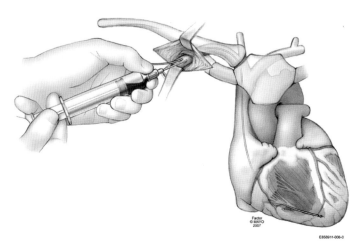

Fig. 5.44 If a second lead is to be used, a second subclavian puncture can be made parallel to the already placed pacing lead, or the second puncture can be accomplished after the first guidewire is in place but before the first pacing lead is inserted. If the second puncture is made after the initial lead is in place, care should be taken to avoid puncturing the indwelling lead. The potential for damage can be minimized by placing the puncture medial to the existing lead. (From Holmes DR, Hayes DL, Furman S. Permanent pacemaker implantation. In: Furman S, Hayes DL, Holmes DR Jr, eds. A Practice of Cardiac Pacing, 2nd edn. Mount Kisco, NY: Futura Publishing Co., 1989: 239–87, by permission of Mayo Foundation.)

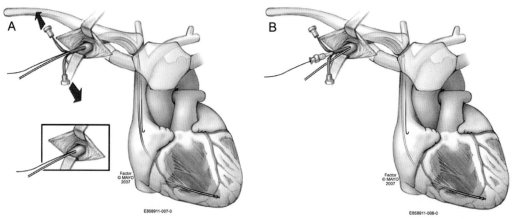

E858911-007-0   E858911-008-0

Fig. 5.45 Two leads can be placed without a second subclavian puncture and without simultaneously passing the leads. (A) As the dilator and guidewire are removed and the initial pacing lead is passed into the right heart, the guidewire is reinserted through the peel-away introducer alongside the pacing lead. The introducer is then peeled away, and the pacing lead and guidewire are left in place. (B) A second introducer is then passed over the reintroduced guidewire, and the second lead is placed. (From Holmes DR, Hayes DL, Furman S. Permanent pacemaker implantation. In: Furman S, Hayes DL, Holmes DR Jr, eds. A Practice of Cardiac Pacing, 2nd edn. Mount Kisco, NY: Futura Publishing Co., 1989: 239–87, by permission of Mayo Foundation.)

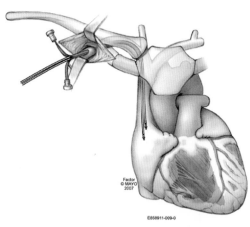

E858911-009-0

Fig. 5.46 If two pacing leads are necessary, they can be inserted simultaneously through a peel-away introducer large enough to accommodate both of them. With straight stylets in place, one lead is staggered 1–2 cm behind the other lead, and they are passed simultaneously into the right heart, whereupon the introducer is peeled away. (From Holmes DR, Hayes DL, Furman S. Permanent pacemaker implantation. In: Furman S, Hayes DL, Holmes DR Jr, eds. A Practice of Cardiac Pacing, 2nd edn. Mount Kisco, NY: Futura Publishing Co., 1989: 239–87, by permission of Mayo Foundation.)

away (Fig. 5.45A); after positioning the first lead, an introducer is placed over the retained guidewire to accommodate the second lead (Fig. 5.45B). In an uncommonly used third variation, two leads (one for atrial and one for ventricular placement) can be advanced through the same introducer sheath into the right side of the heart (Fig. 5.46). (The size of the introducer required to introduce two leads depends on the additive size of the two leads.) Our preference is to position the ventricular lead and then pass the atrial lead. Alternatively, both leads can be passed into the right heart and the atrial lead held in a stable position in the right atrium while the ventricular lead is positioned in the RV apex. After stable ventricular placement is achieved, the atrial lead is positioned.

Although the atrial lead has most commonly been positioned in the right atrial appendage, satisfactory pacing can be achieved from multiple positions within the right atrium. In patients with previous cardiac surgery in whom the appendage has been cannulated or amputated, finding a stable position in the vicinity of the atrial appendage may be difficult and not always possible.

Technique varies, depending on whether a preformed atrial J lead or a nonpreformed lead, i.e., a standard straight lead that can be used in either the atrium or the ventricle, is used. At this time, standard leads (nonpreformed J) are much more commonly used than preformed J leads.

If a preformed J lead is chosen, a straight stylet is placed in the lead to straighten it, and the lead is passed

potential for displacement of one lead while the other is being positioned, but requires two separate venepunctures. In the second variation, one venepuncture is made and one lead is introduced, and the guidewire is reintroduced or retained before the sheath is peeled

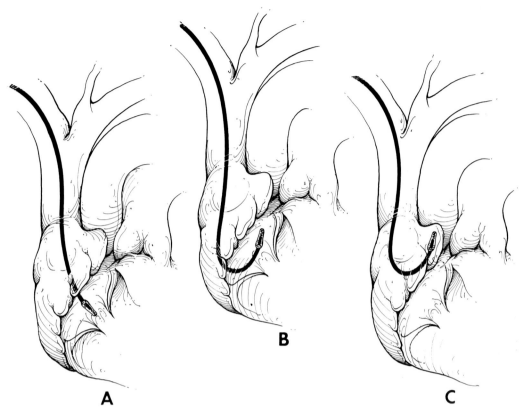

Fig. 5.47 Placement of a preformed atrial J lead. (A) The lead is at the middle of the right atrium with a straight stylet in place. (B) The straight stylet is removed; removal allows the catheter to assume the preformed J configuration. (C) The entire lead is pulled back, and the tip of the electrode is allowed to enter the right atrial appendage. The lead has a characteristic to-and-fro motion when positioned in the right atrial appendage. (From Holmes DR, Hayes DL, Furman S. Permanent pacemaker implantation. In: Furman S, Hayes DL, Holmes DR Jr, eds. A Practice of Cardiac Pacing, 2nd edn. Mount Kisco, NY: Futura Publishing Co., 1989: 239–87, by permission of Mayo Foundation.)

into the middle to low right atrium (Fig. 5.47A). The straight stylet is withdrawn approximately 10 cm, and the lead assumes the J shape (Fig. 5.47B). The lead is gradually withdrawn in an effort to secure the lead tip against the endocardial surface (Fig. 5.47C). If the lead tip is securely against the atrial wall when the J begins to straighten, the lead should again be advanced slowly to allow the appropriate J to occur. If the lead has active fixation, the fixation mechanism should then be secured. Sensing and pacing thresholds should be checked. If they are adequate, the lead should be secured with the sleeve provided, as previously described.

Entry into the atrial appendage is indicated by a rhythmic to-and-fro medial and lateral motion of the J portion of the lead. The posteroanterior fluoroscopic projection may show that the lead is medial or lateral, and a lateral projection shows the lead to be anterior at approximately the same level as a lead in the RV apex.

If the atrial lead is being placed as part of a dual-chamber implant, the ventricular lead should be carefully observed so that it is not inadvertently displaced.

If a straight active fixation lead is used, a J curved stylet is needed to position the lead. J curved stylets are usually provided with the lead. Whether the lead is being positioned in the right atrial appendage or other right atrial site, a stylet with some degree of J shape will usually be required. The stylet is introduced into the atrial lead in the low right atrium, and the lead is pulled into the right atrial appendage. The active fixation lead is fixed in place, and the J guidewire is gently withdrawn to avoid displacing the lead from the point of attachment. Again, sensing and pacing thresholds should be checked. If they are adequate, the lead should be secured with the sleeve provided, as previously described.

Regardless of whether a preformed J or a straight lead is implanted in the atrium, with implantation in the right atrial appendage the J portion of the lead is slightly medial on the posteroanterior projection and anterior on the lateral projection. Optimally, the limits of the J should be no greater than approximately 80° apart. Redundancy proximal to the J within the atrium or SVC should not be seen.

Locations other than the right atrial appendage may be used for atrial lead positioning, and their use is increasing. There are some advocates of routine placement of the right atrial lead on the atrial septum. The right atrium can be explored to find optimal positioning for lead placement. With active fixation leads, the lead can be placed anywhere the lead is stable and good thresholds are obtained (Fig. 5.48).

Atrial leads are occasionally positioned in the CS and adjacent to the CS ostium (os) to prevent recurrent atrial fibrillation and flutter.[31] (Atrial septal lead positioning[32,33] or Bachmann's bundle positioning[34] is also favored by some for the prevention of paroxysmal atrial fibrillation or flutter.) The hemodynamic implications of dual-site atrial pacing are discussed in detail in Chapter 2: Hemodynamics of Cardiac Pacing.

The technical details of introduction of a CS lead have previously been described. Obviously, for atrial

pacing, the CS lead needs to be positioned in a tributary of the CS that will afford adequate and stable atrial pacing and sensing. The ideal position is probably in the vein of Marshall (Fig. 5.49). Once again, because of the individual variability in coronary venous anatomy, not all patients have a true vein of Marshall.

To position an active fixation atrial lead near the CS os, the lead is passed into the CS and then gently withdrawn and secured after exiting the CS. (A straight lead is required; a preformed J should not be used.) Fluoroscopic imaging in a RAO position may allow one to better visualize the posterior and septal position desirable (Fig. 5.50). The LAO fluoroscopic view is helpful subsequently to verify the location of the lead.

Measurement of pacing and sensing thresholds

Knowledge and measurement of pacing and sensing thresholds are integral parts of the placement of a permanent pacemaker, ICD, or CRT system. The equipment used and measurements made vary from laboratory to laboratory. In most institutions, pacing system analyzers available from the pulse generator manufacturers are used. Most centers use an analyzer

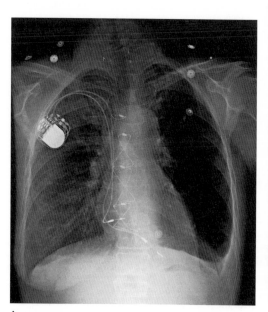
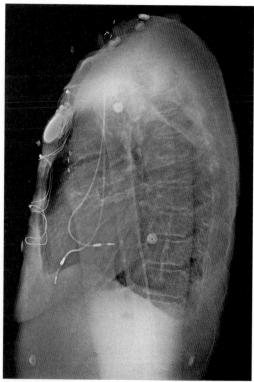

A

B

Fig. 5.48 Posteroanterior (A) and lateral (B) views of placement of an active fixation atrial lead near the coronary sinus ostium.

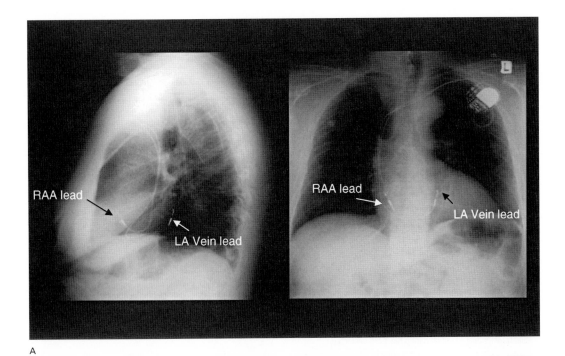

A

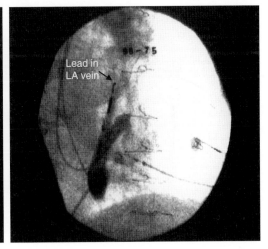

B

Fig. 5.49 Chest radiographs (A) and coronary venograms (B) depicting the vein of Marshall, a coronary venous position for left atrial pacing. LA, left atrial; RAA, right atrial appendage. (Courtesy of Dr. Anthony Tang, Ottawa Heart Institute, Ottawa, Ontario, Canada.)

from a single manufacturer. (Although of historical concern, use of a mismatched pacing system analyzer and pulse generator does not result in any clinical problem.) Measurements necessary during device implantation are listed in Table 5.1.

Determination of pacing threshold
The pacing threshold is the minimal electrical stimulus required to produce consistent cardiac depolarization.

It should be measured with the same electrode configuration (unipolar or bipolar) as the lead and pulse generator that are to be used. During pacing, the output of the pacing system analyzer is gradually decreased from 5 V at 0.5 ms pulse width to the point at which loss of capture is documented. The pacing rate selected during this measurement is important. The rate should be just fast enough (approximately 10 ppm faster) to override the intrinsic rhythm. In some patients, pacing

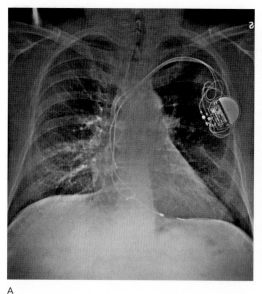
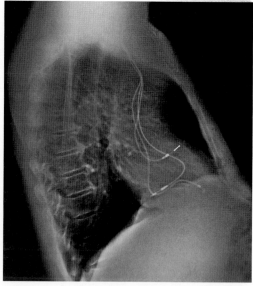

A   B

Fig. 5.50 Posteroanterior (A) and lateral (B) chest radiographs from a patient with paroxysmal atrial fibrillation in whom a dual-chamber pacemaker with dual-site atrial pacing has been implanted.

Table 5.1 Measurements during pacemaker, ICD, and CRT implantation.

- Threshold of stimulation*
- Sensing threshold*
- Measurement of electrogram†
- Defibrillation threshold‡

*Necessary for any lead placed in any transvenous, coronary sinus or epicardial position.
†Electrograms are easily obtained via the pacing system analyzer. We generally assess the electrogram during the implant procedure.
‡For cardioverter-defibrillator implantation only.

during measurement of thresholds suppresses intrinsic rhythm and results in lack of a stable ventricular escape focus, or even asystole, when pacing is discontinued. The lower the stimulation threshold, the better. Acceptable acute thresholds are generally considered to be <1 V for both ventricular and atrial leads at 0.5 ms pulse duration.

If active fixation leads are used, thresholds checked immediately after deployment of the fixation mechanism may not reflect true thresholds. If the lead position looks good and the initial thresholds are high, it is worthwhile waiting for a short time, e.g., 1 min, and repeating the measurements to see whether the thresh-

olds are now acceptable. If the repeat threshold is lower but still not at the desirable level, it may be worthwhile waiting another minute or so and rechecking to see if the trend continues toward a lower threshold, as it often will.

The impedance of the pacing electrode is also measured. Measurement of voltage and current allows calculation of the lead resistance, which varies greatly depending on the lead used. A range of $300-1500\,\Omega$ may be seen, depending on lead type. Impedances should always be measured under standardized conditions of output and pulse duration. The finding of unsuspected low impedance raises the possibility of insulation failure in the lead and that of high impedance the possibility of a poor connection in the connector block, or lead fracture.

Determination of sensing threshold

Measurement of sensing thresholds is equally important. Adequate sensing thresholds are essential to avoid the problem of undersensing or oversensing after implantation. The pulse generator senses intracardiac events, not the events seen on the surface ECG (Fig. 5.51). The intrinsic deflection is that component of the intracardiac electrogram that is sensed.[35] It is the amplitude of this intracardiac signal in the chamber to be paced that is measured. The result is expressed as a voltage. The ventricular electrogram sensed for ade-

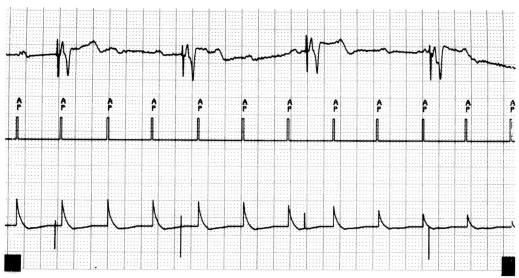

Fig. 5.51 Intracardiac electrograms obtained via the programmer at the time of pacemaker implantation in a patient with complete heart block. Pacemakers sense intracardiac electrograms, specifically intrinsic deflection of either ventricle or atrium. The slew rate is a measure of dV/dt (see text for details).

quate long-term sensing should be >4 mV. More commonly, the ventricular signal is 6–20 mV, a range that provides excellent sensing. Programmable options for ventricular sensing in permanent pacemakers may exist at ≤1 mV. However, the goal for a measured ventricular signal should be ≥5 mV during normal rhythm. This is particularly true for implantable defibrillators, to ensure that the small-amplitude signals during ventricular fibrillation are appropriately sensed.[36]

For atrial sensing, a signal of at least 2 mV is desirable. However, with current pacemakers that offer programmable options for atrial sensing as low as 0.18 mV and with ICDs that incorporate autosensing to vary sensitivity values, lower atrial sensing thresholds can at times be accepted. Still, the goal should be a measured P wave of ≥2 mV. With an atrial lead placed in the appendage, it is common to see a far-field R wave on the electrogram. This results because the large mass of the ventricle generates an electric signal seen by the lead at a distance. The far-field R wave should be significantly smaller than the P wave (ideally one-quarter the size or smaller) to ensure that it is not detected by the device. This is particularly true in defibrillators, because reliable sensing of P waves is important for rhythm discrimination.

In addition to peak amplitude, other aspects of sensing should be considered. The change in voltage with time (dV/dt), the slew rate, of the intrinsic deflection may be clinically important. Usually, this is most important in patients with borderline sensing voltages. In patients with low voltages (<5 mV), the slew rate measurement may be helpful and with current pacing system analyzers is easy to obtain. Some patients with a QRS of 3 mV but a slow slew rate may have undersensing, whereas other patients with a QRS of 3 mV but a normal slew rate may have adequate sensing.

Historically, some implanters would assess the current of injury at the time of lead placement but this is not commonly done at this time. The current, appearing as an increase in the electrical potential that immediately follows the intrinsic deflection, represents a small area of endocardium that reacts to placement of the lead (Fig. 5.52). This finding indicates adequate contact with the endocardium. A large current of injury may be mistaken for an adequate sensed intrinsic electrogram.

Additional measurements

Assessment of AV nodal conduction is necessary if an AAI pacemaker is to be implanted. In this situation, the atrial lead is positioned and the atrium is paced at rates nearly equal to the sinus rate and then at incremental rates up to approximately 150 ppm. A typical sequence might be 80, 100, 120, 140, and 160 ppm. The pacing rate at which Wenckebach, or higher grade, AV block occurs is recorded, as is the AR interval (paced atrial event to intrinsic QRS). To proceed with AAI pacing, the patient should have 1 : 1 conduction to rates of

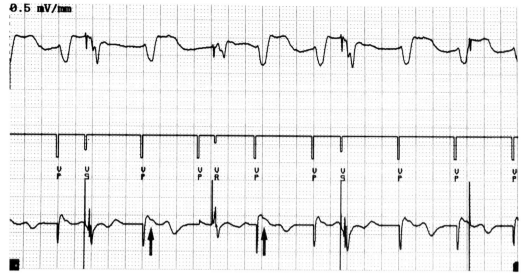

0.5 mV/mm

Fig. 5.52 Intracardiac electrograms obtained via the programmer at the time of pacemaker implantation. In addition to assessment of magnitude and relationship of intrinsic deflection of atrium and ventricle, a current of injury is identified (arrows). This current of injury, manifested as an increase in electrical potential after intrinsic deflection, indicates adequate endocardial contact.

130–140 ppm without any significant prolongation of the AR interval.

Epicardial systems

Epicardial (also called myocardial) systems account for a very small percentage of device implantation procedures. Three groups of patients still undergo placement of epicardial systems.

1 Patients undergoing cardiac surgery for another indication. In these patients, permanent epicardial leads may be placed at the time of surgery. Alternatively, some of these patients have temporary pacing until recovery from open-heart surgery. Before dismissal from the hospital, they may undergo placement of a transvenous pacing system. This latter approach is preferable, because transvenous leads have proven to be more reliable than epicardial leads.

2 Patients with a prosthetic tricuspid valve, a congenital anomaly, or atresia of the tricuspid valve without access to the CS. In these patients, epicardial ventricular leads are usually required. However, bioprosthetic valves are compatible with transvenous implantation. It is difficult to quantify adverse outcomes from placing a transvenous lead across a bioprosthetic valve, and it is certainly in the patient's best interest to protect the bioprosthetic valve as much as possible. If a lead is to be placed across a bioprosthetic valve it is advisable to use the smallest lead possible, i.e., smallest French size.

3 Patients with ventricular septal defects or patients with right-to-left shunts in whom the possibility for systemic embolization exists.

Two surgical procedures have been described for the placement of epicardial leads: (i) subxiphoid, or left costal, approach; and (ii) left lateral thoracotomy. Such procedures obviously require a trained surgeon, and the reader is referred to cardiovascular surgical texts for details of these approaches.

In patients who have either tricuspid atresia or other conditions that preclude entering the RV through the tricuspid valve, the CS and ventricular vein may be used to pace the ventricle. In some types of Fontan correction, the CS continues to drain into the right atrium. If no other shunts at the atrial or ventricular level are present, the CS can be cannulated (as described under Coronary sinus lead placement, above) and the lead placed in a ventricular vein. Care must be taken to ensure that there are no insidious shunts (fenestration of the Fontan patch or unroofing of the CS). Because left ventricular leads tend to be less stable than endocardial screw-in leads, in patients with pacemaker dependence it may be best to proceed with epicardial pacing even when the CS is accessible.

Hardware adaptations

The "connector pin" of the implanted lead connector plugs into an appropriate connector cavity in the "header" of the pulse generator to provide the permanent but reversible connection between the two. The connector cavity in the header holds the proximal (i.e., the extravascular) end of the lead.

Although a few bifurcated bipolar leads may remain in service, the vast majority of contemporary leads, whether unipolar or bipolar and whether coaxial or some other conductor design, employ "inline" connectors. They conform to a formal, international connector standard, published by the International Standards Organization in Brussels, Belgium, known as the "international standard," or IS-1, design.

Older voluntary standard (VS) lead connector designs and the current/IS-1 pacing lead connectors are 3.2 mm in diameter, have sealing rings on the lead, and have a short (0.508 cm) connector pin (Fig. 5.53). The old "VS-1" and the current IS-1 pacing lead connectors fit pacemakers that have 3.2-mm connector cavities. VS-1/IS-1 pacemaker header connector cavities are 3.2 mm in diameter, have no sealing rings, have a short (0.508 cm) cavity bore for the lead's connector pin, and accept only the VS-1/IS-1 pacing lead connectors.

A few pacemakers still exist that have header connector cavities with the designations "VS-1A" and "VS-1B," and are a point of confusion (Fig. 5.54). Pacemaker connector cavities designated VS-1A are 3.2 mm in diameter, have no sealing rings, and have a long (0.851 cm) receptacle for the lead's connector pin. Pacemakers with the VS-1B designation have sealing rings in the header's connector cavities but are otherwise like the VS-1A designation (Fig. 5.54). This terminology need not be confusing. Dimensions are the same for both unipolar and bipolar "VS-1" and "IS-1" leads and pacers. There is only one configuration for VS-1 and IS-1 lead connectors. The VS-1 and IS-1 designs have provisions within the pacer connector for three functional options (Table 5.2).

Older leads with non-IS-1 lead connectors also still remain in use; therefore, as pulse generator replacement is required, adapters may be necessary. Some pulse generators are now made specifically to accommodate pulse generator replacement with such older leads. Some pacemakers are available in a variety of connector formats: (i) inline bipolar, i.e., 3.2 mm; (ii) 3.2 mm IS-1 unipolar; (iii) unipolar to accept an older 5-mm lead only; and (iv) unipolar to accept a 5 or 6-mm lead.

An attempt should be made to match polarity and design of the pacing lead and pulse generator; e.g., a bipolar inline lead connector to a bipolar inline pulse generator connector cavity and a bifurcated 5-mm bipolar lead's two-lead connectors must each be connected into separate 5-mm unipolar connector cavities in a bipolar pulse generator. Special adaptors are necessary to allow use of polarity-mismatched lead connectors and pulse generators. Table 5.3 outlines possible

VS•1/IS-1

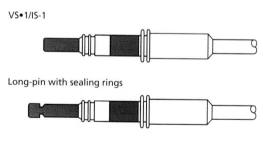

Long-pin with sealing rings

Long-pin without sealing rings

Fig. 5.53 VS-1/IS-1 connectors are intended to restore universal interconnection of all leads and pulse generators via the standardized 3.2-mm connectors. The pin is connected to the negative output and the ring to the positive terminal in the pulse generator header. Unipolar leads of similar configuration exist, but without a positive terminal, and are of the same size as and interchangeable with a bipolar receptacle. The ridges represent the sealing rings, which prevent the ingress of fluid into the header.

VS•1/IS-1

VS•1A

VS•1B

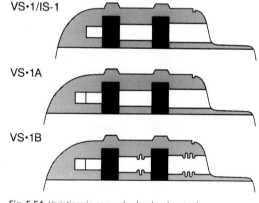

Fig. 5.54 Variations in pacemaker headers (see text).

Table 5.2 Pacemaker header connector cavity variations.

Pacemaker header connector cavity	Lead connector
VS-1/IS-1	Accepts only VS-1/1S-1 lead connectors
VS-1A/IS-1	Accepts VS-1A or 1S-1 leads and 3.2-mm inline leads with a longer pin
VS-1B/IS-1	Accepts VS-1B or IS-1 leads and 3.2-mm inline leads that have a longer pin and sealing rings

Table 5.3 Specific adaptor for specific combination.

Pulse generator connector cavity	Lead connector		
	Unipolar	Inline bipolar	Bifurcated bipolar
Unipolar		Low-profile adaptor sleeve	End cap
Inline bipolar	Low-profile lead to bifurcated pulse generator and an indifferent electrode		Bifurcated lead to in-line generator adaptor
Bipolar with bifurcated connector	Indifferent electrode	Low-profile lead to bifurcated pulse generator adaptor	

Source: from Holmes DR, Hayes DL, Furman S. Permanent pacemaker implantation. In: Furman S, Hayes DL, Holmes DR Jr, eds. A Practice of Cardiac Pacing, 2nd edn. Mount Kisco, NY: Futura Publishing Co., 1989: 276, by permission of Mayo Foundation.

combinations and adaptors necessary. Various adaptors are pictured in Fig. 5.55. Again, every attempt should be made to match lead and pulse generator hardware configuration.

ICD leads currently follow a different international connector standard, known as "DF-1," from that for pacing leads (Fig. 5.56).[35] At present, ICD leads from all US and most European manufacturers utilize lead connectors and ICDs that are compatible with the DF-1 connector standard. The proximal portion of a defibrillation lead is bifurcated or trifurcated, with an IS-1 connector that conducts to the distal pace/sense electrodes, and one or two DF-1 connectors that conduct to the defibrillation coils. The IS-4 connector is the new standard for ICDs that uses a single inline connector for both acing and defibrillation and is discussed in greater detail in Chapter 4: Choosing the Device Generator and Leads.

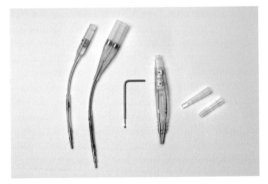

Fig. 5.55 Various adaptors used for pacing lead and pulse generator mismatches. From left to right: DF1 to LV1 lead adaptor; adapt two unipolar leads or a bifurcated lead to a bipolar inline connector; Allen wrench used to place the small screws needed for certain lead adaptors; inline lead to a bifurcated connector; end cap; bipolar inline sleeve adaptor to convert to a unipolar generator.

Special considerations in pediatric patients

Device implantation in the pediatric population raises specific issues, including the size and expected growth of the patients, whether congenital heart disease is associated, the need for long-term pacing, and whether the age and size of the patient should influence the selection of the system implanted.

Transvenous systems are used most frequently in the pediatric population, but epicardial systems remain very important for the pediatric age group, especially the neonate and infant.[37]

Older literature with much earlier designs of epicardial leads demonstrated that survival of endocardial leads was superior to that of epicardial leads in pediatric patients.[38] However, with improvement in epicardial lead design there is probably less difference in lead longevity, although controversy persists.[39,40] The lead for the pediatric patient, be it neonate, infant, or older, should be chosen based on the individual patient.

In the pediatric patient with congenital cardiovascular anomalies who is undergoing device implantation, it is helpful to know before implantation whether the child has an associated persistent left SVC. This can usually be determined echocardiographically. If concern exists, angiography is diagnostic. Advancing the pacing lead into a persistent left SVC results in traversing the CS and entering the heart in the right atrium. This makes ventricular access more difficult to the position and angulation of the lead as it emerges from the CS. To avoid the problems associated with a persistent left SVC, the right subclavian vein should be used if there is any doubt about whether the patient has a persistent left SVC. Even with a left SVC, the patient usually has a right SVC.

For lead placement, there are two potential approaches. The first is to allow more lead redundancy than would usually be left in an adult patient, but oth-

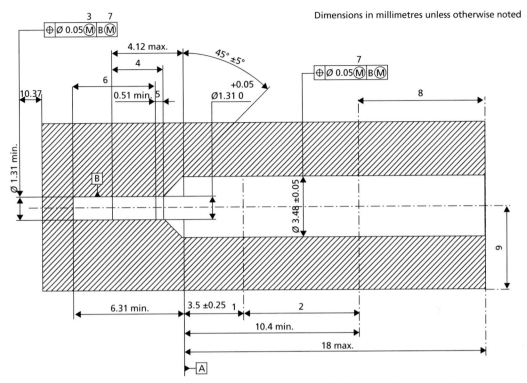

Fig. 5.56 Schematic representation of the DF-1 connector for implantable cardioverter-defibrillator leads. Dimensions in millimeters unless otherwise noted.

erwise to use standard techniques to place the lead, including securing the lead with the sleeve provided. However, instead of securing the sleeve with nonabsorbable suture, as is our usual practice, some believe that the use of absorbable suture may allow the lead to advance as the child grows. Whether or not this makes a long-term difference for the patient is difficult to prove. If the lead were to become fibrosed along the venous route or in an intramyocardial position, the lead could not advance. However, growth of the pediatric patient may minimize fibrosis.

The additional redundancy of the lead allows for growth of the pediatric patient (Fig. 5.57). If this approach is taken, the leads must be evaluated periodically during follow-up. If the child "outgrows" the lead, i.e., there is radiographic evidence of straightening of the lead, it is necessary to place a new lead. Because of entrapment of the lead in the venous system and cardiac chambers, the lead may not "advance" on its own, and lead advancement may not even be possible with a stylet in place after the lead has been implanted for a long period. Although a variety of clinical situations may develop when the patient truly "out-

grows" the pacing system, most commonly, intermittent sensing abnormalities occur as tension develops on the lead at the electrode–tissue interface.

It is of particular importance to select the smallest pulse generator that serves the needs of the pediatric patient. The small weight and dimensions of current pacemakers allow implantation in a prepectoral position in a patient of almost any size. In very small infants, if there is concern that there is not enough subcutaneous tissue to protect the device, consideration may be given to placing the pulse generator in a subpectoral position. In our experience, this placement is not often necessary with pacemakers, but has been necessary at times for ICDs. Before the advent of very small pulse generators, the transvenous lead was occasionally tunneled subcutaneously from the pectoral entry site to an area in the abdomen or flank where the pulse generator could be placed more easily. This approach, too, is rarely necessary with the small size of currently available pulse generators.

Traditional venous routes can be used in the pediatric patient; i.e., the axillary puncture technique with placement of one or two leads via the axillary vein is

A

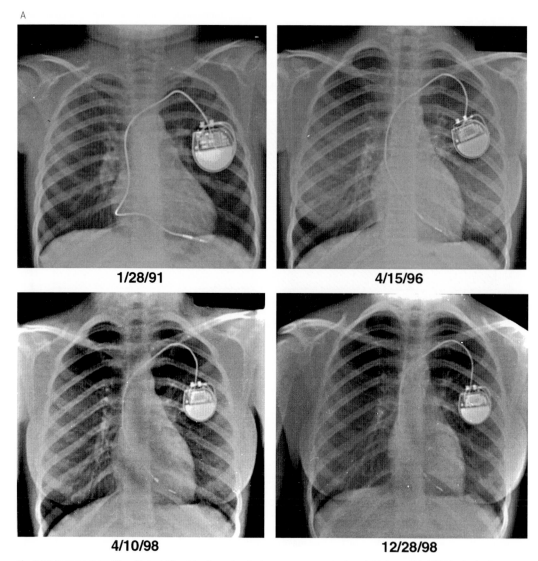

Fig. 5.57 Posteroanterior (A) and lateral (B) serial radiographs of a transvenous pacemaker in a child show which initial lead redundancy decreases with growth.

usually possible. Two leads can often be placed via the cephalic vein as well. Although rarely used, a single-pass VDD pacing system could be considered in the pediatric patient with AV block. Such a system minimizes hardware but still accomplishes AV synchrony and maintains P-synchronous rate adaptation if the sinus node is intact.

Although any standard pacing lead can be used in pediatric patients, active fixation leads are generally preferred for specific reasons. Active fixation may allow additional stability of the lead in the immediate post-

implantation period, when it is difficult to control the activities of a pediatric patient. The pediatric patient may require several pacing systems during the growth years. Although a noninfected lead may be abandoned and left in place, it is reasonable to attempt removal of abandoned leads in the pediatric patient so that an excessive amount of hardware does not accumulate in the patient throughout a lifetime. Some preference has therefore been given to active fixation leads, because they are generally easier to remove than a long-term passive fixation (tined) lead.

B

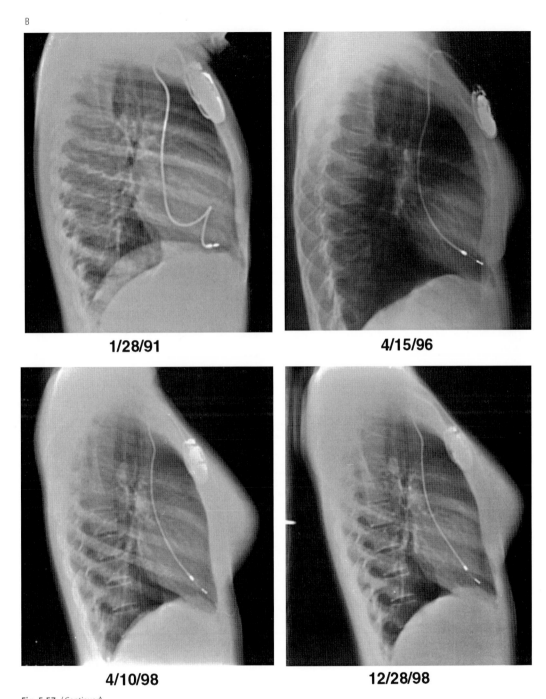

1/28/91

4/15/96

4/10/98

12/28/98

Fig. 5.57 (*Continued*)

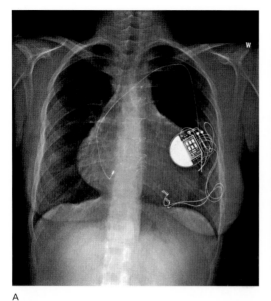
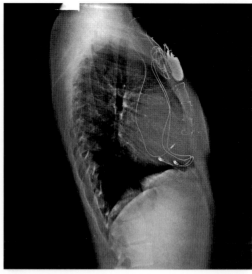

A   B

Fig. 5.58 Posteroanterior (A) and lateral (B) radiographs from a patient with a dual-chamber pacemaker. The ventricle is paced from the epicardial position, and the atrium is paced from the endocardial position. The atrial lead is then tunneled subcutaneously to the site of the pulse generator.

Finally, active fixation leads can be placed in a greater variety of positions than passive fixation leads. This advantage is important in the patient with associated congenital heart disease, because the anatomy may be quite distorted. An active fixation lead allows placement in all portions of the atrium, not the atrial appendage alone. Active fixation leads have been used in patients after the Mustard procedure, with the leads placed across the intra-atrial baffle and pacing in the left atrium.

A specific problem in pediatric pacing involves cardiac pacing after the Fontan procedure. Because the postoperative anatomy precludes transvenous endocardial ventricular pacing, dual-chamber pacing in these patients has been accomplished by placing a ventricular epicardial lead at the time of surgery and subsequently placing an atrial endocardial lead and tunneling the two leads to a common prepectoral position for attachment to a dual-chamber pacemaker (Fig. 5.58).

Device implantation after cardiac transplantation

There are special considerations for device implantation in the patient who has undergone cardiac transplantation. Although dependent on the surgical transplant technique used, often after cardiac transplantation, the donor atrium can no longer receive stimuli from the intrinsic or native (recipient) sinoatrial node. The sinoatrial node remains in continuity with the recipient atrium and may drive the recipient atrium at a normal rate or at a rate more rapid than normal. The suture line between the free wall of the donor atrium and the recipient atrium is a barrier to the passage of stimuli, which normally traverse the atrium to reach the AV node and bundle of His. After transplantation, the patient has two atrial rhythms, that of the donor atrium and that of the recipient atrium, both of which may be visible on the ECG.

Several approaches have been used for pacing in cardiac transplant recipients, some of which are quite complex. We have taken a conservative and simple approach. Because normal AV conduction usually exists between the donor atrium and ventricle, atrial pacing could be used both to preserve the AV sequence and to modulate the rate appropriately. Also, in many transplant recipients, sinus node dysfunction, a potential clinical problem for 1–6 months after transplantation, often resolves. Nevertheless, our approach has been to implant a standard dual-chamber pacemaker and to position the atrial lead in the donor atrium. Even if there is no clinical manifestation of AV conduction disease, we are more comfortable placing a dual-chamber pacemaker for the unlikely event of late AV block.[41,42]

Hospital stay after implantation

The length of time the patient should be kept in hospital after pulse generator implantation varies among institutions. Patients are told to fast after midnight the night prior to the device implantation or pulse generator replacement. They are instructed to take their chronic medications with as little water as possible the morning of the procedure.

No medications are routinely withheld prior to elective pulse generator implantation. If the patient is on aspirin and/or clopidogrel (Plavix) the medications are continued. However, the patient is told that there may be significant ecchymoses following the procedure and there may be a higher risk of hematoma formation. This approach is taken because the risk of aspirin alone is minimal and does not merit discontinuation of the drug and waiting the length of time necessary for platelet function to return to normal. If consideration were to be given to discontinuation of Plavix, the risk of stopping the drug would have to be considered.

We do not reverse warfarin prior to pulse generator implantation. We prefer that the International Normalized Ratio (INR) be ≤2.5. If the patient is chronically anticoagulated and generally has an INR of >2.5, we suggest that the Coumadin be held for 1–2 nights prior to implantation. An INR is rechecked the morning of the procedure to be certain that the INR is ≤2.5. Patients are allowed to resume Coumadin the evening of the implant procedure. We have not appreciated any increase in hematoma formation or bleeding complications with this protocol. Others have described a similar experience with implant procedures in the anticoagulated patient.[43,44] Conversely, unfractionated heparin or low-molecular-weight heparin are always discontinued prior to device implant and ideally avoided for a minimum of 24 h post-implantation.

We currently admit patients on the morning of the procedure and usually dismiss them the next morning. The patient is monitored during the overnight stay. If the patient is pacemaker-dependent, we keep the patient on bed rest overnight after implantation unless a different duration is ordered as an exception. A posteroanterior and lateral chest X-ray is obtained after the bed rest restriction is completed. Before dismissal, thresholds are documented and the pulse generator is programmed to its final settings. When the patient's pulse generator reaches battery depletion, the pulse generator is replaced as an outpatient procedure.

Many institutions perform initial device implantation as an outpatient procedure. Some physicians restrict outpatient implantation to nonpacemaker-dependent patients, whereas others perform outpatient procedures regardless of dependency status. Some third-party payers now insist that device implantation be accomplished as an outpatient procedure or that the hospital stay be <24 h. If the implantation is performed as an outpatient procedure, a mechanism should exist whereby the patient can be seen urgently by caregivers knowledgeable in device management should questions or problems arise.

Pulse generator replacement

Expected battery depletion is the most common cause of pulse generator replacement (Figs 5.59 and 5.60).[45]

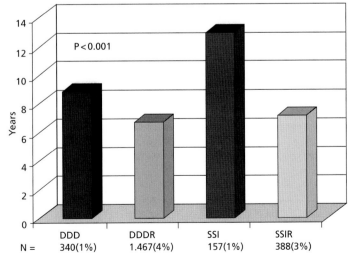

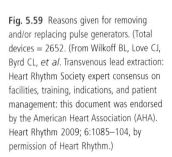

Fig. 5.59 Reasons given for removing and/or replacing pulse generators. (Total devices = 2652. (From Wilkoff BL, Love CJ, Byrd CL, *et al*. Transvenous lead extraction: Heart Rhythm Society expert consensus on facilities, training, indications, and patient management: this document was endorsed by the American Heart Association (AHA). Heart Rhythm 2009; 6:1085–104, by permission of Heart Rhythm.)

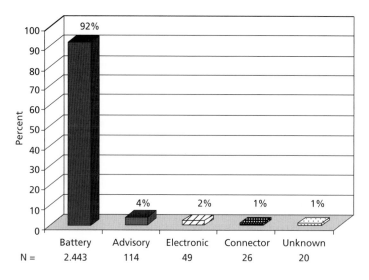

Fig. 5.60 Battery longevity for pulse generators with vs. those without the capability of rate adaptation. The percentages represent proportion of pulse generators that failed prematurely, defined by this registry as ≤3 years [47] (Reprinted from Heart Rhythm with permission.)

When it has been established that a pacemaker or defibrillator has reached elective replacement indicators (ERI), the patient should be notified and plans made to bring the patient in for pulse generator change. Usually, the implanted device will perform reliably for approximately 2–3 months following ERI, although the actual time is a function of the device model, pacing frequency, and other factors. In our practice, we electively replace devices within 2–4 weeks of ERI.

Having completed a focused history and physical examination, reviewed medications and checked basic preoperative laboratory work, i.e., potassium, sodium, creatinine, fasting glucose, complete blood count, the patient is told to fast after midnight the night prior to the procedure. The patient comes to the hospital early the following morning and every attempt is made to complete the pulse generator replacements as the initial cases so the patient may recover early and be dismissed from hospital in the afternoon.

The patient is taken to the implant suite and, if pacemaker-dependent, a temporary pacemaker is placed via the femoral vein. After infiltration with 1% lidocaine, the prior infraclavicular incision is reincised and dissection carried out to the level of the pacemaker, taking care to avoid the permanent leads. Parallel incisions (i.e., a new incision, parallel to the old one) are avoided becuase of compromise of the vascular supply between the new and old incisions; it is preferable to reincise the old scar. The device is explanted and disconnected from the chronic leads and thresholds checked via the pacing system analyzer. If the thresholds are acceptable (see later), the pocket is inspected for hemostasis, any bleeding areas cauterized, and the pocket is copiously irrigated with saline solution. The

new pulse generator is connected to the chronic leads and the leads are gently "tugged" to be certain they are securely in the connector block. The device is then placed in the pocket and we routinely recheck thresholds via the programmer. This assures the implanter that the leads are making good contact in the connector block and the appropriate lead has been placed in the appropriate port. The incision is then closed in our standard fashion.

What is considered acceptable for chronic thresholds will depend on the patient and associated comorbidities. We generally prefer chronic pacing threshold to be <2.0V and there be no significant change in measured intrinsic P or R wave or impedance from the initial implant. In the patient who is very elderly, in whom the longevity of the pulse generator is not a major consideration, or the patient in whom there are comorbidities or other issues that make the patient less likely to tolerate or unwilling to consider any risks inherent in lead replacement, higher chronic thresholds may be accepted.

Whether the pulse generator is being changed for battery depletion or on the basis of a recall or advisory, patients should be informed of the risks of this relatively minor procedure. This is especially important when the pulse generator is being replaced on the basis of an advisory or recall, because the risk of device failure may be lower than the risk of pulse generator change-out; the patients need this information to make an informed decision. Operation-associated complications requiring intervention were noted in 1.24% of our population.[46] Complications included five infections, three hematomas, and one incisional dehiscence. Although this complication rate is lower than that reported in a multicenter survey of pulse generator complications that were seen in 8.1% of patients,[47] generator replacement is not a benign procedure, and associated risks must be weighed in the context of other variables when this is considered on the basis of a recall or advisory.

Post-implant order set

We have established specific order sets that are used for patients following device implantation (Fig. 5.61). This approach not only ensures consistency in postoperative care and management, but also allows for greater efficiency and adds an extra safety measure. If any electronic order that is part of the order set in any way contradicts or significantly alters the standard order set, the RN entering the electronic order set must account for the discrepancy and when the doctor responsible for issuing and signing the orders completes the sign-off, they will again need to recognize and explain any discrepancies. If the patient has an allergy listed in the electronic record, and medications ordered as part of the order set, e.g., antibiotics, include a medication that has been listed as an allergy or has cross-reactivity to a noted medication allergy, the orders cannot be completed until the discrepancy is reconciled or explained.

As noted in Fig. 5.61, we routinely use antibiotics post device implantation. Although good sterile technique is the most important factor in avoiding an implant-related complication of infection and some controversy exists regarding post-implant antibiotic administration, we favor their use. Our antibiotic regimen is shown in Table 5.4.

Homegoing instructions

After implantation, the incision is covered with sterile gauze and tape or a "coverlet." This is generally removed the next morning, and if the incision is dry it is left uncovered. Patients are allowed to bathe 48 h after implantation, but instructed not to scrub the incisional site but to simply allow water to run over the site.

Postoperatively, we recommend that the patient avoid lifting the arm on the side of the pulse generator higher than shoulder level for the first 4 weeks after implantation. This restriction may be overcautious, but it serves to remind the patient to avoid aggressive activities while at the same time not significantly limiting arm or shoulder motion or activities of daily living. Use of a loose sling for the first 5–7 days may serve as a helpful reminder to limit arm and shoulder activities. Patients should be instructed not to overreact to this recommendation and completely restrict the movement of the ipsilateral shoulder. Movement should be encouraged, because immobility may cause pain later when full mobilization is attempted, with consequent further restriction of movement (frozen shoulder) or reflex sympathetic dystrophy. Movement of the shoulder should be encouraged on the first postoperative day. Early movement will not displace a well-placed and secure lead system.

For medicolegal reasons, we recommend that the patient not drive for 2 weeks after receiving a pacemaker or CRT implant. Return to driving after ICD implantation is a more complex issue and depends on the clinical history, rhythm disturbance requiring the ICD, and applicable state or country regulations. Briefly, when ICDs are implanted for prophylactic sudden death prevention, driving restrictions are similar to pacing restrictions. In the setting of syncope or ventricular tachyarrhythmias, patients are advised not to drive for 6 months. This is discussed in greater detail in Chapter 13: Follow-up.

An RN with expertise in patient education and implantable devices meets with the patient and available family members prior to discharge. The RN instructs the patient in post-implant care and assessment of the implant site, basic device function, post-implant restrictions, transtelephonic, and/or remote monitoring of the device, in-clinic follow-up schedule, how and when to contact caregivers in the event of concern related to the implantable device, and any other questions posed by the patient or family. The patient is also given an instructional CD regarding the device and device management and follow-up, as well as educational brochures related to implantable devices.

Lead extraction

Lead extraction is a necessity in some patients, primarily those with infected device systems, but the procedure is not without significant potential risks, including death, and should not be undertaken lightly or without a thorough understanding of the technique and possible difficulties.

Indications for lead extraction

Although some controversy exists about indications for lead extractions, the 2009 Heart Rhythm Society expert consensus on facilities, training, indications, and patient management for transvenous lead extraction provides the following guidelines.[48] CIED stands for cardiac implantable electronic device and the level of recommendation and evidence follows the American Heart Association classification.

Infection

Class I

- Complete device and lead removal is recommended in all patients with definite CIED system

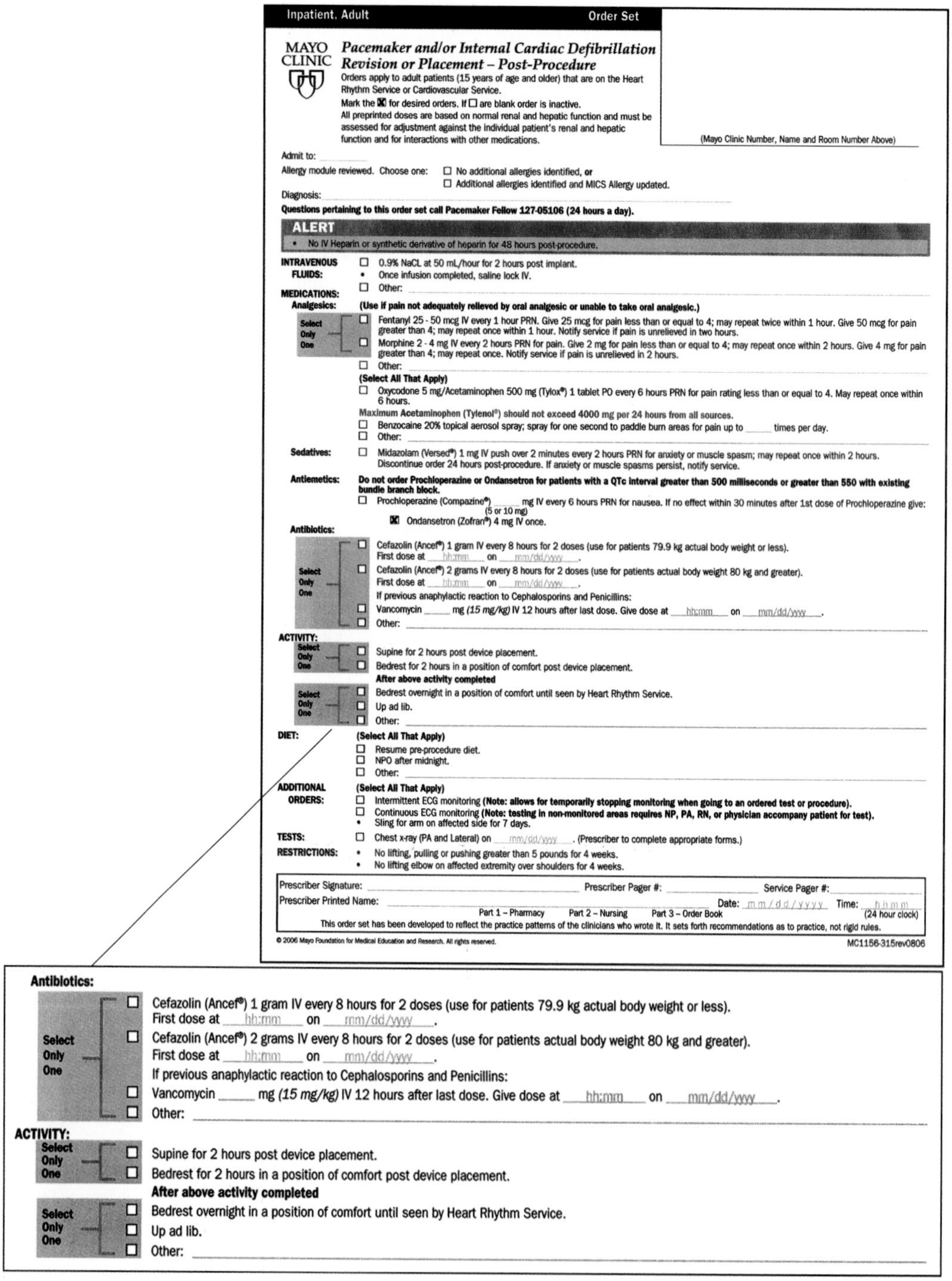

Inpatient. Adult	Order Set

MAYO CLINIC *Pacemaker and/or Internal Cardiac Defibrillation Revision or Placement – Post-Procedure*

Orders apply to adult patients (15 years of age and older) that are on the Heart Rhythm Service or Cardiovascular Service.

Mark the ☒ for desired orders. If ☐ are blank order is inactive.

All preprinted doses are based on normal renal and hepatic function and must be assessed for adjustment against the individual patient's renal and hepatic function and for interactions with other medications.

(Mayo Clinic Number, Name and Room Number Above)

Admit to: _____

Allergy module reviewed. Choose one: ☐ No additional allergies identified, **or**
☐ Additional allergies identified and MICS Allergy updated.

Diagnosis: _____

Questions pertaining to this order set call Pacemaker Fellow 127-05106 (24 hours a day).

ALERT
- No IV Heparin or synthetic derivative of heparin for 48 hours post-procedure.

INTRAVENOUS FLUIDS:
☐ 0.9% NaCL at 50 mL/hour for 2 hours post implant.
- Once infusion completed, saline lock IV.
☐ Other: _____

MEDICATIONS:
Analgesics: (Use if pain not adequately relieved by oral analgesic or unable to take oral analgesic.)

Select Only One
☐ Fentanyl 25 - 50 mcg IV every 1 hour PRN. Give 25 mcg for pain less than or equal to 4; may repeat twice within 1 hour. Give 50 mcg for pain greater than 4; may repeat once within 1 hour. Notify service if pain is unrelieved in two hours.
☐ Morphine 2 - 4 mg IV every 2 hours PRN for pain. Give 2 mg for pain less than or equal to 4; may repeat once within 2 hours. Give 4 mg for pain greater than 4; may repeat once. Notify service if pain is unrelieved in 2 hours.
☐ Other: _____

(Select All That Apply)
☐ Oxycodone 5 mg/Acetaminophen 500 mg (Tylox®) 1 tablet PO every 6 hours PRN for pain rating less than or equal to 4. May repeat once within 6 hours.
Maximum Acetaminophen (Tylenol®) should not exceed 4000 mg per 24 hours from all sources.
☐ Benzocaine 20% topical aerosol spray; spray for one second to paddle burn areas for pain up to ____ times per day.
☐ Other: _____

Sedatives:
☐ Midazolam (Versed®) 1 mg IV push over 2 minutes every 2 hours PRN for anxiety or muscle spasm; may repeat once within 2 hours. Discontinue order 24 hours post-procedure. If anxiety or muscle spasms persist, notify service.

Antiemetics: Do not order Prochlorperazine or Ondansetron for patients with a QTc interval greater than 500 milliseconds or greater than 550 with existing bundle branch block.
☐ Prochlorperazine (Compazine®) ____ mg IV every 6 hours PRN for nausea. If no effect within 30 minutes after 1st dose of Prochlorperazine give: (5 or 10 mg)
☒ Ondansetron (Zofran®) 4 mg IV once.

Antibiotics:
Select Only One
☐ Cefazolin (Ancef®) 1 gram IV every 8 hours for 2 doses (use for patients 79.9 kg actual body weight or less). First dose at ___hh:mm___ on ___mm/dd/yyyy___.
☐ Cefazolin (Ancef®) 2 grams IV every 8 hours for 2 doses (use for patients actual body weight 80 kg and greater). First dose at ___hh:mm___ on ___mm/dd/yyyy___.
If previous anaphylactic reaction to Cephalosporins and Penicillins:
☐ Vancomycin ____ mg (15 mg/kg) IV 12 hours after last dose. Give dose at ___hh:mm___ on ___mm/dd/yyyy___.
☐ Other: _____

ACTIVITY:
Select Only One
☐ Supine for 2 hours post device placement.
☐ Bedrest for 2 hours in a position of comfort post device placement.
After above activity completed
Select Only One
☐ Bedrest overnight in a position of comfort until seen by Heart Rhythm Service.
☐ Up ad lib.
☐ Other: _____

DIET: (Select All That Apply)
☐ Resume pre-procedure diet.
☐ NPO after midnight.
☐ Other: _____

ADDITIONAL ORDERS: (Select All That Apply)
☐ Intermittent ECG monitoring (Note: allows for temporarily stopping monitoring when going to an ordered test or procedure).
☐ Continuous ECG monitoring (Note: testing in non-monitored areas requires NP, PA, RN, or physician accompany patient for test).
- Sling for arm on affected side for 7 days.

TESTS: ☐ Chest x-ray (PA and Lateral) on ___mm/dd/yyyy___. (Prescriber to complete appropriate forms.)

RESTRICTIONS:
- No lifting, pulling or pushing greater than 5 pounds for 4 weeks.
- No lifting elbow on affected extremity over shoulders for 4 weeks.

Prescriber Signature: _____ Prescriber Pager #: _____ Service Pager #: _____
Prescriber Printed Name: _____ Date: __mm/dd/yyyy__ Time: __hh:mm__ (24 hour clock)
Part 1 – Pharmacy   Part 2 – Nursing   Part 3 – Order Book
This order set has been developed to reflect the practice patterns of the clinicians who wrote it. It sets forth recommendations as to practice, not rigid rules.

© 2006 Mayo Foundation for Medical Education and Research. All rights reserved. MC1156-315rev0806

Antibiotics:
Select Only One
☐ Cefazolin (Ancef®) 1 gram IV every 8 hours for 2 doses (use for patients 79.9 kg actual body weight or less). First dose at ___hh:mm___ on ___mm/dd/yyyy___.
☐ Cefazolin (Ancef®) 2 grams IV every 8 hours for 2 doses (use for patients actual body weight 80 kg and greater). First dose at ___hh:mm___ on ___mm/dd/yyyy___.
If previous anaphylactic reaction to Cephalosporins and Penicillins:
☐ Vancomycin ____ mg (15 mg/kg) IV 12 hours after last dose. Give dose at ___hh:mm___ on ___mm/dd/yyyy___.
☐ Other: _____

ACTIVITY:
Select Only One
☐ Supine for 2 hours post device placement.
☐ Bedrest for 2 hours in a position of comfort post device placement.
After above activity completed
Select Only One
☐ Bedrest overnight in a position of comfort until seen by Heart Rhythm Service.
☐ Up ad lib.
☐ Other: _____

Fig. 5.61 Order set used for patients post device implantation. The "inset" highlights a few of the specific orders included.

Table 5.4 Mayo Clinic Rochester antibiotic recommendations for implantable device procedure

- Cefazolin 1 g intravenously if <80 kg or 2 g if >80 kg, within 60 min before the initial incision and every 8 h for two doses in patients staying overnight (For pulse generator change only the initial dose is given)
- If penicillin or cephalosporin-sensitive, 20 mg/kg vancomycin intravenously within 2 h before the initial incision. If patient is staying overnight, 15 mg/kg once 12 h later. Dose is adjusted for renal insufficiency (For pulse generator change only the initial dose is given)
- For prolonged procedures, electrophysiologic or device, same prophylaxis as listed above and repeat cefazolin at 97 h after start of procedure and repeat vancomycin at 12 h.

infection, as evidenced by valvular endocarditis, lead endocarditis, or sepsis. (Level of evidence: B)
• Complete device and lead removal is recommended in all patients with CIED pocket infection as evidenced by pocket abscess, device erosion, skin adherence, or chronic draining sinus without clinically evident involvement of the transvenous portion of the lead system. (Level of evidence: B)
• Complete device and lead removal is recommended in all patients with valvular endocarditis without definite involvement of the lead(s) and/or device. (Level of evidence: B)
• Complete device and lead removal is recommended in patients with occult Gram-positive bacteremia (not contaminant). (Level of evidence: B)

Class IIa
• Complete device and lead removal is reasonable in patients with persistent occult Gram-negative bacteremia. (Level of evidence: B)

Class III
• CIED removal is not indicated for a superficial or incisional infection without involvement of the device and/or leads. (Level of evidence: C)
• CIED removal is not indicated to treat chronic bacteremia due to a source other than the CIED, when long-term suppressive antibiotics are required. (Level of evidence: C)

Chronic pain
Class IIa
• Device and/or lead removal is reasonable in patients with severe chronic pain, at the device or lead insertion site, that causes significant discomfort for the patient, is not manageable by medical or surgical techniques and for which there is no acceptable alternative. (Level of evidence: C)

Thrombosis or venous stenosis
Class I
• Lead removal is recommended in patients with clinically significant thromboembolic events associated with thrombus on a lead or a lead fragment. (Level of evidence: C)
• Lead removal is recommended in patients with bilateral subclavian vein or SVC occlusion precluding implantation of a needed transvenous lead. (Level of evidence: C)
• Lead removal is recommended in patients with planned stent deployment in a vein already containing a transvenous lead, to avoid entrapment of the lead. (Level of evidence: C)
• Lead removal is recommended in patients with SVC stenosis or occlusion with limiting symptoms. (Level of evidence: C)
• Lead removal is recommended in patients with ipsilateral venous occlusion preventing access to the venous circulation for required placement of an additional lead when there is a contraindication for using the contralateral side (e.g. contralateral AV fistula, shunt or vascular access port, mastectomy). (Level of evidence: C)

Class IIa
• Lead removal is reasonable in patients with ipsilateral venous occlusion preventing access to the venous circulation for required placement of an additional lead, when there is no contraindication for using the contralateral side. (Level of evidence C)

Functional leads
Class I
• Lead removal is recommended in patients with life-threatening arrhythmias secondary to retained leads. (Level of evidence: B)
• Lead removal is recommended in patients with leads that, due to their design or their failure, may pose an immediate threat to the patients if left in place (e.g. Telectronics ACCUFIX J wire fracture with protrusion). (Level of evidence: B)
• Lead removal is recommended in patients with leads that interfere with the operation of implanted cardiac devices. (Level of evidence: B)
• Lead removal is recommended in patients with leads that interfere with the treatment of a malignancy (radiation/reconstructive surgery). (Level of evidence: C)

Class IIb
• Lead removal may be considered in patients with an abandoned functional lead that poses a risk of interference with the operation of the active CIED system. (Level of evidence: C)

• Lead removal may be considered in patients with functioning leads that, due to their design or their failure, pose a potential future threat to the patient if left in place (e.g. Telectronics ACCUFIX without protrusion). (Level of evidence: C)

• Lead removal may be considered in patients with leads that are functional but not being used (i.e. RV pacing lead after upgrade to ICD). (Level of evidence: C)

• Lead removal may be considered in patients who require specific imaging techniques (e.g. magnetic resonance imaging [MRI]) that cannot be imaged due to the presence of the CIED system for which there is no other available imaging alternative for the diagnosis. (Level of evidence: C)

• Lead removal may be considered in patients in order to permit the implantation of an MRI conditional CIED system. (Level of evidence: C)

Class III

• Lead removal is not indicated in patients with functional but redundant leads if patients have a life expectancy of less than 1 year. (Level of evidence: C)

• Lead removal is not indicated in patients with known anomalous placement of leads through structures other than normal venous and cardiac structures (e.g., subclavian artery, aorta, pleura, atrial or ventricular wall, or mediastinum) or through a systemic venous atrium or systemic ventricle. Additional techniques including surgical backup may be used if the clinical scenario is compelling. (Level of evidence: C)

Nonfunctional leads

Class I

• Lead removal is recommended in patients with life-threatening arrhythmias secondary to retained leads or lead fragments. (Level of evidence: B)

• Lead removal is recommended in patients with leads that, due to their design or their failure, may pose an immediate threat to the patients if left in place (e.g. Telectronics ACCUFIX J wire fracture with protrusion). (Level of evidence: B)

• Lead removal is recommended in patients with leads that interfere with the operation of implanted cardiac devices. (Level of evidence: B)

• Lead removal is recommended in patients with leads that interfere with the treatment of a malignancy (radiation/reconstructive surgery). (Level of evidence: C)

Class IIa

• Lead removal is reasonable in patients with leads that, due to their design or their failure, pose a threat to the patient, that is not immediate or imminent if

left in place (e.g. Telectronics ACCUFIX without protrusion). (Level of evidence C)

• Lead removal is reasonable in patients if a CIED implantation would require more than four leads on one side or more than five leads through the SVC. (Level of evidence C)

• Lead removal is reasonable in patients who require specific imaging techniques (e.g. MRI) and cannot be imaged due to the presence of the CIED system for which there is no other available imaging alternative for the diagnosis. (Level of evidence C)

Class IIb

• Lead removal may be considered at the time of an indicated CIED procedure, in patients with nonfunctional leads, if contraindications are absent. (Level of evidence C)

• Lead removal may be considered in order to permit the implantation of an MRI conditional CIED system. (Level of evidence: C)

Class III

• Lead removal is not indicated in patients with nonfunctional leads if patients have a life expectancy of less than 1 year. (Level of evidence C)

• Lead removal is not indicated in patients with known anomalous placement of leads through structures other than normal venous and cardiac structures (e.g. subclavian artery, aorta, pleura, atrial or ventricular wall, or mediastinum) or through a systemic venous atrium or systemic ventricle. Additional techniques including surgical backup may be used if the clinical scenario is compelling. (Level of evidence: C)

Class I: procedure/treatment should be performed or administered.

Class IIa: it is reasonable to perform procedure/ administer treatment

Class IIb: procedure/treatment may be considered

Class III: procedure/treatment should not be administered because it is not helpful and may be harmful

Level of evidence A: data derived from multiple randomized trials or meta-analyses

Level of evidence B: data derived from a single randomized trial or nonrandomized study

Level of evidence C: only consensus opinion of experts, case studies or standard of care

If the lead can potentially harm the patient, extraction should be considered. Infection and mechanical complications of retained leads have been the obvious lead complications with the potential to harm the patient. Of the multiple lead advisories issued in the past decade, most have been for leads with unacceptably high pacing or sensing failure rates due to insulation problems. Although these failed leads may have required abandonment and implantation of a new lead, extraction of the defective lead has not usually been necessary.

The recall of the Accufix atrial J lead that occurred in the 1990s differed significantly, because simply abandoning the lead and placing a new atrial lead did not protect the patient.[49] This lead is largely of historical interest, but some centers, including ours, are still following patients with this problem lead. The Accufix lead incorporated a small wire to retain the J shape of the atrial lead. The wire has been shown to have the potential to fracture, and if the wire breaks and extrudes through the insulation, it can lacerate the aorta or perforate the atrial myocardium, injuries leading to fatal bleeding or cardiac tamponade.

The indications for lead extraction listed above are meant to be used as a guideline. Each patient's situation must be individualized, and the procedure and potential complications should be discussed in detail with the patient. The Heart Rhythm Society (HRS) policy statement lists the following clinical factors that should be taken into consideration:
• Patient's age
• Patient's sex (published complication rates are higher in women)
• Patient's overall health, both physical and mental
• Calcification involving the lead or leads
• Vegetations in the heart
• Number of leads in the intravascular space
• Length of time the lead or leads have been in place
• Fragility, condition, and physical characteristics of the lead
• Experience of the physician
• Patient's preference, i.e., extraction or not.

Facility requirements for lead extraction
Lead extraction should generally not be considered if the necessary equipment is not available, the patient is not a candidate for emergency thoracotomy should a complication require surgery, or there is known anomalous placement of the lead or leads through structures other than the normal venous and right-sided cardiac chambers (e.g., the leads are in an arterial position, left-sided cardiac chambers, pericardial space).

Who should perform extraction once the decision has been made to extract a lead? Less experienced operators have less successful outcomes, and the incidence of complications is higher and the procedure time is longer. There appears to be a significant improvement in success rate and decline in complications following the first 20 extraction procedures.[50,51] What qualifications are necessary for performance of lead extraction? Although guidelines are established for a minimum of 25 procedures for each of pacemakers, ICD, and CRT device implantation,[35] they are vague in referring to

appropriate training for lead extraction.[52] The HRS consensus statement recommends training in lead extraction procedures similar in number to those required for device implantation.[48] More rigorous guidelines for training requirements in lead extraction are needed. Ideally, lead extraction procedures require specialized training in a center that frequently performs extraction. If a trainee cannot learn such techniques during the training period and wants to perform the procedure at a later date, that experience should be sought with someone expert in extraction.

Outcomes of lead extraction

Defining success
The HRS consensus statement on lead extraction provides the following definitions for assessing and reporting outcomes in a uniform fashion.[48]

Complete procedural success: Removal of all targeted leads and all lead material from the vascular space, with the absence of any permanently disabling complication or procedure related death.

Clinical success: Removal of all targeted leads and lead material from the vascular space, or retention of a small portion of the lead that does not negatively impact the outcome goals of the procedure. This may be the tip of the lead or a small part of the lead (conductor coil, insulation, or the latter two combined) when the residual part does not increase the risk of perforation, embolic events, perpetuation of infection, or cause any undesired outcome. The clinical goals of the procedure will vary based on the indication for extraction. While retention of any device fragment will be a clinical failure in CIED infection, retention of a small portion such as the tip may still be a clinical success in nonfunctional leads.

Failure: Inability to achieve either complete procedural or clinical success, or the development of any permanently disabling complication or procedure related death.

Complications of lead extraction
The HRS consensus statement classifies potential complications into major and minor.[53]

Major complications
• Death
• Cardiac avulsion or tear requiring thoracotomy, pericardiocentesis, chest tube, or surgical repair
• Vascular avulsion or tear (requiring thoracotomy, pericardiocentesis, chest tube, or surgical repair)

• Pulmonary embolism requiring surgical intervention
• Respiratory arrest or anesthesia-related complication leading to prolongation of hospitalization
• Stroke
• Pacing system related infection of a previously non-infected site.

Minor complications

• Pericardial effusion not requiring pericardiocentesis or surgical intervention
• Hemothorax not requiring a chest tube
• Hematoma at the surgical site requiring reoperation for drainage
• Arm swelling or thrombosis of implant veins resulting in medical intervention
• Vascular repair near the implant site or venous entry site
• Hemodynamically significant air embolism
• Migrated lead fragment without sequelae
• Blood transfusion related to blood loss during surgery
• Pneumothorax requiring a chest tube
• Pulmonary embolism not requiring surgical intervention.

In various analyses success and complication rates have been correlated to: (i) time from implant; (ii) presence of infection; (iii) female gender; (iv) body mass index (BMI) <25 kg/m^2; and (v) institutional procedural volume.

The advent of powered sheaths for lead extraction has resulted in better success rates and similar rates of complications. The Pacemaker Lead Extraction with the Laser Sheath (PLEXES) study randomized patients to extraction using a laser sheath or a mechanical sheath.[54] The laser sheath was associated with a greater rate of complete lead removal (94 vs. 64%) and shorter extraction time (mean 10.1 vs. 12.9 minutes). Failed nonlaser extraction was completed with laser in 88%. Major complications occurred in 2% of the laser group (including one death and two major bleeds) compared with 0.9% in the nonlaser group. Subsequently, Byrd et al.[55] published the US experience with laser sheath extraction in a cohort of 1684 patients with 2561 leads. Complete and partial lead removal was achieved in 90% and 3%, respectively. A total of 1.9% experienced a major complication including tamponade, hemothorax, pulmonary embolism, lead migration, and death (0.8%). The LEXiCon study reported the contemporary experience with laser-assisted extraction achieving complete lead removal in 96.5%, major complications in 1.4%, and death in 0.28%.[53] Thus, the laser sheath has greatly improved success of lead extraction to >90% with an expected major complication rate of <2% and death rate of <1%. Similarly high rates of success have

been reported with the electrosurgical dissection sheath (93%)[56] and the Evolution sheath (Cook vascular) (86%).[57]

Extraction techniques

Several approaches to lead extraction have been described, including simple traction, locking stylet, and telescoping sheaths with countertraction, an inferior approach with various catheter techniques to snare the lead,[58] laser-lead extraction,[54] extraction with electrosurgical dissection sheaths,[56] and open surgical techniques. Although individual operators may have definite biases about technique,[54,58,59] it is important that the operator has a thorough understanding of the equipment and options at their disposal, allowing the approach to be defined by comfort level and expertise.

Before any attempt at extraction, the lead must be freed from underlying tissue in the pocket, and any sleeve around the lead securing it to underlying tissue must be released. A stylet should be placed in the lead before any traction is applied. Traction should be gentle. Fluoroscopic observation may indicate the extent of fibrosis holding the lead to the underlying vascular structures. Figure 5.62 shows how fibrous tissue surrounds the lead. Fibrosis may occur in specific areas such as the subclavian vein entry site, the SVC, tricuspid valve, and ventricular myocardium or along the entire course of the lead and between the leads. As traction is applied (Fig. 5.63), the ECG should be monitored for ectopy, and the patient's blood pressure should be observed for hypotension. Traction is often successful in leads less than 6 months old. With increasing length of implantation, there is a greater chance of fibrosis of the lead and hence complications with simple traction. In the presence of fibrosis there are three simultaneous thresholds at play during application of manual traction. The first is the strength of the adhesion and the force required to break it, the second is the tensile strength of the lead body, and the third is the tensile strength of the vessel or cardiac wall. The tensile strength of the fibrous tissue is often greater than that of the vessel or cardiac wall leading to shearing or avulsion with application of excess force. Similarly, in leads with low tensile strength, any sign of separation of the lead or insulation damage should prompt cessation of simple traction.

The helix in active fixation leads should be retracted when possible. However, a fractured lead will not transmit torque well and a stylet should be introduced before attempting further rotation to avoid closing the central lumen. In cases where the helix cannot be withdrawn, the entire lead can be rotated after releasing all fibrotic adhesions. Helix retraction may not be possible

A

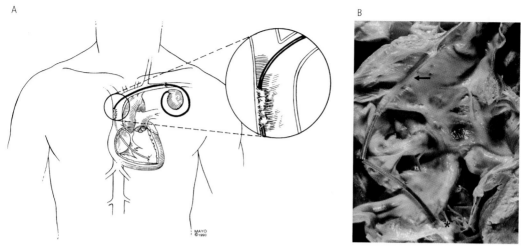

B

Fig. 5.62 (A) Drawing of a chronically implanted pacing lead. The enlarged inset depicts fibrosis that occurs around the lead where it abuts the superior vena cava. Fibrosis may be minimal or extend throughout the entire course of the lead. (From Spittell PC, Hayes DL. Venous complications after insertion of a transvenous pacemaker. Mayo Clinic Proc 1992; 67:258–65. Copyrighted and used with permission of Mayo Foundation for Medical Education and Research.) (B) Fibrosis of lead to the SVC (arrow) and perforation through the tricuspid valve (*).

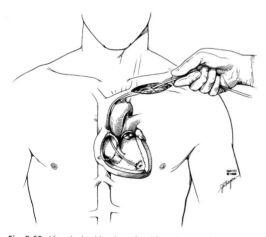

Fig. 5.63 After the lead has been freed from the underlying tissue, a stylet is placed in the lead and gentle traction is applied while the ECG and blood pressure are monitored. (Copyrighted and used with permission of Mayo Foundation for Medical Education and Research.)

in some leads despite these techniques. Removal of the lead without helix retraction is more of a concern in the atrium where the wall is significantly thinner.

If traction fails, our next approach is to transect the lead just beyond the connector pin in a nonisodiametric portion of the lead, trying to leave as much as possible with which to work. A locking stylet placed in the inner conduction coil is used to maintain lead integrity

and transmit traction forces to the lead tip. There are now several varieties of locking stylets (Fig. 5.64). Ideally, the locking stylet can be locked and unlocked if necessary. We also advocate tying a securing suture to the outer insulation and leading it back through the loop in the locking stylet, especially when running through a sheath where at the initial stages the lead may not be able to be grasped directly. This aids in placing tension along the whole lead rather than just on the inner or outer components. This is thought to reduce the chances of "snow-plowing" or tear of the insulation which can make the passage of sheaths difficult.

The next step is often the advancement of nonpowered telescoping sheaths over the lead which acts as a rail. Countertraction is applied to the sheath as traction is being applied to the lead to break adhesions at each binding site. Once the sheath has been passed to the tip of the lead, it is used to steady against the endocardium so that traction is confined to the lead tip. This reduces the chance of venous wall tears and cardiac avulsion. Adequate traction on the lead and coaxial alignment of the sheath over the lead should be maintained to maximize the removal of fibrotic adhesions and minimize trauma to vascular structures. Inadequate traction can result in the sheath passing outside the line created by the lead itself and laceration of cardiovascular structures.

If countertraction using nonpowered sheaths is unsuccessful, powered sheaths are used. Powered sheaths have tips that can cut through fibrous tissue,

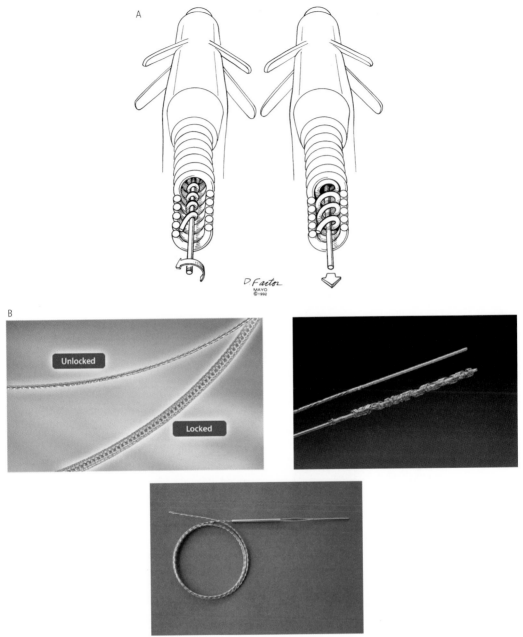

Fig. 5.64 (A) The locking stylet functions by a mechanism that results in the stylet being caught or entwined in the inner electrode coil. In the original Cook locking stylet, after the lead was sized and the appropriately sized locking stylet chosen, the stylet was advanced as far as possible, ideally the length of the lead, and counterclockwise turning of the stylet "locked" it into place (left panel). Traction could then be applied (right panel). (From Furman S. Troubleshooting. In: Furman S, Hayes DL, Holmes DR Jr, eds. A Practice of Cardiac Pacing, 3rd edn. Mount Kisco, NY: Futura Publishing Co., 1993:685–723, by permission of Mayo Foundation.) (B) Locking stylets and Bulldog lead extender. (B-A) Lead locking device Ez (LLD Ez) (Spectranectics) undeployed (above) and deployed (below). When deployed in the central lumen of the lead, the LLD Ez locks the lead throughout its length. Used with permission from Spectranectics. (B-B) Liberator locking stylet (Cook Medical) shown undeployed (above) and deployed (below). This stylet locks the lead at the tip. Used with permission from Cook Medical. (B-C) Bulldog lead extender (Cook Medical) can be used to stabilize leads that cannot take a locking stylet due to damage to the conductor lumen and lumenless leads. The lead is passed through the loop at the end and a metal sleeve passed over the lead to lock it. Used by permission of Cook Medical.

which significantly reduces the amount of traction and countertraction needed to extract the lead. This has resulted in greater success rate and fewer lead breakages. The commonly used powered sheaths are laser sheaths, electrosurgical dissection sheath, and the Evolution mechanical sheath (Cook Medical) (Fig. 5.65). The Excimer laser sheath (Spectranectics, Colorado Springs) has circumferential fiber-optic cables delivering pulses of wavelength 308 nm in the ultraviolet spectrum which leads to photoablation of fibrous adhesions by vaporization of water. The tissue penetration with the laser sheath is 50 μm. The electrosurgical dissection sheath uses radiofrequency energy from two tungsten electrodes at the tip of a Teflon sheath. Because the dissection plane from the radiofrequency energy is limited to a small arc along the radius of the sheath, catheter rotation may be required to free the lead circumferentially. Use of electrosurgical dissection sheaths has been associated with similar success rates to the

laser sheath. Both sheaths use an outer sheath for support, countertraction against the endocardium, and serves as a work station. Both the laser and electrosurgical dissection sheaths are not effective in separating some materials such as calcification, suture material, sleeves, and bunching of insulation material. In the event that failure to progress occurs it is essential to re-evaluate the area visually. If bunching of insulation or "snow-plowing" is thought to be the issue, upsizing to a larger French sheath is often helpful. The Evolution sheath has a handle-trigger driven, stainless steel treaded barrel rotational tip at the end of a flexible sheath designed to drill through fibrosis, calcification, sleeve, and suture material.

Approach to extraction

The majority of leads are extracted through the vein through which the lead was implanted. Lead extraction using multiple venous access sites such as the internal

A
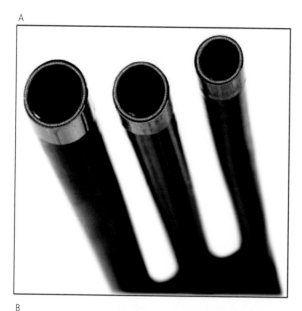

B
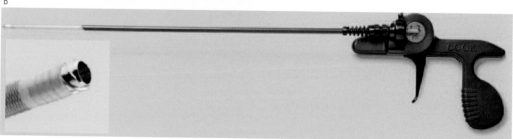

Fig. 5.65 Powered extraction sheaths (A) The Excimer Laser Sheath (Spectranectics) showing circumferential arrangement of the fiberoptic fibers at the tip. Used with permission from Spectranectics. (B) Evolution lead extraction system (Cook Medical). Used by permission of Cook Medical.

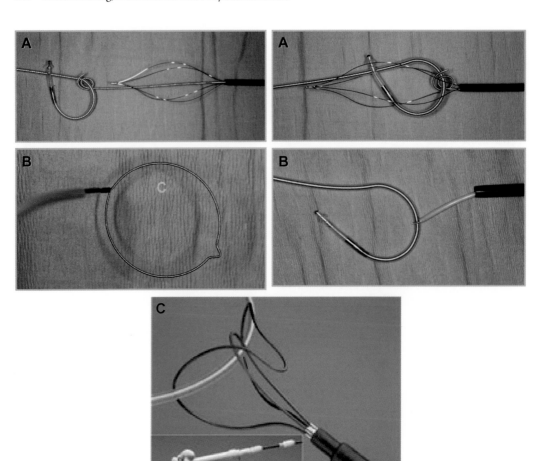

Fig. 5.66 Snares used for femoral lead extraction. (A) Lead deflecting wire and Dotter basket; (B) Loop snare; and (C) Needle's eye snare (Cook Medical). Used by permission of Cook Medical.

jugular vein and vein of implantation have also been described.[60]

Lead extraction through the femoral vein is commonly performed as a rescue procedure when the lead is inaccessible from the vein of implantation, for disrupted leads with free floating ends, and for leads that cannot be freed from the endocardium. This approach can also be used when there is excessive venous scar or due to operator preference. Because traction is applied from an inferior approach, the femoral approach is thought to have lower propensity for perforation, venous tear, and cardiac avulsion. There are a number of tools currently available for femoral lead extraction including the Byrd Femoral Work Station (BFWS) (Cook Medical). Equipment that

is often used include long sheaths that act as a workstation, tip deflecting wire, Dotter retriever snare, needle eye's snare, loop snare, Amplatz goose neck snare, and pigtail catheter (Fig. 5.66).

The basic approach varies based on whether the lead tip has been freed or not (Fig. 5.67). If the lead tip has been freed, the femoral venous sheath is positioned in the right atrium. The lead is amputated proximally at the venous entry site. The free end is snared in the right atrium or in the inferior vena cava after pulling the lead into the inferior vena cava. It can then be removed by traction. If the lead tip is still attached to the endocardium, the femoral venous sheath is positioned in the right atrium and a loop of the lead is snared and brought into the sheath. The proximal end is ampu-

A

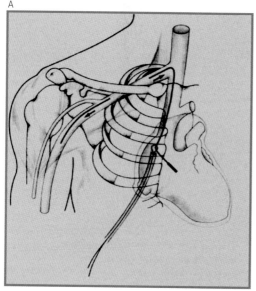

B

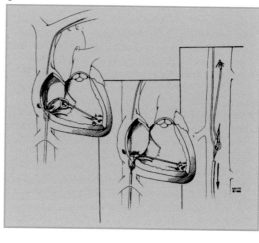

Fig. 5.67 Femoral venous lead extraction when (A) the lead tip has been freed; (B) when the lead tip is adherent to the endocardium.

tated and the lead tip freed with traction and counter-traction. Both techniques involve some form of snaring device. It is important to ensure that when the lead is snared, the process is reversible. If the lead is grabbed but cannot be reversed, thoracotomy may be required to remove the lead and the extraction device.

Surgical extraction by thoracotomy is currently reserved for larger vegetations or for cases where surgical intervention is required for other reasons. Although most leads can be extracted by a percutaneous technique, some cannot, and thoracotomy or some other limited surgical approach may be the best option for the patient.[61] Surgical extraction should also be considered for extraction of epicardial leads and unusual implants such as azygous leads.

If lead revision or reimplantation is planned following extraction, and the vein of implantation is found to be occluded, the operator has one of several options: (i) venoplasty of the vein of implantation; (ii) implantation of the new lead on the opposite side with or without tunneling of the lead; (iii) alternate venous access such as the iliac vein; and (iv) maintenance of venous access by passing a guidewire through the laser sheath used for extraction.

At times, a combination of techniques is required to effect complete lead extraction. For example, laser extraction is required for the subclavian and SVC portion of an adherent pacing or ICD lead. However, if the lead continues to be adherent within the ventricle

itself, particularly at the tip, simple traction may continue to be effective, and it is generally inadvisable to continue to lase into the ventricular myocardium. At this point, a femoral route can be used to snare the heel of the lead and apply traction from this femoral route. Any stylets that were placed in the lead from above are removed and the leads cut in the infraclavicular pocket. With continued traction, the lead can often be removed in its entirety via the femoral vein. Another example of combined approaches is the application of radiofrequency energy through a standard ablation catheter for portions of retained lead fragments or intramyocardial adherent portions of the lead where laser is inaccessible. The lead now free can be snared and then removed via the femoral route.

The most recent challenge in lead extraction is the increasing requirement for experience in extraction of CS leads. Although clinical experience remains limited regarding extraction of chronically implanted leads in the coronary venous system, multiple techniques have been employed.[62] Extraction techniques will continue to evolve and improve. For now and the foreseeable future, this procedure must be approached with great respect by personnel committed to developing expertise.

References

1 Hayes D, Holmes DJ, Furman S. Permanent pacemaker implantation. In Furman S, Hayes D, Holmes DJ, eds. A

Practice of Cardiac Pacing. Mount Kisco, NY: Future Publishing Co., 1993: 261–307.

2 Bubien RS, Fisher JD, Gentzel JA, et al. NASPE expert consensus document: use of i.v. (conscious) sedation/analgesia by nonanesthesia personnel in patients undergoing arrhythmia specific diagnostic, therapeutic, and surgical procedures. Pacing Clin Electrophysiol 1998; 21:375–85.

3 Byrd CL. Clinical experience with the extrathoracic introducer insertion technique. Pacing Clin Electrophysiol 1993; 16:1781–4.

4 Burri H, Sunthorn H, Dorsaz PA, Shah D. Prospective study of axillary vein puncture with or without contrast venography for pacemaker and defibrillator lead implantation. Pacing Clin Electrophysiol 2005; 28(Suppl 1):280–3.

5 Calkins H, Ramza BM, Brinker J, et al. Prospective randomized comparison of the safety and effectiveness of placement of endocardial pacemaker and defibrillator leads using the extrathoracic subclavian vein guided by contrast venography versus the cephalic approach. Pacing Clin Electrophysiol 2001; 24:456–64.

6 Ramza BM, Rosenthal L, Hui R, et al. Safety and effectiveness of placement of pacemaker and defibrillator leads in the axillary vein guided by contrast venography. Am J Cardiol 1997; 80:892–6.

7 Chan NY, Liem LB, Mok NS, Wong W. Clinical experience of contrast venography guided axillary vein puncture in biventricular pacing R1. Int J Cardiol 2003; 92:55–8.

8 Higano ST, Hayes DL, Spittell PC. Facilitation of the subclavian-introducer technique with contrast venography. Pacing Clin Electrophysiol 1990; 13:681–4.

9 Magney JE, Staplin DH, Flynn DM, Hunter DW. A new approach to percutaneous subclavian venipuncture to avoid lead fracture or central venous catheter occlusion. Pacing Clin Electrophysiol 1993; 16:2133–42.

10 Furman S. Venous cutdown for pacemaker implantation. Ann Thorac Surg 1986; 41:438–9.

11 Ching CK, Elayi CS, Di Biase L, et al. Transiliac ICD implantation: defibrillation vector flexibility produces consistent success. Heart Rhythm 2009; 6:978–83.

12 Erdogan O, Augostini R, Saliba W, Juratli N, Wilkoff BL. Transiliac permanent pacemaker implantation after extraction of infected pectoral pacemaker systems. Am J Cardiol 1999; 84:474–5.

13 Ellestad MH, French J. Iliac vein approach to permanent pacemaker implantation. Pacing Clin Electrophysiol 1989; 12:1030–3.

14 Garcia Guerrero JJ, De La Concha Castaneda JF, Fernandez Mora G, et al. Permanent transfemoral pacemaker: a single-center series performed with an easier and safer surgical technique. Pacing Clin Electrophysiol 2005; 28:675–9.

15 Giudici MC, Karpawich PP. Alternative site pacing: it's time to define terms. Pacing Clin Electrophysiol 1999; 22:551–3.

16 Vlay SC. Right ventricular outflow tract pacing: practical and beneficial: a 9-year experience of 460 consecutive implants. Pacing Clin Electrophysiol 2006; 29:1055–62.

17 Bardy GH, Lee KL, Mark DB, et al. Amiodarone or an implantable cardioverter-defibrillator for congestive heart failure. N Engl J Med 2005; 352:225–37.

18 Kroll MW, Efimov IR, Tchou PJ. Present understanding of shock polarity for internal defibrillation: the obvious and non-obvious clinical implications. Pacing Clin Electrophysiol 2006; 29:885–91.

19 Denman RA, Umesan C, Martin PT, et al. Benefit of millisecond waveform durations for patients with high defibrillation thresholds. Heart Rhythm 2006; 3:536–41.

20 Kuhlkamp V, Dornberger V, Khalighi K, et al. Effect of a single element subcutaneous array electrode added to a transvenous electrode configuration on the defibrillation field and the defibrillation threshold. Pacing Clin Electrophysiol 1998; 21:2596–605.

21 Cooper JA, Latacha MP, Soto GE, et al. The azygos defibrillator lead for elevated defibrillation thresholds: implant technique, lead stability, and patient series. Pacing Clin Electrophysiol 2008; 31:1405–10.

22 Faheem O, Padala A, Kluger J, Zweibel S, Clyne CA. Coronary sinus shocking lead as salvage in patients with advanced CHF and high defibrillation thresholds. Pacing Clin Electrophysiol 2010; 33:967–72.

23 Gerber TC, Kantor B, Keelan PC, Hayes DL, Schwartz RS, Holmes DR. The coronary venous system: an alternate portal to the myocardium for diagnostic and therapeutic procedures in invasive cardiology. Curr Interv Cardiol Rep 2000; 2:27–37.

24 Giudici M, Winston S, Kappler J, et al. Mapping the coronary sinus and great cardiac vein. Pacing Clin Electrophysiol 2002; 25:414–9.

25 Ortale JR, Gabriel EA, Iost C, Marquez CQ. The anatomy of the coronary sinus and its tributaries. Surg Radiol Anat 2001; 23:15–21.

26 Hayes DL, Wang P, Sackner-Bernstein J, Asirvatham S. Resynchronization and Defibrillation for Heart Failure: A Practical Approach. Oxford: Blackwell Publishing, 2004.

27 Yu C, Hayes DL, Auricchio A. Cardiac Resynchronization Therapy. Oxford: Blackwell Publishing, 2006.

28 Alonso C, Leclercq C, d'Allonnes FR, et al. Six year experience of transvenous left ventricular lead implantation for permanent biventricular pacing in patients with advanced heart failure: technical aspects. Heart 2001; 86:405–10.

29 Walker S, Levy T, Paul VE. Dissection of the coronary sinus secondary to pacemaker lead manipulation. Pacing Clin Electrophysiol 2000; 23:541–3.

30 Auricchio A, Stellbrink C, Sack S, et al. The Pacing Therapies for Congestive Heart Failure (PATH-CHF) study: rationale, design, and endpoints of a prospective randomized multicenter study. Am J Cardiol 1999; 83: 130D–5D.

31 Delfaut P, Saksena S, Prakash A, Krol RB. Long-term outcome of patients with drug-refractory atrial flutter and fibrillation after single- and dual-site right atrial pacing for arrhythmia prevention. J Am Coll Cardiol 1998; 32: 1900–8.

32 Padeletti L, Michelucci A, Pieragnoli P, Colella A, Musilli N. Atrial septal pacing: a new approach to prevent atrial fibrillation. Pacing Clin Electrophysiol 2004; 27:850–4.

33 Spencer WH 3rd, Zhu DW, Markowitz T, Badruddin SM, Zoghbi WA. Atrial septal pacing: a method for pacing both

atria simultaneously. Pacing Clin Electrophysiol 1997; 20:2739–45.

34 Bailin SJ: Is Bachmann's Bundle the only right site for single-site pacing to prevent atrial fibrillation? Results of a multicenter randomized trial. Card Electrophysiol Rev 2003; 7:325–8.

35 Cardiac defibrillators: connector assembly or implantable defibrillators-dimensional and test requirements. ISO 11318:1993/Amd. 1:1996(E).

36 Furman S. Sensing and timing the cardiac electrogram. In Furman S, Hayes DL, Holmes DR, eds. A Practice of Cardiac Pacing. Mount Kisco, NY: Futura Publishing Co., 1993; 89–133.

37 Ector B, Willems R, Heidbuchel H, et al. Epicardial pacing: a single-centre study on 321 leads in 138 patients. Acta Cardiol 2006; 61:343–51.

38 Hayes DL, Holmes DR Jr, Maloney JD, Neubauer SA, Ritter DG, Danielson GK. Permanent endocardial pacing in pediatric patients. J Thorac Cardiovasc Surg 1983; 85:618–24.

39 Silvetti MS, Drago F, Grutter G, De Santis A, Di Ciommo V, Rava L. Twenty years of paediatric cardiac pacing: 515 pacemakers and 480 leads implanted in 292 patients. Europace 2006; 8:530–6.

40 Tomaske M, Harpes P, Pretre R, Dodge-Khatami A, Bauersfeld U. Long-term experience with AutoCapture-controlled epicardial pacing in children. Europace 2007; 9:645–50.

41 Meyer SR, Modry DL, Bainey K, et al. Declining need for permanent pacemaker insertion with the bicaval technique of orthotopic heart transplantation. Can J Cardiol 2005; 21:159–63.

42 Zieroth S, Ross H, Rao V, et al. Permanent pacing after cardiac transplantation in the era of extended donors. J Heart Lung Transplant 2006; 25:1142–7.

43 al-Khadra AS. Implantation of pacemakers and implantable cardioverter defibrillators in orally anticoagulated patients. Pacing Clin Electrophysiol 2003; 26:511–4.

44 Giudici MC, Paul DL, Bontu P, Barold SS. Pacemaker and implantable cardioverter defibrillator implantation without reversal of warfarin therapy. Pacing Clin Electrophysiol 2004; 27:358–60.

45 Hauser RG, Hayes DL, Kallinen LM, et al. Clinical experience with pacemaker pulse generators and transvenous leads: an 8-year prospective multicenter study. Heart Rhythm 2007; 4:154–60.

46 Kapa S, Hyberger L, Rea RF, Hayes DL. Complication risk with pulse generator change: implications when reacting to a device advisory or recall. Pacing Clin Electrophysiol 2007; 30:730–3.

47 Gould PA, Krahn AD. Complications associated with implantable cardioverter-defibrillator replacement in response to device advisories. Jama 2006; 295:1907–11.

48 Wilkoff BL, Love CJ, Byrd CL, et al. Transvenous lead extraction: Heart Rhythm Society expert consensus on facilities, training, indications, and patient management: this document was endorsed by the American Heart Association (AHA). Heart Rhythm 2009; 6:1085–104.

49 Smith HJ, Fearnot NE, Byrd CL, Wilkoff BL, Love CJ, Sellers TD. Five-years experience with intravascular lead extraction. US Lead Extraction Database. Pacing Clin Electrophysiol 1994; 17:2016–20.

50 Bracke FA, Meijer A, Van Gelder B. Learning curve characteristics of pacing lead extraction with a laser sheath. Pacing Clin Electrophysiol 1998; 21:2309–13.

51 Byrd CL, Wilkoff BL, Love CJ, et al. Intravascular extraction of problematic or infected permanent pacemaker leads: 1994–1996. US Extraction Database, MED Institute. Pacing Clin Electrophysiol 1999; 22:1348–57.

52 Naccarelli GV, Conti JB, DiMarco JP, Tracy CM. Task force 6: training in specialized electrophysiology, cardiac pacing, and arrhythmia management endorsed by the Heart Rhythm Society. J Am Coll Cardiol 2008; 51:374–80.

53 Wazni O, Epstein LM, Carrillo RG, et al. Lead extraction in the contemporary setting: the LExICon study: an observational retrospective study of consecutive laser lead extractions. J Am Coll Cardiol 2010; 55:579–86.

54 Wilkoff BL, Byrd CL, Love CJ, et al. Pacemaker lead extraction with the laser sheath: results of the pacing lead extraction with the excimer sheath (PLEXES) trial. J Am Coll Cardiol 1999; 33:1671–6.

55 Byrd CL, Wilkoff BL, Love CJ, Sellers TD, Reiser C. Clinical study of the laser sheath for lead extraction: the total experience in the United States. Pacing Clin Electrophysiol 2002; 25:804–8.

56 Neuzil P, Taborsky M, Rezek Z, et al. Pacemaker and ICD lead extraction with electrosurgical dissection sheaths and standard transvenous extraction systems: results of a randomized trial. Europace 2007; 9:98–104.

57 Hussein AA, Wilkoff BL, Martin DO, et al. Initial experience with the Evolution mechanical dilator sheath for lead extraction: safety and efficacy. Heart Rhythm 2010; 7: 870–3.

58 Espinosa RE, Hayes DL, Vlietstra RE, Osborn MJ, McGoon MD. The Dotter retriever and pigtail catheter: efficacy in extraction of chronic transvenous pacemaker leads. Pacing Clin Electrophysiol 1993; 16:2337–42.

59 Love CJ. Current concepts in extraction of transvenous pacing and ICD leads. Cardiol Clin 2000; 18:193–217.

60 Bongiorni MG, Soldati E, Zucchelli G, et al. Transvenous removal of pacing and implantable cardiac defibrillating leads using single sheath mechanical dilatation and multiple venous approaches: high success rate and safety in more than 2000 leads. Eur Heart J 2008; 29:2886–93.

61 Vogt PR, Sagdic K, Lachat M, Candinas R, von Segesser LK, Turina MI. Surgical management of infected permanent transvenous pacemaker systems: ten year experience. J Card Surg 1996; 11:180–6.

62 Burke MC, Morton J, Lin AC, et al. Implications and outcome of permanent coronary sinus lead extraction and reimplantation. J Cardiovasc Electrophysiol 2005; 16: 830–7.

6 Implant-Related Complications: Relevant Anatomy and an Approach for Prevention

Seth H. Sheldon, David L. Hayes, Paul A. Friedman, Samuel J. Asirvatham

Mayo Clinic, Rochester, MN, USA

Complications related directly to the implant procedure 220
Lead dislodgement 220
Pneumothorax 223
Lead perforation 225
Pericarditis 228
Arrhythmias 228
Pulse generator pocket complications 229
Pain 230
Inadvertent left ventricular lead placement 232
Thrombosis 232
Loose connector block connection 234
Lead damage 234
Infection 235
Abandoned and nonfunctioning, noninfected leads 238
Twiddler's syndrome 240

New symptoms secondary to pacemaker placement 245
Extracardiac stimulation 245
Pacemaker syndrome 245
Tricuspid regurgitation 245
Battery depletion 246
Implant or hardware-related complications that may result in recurrence of preimplantation symptoms 246
Loss of circuit integrity 246
Lead fracture and insulation defect 248
Exit block 248
References 252

Cardiac Pacing, Defibrillation and Resynchronization: A Clinical Approach, Third Edition.
David L. Hayes, Samuel J. Asirvatham, and Paul A. Friedman.
© 2013 Mayo Foundation for Medical Education and Research. Published 2013 by John Wiley & Sons, Ltd.

Although pulse generator implantation is usually straightforward and free of adverse events, there are multiple potential complications that can occur. Prior to device implant, not only should the procedure be explained in detail to the patient, but potential complications should be discussed and that discussion documented in the permanent medical record. Our practice is to routinely discuss the complications that are the most common or that carry the greatest threat to the patient. This includes lead dislodgement, pocket bleeding, pneumothorax, infection, and cardiac perforation with tamponade. With implantable cardioverter-defibrillator (ICD) implantation we also discuss complications associated with defibrillation threshold (DFT) testing, as well as the potential need for additional hardware in order to achieve an adequate DFT. If a cardiac resynchronization therapy (CRT) system is being implanted, additional time should be spent discussing problems that can arise with placement of the coronary sinus (CS) lead.

Complications related directly to the implant procedure

Complications of lead placement result from cannulation of the vein, catheterization of the heart, and from placement of a permanent lead.

Lead dislodgement

Historically, the most common complication of transvenous pacing has been lead dislodgement. Improved fixation mechanisms have substantially reduced the frequency of this complication for both atrial and ventricular pacing leads. Secondary intervention rates for all reasons should be <2% for ventricular leads and <3% for atrial leads. Some experienced implanters would argue that dislodgement rates should be even lower, e.g., 1% for right ventricular (RV) leads and 2% for atrial leads. In the Pacemaker Selection in the Elderly (PASE) trial, lead dislodgement was the most common complication, occurring in 9 of the 407 patients, or 2.2%.[1] In the REPLACE registry of patients undergoing pacemaker or ICD generator replacements, lead dislodgement was the most common major complication with a 6-month incidence of 1.0% in patients undergoing generator replacement alone vs. 7.9% in patients undergoing generator replacement and lead implantation (the majority of patients had an upgrade to a CRT device).[2] Procedures involving placement of additional leads (upgrade) may be complex as a result of obstructed veins or thrombosis, and extensive manipulation may result in either dislodgement of the previously existing lead or lead damage. These data

suggests that lead dislodgement rates for CS leads may be even higher. Slightly higher dislodgement rates may also be tolerable in pediatric patients, whose activity is more difficult to control, and in patients with unusual anatomy, such as congenital cardiac anomalies.

Dislodgement is often classified as "macrodislodgement" or "microdislodgement." Macrodislodgement is radiographically evident, but microdislodgement is not (Fig. 6.1). Adequate lead position is assessed by posteroanterior and lateral chest radiographs (see Chapter 11: Radiography of Implantable Devices). Lead placement by chest radiography may appear excellent in the patient with microdislodgement, but the tip has moved sufficiently to impair myocardial contact and function. Due to beat-to-beat variability in cardiac and lead position, only gross lead movement is identified as macrodislodgement.

The atrial lead dislodgement rate has traditionally been higher than the ventricular dislodgement rate (Fig. 6.2). The optimal atrial lead design remains uncertain. A retrospective study found the lowest rate of lead dislodgement with straight "J-post shaped" active fixation atrial leads compared with active and passive fixation J-shaped leads.[3] A prospective study, contrastingly, found that straight leads, as compared with preformed J leads, are more likely to dislodge but less likely to malfunction.[4] In another prospective comparison of atrial passive and active fixation J-shaped leads, both performed well. Passive fixation leads, however, required less fluoroscopy at implantation, had better thresholds, and had a considerably lower rate of pericardial irritation or effusion.[5] As newer, smaller leads become available, performance characteristics will further evolve. Atrial lead dislodgement may be related more to implanter experience than the fixation mechanism or shape. The geometry and pathology of the atrium may also dictate atrial lead type. In general, preformed atrial leads may be difficult to use when a large atrium or surgical scarring requires shaping the lead (stylet) to access a particular location. In unusual circumstances, a lead delivery system similar to those used for cardiac resynchronization may be necessary to place a nonpreformed lead.

The dislodgement rate of CS leads tends to be higher for several reasons. In addition to microdislodgement and macrodislodgement giving rise to inadequate thresholds being made more likely with the complex venous system, even with adequate thresholds, phrenic nerve stimulation or inadequate resynchronization may occur as a result of lead dislodgement. A novel active fixation CS lead has a low dislodgement rate, although it may potentially be more difficult to extract.[6] Patients scheduled to receive a CS lead should be counseled regarding the importance of checking for

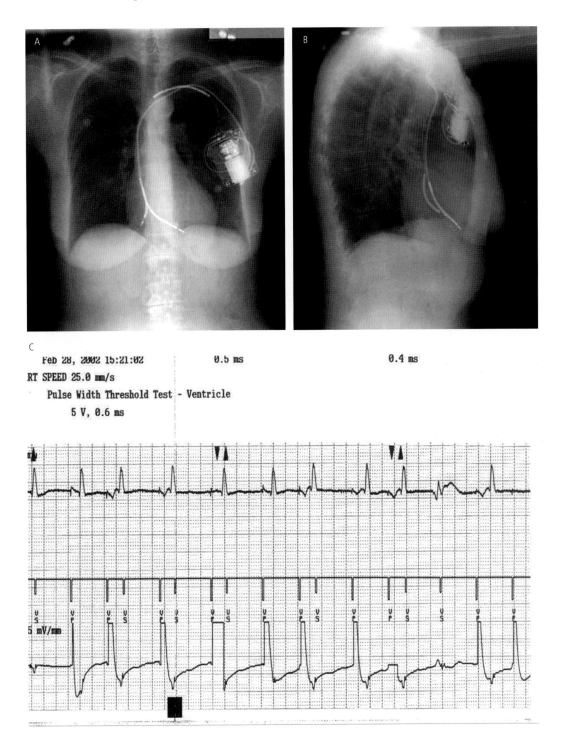

Fig. 6.1 Posteroanterior (A) and lateral (B) chest radiographs on the day after implantable cardioverter-defibrillator (ICD) implantation. The fluoroscopic image at the end of the implant had demonstrated a right ventricular apical position and adequate "J" on the atrial lead. However, on the X-ray shown, both atrial and ventricular lead positioning is suboptimal due to gross dislodgment. It appears that neither was adequately secured and have pulled back to a more shallow position. (C) The tracing was obtained when the ICD was programmed to the VVI pacing mode. Note complete failure to capture.

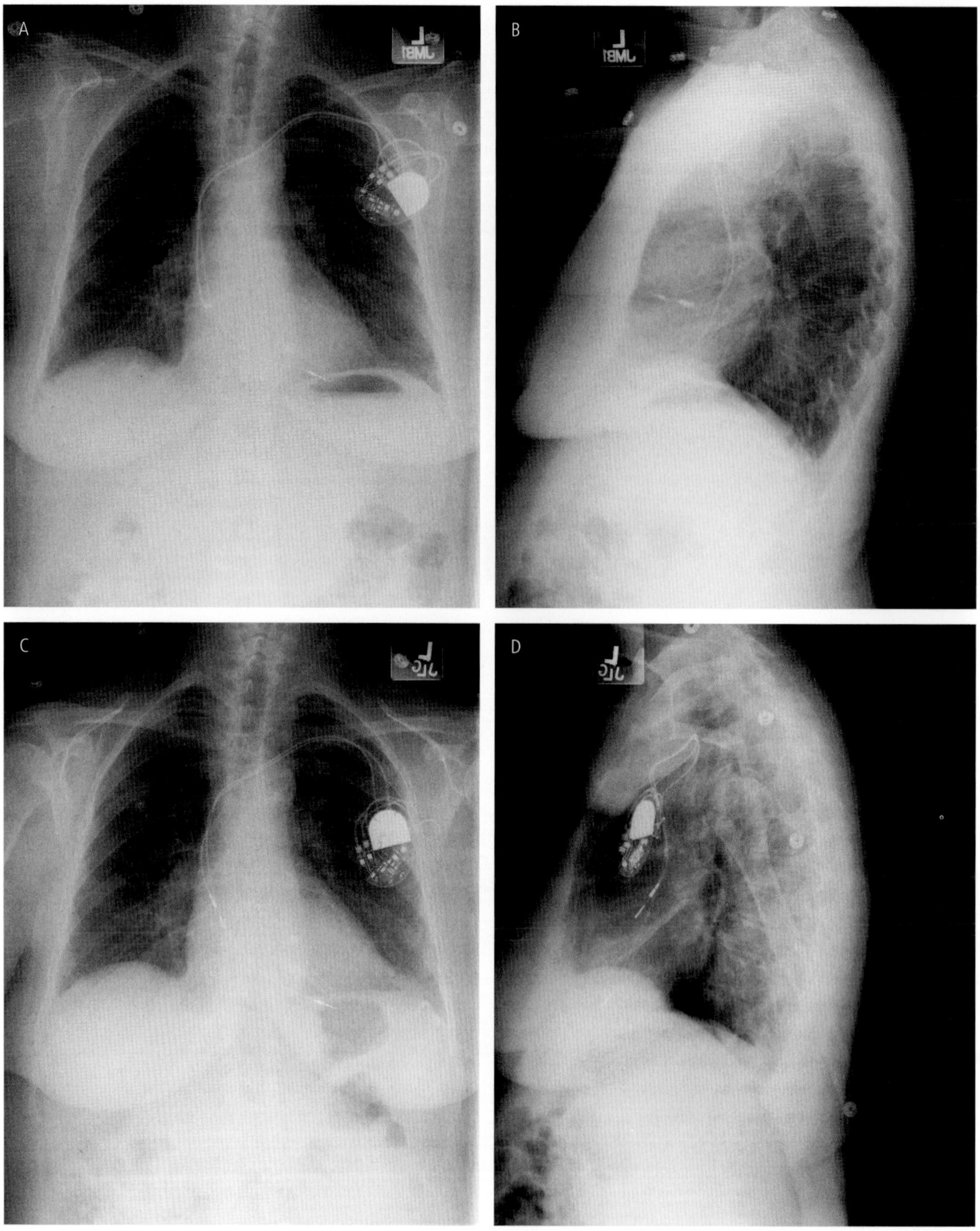

Fig. 6.2 (A) Posteroanterior (PA) and (B) lateral radiographs on the morning after implantation of a dual-chamber pacemaker. The active-fixation atrial lead appears to be somewhat shallow on the PA film but reasonable "J" configuration of the lead is noted on the lateral film. Atrial thresholds were excellent. (C) PA and (D) lateral radiographs obtained a few days later when the patient presented with vague fatigue. The atrial lead has clearly dislodged, being most evident on the lateral view.

adequate resynchronization (EKG, echo) in addition to the need for DFT testing, if applicable. Furthermore, they should be informed of a higher necessity for lead revision.

Complications of CS lead placement, including dislodgement, from MUSTIC, CONTAK-CD, and MIRACLE-ICD trials, have been summarized in an Expert Consensus Statement: Resynchronization Therapy for Heart Failure from the Heart Rhythm Society.[7] A table from that consensus statement summarizing CS lead implantation success rates, implant problems, complications, and thresholds is shown in Table 6.1.

Pneumothorax

Complications of venous entry, inherent in any approach to venous structures, include damage to associated arterial or neural structures, extensive bleeding, air embolism, and thrombosis. With the subclavian approach, the potential for pneumothorax also exists. This can be minimized by knowledge of the patient's anatomy, attention to detail, and contrast venography (Fig. 6.3). In an older multicenter trial, pneumothorax occurred in 2.0% of patients and was more common in older patients and patients with lower body mass indices ($<20 \, kg/m^2$).[1] A recent system-atic review reported a 0.9% incidence of pneumothorax with either ICD or CRT implantation.[8]

It has been reported that when experienced implanters use the subclavian puncture technique, the incidence of pneumothorax approaches 1%.[9] As noted in Chapter 5: Implantation techniques, peripheral injection of contrast media and fluoroscopic guidance of the subclavian puncture may help to minimize complications (Figs 5.6 and 5.7).[10] In addition, the regional anatomy must be considered before subclavian puncture is undertaken. In a patient with unusual anatomy of the chest wall or clavicle, the subclavian vein can be displaced, and the usual subclavian puncture landmarks can be altered. Care must also be taken in the kyphotic patient in whom the venous anatomy may be displaced. Subclavian arterial dilatation or aneurysm may displace the targeted veins. Direct ultrasound visualization using a handheld device can help avoid contrast and yet identify the vein before it enters the thorax. However, caution is necessary to avoid contamination of the field, and placing the needle into the vein while continuing to visualize the vessel after a relatively small pocket has been created can be challenging. Excessive contrast use (obviated with this technique) has been linked with poorer outcomes including transient renal insufficiency.[11]

Table 6.1 Complications of coronary sinus lead placement. (Reproduced with permission from Saxon LA, De Marco T, Prystowsky EN, et al. www.hrsonline.org/ClinicalGuidance/upload/resynch_therapy_HF.pdf. [accessed 14 September 2012]

	MUSTIC	CONTAK-CD	MIRACLE-ICD
N	64	286	421
Successful			
• First attempt	90%	87%	NA
• Total	92%	NA	88%
Implantation problems			
• Failure	8%	13%	12%
• Coronary sinus trauma	NA	2%	4%
• Deaths	0%	0%	0%
• Others	4.5%	15.2%	38%
Late complications			
• Dislodgment	13.6%	6.8%	8.6%
• Extracardiac stimulation	12%	1.6%	3.0%
• Pocket infection	3.4%	0%	0%
• Loss of capture	0%	0%	0%
• Deaths	0%	0%	0%
• Others	3.4%	1.8%	1.3%
Pacing thresholds (Ldts)			
• At implantation	1.36 ± 0.96	NA	1.5–1.7 (Model 4189)
• Chronic	2.4(3 mo)	1.8 ± 1.2 (13 mo)	1.7–2.3 (Models 218 7/8)

NA – not available.

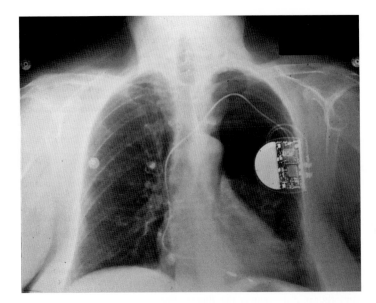

Fig. 6.3 Posteroanterior radiograph taken within a few hours after implantation in a patient complaining of mild dyspnea and left-sided chest discomfort. The patient has a substantial pneumothorax on the left as a complication of subclavian puncture.

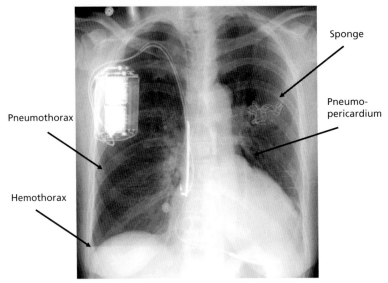

Sponge

Pneumo-pericardium

Pneumothorax

Hemothorax

Fig. 6.4 Posteroanterior chest radiograph from a patient with an internal cardioverter-defibrillator implanted on the right side. There are multiple complications that are evident radiographically. The patient initially had a device on the left side, which was removed, but there is a retained sponge in the abandoned pocket. Close inspection at the left upper cardiac border reveals air in the pericardial space. The arrow points to a faint line which represents the pericardium that is separated from the cardiac surface by a pneumopericardium. On the right side of the chest the upper arrow points to a pneumothorax. The lower arrow on the right side of the chest points to a fluid level that represents an accumulation in the chest, most likely a hemothorax.

If a pneumothorax develops, it may manifest during the pacemaker procedure or as late as 48 h after implantation. Indications of pneumothorax are aspiration of air during subclavian puncture when the exploring needle is either introduced or removed, unexplained hypotension, chest pain, or respiratory distress.

If the subclavian artery is lacerated, hemopneumothorax may occur (Fig. 6.4), or bleeding may occur into the tissues, resulting in hematoma formation (Fig. 6.5). Other potential complications of subclavian venous entry are air embolism, arteriovenous fistula, thoracic duct injury, and brachial plexus injury. Although all are

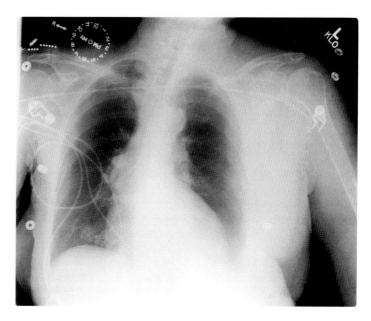

Fig. 6.5 Posteroanterior chest radiograph of a patient following attempted pacemaker implantation. During the procedure the subclavian artery was inadvertently punctured. On the radiograph shown, there is fullness of the axillary and left lateral chest and a density can be appreciated above the left breast. This represents hematoma formation which corresponded to a substantial fall in the patient's hemoglobin.

uncommon, it is essential that the implanter using the subclavian puncture technique be familiar with the potential problems.

After puncture of the subclavian or axillary vein, a chest radiograph should be obtained and inspected specifically for pneumothorax. A pneumothorax estimated to involve <10% of the pleural space can probably be observed without chest tube placement. A chest tube should be considered if >10% of the lung is involved, the patient has continued respiratory distress, or hemopneumothorax is present.

Lead perforation

Cardiac perforation during lead implantation is among the most potentially serious complications that occur with device procedures. Anatomically, the free wall of the right atrium and right ventricle as well as the distal coronary venous system is extremely thin and prone to perforation. CT scan studies have revealed a high rate of asymptomatic and otherwise clinically unrecognized perforations. Care with avoiding the free wall and placing leads whenever possible onto the septum decreases the chance of significant perforation.

The true frequency of lead perforation is difficult to determine and varies widely depending on the series and types of leads evaluated. Perforation has been shown to occur in 0.1–0.8% of patients undergoing pacemaker implantation and 0.6–5.2% in patients undergoing ICD implantation.[2,10,12] The incidence of coronary vein dissection and coronary vein perforation with CS lead placement has each been reported at 1.3%.[8]

Perforations are more common in elderly patients in whom the RV wall may be thinner. Anecdotally, the risk is higher in elderly women than men. In patients in whom a post-implant pericardial effusion was present and was believed to be a consequence of perforation, risk factors included the presence of a temporary pacemaker, helical screw leads, and systemic steroid use (Fig. 6.6). The only protective factor was RV systolic pressure >35 mmHg.[12]

Diagnosis of a perforation is usually based on clinical findings. Echocardiography may suggest perforation, but unless the lead is completely through the myocardium, the study may be inconclusive. More recently, computed tomography (CT) has been reported as a method of diagnosing myocardial perforation (Fig. 6.7).[13] In a retrospective review of CT scans obtained in 100 patients with prior device implantation, there was a surprisingly high incidence of radiographically evident perforations. Overall, 15% of patients had a myocardial perforation. Rates of perforation were 15% for atrial leads and 6% for ventricular leads. There was perforation of 14% of RV ICD leads and 3% of RV pacemaker leads. Active fixation right atrial leads had a 12% perforation rate, and passive fixation atrial leads had a 25% perforation rate. Of RV pacemaker leads, 7% of active fixation and 5% of passive fixation leads demonstrated perforation. When correlated with measured pacing values, there was no difference in impedance between perforated and nonperforated leads. Only one perforated ventricular lead was said to have a "high" threshold.[14] In an older autopsy study, lead perforation

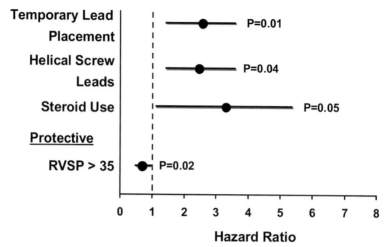

Fig. 6.6 Multivariate hazard ratios for development of pericardial effusion and symptoms consistent with cardiac perforation following permanent pacemaker placement. RVSP, right ventricular systolic pressure. (Reprinted from Mahapatra S, Bybee KA, Bunch TJ, *et al.* Incidence and predictors of cardiac perforation after permanent pacemaker placement. Heart Rhythm 2005; 2:907–11, with permission.)

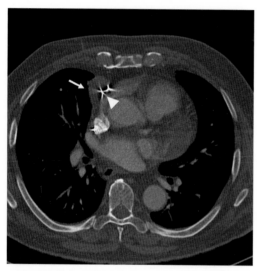

Fig. 6.7 Axial image from a 64-detector ECG gated computed tomography with IV contrast material in a 73-year-old man. There is a circumscribed mass adjacent to the right atrial appendage presumed to be a hematoma (arrow). A portion of the pacemaker lead (arrowhead) is seen outside of the right atrial appendage in the presumed mediastinal hematoma.

was seen in 27% of patients with right atrial leads.[15] The high incidence of asymptomatic radiographic and autopsy identified myocardial perforations suggests that they are not uniformly detrimental.

Perforation can present in multiple ways. It may potentially be asymptomatic and detected radiographi-

cally or by a rising stimulation threshold. In other patients, signs may include right bundle branch block (RBBB)-paced rhythm in a patient in whom the lead is placed in the RV (Fig. 6.8), intercostal muscle, or diaphragmatic stimulation, friction rub after implantation, pericarditis, pericardial effusion, and cardiac tamponade. (Note: When the lead is placed in the RV, because left ventricular (LV) activation is late, a left bundle branch block (LBBB) pattern is expected. However, even in the absence of cardiac perforation and LV stimulation which routinely results in RBBB pattern when the RV is abnormal or the heart is rotated, apical RV pacing may result in RBBB pattern during stimulation even in the absence of perforation.) Hemodynamic deterioration may occur at the time of perforation, but a "slow" pericardial leak may also arise, and symptoms may not appear for 24–48 h. Delayed perforation, i.e., >1 month, although rare, has also been described.[16]

If the patient has mild symptoms or signs compatible with lead perforation, such as pericardial pain and friction rub, but a persistent perforation cannot be identified, observation is reasonable. If the symptoms or signs resolve within 24–48 hours, lead repositioning may not be necessary. If an echocardiogram reveals a small pericardial effusion but no definite perforation, serial echocardiograms should be obtained to be certain that the effusion is not hemodynamically significant or enlarging.

Management of lead perforation depends, in part, on the clinical sequelae. Perforation associated with hemo-

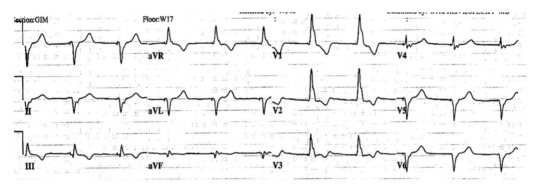

Fig. 6.8 Twelve-lead electrocardiogram obtained immediately after VVI pacemaker implantation. The paced ventricular complex has a right bundle branch block configuration compatible with left ventricular lead placement.

dynamic compromise must be dealt with as an emergency. If clinical and echocardiographic findings are consistent with tamponade, echocardiographically guided pericardiocentesis should be performed. Usually, placing an indwelling pigtail catheter is reasonable to avoid recurrent hemodynamic compromise and to measure drainage accurately. If neither significant additional drainage nor reaccumulation occurs by echocardiography, the catheter can be removed in 48–72 hours and the patient managed by observation and reimaging. If no reaccumulation occurs, the leads may not have to be repositioned so long as thresholds remain stable. With acute perforation, any significant rise in threshold necessitates lead withdrawal and repositioning. With delayed perforation and a rising lead threshold, depending on the lead position, one might consider a conservative approach with placement of a new lead rather than withdrawal or repositioning of the perforated lead.[17] Any time a lead suspected of perforation is withdrawn, there is the potential for pericardial bleeding. In our institution, we do this in our usual pacemaker implant suite with the echocardiographer and necessary equipment for echocardiographic-guided pericardiocentesis standing by. Others prefer to retract the lead suspected of perforation in an operating room with a cardiac surgeon on standby.[18]

Late complications of lead perforation may occur if lead extraction is required. As discussed above, lead perforation is probably more common than realized, and patients may do well over the long term unless lead extraction is required. If there has been transmyocardial perforation or perforation and/or dissection of the venous system with re-entrance into the circulation at the time of implant, catastrophic results may occur when trying to extract these leads either with traction

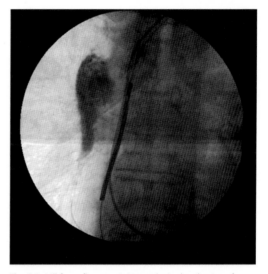

Fig. 6.9 Still-frame fluoroscopic image obtained at the time of upgrade from a dual-chamber pacemaker to a CRT-D system. As the new ventricular lead was passed through the venous system, the lead perforated, probably at the level of the superior vena cava. Because of uncertainty of the lead position, a contrast injection was performed and contrast is apparent in the mediastinum. The patient remained asymptomatic and hemodynamically stable. The lead was withdrawn and the procedure successfully completed.

or a laser extraction system. Careful review of the patient's implantation and associated images (however remote) is recommended when questions arise prior to performing lead extraction.

Perforation of the great vessels may also occur as a procedural complication. Management would be dependent on the patient's symptoms and hemodynamic stability (Fig. 6.9).

Pericarditis

Clinical findings of pericarditis, as mentioned, may be associated with lead perforation. However, pericarditis may occur with or without any other clinical evidence of perforation. It is possible for the tip of an active fixation lead to irritate the pericardium, most commonly a right atrial active fixation lead.[19,20] If there is no evidence of tamponade or symptomatic pericardial effusion, it is reasonable initially to treat the patient conservatively, i.e., observation and pain medications. Anti-inflammatory medications, e.g., nonsteroidal anti-inflammatory drugs or steroids, may relieve symptoms. However, if the medications cannot be withdrawn without symptom recurrence, it may be necessary to remove and reposition the lead.

Arrhythmias

A frequent complication during lead implantation is development of supraventricular or ventricular arrhythmias related to lead manipulation. These effects are usually transient, ending promptly when the lead position is changed. Rarely, they may be sustained. Atrial manipulation may rarely result in sustained atrial tachycardia, fibrillation, or flutter, which complicates placement of a permanent atrial lead. Atrial tachycardia or flutter may revert to normal sinus rhythm with gentle manipulation of the electrode against the atrial wall or by overdrive pacing. Commonly used pacing system analyzers have a "temporary" overdrive-pacing mode available that allows rapid pacing. If the patient is in atrial tachycardia or flutter, burst overdrive pacing via the pacing system analyzer may interrupt the tachyarrhythmia and restore normal sinus rhythm.

Management of atrial fibrillation is more difficult and may require cardioversion to restore normal sinus rhythm during the implant procedure. Prior to cardioversion, the patient's arrhythmia history and anticoagulation history should be reviewed to be certain cardioversion is safe. We routinely place transcutaneous "pacing pads" which can be used for cardioversion in the event that cardioversion is

necessary. Moreover, we routinely perform device implantation in anticoagulated patients, as long as the international normalized ratio (INR) is <2.5. Patients who are not anticoagulated and who have been in atrial fibrillation or flutter for >48 hours are generally not cardioverted because of the potential risk of thromboembolism and stroke.[21] Brief ventricular arrhythmias are also common, particularly during ventricular lead manipulation. They are usually easily controlled. However, in patients with a history of spontaneous sustained ventricular tachycardia, manipulation of the lead may initiate ventricular tachyarrhythmias. Occurrence is obviously more likely during implantation of an ICD. For this reason, all pacemaker and ICD recipients are monitored, and life-support equipment and an external defibrillator are immediately available.

Ventricular extrasystoles may occur in the early post-implantation period as a result of irritation at the electrode–myocardium interface. These premature beats, termed "tip extrasystoles," are usually of the same morphology as the paced ventricular beat (Fig. 6.10). They usually subside within 24 hours after implantation and rarely, if ever, require treatment. In patients receiving a defibrillator with frequent lead-related ectopy or nonsustained VT seen at the end of the procedure or during post-procedure observation, device detections and therapies may be programmed off temporarily and the patient observed to see that lead-related ectopy and arrhythmia have subsided. If they do not subside in a day, consideration for moving the lead to an alternate location should be given.

In addition to tachyarrhythmias, bradyarrhythmias may occur during implant. In patients with intermittent atrioventricular (AV) block and LBBB, catheter trauma to the right bundle may result in AV block. More commonly, bradycardia follows overdrive suppression of an escape ventricular focus during threshold testing. In a patient at high risk for development of asystole or complete heart block during the procedure, a temporary pacemaker may be placed before implantation. Alternatively, external pacing pads

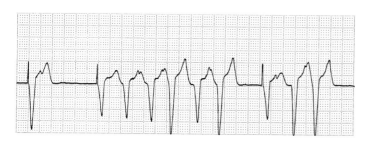

Fig. 6.10 Electrocardiographic tracing obtained within hours after VVI pacemaker implantation. The pacemaker is programmed to a lower rate of 50 ppm. There are frequent ventricular extrasystoles morphologically similar to the paced beats, and at least one of the premature beats is undersensed.

can be placed during the procedure should temporary pacing be needed. This method may obviate adjunctive transvenous temporary pacing. At our institution we routinely place external pacing pads.

Pulse generator pocket complications

Pocket hematomas are a frequent complication of permanent pacemaker and ICD implantation, occurring in 4.9–9.5% of patients.[22–24] Bleeding complications are more likely to occur in patients on antiplatelet agents or anticoagulants. While aspirin alone does not appear to increase the risk for pocket hematomas, the combination of aspirin and clopidogrel increases the incidence of hematomas to 7.2–24.2%.[22,23] Renal dysfunction also increases the risk for periprocedureal bleeding.[25] Patients should be informed of the risk for bleeding complications related to device implantation.

The provider must consider the indications for antiplatelet agents and anticoagulants prior to device implantation. It is not our routine practice to discontinue antiplatelet agents. In patients at high risk for thromboembolism, continuing oral anticoagulation with warfarin is preferred to bridging with low-molecular-weight and unfractionated heparin.[26] A retrospective study found a substantially higher risk for hematoma with no difference in thromboembolism in patients on bridging anticoagulation vs. continued warfarin (mean INR 2.57).[27,28] A prospective study in patients undergoing implantation of CRT devices found a four times higher risk for pocket hematoma in patients on bridging anticoagulation compared with continued warfarin (mean INR 2.39).[29] In patients requiring oral anticoagulants (warfarin), we like the INR to be <2.5 at the time of implantation. For many patients, this may not require any alteration in therapy. If the patient is maintained at a higher INR, holding the warfarin for one to two nights prior to implantation will generally result in the INR being at acceptable levels to proceed. As noted previously in this chapter, unfractionated heparin or low-molecular-weight heparin are always discontinued prior to device implant and ideally avoided for a minimum of 24 hours post-implantation. Periprocedural management of newer oral anticoagulants, such as dabigatran, remains uncertain.

Careful local hemostasis during implantation is essential. Special steps can be considered at the time of implant in patients with excessive "oozing" within the pocket. Materials that can be used in patients with excessive oozing refractory to electrocautery include Gelfoam, thrombin-treated biodegradable mesh, and topical application of thrombin, which can be highly effective in stopping the bleeding. If topical thrombin is used, it may interfere with subsequent INR measurements.

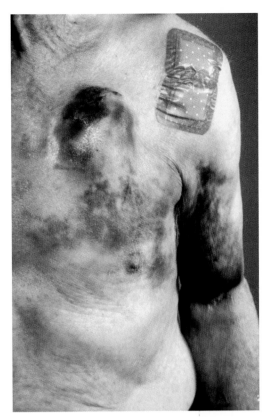

Fig. 6.11 Extensive ecchymoses following device implantation. The patient was on aspirin therapy at the time of the procedure. A portion of the left arm ecchymoses was secondary to an earlier unrelated procedure. The ecchymoses resolved without any adverse effects.

Because local ecchymoses are common after pacemaker implantation, an ecchymosis, regardless of size, that is not expanding is treated by observation only. Discrete hematoma formation at the site must be dealt with on the basis of its secondary consequences (Figs 6.11 and 6.12). Should a substantial hematoma occur, conservative treatment is preferred, if possible. If bleeding continues, pain cannot be managed with mild analgesics, or the integrity of the incision is threatened, evacuating the hematoma should be considered. Aspiration of the hematoma or placement of a drain should not be attempted, because it is often ineffective, and regardless of the care taken to maintain sterile technique, increases the risk of infection. If hematoma evacuation is required, the procedure should be thoroughly sterile.

Late complications, including erosion and migration, are often the result of suboptimal initial surgery

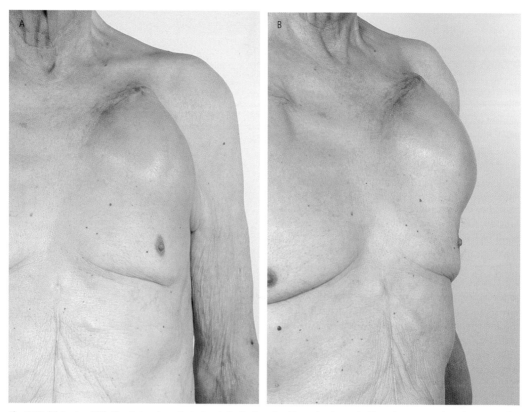

Fig. 6.12 (A) Front and (B) side photos of a patient after device implantation. The patient has a significant hematoma. Discomfort was easily managed with analgesics and there was no threat to the integrity of the incision. The hematoma gradually resolved without consequence.

or infection (Figs 6.13 and 6.14). These can be minimized by careful technique at the time of initial pacemaker implantation and by the formation of an adequate pocket. A painful pocket may also result from inadequate positioning of the pacemaker below the subcutaneous tissues, and the pulse generator may have to be repositioned.

Pain

Patients should be told to expect some local discomfort at the pacemaker implantation site. This gradually subsides and can usually be managed with mild analgesics, such as acetaminophen. A painful pacemaker site, commonly called a "painful pocket," can occur for several reasons and should be taken seriously. The differential diagnosis includes:

- Infection
- Pacemaker implanted too superficially
- Pacemaker implanted too laterally
- Pacemaker allergy.

An indolent infection may manifest as a painful pocket long before any other signs of infection. This

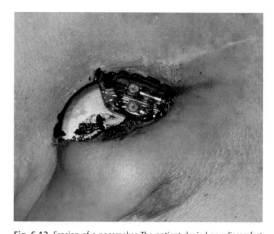

Fig. 6.13 Erosion of a pacemaker. The patient denied any discomfort and stated that he had been able to see some portion of the device for at least 3 months prior to seeking medical attention.

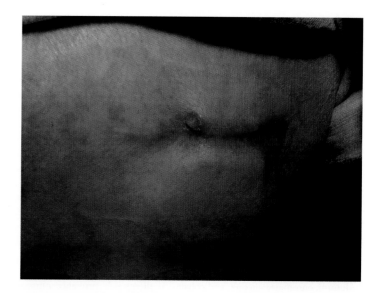

Fig. 6.14 Erosion of a previously abandoned and capped lead.

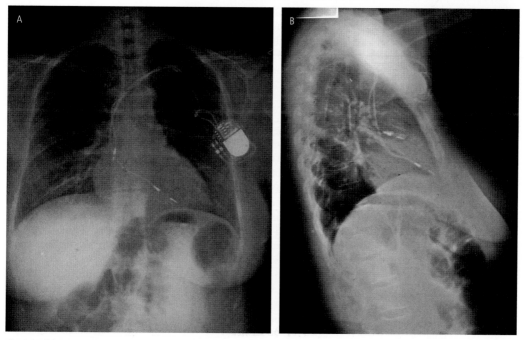

Fig. 6.15 (A) Posteroanterior and (B) lateral radiograph from a patient with chronic pain and arm limitation after pacemaker implantation. An attempt had been made to place the pacemaker in an axillary position for cosmetic reasons. From this single view it also appears that both leads are "shallow," i.e., suboptimal redundancy on the ventricular lead and suboptimal "J" on the atrial lead.

diagnosis can be difficult. Needle aspiration of a pacemaker site is not advised for fear of introducing infection. However, if a painful pocket is explored for any reason, culture specimens should be obtained.

The pacemaker pocket should be formed in the prepectoralis fascia, i.e., deep to adipose tissue in the subcutaneous space. If it is placed anterior to the adipose layer, i.e., within subcutaneous tissues, significant pain may result. This is one of the most common causes of a painful pocket and justifies revision of the pacemaker pocket.

If the pacemaker is positioned too laterally, impingement on the axillary space may cause discomfort (Fig. 6.15). Although there are published series on axillary pocket placement, substantial experience is required to position the pacemaker in such a way that there is no discomfort.[30]

Allergic reaction to the pacemaker can or other components of the pacing system is a rare but reported complication.[31] Pain at the pocket site may occur if the allergic reaction is to the pacemaker can or other component located within the pocket site. Proof of such an allergy requires sophisticated allergy testing, and correction of the problem may require changing certain components of the hardware. Some of the instances of "allergy" are, in reality, low-grade infections, which should be treated as infections rather than allergies. Diagnosis of allergy should not be made until infection has been ruled out.

Pacing system components to which there have been documented allergic reactions include: titanium, polychloroparaxylene, nickel, polyurethane, epoxy, mercury, cadmium, chromate, silicone, and cobalt.[31] If allergy is a likely consideration in a patient with a painful pocket or other symptoms that may suggest an unusual allergic reaction, the manufacturer of the patient's pulse generator and lead(s) should be contacted and a testing kit requested. The manufacturer should be able to provide a sample of all components that a dermatologist or allergist can use for skin testing.

Inadvertent left ventricular lead placement
Inadvertent placement of the transvenous lead in the LV cavity is not uncommon. This most often occurs when a lead is passed across an atrial septal defect (ASD) or ventricular septal defect (VSD) that is not known to exist (Fig. 6.16). It can also occur by inadvertent puncture and cannulation of the subclavian artery (Fig. 6.17). A left-sided position of the lead can be suspected from an unusually high "takeoff" of the ventricular lead, with the lead passing to the left side of the heart at a point higher than the lowermost portion of the atrial J. If lateral fluoroscopy or lateral chest radiography is performed, the LV position is fairly obvious because the lead is directed posteriorly.

The right anterior oblique (RAO) and left anterior oblique (LAO) fluoroscopic views performed either at the time of implant or requested at the time of later chest X-ray can be extremely useful in understanding the exact route of a ventricular pacing lead, especially when systemic circulation pacing is a concern. The LAO projection demonstrates the relationship of the lead tip to the interventricular septum (left or right of). Once left-sided pacing is established from the LAO projection, the RAO projection can distinguish between CS pacing, entrance via an ASD, entrance via a VSD, or epimyocardial pacing following perforation. With CS pacing, the characteristic entrance into the CS in the

region of the epicardial fat pad at the annulus (where the diaphragm crosses the cardiac silhouette) will be seen with a relatively straight course of the pacing lead before the lead turns towards the sternum (ventricular) to reach its pacing location. When the pacing lead in the RAO projection is not near the region of the posterior fat pad/diaphragm, then either an ASD or VSD (or equivalent) is present. The distinction between these two entities can again be made with a quick RAO view. ASDs will be found closer to the vertebral column (atrial) and VSDs closer to the sternum (ventricular). With myocardial perforations in either the RAO or LAO view, the lead will be seen traversing outside the cardiac silhouette, and, at implant, excessive mobility of the lead following perforation is characteristic.

LV lead placement is concerning, given the potential for thromboembolism. Small thromboemboli arising from the pacing leads on the right side of the heart are probably common but are rarely of clinical significance. In contrast, a small thromboembolism in the systemic circulation can be catastrophic. If such a position is realized within the first few days after implantation, the lead should be withdrawn and repositioned if the patient does not have a right-to-left shunt across the defect that allows the lead to cross. With a shunt, epimyocardial lead placement is recommended.

If LV lead position is not recognized in the early post-implant period, it is not likely to be realized for some time. If months have passed, the approach must be individualized for the patient. If the lead is to remain in the system circulation, the patient should receive anticoagulation with warfarin and be told of the potential risk of embolic phenomena. Lead extraction can be considered, although controversy exists. Because of the potential for embolization of small clots during extraction, some physicians opt for removal of the leads only during an open chest approach. Many extraction procedure experts believe that the risk of embolization is small and proceed with standard extraction techniques. Regardless, options should be discussed with the patient.

Thrombosis
Symptomatic thromboembolic complications after permanent pacemaker implantation are uncommon, estimated to occur in 0.6–3.5% of implants.[32,33] Asymptomatic lead-associated thrombosis is more frequent. A prospective study with transesophageal echocardiography, transthoracic echocardiography, and venography at 6 months reported a 9% incidence of right atrial or superior vena cava thrombus and 20% incidence of subclavian or innominate vein thrombi (Fig. 6.18).[34] If thrombosis involves the superior vena cava, axillary

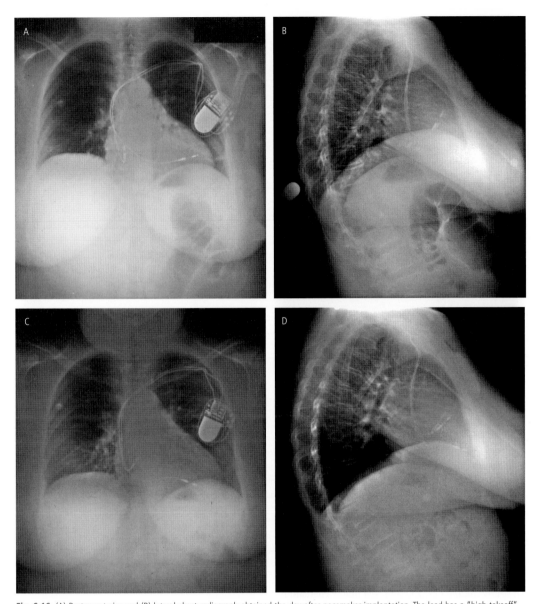

Fig. 6.16 (A) Posteroanterior and (B) lateral chest radiograph obtained the day after pacemaker implantation. The lead has a "high takeoff" as it begins to cross to the left from the atrial position. This lead had been passed across an unknown patent foramen ovale and positioned in the left ventricle. (C) Posteroanterior and (D) lateral chest radiograph obtained the day after the lead had been withdrawn and repositioned in the right ventricular apex.

vein, or area around the pacemaker lead in the right atrium or RV, several problems can develop (Fig. 6.19). These include occlusion of the superior vena cava and superior vena cava syndrome; thrombosis of the superior vena cava, right atrium, or RV, with hemodynamic compromise or pulmonary embolism; and symptomatic thrombosis of the subclavian vein with an edematous painful upper extremity (Fig. 6.20).

Partial or silent thrombosis is common and usually clinically insignificant except at the time of pacing system revision; an alternative venous access may be required. Venoplasty has been used when partial thrombosis limits venous access and a new lead must be placed (Fig. 6.21).[35] Venoplasty may also be performed in a coronary vein if a stenosis limits CS lead placement (Fig. 6.22).[36]

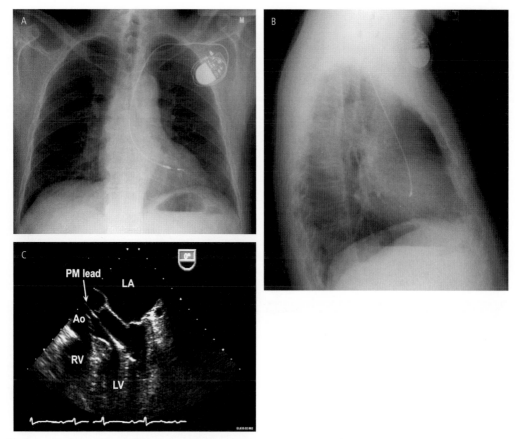

Fig. 6.17 Posteroanterior (A) and (B) lateral chest radiograph of a patient with a single-chamber pacing system. Note that the lead takes an unusual course and remains to the left of the vertebral column and on the lateral image the lead is in a shallow ventricular position and oriented slightly posteriorly. (C) Still-frame from a 2-D echocardiogram of the same patient. The pacing lead (PM lead) noted by the arrow goes through the aortic (Ao) valve and into the left ventricle (LV). The lead had been inadvertently placed by subclavian artery puncture. LA, left atruim; RV, right ventricle.

If a patient presents with symptomatic venous thrombosis, several therapeutic approaches can be considered. The most common presentation is a mildly edematous arm and complaints of "aching" or a "heavy" sensation in the arm. Conservative treatment with bed rest, arm elevation, and therapeutic anticoagulation often results in symptom relief. There are reports of thrombolytic therapy for symptomatic thrombosis after device implantation. Although this method may work well, the patient should be advised that, in addition to systemic risks, there is some risk of bleeding within the pocket if the procedure has been recently performed. We generally favor the use of warfarin for at least 3 months after initial treatment with unfractionated heparin or low-molecular-weight heparin.[37] The need for subsequent long-term anticoagulation is variable. In the patient with more extensive thrombosis, such as superior vena cava syndrome, other interventions may be required (Fig. 6.23).

Loose connector block connection

Intermittent or complete failure of output can occur because of a loose connection at the pacing lead–connector block interface. This failure usually occurs because the lead was inadequately secured at the time of pacemaker implantation. When there is a loose connection, manipulating the pacemaker may reproduce the problem. The poor connection may be evident radiographically (Fig. 6.24).

Lead damage

Lead damage during pacemaker implantation may be under-recognized. Inadvertent damage to pacing leads by scissors or scalpel may go unnoticed. Polyurethane

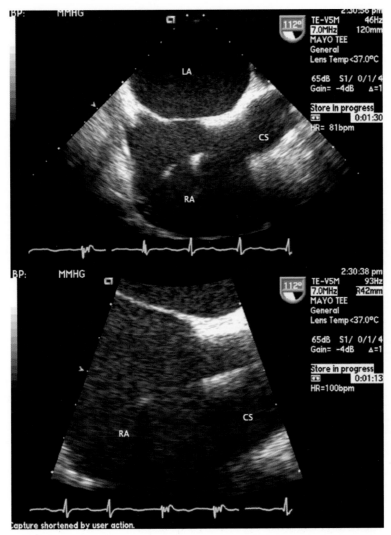

Fig. 6.18 (A) A transesophageal echocardiogram in a patient with a coronary sinus lead vegetation. The left atrium is at the top portion of the image and the right atrium below. The coronary sinus extends to the right and the vegetation is present on the right atrial aspect of the coronary sinus lead. (B) A magnified view of the lead vegetation.

leads can be easily damaged by placement of a ligature directly around the lead itself (Figs 6.25 and 6.26). A protector sleeve, which is provided on or with the leads, should be used to secure the lead to the underlying support structures.

Rarely, the lead may be damaged by the stylet during implantation. This may occur if the stylet is forced at an angle through the conductor and the surrounding insulating material. If this is recognized during the procedure, the lead should be removed and discarded.

Infection

Cardiovascular implantable electronic device (CIED) infections are an infrequent occurrence with significant morbidity and mortality.[38] The incidence of infection after pacemaker implantation should be <2%. In an earlier trial, erosion and pocket infection occurred in 0.5% of patients.[1] Similarly, the incidence of infection after 6-month follow-up in the REPLACE registry was 1.3%, with 0.6% of patients requiring device extraction.[2] Independent risk factors for pacemaker infection include long-term corticosteroid use and the presence of more than two pacing leads vs. two leads.[39]

CIED infections are predominantly caused by Gram-positive organisms. In a retrospective review of patients with infected CIEDs at our institution, the majority were caused by coagulase-negative staphylococci and *Staphylococcus aureus* (42% and 29%, respectively;

Fig. 6.27).[40] Early infections are most commonly caused by *S. aureus*, are more aggressive, and are often associated with fever and systemic symptoms. Late infections are frequently caused by coagulase-negative staphylococci (such as *Staphylococcus epidermidis*) and are more indolent, usually without fever or systemic manifestations.

Local pocket-site infections or systemic/blood stream infections can be seen with CIEDs. Early, superficial infections, including cellulitis and incisional infections,

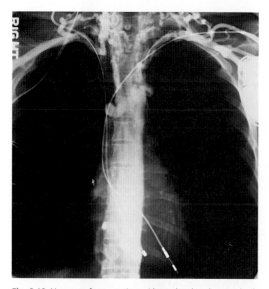

Fig. 6.19 Venogram from a patient with an abandoned pacing lead on the left and a functional but failing pacemaker lead through the left subclavian vein. Extensive thrombosis is present in the subclavian vein with bilateral inominate vein occlusion.

do not necessitate CIED removal and are frequently managed with oral or intravenous antibiotics. If deeper infection is suspected, percutaneous pocket aspiration should not be performed given the risk of introducing infection to the entire CIED. Any invasive CIED site evaluation should be performed in an operating suite using full aseptic techniques. All patients with pocket infections require complete CIED removal.[38]

Pocket-site infections can be subtle. Adherence of the pulse generator to the skin strongly suggests an infection, and salvage of the site may not be possible. Impending erosion (skin thinned to the point of transparency) should be dealt with as an emergency. Once the skin is broken, the CIED is contaminated; while it is still closed, the CIED is protected. If infection is not present and revision is accomplished before the CIED has fully eroded, the original site can be revised and CIED reused. Culture specimens should be obtained in all such circumstances.

Although erosion of the pulse generator through the skin usually occurs long after implantation, it is often related to the implantation technique (Figs 6.13 and 6.14). Erosion is an uncommon complication that may occur in five situations:

1 The patient has an indolent infection

2 The pacemaker pocket formed at the time of surgery is too small for the implanted pulse generator

3 The pulse generator is implanted too superficially, especially in children and small-framed adults, in who lack of adipose tissue results in "tightness" of the pacemaker despite adequate pocket size

4 The generator is implanted too far laterally in the anterior axillary fold

5 The lead has been sutured to the subcutaneous or subcuticular tissue.

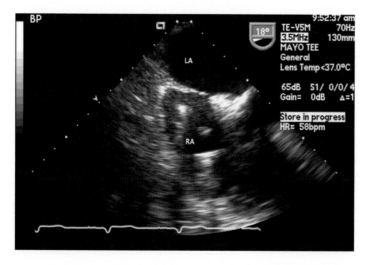

Fig. 6.20 Transesophageal echocardiogram image showing a vegetation on the right atrial aspect of a right ventricular lead.

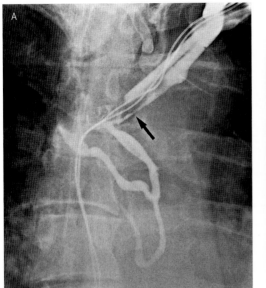
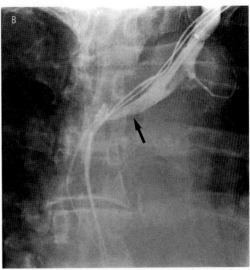

Fig. 6.21 (A) Initial venogram reveals high-grade stenosis of the left innominate vein and large bridging collateral venous channels around the area of stenosis (arrow). (B) Venogram after venoplasty shows large opening in area of previously noted stenosis (arrow). Dilatation was sufficient to allow passage of the pacemaker lead. (From Spittell and Hayes,[32] by permission of Futura Publishing Co.)

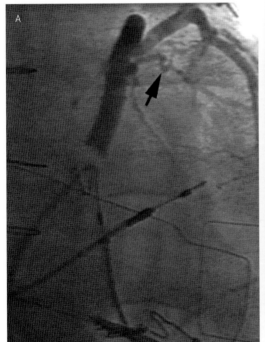
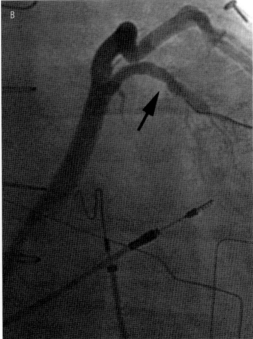

Fig. 6.22 Images obtained during coronary venous lead placement. (A) Initial coronary venogram reveals significant venous stenosis and inability to pass pacing lead. (B) Venoplasty performed and lead advanced without difficulty. (Figures courtesy of Seth J. Worley, Lancaster, PA, USA.)

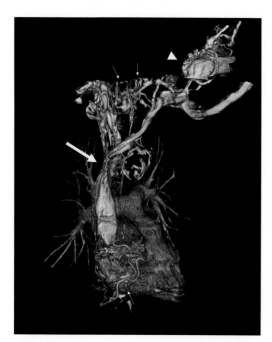

Fig. 6.23 3-D volume rendered reconstruction from a 64-detector computed tomography scan of the chest in a patient with a dual-lead pacemaker. The pacemaker device is visible (arrowhead). Narrowing of the superior vena cava is seen (large arrow). Small collateral veins are visible in the midline (small arrows).

Erosion, whether secondary to underlying infection or not, results in contamination of the entire cardiac device. The entire system (both pulse generator and leads) should be extracted.[38]

Retrospective review at our institution found that the majority of CIED infections were pocket infections without bacteremia (52%). The remainder were systemic infections, including pocket infection with bacteremia, bacteremia without localizing signs of infection in the CIED pocket, and CIED-related endocarditis.[40] A high index of suspicion for CIED infection should be present when patients with CIED present with fever and positive blood cultures without another likely source for infection.

Prevention of CIED infection at implantation is paramount. Careful attention to surgical details and adherence to sterile technique during implantation are critical. Preimplantation antibiotic prophylaxis has been shown to reduce the incidence of CIED infection.[40] As noted in Chapter 5: Implantation techniques, we use antibiotic prophylaxis at the time of implant (details are described in Box 5.2). Prophylactic antibiotics are not, however, indicated prior to dental or other invasive procedures in patients with a CIED.[38]

Management of suspected CIED infection begins with obtaining at least two sets of blood cultures prior to initiating antimicrobial therapy. A transesophageal echocardiogram should be performed if cultures are positive, blood cultures were obtained after initiation of antimicrobial therapy, or if endocarditis is suspected. If the CIED is extracted, cultures should be performed on a swab from the pocket site and lead-tip.

Antimicrobial therapy should initially cover the predominant organisms and then be tailored to results from pathogen identification. Duration of antimicrobial therapy should be at least 10–14 days after CIED removal for pocket-site infections, 14 days after CIED removal for blood stream infections, and 4–6 weeks for complicated infection. Repeat blood cultures should be obtained post-extraction in patients with positive cultures prior to extraction. In patients with continued necessity for CIED after extraction, reimplantation should occur in a site contralateral to the extraction site or another alternative location. New CIED implantation should be after 72 hours of negative post-extraction blood cultures and at least 14 days after CIED system removal if there was valvular endocarditis.[38] An algorithm for management of the patient with an infected pacing or ICD system is shown in Fig. 6.28. The guidelines for the diagnosis and management of device infections are listed in Table 6.2.

Abandoned and nonfunctioning, noninfected leads

Abandoned leads must be removed if they are part of an infected system. Whether abandoned or nonfunctioning, noninfected leads should be extracted is, however, controversial. In certain situations, extraction may be desirable. Specific situations include the following:

• Tricuspid regurgitation (TR) felt to be caused by or exacerbated by multiple leads across the valve (see discussion below; Fig. 6.29)
• Symptomatic thrombosis[41,42]
• The abandoned lead(s) is an impediment to placement of a new pacing lead
• There is an interaction between abandoned and active lead(s), e.g. the functioning lead senses "noise" from contact with the abandoned lead
• Pediatric patients in whom multiple lead changes will be required and in whom abandonment would result in excessive hardware.

If none of these conditions exists, it may be reasonable to abandon leads in place while taking into consideration abandoned hardware that may already exist (Fig. 6.30).[43]

At the time of lead extraction, a portion of the lead, specifically, portions of the "tines," may be left in an

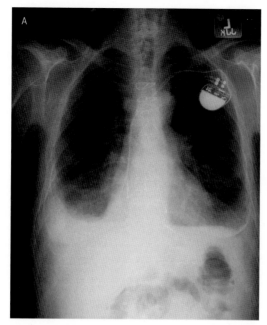

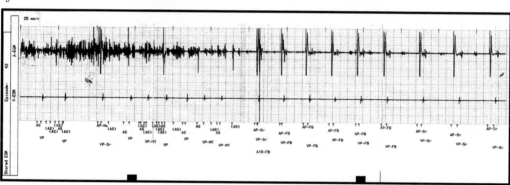

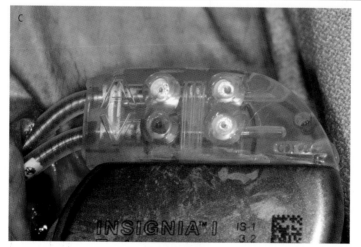

Fig. 6.24 (A) Close-up of the pacemaker on a posteroanterior chest X-ray. Note that the atrial lead (top lead) is not completely inserted into the connector block. Comparing it with the ventricular lead, where the pin is visible coming through the connector block, the pin is not visible on the atrial lead. (B) The corresponding tracing shows substantial "noise" on the atrial lead, which is common if the lead is not secure in the connector block. (C) Photograph obtained at the time of revision. Again, the pin of the ventricular lead can be seen through the connector block, but the atrial pin cannot.

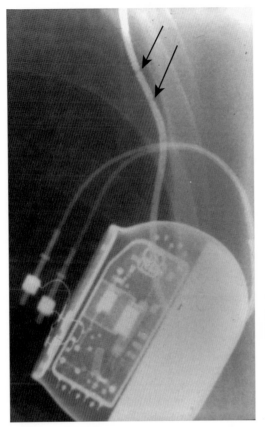

endocardial position. A distal electrode also may not be removed and be left somewhere within the vascular tree (Fig. 6.31). A clinical problem usually does not result from these retained fragments. In a retrospective study of ICD recipients, we found that capping and abandoning leads does not generally affect sensing function or DFTs.[44]

Twiddler's syndrome

Purposeful or absent-minded "twiddling" – manipulation of the pulse generator by the patient – has been named "twiddler's syndrome." Manipulation may cause axial rotation of the pacemaker, twisting of the lead, and eventual fracture or dislodgement of the lead. The syndrome commonly occurs when the pacemaker sits loosely in the pacemaker pocket (Fig. 6.32), either because the pocket is too large or because the

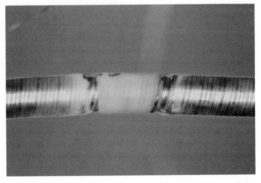

Fig. 6.25 Close-up view from a posteroanterior radiograph shows a pacemaker and the proximal portion of a lead. At two sites (arrows), the insulation is compressed by ligatures placed around a securing sleeve. (From Hayes DL. Pacemaker radiography. In: Furman S, Hayes DL, Holmes DR Jr, eds. A Practice of Cardiac Pacing. Mount Kisco, NY, Futura Publishing Company, 1989: 323–68. Copyrighted and used by permission of Mayo Foundation for Medical Education and Research.)

Fig. 6.26 An explanted lead. There is evidence of the contour of the lead being permanently altered by the ligatures placed on the sleeve, not on the lead directly. However, it cannot be determined from the photograph that there was evidence of loss of integrity of the lead insulation.

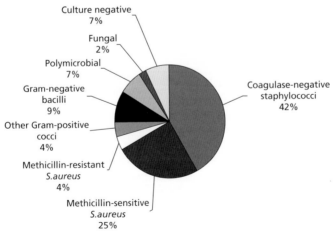

Fig. 6.27 Microbiology of PPM/ICD infections. ICD, implantable cardioverter-defibrillator; PPM, permanent pacemaker. (From Sohail MR, Uslan DZ, Khan AH, *et al*. Risk factor analysis of permanent pacemaker infection. Clin Infect Dis 2007; 45:166–73, with permission.)

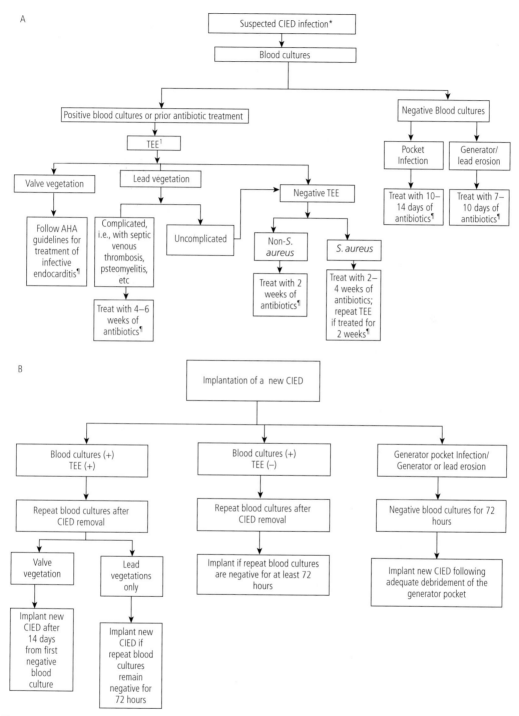

Fig. 6.28 American Heart Association (AHA) 2010 recommendations for the diagnosis and management of cardiac implantable electronic device (CIED) infections (From Baddour LM, Epstein AE, Erickson CC, *et al.* Update on cardiovascular implantable electronic device infections and their management: a scientific statement from the American Heart Association. Circulation 2010; 121:458–77, by permission of Lippincott Williams and Wilkins.)

Table 6.2 Summary of recommendations. (From Baddour LM, Epstein AE, Erickson CC, *et al*. Update on cardiovascular implantable electronic device infections and their management: a scientific statement from the American Heart Association. Circulation 2010; 121:458–77, by permission of Lippincott Williams and Wilkins.)

Recommendation	Class and Level of Evidence
A. Recommendations for diagnosis of CIED infection and associated complications	
1. All patients should have at least 2 sets of blood cultures drawn at the initial evaluation before prompt initiation of antimicrobial therapy for CIED infection.	IC
2. Generator-pocket tissue Gram stain and culture and lead-tip culture should be obtained when the CIED is explanted.	IC
3. Patients with suspected CIED infection who either have positive blood cultures or have negative blood cultures but have had recent antimicrobial therapy before blood cultures were obtained should undergo TEE for CIED infection or valvular endocarditis.	IC
4. All adults suspected of having CIED-related endocarditis should undergo TEE to evaluate the left-sided heart valves, even if transthoracic views have demonstrated lead-adherent masses. In pediatric patients with good views, TTE may be sufficient.	IB
5. Patients should seek evaluation for CIED infection by cardiologists or infectious disease specialists if they develop fever or bloodstream infection for which there is no initial explanation.	IIaC
6. Percutaneous aspiration of the generator pocket should not be performed as part of the diagnostic evaluation of CIED infection.	IIIC
B. Recommendations for antimicrobial management of CIED infection	
1. Choice of antimicrobial therapy should be based on the identification and in vitro susceptibility results of the infecting pathogen.	IB
2. Duration of antimicrobial therapy should be 10 to 14 days after CIED removal for pocket-site infection.	1C
3. Duration of antimicrobial therapy should be at least 14 days after CIED removal for bloodstream infection.	1C
4. Duration of antimicrobial therapy should be at least 4 to 6 weeks for complicated infection (ie, endocarditis, septic thrombophlebitis, or osteomyelitis or if bloodstream infection persists despite device removal and appropriate initial antimicrobial therapy).	1C
C. Recommendations for removal of infected CIED	
1. Complete device and lead removal is recommended for all patients with definite CIED infection, as evidenced by valvular and/or lead endocarditis or sepsis.	IA
2. Complete device and lead removal is recommended for all patients with CIEM pocket infection, as evidenced by abscess formation, device erosion, skin adherence, or chronic draining sinus without clinically evident involvement of the transvenous portion of the lead system.	1B
3. Complete device and lead removal is recommended for all patients with valvular endocarditis without definite involvement of the lead(s) and/or device.	1B
4. Complete device and lead removal is recommended for patients with occult staphylococcal bacteremia.	1B
5. Complete device and lead removal is reasonable in patients with persistent occult Gram-negative bacteremia despite appropriate antibiotic therapy.	IIaB
6. CIED removal is not indicated for a superficial or incisional infection without involvement of the device and/or leads.	IIIC
7. CIED removal is not indicated for relapsing bloodstream infection due to a source other than a CIED and for which long-term suppressive antimicrobials are required.	IIIC
D. Recommendations for new CIED implantation after removal of an infected CIED	
1. Each patient should be evaluated carefully to determine whether there is a continued need for a new CIED.	IC
2. The replacement device implantation should not be ipsilateral to the extraction site. Preferred alternative locations include the contralateral side, the iliac vein, and epicardial implantation.	1C
3. When positive before extraction, blood cultures should be drawn after device removal and should be negative for at least 72 hours before new device placement is performed.	IIaC
4. New transvenous lead placement should be delayed for at least 14 days after CIED system removal when there is evidence of valvular infection.	IIaC

Table 6.2 (*Continued*)

Recommendation	Class and Level of Evidence
E. Recommendations for use of long-term suppressive antimicrobial therapy	
1. Long-term suppressive therapy should be considered for patients who have CIED infection and who are not candidates for complete device removal.	IIbC
2. Long-term suppressive therapy should not be administered to patients who are candidates for infected CIED removal.	IIIC
F. Recommendations for antimicrobial prophylaxis at the time of CIED placement	
1. Prophylaxis with an antibiotic that has in vitro activity against staphylococci should be administered. If cefazolin is selected for use, then it should be administered intravenously within 1 hour before incision; if vancomycin is given, then it should be administered intravenously within 2 hours before incision.	IA
G. Recommendations for antimicrobial prophylaxis for invasive procedures in patients with CIEDs	
1. Antimicrobial prophylaxis is not recommended for dental or other invasive procedures not directly related to device manipulation to prevent CIED infection.	IIIC
H. Recommendations to avoid microbiological studies in cases of CIED removal for noninfectious reasons	
1. Routine microbiological studies should not be conducted on CIEDs that have been removed for noninfectious reasons.	IIIB

TTE indicates transthoracic echocardiography.

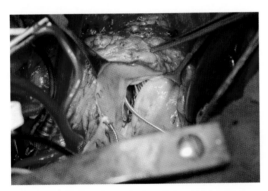

Fig. 6.29 Photograph taken at the time of tricuspid valve surgery. The pacing lead has "creased" the anterior leaflet of the tricuspid valve and caused rolling of the free edge.

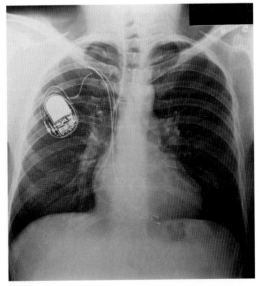

Fig. 6.30 Posteroanterior chest radiograph shows three ventricular leads in place. All three leads are fractured. Two of the leads were transected at the time they were replaced. At the time of this radiograph, the patient presented with fracture of the third lead. No clinical problems could be attributed to the excessive abandoned hardware. (From Hayes DL. Pacemaker radiography. In: Furman S, Hayes DL, Holmes DR Jr, eds. A Practice of Cardiac Pacing, 3rd edn. Mount Kisco, NY: Futura Publishing Co., 1993: 361–400, by permission of Mayo Foundation.)

pacemaker has migrated. Obesity and neuropsychiatric illnesses may predispose patients to this complication.

If the problem has occurred because of pacemaker migration or a poorly fashioned pacemaker pocket, the pocket should be revised. Avoiding the creation of an excessively large pocket, fixing the pulse generator by an anchoring suture, anchoring the lead to the prepectoral fascia by a sleeve, or placing the pulse generator in a subpectoral position may prevent this problem. Another technique that is more of historical interest is to place the pacemaker in a snugly fitting Dacron pouch to reduce migration and torsion of the pacing system by promoting tissue in-growth and stabilization of the pacemaker. Although these Dacron pouches are still available, they are rarely used.

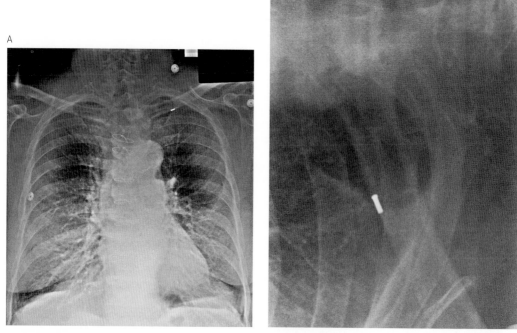

Fig. 6.31 (A) Posteroanterior chest radiograph and (B) close-up view of a retained lead fragment, the distal electrode, after partial lead extraction. The fragment is wedged in an infraclavicular portion of the subclavian vein. The retained fragment has not produced long-term complications.

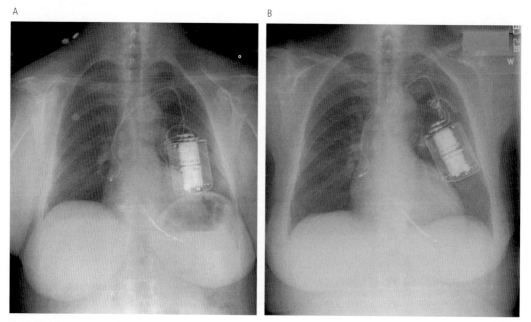

Fig. 6.32 (A) Posteroanterior (PA) chest radiograph from a patient with an earlier generation internal cardioverterdefibrillator. The X-ray was obtained the day after implant. (B) PA chest radiograph from the same patient obtained at the 3-month follow-up visit. Note that lead positions are now more shallow, and there is gross twisting of the leads above the pulse generator. This is consistent with "twiddler's syndrome" regardless of the etiology of the lead entanglement.

New symptoms secondary to pacemaker placement

Extracardiac stimulation

Extracardiac stimulation usually involves the diaphragm, pectoral muscle, or, less commonly, the intercostal muscles. Diaphragmatic stimulation may be caused by direct stimulation of the diaphragm (usually stimulation of the left hemidiaphragm) or stimulation of the phrenic nerve (usually stimulation of the right hemidiaphragm). Diaphragmatic stimulation is particularly problematic with CS leads, because of the course of the left phrenic nerve along the left lateral cardiac border.

The potential for diaphragmatic stimulation should be tested at implantation. If any stimulation is noted with 10V, the pacing lead should be repositioned. Testing is usually performed in a supine position. Thus, there remains a possibility of diaphragmatic stimulation when the patient is upright. Diaphragmatic stimulation occurring during the early post-implantation period may be caused by microdislodgement of the pacing lead, macrodislodgement of the pacing lead, or myocardial perforation. In some circumstances, extracardiac stimulation may be diminished or alleviated by decreasing the voltage output or the pulse width. (An adequate pacing margin of safety must be maintained after the output settings are decreased.) The use of bipolar pacemaker leads rather than unipolar leads can also help reduce local muscle stimulation.

In CRT devices, a programming change of the pacing configuration can help not only in identifying a lower pacing threshold, but also with avoiding phrenic nerve stimulation. In one study, phrenic nerve stimulation occurred in 12% of patients who had a device with a programmable pacing configuration and was corrected by a change in pacing configuration in all patients.[45]

Pectoral muscle stimulation may also be caused by an insulation defect of the pacing lead, current leakage from the connector or sealing plugs, erosion of the pacemaker's protective coating, or rapid high-amplitude atrial output in a unipolar dual-chamber pacemaker. If the problem is due to an insulation defect on either a unipolar pacemaker or the pacemaker lead, decreasing the voltage output or the pulse width (or both) may minimize stimulation until the defective portion of the system is replaced. In addition to symptoms of pectoral muscle stimulation, a patient with pectoral muscle stimulation and an activity-sensing rate-adaptive pacemaker may have inappropriate sensor activation and inappropriately rapid pacing rates for a given level of activity. If pectoral muscle stimulation occurs in a polarity-programmable pacemaker, reprogramming to the alternate polarity configuration may alleviate the problem.

Pacemaker syndrome

Pacemaker syndrome, described in Chapter 2: Hemodynamics of Cardiac Pacing, implies adverse hemodynamics associated with loss of AV synchrony. It can occur as a hardware-related complication if the atrial lead becomes nonfunctional for any reason and results in loss of AV synchrony. A classic example would be dislodgement of the atrial lead so that it either fails to capture or captures the ventricle; in either event, the patient has functional ventricular pacing only. Pacemaker syndrome can also occur in the absence of a hardware-related complication.

Tricuspid regurgitation

New-onset or worsened triscuspid regurgitation (TR) can be associated with transvenously placed RV leads. Retrospective analyses of patients with an echocardiogram before and after pacemaker or ICD implantation demonstrate worsening or new TR in 18–24% of patients. Prospective studies with an echocardiogram before and after lead implantation (<6 months' follow-up) showed worsened TR in 4 out of 35 patients in one study[46] and 8 out of 61 patients in another.[47] Older patients and those with ICD leads were more likely to develop TR.[48,49]

The mechanism of lead-associated TR can vary, including both mechanical and functional causes (Fig. 6.33). In a series of 41 patients with morphologically normal tricuspid valves and severe lead-associated TR undergoing tricuspid surgery, the mechanism of regurgitation was: lead impingement of the valve (16 patients); lead adherence to the valve (14 patients); valve perforation by the lead (7 patients); and lead entanglement (4 patients).[50] A study of 23 patients without primary dysfunction of the tricuspid valve in whom an echocardiogram was performed with and without active RV pacing showed worsening of TR with active RV pacing and thus demonstrated a functional cause for lead-associated TR.[51]

Imaging studies are helpful in the evaluation of a patient with clinically suspected lead-associated TR. Although traditional transthoracic and transesophageal echocardiograms may be helpful in the initial assessment, evaluation of TR is limited by acoustic shadowing from the pacemaker lead. However, 3-D echocardiography can be helpful in determining the lead route through the tricuspid valve and cause of TR (Fig. 6.34).[52]

Lead-induced TR can be minimized by the use of smaller diameter leads and alternative lead locations (i.e., CS, RV outflow tract, pericardial). It has been suggested that placing a smaller diameter lead in the commissures of the tricuspid valve will minimize TR. The ability to reliably place a lead in such a way that it will

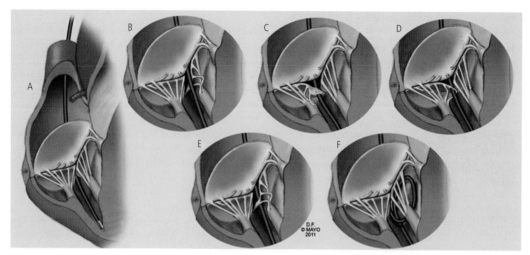

Fig. 6.33 Images of tricuspid valve complications as a result of a right ventricular (RV) pacing lead. (A) Optimal lead position between the septal and posterior leaflets with intact coaptation. (B) RV pacing lead impingement on the septal leaflet causing tricuspid regurgitation (TR). (C) RV pacing lead adhering to the posterior tricuspid leaflet causing TR. (D) RV pacing lead interfering with the tricuspid chordae tendineae causing TR. (E) RV pacing lead perforation through the septal leaflet of tricuspid valve causing TR. (F) A redundant loop of the RV pacing lead between the ventricular septum and septal leaflet of the tricuspid valve resulting in tricuspid stenosis.

securely stay in the commissure, however, is more theoretical than practical. Lead designs that do not cross the tricuspid valve, such as a novel dual-electrode intramyocardial lead, would be ideal for avoiding TR.[53,54]

The treatment for lead-induced TR depends on the associated symptoms and patient-specific factors. Options include lead repositioning, lead removal and placement in an alternative location, and surgical tricuspid valve repair or replacement.

Although rare, lead-associated tricuspid stenosis has also been reported secondary to a subvalvular loop and subsequent adhesion.[55]

Battery depletion

Battery depletion is expected and should not be considered a complication in most patients. Nevertheless, battery depletion is the most common reason for pulse generator removal (see Chapter 10: Troubleshooting; Fig 10.4).[56] If the pulse generator displays end-of-life characteristics earlier than expected, potential problems should be explored. Early battery depletion may be caused by inappropriate programming of unnecessarily high output; excess current drain caused by a loss of lead integrity; or internal current loss because of pulse generator component malfunction. The manufacturer should also be consulted for data on performance of the pulse generator, i.e., pulse generator longevity predicted or observed in other patients.

From a pacemaker registry at 8 years of prospective follow-up, battery depletion was the most common cause of pulse generator removal. Of the pulse generators displaying battery depletion indicators, 95% exhibited normal elective replacement, i.e., >3 years post-implant. In the remaining 5% of patients, depletion occurred at <3 years post-implant and was designated as "severe" battery depletion. These depletions presented primarily as loss of telemetry or no or low output.[56] If battery depletion is advanced, it may not be possible to program the pacemaker (see Chapter 10: Troubleshooting). At other times, attempting to program a pacemaker at an advanced stage of battery depletion may result in sudden complete loss of output (Fig. 6.35).

Implant or hardware-related complications that may result in recurrence of preimplantation symptoms (see also Chapter 10: Troubleshooting)

Loss of circuit integrity

Any abnormality that can permanently or intermittently interrupt the integrity of the pacing circuit can allow recurrent bradycardia and therefore recurrence of symptoms. Likewise, interruption of the circuit in an ICD can result in recurrent bradyarrhythmia or tachyarrhythmia. Circuit interruption in a CRT system

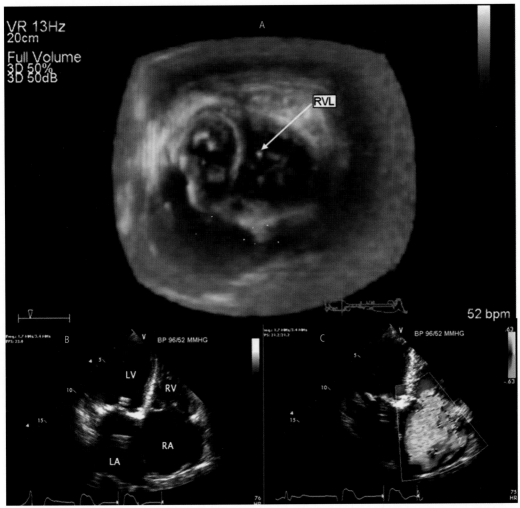

Fig. 6.34 (A) A short-axis 3-D echocardiogram still image of the tricuspid valve apparatus on the right with an arrow pointing to the right ventricular lead (RVL) entering the right ventricle between the septal and anterior cusps. It is impinging on the cusps leading to poor coaptation. (B) A four-chamber 2-D echocardiogram image with the right ventricle on the top right and the right ventricular lead traversing the tricuspid valve with poor coaptation. (C) A Doppler 2-D echocardiogram showing extensive lead-associated tricuspid regurgitation. (Images courtesy of Dr. Grace Lin, Mayo Clinic, Rochester.)

could result in the lack of biventricular pacing and recurrent symptoms. This can occur with fracture of the lead conductor coil, breach of lead insulation, defect in a lead adaptor (Fig. 6.36), or loose connection where the lead pin joins the connector block (Fig. 6.24). Failure of the pacemaker circuitry, which would also allow recurrent bradycardia, is extraordinarily rare unless the pacemaker is exposed to some external source (see Chapter 12: Electromagnetic Interference). For example, exposure to a strong electrical source, such as defibrillation, can result in circuit failure. Design improvements, including bipolar leads and use of bipolar external defibrillators, have reduced the risk of circuit failure with external defibrillation.[57]

A component failure is a diagnosis of exclusion. In this situation, the specific problem may not be clear until the device has been removed, returned to the manufacturer, and subjected to destructive analysis. Determining the cause of system malfunction is discussed extensively in Chapter 10: Troubleshooting.

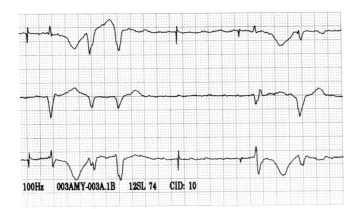

Fig. 6.35 Tracing from a patient with a 10-year-old pacemaker and failure to capture. The pacemaker was nearing total battery depletion and was generating insufficient voltage to maintain capture.

Exposing a pacemaker, ICD, or CRT to therapeutic radiation may also result in unpredictable component failure and a "runaway" or "sudden no output" response (see Chapter 12: Electromagnetic Interference). A pacemaker in or very near the field of therapeutic radiation should be moved to avoid damage to the circuitry and to prevent compromise of the field as defined by the radiation oncologist. This situation is most common in a woman with a breast malignancy on the same side as the pacemaker or ICD. The simplest and least invasive approach is to explant the device, form a new pocket on the contralateral side, and tunnel the leads subcutaneously to the other side. If the leads are not long enough to reach, "lead extenders" can be connected to span the additional distance (Fig. 6.37). Alternatively, the pulse generator could be removed, leads capped, and a new system placed on the contralateral side.

Lead fracture and insulation defect

Lead malfunction resulting from fracture or insulation defect is most commonly seen in the late post-implantation period (Fig. 6.38). Lead fractures most often occur adjacent to the pulse generator or near the site of venous access, i.e., at a stress point, although fracture has also been reported of more distal portions of the pacing lead. Although uncommon, direct trauma may result in damage to the pacing lead. When lead fracture does occur, it is usually necessary to replace the lead. If the fracture is in a bipolar lead and the pacemaker is polarity programmable, it may be possible to restore pacing by reprogramming to the unipolar configuration. This is a short-term solution and should not be a substitute for replacing the lead (Fig. 6.39). In ICDs, lead fractures often manifest as inappropriate shocks due to "make-break" noise at the fracture site detected as ventricular fibrillation.

Polyurethane and silicone are used as insulating materials for most permanent pacing leads. Insulation defects in polyurethane leads have been described at stress points. This occurs most commonly with crush injury, especially at the costoclavicular space after placement by the subclavian puncture technique (Fig. 6.40), and at the site of ligatures, even with a suture sleeve. In bipolar coaxial leads, the insulation defect often occurs internally, in the layer of insulation between coils, rather than externally, on the outer surface.

Exit block

Exit block has been defined in several ways. A commonly accepted clinical definition is high pacing thresholds, often progressive, that cannot be explained by radiographic dislodgement or perforation. (If normal thresholds are achieved and maintained after repositioning of the lead, the term "exit block" does not apply.) In true exit block, stimulation thresholds are often excellent at the time of implantation, but instead of the usual early rise at 3–6 weeks with a subsequent decrease and plateau, the threshold remains high. Exit block is uncommon and appears to represent an abnormality at the myocardial tissue–electrode interface. The cause is controversial. Some believe that the problem is with the lead design, and others that it is intrinsic to the patient's myocardium, resulting in excessive reaction to the electrode. Steroid-eluting leads are often effective in preventing exit block.

With ventricular epicardial or CS pacing leads, exit block and exit delay is more prevalent. Exit block with CS leads often results from the lead pacing near diseased and/or ischemic LV myocardium, resulting in excessive delay from the pacing site despite adequate thresholds. This can result in failure of resynchronization

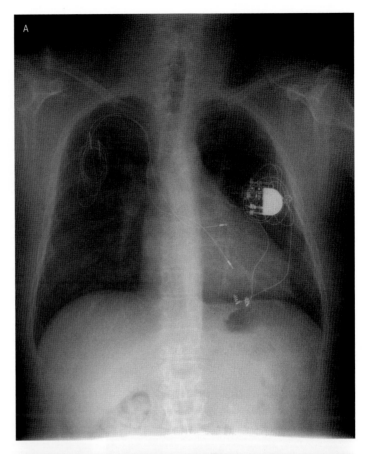

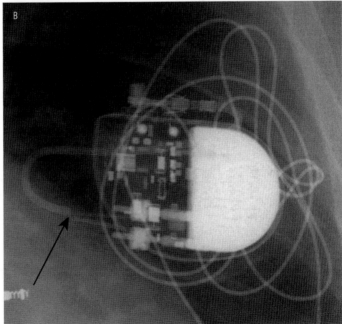

Fig. 6.36 (A) Posteroanterior chest radiograph and (B) close-up from a patient in whom a "Y-adaptor" has been used to adapt two unipolar epicardial leads to an inline bipolar lead. The arrow on the close-up notes a defect (fracture) of the Y-adaptor which led to intermittent failure to pace.

A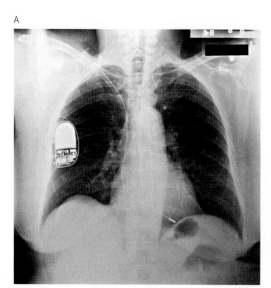

B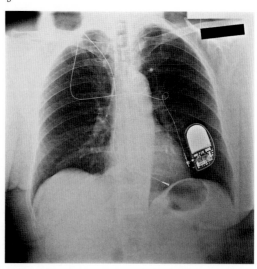

Fig. 6.37 Posteroanterior chest radiographs of a VVIR pacing system. (A) The pacemaker is located in the right prepectoral position. (B) The pacemaker is now located on the left, and the previous wire has been tunneled subcutaneously across the chest. This relocation removed the pacemaker from the field for therapeutic radiation.

A

B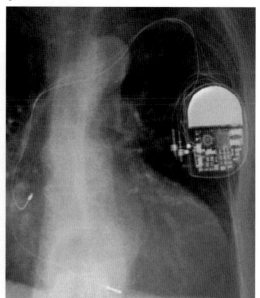

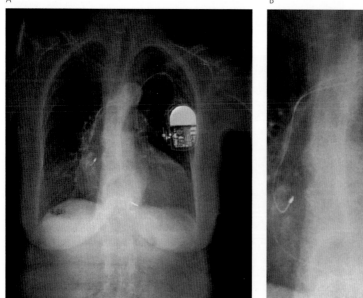

Fig. 6.38 (A) Posteroanterior chest radiograph and (B) close-up view of a fractured atrial lead. What appears to be complete fracture of the conductor coil was accompanied by failure to pace in the atrium. Atrial sensing, however, remained intact. The most likely explanation is that intact insulation and a fluid column between the fractured ends of the conductor coil allowed maintenance of sensing function.

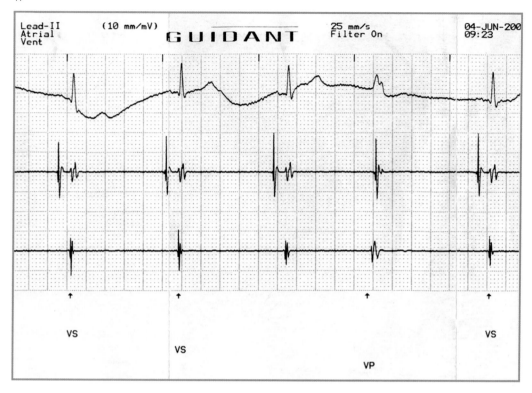

A

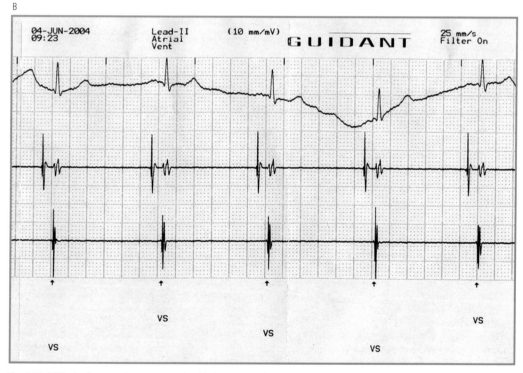

B

Fig. 6.39 (A) Tracing from a patient programmed to bipolar pacing and sensing at a pacing rate of 30 ppm. There is failure to sense of the third ventricular complex. Note that this beat is not labeled by the "marker channel" because it was not sensed. This is the first sign of an insulation effect. (B) The pacemaker is reprogrammed to unipolar pacing and sensing is normal.

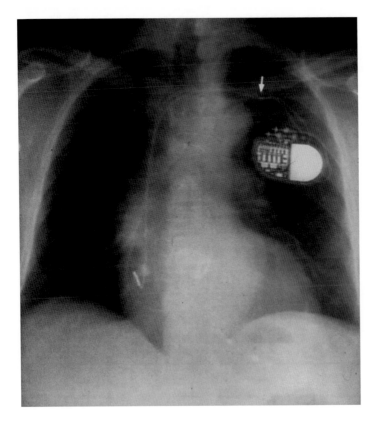

Fig. 6.40 Posteroanterior chest radiograph in a patient with kinking or crushing of the lead as it passes under the clavicle. The patient presented with evidence of lead-insulation failure. Close inspection of the distal tip of the lead identified three poles, and inspection of the connector block of the pulse generator also identified a third port. The third "pole" was required for a special rate-adaptive sensor. (Reproduced with permission from Hayes DL. Radiography of implantable arrhythmia management devices. In: Kusumoto F, Goldschlager N, eds. Cardiac Pacing for the Clinician. New York, NY: Springer Science and Business Media LLC. 2008: 627.)

despite simultaneous biventricular stimulation. When exit delay or block exists, pacing at higher than threshold output, setting an offset for the CS lead to be paced ahead of the RV lead, and possibly varying the pacing vector should be attempted before considering lead revision.

References

1 Link MS, Estes NA 3rd, Griffin JJ, et al. Complications of dual chamber pacemaker implantation in the elderly. Pacemaker Selection in the Elderly (PASE) Investigators. J Interv Card Electrophysiol 1998; 2:175–9.

2 Poole JE, Gleva MJ, Mela T, et al. Complication rates associated with pacemaker or implantable cardioverter-defibrillator generator replacements and upgrade procedures: results from the REPLACE registry. Circulation 2010; 122:1553–61.

3 Zoppo F, Zerbo F, Brandolino G, Bacchiega E, Lupo A, Bertaglia E. Straight screw-in atrial leads "j-post shaped" in right appendage versus j-shaped systems for permanent atrial pacing: a safety comparison. Pacing Clin Electrophysiol 2011; 34:325–30.

4 Luria D, Bar-Lev D, Gurevitz O, et al. Long-term performance of screw-in atrial pacing leads: a randomized com-

parison of J-shaped and straight leads. Pacing Clin Electrophysiol 2005; 28:898–902.

5 Luria DM, Feinberg MS, Gurevitz OT, et al. Randomized comparison of J-shaped atrial leads with and without active fixation mechanism. Pacing Clin Electrophysiol 2007; 30:412–7.

6 Crossley GH, Exner D, Mead RH, et al. Chronic performance of an active fixation coronary sinus lead. Heart Rhythm 2010; 7:472-8.

7 Resynchronization therapy for heart failure. (Accessed July 17, 2011, at http://www.hrsonline.org/ClinicalGuidance/upload/resynch_therapy_HF.pdf)

8 van Rees JB, de Bie MK, Thijssen J, Borleffs CJ, Schalij MJ, van Erven L. Implantation-related complications of implantable cardioverter-defibrillators and cardiac resynchronization therapy devices a systematic review of randomized clinical trials. J Am Coll Cardiol 2011; 58:995–1000.

9 Trigano AJ, Taramasco V, Paganelli F, Gerard R, Levy S. Incidence of perforation and other mechanical complications during dual active fixation. Pacing Clin Electrophysiol 1996; 19:1828–31.

10 Higano ST, Hayes DL, Spittell PC. Facilitation of the subclavian-introducer technique with contrast venography. Pacing Clin Electrophysiol 1990; 13:681–4.

11 Tester GA, Noheria A, Carrico HL, *et al.* Impact of radiocontrast use during left ventricular pacemaker lead implantation for cardiac resynchronization therapy. Europace 2012; 14:243–8.

12 Mahapatra S, Bybee KA, Bunch TJ, *et al.* Incidence and predictors of cardiac perforation after permanent pacemaker placement. Heart Rhythm 2005; 2:907–11.

13 Henrikson CA, Leng CT, Yuh DD, Brinker JA. Computed tomography to assess possible cardiac lead perforation. Pacing Clin Electrophysiol 2006; 29:509–11.

14 Hirschl DA, Jain VR, Spindola-Franco H, Gross JN, Haramati LB. Prevalence and characterization of asymptomatic pacemaker and ICD lead perforation on CT. Pacing Clin Electrophysiol 2007; 30:28–32.

15 Ishikawa K, Chida K, Taniguchi T, *et al.* Myocardial perforation and/or penetration by a permanent endocardial electrode of the pacemaker in autopsy cases. J Arrhythmia 1999; 15:39–44.

16 Khan MN, Joseph G, Khaykin Y, Ziada KM, Wilkoff BL. Delayed lead perforation: a disturbing trend. Pacing Clin Electrophysiol 2005; 28:251–3.

17 Refaat MM, Hashash JG, Shalaby AA. Late perforation by cardiac implantable electronic device leads: clinical presentation, diagnostic clues, and management. Clin Cardiol 33:466–75.

18 Laborderie J, Barandon L, Ploux S, *et al.* Management of subacute and delayed right ventricular perforation with a pacing or an implantable cardioverter-defibrillator lead. Am J Cardiol 2008; 102:1352–5.

19 Sivakumaran S, Irwin ME, Gulamhusein SS, Senaratne MP. Postpacemaker implant pericarditis: incidence and outcomes with active-fixation leads. Pacing Clin Electrophysiol 2002; 25:833–7.

20 Levy Y, Shovman O, Granit C, *et al.* Pericarditis following permanent pacemaker insertion. Isr Med Assoc J 2004; 6:599–602.

21 Fuster V, Ryden LE, Cannom DS, *et al.* ACC/AHA/ESC 2006 Guidelines for the Management of Patients with Atrial Fibrillation: a report of the American College of Cardiology/American Heart Association Task Force on Practice Guidelines and the European Society of Cardiology Committee for Practice Guidelines (Writing Committee to Revise the 2001 Guidelines for the Management of Patients With Atrial Fibrillation): developed in collaboration with the European Heart Rhythm Association and the Heart Rhythm Society. Circulation 2006; 114:e257–354.

22 Kutinsky IB, Jarandilla R, Jewett M, Haines DE. Risk of hematoma complications after device implant in the clopidogrel era. Circ Arrhythm Electrophysiol 2010; 3:312–8.

23 Tompkins C, Cheng A, Dalal D, *et al.* Dual antiplatelet therapy and heparin "bridging" significantly increase the risk of bleeding complications after pacemaker or implantable cardioverter-defibrillator device implantation. J Am Coll Cardiol 2010; 55:2376–82.

24 Wiegand UK, LeJeune D, Boguschewski F, *et al.* Pocket hematoma after pacemaker or implantable cardioverter defibrillator surgery: influence of patient morbidity, operation strategy, and perioperative antiplatelet/anticoagulation therapy. Chest 2004; 126:1177–86.

25 Tompkins C, McLean R, Cheng A, *et al.* End-stage renal disease predicts complications in pacemaker and ICD implants. J Cardiovasc Electrophysiol 2011; 22:1099–104.

26 Tischenko A, Gula LJ, Yee R, Klein GJ, Skanes AC, Krahn AD. Implantation of cardiac rhythm devices without interruption of oral anticoagulation compared with perioperative bridging with low-molecular weight heparin. Am Heart J 2009; 158:252–6.

27 Ahmed I, Gertner E, Nelson WB, *et al.* Continuing warfarin therapy is superior to interrupting warfarin with or without bridging anticoagulation therapy in patients undergoing pacemaker and defibrillator implantation. Heart Rhythm 2010; 7:745–9.

28 Li HK, Chen FC, Rea RF, *et al.* No increased bleeding events with continuation of oral anticoagulation therapy for patients undergoing cardiac device procedure. Pacing Clin Electrophysiol 2011; 34:868–74.

29 Ghanbari H, Feldman D, Schmidt M, *et al.* Cardiac resynchronization therapy device implantation in patients with therapeutic international normalized ratios. Pacing Clin Electrophysiol 2010; 33:400–6.

30 Gadhoke A, Roth JA. Retromammary implantation of an ICD using a single lead system: an alternative approach to pectoral implantation in women. Pacing Clin Electrophysiol 1997; 20:128–9.

31 McManus DD, Mattei ML, Rose K, Rashkin J, Rosenthal LS. Inadvertent lead placement in the left ventricle: a case report and brief review. Indian Pacing Electrophysiol J 2009; 9:224–8.

32 Spittell PC, Hayes DL. Venous complications after insertion of a transvenous pacemaker. Mayo Clin Proc 1992; 67:258–65.

33 Barakat K, Robinson NM, Spurrell RA. Transvenous pacing lead-induced thrombosis: a series of cases with a review of the literature. Cardiology 2000; 93:142–8.

34 Worley SJ, Gohn DC, Pulliam RW, Raifsnider MA, Ebersole BI, Tuzi J. Subclavian venoplasty by the implanting physicians in 373 patients over 11 years. Heart Rhythm 2011; 8:526–33.

35 Spittell PC, Vlietstra RE, Hayes DL, Higano ST. Venous obstruction due to permanent transvenous pacemaker electrodes: treatment with percutaneous transluminal balloon venoplasty. Pacing Clin Electrophysiol 1990; 13:271–4.

36 Worley S, Ellenbogen KA. Application of interventional procedures adapted for device implantation: new opportunities for device implanters. Pacing Clin Electrophysiol 2007; 30:938–41.

37 Hirsh J, Guyatt G, Albers GW, Harrington R, Schunemann HJ. Executive summary: American College of Chest Physicians Evidence-Based Clinical Practice Guidelines, 8th edn. Chest 2008; 133:71S–109S.

38 Baddour LM, Epstein AE, Erickson CC, *et al.* Update on cardiovascular implantable electronic device infections and their management: a scientific statement from the American Heart Association. Circulation 2010; 121:458–77.

39 Sohail MR, Uslan DZ, Khan AH, *et al.* Risk factor analysis of permanent pacemaker infection. Clin Infect Dis 2007; 45:166–73.

40 Sohail MR, Uslan DZ, Khan AH, *et al.* Management and outcome of permanent pacemaker and implantable cardioverter-defibrillator infections. J Am Coll Cardiol 2007; 49:1851–9.

41 Suga C, Hayes DL, Hyberger LK, Lloyd MA. Is there an adverse outcome from abandoned pacing leads? J Interv Card Electrophysiol 2000; 4:493–9.

42. Silvetti MS, Drago F. Outcome of young patients with abandoned, nonfunctional endocardial leads. Pacing Clin Electrophysiol 2008; 31:473–9.

43 Furman S, Behrens M, Andrews C, Klementowicz P. Retained pacemaker leads. J Thoracic Cardiovasc Surg 1987; 94:770–2.

44 Martin ML GM, Hodge DO, *et al.* Do abandoned leads pose risk to implantable defibrillator patients? J Am Coll Cardiol 2004; 43(Suppl. A):140A.

45 Gurevitz O, Nof E, Carasso S, *et al.* Programmable multiple pacing configurations help to overcome high left ventricular pacing thresholds and avoid phrenic nerve stimulation. Pacing Clin Electrophysiol 2005; 28:1255–9.

46 Leibowitz DW, Rosenheck S, Pollak A, Geist M, Gilon D. Transvenous pacemaker leads do not worsen tricuspid regurgitation: a prospective echocardiographic study. Cardiology 2000; 93:74–7.

47 Kucukarslan N, Kirilmaz A, Ulusoy E, *et al.* Tricuspid insufficiency does not increase early after permanent implantation of pacemaker leads. J Cardiac Surg 2006; 21:391–4.

48 Kim JB, Spevack DM, Tunick PA, *et al.* The effect of transvenous pacemaker and implantable cardioverter defibrillator lead placement on tricuspid valve function: an observational study. J Am Soc Echocardiogr 2008; 21: 284–7.

49 Klutstein M, Balkin J, Butnaru A, Ilan M, Lahad A, Rosenmann D. Tricuspid incompetence following permanent pacemaker implantation. Pacing Clin Electrophysiol 2009; 32(Suppl 1):S135–7.

50 Lin G, Nishimura RA, Connolly HM, Dearani JA, Sundt TM 3rd, Hayes DL. Severe symptomatic tricuspid valve regurgitation due to permanent pacemaker or implantable cardioverter-defibrillator leads. J Am Coll Cardiol 2005; 45:1672–5.

51 Vaturi M, Kusniec J, Shapira Y, *et al.* Right ventricular pacing increases tricuspid regurgitation grade regardless of the mechanical interference to the valve by the electrode. Eur J Echocardiogr 2010; 11:550–3.

52 Seo Y, Ishizu T, Nakajima H, Sekiguchi Y, Watanabe S, Aonuma K. Clinical utility of 3-dimensional echocardiography in the evaluation of tricuspid regurgitation caused by pacemaker leads. Circ J 2008; 72:1465–70.

53 Asirvatham SJ, Bruce CJ, Danielsen A, *et al.* Intramyocardial pacing and sensing for the enhancement of cardiac stimulation and sensing specificity. Pacing Clin Electrophysiol 2007; 30:748–54.

54 Henz BD, Friedman PA, Bruce CJ, *et al.* Synchronous ventricular pacing without crossing the tricuspid valve or entering the coronary sinus: preliminary results. J Cardiovasc Electrophysiol 2009; 20:1391–7.

55 Taira K, Suzuki A, Fujino A, Watanabe T, Ogyu A, Ashikawa K. Tricuspid valve stenosis related to subvalvular adhesion of pacemaker lead: a case report. J Cardiol 2006; 47: 301–6.

56 Hauser RG, Hayes DL, Kallinen LM, *et al.* Clinical experience with pacemaker pulse generators and transvenous leads: an 8-year prospective multicenter study. Heart Rhythm 2007; 4:154–60.

57 Gammage MD. External cardioversion in patients with implanted cardiac devices: is there a problem? Eur Heart J 2007; 28:1668–9.

7 Timing Cycles

David L. Hayes[1], Paul J. Wang[2], Samuel J. Asirvatham[1], Paul A. Friedman[1]

[1]Mayo Clinic, Rochester, MN, USA

[2]Stanford School of Medicine, Stanford University, Stanford, CA, USA

Basic approach 256
Pacing modes 257
  Ventricular asynchronous pacing, atrial asynchronous pacing, and atrioventricular sequential asynchronous pacing 257
  Ventricular inhibited pacing 257
Atrial inhibited pacing 257
Single-chamber triggered-mode pacing 259
Rate-modulated pacing 259
  Single-chamber rate-modulated pacing 259
  Rate-modulated asynchronous pacing 261
Atrioventricular sequential, ventricular inhibited pacing (DVI) 261
Atrioventricular sequential, non-P-synchronous pacing with dual-chamber sensing (DDI) 261
Atrioventricular sequential, non-P-synchronous, rate-modulated pacing with dual-chamber sensing (DDIR) 262
Atrial synchronous (P-tracking/P-synchronous) pacing (VDD) 262
Dual-chamber pacing and sensing with inhibition and tracking (DDD) 262
Portions of pacemaker timing cycles 264
Atrioventricular interval 264
  Differential atrioventricular interval 268
  Rate-variable or rate-adaptive atrioventricular interval 268
  Atrioventricular interval hysteresis 268
Comparison of atrial with ventricular-based timing 268
Dual-chamber rate-modulated pacemakers: effect on timing cycles 272
Mode switching 276
Avoiding atrial pace/sense competition 276
Timing components of ventricular avoidance pacing algorithms 278
  Managed Ventricular Pacing (MVP)™ Medtronic, Inc. 279
  SafeR™, Sorin Medical 279

Endless-loop tachycardia 279
Timing cycles with algorithms responding to sudden bradycardia 280
Timing cycles unique to biventricular pacing 281
  Achieving consistent biventricular pacing 281
  Cardiac resynchronization therapy lower rate behavior 284
  Univentricular sensing and biventricular pacing 284
  Upper rate behavior in biventricular pacing 285
  Premature beats and biventricular timing cycles 286
  Refractory periods and biventricular pacing 286
Timing cycles in ICDs 287
Initial electrocardiographic interpretation 288
Response to magnet application 289
Single-chamber pacemakers 291
Dual-chamber pacemakers 292
  Atrioventricular interval 292
  Upper rate behavior 295
  Rate smoothing 295
    Ventricular rate regularization 295
  Fallback 296
Biventricular paced electrocardiogram: position, adequacy, and timing 296
  Assessing pacemaker lead position 298
  The cardiac vector principle 298
  The left lateral leads 298
  Right-sided leads 298
  Anterior/posteroinferior leads 298
  Base vs. apex 298
Characteristic electrocardiographic patterns with specific lead locations 299
  Right ventricular apical pacing 299
  Nonapical right ventricular site pacing 300
  Left ventricular lateral wall pacing – the "ideal" pacing location 300
  Anterior and posterior left ventricular pacing 300
  Biventricular paced ECG 300

Cardiac Pacing, Defibrillation and Resynchronization: A Clinical Approach, Third Edition.
David L. Hayes, Samuel J. Asirvatham, and Paul A. Friedman.
© 2013 Mayo Foundation for Medical Education and Research. Published 2013 by John Wiley & Sons, Ltd.

Timing intervals and the ECG 302
    Capture latency and the stimulus–QRS interval 303
    Clues to electrical resynchronization from the
        12-lead ECG 304
        QRS duration 304
        QRS vector fusion 304
        V-V interval 305
    Atrioventricular interval programming 307

Electrocardiographic considerations in the patient
    not responding to CRT 316
    Inappropriate lack of left ventricular pacing 316
    Anodal stimulation 316
    Ventricular ectopy 316
Conclusions 316
References 316

An understanding of the basic concepts of cardiac pacing (see Chapter 1: Pacing and Defibrillation) and comprehension of the pacemaker timing cycles of cardiac pacing are important as one approaches the paced electrocardiogram (ECG). The first portion of this chapter provides a detailed description of "timing cycles" and approaches the subject by pacing mode and descriptions of other features that are used with some frequency that can alter the timing cycle. The second portion of the chapter outlines assessment of the paced ECG.

Basic approach

Paced electrocardiography must be approached systematically, much as nonpaced electrocardiography, chest radiography, or any other diagnostic procedure. Knowing the type of pacemaker, the programmed parameters, and the underlying rhythm necessitating pacing is important in interpreting the paced ECG. Obviously, this information makes the interpretation much easier, but it is frequently not available.

A sensed event occurs when a pacemaker registers activity deemed to be electrical cardiac events; a paced event occurs when the pulse generator delivers current to stimulate the heart. Paced events are followed by blanking periods, during which amplifiers are switched off and no electrical activity is registered. Blanking periods are followed by refractory periods, during which cardiac electrical activity is normally sensed, but the response of the device to the event is limited. For example, atrial events occurring during an atrial refractory period will not be tracked (i.e., followed by a ventricular paced event), but are used to determine whether mode switching should occur. Blanking and refractory periods serve to prevent oversensing of physiologic signals (such as T waves) and cross-chamber sensing. There is some variation among manufacturers as to how blanking and refractory periods are defined and implemented; their role in timing cycles is discussed further below. In defibrillators and in mode switch operation in

pacemakers, a series of sensed events augment counters, leading to arrhythmia detection, which may then result in therapy delivery or mode switch. Defibrillator sensing and detection are discussed in greater detail in Chapter 8: Programming.

Pacemaker timing cycles include all potential variations of a single complete pacing cycle (Table 7.1). This could mean the time from paced ventricular beat to paced ventricular beat (VV); from paced ventricular beat to an intrinsic ventricular beat (VR), whether it be a conducted R wave or a premature ventricular contraction; from paced atrial beat to paced atrial beat (AA); from intrinsic atrial beat to paced atrial beat (PA); and so forth. Various aspects of each of these cycles include

Table 7.1 Abbreviations for native and paced events and portions of the timing cycle.

P	Native atrial depolarization
A	Atrial paced event
R	Native ventricular depolarization
V	Ventricular paced event
I	Interval
AV	Sequential pacing in the atrium and ventricle
AVI	Programmed atrioventricular pacing interval
AR	Atrial paced event followed by intrinsic ventricular depolarization
ARP	Atrial refractory period
PV	Native atrial depolarization followed by a paced ventricular event, P synchronous pacing
LRL	Lower rate limit
URL	Upper rate limit
MTR	Maximum tracking rate
MSR	Maximum sensor rate
PVARP	Post-ventricular atrial refractory period
RRAVD	Rate-responsive atrioventricular delay
VA interval	Interval from a ventricular sensed or paced event to an atrial paced event
VRP	Ventricular refractory period

events sensed, events paced, and periods when the sensing circuit or circuits are refractory or blanked. Each portion of the pacemaker timing cycle should be considered in milliseconds (ms) and not in paced beats per minute (ppm). Although it may be easier to think of the patient's pacing rate in paced beats per minute, portions of the timing cycle are too brief to be considered in any unit but milliseconds.

If one knows the relationship between the various elements of the paced ECG, understanding pacemaker rhythms becomes less complicated. Although a native rhythm may be affected by multiple unknown factors, each timing circuit of a pacemaker can function in only one of two states. A given timer can proceed until it completes its cycle; completion results in either the release of a pacing stimulus or the initiation of another timing cycle. Alternatively, a given timer can be reset by a sensed event, at which point it reinitiates the timing cycle.

Pacing modes

Ventricular asynchronous pacing, atrial asynchronous pacing, and atrioventricular sequential asynchronous pacing

Ventricular asynchronous (VOO) pacing is the simplest of all pacing modes, because there is no sensing and no mode of response. The timing cycle is shown in Fig. 7.1. Irrespective of any other events, the ventricular pacing artifacts occur at the programmed rate. The timing cycle cannot be reset by any intrinsic event. Without sensing, there is no defined refractory period. Atrial asynchronous (AOO) pacing behaves exactly like VOO except that the pacing artifacts occur in the atrial chamber.

Dual-chamber, or atrioventricular (AV) sequential asynchronous (DOO), pacing has an equally simple timing cycle. The interval from atrial artifact to ventricular artifact (atrioventricular interval [AVI]) and the interval from the ventricular artifact to the subsequent atrial pacing artifact (ventriculoatrial, or atrial escape, interval [VA interval]) are fixed. The intervals never change, because the pacing mode is insensitive to any atrial or ventricular activity, and the timers are never reset (Fig. 7.2).

Ventricular inhibited pacing

By definition, ventricular inhibited (VVI) pacing (also referred to as inhibited demand pacing) incorporates sensing on the ventricular channel, and pacemaker output is inhibited by a sensed ventricular event (Fig. 7.3). VVI pacemakers are refractory for a period after a paced or sensed ventricular event, the ventricular refractory period (VRP). Ventricular events occurring within the VRP do not reset the ventricular timer (Fig. 7.4). (Every pacemaker capable of sensing and all defibrillators must include a refractory period in their basic timing cycles. Refractory periods prevent the sensing of early inappropriate signals, such as the evoked potential and repolarization [T wave].)

Atrial inhibited pacing

Atrial inhibited (AAI) pacing, the atrial counterpart of VVI pacing, incorporates the same timing cycles, with the obvious difference that pacing and sensing occur from the atrium and pacemaker output is inhibited by a sensed atrial event (Fig. 7.5). An atrial paced or sensed event initiates a refractory period during which electrical signals are ignored by the pacemaker. Because we are most accustomed to devices with ventricular sensing, confusion can arise when ventricular events are appropriately ignored [not seen] in the AAI/AAIR pacing mode. For example, in addition to the intrinsic QRS that follows a paced atrial beat, if a premature ventricular beat occurs, it does not inhibit an atrial

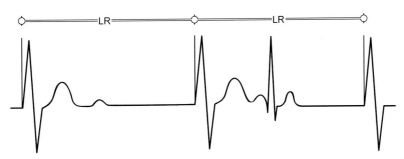

Fig. 7.1 The VOO timing cycle consists of only a defined rate. The pacemaker delivers a ventricular pacing artifact at the defined rate regardless of intrinsic events. In this example, an intrinsic QRS complex occurs after the second paced complex, but because there is no sensing in the VOO mode, the interval between the second and the third paced complex remains stable. LR, lower rate (limit).

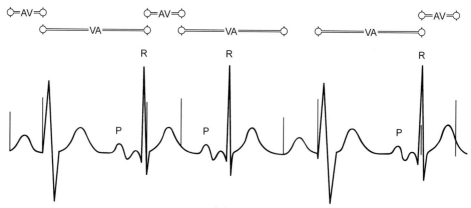

Fig. 7.2 The DOO timing cycle consists of only defined atrioventricular (AV) and VV intervals. The ventriculoatrial (VA) interval is a function of the AV and VV intervals. An atrial pacing artifact is delivered, and the ventricular artifact follows at the programmed AV interval. The next atrial pacing artifact is delivered at the completion of the VA interval. There is no variation in the intervals because no activity is sensed, i.e., nothing interrupts or resets the programmed cycles. (From Hayes DL, Levine PA: Pacemaker timing cycles. In Cardiac Pacing, Ellenbogen KA, ed. Boston, Blackwell Scientific Publications, 1992: 263–308.)

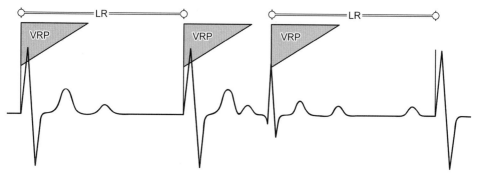

Fig. 7.3 The VVI timing cycle consists of a defined lower rate (LR) limit and a ventricular refractory period (VRP, represented by triangle). When the LR limit timer is complete, a pacing artifact is delivered in the absence of a sensed intrinsic ventricular event. If an intrinsic QRS occurs, the LR limit timer is started from that point. A VRP begins with any sensed or paced ventricular activity.

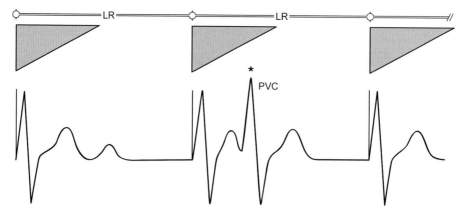

Fig. 7.4 If, in the VVI mode, an intrinsic ventricular event (*) occurs during the ventricular refractory period (VRP, represented by triangle), it is not sensed and therefore does not reset the lower rate (LR) limit timer. PVC, premature ventricular contraction.

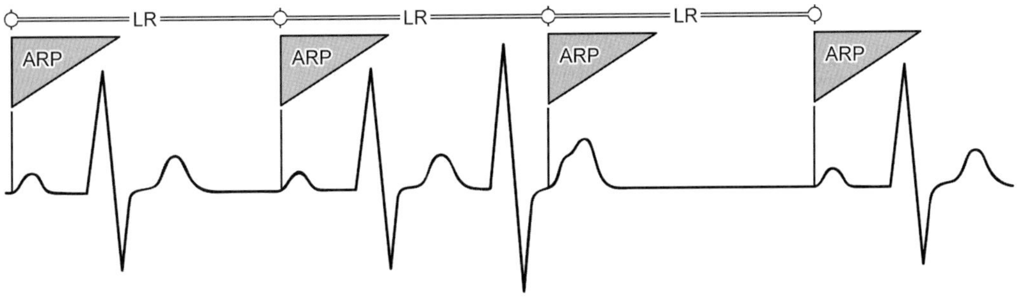

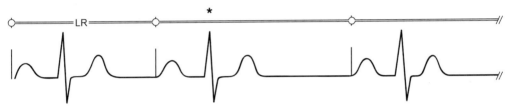

Fig. 7.5 The AAI timing cycle consists of a defined lower rate (LR) limit and an atrial refractory period (ARP). When the LR limit timer is complete, a pacing artifact is delivered in the atrium in the absence of a sensed atrial event. If an intrinsic P wave occurs, the LR limit timer is started from that point. An ARP begins with any sensed or paced atrial activity. In the AAI mode, only atrial activity is sensed. In this example, it may appear unusual for paced atrial activity to occur so soon after intrinsic ventricular activity. Because sensing occurs only in the atrium, ventricular activity would not be expected to reset the pacemaker's timing cycle.

Fig. 7.6 In this example of AAI pacing, the AA interval is 1000 ms (60 ppm). The interval between the second and the third paced atrial events exceeds 1000 ms. The interval from the second QRS complex to the subsequent atrial pacing artifact is 1000 ms. This occurs because the second QRS complex (*) has been sensed on the atrial lead (far-field sensing) and has inappropriately reset the timing cycle. LR, lower rate (limit).

pacing artifact from being delivered. When the AA timing cycle ends, the atrial pacing artifact is delivered regardless of ventricular events, because an AAI pacemaker should not sense anything in the ventricle. If a ventricular event is large enough that it is inappropriately sensed on the atrial lead, the event is termed far-field sensing (Fig. 7.6). In this situation, the atrial timing cycle is reset, leading to a pacing rate slower than the programmed lower rate limit (Fig. 7.6). Sometimes this anomaly can be corrected by making the atrial channel less sensitive or by lengthening the refractory period. Interpretation can be made easier in some devices when a programmable ADI mode is available. This mode is operationally the same as AAI pacing mode, but ventricular events are recorded on the diagnostic channels (Fig. 7.7).

Single-chamber triggered-mode pacing
Initially developed as a way to defeat the problem associated with oversensing in the inhibited demand mode,

the single-chamber triggered mode (AAT, VVT) has its own unique advantages as well as disadvantages. In single-chamber triggered-mode pacing, the pacemaker releases an output pulse every time a native event is sensed (Fig. 7.8). This feature increases the current drain on the battery, accelerating its rate of depletion. This mode of pacing also deforms the intrinsic depolarization, compromising interpretation of the ECG. However, it can serve as an excellent marker for the site of sensing within a complex. It can also prevent inappropriate inhibition from oversensing when the patient does not have a stable native escape rhythm.

Rate-modulated pacing

Single-chamber rate-modulated pacing
Single-chamber pacemakers capable of rate-modulated (SSIR) pacing can be implanted in the ventricle (VVIR) or atrium (AAIR). The timing cycles for SSIR pacemakers are not significantly different from those of their non-rate-modulated counterparts. The timing cycle

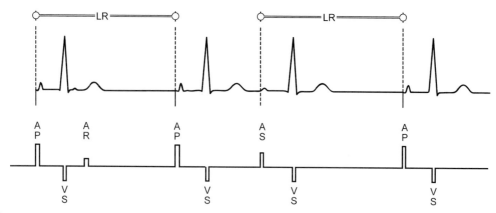

Fig. 7.7 Although an AAI pacemaker is incapable of responding to ventricular events, interpretation is easier if the ventricular events are identified. One manufacturer has a programmable ADI mode in dual-chamber pacemakers. This mode is operationally the same as AAI, but events sensed in the ventricle are recorded on the diagnostics. (Reproduced with permission from Medtronic Adapta Technical Manual.)

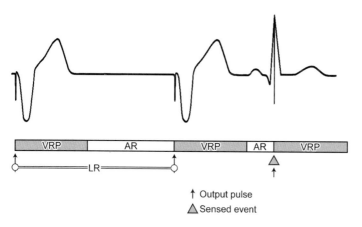

↑ Output pulse
△ Sensed event

Fig. 7.8 In the VVT mode, when an intrinsic atrial event occurs a pacing artifact is delivered at the point of sensing (TP). If the lower rate limit timer is completed, a pacing artifact is delivered with paced depolarization.

includes the basic VV or AA interval and a refractory period from the paced or sensed event. The difference lies in the variability of the VV or AA interval (Fig. 7.9). Depending on the sensor incorporated and the level of exertion of the patient, the basic interval shortens from the programmed lower rate limit (LRL). An upper rate limit (URL) must be programmed to define the absolute shortest cycle length allowable. Some SSIR pacemakers incorporate a fixed refractory period; that is, regardless of whether the pacemaker is operating at the LRL or URL, the refractory period remains the same. Thus, at the higher rates under sensor drive, the pacemaker may effectively become asynchronous, i.e., SOOR, because the period during which sensing can occur is so abbreviated. Native beats falling during the refractory period do not reset timing cycles.

In the VVIR pacing mode the refractory period should be programmed to a short interval to maximize the sensing interval at both the low and high sensor-driven rates. In an AAIR pacing mode, the refractory period should be programmed long enough to avoid far-field sensing and short enough to allow sensing of native atrial events at rates up to the programmed upper sensor rate. Rate-variable or rate-adaptive refractory period as a programmable option, i.e., as the cycle length shortens, the refractory period shortens appropriately, analogous to the QT interval of the native ventricular depolarization, is often available.

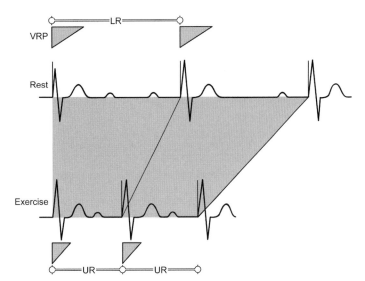

Fig. 7.9 The VVIR timing cycle consists of a lower rate (LR) limit, an upper rate (UR) limit, and a ventricular refractory period (VRP, represented by triangle). As indicated by sensor activity, the VV cycle length shortens accordingly. (The shaded area represents the range of sensor driven VV cycle lengths.) In some VVIR pacemakers, the VRP remains fixed despite the changing VV cycle length and in others the VRP shortens as the cycle length shortens.

Rate-modulated asynchronous pacing

If rate modulation is incorporated in an asynchronous pacing mode, the basic cycle length is altered by sensor activity. In the single-chamber rate-modulated asynchronous (AOOR and VOOR) pacing modes, any alteration in cycle length is due to sensor activity and not to the sensing of intrinsic cardiac depolarizations. In the dual-chamber rate-modulated asynchronous (DOOR) pacing mode, the pacing rate changes in response to the sensor input signal, but not to the native P or R wave.

Atrioventricular sequential, ventricular inhibited pacing (DVI)

AV sequential, ventricular inhibited (DVI) pacing is rarely used as the programmed pacing mode of choice, but remains a programmable option in some pacemakers. It is helpful to understand the timing cycles for DVI pacing.

By definition, DVI provides pacing in both the atrium and the ventricle (D), but sensing only in the ventricle (V). The pacemaker is inhibited and reset by sensed ventricular activity but ignores all intrinsic atrial complexes.

The timing cycle (VV) consists of the AVI and the VA interval. The basic cycle length (VV), or LRL, is programmable, as is the AVI. The difference, VV − AV, is the VA interval. During the initial portion of the VA interval, the sensing channel is refractory. After the refractory period, the ventricular sensing channel is again operational, or "alert." If ventricular activity is not sensed by the expiration of the VA interval, atrial pacing occurs, followed by the AVI. If intrinsic ventricular activity occurs before the VA interval is completed, the timing cycle is reset.

Atrioventricular sequential, non-P-synchronous pacing with dual-chamber sensing (DDI)

AV sequential pacing with dual-chamber sensing, non-P-synchronous (DDI) pacing can be thought of as DDD pacing without atrial tracking. As opposed to the DVI mode just described, DDI incorporates atrial sensing as well as ventricular sensing, which prevents competitive atrial pacing. The DDI mode of response in the atrium is inhibition only; that is, no tracking of P waves can occur. Therefore, the paced ventricular rate cannot be greater than the programmed LRL in the non-rate-adaptive mode. (In the DDI mode there is only one programmable rate; in the DDIR mode there would be, by definition for any sensor-driven mode, a lower rate limit and an upper sensor rate.) The timing cycle consists of the LRL, AVI, post-ventricular atrial refractory period (PVARP), and VRP. The PVARP is the period after a sensed or paced ventricular event during which the atrial sensing circuit is refractory. Any atrial event occurring during the PVARP will not reset timing cycles. If a P wave occurs after the PVARP and is sensed, the subsequent ventricular pacing artifact cannot occur until the VV interval has been completed; i.e., the LRL cannot be violated (Fig. 7.10).

It bears repeating that because P wave tracking does not occur with the DDI mode, the paced rate is never greater than the programmed base rate (i.e., the LRL). A slight exception to this statement may occur, depending on the timing system incorporated in

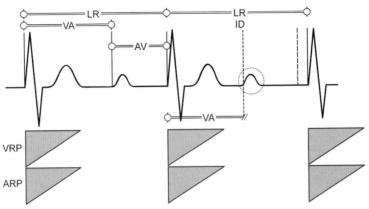

Fig. 7.10 The timing cycle in DDI consists of a lower rate (LR) limit, an atrioventricular (AV) interval, a ventricular refractory period (VRP), and an atrial refractory period (ARP). The VRP is initiated by any sensed or paced ventricular activity, and the ARP is initiated by any sensed or paced atrial activity. DDI can be thought of as DDD pacing without the capability of P wave tracking or DVI without the potential for atrial competition by virtue of atrial sensing. The LR limit cannot be violated even if the sinus rate is occurring at a faster rate. For example, the LR limit is 1000 ms, or 60 ppm, and the AV interval is 200 ms. If a P wave occurs 500 ms after a paced ventricular complex, the AV interval is initiated; but at the end of the AV interval, 700 ms from the previous paced ventricular activity, a ventricular pacing artifact cannot be delivered, because it would violate the LR limit. ID, intrinsic deflection; UR, upper rate (limit); VA, ventriculoatrial (interval).

the pulse generator, when an intrinsic ventricular complex takes place after the paced atrial beat (AR) and inhibits paced ventricular output before completion of the programmed AVI; i.e., AR < AV. In this situation, the cycle length from A to A is shorter than the programmed LRL by the difference between the AR and the programmed AVI.

Atrioventricular sequential, non-P-synchronous, rate-modulated pacing with dual-chamber sensing (DDIR)

The timing cycles for non-P-synchronous, rate-modulated AV sequential (DDIR) pacing are the same as those described above for DDI pacing, except that paced rates can exceed the programmed LRL through sensor-driven activity.

Atrial synchronous (P-tracking/P-synchronous) pacing (VDD)

Atrial synchronous (P-tracking/P-synchronous) (VDD) pacemakers pace only in the ventricle (V), sense in both atrium and ventricle (D), and respond both (D) by inhibition of ventricular output by intrinsic ventricular activity (I) and by ventricular tracking of P waves (T). The VDD mode is available as a single-lead pacing system. In this system, a single lead is capable of pacing in the ventricle in response to sensing atrial activity by way of a remote electrode(s) situated on the

intra-atrial portion of the ventricular pacing lead. (Single-lead VDD systems are not commonly used.)

The timing cycle is composed of LRL, AVI, PVARP, VRP, and URL. A sensed atrial event initiates the AVI. If an intrinsic ventricular event occurs before the termination of the AVI, ventricular output is inhibited and the LRL timing cycle is reset. If a paced ventricular beat occurs at the end of the AVI, this beat resets the LRL. If no atrial event occurs, the pacemaker escapes with a paced ventricular event at the LRL; i.e., the pacemaker displays VVI activity in the absence of a sensed atrial event (Fig. 7.11).

Dual-chamber pacing and sensing with inhibition and tracking (DDD)

Although it involves more timers, standard dual-chamber pacing and sensing with inhibition and tracking (DDD) is reasonably easy to comprehend if one understands the timing cycles already discussed. The basic timing circuit associated with LRL pacing is divided into two sections. The first is the interval from a ventricular sensed or paced event to an atrial event. This is the VA interval. The second interval begins with an atrial sensed or paced event and extends to a ventricular event. This interval may be defined as paced in both chambers (AV), intrinsic in both chambers (PR), atrial paced/ventricular intrinsic (AR), or intrinsic atrial/paced ventricular (PV). A sensed atrial event that

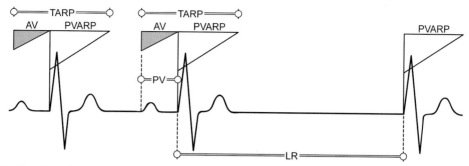

Fig. 7.11 The timing cycle of VDD consists of a lower rate (LR) limit, an atrioventricular interval (AV), a ventricular refractory period, a post-ventricular atrial refractory period (PVARP), and an upper rate limit. A sensed P wave initiates the AVI (during the AVI, the atrial sensing channel is refractory). At the end of the AVI, a ventricular pacing artifact is delivered if no intrinsic ventricular activity has been sensed, i.e., P wave tracking. Ventricular activity, paced or sensed, initiates the PVARP and the ventriculoatrial interval (the LR limit interval minus the AVI). If no P wave activity occurs, the pacemaker escapes with a ventricular pacing artifact at the LR limit. PV, native atrial depolarization followed by paced ventricular event; TARP, total atrial refractory period.

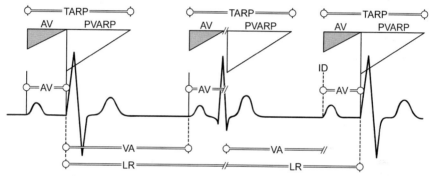

Fig. 7.12 The timing cycle in DDD consists of a lower rate (LR) limit, an atrioventricular (AV) interval, a ventricular refractory period, a post-ventricular atrial refractory period (PVARP), and an upper rate limit. If intrinsic atrial and ventricular activity occur before the LR limit times out, both channels are inhibited and no pacing occurs. In the absence of intrinsic atrial and ventricular activity, AV sequential pacing occurs (first cycle). If no atrial activity is sensed before the ventriculoatrial (VA) interval is completed, an atrial pacing artifact is delivered, which initiates the AV interval. If intrinsic ventricular activity occurs before the termination of the AV interval, the ventricular output from the pacemaker is inhibited, i.e., atrial pacing (second cycle). If a P wave is sensed before the VA interval is completed, output from the atrial channel is inhibited. The AV interval is initiated, and if no ventricular activity is sensed before the AV interval terminates, a ventricular pacing artifact is delivered, i.e., P-synchronous pacing (third cycle). ID, intrinsic deflection; TARP, total atrial refractory period.

occurs before completion of the VA interval terminates this interval and initiates the PV interval, and the result is P wave synchronous ventricular pacing. If the intrinsic sinus rate is less than the programmed LRL, AV sequential pacing at the programmed rate or functional single-chamber atrial (AR) pacing occurs (Fig. 7.12).

In a DDD system, a sensed or paced atrial event initiates an atrial blanking period, a ventricular blanking period, an atrial refractory period (ARP) and also initiates the AVI (Fig. 7.13). During this portion of the timing cycle, the atrial channel is refractory to any sensed events; nor will atrial pacing occur during this period. The ventricular blanking period initiated by an atrial event prevents ventricular inhibition or initiation of ventricular safety pacing as a result of sensing the atrial event on the ventricular lead.

A sensed or paced ventricular event initiates a ventricular blanking period, and a VRP. (A VRP is always part of the timing cycle of any pacing system with ventricular pacing and sensing.) The ventricular blanking

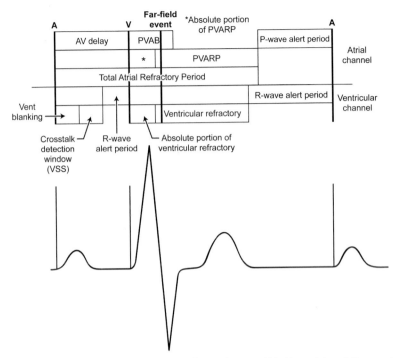

Fig. 7.13 Schematic representation of the timing cycle interactions of most refractory and blanking periods available on contemporary dual-chamber pacemakers. (Figure is courtesy of and copyrighted by St. Jude Medical.)

period prevents any sensing on the ventricular sensing channel in the period immediately following the ventricular pacing output or sensing of an intrinsic event. The VRP prevents sensing of the evoked potential and the resultant T wave on the ventricular channel of the pacemaker. A sensed or paced ventricular event also initiates a post-ventricular atrial blanking period (PVAB) and a PVARP. (By definition, the sensing circuit is "off" during a blanking period, but conceptually the PVAB as the interval immediately after the ventricular event can be thought of as the "absolute refractory" portion of the PVARP.) The PVAB prevents sensing of far-field R waves and ventricular pacing events on the atrial channel. The PVARP prevents atrial sensing of a retrograde P wave (see Endless-loop tachycardia, below) and also prevents sensing of far-field ventricular events.

A dual-chamber pacemaker can track the atrial rhythm to a defined maximum tracking rate (MTR). The combination of the PVARP and the AVI forms the total atrial refractory period (TARP) (Fig. 7.14). The TARP, in turn, is the limiting factor for the maximum sensed atrial rate that the pacemaker can reach. For example, if the AVI is fixed at 150 ms and the PVARP is fixed at 250 ms, the TARP is 400 ms, or 150 ppm. In this case, a paced ventricular event initiates the 250-ms

PVARP, and only after this interval has ended can an atrial event be sensed. If an atrial event is sensed immediately after the termination of the PVARP, the sensed atrial event initiates the AVI of 150 ms. On termination of the AVI, in the absence of an intrinsic R wave, a paced ventricular event occurs, resulting in a VV cycle length of 400 ms, or 150 ppm. Programming a long PVARP limits the upper rate by limiting the maximum sensed atrial rate (Fig. 7.15, top). If the native atrial rate were 151 bpm, every other P wave would coincide with the PVARP, not be sensed, and hence not be tracked, so that the effective paced rate would be approximately 75 ppm, or half the atrial rate (Fig. 7.15, bottom). Pseudo-Wenckebach behavior (Fig. 7.15, top) will result in variable PV intervals that can be quantitated by mathematical equations (Fig. 7.16).[1] Figure 7.17 schematically displays the relationship of the effective paced ventricular rate and the atrial rate.

Portions of pacemaker timing cycles
Atrioventricular interval
The AVI is initiated by a sensed or paced event (Fig. 7.18A). A ventricular blanking period, usually programmable (ranging from 12 to 125 ms), accounts for

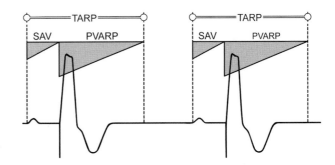

Fig. 7.14 The total atrial refractory period (TARP) is the sum of the atrioventricular (AV) delay and the post-ventricular atrial refractory period (PVARP). SAV, sensed AV interval.

Fig. 7.15 When the sinus rate exceeds the programmed maximum tracking rate, several upper rate (UR) behaviors can occur. In the top panel, pseudo-Wenckebach behavior is seen. If a P wave occurs outside the post-ventricular atrial refractory period (PVARP) and is sensed, the atrioventricular interval (AVI) is initiated. However, a ventricular pacing artifact cannot be delivered at the end of the programmed AVI if this would violate the programmed maximum tracking rate. Instead, the AVI would be lengthened and the ventricular pacing artifact would occur when the maximum tracking rate had "timed out." For example, if the maximum tracking rate is 120 ppm, or an interval of 500 ms, the AVI is 150 ms, the PVARP is 250 ms and the P wave is sensed 10 ms after completion of the PVARP, or 260 ms after the preceding ventricular event, the next ventricular pacing artifact could not be delivered for 240 ms (500–260 ms). In the bottom panel, 2 : 1 UR behavior occurs when every other sinus beat falls in the PVARP. ID, intrinsic deflection. (From Hayes DL. DDDR timing cycles: upper rate behavior. In: Barold SS, Mugica J, eds. New Perspectives in Cardiac Pacing, 3rd edn. Mount Kisco, NY: Futura Publishing Co., 1993: 33–57, by permission of Futura Publishing Co.)

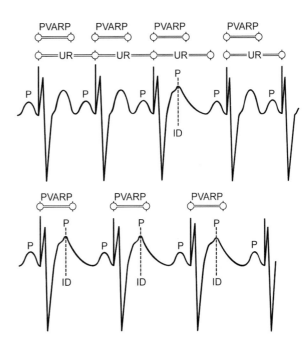

the earliest portion of the AVI. If the atrial pacing artifact were sensed by the ventricular sensing circuit, ventricular output inhibition would result. This is termed "crosstalk." To prevent this, the leading edge of the atrial pacing artifact is masked, or blanked, by essentially turning "off" the ventricular sensing circuit refractory during the very early portion of the AVI (Fig. 7.18B). The blanking period is traditionally of short duration because it is important for the ventricular sensing circuit to be returned to the "alert" state relatively early during the AVI so that intrinsic ventricular activity can inhibit pacemaker output if it occurs before the AVI times out. The potential exists for signals other than those of intrinsic ventricular activity to be sensed and

to inhibit ventricular output. Even though the leading edge of the atrial pacing artifact is effectively ignored because of the blanking period, the trailing edge of the atrial pacing artifact can at times persist beyond the blanking period so that it is sensed on the ventricular channel. In a pacemaker-dependent patient, inhibition of ventricular output by crosstalk would result in asystole. A safety mechanism is present to prevent such an outcome.

If activity is sensed on the ventricular sensing circuit in a given portion of the AVI immediately after the blanking period (the second portion of the AVI has been called the "ventricular triggering period" or the "crosstalk sensing window"), it is assumed that

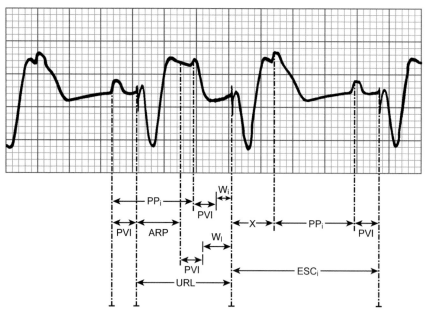

Fig. 7.16 Electrocardiographic tracing from a patient with pseudo-Wenckebach upper rate behavior. ARP, atrial refractory period; ESC_i, escape interval; PP_i, atrial rate; PVI, interval from P wave to ventricular stimulus; URL, upper rate limit; W_i, interval from beat to beat prolongation of the P wave to ventricular stimulus; W_l, URL TARP (total atrial refractory period), representing the theoretical maximum increment in PV interval allowed; X, time from the ventricular stimulus to the first P wave that has fallen in the post-ventricular atrial refractory period. (From Higano ST, Hayes DL. Quantitative analysis of Wenckebach behavior in DDD pacemakers. Pacing Clin Electrophysiol 1990; 13:1456–65, by permission of Futura Publishing Co.)

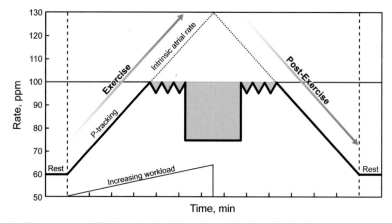

Fig. 7.17 Schematic of the rate response of a DDD pacemaker with pseudo-Wenckebach type block at the upper rate limit (100 ppm). The dotted line represents the intrinsic atrial rate, and the heavy black line represents the ventricular paced rate, assuming pseudo-Wenckebach block as the atrial rate exceeds the maximum tracking rate. (Modified from Higano ST, Hayes DL, Eisinger G. Sensor-driven rate smoothing in a DDDR pacemaker. Pacing Clin Electrophysiol 1989; 12:922–9, by permission of Futura Publishing Co.)

crosstalk cannot be differentiated from intrinsic ventricular activity. To prevent catastrophic ventricular asystole, in most pulse generators a ventricular pacing artifact is delivered early, i.e., at an AVI of 100–120 ms, although in some pacemakers this interval is program-mable for 50–150 ms (Fig. 7.18C). If the signal sensed is indeed something other than a ventricular event, a paced ventricular complex at the abbreviated interval prevents ventricular asystole. If, on the other hand, intrinsic ventricular activity occurs during the crosstalk

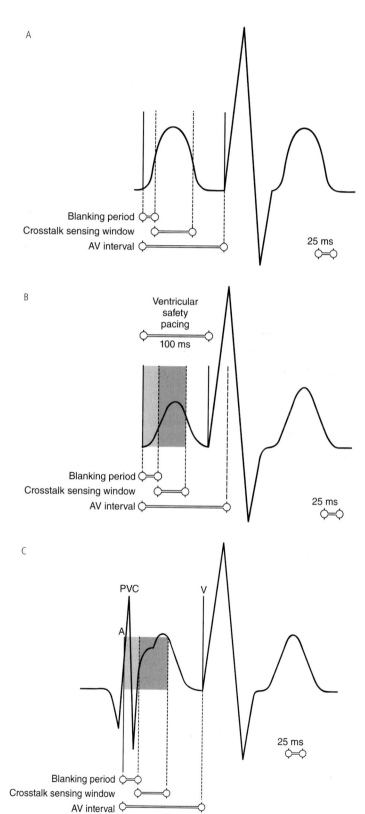

Fig. 7.18 (A) The atrioventricular (AV) interval should be considered as a single interval with two subportions. The entire AV interval corresponds to the programmed value, i.e., the interval following a paced or sensed atrial beat allowed before a ventricular pacing artifact is delivered. The initial portion of the AV interval is the blanking period. This interval is followed by the crosstalk sensing window. (B) If the ventricular sensing circuit senses activity during the crosstalk sensing window, a ventricular pacing artifact is delivered early, usually at 100–110 ms after the atrial event. This has been referred to as "ventricular safety pacing," "110 ms phenomenon," and "nonphysiologic AV delay." (C) The initial portion of the AVI in most dual-chamber pacemakers is designated as the blanking period. During this portion of the AVI, sensing is suspended. The primary purpose of this interval is to prevent ventricular sensing of the leading edge of the atrial pacing artifact. Any event that occurs during the blanking period, even if it is an intrinsic ventricular event, as shown in this figure, is not sensed. In this example, the ventricular premature beat that is not sensed is followed by a ventricular pacing artifact delivered at the programmed AV interval and occurring in the terminal portion of the T wave. PVC, premature ventricular contraction.

sensing window of the AVI, the safety mechanism results in delivery of a ventricular pacing artifact within or immediately after the intrinsic beat. This delivery is safe because the ventricle is still refractory, so that no depolarization results from the pacing artifact, and the pacing artifact is delivered too early to coincide with ventricular repolarization or a vulnerable period. This is referred to as "ventricular safety pacing," "nonphysiologic AV delay," or the "110-ms phenomenon." The actual safety pacing duration varies from approximately 70 to 120 ms depending on the device manufacturer and model. One manufacturer does not have "safety pacing" but instead uses a "noise-rejection" interval of 40–60 ms that begins with an atrial pace but is retriggerable and can be retriggered to a maximum of the programmed AV delay, i.e., at the end of that period, even if noise is being detected and retriggering the noise-rejection interval, a pacing output will be delivered.

Differential atrioventricular interval

If there is a consistent difference between an AVI initiated by a sensed event and those triggered by a paced event, the most likely explanation is a differential AVI. This is an attempt to provide an interatrial conduction time of equal duration irrespective of whether the atrial contraction is paced or sensed. The PV interval initiated with atrial sensing begins at the time of atrial depolarization. Conversely, the AVI initiated with atrial pacing commences with the pacing artifact, not with atrial depolarization. The AVI following a sensed atrial event should therefore be shorter than that following a paced atrial event (Fig. 7.19). The differential between AV and PV is programmable.

Rate-variable or rate-adaptive atrioventricular interval

Most DDDR pacemakers may have the capability of shortening the AVI as the heart rate increases to allow

for both tracking and sensor-driven operation.[2–4] Rate-adaptive or rate-variable AVI is intended to optimize cardiac output by mimicking the normal physiologic decrease in the PR interval that occurs in the normal heart as the atrial rate increases(Fig. 7.20). The rate-related shortening of the AVI may also improve atrial sensing by shortening the TARP and thereby giving more time for the atrial sensing window. Thus, use of a rate-adaptive AVI permits programming a higher upper rate limit.

There are many variations of rate-adaptive AVI, but linear shortening of the AVI from a programmed baseline AVI to a programmed minimum AVI is common (Fig. 7.21).

Atrioventricular interval hysteresis

This term is most commonly used to note an alteration of the AVI depending on the patient's native AV conduction. The term is not used uniformly by manufacturers or caregivers.

Historically, the term "positive" AVI hysteresis was often used to describe a lengthening of the AVI in an effort to maintain intrinsic AV nodal conduction. It basically involves a gradual lengthening of the programmed AVI to determine if an intrinsic ventricular depolarization will occur within a certain interval. If criteria are met, the extended AVI persists unless there is lengthening of the AR or PR interval beyond preset limits, which would once again invoke the programmed AVI (Fig. 7.22). As discussed below and in Chapter 8: Programming, this feature is useful for minimizing the frequency of right ventricular (RV) pacing, thus minimizing the potential adverse hemodynamic effect of RV pacing.[2,5,6]

"Negative" AVI hysteresis is usually used to describe a shortening of the AVI in an effort to maintain paced ventricular depolarization (Fig. 7.23). This was at one time felt to have potential hemodynamic benefits for specific patients where it was important to achieve a high percentage of ventricular pacing, and remains useful in cardiac resynchronization devices to ensure that a high percentage of biventricular pacing is achieved.

Table 7.2 lists the type of AVI hysteresis by manufacturer with a brief definition and programmable values.

Comparison of atrial with ventricular-based timing

The way the timing of the pacemaker behaves in response to a sensed atrial and/or ventricular signal varies among manufacturers and among devices from the same manufacturer. Dual-chamber pacemakers may have a ventricular-based timing system, an atrial-based timing system, or a hybrid of these two systems.[3,4] The

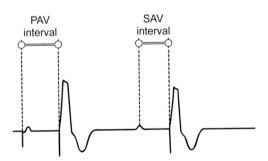

Fig. 7.19 Differential atrioventricular (AV) interval timing represents the difference in the AV delay that is dependent on whether it is initiated by an atrial sensed (SAV) or atrial paced (PAV) event.

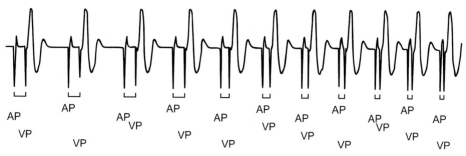

AP
AP
VP
VP
AP
VP
AP
VP
AP
VP
AP
VP
AP
VP
AP
VP
AP
VP
AP
VP

Fig. 7.20 Schematic representation of rate-adaptive atrioventricular (AV) interval. As the ventricular rate increases, the AV interval progressively shortens.

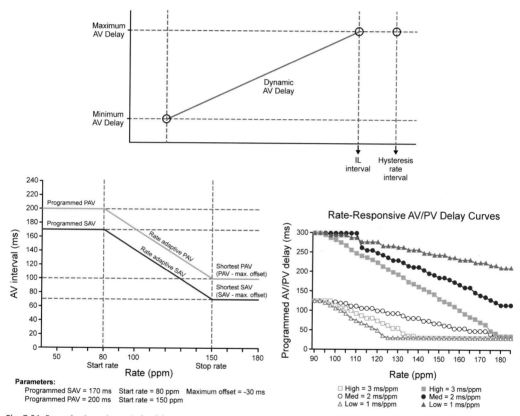

Fig. 7.21 Rate-adaptive atrioventricular delay response curves vary between manufacturers. This figure includes a combination of curve responses from various manufacturers. (Reproduced with permission from: upper, Boston Scientific Corp.; bottom left, Medtronic, Inc.; bottom right, St Jude Medical.)

difference between contemporary atrial and ventricular-based dual-chamber pacemakers is of little clinical importance, although the difference may create confusion in interpretation of paced ECGs. Regardless of the timing system used, most manufacturers have modified the timing systems in such a way that the function and ECG manifestations are very similar.

In earlier pacing systems that were pure ventricular-based timing systems, the VA interval was "fixed." In a pure ventricular-based timing system, a ventricular

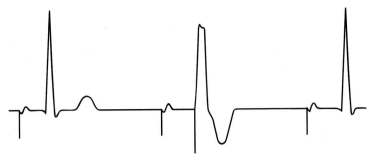

Fig. 7.22 Simulated electrocardiographic tracing demonstrating "positive" atrioventricular interval (AVI) hysteresis. The AVI is prolonged to allow intrinsic atrioventricular nodal conduction.

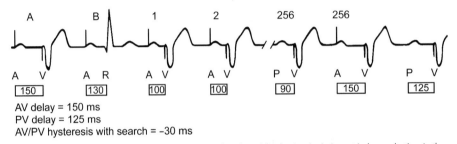

AV delay = 150 ms
PV delay = 125 ms
AV/PV hysteresis with search = –30 ms

Fig. 7.23 In the cycle labeled "B," a sensed R-wave occurs 130 ms after the atrial pulse, i.e., intrinsic ventricular conduction. In the next cycle, the algorithm subtracts the programmed hysteresis value (30 ms) from the measured A-R interval (130 ms), i.e., 130 − 30 = 100 ms AV delay. This is labeled as "1" because it is the first cycle with the shortened AV delay. After 32 cycles, at the shortened AV delay of 100 ms, the programmed AV delay is restored because no R waves have been detected in the AV delay. (Figure is courtesy of and copyrighted by St. Jude Medical.)

sensed event occurring during the VA interval resets this timer, causing it to start all over again. A ventricular sensed event occurring during the AVI both terminates the AVI and initiates a VA interval (Fig. 7.24). If there is intact conduction through the AV node after an atrial pacing stimulus such that the AR interval (atrial stimulus to sensed R wave) is shorter than the programmed AVI, the resulting paced rate accelerates. When this occurs at the LRL the rate acceleration would be minimal, e.g., if the pacemaker is programmed to an LRL of 60 ppm (a pacing interval of 1000 ms). With a programmed AVI of 200 ms, the VA interval is 800 ms (VA interval = LRL − AVI). If AV nodal function permits conduction in 150 ms (AR interval = 150 ms), the conducted or sensed R wave inhibits the ventricular output. This, in turn, resets the VA interval, which remains stable at 800 ms. The resulting interval between consecutive atrial pacing stimuli is 950 ms (VA interval + AR interval). This is equivalent to a rate of 63 ppm, which is slightly faster than the programmed LRL (Fig.

7.24). When a native R wave occurs – e.g., a ventricular premature beat during the VA interval – the VA interval is also reset. The pacemaker timing cycle is reset, and the result is a rate defined by the sum of the VA interval and the AVI. This escape interval is therefore equal to the LRL. In both cases, the sensed ventricular event, an R wave, regardless of where it occurs, resets the VA interval.

In contrast, in a pure atrial-based timing system, the AA interval is fixed. As long as there is stable LRL pacing, there will be no discernible difference between the two timing systems.

In a system with pure atrial-based timing, a sensed R wave occurring during the AVI inhibits the ventricular output, but does not alter the basic AA timing (Fig. 7.25). Hence, the rate stays at the programmed LRL during effective single-chamber atrial pacing. When a ventricular premature beat is sensed during the VA interval, the timers are also reset, but now it is the AA interval rather than the VA interval that is reset. The

Table 7.2 Manufacturer-specific atrioventricular (AV) hysteresis options.

Manufacturer	Terminology	Operation
Biotronik	AV hysteresis	Encourages intrinsic conduction and is programmable as a "repetitive" or "scan" option. In AV repetitive hysteresis the AVD is extended by a defined value when an intrinsic ventricular beat is sensed. When a paced ventricular event occurs, a long AV delay (AVD) is employed for a programmed number of pacing cycles. If an intrinsic event occurs during one of these cycles then the long AVD remains in operation, but if no intrinsic events occur then the original AVD is resumed. With AV scan hysteresis, after 180 consecutive cycles, the AVD is extended for a programmed number of pacing cycles and if an intrinsic event is detected when it is extended, the longer AVD remains in operation. If an intrinsic event is not detected, the original AVD is resumed. A negative AV hysteresis can be initiated whereby the AVD is decreased by a programmed value after an intrinsic ventricular event. The normal AVD will resume after the programmed number of consecutive ventricular paced cycles has elapsed
Boston Scientific	AV search hysteresis	When enabled, the AVI will lengthen periodically for up to eight consecutive cycles. It will remain active as long as the intrinsic PR interval is shorter than the hysteresis AV delay. When the first ventricular pace occurs at the hysteresis AV delay, or when the eight-cycle search expires without sensing an intrinsic ventricular event, the device reverts to the programmed AVD
Medtronic	Search AV +	The pacemaker tracks the 16 most recent AV conduction sequences (start with nonrefractory atrial senses or paces in atrial tracking modes and start only with atrial paces in DDI[R] and DVI[R] modes) and adjusts PAV/SAV delays (up by 62 ms or down by 8 ms) to keep intrinsic conducted events in an "AV" delay window that precedes scheduled paced events (by 15–55 ms). The AV delay window is set to promote intrinsic conduction to the ventricles, but ends early enough to avoid fusion or pseudo-fusion beats if pacing is necessary
Sorin	Dplus Mode (DDD AV Hyst mode)	Dplus pacing mode is an automatic AVD hysteresis algorithm, designed to promote spontaneous AV conduction. The algorithm uses an automatic extended AVD equal to the PR interval plus a 50-ms window that will allow intrinsic AV conduction (pseudo-AAI). Dplus will switch to DDD during loss of AV conduction (no V sensed event during hysteresis window) and will use the auto adjusted AV delays. While in DDD mode, Dplus periodically (every 100 V-V cycles) extends the AVD to promote the spontaneous AV conduction
St. Jude Medical	AV/PV hysteresis with search	The pacemaker will search for intrinsic ventricular conduction every 256 cycles by adding or subtracting the AV/PV hysteresis with search to programmed AV/PV delay. If a ventricular event is not sensed during the extension the programmed AV/PV delay is resumed for another 256 cycles. If it is sensed, the delay remains extended until the interval times out, i.e., no intrinsic event occurs and a ventricular pacing output is delivered. If a "negative" search is programmed then a sensed ventricular event initiates the hysteresis interval being subtracted from the programmed AV/PV delay and the shorter interval will stay in effect for 256 cycles or until another sensed event occurs. (Newest generation of devices have Ventricular Intrinsic Preference [VIP]; see text)
	Ventricular Intrinsic Preference (VIP)	Search intervals and search cycles are programmable. When three consecutive R waves are sensed during the search interval the algorithm is activated. It is deactivated when the number of ventricular paced events equals the programmed number of cycle counts

pacemaker counts out an AA interval and then adds the programmed AVI, attempting to mimic the compensatory pause commonly seen in normal sinus rhythm with ventricular ectopy. For example, if the pacemaker was programmed to 60 ppm, 1000 ms cycle length, and an AV delay of 200 ms, AV sequential pacing occurs and is followed by an atrial paced event at 1000 ms from the previous paced atrial event. However, if intrinsic ventricular conduction occurs at 150 ms, i.e., truncates the AV delay by 50 ms, it would result in an effective ventricular rate of 950 ms, or 63 ppm, i.e., an 800-ms VA interval plus a 150-ms AR interval. The next paced atrial event is still delivered at 1000 ms after the preceding paced atrial event, as defined by atrial-based timing.

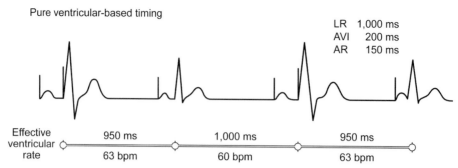

Pure ventricular-based timing

LR 1,000 ms
AVI 200 ms
AR 150 ms

Effective ventricular rate

950 ms	1,000 ms	950 ms
63 bpm	60 bpm	63 bpm

Fig. 7.24 With ventricular-based timing in patients with intact atrioventricular (AV) nodal conduction after atrial (AR) pacing, the sensed R wave resets the ventriculoatrial (VA) interval. The base pacing interval consists of the sum of the AR and the VA intervals; thus, it is shorter than the programmed minimum rate interval.

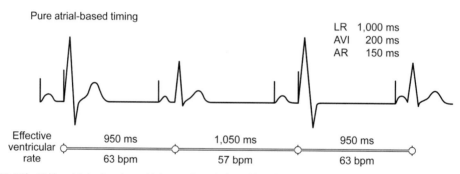

Pure atrial-based timing

LR 1,000 ms
AVI 200 ms
AR 150 ms

Effective ventricular rate

950 ms	1,050 ms	950 ms
63 bpm	57 bpm	63 bpm

Fig. 7.25 With atrial-based timing in patients with intact atrioventricular nodal conduction after AR pacing, the sensed R wave inhibits the ventricular output but does not reset the basic timing of the pacemaker. There is AR pacing at the programmed base rate. ARI, interval from paced atrial event to intrinsic QRS; AVI, atrioventricular interval; LR, lower rate limit.

This time, the programmed AVI expires and a paced ventricular complex occurs. This results in an effective ventricular rate of 850 ms; the VA interval, which was lengthened by 50 ms because of the preceding intrinsic ventricular activity, and the 200-ms AVI, for a cycle length of 1050 ms, or 57 ppm.

Most contemporary pacemakers are hybrid timing systems. The best source of information for the timing cycle of a specific pulse generator is the technical manual for the device in question. A summary of the timing systems in the most recent generation of pacemakers from each company is shown in Table 7.3.

Dual-chamber rate-modulated pacemakers: effect on timing cycles

DDDR pacing systems further increase the complexity of the upper rate behavior because the pacemaker can be driven by intrinsic atrial activity to cause PV (native atrial depolarization followed by a paced ventricular event) pacing or by a sensor whose input signal is not identifiable on the ECG, or by both, to result in AV or AR pacing. The eventual upper rate also depends on the type of sensor incorporated in the pacemaker and how the sensor is programmed. Between the programmed LRL and the programmed URL, there may be stable P wave synchronous pacing, P wave synchronous pacing alternating with AV sequential pacing, or stable AV sequential pacing at rates exceeding the base rate (Fig. 7.26). AV sequential pacing rates may increase to the programmed maximum sensor rate (MSR).

Although the MSR and MTR are closely related, they are not identical. The tracking rate refers to the rate when the pacemaker is sensing and tracking intrinsic atrial activity. The MTR is the maximum ventricular paced rate that is allowed in response to sensed atrial rhythms. This may result in fixed-block, pseudo-

Table 7.3 Summary of the timing systems in the most recent generation of pacemakers from each company.

Manufacturer	Timing system
Biotronik	The DDI mode is a ventricular-based mode. The lower rate timer is triggered off of Vs, Vp, and PVC events. A VA timer is calculated by subtracting the programmed AVD from the lower rate timer. This system "assumes" that the full AVD is being utilized, and thus if Vs occurs then atrial pacing may be observed above the current indicated rate. Example: lower rate timer = 1000 ms, AVD = 300 ms, thus the VA timer = 700 ms. The patient's intrinsic PR interval is 180 ms. Vs to Ap = 700 ms. Ap to Vs = 180 ms. Thus, Vs to Vs = 880 ms, which is faster than the current indicated rate
Boston Scientfic	If the ventricle is being paced, the escape interval timing occurs from one ventricular event to the next. If a sensed ventricular event occurs, i.e., the AV interval is truncated by an intrinsic R, the timing system switches to one of atrial-based timing to maintain rates that are true to the programmed rates. However, conducted atrial pacing or As Vs intrinsic cycles could result in ventricular rates slightly below the LRL
Medtronic	A-to-A timing is used on all current bradycardia treatment devices (IPGs) for all dual-chamber modes that include atrial pacing (i.e. not for VDI[R]). The pacemaker will lengthen the subsequent V-A timing to adjust for a prior shortened A-V delay due to native R waves being sensed or due to rate-adaptive AV adjustments, etc. This strategy will, by design, promote tracking of intrinsic atrial activity and provide consistent A-to-A intervals at the expense of producing V-to-V delays that may be somewhat slower than the programmed lower rate (e.g., V-to-V rate may be as slow as 60,000/[lower rate interval + PAV − measured AV]) and sometimes seen as such in ventricular rate histograms. Some possible exceptions to A-A timing include cycles with PAC, PVC, ventricular safety pacing (VSP) and NCAP delayed AP events as well as R waves sensed in the V-A delay for DVI[R] mode
Sorin	Modified atrial-based timing system; basic intervals are determined by the atrial channel in tracking modes. PVCs (ventricular events not preceded by an atrial event) will reset all clocks as well as automatically add a nonprogrammable 500-ms atrial refractory period to prevent pacemaker-mediated tachycardia
St. Jude Medical	Ventricular based timing if: VDD; DDI; DDD when PV >MTR; DDD with safety pacing; VDD/DDD with PVC. Modified* atrial-based timing if: DDD; DDD with PV <MTR or AV events; DOO)

*Change to ventricular-based timing when atrial events are faster than MTR but still in alert.

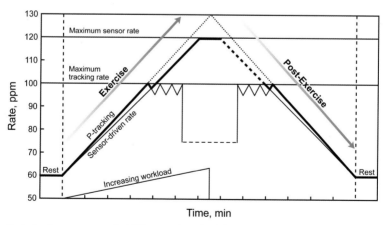

Fig. 7.26 Diagram illustrating the rate response of a DDDR pacemaker and its behavior at both the maximum tracking and the maximum sensor rates. The dotted line represents the intrinsic atrial rate, during progressively increasing workloads and as the intrinsic atrial rate decrements when exercise is stopped. The dashed line indicates sensor-driven pacing dominating until it decrements to the maximum tracking rate at which point ventricular pacing is again driven by the intrinsic atrial rate. The heavy black line shows the ventricular paced rate, assuming complete heart block as it progresses from the P-tracking mode to atrioventricular (AV) sequential pacing through a period of pseudo-Wenckebach block. Note that the DDD pseudo-Wenckebach interval is shortened by sensor-driven pacing. Maximal shortening of the pseudo-Wenckebach period is accomplished by optimal programming of the sensor rate-adaptive variables. (From Higano ST, Hayes DL, Eisinger G. Sensor-driven rate smoothing in a DDDR pacemaker. Pacing Clin Electrophysiol 1989; 12:922–9, by permission of Futura Publishing Co.)

Wenckebach, fallback, or rate-smoothing responses, depending on the design of the system.[1] The sensor-controlled rate is the rate of the pacemaker that is determined by the sensor input signal. The MSR is the maximum rate that the pacemaker is allowed to achieve under sensor control. In some pulse generators in which the MTR and MSR can be independently programmed, the ventricular paced rate under sensor drive might exceed that attained when intrinsic atrial activity is being tracked.

Whether at the MTR or during rate acceleration below the MTR, the rhythm that results may be in part sensor-driven and in part sinus-driven (P wave tracking) and not purely one or the other (Fig. 7.27). Which of these mechanisms predominates depends on the integrity of the sinus node and programming of the rate-adaptive sensor. If the sensor is optimally programmed, as the atrial rate exceeds the MTR, the RR interval will display minimal variation between sinus-

driven and sensor-driven pacing (Fig. 7.28).[7] If the rate-responsive circuitry is programmed to mimic the native atrial rate, the paced ventricular rate will not demonstrate the 2:1, or pseudo-Wenckebach-type, behavior. Conversely, if the rate-responsive circuitry is programmed in such a way that the sensor does not allow the patient to achieve sensor-driven rates above the MTR, upper rate behavior will be the same as with DDD pacing, i.e., the patient will experience pseudo-Wenckebach and/or 2:1 AV block when the programmed upper rate is reached.

Optimal programming of the rate-adaptive sensor is required to minimize cycle length variations between sinus-driven and sensor-driven pacing. As shown in Fig. 7.28, the variation in RR interval is markedly lessened with the sensor "on" (DDDR) rather than "passive" (DDD). In the DDDR mode, the RR interval is allowed to lengthen only as much as the difference between the MTR and the current sensor-indicated rate. For

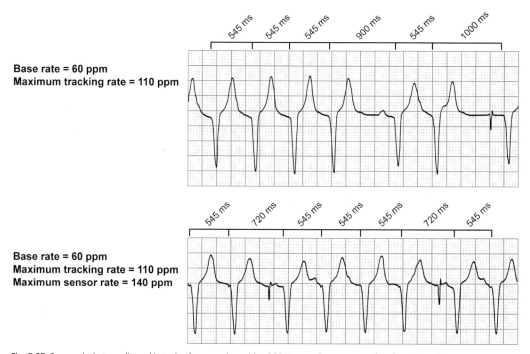

Fig. 7.27 Top panel: electrocardiographic tracing from a patient with a DDDR pacemaker programmed to the DDD mode. During exercise, when the maximum tracing rate is exceeded, there are marked variations in VV cycle length as the pacemaker either waits until the ventriculoatrial interval "times out" to deliver an atrial pacing artifact or tracks an intrinsic atrial event that occurs. Bottom panel: electrocardiographic tracing from the same patient, whose pacemaker is now programmed to the DDDR mode. Sensor-driven pacing during exercise minimizes the variation in VV cycle length. This effect has been called "sensor-driven rate smoothing." (From Hayes DL, Higano ST, Eisinger G. Electrocardiographic manifestations of a dual-chamber, rate-modulated (DDDR) pacemaker. Pacing Clin Electrophysiol 1989; 12:555–62, by permission of Futura Publishing Co.)

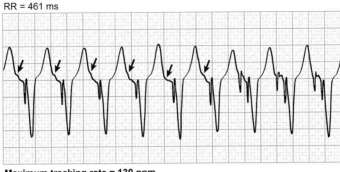

RR = 461 ms

Maximum tracking rate = 130 ppm
Maximum sensor rate = 130 ppm

Fig. 7.28 Electrocardiographic tracing from a patient with a DDDR pacemaker programmed to maximum sensor and tracking rates of 130 ppm. The tracing initially demonstrates P-synchronous pacing (arrows indicate P waves), which is followed by atrioventricular sequential or sensor-driven pacing at an almost identical rate. Minimizing the variation in cycle length between sinus-driven and sensor-driven pacing is the goal of optimal programming, i.e., "sensor-driven rate smoothing." (From Hayes DL, Higano ST, Eisinger G. Electrocardiographic manifestations of a dual-chamber, rate-modulated (DDDR) pacemaker. Pacing Clin Electrophysiol 1989; 12:555–62, by permission of Futura Publishing Co.)

example, if a device is programmed to a P wave tracking limit of 120 ppm and the patient's atrial rate exceeds this, the pacemaker will operate in a pseudo-Wenckebach-type block. If the sensor-indicated rate at this time is 100 ppm, the paced rate will drop from 120 ppm (500 ms) to an AV sequential paced rate of 100 ppm (600 ms) for the pseudo-Wenckebach cycle and then return to P wave tracking at a rate of 120 ppm. This situation usually shortens the DDD pseudo-Wenckebach interval, but this interval depends on the atrial rate and the programmed values for the MTR and the TARP.

The portion of the RR cycle that is not part of the PVARP or the AVI is the period during which the atrial sensing channel is not refractory and atrial senses will inhibit scheduled atrial paces and start the SAV for tracking modes of operation. This interval can be designated as the atrial sensing window (ASW). Intrinsic atrial events in the ASW are tracked; atrial events that occur during the TARP are not tracked, but may affect mode switch, tachyarrhythmia detection and diagnostic information. If the PVARP or AVI (or both) is extended, the ASW may essentially be eliminated, so that a DDD pacemaker functions effectively as a DVI system.

Conversely, if a DDDR pacemaker is pacing at sensor triggered rates faster than the MTR (also abbreviated at times as UTR for "upper tracking rate"), P waves falling into the ASW will inhibit the sensor-driven atrial pacing, giving the appearance of P wave tracking at rates greater than the MTR (Fig. 7.29).

Although the MTR is programmed to a single value in DDDR pacing, it behaves as if it were variable and

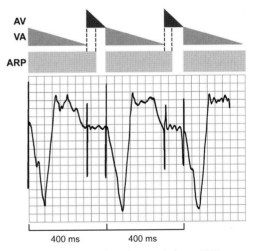

Fig. 7.29 In this electrocardiographic example from a DDDR pacemaker, the maximum sensor rate is 150 ppm (400 ms), the atrial refractory period (ARP) is 350 ms, and the atrioventricular (AV) interval is 100 ms. As illustrated in the block diagrams above the electrocardiogram, the two sensor-driven atrial pacing artifacts both occur during the terminal portion of the post-ventricular atrial refractory period (PVARP). Even though no atrial sensing can occur during the PVARP, as can be seen in this example by the intrinsic P wave that occurs immediately after the first paced ventricular depolarization, a sensor-driven atrial pacing artifact is not prevented by the PVARP. Whether a sensor-driven atrial pacing artifact is delivered depends on the sensor indicated rate at that time and not on the PVARP. VA, ventriculoatrial. (From Higano ST, Hayes DL. Quantitative analysis of Wenckebach behavior in DDD pacemakers. Pacing Clin Electrophysiol 1990; 13:1456–65, by permission of Futura Publishing Co.)

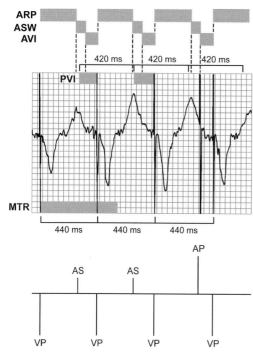

Fig. 7.30 Diagram showing how an appropriately timed P wave can inhibit the sensor-driven A spike and result in apparent P wave tracking above the maximum tracking rate (MTR). In this example, the MTR is 100 ppm, or 600 ms. The second and third complexes are preceded by intrinsic P waves that occurred during the atrial sensing window (ASW). This resulted in A spike inhibition, or P wave tracking above the MTR. The fourth complex was initiated by atrial pacing, because the preceding native P wave occurred outside the ASW in the atrial refractory period (ARP, 275 ms). Note the short P stimulus interval produced by the subsequent atrial spike. Also shown are the ASW (65 ms), atrioventricular interval (AVI, 100 ms), and variable PV interval. The intrinsic atrial rate is 143 bpm (420 ms). The sensor rate is 136 ppm (440 ms). A marker-channel diagram demonstrates the electrocardiographic findings. AP, atrial paced event; AS, atrial sensed event; VP, ventricular paced event. (From Higano ST, Hayes DL. P wave tracking above the maximum tracking rate in a DDDR pacemaker. Pacing Clin Electrophysiol 1989;1044–8, by permission of Futura Publishing Co.)

equal to the sensor-driven rate when the sensor-driven rate exceeds the programmed MTR (if a P wave occurs during the ASW to inhibit output of an atrial pacing artifact) (Fig. 7.30).

Mode switching

Mode switching refers to the ability of the pacemaker to change automatically from one mode to another in response to an atrial tachyarrhythmia. This may alter the ECG "timing" in a significant way.[8] When the pacemaker is programmed to a pacing mode with ventricular tracking of atrial events, mode-switching algorithms automatically reprogram the device to a nontracking mode when an atrial tachyarrhythmia occurs and meets detection criteria (Fig. 7.31).[9] In the absence of mode switch, with the DDD or DDDR pacing modes a supraventricular arrhythmia may result in rapid ventricular pacing (Fig. 7.32). Permanently programming the device to a nontracking mode, e.g., DDI, DDIR, VVIR, eliminates rapid paced rates during tachyarrhythmias, but also eliminates the ability to track normal sinus rhythm, which is disadvantageous in patients with paroxysmal arrhythmia. Mode switching avoids this limitation by permitting tracking of atrial events only during normal sinus rhythm.

Atrial flutter may not be detected by some mode-switch algorithms, requiring additional options. With a blanked atrial flutter search, if the algorithm determines that every other atrial event is being "blanked" the pacemaker will extend the PVARP and the VA interval in an effort to uncover any atrial sensed events that have been blanked.[10] If criteria are met, a diagnosis of atrial flutter is made by the pulse generator and a mode switch will occur.

Avoiding atrial pace/sense competition

There are features intended for prevention of an atrial tachycardia being initiated by pacing within the atrium's relative refractory period, e.g., "Non-Competitive Atrial Pacing™") This feature may affect both atrial and ventricular timing. If a refractory sensed atrial event occurs within the PVARP, a 300-ms interval is initiated during which no atrial pacing may occur (Fig. 7.33). If the timing cycle should have resulted in release of a sensor-driven atrial stimulus or lower pacing rate atrial stimulus during the 300-ms noncompetitive atrial pacing (NCAP) extension, the VA interval is extended until the NCAP expires. If timers do not indicate that an atrial paced event should occur during the 300-ms NCAP extension, atrial pacing occurs at the end of NCAP period. If an atrial sense occurs during the NCAP, a new NCAP is initiated.

If delivery of an atrial pacing stimulus is delayed by the NCAP, the pacemaker will attempt to keep the ventricular rate stable by shortening the PAV interval that would follow the NCAP. If the pacemaker is programmed so that the lower rate is relatively high and the PVARP relatively long, NCAP could result in ventricular pacing at a rate slightly below the lower rate limit.

Another manufacturer includes Atrial Protection Interval (API™), which shortens the PVARP for each interval where the pseudo-Wenckebach window is

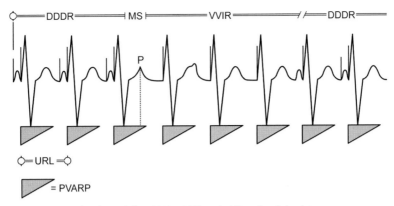

Fig. 7.31 Schematic representation of mode-switch from DDDR to VVIR mode. MS, mode switch point.

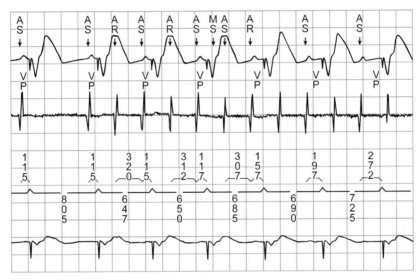

Fig. 7.32 Mode switch from DDDR to DDDIR mode. MS, mode switch.

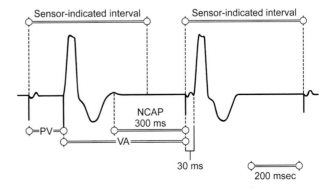

Fig. 7.33 Noncompetitive atrial pacing (NCAP) is a feature designed to prevent initiation of an atrial tachyarrhythmia by an atrial pacing artifact occurring in a vulnerable portion of the timing cycle. (Reproduced with permission from Medtronic Adapta Technical Manual.)

<125 ms. This provides a noncompetitive pacing window of 125 ms.

Another feature, the atrial upper rate (AUR), essentially prevents atrial pacing when the atrial tissue is refractory and potentially vulnerable. AUR prevents atrial pacing from occurring in the vulnerable phase after an atrial sensed event during the PMT protection interval, and ensures that the next atrial paced event occurs after the heart's natural atrial refractory period. To avoid this, an atrial upper rate of 240 ppm (atrial upper interval [AUI], 250 ms) is started after a PMT-atrial sensed (As) event. The next atrial paced event (Ap) can only be emitted after the expiration of the AUI. When there are high sensor rates, the atrial pacing is shifted.

Timing components of ventricular avoidance pacing algorithms

Data demonstrating the potential adverse hemodynamic effects of RV pacing have led to a variety of ventricular avoidance pacing algorithms (see Chapter 2: Hemodynamics).

The "timing" aspects of these algorithms vary significantly between manufacturers, best explained in a combination of manufacturer-specific and generic descriptions.

The most common feature used to promote intrinsic AV conduction is AV search hysteresis. Although each of the manufacturers that use this approach has slight differences in their algorithms, the basic operation is that of a programmed AV delay being extended to a programmed extension if a sensed ventricular event occurs. The extended AV delay persists until a paced ventricular event and the programmed AV delay is then re-established. Depending on the algorithm, the pacemaker may periodically invoke the extended AV delay to "search" for intrinsic AV conduction. At the present time, variations of this approach are used by multiple manufacturers (Figs 7.34–7.36).

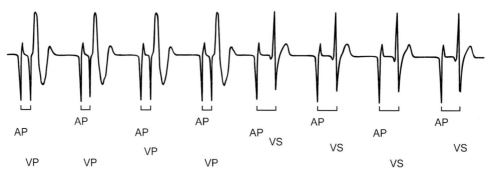

Fig. 7.34 Schematic example of AV search hysteresis which successfully allows intrinsic AV conduction.

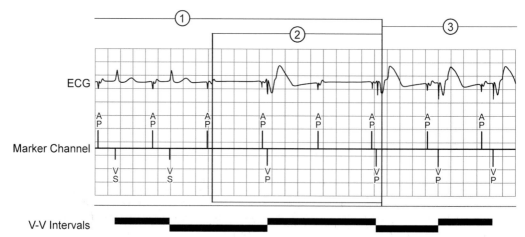

Fig. 7.35 Example of managed ventricular pacing (MVP). Initially AAIR pacing is seen and if an atrial pace event occurs without a ventricular sensed event, a ventricular back-up output occurs and the pacemaker then switches to DDDR mode. (With permission from Medtronic Adapta Manual, pp. 5–12; Figure 5–10.)

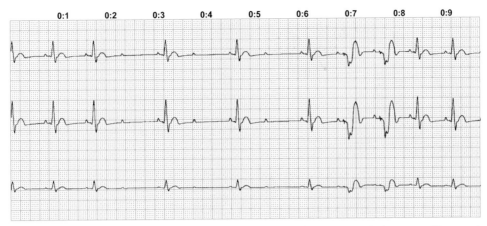

Fig. 7.36 Example of SafeR. The SafeR algorithm has the capability to provide ventricular pacing support in the presence of first, second or third degree AV block. This strip illustrates the response to second degree AV block; reversion to pacing support when 3 of the last 12 P-waves were not conducted.

Some algorithms used to promote intrinsic AV conduction warrant more detailed description in order to understand their potential impact on the timing cycle of the pacemaker.

Managed Ventricular Pacing (MVP)™ Medtronic, Inc.

There are two available modes, AAIR ⇔ DDDR and AAI ⇔ DDD, meaning that atrial pacing is delivered allowing intrinsic AV conduction with continuous monitoring of AV conduction. If there is persistent loss of AV conduction, the mode will switch to the corresponding dual-chamber mode, i.e., DDDR or DDD (Fig. 7.35). When the pacemaker detects the return of AV conduction, the atrial pacing mode is resumed.

If there is transient loss of AV conduction, the pacemaker delivers a backup ventricular pacing output in response to an A-A interval that does not contain a ventricular sensed event.

Persistent loss of AV conduction is defined as two of the four most recent nonrefractory A-A intervals missing a ventricular event. This results in a switch to the DDD or DDDR mode.

Following a mode change to DDD or DDDR, the pacemaker does periodic single-cycle assessments for AV conduction and, if present, will resume AAIR or AAI pacing mode.

SafeR™, Sorin Medical

When this algorithm is active and the device is functioning in AAI or AAIR mode, an AV delay is not initiated after sensed or paced atrial events. The device will tolerate first, second and third-degree AV block up to a specific number of long PR intervals or consecutively blocked P waves before the mode changes to DDD or DDDR mode. PR and AR intervals are permanently monitored (Fig. 7.36). If the PR interval exceeds 350 ms or the AR interval exceeds 450 ms the mode switches to the DDD or DDDR mode and invokes the programmed AV delay.

The mode will return to AAI or AAIR mode if there is sensing of 12 consecutive R waves or after 100 cycles in DDD(R) mode. If there have been more than five switches to DDD(R) mode per day on three consecutive days or ≥15 switches occur within 24 hours, a change back to the AAI(R) mode will not occur until the device is reprogrammed.[11–13]

Endless-loop tachycardia

Endless-loop tachycardia (ELT) is not a portion of the timing cycle, but understanding the timing cycle of dual-chamber pacing is crucial to understanding ELT and vice versa. ELT, also referred to as "pacemaker-mediated tachycardia," "pacemaker-mediated reentry tachycardia," and "pacemaker circus movement tachycardia," is defined as a re-entry arrhythmia in which the dual-chamber pacemaker acts as the antegrade limit of the tachycardia and the natural conduction pathway acts as the retrograde limit (Fig. 7.37).

If AV synchrony is uncoupled, i.e., if the P wave is displaced from its normal relation to the QRS complex, the subsequent ventricular event may result in retrograde atrial excitation if retrograde or VA conduction is intact. If the retrograde P wave is sensed, the AVI of the pacemaker is initiated. On termination of the AVI and MTR interval, a ventricular pacing pulse is delivered, which could once again be conducted in a retrograde fashion. Once established, this re-entrant mechanism continues until interrupted or until the

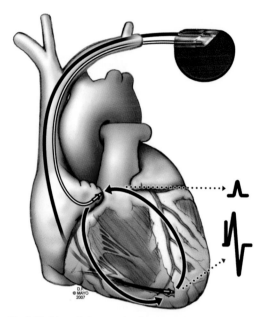

Fig. 7.37 Schematic diagram of endless loop tachycardia. When AV synchrony is lost for whatever reason with a dual-chamber pacemaker with atrial sensing, the paced ventricular beat may result in retrograde conduction. If the retrograde conduction results in a retrograde atrial event which is sensed by the device, the AV interval is again initiated resulting in another paced ventricular event, at or near maximum tracking limit. (Reproduced with permission from the Mayo Clinic.)

retrograde limb of the circuit is exhausted (Fig. 7.38). The paced VV interval cannot violate the programmed maximum limit, or URL, of the pacemaker, and the ELT often occurs at the URL.

There are two basic mechanisms that have been adopted to prevent or minimize ELT. If the pacemaker detects a programmable number of consecutive AS-VP cycles at the maximum tracking rate with a constant VP to AS interval, the pacemaker will extend the PVARP for at least one cycle. The next retrograde P wave will fall into the PVARP and terminate the tachycardia. In some devices the detect rate may be programmed at a rate less than the MTR (Fig. 7.39).

Because a premature ventricular event may commonly be the initiator of ELT, many pacemakers extend the PVARP when a premature ventricular contraction (PVC) is detected. (A PVC is defined as two consecutive ventricular sensed events without an intervening atrial event.) Once again, by extending the PVARP, a retrograde atrial event that occurs as a result of a PVC would occur in refractory and be ignored.

Timing cycles with algorithms responding to sudden bradycardia

Algorithms used in patients paced for neurocardiogenic syncope with clinically significant cardio-inhibition and vasodepression may alter timing cycles by introducing a sudden increase in pacing rate. If a patient's heart

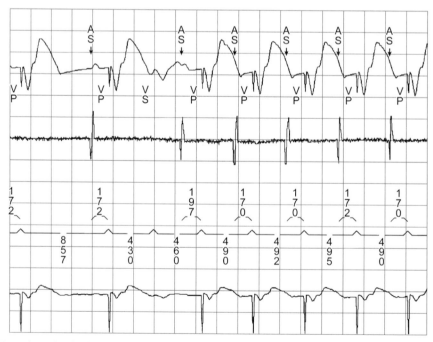

Fig. 7.38 Pacemaker-mediated tachycardia (PMT) initiated by a premature ventricular event (VS).

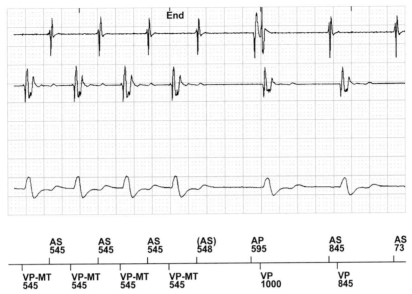

Fig. 7.39 Tracing demonstrating the termination of a pacemaker-mediated tachycardia. In this example the pacemaker-mediated tachycardia algorithm is satisfied on the 4th ventricular complex on this tracing. At that point the PVARP is extended, the atrial event falls into refractory as noted by (AS). The VP-MT designation indicates that the device is at the "maximum tracking" rate. (From Friedman PA, Rott MA, Wokhlu A, Asirvatham SJ, Hayes DL. A Case-based approach to pacemakers, ICDs, and cardiac resynchronization: Advanced questions for exam review and clinical practice. Minneapolis: Cardiotext. 2011. Used with permission of Mayo Foundation for Medical Education and Research.)

rate occurs in a manner that meets the criteria of the algorithm, the device responds with pacing at a programmable faster rate, most commonly 90–100 ppm, in an attempt to blunt the patient's symptoms (Fig. 7.40). Figures 7.41 and 7.42 demonstrate features from two manufacturers in a diagrammatic fashion.

Timing cycles unique to biventricular pacing

Programmable pacing modes in cardiac resynchronization therapy (CRT) devices are the same as those described for standard pacemakers, and the general criteria for mode selection are similar to those for standard pacing.

Additional features that add complexity to biventricular pacemakers include the need to maintain a high frequency of ventricular pacing, and the need to tailor interventricular timing and pace/sense vectors in many patients.[14–18]

In contemporary cardiac resynchronization devices, ventricular sensing (Fig. 7.43) mechanisms vary between manufacturers as follows:
• Biotronik: CRT devices provide sensing from RV and LV leads and triggering from RVs to LVP or RVES (RV extrasystole or RV PVC) to LVP.

• Boston Scientific: Sense on both leads but only RV is used for timing and detection. LV sense is strictly for counters and histograms.
• Medtronic: CRT-P can be programmed to sense RV or LV, unipolar or bipolar. Unipolar sensing is not used for CRT-D.
• Sorin: No sense input but EGM available from LV lead.
• St. Jude Medical: In permanently programmed mode, CRT devices sense only from the RV lead. For testing purposes, temporary sensing is possible, either LV Bipolar or LV Unipolar-Tip.

Because the paced V-V interval is programmable, biventricular stimulation may occur simultaneously, or with an offset with one ventricle preceding the other. This must be considered when interpreting the timing cycle (Fig. 7.44).

Achieving consistent biventricular pacing

Benefits will not be realized from biventricular stimulation if resynchronization is not maintained. Resynchronization requires pacing and capture from the left ventricular (LV) lead. In many patients, the AV delay must be relatively short in order to maintain consistent

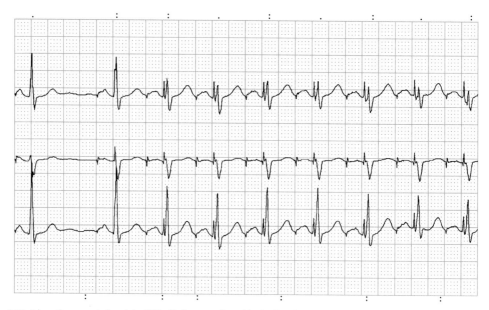

Fig. 7.40 Schematic representation of the ECG with the onset of a sudden bradycardia response algorithm. The rate of 60 ppm at the onset of this tracing actually represents dramatic slowing which triggers the algorithm and results in a pacing rate of 100 ppm.

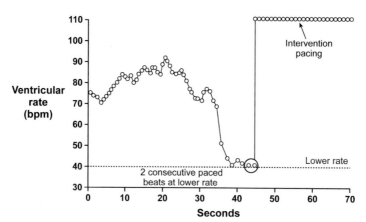

Fig. 7.41 Schematic diagram of "rate-drop response." (Reproduced with permission from Medtronic.)

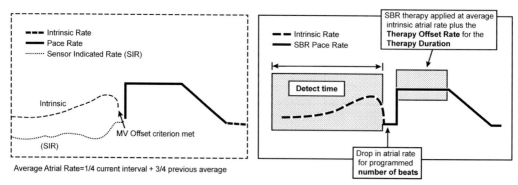

Average Atrial Rate=1/4 current interval + 3/4 previous average

Fig. 7.42 Schematic diagram of "sudden-brady response" (SBR). The left panel demonstrates SBR response if minute ventilation sensor (MV) is programmed "on" and the rate and duration criteria for rate drop are met but the sensor indicates a lower rate. By comparing the current MV sensor value with a stored comparison value, if the stored value is greater then SBR will be initiated. The right panel demonstrates a standard SBR response. If rate and duration criteria are met the pacemaker paces at a faster rate determined by the average intrinsic atrial rate plus the "therapy offset rate" for a programmed duration. (Reproduced with permission from Boston Scientific Corp.)

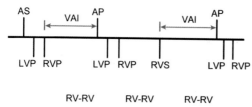

Fig. 7.43 Right ventricular-based timing. Right ventricular sensed or paced events are used to reset the timing, resulting in a new VA interval (VAI). (From Wang P, Kramer A, Estes NA 3rd, Hayes DL. Timing cycles for biventricular pacing. Pacing Clin Electrophysiol 2002; 25:62–75, by permission of Blackwell Publishing.)

ventricular pacing and avoid fusion with intrinsic conduction.[19] However, the AV delay must be long enough to allow adequate ventricular diastolic filling (see Chapter 2: Hemodynamics).

The goal should be to achieve as close as possible to 100% biventricular pacing.[20] Several algorithms have been designed to maintain biventricular pacing and prevent inhibition by intrinsic rhythm.

AV hysteresis, discussed above, is used to promote intrinsic ventricular conduction (positive AV hysteresis) in non-CRT systems. In CRT systems, the opposite, or negative AV hysteresis maintains a paced ventricular

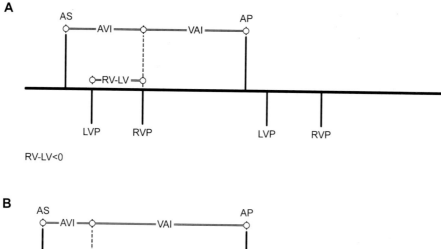

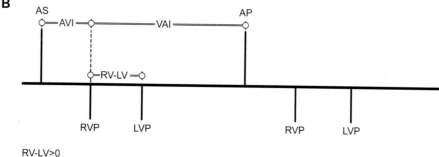

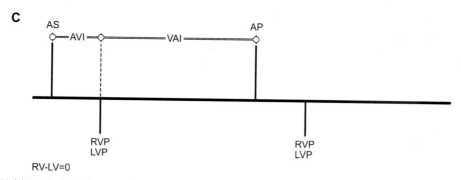

Fig. 7.44 (A) Negative RV-LV. The LV paced event occurs before the RV paced event. (B) Positive RV-LV. The right ventricular paced event occurs before the left ventricular paced event. (C) Zero RV-LV. The right and left ventricular paced events occur simultaneously. (From Wang P, Kramer A, Estes NA 3rd, Hayes DL. Timing cycles for biventricular pacing. Pacing Clin Electrophysiol 2002; 25:62–75, by permission of Blackwell Publishing.)

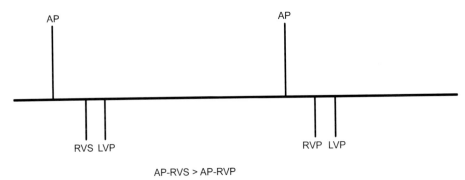

AP-RVS > AP-RVP

Fig. 7.45 Biventricular RV-LV hysteresis may be used to force biventricular pacing. RV, right ventricular; LV, left ventricular; LVP, left ventricular paced; RVP, right ventricular paced; RVS, right ventricular sensed. (From Wang P, Kramer A, Estes NA 3rd, Hayes DL. Timing cycles for biventricular pacing. Pacing Clin Electrophysiol 2002; 25:62–75, by permission of Blackwell Publishing.)

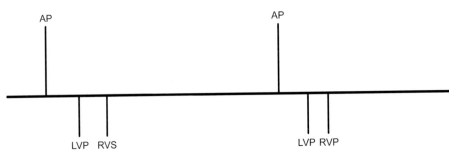

Fig. 7.46 Biventricular hysteresis. Because conduction resulted in RVS event, negative hysteresis would be used to maintain biventricular pacing. LVP, left ventricular paced; RVP, right ventricular paced; RVS, right ventricular sensed. (From Wang P, Kramer A, Estes NA 3rd, Hayes DL. Timing cycles for biventricular pacing. Pacing Clin Electrophysiol 2002; 25:62–75, by permission of Blackwell Publishing.)

rhythm because a sensed ventricular event results in shortening of the subsequent AV interval. Although algorithms for negative AV hysteresis vary among manufacturers, most algorithms periodically lengthen the AV delay. If the ventricular event that follows is paced, the longer AV delay is maintained (promoting filling) until a sensed ventricular event occurs, at which time the AV delay is again shortened (Figs 7.45 and 7.46).

The Ventricular Sense Response™ algorithm maintains resynchronization by immediately pacing the LV in response to a sensed event in the RV (Fig. 7.47). Similarly, in some CRT devices the DDT mode allows triggered pacing when a ventricular sensed event occurs (Fig. 7.48).

In addition to lack of ventricular stimulation secondary to inhibition by intrinsic ventricular events, successful biventricular stimulation may also be lost if LV capture thresholds exceed the programmed output

parameters. Some biventricular devices have a feature that will periodically assess LV pacing thresholds and adjust the outputs to ensure LV capture.[21] Loss of LV capture during testing, however, could lead to scenarios with transient inhibition of biventricular pacing.

Cardiac resynchronization therapy lower rate behavior
Lower rate behavior in CRT systems is similar to dual-chamber pacemaker function.

Univentricular sensing and biventricular pacing
Whenever pacing without sensing occurs in a specific cardiac chamber, there is theoretical concern that competitive pacing could result in the induction of a tachyarrhythmia. To date, this has not been a significant clinical problem with CRT devices. Physiologically, if activation of the LV occurs before LV pacing, the ven-

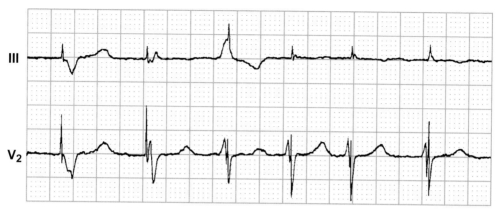

Fig. 7.47 Ventricular Sense Response™ is demonstrated in a telemetry tracing which demonstrates ventricular pacing occurring after the onset of the QRS. This is due to the Ventricular Sense Response™ algorithm, which introduces a triggered biventricular pacing pulse each time a sensed RV event is seen. (Reproduced with permission from Swerdlow CD, Friedman PA. Advanced ICD troubleshooting: Part I. Pacing Clin Electrophysiol 2005; 28:1322–46.)

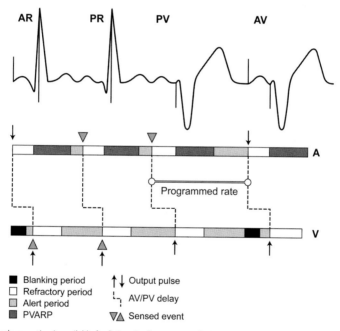

Fig. 7.48 In the DDT mode an option is available for "triggering" to occur on the P wave, R wave, or both P and R waves. R wave triggering can provide simultaneous right and left ventricular stimulation. (Figure is courtesy of and copyrighted by St. Jude Medical.)

tricle should be refractory and the LV pacing stimulus would be ineffective (Fig. 7.49). However, because there are situations where competitive LV pacing could possibly result in competitive pacing and induction of a ventricular tachyarrhythmia (Fig. 7.50), devices may incorporate a protective feature. Features such as Left Ventricular Protection Period (LVPP™) and LV-T wave

Protection are designed to prevent pacing during the LV vulnerable period (T wave) (Fig. 7.51).

Upper rate behavior in biventricular pacing
Specific to biventricular pacing is an understanding of how upper rate behavior could impact consistent ventricular stimulation. The majority of patients

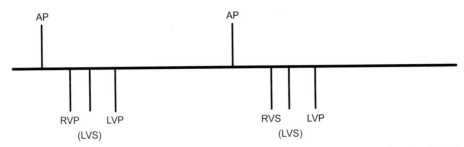

Fig. 7.49 Right ventricular sensing with biventricular pacing. The left ventricular event, resulting from conduction from the right to left ventricle, is not sensed. Therefore, because the RV-LV interval is positive, the LV paced event follows the LV event. In this theoretical schematic, it is unlikely that the LVP would result in effective capture. The second output pulse, i.e., the LVP in this example, would either encounter physiologically refractory tissue or in the setting of a very delayed interventricular conduction, true fusion would result. It is unlikely that this type of competitive pacing would induce a repetitive rhythm. (From Wang P, Kramer A, Estes NA 3rd, Hayes DL. Timing cycles for biventricular pacing. Pacing Clin Electrophysiol 2002; 25:62–75, by permission of Blackwell Publishing.)

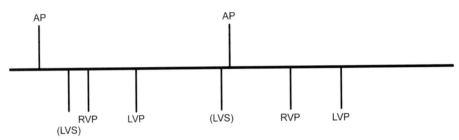

Fig. 7.50 In this hypothetical scenario a left ventricular sensed (LVS) event precedes the RV paced event. When a long RV-LV interval is present, and LV-RV conduction is very prolonged, the LV paced event may occur when the LV is no longer refractory. (From Wang P, Kramer A, Estes NA 3rd, Hayes DL. Timing cycles for biventricular pacing. Pacing Clin Electrophysiol 2002; 25:62–75, by permission of Blackwell Publishing.)

receiving biventricular pacing have intact AV conduction. Therefore, upper rate behavior that would result in pseudo-Wenckebach behavior should be avoided, because extension of the AV delay would allow a sensed ventricular event to occur and inhibit biventricular pacing (Fig. 7.52). Once ventricular sensing occurs, it is possible for inhibition to persist until the sinus cycle length becomes longer than the PR + PVARP, the so-called intrinsic TARP. The upper rate could also be affected by atrial tachyarrhythmias that are frequently seen in this population of patients. In order to maintain consistent biventricular pacing, ideally at or near 100% pacing, the TARP should be sufficiently short and the MTR should be sufficiently high. Sensor-driven pacing can also be used to permit continued biventricular pacing.

Atrial premature beats with conduction may cause a similar phenomenon by causing atrial undersensing and loss of biventricular pacing.[22]

Premature beats and biventricular timing cycles
In a dual-chamber pacemaker a PVC is usually defined as two consecutive ventricular events without an intervening atrial event. In a dual-chamber pacemaker the presence of an event identified as a PVC would reset the timing cycle and potentially uncouple AV synchrony. In addition, a PVC may trigger an extension of the PVARP to prevent the occurrence of pacemaker-mediated tachycardia.

In a CRT system, a PVARP extension and the subsequent functional atrial undersensing that may occur along with uncoupling of AV synchrony may result in loss of biventricular pacing. Thus, the PVC-PVARP extension function, if an option, should usually be deactivated in a CRT system.

Refractory periods and biventricular pacing
After pacing in one ventricular chamber, a cross-chamber refractory period may be created. If there is

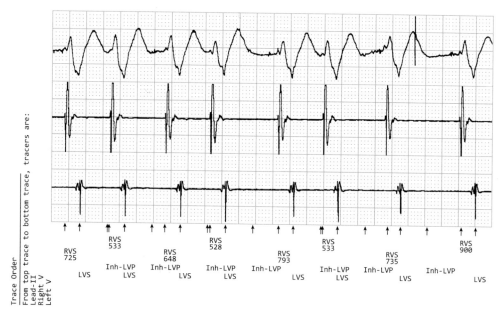

Fig. 7.51 In this tracing there is a notation in the marker channel of "Inh-LVP" which represents inhibition of left ventricular (LV) pacing. This is due to the LV protection period algorithm, which is designed to prevent pacing during the LV vulnerable period (T wave). (Reproduced with permission from Swerdlow CD, Friedman PA. Advanced ICD troubleshooting: Part I. Pacing Clin Electrophysiol 2005; 28:1322–46.)

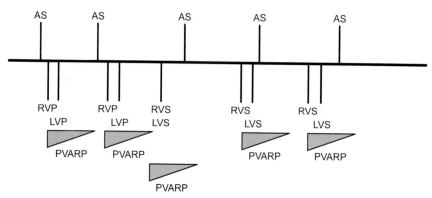

Fig. 7.52 Biventricular pacing and sensing with loss of atrioventricular synchrony and biventricular pacing. The premature right ventricular sensed event places the next P wave within the post-ventricular atrial refractory period (PVARP). Since the intrinsic PR is long, the next atrial event falls again in PVARP. (From Wang P, Kramer A, Estes NA 3rd, Hayes DL. Timing cycles for biventricular pacing. Pacing Clin Electrophysiol 2002; 25:62–75, by permission of Blackwell Publishing.)

a programmed offset between LV and RV pacing, the total ventricular refractory period may be prolonged. If the device is programmed so that LV stimulation precedes RV stimulation, the total ventricular refractory period may be quite long. In a CRT-D system the prolonged sensing refractoriness could theoretically compromise detection of ventricular tachyarrhythmias.

Timing cycles in ICDs

The timing cycles of pacemakers apply to ICDs as well. However, there are timing cycle issues and "lock-outs" that are specific to ICDs. These features are discussed in detail in Chapter 10: Troubleshooting.

Initial electrocardiographic interpretation

In reviewing an ECG from a patient with an implanted pacemaker, one should carefully assess the underlying rhythm and its relationship to the pacemaker artifacts. The first step is to find any portion of the ECG during which intrinsic cardiac rhythm can be identified. That portion of the ECG should be interpreted as any ECG would be: PR, QRS, and QT intervals; rate; axis; voltage; and so forth. If no intrinsic rhythm is apparent, the patient may be pacemaker dependent or the pacemaker may be programmed to stimulate faster (i.e., at a shorter cycle length) than the intrinsic rate. After determining the spontaneous atrial and ventricular rhythms, one should look for any relationship between the two; e.g., does a P wave result in a QRS complex, indicating intact AV conduction? After the intrinsic rhythm has been carefully scrutinized, pacemaker activity should be assessed. If pacemaker activity is present, is there one stimulus or are there two stimuli? If only one stimulus is present, does it result in atrial (Fig. 7.53) or ventricular (Fig. 7.54) depolarization? Is there an

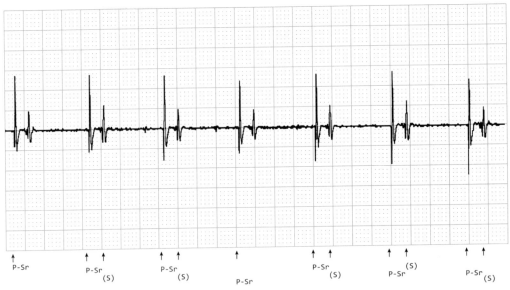

Fig. 7.53 Programmer-derived tracing of a patient programmed to AAIR pacing mode. The atrial events are paced (P, paced; Sr, sensor-driven). However, there are also events that are sensed on the atrial channel but occurring within the refractory period and corresponding to the ventricular events on the tracing, with the exception of the first and fourth ventricular events. (This manufacturer designates a sensed event as "S" and the ( ) indicate that it has occurred in the refractory period.) Therefore, there is atrial far-field sensing, but because the events fall in refractory, they do not alter the timing cycle.

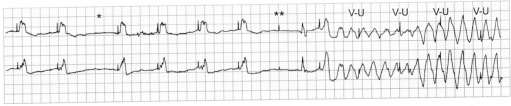

Fig. 7.54 ECG tracing from a patient with a pacemaker programmed to VVI at approximately 70 ppm. There is a longer V-V interval representing oversensing (*); there is a subsequent pacing spike with failure to capture (**); and in the terminal portion of the tracing the patient develops ventricular tachycardia and the pacemaker does not sense the tachyarrhythmia. Pacing artifacts can be seen to march through the tachyarrhythmia, labeled as V-U (ventricular undersensing).

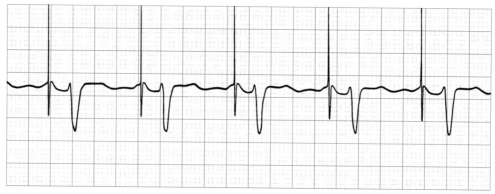

Fig. 7.55 ECG tracing demonstrating AAT pacing mode with a pacing artifact occurring within each intrinsic atrial event. In the absence of an intrinsic atrial event, a pacing artifact is delivered at the same interval and atrial depolarization follows the pacing artifact.

apparent relationship between pacemaker activity and atrial activity or ventricular activity, or both? If pacing artifacts are occurring only in the ventricle, there is no relationship between the pacemaker stimulus and a preceding P wave and the pacemaker stimulus follows the intrinsic QRS complex at a consistent cycle length, ventricular sensing as part of ventricular inhibited (VVI) pacing is present (Fig. 7.54). If a pacemaker artifact is consistently found within intrinsic P or QRS complexes, a triggered pacing mode (AAT or VVT) exists (Fig. 7.55).

It is usually not possible to determine from the ECG whether the pacemaker is operating in a bipolar or a unipolar configuration. With analog recording systems, it may be possible to assess the size of the pacemaker stimulus in an effort to determine polarity. If the pacemaker artifact is large, it is most likely of the unipolar configuration; if a very small pacemaker artifact is present, it is most likely of the bipolar configuration. With the more commonly used digital recording systems, which artificially simulate the pacemaker artifact, the size of pacing artifacts is meaningless. There may even be situations in which all cardiac activity is paced and no artifacts are visualized or artifacts are only intermittently present even though all activity is paced (Fig. 7.56).

Response to magnet application
Assessing the magnet response of the pacemaker provides additional information about pacemaker function and may be helpful in interpretation of the paced ECG. Magnet response may also help identify the pacing mode and often the specific pulse generator, and is equally useful for single-chamber and dual-chamber pacing.

Application of a magnet to a single-chamber pacemaker always results in single-chamber asynchronous pacing (Fig. 7.57). In dual-chamber pacemakers, magnet application almost always results in asynchronous pacing in both the atrial and the ventricular chambers (DOO mode) (Fig. 7.58). There are pacemakers that have a programmable option of turning the magnet response "off" and some with an option of having asynchronous operation for a specified number of beats followed by return of synchronous behavior. If magnet application fails to result in asynchronous behavior, programmed parameters should be checked to see if the magnet has been programmed "off." Also, some pacemakers, when in a "reset" mode, will not display a magnet response. Historically there have been exceptions, e.g., pacemakers with a VOO magnet response even when programmed to the DDD mode, but few, if any, remain in service.

The pacing rate should be determined during magnet application. Is the magnet rate faster or slower than or the same as the programmed pacemaker rate? If the pacemaker is a single-chamber pacemaker, does it result in atrial or ventricular depolarization? Having determined what chamber is being paced, one can assess the pacemaker artifact and subsequent depolarization to ensure proper capture. It should be remembered that pacemakers of different manufacturers respond differently to magnet application. Some continue to pace asynchronously for a specific number of beats after removal of the magnet and may do so at more than one rate. The magnet response of a particular pacemaker may vary depending on the programmed parameters, i.e., the mode, of the pacemaker.

It is important that few assumptions be made about the details of the magnet mode of operation

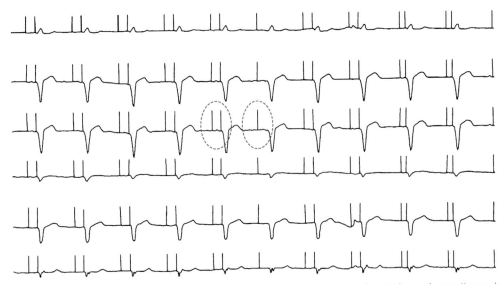

Fig. 7.56 Twelve-lead electrocardiogram (insert is close-up of the area described) that demonstrates all ventricular paced events. However, in the area circled, there is a ventricular paced event without a discernible pacing artifact. The ventricular event is paced in this completely dependent patient and the absence of the pacing artifact is a function of the digital recording system.

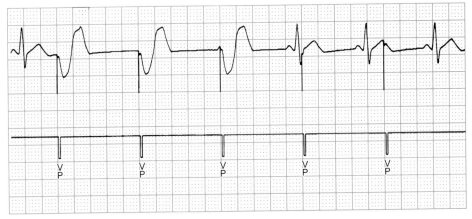

Fig. 7.57 VVI pacemaker with magnet application resulting in VOO pacing and competition with the underlying rhythm.

and that one be aware of the specifics of the magnet response in a particular unit; otherwise, an erroneous interpretation of inappropriate operation may be made. The magnet mode is usually (but not always) free of sensing any events and is often at a specific rate independent of the programmed rate and sensitivity settings. In the presence of a puzzling or unusual ECG, magnet application may allow determination of whether the pulse generator is capable of operating normally.

When a single cardiac chamber is being paced, the effect of the paced chamber on the remaining chamber should be determined. For example, if an atrial pacemaker is present, does atrial depolarization result in AV conduction and an intrinsic QRS complex, demonstrating intact AV conduction (Fig. 7.59)? Alternatively, if a ventricular pacemaker is present, is there retrograde activation of the atrium, resulting in retrograde P wave activity following the paced ventricular complex (Fig. 7.60)?

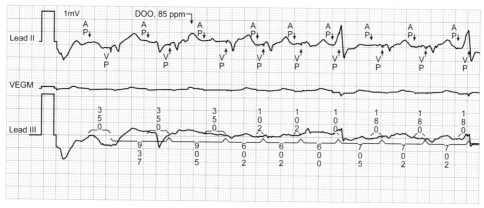

Fig. 7.58 DDD pacemaker with "magnet test" performed via the pacemaker. This results in DOO operation with competition between asynchronous pacing and underlying intrinsic rhythm.

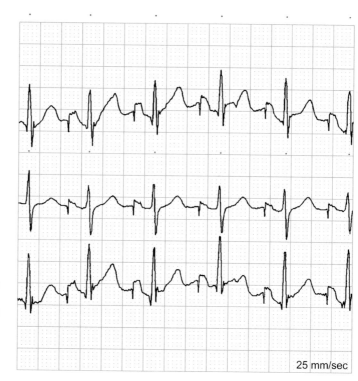

Fig. 7.59 From inspection of the ECG tracing one can discern that there is atrial pacing with subsequent atrial depolarization and intrinsic ventricular depolarization. Based on this one can assume that the pacing mode could be AAI or AAIR, or possibly DDD or DDDR, with a programmed AV interval that is longer than the measured AR interval, or the patient may have a feature such as positive AV hysteresis or another ventricular pacing avoidance algorithm.

25 mm/sec

Single-chamber pacemakers

By following the preceding steps, one will have determined whether a single-chamber or dual-chamber pacemaker is present and whether the pacemaker stimuli result in atrial or ventricular depolarization (or both). If a single-chamber atrial pacemaker is present,

if stimulation produces atrial capture, and if the pacemaker artifact is inhibited by intrinsic P waves, the pacemaker is in the atrial inhibited (AAI) mode (Fig. 7.53). In the AAI mode, paced ventricular activity is never seen, with or without magnet application, and with normal function a pacemaker artifact does

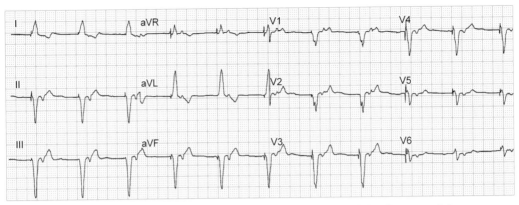

Fig. 7.60 Twelve-lead ECG with consistent ventricular pacing and each ventricular paced event is followed by a retrograde P wave.

not occur within the intrinsic P waves. If a stimulus occurs that results in ventricular capture with inhibition by QRS complexes, the pacemaker is in the ventricular inhibited mode (VVI). If the pacemaker is pacing asynchronously without sensing or capture of either the atrium or the ventricle, the mode cannot be determined. Similarly, with a single-chamber pacemaker, either atrial or ventricular, if intrinsic activity is never seen and every complex is paced, either the patient is pacemaker-dependent or the pacemaker has been programmed to a rate faster than the intrinsic cardiac rate.

If a single stimulus falls consistently into the spontaneous P wave or QRS complex, the mode is of the triggered variety (AAT/VVT) (Fig. 7.55). Although this mode of pacing is available in many multimodal programmable pacemakers, it is rarely used as a long-term pacing mode. Programming a pacemaker to the triggered mode is sometimes helpful to determine exactly where on the surface ECG sensing occurs.

An exception to the rule of the timing cycles in AAI and VVI pacing and a long-standing source of confusion is hysteresis. This programmable feature allows the escape interval for the initial paced beat to be at a longer cycle length than subsequent paced intervals (Fig. 7.61). For example, if a patient has sinus node dysfunction with episodes of sinus bradycardia or sinus arrest, the pacemaker can be programmed to pace continuously at an interval of 1000 ms (rate of 60), but hysteresis takes place at a rate of 40, i.e., 1500 ms without a paced event is allowed before pacing is initiated at the programmed rate. If one does not know that hysteresis is "on," the two different intervals may give the appearance of over-sensing. However, if the intervals are repetitive and the longer interval always follows an intrinsic beat, hysteresis is the most likely explanation.

Dual-chamber pacemakers

If a dual-chamber pacemaker is present, the steps already outlined should be followed, including determination of the AVI and the status of AV and VA conduction.

The next step in interpretation of an ECG with dual-chamber pacing should be to determine the pacing mode. During the free-running (nonmagnet) pacemaker mode, it should be determined whether ventricular sensing, ventricular pacing, atrial pacing, or ventricular tracking of atrial activity occurs.

If P wave activity is being sensed, does each P wave begin a pacemaker cycle? If each spontaneous P wave results in a paced ventricular complex at a consistent preset AV delay, the pacemaker is P synchronous and may be in the DDD or VDD mode (Fig. 7.62). There are several ways to differentiate VDD from DDD pacing. Intermittent atrial pacing indicates DDD pacing; the absence of atrial activity followed by ventricular pacing at the lower rate or sensor-indicated rate is consistent with VDD pacing (Fig. 7.63). With magnet application, DDD pacemakers usually respond with DOO pacing and VDD pacemakers with VOO pacing.

If each sensed P wave inhibits pacemaker output but initiates synchronous ventricular pacing, the pacemaker is in the DDI mode (Fig. 7.64). Sensed atrial activity inhibits atrial output but does not result in a ventricular stimulus after the AV delay. AV sequential pacing at the programmed rate is provided if intrinsic activity is absent. Intrinsic ventricular activity occurring during the atrial escape interval or AV delay inhibits the pacemaker and resets the timing cycle.

Atrioventricular interval

The components and potential variations of the AVI have already been discussed. As the ECG is analyzed,

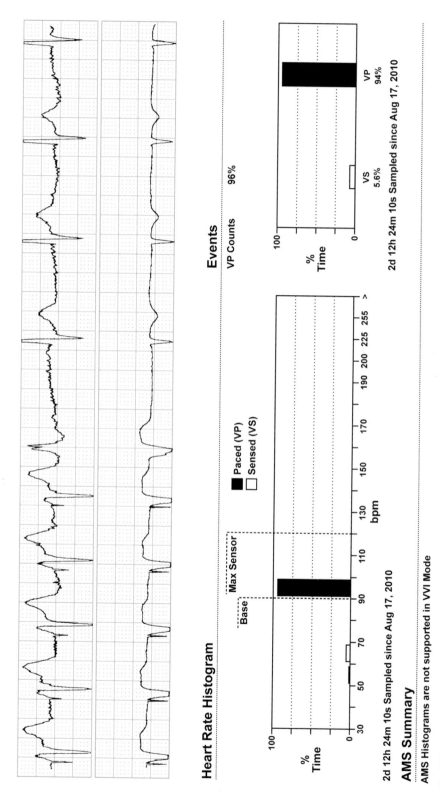

Heart Rate Histogram

Max Sensor

Base

100

%
Time

0

30   50   70   90   110   130   150   170   190   200   225   255 >

bpm

■ Paced (VP)
□ Sensed (VS)

2d 12h 24m 10s Sampled since Aug 17, 2010

AMS Summary

AMS Histograms are not supported in VVI Mode

Events

VP Counts   96%

100

%
Time

0

VS   VP
5.6%   94%

2d 12h 24m 10s Sampled since Aug 17, 2010

Fig. 7.61 ECG tracing from a patient with a pacemaker programmed to VVIR pacing with a lower rate of 90 ppm and a hysteresis rate of 50 ppm. The tracing begins with pacing at a rate of 90 ppm (666 ms) but when an intrinsic ventricular event occurs (VS) pacing at a rate of 90 ppm is no longer evident because the pacemaker will not reinitiate pacing at a rate of 90 ppm until the lower rate times out at the hysteresis interval of 50 ppm or 1200 ms. (From Friedman PA, Rott MA, Wokhlu A, Asirvatham SJ, Hayes DL. A Case-based approach to pacemakers, ICDs, and cardiac resynchronization: Advanced questions for exam review and clinical practice. Minneapolis: Cardiotext. 2011. Used with permission of Mayo Foundation for Medical Education and Research.)

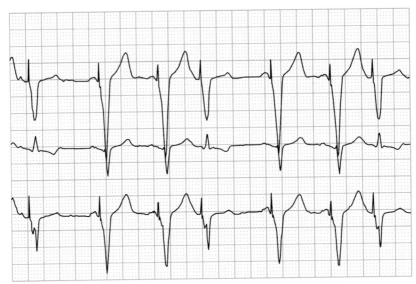

Fig. 7.62 ECG tracing in which only one pacing artifact is present for each cardiac cycle and it consistently depolarizes the ventricle. However, one can assume that the pacemaker is functioning in a VDD or DDD mode, because every paced ventricular event is preceded by an intrinsic P wave.

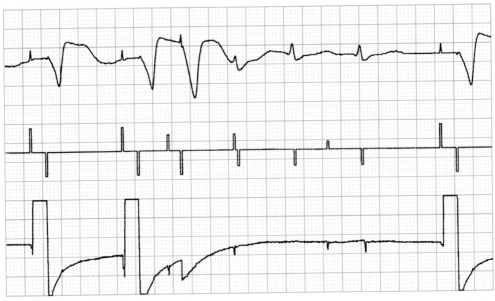

Fig. 7.63 ECG tracing from a patient with atrial and ventricular sensing and pacing. This can only be compatible with DDD or DDDR pacing mode. Pacing artifacts are detectable in this example. However, in addition to looking for and at the pacing artifacts, note the marker channel (middle tracing). Marks going up from baseline represent atrial events and downward marks are ventricular events. The "longer" marks correspond to paced events, the intermediate sized marks represent sensed events and the shortest mark. represents an event that occurs in a refractory period. Even if the pacing artifacts were not easily seen and even if the marker channel was not labeled, it is still possible to identify events by the direction and length of the "marks" provided on the marker channel.

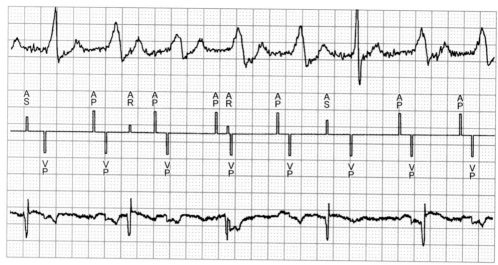

Fig. 7.64 ECG tracing in which both atrial and ventricular pacing artifacts are present. In addition to looking at the artifacts, look for relationships between the atrial and ventricular events. It is striking that although the atrial pace (AP) to ventricular pace (VP) is constant, there is variation between the native P waves (AS) and the subsequent paced ventricular event (VP). This is because the device is programmed to the DDI mode and, although the atrial events are sensed, they are not tracked. In addition, there is an AP event with failure to capture followed by an intrinsic atrial event that falls in refractory (AR). The VP event occurs essentially simultaneously with the AR event and is triggered by the programmed paced AV interval that is initiated with the AP that fails to capture.

the AVI should be assessed for any variations. The possible explanations for a variant AVI include:

- Ventricular safety pacing
- PV vs. AV interval (differential AV delay)
- AVI hysteresis – either "positive" or "negative"
- Rate-variable or rate-adaptive AVI
- Ventricular pacing avoidance algorithm.

Upper rate behavior

Descriptions have already been provided for 1:1 P synchronous pacing at the MTR, pseudo-Wenckebach, and 2:1 upper rate behavior (Fig. 7.65). Other variations are fallback and rate smoothing.

Rate smoothing

Rate smoothing avoids abrupt changes in pacing rate, such as those that can occur during a sudden transition to pseudo-Wenckebach or 2:1 upper rate behavior, sinus pause or sinus arrest, premature ventricular and/or atrial contractions, paroxysmal supraventricular tachyarrhythmias, and may eliminate patient symptoms associated with sensed rhythm disturbances.

Rate smoothing controls sudden changes in ventricular cycle length by monitoring the interval between ventricular events (both paced and sensed) and storing the most recent RR interval in memory (Fig. 7.66). On

the basis of this RR interval and the programmed rate-smoothing percentage, the pulse generator sets up two rate-control windows for the next cycle – one for the atrium and one for the ventricle (Fig. 7.67). For example, if the monitored VV interval is 800 ms and 6% rate smoothing is programmed, the algorithm allows the upcoming VV cycle length to increase or decrease a maximum of 6%, or ±48 ms (752–848 ms).

The rate-smoothing algorithm determines the atrial control window in a manner analogous to the basic ventricular timing cycle: VV = VA + AV. To determine the VA interval from this equation if the VV interval and AVI are known, one simply subtracts the AVI from the VV interval. Rate smoothing does likewise by subtracting the AVI value from the ventricular control window, and the result is a "rate-controlled VA interval." Extending the previous example, if the AVI is 150 ms, the atrial control window is also ±48 ms (602–698 ms). Atrial pacing is observed at the maximum calculated VA interval of 698 ms if no sensed event occurs before the end of the VA interval.

Ventricular rate regularization This feature is useful in patients with chronic atrial fibrillation or frequent atrial tachyarrhythmias. The purpose of the algorithm is to reduce variability in V-V cycle length when atrial

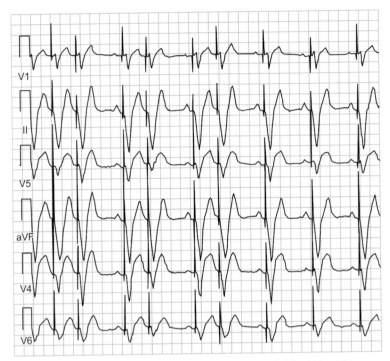

Fig. 7.65 ECG example of upper rate behaviors including transient pseudo-Wenckebach on the left, which rapidly progresses to 2:1 upper rate behavior as the atrial rate continues to increase.

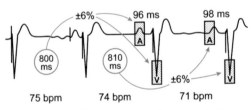

Fig. 7.66 Example of how two rate-smoothing synchronization windows are calculated. If the heart rate is 75 ppm (800 ms) and rate smoothing is programmed "on" at 6%, the next cycle length may vary by 48 ms, a range from 752 to 848 ms. The subsequent cycle would be calculated as ±6% of 752 or 848 ms, depending on whether the atrial rate was increasing or decreasing.

arrhythmias are conducted. Pacing during AF may also modestly slow the ventricular response by means of concealed conduction into the AV node. Specific algorithms vary between manufacturers, but similar to "rate-smoothing" described above a regularization algorithm will calculate the differences between cycle lengths and pace as necessary to minimize ventricular cycle length variation.

Fallback

In a generic sense this feature can be thought of as a mechanism to decrease the paced rate gradually, but the specific "fallback" feature may vary between manufacturers. Fallback operation refers to the decrement in paced rate that occurs after criteria for mode-switch have been met. Once the mode has switched, the pacing rate will "fallback" to either the sensor-indicated rate or the programmed lower rate that is specific to the mode-switch algorithm (Fig. 7.68).

A different type of paced rate "fallback" may be an option for the patient's hours of sleep. A "sleep" function allows a lower rate to be used during the sleeping hours. In some devices the patient's usual hours of bedtime and arising are programmed into the pacemaker and the desired lower rate during "sleep." In other devices the sleep function may be tied to the rate-adaptive sensor. If the sensor detects no activity for a given period of time, the lower "sleep" rate would go into effect until activity is again recognized.

Biventricular paced electrocardiogram: position, adequacy, and timing

Along with clinical examination, device interrogation, and echocardiography, the biventricular paced ECG

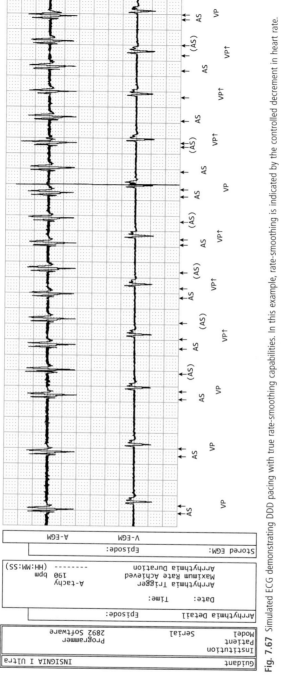

Fig. 7.67 Simulated ECG demonstrating DDD pacing with true rate-smoothing capabilities. In this example, rate-smoothing is indicated by the controlled decrement in heart rate.

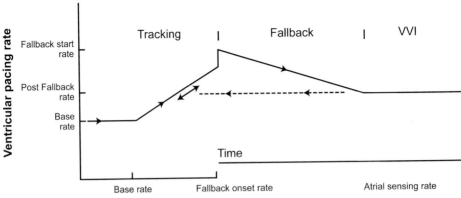

Fig. 7.68 Schematic representation of "fallback" behavior. (Figure is courtesy of and copyrighted by St. Jude Medical.)

provides important and, at times, unique insights into adequacy of lead position and device function. In addition, appropriate adjustments made to the biventricular device based on knowledge of the relevant timing cycles and ECG findings may optimize device function.

The caregiver should interpret the ECG from a patient with a CRT device with two broad questions in mind. First, what can be said about the location and adequacy of LV lead capture, and the second, whether clues as to why a specific patient may not be benefiting from CRT therapy are present.[23–27]

Assessing pacemaker lead position
With careful analysis of the 12-lead ECG, one should be able to comment on whether the LV lead is capturing and the exact location of the LV lead.

The cardiac vector principle
When the wave front of depolarization (cardiac activation) proceeds towards the positive electrode of an ECG lead, a positive deflection is inscribed (R wave) on that ECG lead recording.[28–30]

It follows that when cardiac activation moves away from the positive electrode of that ECG lead, a negative deflection or S wave is inscribed. This simple principle allows highly accurate interpretation of pacemaker lead location and adequacy of capture.

All that remains to obtain full appreciation of device and lead function from the ECG is for one to know where the positive poles for the various ECG leads are located (Fig. 7.69).[31–34]

The left lateral leads
Leads I, aVL, V5, and V6 all have their positive electrode equivalent on the left side of the heart. Thus, right ventricular pacing typically results in an R wave on these leads while LV lateral wall pacing causes a predominant S wave in these leads.

Right-sided leads
Leads V1, aVR, and lead III have their positive electrodes on the right side of the body, and in these leads an S wave is generated with right ventricular pacing, etc.[35]

Anterior/posteroinferior leads
ECG leads II, III, and aVF all have their positive electrodes inferiorly (feet leads). The primary use of interpreting the ECG vector in these leads is to define whether the pacing lead is located anteriorly (tributaries of these anterior intraventricular vein, right ventricular outflow tract position, etc.) or on the inferior wall of the heart (middle cardiac vein, posterior cardiac vein, or RV apical location). Thus, a tall R wave in leads II, III, and aVF suggests lead location and origin of activation on the anterior surface of the heart while deep S waves in II, III, and aVF are typical of RV apical or middle cardiac vein pacing location.

Base vs. apex
Also of interest to determine adequacy of lead position is to know whether the LV pacing lead is apically or basally (near the mitral annulus) located.[36–38] Analysis of several leads in conjunction is required to make this determination. Most precordial leads (lead II–V6) have their positive electrodes located near the cardiac apex, and thus basally located leads tend to be positive (R wave) in the precordial chest leads whereas apical lead location is reflected by S waves inscribed in these leads.[39] Leads aVR and aVL are high superior leads on the right and left side of the heart, respectively, and will be negative (S wave) with basal lead location and posi-

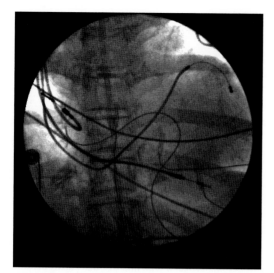

Fig. 7.69 Pacemaker leads in the right atrial appendage and right ventricular apex are positioned in the usual fashion. The left ventricular lead courses through the coronary sinus and is placed in a lateral cardiac vein midway between the base and apex. Pacing from this left ventricular stimulation site will result in a vector that moves away from lead I and aVL and toward leads V1 and aVR.

tive with more apical lead location. For example, if the LV pacing lead has been placed in a lateral cardiac vein and advanced all the way to the apex, lead V4, V5, and V6 will show predominantly S waves, but lead aVR will be positive.[40]

For a given lead, the reader will note that it certainly serves more than one purpose, e.g., V4, V5, and V6 help define apical as well as lateral location, and lead III is both a right-sided lead and an inferior lead.

Similarly, one set of leads like the inferior leads (II, III, aVF) can be analyzed to have an idea of whether the pacing lead is located in the right inferior or left inferior location. For example, middle cardiac vein pacing will result in a negative deflection in all three of these inferior leads, but lead II will be more negative than lead III, whereas with right ventricular apical pacing lead III tends to be more negative than lead II.

Characteristic electrocardiographic patterns with specific lead locations

Right ventricular apical pacing

Typical RV apical pacing is readily recognized on the ECG (Fig. 7.70).[41] The rightward lead, V1, shows an S wave and thus mimics left bundle branch block. Leads II, III, and aVF show deep S waves because the vector proceeds from this inferior pacing site away from these

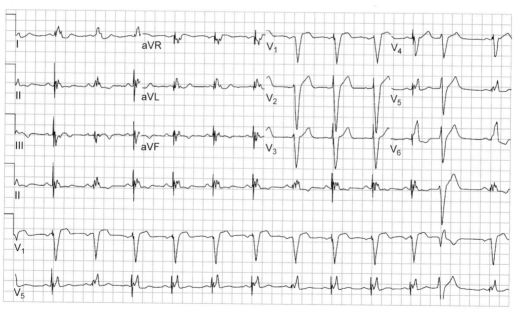

Fig. 7.70 Pacing from the standard right ventricular position. This site is characterized by the left bundle branch block pattern in lead V1 and positive deflections in leads I and aVL. Note that lead aVR may be negative or positive depending on how apical the lead is located. In this instance, the lead is about 1 cm proximal to the apex, as evidenced by small positive deflections in leads II and aVF.

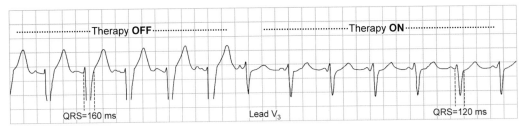

Fig. 7.71 When biventricular stimulation therapy is turned on, the QRS duration markedly narrows. This is the anticipated result of simultaneous stimulation of the right and left ventricles. As noted in the text, stimulation from a single site on the ventricular septum may result in a narrow QRS complex. Conversely, biventricular stimulation when there is marked exit delay as well as interventricular conduction delay will not result in a narrow QRS complex despite simultaneous biventricular pacing.

leads. Lead I (a left-sided lead) shows an R wave, and lead III (a rightward inferior lead) is invariably negative (deep S wave).[42,43]

Nonapical right ventricular site pacing

When analyzing the biventricular electrogram, it is important to know where the right ventricular lead is placed and appreciate the typical ECG vector from RV pacing alone from these locations.

When the pacing lead is placed in the RVOT, V1 shows a negative deflection (left bundle branch block-like pattern as with RV apical pacing). However, leads II, III, and aVF show strongly positive R waves.

Septal locations for the RV pacing lead often have a relatively narrow QRS complex (Figs 7.71 and 7.72)[44] because bipolar capture on the septum may result in near-simultaneous depolarization of LV and RV myocardium. All RV free wall locations would be associated with wider QRS complexes and a tall R wave in lead I.

Left ventricular lateral wall pacing – the "ideal" pacing location

It is important to be familiar with the ECG pattern associated with LV free wall (lateral wall) pacing midway between the base and apex. Most studies support the premise that LV lead placement in this location (assuming there are good thresholds, no phrenic nerve stimulation, and no lateral wall myocardial infarction) is optimal for CRT benefit.[45–56] The main branches of the coronary sinus may all allow LV free wall pacing (lateral branches of the anterior intraventricular vein, posterolateral vein, and lateral branches of the middle cardiac vein) (Figs 7.73 and 7.74).

As with most LV pacing sites, this "ideal" location produces an R wave in V1 (right bundle morphology), but, in addition, lead I is either all negative or mostly an S wave when the lateral wall of the LV is the site of

pacing origin. Leads aVR and leads V4/V5 will have an overall similar vector with mid free wall pacing because the cardiac activation goes both towards the apex (leads V4, V5, V6) as well as towards the base (aVR). Of these criteria, lead I being negative is a simple and clinically useful ECG tool to recognize adequate position on the free wall of the LV. RV and LV pacing sites that are too close to the septum will have an initial vector that goes towards lead I and thus an initial R wave.

Anterior and posterior left ventricular pacing

Lateral branches of the anterior or middle cardiac vein when used for pacing produces an ECG pattern very similar to that seen with LV free wall pacing – the "ideal" location described above. When the lead is located more anteriorly, however, leads II, III, and aVF tend to be positive (Figs 7.75–7.77), but with middle cardiac vein or posterior vein pacing, leads II, III, and aVF will be more negative (deeper S waves).

Middle cardiac vein pacing can be difficult to distinguish from RV apical pacing on the limb lead access. However, because the LV is more posterior than the RV and the middle cardiac vein is located on the epicardial inferior wall of the LV (Fig. 7.78), there will usually be a tall R wave in lead V1 (a right anterior lead) giving rise to a right bundle branch block morphology rather than the left bundle morphology seen with RV apical pacing.

Biventricular paced ECG

With both RV and LV lead pacing, a hybrid ECG pattern is produced. Once the interpreting healthcare provider is thoroughly familiar with the RV apical pacing ECG, then by appreciating where the vector deviates from this known pattern (RV apical), the location of the LV pacing lead can be deduced. For example, in a patient with biventricular stimulation and the RV lead known to be located in the RV apex, if lead I is

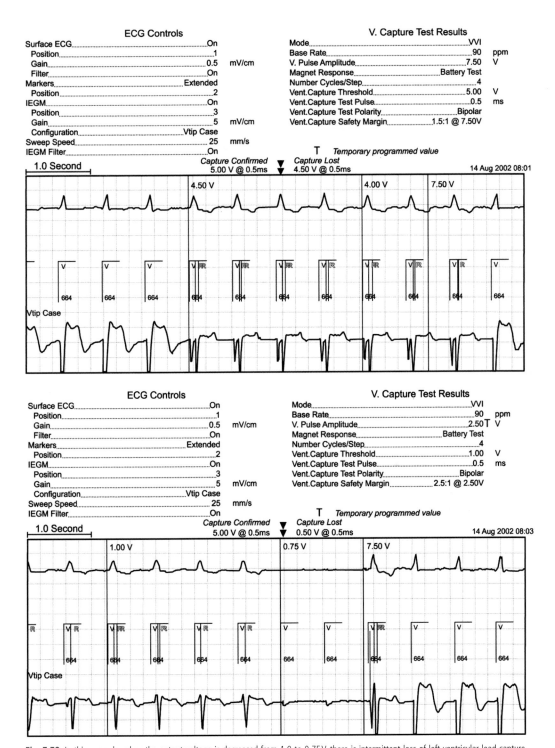

Fig. 7.72 In this example, when the output voltage is decreased from 1.0 to 0.75V, there is intermittent loss of left ventricular lead capture. This is evidenced by the appearance of the sensed electrogram on the ventricular pacing lead. In addition, a change in QRS duration is seen intermittently. With further decrease in voltage at 0.5V, complete loss of capture is noted. In this particular device, the presence or absence of the sensed electrogram is also useful in determining capture.

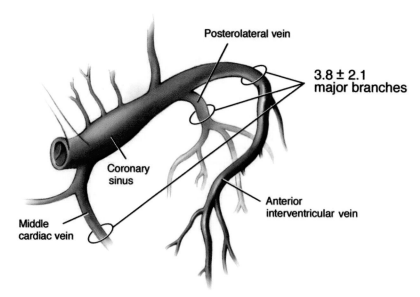

Fig. 7.73 Typical coronary venous anatomy. Usually three to five major branches of the coronary sinus are visible at angiography and can be used for left ventricular stimulation. The three most consistent branches are the middle cardiac vein, the posterolateral or lateral vein, and the anterior interventricular vein.

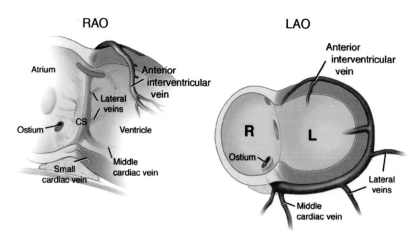

Fig. 7.74 Typical right anterior oblique (RAO) and left anterior oblique (LAO) projections of the coronary sinus (CS) and ventricular veins. Note that the lateral veins as well as lateral branches of the anterior intraventricular vein drain the free wall of the left ventricle. Pacing from these sites results in a negative deflection in leads I and aVL.

negative, then one can be fairly certain that the LV lead is located on the lateral wall of the LV (Fig. 7.79).[29–47]

Timing intervals and the ECG

ECG analysis in the patient with a CRT device can help assess ventricular synchrony and sometimes point to necessary changes in timing intervals to optimize device function (Table 7.4).[48,49]

The premise for biventricular pacing benefit is that simultaneous stimulation of the RV and LV leads gives rise to near-equal electrical activation wave fronts that in turn leads to mechanical synchronization of ventricular function. While equal and simultaneous stimulation should clearly shorten the total QRS duration, the relationship between electrical and mechanical synchronization is not straightforward.[49]

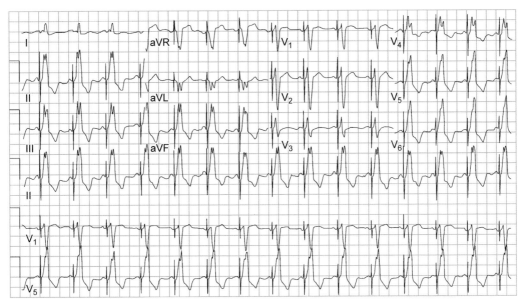

Fig. 7.75 Biventricular pacing with left ventricular lead in anterior vein. This ECG demonstrates features of both right and left ventricular pacing. In lead V1, there is a small initial deflection that is positive; otherwise, the morphology appears like left bundle branch block. This suggests biventricular pacing with early activation of the left ventricle giving rise to the initial positive R wave. The left ventricular lead is likely to be in a branch of the anterior interventricular vein, as evidenced by the tall positive R waves in leads II, III, and aVF. In this example, leads I and aVL have opposite deflections. This suggests that the lead is located very basally in the anterior interventricular vein at a more septal location.

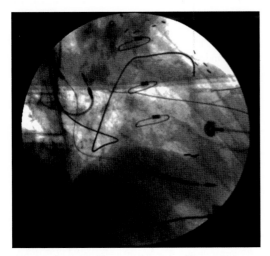

Fig. 7.76 Fluoroscopic image in right anterior oblique projection showing the coronary sinus lead being placed in a lateral branch of the anterior interventricular vein.

Once it is determined that both the RV and LV leads do capture at the programmed output, there are several factors that may yet lead to unequal contributions toward electrical and mechanical activation from each of these leads. Measurement of intracardiac intervals and assessing the differences in the 12-lead ECG with biventricular stimulation vs. single-lead stimulation (RV and LV) allows the caregiver to make these assessments.

Capture latency and the stimulus–QRS interval

In the diseased heart, there can be significant capture latency. Thus, even if both leads activate simultaneously, if there is significant capture latency from the left-sided lead, the onset of electrical activation in the myocardial tissue may occur later and thus contribute less to global ventricular electrical and mechanical activation (Fig. 7.80). Measuring the stimulus–QRS interval with single site stimulation will help make the determination whether adjustments for unusually long capture latency are needed.

In addition to true capture latency, a more common scenario is exit delay. Here, following the stimulation spike, the local ventricular electrogram is captured normally (normal capture latency); however, for electrical activation to propagate from this area of abnormal tissue to the rest of the ventricle and thus start the inscription of the surface 12-lead QRS complex may be unduly prolonged. In an extreme case, this prolongation can be so severe that entire ventricular activation

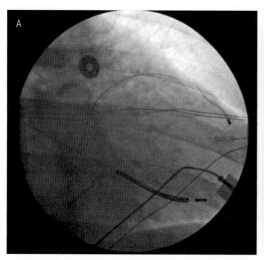 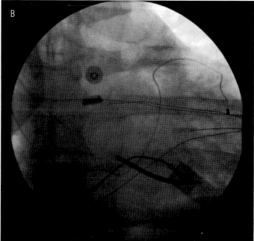

Fig. 7.77 Right and left anterior oblique projections showing coronary sinus lead placement in the lateral branch of the anterior interventricular vein. Note that on the right anterior oblique projection it is not possible to determine whether the lead is septal or lateral. However, this is easily seen in the left anterior oblique projection.

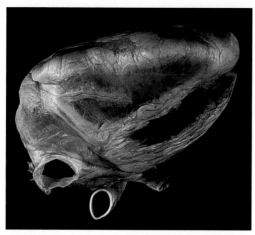

Fig. 7.78 Autopsy specimen showing the course of the middle cardiac vein (MCV) along the posterior interventricular septum. Pacing from this site results in a vector moving away from the feet. Thus, the ECG is characterized by negative deflections in leads II, III, and aVF.

is from the RV lead, and there is no contribution from an otherwise well-positioned LV lead.

The operator can determine whether this is likely to happen during the implant procedure by measuring the pacing stimulus to local ventricular ECG interval (capture latency estimation) and the stimulus to surface ECG interval (capture latency and exit delay) for each lead position. If this interval is greater than 80 ms,[50,51] either a device capable of a similar offset with V-V timing (see later) should be chosen or another lead position tried.

Clues to electrical resynchronization from the 12-lead ECG

QRS duration: One would expect the QRS duration to decrease when there is simultaneous biventricular electrical stimulation and was initially thought to be a simple predictor of likely resynchronization success (Fig. 7.71).[25,52,53] However, the electromechanical coupling interval at each ventricular site, particularly in diseased hearts, can vary significantly. As a result, even with ideal electrical stimulatory wave fronts from biventricular pacing, some sites may contract earlier and others may contract late, giving rise to significant mechanical dyssynchrony.[49] In addition, when only a few ECG leads are being assessed, there may be isoelectric intervals as a result of opposing wave front vectors relative to that particular lead and give a false impression of a narrow QRS. Thus, while QRS duration can be looked at as a very approximate surrogate for adequate resynchronization, further insights from the 12-lead ECG and mechanical activation patterns are usually required.

QRS vector fusion: The biventricular paced ECG should approximately be a hybrid pattern from RV and LV pacing. An ECG should be obtained with RV pacing alone and with LV pacing alone and then with simultaneous biventricular stimulation (Figs 7.81 and 7.82). If the resulting ECG shows a pattern that in most leads is an arithmetic sum of the positive and negative deflections with individual pacing, there is probably near-equal contribution to ventricular activation from these two leads. For example, if with LV pacing alone there is

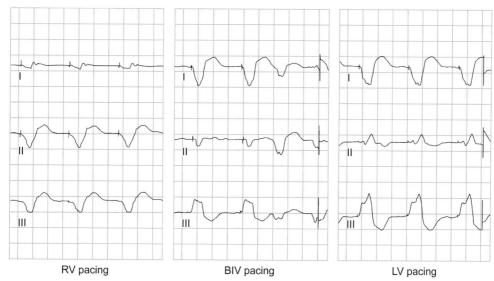

| RV pacing | BIV pacing | LV pacing |

Fig. 7.79 Although it is ideal to have a 12-lead ECG to analyze completely biventricular (BiV) pacemaker function, often a limited number of leads are available for review. In this example right ventricular (RV) pacing is associated with the expected negative deflections in leads II and III. However, lead I is isoelectric. Left ventricular (LV) pacing is likely from a lateral branch of the anterior inverventricular vein. Leads II and III are positive, suggesting an anterior stimulation site, and lead I is negative, suggesting a lateral stimulation site. In reviewing the BiV pacing ECG, no difference is discernible between BiV pacing and LV pacing on lead I. This is because of the minimal contribution to the vector in lead I from RV pacing. However, in analyzing lead II, a clear difference is seen. Also to be noted on this tracing is the minimal change in QRS width with BiV pacing. A clue to the reason for this lack of change can be deduced from the wide QRS also seen with the premature ventricular complex likely from the LV apex (negative lead I, negative leads II and III). With the wide QRS seen with these multiple stimulation sites, this patient is likely to have prominent intraventricular conduction delay.

Table 7.4 Approach to electrocardiographic (ECG) assessment of cardiac resynchronization therapy (CRT) devices.

Step	Action
1. Obtain 12-lead ECG RV pacing alone	
2. Obtain 12-lead ECG LV pacing alone	If stimulation to QRS onset >60 ms, consider reposition or device with V-V timing option
3. Obtain 12-lead ECG with simultaneous biventricular pacing	
4. Does the 12-lead ECG with biventricular pacing resemble RV pacing?	Program offset with LV early
5. Does the 12-lead ECG with biventricular pacing resemble LV pacing?	Program offset with RV early
6. Is LV pacing percentage adequate?	Assess for ventricular ectopy and enhanced intrinsic conduction via the AV node
7. Assess for evidence of anodal stimulation	Program to closely spaced bipolar pacing

AV, atrioventricular; LV, left ventricular; RV, right ventricular.

a tall R wave in lead V1 but with RV pacing alone there is a predominant S wave (left bundle morphology) in lead V1, biventricular stimulation should give either a biphasic pattern or a small amplitude QRS (isoelectric) in lead V1.

V-V interval: Analysis for vector fusion on the 12-lead ECG can be used at implant to help position the LV lead at a site where with simultaneous stimulation, a fused vector can be obtained (no inordinate exit delay from LV site). However, ECG utility is most commonly

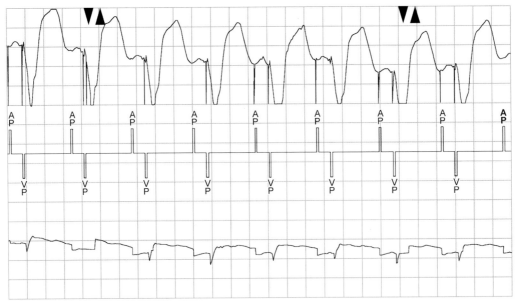

Fig. 7.80 Subtle changes in the QRS morphology can sometimes be seen on careful analysis without change in the pacing output. This is usually seen at or near threshold. Reasons for this include anodal stimulation where there is a transient change in the vector of stimulation, and in severely diseased hearts, variable degrees of exit delay from the left ventricular pacing site (presumably within markedly diseased tissue) result in varying degrees of fusion.

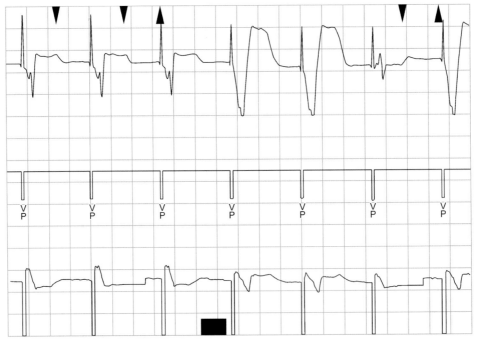

Fig. 7.81 Biventricular, posterolateral vein to right ventricle only. Lead III QRS complexes are seen while pacing output is being decreased. The first three complexes show biventricular capture. The next two complexes show loss of capture from the left ventricular lead, giving rise to right ventricular stimulation only. The next complex is a fusion beat between right ventricular pacing and intrinsic conduction. Note widening of the QRS complex when biventricular capture is lost. Lead III continues to be negative with or without biventricular stimulation. This suggests that the left ventricular pacing lead is located in a posterior or posterolateral location, i.e., the middle cardiac or posterolateral vein. However, the degree of QRS narrowing during biventricular stimulation suggests that the lead is in fact in the posterolateral vein, resulting in better synchronization and shortening of the QRS complex than is likely from the middle cardiac vein.

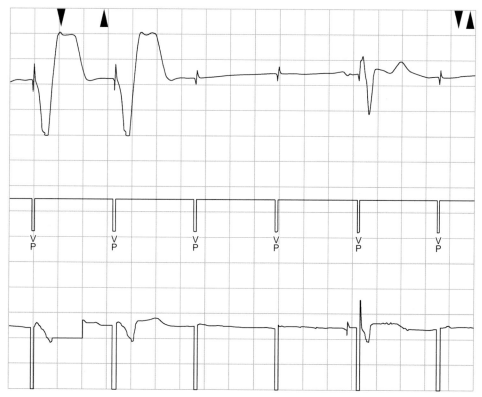

Fig. 7.82 Further decrease in the output results in loss of right ventricular capture, and the intrinsic complex can be seen. Often, the intrinsic complexes seen soon after loss of capture are narrow compared with the native QRS complexes seen before pacing was initiated. This is probably due to retrograde penetration bilaterally of the bundle branch system giving rise to equal delay when intrinsic conduction comes through, relatively normalizing the QRS complex.

utilized in practice at follow-up. Especially if patients have experienced less than optimal benefit from CRT lead placement, then a 12-lead ECG with RV pacing alone, LV pacing alone, and biventricular simultaneous stimulation can be obtained. Most devices now allow V-V timing options; i.e., setting an offset that allows one of the leads to stimulate before the other.

If the biventricular paced ECG shows a morphology very similar to RV pacing alone, then progressively longer offsets with LV early should be programmed and ECGs obtained until a fused/hybrid pattern is seen. On the other hand, if the biventricular simultaneous stimulation ECG looks mostly like LV pacing alone, then an offset with RV early should be programmed on and ECGs obtained an analyzed in an iterative fashion until adequate vector fusion is noted.

Because electromechanical coupling intervals may be quite disordered and hard to predict in diseased hearts, ECG based V-V timing can be carried out in conjunc-

tion with echocardiography using techniques that allow high sampling or frame rates.[54-56]

Atrioventricular interval programming

In patients with cardiac disease, atrial conduction may be abnormal.[57] As a result, with right atrial pacing and biventricular stimulation, the left atrium may be activated quite late and simultaneous or even after LV activation. This situation may create an equivalent of left-sided pacemaker syndrome and lead to increased pulmonary venous pressures, etc. While the situation can be detected and appropriate AV interval programming performed with echocardiographic guidance,[58,59] the 12-lead ECG may also be of value. Here, the P wave duration is noted, and if ventricular stimulation occurs even before inscription of the terminal P wave, the AV interval is likely programmed too short and optimal atrial filling is unlikely to occur (Figs 7.83–7.86). Left atrial pacing via the coronary sinus can be considered

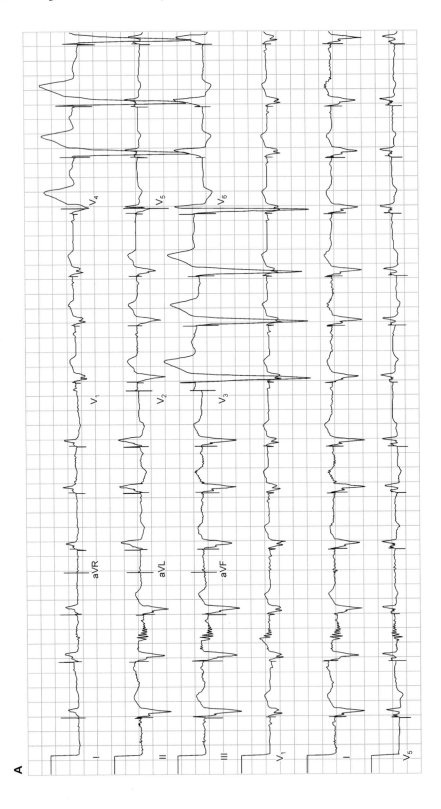

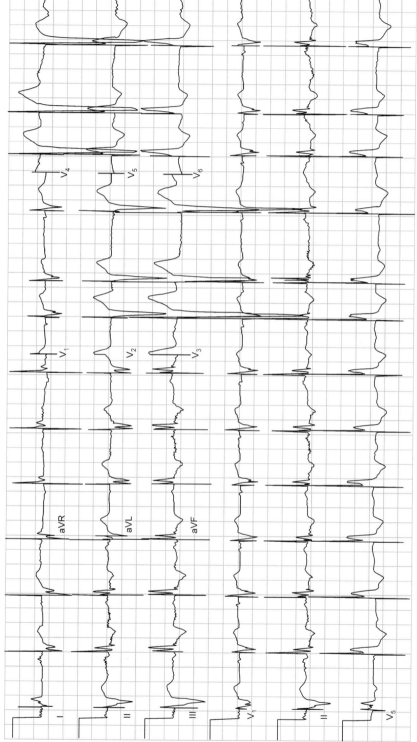

Fig. 7.83 The classic pattern with right ventricular pacing from the right ventricular apex is shown in (A). A left bundle branch block morphology with negative deflections in leads II, III and aVF and a tall R wave in leads I and aVL all signify right ventricular apical pacing. Biventricular capture is seen in (B) (after the first beat). There is a dramatic shortening in the QRS complex and a marked change in the vector. Lead I now becomes negative, suggesting lateral ventricular stimulation, and leads II, III, and aVF become positive, suggesting an anterior location. Note that despite the anterolateral rather than straight lateral location, excellent shortening of the QRS duration is seen. The 9th, 11th and 12th beats in (B) are premature atrial contractions with biventricular capture. Note that the QRS complex is slightly more prolonged with the faster pacing rate triggered by the premature atrial contractions in patients with ventricular conduction abnormalities or those taking antiarrhythmic drugs. This effect can be pronounced. This is one of the limitations to biventricular pacing in patients with atrial fibrillation and relatively rapid ventricular responses necessitating rapid pacing rates.

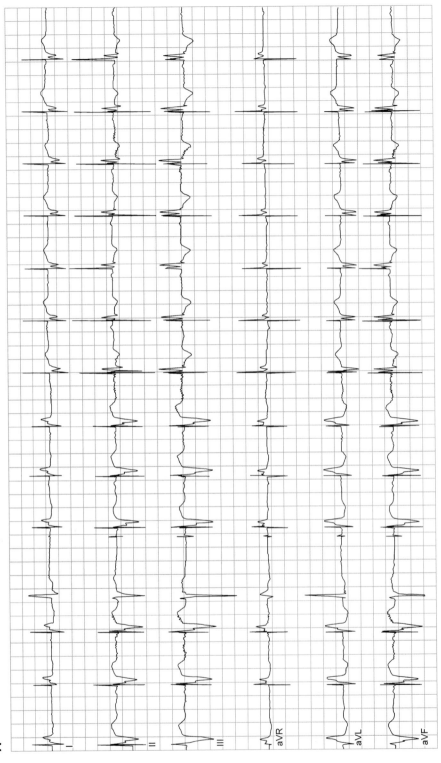

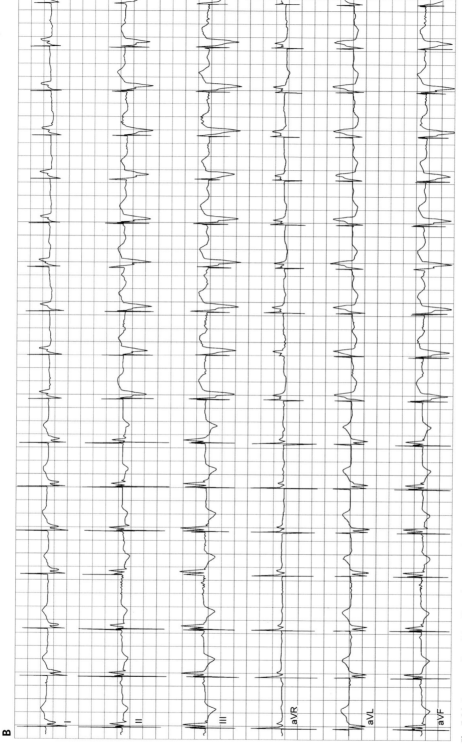

Fig. 7.84 Demonstration of the effect of increasing the pacing output (A) and then decreasing it (B). Because of the given lead position in this example, any one of the leads can be used to quickly see whether biventricular stimulation is occurring. For example, the negativity in lead I and the positivity in lead III are easily observed when increasing the output and obtaining left ventricular stimulation.

I

II

III

aVR

aVL

aVF

B

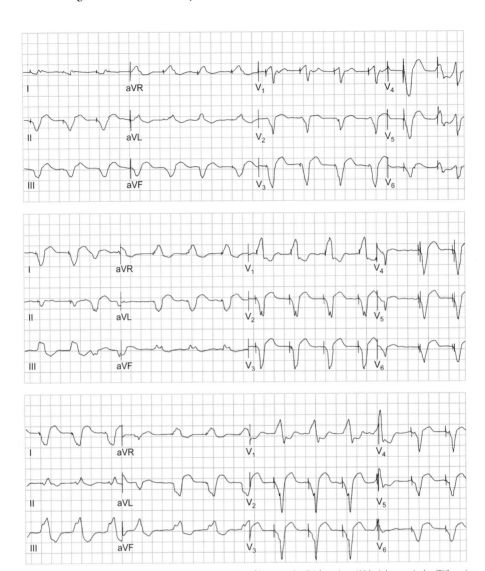

Fig. 7.85 This example illustrates the importance of systematic analysis of biventricular (BiV) tracings. With right ventricular (RV) pacing, a relatively characteristic morphology is seen, with a left bundle branch block pattern and negative deflections in leads II, III, and aVF. However, careful analysis shows an early small positive deflection in lead V1 and varying degrees of QRS widening, especially evident in lead V2. Both these findings suggest conduction abnormalities at the RV exit site. With left ventricular (LV) pacing, a characteristic right bundle branch block pattern with negative deflections in leads I and aVL is seen. The QRS vector is upright in the inferior leads (leads II, III, and aVF). This suggests that the LV pacing lead has been placed in a lateral vein in a slightly anterior location. BiV pacing results in an ECG that is very similar to LV pacing alone. This suggests that the RV lead is contributing little to the overall pacing vector. Thus, there is no added shortening of the QRS complex duration, a surrogate for resynchronization when adding RV pacing to LV pacing alone. In such instances, the availability of varying the ventricle-to-ventricle stimulation interval (VV timing) will allow better QRS shortening. In this instance, stimulating the RV earlier than the LV lead will approximate simultaneous stimulation of the ventricles. This ability to vary the VV timing may be more important when there is LV delay and the BiV-paced QRS morphology resembles RV pacing alone. This is because QT dynamic data show similar benefits with LV pacing and BiV stimulation.

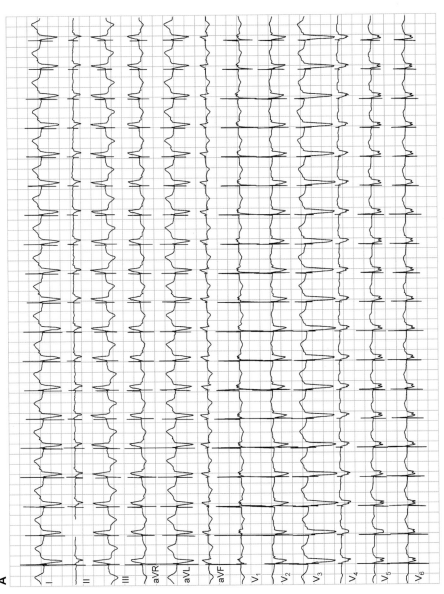

Fig. 7.86 (A–C) This series of ECGs illustrates the difficulty with using a single lead to assess left ventricular capture thresholds. Biventricular stimulation is seen in (A). (B) shows that with decreasing the output of this biventricular system, a change in morphology occurs after the first two QRS complexes. The question is, which lead has lost capture? Is it the right ventricular or the left ventricular pacing lead? (C) shows that further decrease in the output voltage results in the loss of capture altogether, and intrinsic rhythm with left bundle branch block ensues. If one is asked to assess whether the right or left ventricular lead has lost capture (B), it would be nearly impossible to answer this question from analysis of lead III alone, because lead III continues to be positive. This suggests that the right ventricular lead (usually resulting in negative complexes in lead III) has lost capture. However, in lead V1, the resulting QRS complexes are negative (left bundle branch block pattern). In fact, the loss of capture was in the left ventricular lead. However, because the right ventricular lead had been placed in the high interventricular septum, the QRS complex is positive in lead III. Accurate knowledge of the position of the right ventricular lead and analysis of the entire 12-lead ECG are necessary in atypical situations.

(Continued)

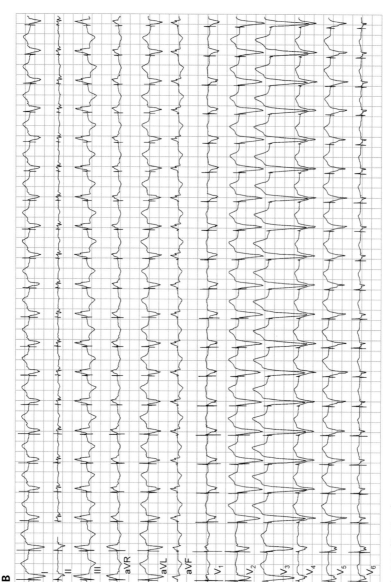

Fig. 7.86 (Continued)

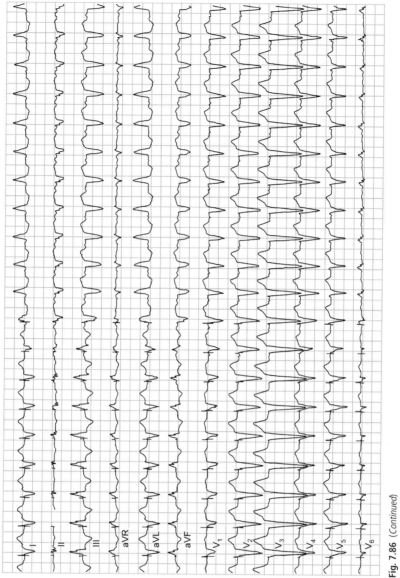

Fig. 7.86 (*Continued*)

in some cases because simply prolonging a long AV interval may inadvertently give rise to diastolic tricuspid regurgitation or inappropriately long AV intervals between the right atrium and RV.[60]

Electrocardiographic considerations in the patient not responding to CRT

Inappropriate lack of left ventricular pacing

Device interrogation should be performed to see what the percentage of LV pacing is. If this is lower than 95%, consider appropriate inhibition as a result of enhanced AV nodal conduction, especially with atrial fibrillation or inappropriately prolonged long AV intervals. Using AV nodal blocking pharmacologic agents and shortening the AV interval will usually suffice. Programming that prolongs AV intervals such as those designed to minimize ventricular pacing should not be used with biventricular pacing systems. Ventricular Sensed Response™ (Medtronic, Minneapolis, MN) or similar algorithms that pace to promote CRT soon after detection of intrinsic conduction may provide additional resynchronization benefit when AV nodal conduction is rapid.

However, the device assessment of percentage biventricular pacing may be inaccurate in a few instances. For example, pseudo-fusion with either intrinsic conduction or PVCs will result in overestimation of true biventricular pacing. A 12-lead ECG or, more appropriately, 24-hour Holter monitoring with visual assessment of QRS complexes will allow the caregiver to recognize pseudo-fusion and make appropriate programming interventions.

Anodal stimulation

Even with an adequately placed LV pacing lead and ideal thresholds and stimulation wave fronts, etc., if a bipolar configuration with LV tip as cathode and the RV coil or ring electrode as the anode, anodal stimulation can occur and take away potential benefit with the CRT device. The ECG readily and reliably allow recognition of anodal stimulation.

The biventricular paced ECG will look very similar to RV pacing alone despite adequate LV lead thresholds and appropriate V-V timing.

When recognized options available to remedy the situation include changing the pacing vector to true bipolar pacing from the LV lead or changing the output for pacing, i.e., distinct threshold for capture as well as for anodal stimulation may be seen, and if a margin is available between these two thresholds, programming could be performed whereby there is an appropriate output for LV lead capture but anodal stimulation does not occur.

Ventricular ectopy

Frequent ventricular ectopy can complicate CRT device and patient management in several ways. Frequent ectopy by itself may be a cause of worsening cardiomyopathy and thus offset potential benefits from resynchronization.

Sensing for CRT devices is typically off the RV lead, but PVCs in diseased hearts often arise from the LV. Thus, by the time a PVC fires and activates the ventricle near the RV lead, RV and/or biventricular pacing may result. In most cases, this gives rise to pseudo-fusion, and there is no real resynchronization benefit. In some instances, if there is more significant delay from the PVC site of origin to the RV lead, true fusion with RV and LV pacing along with the PVC may occur. In these instances, the true extent of biventricular stimulation and potential for resynchronization benefit is significantly less than the percentage of biventricular pacing would suggest.

PVCs also result in appropriate inhibition of pacing, and in patients with intrinsic conduction and long antegrade AV nodal conduction times, a single PVC may result in inhibition of pacing for several beats and decrease potential resynchronization benefit.[32]

The Ventricular Sense Response™ feature (Medtronic, Minneapolis, MN), or similar responses where ventricular pacing is triggered following a PVC, may promote fusion and at least partially offset the negative impact of PVCs on adequate resynchronization.

Conclusions

Careful analysis of the biventricular paced 12-lead ECG performed both at implant and follow-up can assist the operator and follow-up caregivers to assess lead position, adequacy of biventricular stimulation, and optimize device function. ECG information, once understood and appreciated, should be used in conjunction with echocardiographic and clinical data to make appropriate changes in biventricular device programming.

References

1 Higano ST, Hayes DL. Quantitative analysis of Wenckebach behavior in DDD pacemakers. Pacing Clin Electrophysiol 1990; 13:1456–65.

2 Olshansky B, Day JD, Lerew DR, Brown S, Stolen KQ; INTRINSIC RV Study Investigators. Eliminating right ventricular pacing may not be best for patients requiring implantable cardioverter-defibrillators. Heart Rhythm 2007; 4:886–91.

3 Barold SS. Ventricular- versus atrial-based lower rate timing in dual chamber pacemakers: does it really matter? Pacing Clin Electrophysiol 1995; 18:83–96.

4 Barold SS, Fredman CS. Pure atrial-based lower rate timing of dual chamber pacemakers: implications for upper rate limitation. Pacing Clin Electrophysiol 1995; 18: 391–400.

5 DAVID Trial Investigators. Dual-chamber pacing or ventricular backup pacing in patients with an implantable defibrillator (DAVID) trial. JAMA 2002; 288:3115–23.

6 Sweeney MO, Hellkamp AS. Heart failure during cardiac pacing. Circulation 2006; 113:2082–8.

7 Higano ST, Hayes DL, Eisinger G. Sensor-driven rate smoothing in a DDDR pacemaker. Pacing Clin Electrophysiol 1989; 12:922–9.

8 Stroobandt RX, Barold SS, Vandenbulcke FD, Willems RJ, Sinnaeve AF. A reappraisal of pacemaker timing cycles pertaining to automatic mode switching. J Interv Card Electrophysiol 2001; 5:417–29.

9 Lam CT, Lau CP, Leung SK, Tse HF, Ayers G. Improved efficacy of mode switching during atrial fibrillation using automatic atrial sensitivity adjustment. Pacing Clin Electrophysiol 1999; 22:17–25.

10 Barold SS, Israel CW, Herweg B. Mode switching of dual chamber pacemakers from activation of a blanked flutter search algorithm by a single atrial event. Pacing Clin Electrophysiol 2005; 28:917–20.

11 Fröhlig G, Gras D, Victor J, et al. Use of a new cardiac pacing mode designed to eliminate unnecessary ventricular pacing. Europace 2006; 8:96–101.

12 Gillis AM, Pürerfellner H, Israel CW, et al.; Medtronic Enrhythm Clinical Study Investigators. Reducing unnecessary right ventricular pacing with the managed ventricular pacing mode in patients with sinus node disease and AV block. Pacing Clin Electrophysiol 2006; 29:697–705.

13 Sweeney MO, Ellenbogen KA, Casavant D, et al.; Marquis MVP Download Investigators. Multicenter, prospective, randomized safety and efficacy study of a new atrial-based managed ventricular pacing mode (MVP) in dual chamber ICDs. J Cardiovasc Electrophysiol 2005; 16:811–7.

14 Barold SS, Herweg B, Giudici M. Electrocardiographic follow-up of biventricular pacemakers. Ann Noninvasive Electrocardiol 2005; 10:231–55.

15 Barold SS, Herweg B. Upper rate response of biventricular pacing devices. J Intervent Card Electrophysiol 2005; 12: 129–36.

16 Chang KC, Chen JY, Lin JJ, Hung JS. Unexpected loss of atrial tracking caused by interaction between temporary and permanent right ventricular leads during implantation of a biventricular pacemaker. Pacing Clin Electrophysiol 2004; 27:998–1001.

17 Akiyama M, Kaneko Y, Taniguchi Y, Kurabayashi M. Pacemaker syndrome associated with a biventricular pacing system. J Cardiovasc Electrophysiol 2002; 13:1061–2.

18 Wang P, Kramer A, Estes NA 3rd, Hayes DL. Timing cycles for biventricular pacing. Pacing Clin Electrophysiol 2002; 25:62–75.

19 Riedlbauchova L, Kautzner J, Fridl P. Influence of different atrioventricular and interventricular delays on cardiac output during cardiac resynchronization therapy. Pacing Clin Electrophysiol 2005; 28(Suppl. 1):19–23.

20 Hayes DL, Boehmer JP, Day JD, et al. Cardiac resynchronization therapy and the relationship of percent biventricular pacing to symptoms and survival. Heart Rhythm 2011; 8:1469–75.

21 Mead H, Kleckner K, Sheldon T, et al.; LVCM Study Investigators. Automated left ventricular capture management. Pacing Clin Electrophysiol 2007; 30:1190–200.

22 Lipchenca I, Garrigue S, Glikson M, Barold SS, Clementy J. Inhibition of biventricular pacemakers by oversensing of far-field atrial depolarization. Pacing Clin Electrophysiol 2002; 25:365–7.

23 Abraham WT. Cardiac resynchronization therapy for heart failure: biventricular pacing and beyond. Curr Opin Cardiol 2002; 17:346–52.

24 Gras D, Leclercq C, Tang AS, Bucknall C, Luttikhuis HO, Kirstein-Pedersen A. Cardiac resynchronization therapy in advanced heart failure: the multicenter InSync clinical study. Eur J Heart Fail 2002; 4:311–20.

25 Hayes DL, Ketelson A, Levine PA, Markowitz HT, Sanders R, Schaney G. Understanding timing systems of current DDDR pacemakers. Eur J Cardiac Pacing Electrophysiol 1993; 3:70–86.

26 Kay GN, Bourge RC. Biventricular pacing for congestive heart failure: questions of who, what, where, why, how, and how much. Am Heart J 2000; 140:821–3.

27 Tamborero D, Vidal B, Tolosana JM, et al. Electrocardiographic versus echocardiographic optimization of the interventricular pacing delay in patients undergoing cardiac resynchronization therapy. J Cardiovasc Electrophysiol 2011; 22:1129–34.

28 Thompson C, Tsiperfal A. Why does the QRS morphology of the paced beat change in patients with biventricular cardiac pacing systems? Prog Cardiovasc Nurs 2002; 17:101–3.

29 Alonso C, Leclercq C, Victor F, et al. Electrocardiographic predictive factors of long-term clinical improvement with multisite biventricular pacing in advanced heart failure. Am J Cardiol 1999; 84:1417–21.

30 Daoud EG, Kalbfleisch SJ, Hummel JD, et al. Implantation techniques and chronic lead parameters of biventricular pacing dual-chamber defibrillators. J Cardiovasc Electrophysiol 2002; 13:964–70.

31 Willems JL, Lesaffre E. Comparison of multigroup logistic and linear discriminant ECG and VCG classification. J Electrocardiol 1987; 20:83–92.

32 Willems JL, Lesaffre E, Pardaens J. Comparison of the classification ability of the electrocardiogram and vectorcardiogram. Am J Cardiol 1987; 59:119–24.

33 Bortolan G, Willems JL. Diagnostic ECG classification based on neural networks. J Electrocardiol 1993; 26 (Suppl.):75–9.

34 Brohet CR, Robert A, Derwael C et al. Computer interpretation of pediatric orthogonal electrocardiograms: statistical and deterministic classification methods. Circulation 1984; 70:255–62.

35 Kulbertus HE, de Laval-Rutten F, Casters P. Vectorcardiographic study of aberrant conduction anterior displacement of QRS: another form of intraventricular block. Br Heart J 1976; 38:549–57.

36 Mehta S, Asirvatham SJ. Rethinking QRS Duration as an indication for CRT. J Cardiovasc Electrophysiol 2012; 23:169–71.

37 Merchant FM, Heist EK, McCarty D, et al. Impact of segmental left ventricle lead position on cardiac resynchronization therapy outcomes. Heart Rhythm 2010; 7:639–44.

38 Becker M, Altiok E, Ocklenburg C, et al. Analysis of LV lead position in cardiac re-synchronization therapy using different imaging modalities. JACC Cardiovasc Imaging 2010; 3:472–81.

39 Wyman BT, Hunter WC, Prinzen FW, Faris OP, McVeigh ER. Effects of single- and biventricular pacing on temporal and spatial dynamics of ventricular contraction. Am J Physiol Heart Circ Physiol 2002; 282:H372–9.

40 Kornreich F, Block P, Brismee D. The missing waveform information in the orthogonal electrocardiogram (Frank leads): IV. Computer diagnosis of biventricular hypertrophy from "maximal" surface waveform information. Circulation 1974; 49:1123–31.

41 Farrar DJ, Chow E, Wood JR, Hill JD. Anatomic interaction between the right and left ventricles during univentricular and biventricular circulatory support. ASAIO Trans 1988; 34:235–40.

42 Jain A, Chandna H, Silber EN, Clark WA, Denes P. Electrocardiographic patterns of patients with echocardiographically determined biventricular hypertrophy. J Electrocardiol 1999; 32:269–73.

43 Igarashi M, Shiina Y, Tanabe T, Handa S. Significance of electrocardiographic QRS width in patients with congestive heart failure: a marker for biventricular pacing. J Cardiol. 2002; 40:103–9.

44 Cazeau S, Ritter P, Lazarus A, et al. Multisite pacing for end-stage heart failure: early experience. Pacing Clin Electrophysiol 1996; 19:1748–57.

45 Blanc JJ, Etienne Y, Gilard M, et al. Evaluation of different ventricular pacing sites in patients with severe heart failure: results of an acute hemodynamic study. Circulation 1997; 96:3273–7.

46 Yong P, Duby C. A new and reliable method of individual ventricular capture identification during biventricular pacing threshold testing. Pacing Clin Electrophysiol 2000; 23:1735–7.

47 Ansalone G, Giannantoni P, Ricci R, Trambaiolo P, Fedele F, Santini M. Doppler myocardial imaging to evaluate the effectiveness of pacing sites in patients receiving biventricular pacing. J Am Coll Cardiol 2002; 39:489–99.

48 Asirvatham SJ. Cardiac resynchronization: is electrical synchrony relevant? J Cardiovasc Electrophysiol 2007; 18:1028–31.

49 O'Cochlain B, Delurgio D, Leon A, Langberg J. The effect of variation in the interval between right and left ventricular activation on paced QRS duration. Pacing Clin Electrophysiol 2001; 24:1780–2.

50 Contini C, Berti S, Levorato D, et al. Histologic evidence of myocardial damage in apparently healthy subjects with ventricular arrhythmias and myocardial dysfunction. Clin Cardiol 1992; 15:529–33.

51 De Guillebon M, Thambo JB, Ploux S, et al. Reliability and reproducibility of QRS duration in the selection of candidates for cardiac resynchronization therapy. J Cardiovasc Electrophysiol 2010; 21: 890–2.

52 Yip GW, Fung JW. Cardiac resynchronisation therapy for heart failure with narrow or normal QRS. Heart 2011; 97:1029–31.

53 Duvall WL, Hansalia R, Wijetunga MN, Buckley S, Fischer A. Advantage of optimizing V-V timing in cardiac resynchronization therapy devices. Pacing Clin Electrophysiol 2010; 33:1161–8.

54 Parreira L, Santos JF, Madeira J, et al. Cardiac resynchronization therapy with sequential biventricular pacing: impact of echocardiography guided VV delay optimization on acute results. Rev Port Cardiol 2005; 24:1355–65.

55 Rao RK, Kumar UN, Schafer J, et al. Reduced ventricular volumes and improved systolic function with cardiac resynchronization therapy: a randomized trial comparing simultaneous biventricular pacing, sequential biventricular pacing, and left ventricular pacing. Circulation 2007; 115:2136–44.

56 Bouchardy J, Therrien J, Pilote L, et al. Atrial arrhythmias in adults with congenital heart disease. Circulation 2009; 120:1679–86.

57 Melzer C, Borges AC, Knebel F, et al. Echocardiographic AV-interval optimization in patients with reduced left ventricular function. Cardiovasc Ultrasound 2004; 2:30.

58 Meluzin J, Novák M, Müllerová J, et al. A fast and simple echocardiographic method of determination of the optimal atrioventricular delay in patients after biventricular stimulation. Pacing Clin Electrophysiol 2004; 27: 58–64.

59 Baker JH 2nd, McKenzie J 3rd, Beau S, et al. Acute evaluation of programmer-guided AV/PV and VV delay optimization comparing an IEGM method and echocardiogram for cardiac resynchronization therapy in heart failure patients and dual-chamber ICD implants. J Cardiovasc Electrophysiol 2007; 18:185–91.

60 Min X, Meine M, Baker JH, et al. Estimation of the optimal VV delay by an IEGM-based method in cardiac resynchronization therapy. Pacing Clin Electrophysiol 2007; 30: S19–22.

8 Programming: Maximizing Benefit and Minimizing Morbidity Programming

Paul A. Friedman¹, Charles D. Swerdlow², Samuel J. Asirvatham¹, David L. Hayes¹

¹Mayo Clinic, Rochester, MN, USA

²Cedars-Sinai Heart Center at Cedars-Sinai Medical Center; David Geffen School of Medicine, University of California, Los Angeles, CA, USA

Programmers 320
Pacemaker programming 320
  Interrogation 321
  Emergency programming 321
  Programmed parameters 321
  Measured data 322
  Specific programmable parameters to consider in all patients 322
    Mode programming 327
    Rate programmability 328
    Programming hysteresis, AV search hysteresis, ventricular pacing avoidance algorithms, and sudden bradycardia response algorithms 331
    Programming output (pulse width and voltage amplitude) 333
    Programming sensitivity 339
    Polarity programmability 341
    Refractory and blanking periods 346
      Single-chamber pacemakers 346
      Dual-chamber pacemakers 346
    Mode switching 348
    Programming rate-adaptive parameters 350
    Diagnostics – set-up and assessment 350
  Unexpected programming 350
  Programming during routine follow-up 357
Defibrillator programming 360
  Implantable cardioverter-defibrillator sensing 362
    Sensing sources 365
    Programming sensing 365
  Implantable cardioverter-defibrillator detection 366
    Rate cut-off, duration, and zones 367
    Detection zone boundaries 372

Committed and noncommitted shocks 372
Redetection 373
SVT-VT discriminators 373
  Single-chamber SVT-VT discriminators 376
    Morphology 376
    Stability 377
    Onset 382
  SVT-VT discriminator timers 382
  Dual-chamber SVT-VT discriminators 382
    Comparison of atrial and ventricular rates 383
    Enhanced onset and stability and Rhythm ID (Boston Scientific) 387
    PR Logic™ + Wavelet (Medtronic) 388
    St. Jude Rate Branch™ 388
Ventricular therapies 390
  Antitachycardia pacing 390
  Defibrillation 393
  Low-energy cardioversion 393
  Interactions of antibradycardia pacing with tachycardia programming 393
  Atrial defibrillators: detection and therapies 393
  Optimizing programming 394
Cardiac resynchronization programming 395
  Algorithms to promote continuous tracking 395
  Algorithms to manage premature ventricular complexes 398
  Algorithms to manage atrial fibrillation 399
  Device-based optimization for cardiac resynchronization 399
Conclusions 400
References 401

Cardiac Pacing, Defibrillation and Resynchronization: A Clinical Approach, Third Edition.
David L. Hayes, Samuel J. Asirvatham, and Paul A. Friedman.
© 2013 Mayo Foundation for Medical Education and Research. Published 2013 by John Wiley & Sons, Ltd.

Programmability is defined as the ability to make non-invasive, stable but reversible changes in device function. The first truly programmable pacemakers were introduced in 1972 in which a magnetic code was introduced from an external programmer to manipulate four levels of output and six variations of pacing rate. Radiofrequency signals are now exclusively used to communicate between the device and the programmer. The number of programmable features and the variability of each feature have dramatically expanded and offer the ability to uniquely alter device function to meet the specific needs of the patient.

Programmers

Although all programmers allow completion of similar tasks, there is considerable difference among manufacturers in implementation with regard to screen layout, use of touch screen and stylus, number of automatic "measurement" functions, position and operation of emergency programming options, and so on.[1] Thus, programmer-specific familiarity is required for device programming.

Pacemaker programming

All contemporary devices are programmable. The North American Society of Pacing and Electrophysiology/British Pacing and Electrophysiology Group (NASPE/BPG) code designates the degree of programmability.[2] The first letter indicates the chamber(s) paced, the second the chamber(s) sensed, and the third the response. Thus, VVI indicates the ventricle is paced and sensed, and an intrinsic event inhibits output. A fourth letter code describes rate modulation. An "R" in the fourth position indicates that the pacemaker has a sensor to control the rate independent of intrinsic electrical activity of the heart, typically used to increase the heart rate during exertion.

It is important to have a systematic approach to programming. Although the manufacturer-specific approaches differ, a programming sequence should include specific assessments, data collection, and interpretation and optimization if needed.

Most programmable parameters have been discussed in Chapter 7: Timing Cycles, and it is not the purpose of this chapter to discuss each programmable value individually. Nor is there an attempt to cover nuances of specific manufacturers or models. As always, it is important to consult the technical manual and/or the manufacturer's technical services helpdesk for further information about a specific pulse generator or specific feature. Table 8.1 attempts to include most available

Table 8.1 Pacing modes.*

VOO	Ventricular pacing; no sensing	DOO	Dual-chamber pacing; no sensing
VVI	Ventricular pacing; ventricular sensing and inhibition	DVI	Dual-chamber pacing; ventricular sensing and inhibition; no tracking of the atrium
VVT	Ventricular pacing; ventricular sensing and triggering	DVIR	Dual-chamber pacing; ventricular sensing and inhibition; no tracking of the atrium; AV sequential rate modulation
VVIR	Ventricular pacing; ventricular sensing with inhibition; rate-modulated pacing	DDI	Dual-chamber pacing; dual-chamber sensing and inhibition; no tracking of the atrium
VOOR	Ventricular pacing; no sensing; rate-modulated pacing	DDIR	Dual-chamber pacing; dual-chamber sensing and inhibition; no tracking of the atrium; AV sequential rate modulation
AOO	Atrial pacing; no sensing	VDD	Ventricular pacing; dual-chamber sensing; tracking of the atrium with ventricular inhibition
AAI	Atrial pacing; atrial sensing and inhibition	VDDR	Ventricular pacing; dual-chamber sensing; tracking of atrium with ventricular inhibition and ventricular rate modulation
AAT	Atrial pacing; atrial sensing and triggering	DDD	Dual-chamber pacing; dual-chamber sensing and inhibition; tracking of the atrium
AAIR	Atrial pacing; atrial sensing with inhibition; rate-modulated pacing	DDDR	Dual-chamber pacing; dual-chamber sensing and inhibition; tracking of the atrium; AV sequential rate modulation
		OOO	Pacemaker is programmed "off" (allows assessment of underlying rhythm)

AV, atrioventricular.

*Reference is sometimes made to the SSI, SSIR, SST, or SOO mode. Manufacturers use "S" in both the first and the second positions of the pacemaker code to indicate that the device is capable of pacing a single cardiac chamber. Once the device is implanted and connected to a lead in either the atrium or the ventricle, "S" should be changed to either "A" or "V" in the clinical record to reflect the chamber in which pacing and sensing are occurring.

Source: Hayes DL, Lloyd MA, Friedman PA. Cardiac Pacing and Defibrillation: A Clinical Approach. Armonk, NY: Futura Publishing Co., Inc., 2000: 247–323, by permission of Mayo Foundation for Medical Education and Research.

programmable features and a general range of the programmable values for each parameter.

The chapter is structured by major programmable parameters and programming considerations for each. Programmer "screen shots" will be used to demonstrate the type of information available and steps to assessment and optimization when needed.

Interrogation

Interrogation is performed by placing the programming head over or near the pulse generator to establish a communication; in devices equipped with a radiofrequency link the programmer can be within 6–10 feet of the patient, with minor variation among manufacturers. Most contemporary pulse generators are automatically recognized by the programmer and a full interrogation or a display of programmed parameters will be generated.

The initial screen usually displays key programmed parameters, alerts that have occurred since the last interrogation, and options to access other data (Fig. 8.1).

Emergency programming

In order to avoid asystole during the course of programming in a pacemaker-dependent patient, every programmer is equipped with an emergency or "stat set" button that restores nominal pacing parameters when activated. However, there may be a delay between activation of the stat set parameters and actual restoration of nominal pacing parameters. It is important that the caregiver using the programmer be familiar with the specific programmer steps necessary to activate stat set or emergency backup parameters.[1]

Programmed parameters

One or more screens specifically display the programmed parameters. Drop-down menus or other paths display less commonly used programmable parameters or "advanced" programmable parameters.

Parameters may be reprogrammed either directly from the "parameter" screen or from "temporary programming" screens that permit routine programming sequences or troubleshooting without changing permanently programmed values (Fig. 8.2).

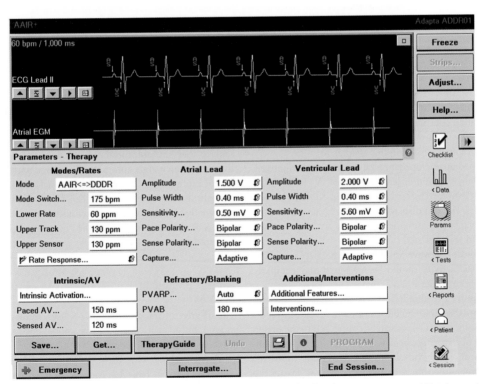

Fig. 8.1 Programmer screen demonstrating primary programmable parameters and other drop-down menus to access additional parameters. There are also other icons to the right to connect to stored data, tests that can be accomplished via the programmer, reports and patient information.

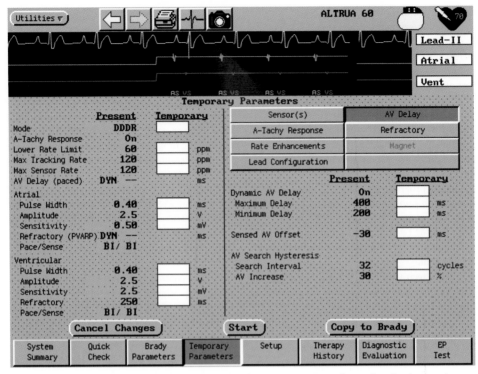

Fig. 8.2 Programmer screen demonstrating temporary programmability. The permanent settings at "present" are listed next to the "temporary" column. Temporary programming allows testing and specific programming sequences to be accomplished without having to alter the prior settings.

Measured data

Measured data are used to modify or verify the appropriateness of programmed parameters and are therefore briefly discussed in this chapter.

• **Impedance:** Impedance values for atrial, right ventricular (RV), and/or left ventricular (LV) leads should be measured to assess lead function. Some pulse generators will also display prior value(s) or a "trend" of impedance measurements, which is diagnostically helpful (Fig. 8.3).

• **P and/or R wave amplitudes:** The size, in mV, of intrinsic activity should be measured and compared with prior values when available (Fig. 8.4).

• **Capture threshold(s):** There are multiple ways the capture threshold can be determined. An autothreshold is usually available and can be configured to the preferences of a specific caregiver or institution. We generally perform capture thresholds at a fixed pulse width and decrement the voltage amplitude. (In some devices this may not be an option.) Some manufacturers require that a touch-sensitive area on the programming screen be held down during autothreshold measurement

(during which pacing outputs are progressively decremented), so that upon loss of capture the operator simply removes pressure to restore pacing. Others only require that the autothreshold be initiated and the threshold search ends automatically upon detection of loss of capture (Fig. 8.5). In some pacemakers a screen may also be available that will display prior values for capture thresholds and other previously measured data (Fig. 8.6). (Chapter 1 reviews the concepts of pacing capture and sensing.)

Specific programmable parameters to consider in all patients

The degree of programmability varies significantly among pulse generators. Pacing mode options are listed in Table 8.1 and commonly used programmable parameters along with their definitions and typical values are listed in Table 8.2. The chapter is written with regard to current generation pulse generators, recognizing that the degree of programmability and the sophistication of programmable parameters may be

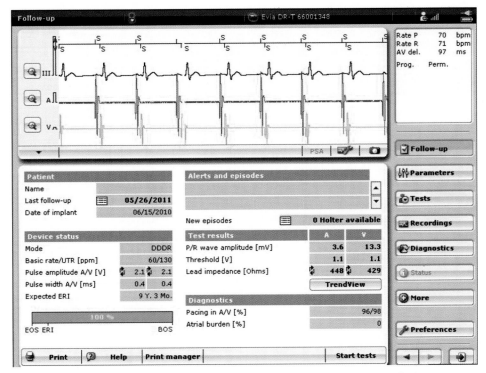

Fig. 8.3 Follow-up screen giving an "overall" view of device status. Basic programmed values are shown in the left column. Battery status and percent pacing are also shown. Measured impedance values are provided, in this example atrial impedance = 448 Ω; ventricular impedance = 429 Ω. In addition, the measured intrinsic P and R waves are shown.

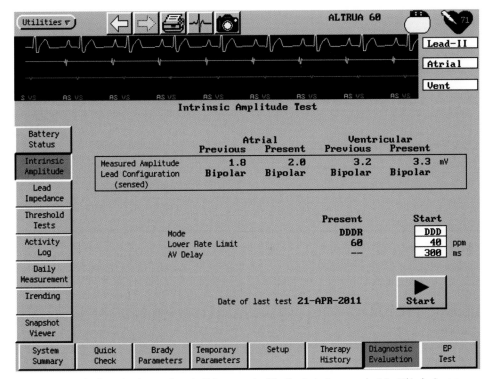

Fig. 8.4 An intrinsic amplitude test has been performed which measured a 2.8-mV unipolar P wave and a 3.3-mV bipolar R wave.

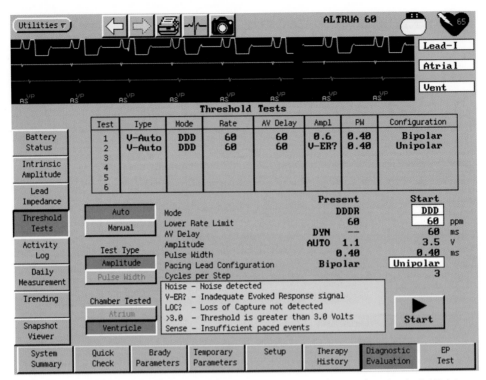

Fig. 8.5 Programmer screen from which threshold testing can be accomplished. In this example ventricular pacing threshold is being performed by decrementing the voltage amplitude at a fixed pulse width of 0.4 ms. The voltage threshold was 0.6 V in a bipolar configuration. The pacemaker is "auto" programmed to 1.1 V and 0.4 ms pulse width. The unipolar pacing threshold could not be determined because of an inadequate evoked potential signal.

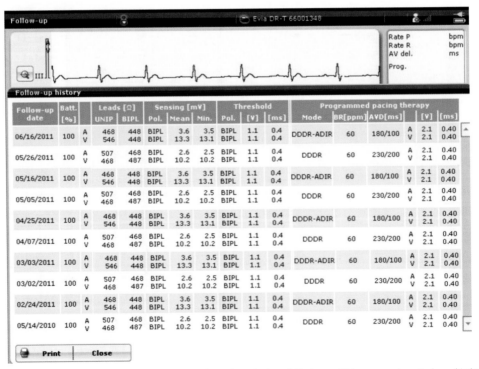

Fig. 8.6 Programmer screen demonstrating stored follow-up data. Information is available from multiple programming episodes and includes battery status, lead impedances, intrinsic P- and R-wave amplitude, atrial and ventricular pacing thresholds and programmed values.

Table 8.2 Common programmable options for pacemakers.

Parameter	Description	Potential programmable values
Atrial refractory period	An interval of the atrial channel timing cycle during which the atrial sensing amplifier is designed to be unresponsive to input signals. In some pacemakers, however, the sensing circuitry is alert for extraneous or noncardiac signals during a portion of the atrial refractory period. In single-chamber atrial pacing modes, the atrial refractory period occurs after a sensed or paced atrial event	150–500 ms
Atrioventricular interval	Period between the initiation of the paced or sensed atrial event and the delivery of a consecutive ventricular output pulse	PAV (Paced AV) also "AV": 25–350 ms SAV (Sensed AV) also "PV": 25–325 ms
Circadian lower rate limit or sleep rate	Reduces the lower rate limit during sleeping or resting hours	Lower rates during sleep, programmable from as low as 30 ppm
Differential AVI	Feature that permits a longer AVI after a paced atrial event (PAV) than after a sensed AVI (SAV). In many pacemakers these are independently programmable (see immediately above). In some the differential is fixed; and in others, it is programmable as a single AV interval with an "offset"	Offset from 0 to 100 ms
Fallback	An upper rate response in which the ventricular paced rate decelerates to, and is maintained at, a programmable fallback rate that is lower than the original programmed MTR. Fallback mechanisms vary among pacemakers. Fallback may also be a programmable parameter related to the mode-switch algorithm indicating the paced rate that will be implemented when mode-switching criteria are met	May be programmable on or off; if on, the rate to which the fallback occurs may be fixed or programmable, i.e., 50–80 ppm
Lower rate limit	Preset or programmed rate at which a pacemaker emits an output pulse without intrinsic cardiac activity	30–170 ppm (options faster than 150 ppm available in some pulse generators)
Magnet response	The response of a permanent pacemaker to magnet application is generally asynchronous pacing, and the behavior of an implantable cardioverter-defibrillator varies among manufacturers and possibly among models or generations of a specific manufacturer	Off, On, EGM storage, i.e., when magnet applied the pulse generator is triggered to store an EGM
Maximum sensor rate (MSR)	The fastest sensor-driven pacing rate that can be achieved in a rate-adaptive pacing system. In a single-chamber demand pacemaker with rate-adaptive capability (SSIR), the maximum sensor rate is the same as the programmed upper rate limit. In a dual-chamber rate-adaptive pacemaker (DDDR), the maximum sensor rate is not necessarily equal to the maximum tracking rate	80–180 ppm
Maximum tracking rate (MTR)	The fastest atrial rate at which consecutively paced ventricular complexes maintain 1:1 synchrony with sensed atrial events. The maximum tracking rate is a function of dual-chamber pacing modes and can be defined as a preset or programmable value. The maximum tracking rate is limited to the total atrial refractory period (TARP)	80–210 ppm
Mode (see Table 8.1)	Preset or programmed response from a pacemaker with or without intrinsic cardiac events	VOO, AOO, VVI, AAI, VDD, DVI, DDD, DDI, DOO, VVT, AAT (all could also have "R" (rate-adaptive) capability
Mode switch	Capability of a dual-chamber pacemaker to automatically switch from an atrial tracking (P synchronous) mode to a non-atrial-tracking mode when an atrial rhythm occurs that the pacemaker determines to be pathologic. When the atrial rhythm meets the criteria for a physiologic rhythm, the mode switches back to an atrial-tracking mode	On or off; if on, the detection rates are often programmable for rates 110–300 ppm; many variables other than the atrial tachycardia detection rate may be programmable depending on the specific mode-switching algorithm

(Continued)

Table 8.2 (*Continued*)

Parameter	Description	Potential programmable values
PMT (Pacemaker Mediated Tachycardia) algorithms	A function of dual-chamber pacemakers that minimizes the initiation or continuation of a PMT. PMT algorithms vary in different pacemakers and usually are a programmable function. Examples of pacemaker-mediated tachycardia protection algorithms include lengthening of the programmed PVARP, an automatic extension of the atrial refractory period after a sensed premature ventricular contraction, and a dropped ventricular output pulse after a predetermined number of beats at a specified rate or upper rate limit	On or off; in others, can choose how long the MTR must persist before detection criteria are met
Polarity	Stimulating electrode typically is the cathode, which has negative polarity relative to the indifferent electrode (anode). If the anode is the "ring" of the pacing lead then a "bipolar" configuration is in use. If the anode is the pulse generator "can," then a "unipolar" configuration is present	Options variable. Older pulse generators may simply be programmable to unipolar or bipolar and applies to any mode programmed and both pacing and sensing configuration. In many devices the sensing and pacing polarity configurations are independently programmable and in many dual-chamber devices the atrial and ventricular channel are independently programmable
Postventricular atrial blanking period (PVAB)	A programmable feature in some dual-chamber pulse generators. During the period specified (in milliseconds), the atrial events are blanked from the atrial channel and therefore not considered when the atrial rate interval is calculated. The postventricular atrial blanking period is initiated with a ventricular paced or sensed event	60–200 ms
Post-ventricular atrial refractory period (PVARP)	In dual-chamber pacemakers, that portion of the timing cycle during which the atrial channel is refractory after a paced or sensed ventricular event. The PVARP prohibits the atrial channel of the pacemaker from sensing the far-field ventricular depolarization or the afterpotential of the ventricular pacing impulse. If the PVARP is sufficiently long, it can prevent pacemaker-mediated tachycardia by prohibiting sensing of premature atrial beats or retrograde atrial depolarizations after ventricular ectopic or paced ventricular beats. However, extension of the PVARP limits the maximum tracking rate unless there is a rate-related shortening of the PVARP	150–500 ms; in some devices, auto-PVARP adjusts with cycle length
Pulse amplitude	Magnitude of the voltage level reached during a pacemaker output pulse, usually expressed in volts	0.25–8.4 V
Pulse width	Duration, in milliseconds, over which the voltage output is delivered	0.05–1.5 ms
PVARP extension	Lengthening of the PVARP after a sensed premature ventricular contraction to prevent sensing of a retrograde P wave	On or off in some; others may program length of extension to as long as 500 ms
Rate hysteresis	Extension of the escape interval after a sensed intrinsic event	Off, 30–130 ppm. (Most commonly used is in SSI device with rates 30–60 ppm. However, in some, if N = the base rate, hysteresis is available at N – 5 or 10 ppm up to as the programmable base rate
Rate smoothing	Prevents atrial or ventricular paced rate from changing by more than a programmed percentage from one cardiac cycle to the next. This prevents large cycle-to-cycle intervals that can be seen at the upper rate limit or during rapid acceleration of atrial rate	On or off; when on options of percent smoothing, i.e., 3%, 6% and 24% change per cycle length allowed; may also have option of being on or off for rate increments or decrements, or both

Table 8.2 (Continued)

Parameter	Description	Potential programmable values
Rate-adaptive AVI	Shortens the AVI as the heart rate increases	On or off only in some devices; in others, able to set the minimum AV delay to as short as 30 ms and in others there is a manufacturer-determined "scale," e.g., low, medium, high that determines how aggressive the AVI shortening will be
Reaction time	A programmable parameter in some rate-adaptive pacemakers which determines how quickly the pacing rate will increase via sensor activation	15–60 s
Recovery time	A programmable parameter in some rate-adaptive pacemakers that determines how quickly the sensor-driven pacing rate will decrease once the sensor is no longer activated	2.5–16 min
Sensitivity	Ability to sense an intrinsic electrical signal, which depends on the amplitude, slew rate, and frequency of the signal	Atrial: 0.1–8 mV; ventricular: 0.5–14 mV
Sensor slope	A programmable value that determines the pacing increment over the base rate which will occur with different levels of sensor signal input	Usually a scale unique to the manufacturer, e.g., 1–10, 1–16
Sensor threshold	A programmable value for rate-adaptive pacemakers which determines, in part, the level of activity necessary to activate the sensor. Programming the sensor threshold is not consistent across manufacturers. In some devices, the higher the sensor threshold is set, the greater the level of activity required to increase the pacing rate, and vice versa in others	Low, medium, high
Ventricular blanking period	A short preset or programmable interval in dual-chamber pacemakers during which the ventricular sensing amplifiers are disabled. Ventricular blanking is initiated by an atrial output pulse and is designed to eliminate ventricular sensing of the atrial stimulus (crosstalk)	Ventricular blanking: 20–50 ms
Ventricular refractory period	An interval of the timing cycle following a sensed or paced ventricular event. The ventricular channel is totally unresponsive to incoming signals or waveforms during the majority of the ventricular refractory period. However, in some pacemakers, the sensing circuitry is alert for extraneous signals during a portion of the ventricular refractory period. The ventricular refractory period also may be referred to as the ventricular refractory interval	125–500 ms
Ventricular safety pacing (VSP)	Delivery of a ventricular output pulse after atrial pacing if a signal is sensed by the ventricular channel during the crosstalk sensing portion of the AVI	On or off in most pulse generators. When on the VSP interval is usually in the range of 90–120 ms. One manufacturer does not have VSP as a programmable option, but as a function of a noise detection algorithm

significantly lower in earlier generation devices that remain in service. Although an attempt is made to discuss programming generically, this is not always possible. Specific programmable parameters may be protected by trademark and available from only one manufacturer. Therefore, it is necessary at times to refer to specific manufacturers and algorithms.

Mode programming

Pacing modes have been discussed in detail in Chapter 7: Timing Cycles.

While there are many programmable mode options listed in Table 8.1, many are particularly useful for specific clinical scenarios, either as a permanent or temporary mode:

- **VVI:** determination of ventricular pacing threshold
- **VVT:** determination of ventricular sensing threshold; determine site of ventricular sensing; for temporary diagnostic use in the evaluation and management of arrhythmias performed by triggering the device output through chest wall stimulation
- **AAI:** determination of atrial pacing threshold
- **AAT:** determination of atrial sensing threshold; determine site of atrial sensing
- **DDI:** allow intrinsic ventricular activity to occur, e.g., during an automated search for underlying ventricular rhythm, DDI may allow the appearance of an intrinsic ventricular rhythm; to avoid tracking atrial tachycardias that are too slow for mode switch to detect
- **ADI*:** display ventricular diagnostics when programmed to the AAI mode
- **VDI*:** display atrial diagnostics when programmed to the VVI mode
- **DAT*:** potentially useful when there is a need for dual-chamber stimulation in the absence of ventricular activity
- **ODO, OVO, OAO:** temporary diagnostic evaluation of underlying rhythm and when a record of the intrinsic activity is needed.

Rate programmability

During programming for pacemaker follow-up, if the patient's intrinsic rate is greater than the programmed rate, the pacing rate is increased to assess the threshold of stimulation. If pacing is occurring at the programmed lower rate, the rate is decreased to determine the status of the patient's underlying rhythm. Ideally, this should be known prior to checking a stimulation threshold; e.g., if a patient is pacemaker-dependent and has no reliable ventricular escape rhythm, loss of capture during threshold determination could have clinical consequences. If thresholds are being obtained with an automated method this is less of a concern than if thresholds are determined manually (Fig. 8.7).

The nominal lower rate, i.e., the manufacturer preprogrammed lower rate, is frequently 60 ppm. Programming to a slower rate may be helpful in an attempt to allow a patient with rare episodes of bradycardia to remain in sinus rhythm rather than in paced rhythm. Programming a rate of 50 ppm or even one as low as 40 ppm may allow the patient's intrinsic rhythm to exist much of the time, with pacing occurring only in the event of a more profound sinus bradycardia or asystole. Hysteresis (see later) and ventricular avoidance pacing algorithms (see Chapter 7: Timing Cycles) allow an even greater ability to promote intrinsic rhythm.

*Manufacturer specific.

More rapid "lower" pacing rates, i.e., >70 ppm, are used most commonly in pediatric patients and are sometimes useful when faster pacing rates may be necessary to enhance cardiac output, e.g., postoperatively. In an occasional patient, a faster rate may be used to suppress an atrial or ventricular arrhythmia.

An option for "circadian response," or "sleep rate," is available in many devices (Fig. 8.8).[2] This feature allows a lower rate to be programmed for the approximate time during which the patient is sleeping. A separate, potentially faster lower rate limit may then be programmed for waking hours. (For example, the lower rate limit may be programmed to 60 ppm during waking hours and 40 ppm during sleeping hours.) In some devices, this feature is tied to a "clock," and the usual waking and sleeping hours are programmed into the device. In other devices, the sleep rate is also set on the basis of waking and sleeping hours, but verification by a sensor is required to allow rate changes to occur.

In rate-adaptive pacemakers and in dual-chamber devices capable of atrial tracking, an upper rate limit must also be programmed. The upper rate defines the fastest paced ventricular rate allowed. Determining the appropriate upper rate depends on the patient's age, exercise requirements, and associated cardiac and noncardiac morbidities. From a programming standpoint, the total atrial refractory period (TARP), which is the post-ventricular atrial refractory period (PVARP) plus the atrioventricular (AV) interval, effectively determines the maximum achievable tracking rate (see Chapter 7: Timing Cycles). In dual-chamber rate-adaptive pacemakers, the upper rate limit may be a single programmable value, or two independently programmed values: one for maximum tracking rate and one for maximum sensor-driven rate (see Chapter 7: Timing Cycles).

The nominal upper rate limit, i.e., the upper rate programmed by the manufacturer, is often in the range of 120–130 ppm. For many active individuals a more aggressive upper rate limit should be considered. In Chapter 9: Rate-Adaptive Pacing, we discuss exercise assessment for patients with rate-adaptive pacemakers. At times it is helpful to assess the patient's rate during ambulatory monitoring, informal exercise[3] or a formal treadmill exercise test.[4,5] Symptoms present during pseudo-Wenckebach or 2:1 upper rate behavior inform programming the upper rate limit and other parameters that impact the upper rate (such as AV delay and PVARP). For example, if the patient has normal sinus node function but the upper rate limit is limited by the TARP, shortening the AV interval and/or the PVARP may be required (Fig. 8.9).

ECG Controls

Surface ECG	On
Position	1
Gain	0.25 mV/cm
Filter	On
Markers	On
Position	2
IEGM	On
Position	1
Gain	2.5 mV/cm
Configuration	Atip-Aring
Sweep Speed	25 mm/s
IEGM Filter	On

V. Capture Test Results

Mode	DDDR
Base Rate	90 **T** ppm
AV Delay	170 ms
PV Delay	150 ms
V. Pulse Amplitude	1.50 **T** V
Magnet Response	Battery Test
Number Cycles/Step	4
Vent. Capture Threshold	1.25 V
Vent. Capture Test Pulse Width	0.5 ms
Vent. Capture Test Polarity	Unipolar

T *Temporary programmed value*

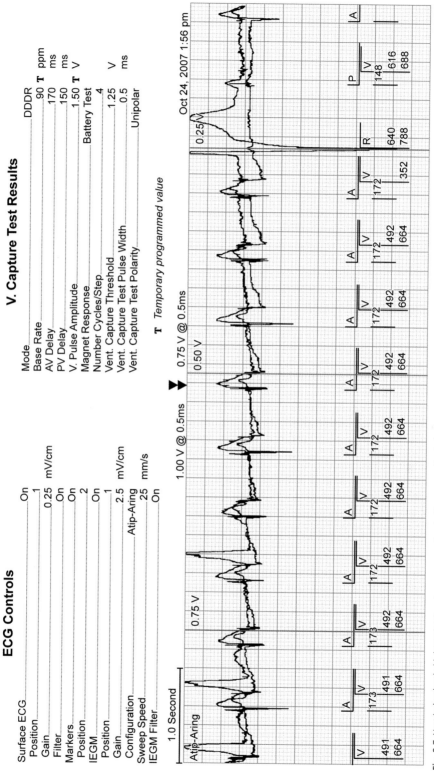

Fig. 8.7 Ventricular threshold determination via programmer threshold sequence. On the surface tracing the atrial depolarization following the atrial pacing artifact is quite large and makes is more difficult to see the ventricular depolarization. In this example ventricular capture is present in the first two beats, lost on the third, regained on the fourth while at 0.75V and then followed by six beats with loss of capture, followed by a ventricular escape beat. (Courtesy and copyrighted by St. Jude Medical.)

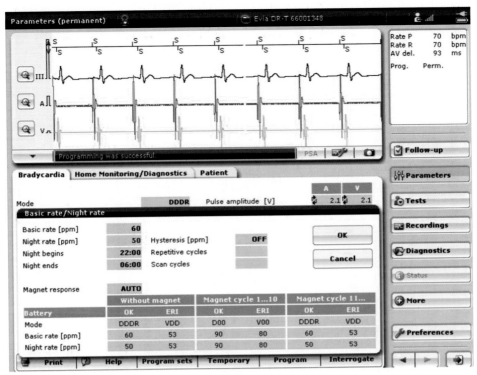

Fig. 8.8 Programmer screen from which the "Basic rate" and "Night rate" can be programmed. In this example the base rate is 60 ppm and the sleep rate is programmed to 50 ppm. Tied to the "clock" in the pulse generator the lower rate will change to 50 ppm at 22.00 h and back to 60 ppm at 06.00 h.

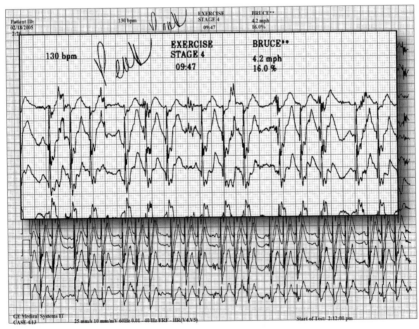

Fig. 8.9 Electrocardiographic tracing obtained during a treadmill exercise test in a 17-year-old patient complaining of sudden onset fatigue during intense exercise. In this example the patient had reached the programmed maximum tracking rate and displays pseudo-Wenckebach behavior. The sensor-indicated rate was not fast enough to prevent a significant alteration in V-V cycle length. The effective sudden decrease in ventricular rate paired with the irregular cycle length resulted in the patient's exertional symptoms.

Programming hysteresis, AV search hysteresis, ventricular pacing avoidance algorithms, and sudden bradycardia response algorithms

Hysteresis has been available for decades but remains a source of confusion. Hysteresis permits prolongation of the first paced escape interval after a sensed event. A ventricular pacemaker programmed at a cycle length of 1000 ms (60 ppm) and a hysteresis rate of 1500 ms (40 ppm) allows 500 ms more after a sensed QRS for another sensed QRS complex. Should another QRS complex not occur, the pacemaker returns to the programmed rate of 60 ppm, an escape interval of 1000 ms (see Chapter 7: Timing Cycles, Fig. 7.62), until once again a sensed event restarts the cycle. The advantage of hysteresis in a single-chamber pacing mode is the ability to maintain spontaneous AV synchrony if the intrinsic rate is below the lower rate limit. In patients with VVI pacing and pacemaker syndrome, hysteresis may prevent symptomatic retrograde ventriculoatrial (VA) conduction and increases the potential for intrinsic conduction.

Several types of AV search hysteresis and ventricular pacing avoidance algorithms are programmable options in dual-chamber pacemakers (detailed in Chapter 7: Timing Cycles). The purpose of these algorithms is to minimize ventricular pacing to promote intrinsic ventricular conduction (Fig. 8.10). Minimizing RV apical pacing (i.e., avoiding pacing in nonresynchronization systems) lowers the risk of pacemaker-induced dyssynchrony, and consequent atrial fibrillation and heart failure.[6–8]

When programming AV intervals, it is reasonable to extend the AV interval to the maximum programmable value or, if available, to program algorithms that promote intrinsic conduction "on" in order to to assess intrinsic conduction (Fig. 8.11). If intrinsic AV nodal conduction is present, then algorithms to minimize ventricular pacing are activated. The often asked question is, "How long can the AV interval be extended before there are adverse consequences?" One study determined the maximal AR interval to be ≥230 ms before negative consequences were seen.[9] We will frequently allow both paced (PAV) and sensed (SAV) intervals to extend to 300 ms. At longer intervals one needs to be certain that AV synchrony is not compromised. Occasionally, it is helpful to use echocardiographic

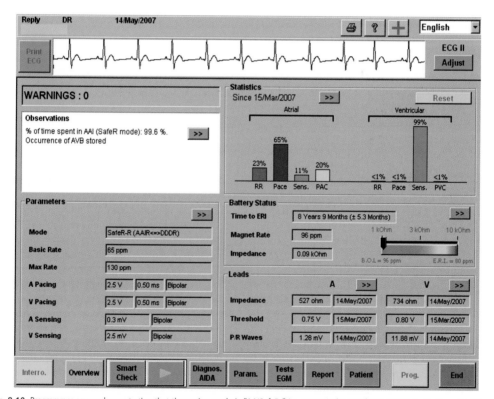

Fig. 8.10 Programmer screen demonstrating that the pacing mode is "AAISafeR," i.e. a ventricular avoidance pacing mode. The patient has been maintained in the AAI pacing mode 99.6% of the time monitored.

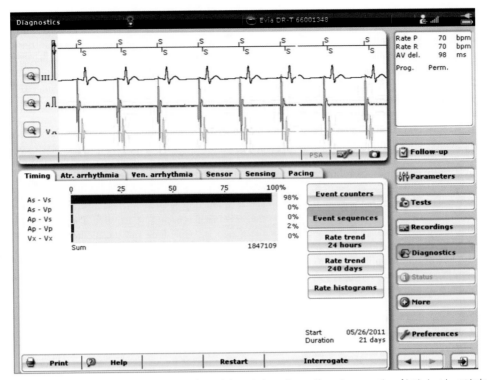

Fig. 8.11 Programmer screen that depicts the outcome of intended ventricular pacing avoidance, i.e., promotion of intrinsic atrioventricular conduction. This example summarizes a 21-day period during which intrinsic ventricular events were present 98% of the time.

techniques to optimize the AV interval in pacemaker patients. The goal of echocardiographic guidance is to optimize atrial contribution to ventricular filling and to minimize or at least limit diastolic mitral insufficiency. Marked prolongation of AR or AV intervals limits the upper tracking rate and may lead to more frequent episodes of pacemaker and/or pacemaker-mediated tachycardia as a result of effective uncoupling of atrial and ventricular activity.

Available AV search hysteresis and ventricular pacing avoidance algorithms are well designed and can be safely turned on in patients with evidence of some degree of intrinsic AV conduction.

In addition to minimizing ventricular pacing, there are patients who will benefit by allowing their native sinus activity to have preference over paced atrial activity. Several manufacturers have algorithms to maximize the presence of the native atrial rhythm.[9] Criteria are programmed that periodically slow the paced rate to a preset level to determine whether or not sinus activity is present. If sinus activity is present, and if the intrinsic atrial rate meets criteria, atrial pacing is inhibited until the patient's intrinsic rate falls to a rate that trig-

gers atrial pacing (Fig. 8.12). Algorithms are also available to allow the converse, i.e., a preference for atrial pacing, to lower the risk of atrial fibrillation (Fig. 8.13).[10]

Another feature that may impact the pacing rate is one that responds to a sudden bradycardia. Most manufacturers have some algorithm whereby, if a significant decrease in heart rate occurs, the device intervenes with pacing at an increased rate in both chambers for a specific, programmed duration (Fig. 8.14). These algorithms were designed to treat vasovagal syncope, although their clinical utility has been modest. At the conclusion of the programmed duration of more rapid pacing, the pacing rate gradually returns to the programmed lower rate. This feature varies between manufacturers. In one algorithm the pacemaker monitors a drop in heart rate that must satisfy a programmable degree of rate decrease, the number of beats the rate must fall, and the duration of time over which the drop in rate occurs. The lower rate limit needs to be programmed slow enough to measure the magnitude of rate drop required for intervention at the faster paced rate. Setting the parameters in a very liberal manner

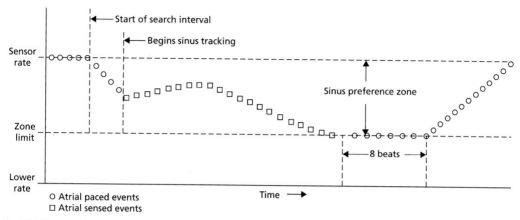

Fig. 8.12 Diagrammatic representation of an algorithm that allows intrinsic sinus rhythm to dominate when preset criteria for the algorithm are met. The rate is allowed to drop below the sensor-indicated rate and, if sinus activity is present within a specific rate "zone," sinus activity is allowed until the rate falls to a specific rate and is maintained at or below that rate for a specified number of beats. If the intrinsic rate does not return to the preferred "rate zone" the pacing rate is gradually incremented back to the sensor-indicated rate. (Reproduced with permission from Medtronic Adapta technical manual, pp. 5–25.)

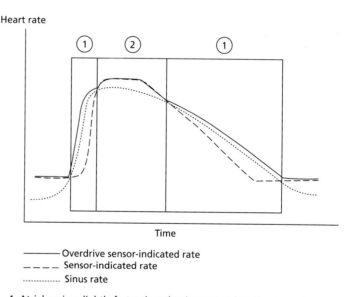

Fig. 8.13 If an atrial pacing preference algorithm is activated the pacemaker will increase the atrial pacing rate when intrinsic activity is sensed in an attempt to maintain a paced rhythm that is just faster than the intrinsic activity. (Reproduced with permission from Medtronic Adapta technical manual, pp. 5–29.)

———— Overdrive sensor-indicated rate
– – – – Sensor-indicated rate
·············· Sinus rate

1 Atrial pacing slightly faster than the sinus rate when the sinus rate exceeds the sensor-indicated rate.
2 Atrial pacing at the sensor-indicated rate when that rate exceeds the sinus rate.

may result in frequent triggering of the algorithm and annoying and unnecessary symptoms (Figs 8.14 and 8.15; see Chapter 7: Timing Cycles).[11-13]

In another algorithm, therapy is triggered when pacing occurs at the programmed lower rate for the programmable consecutive number of "detection beats" (Fig. 8.16).[14] The "antisyncope" algorithms inter-act with sensor use (Medtronic) and the programmed lower rate (Boston Scientific).

Programming output (pulse width and voltage amplitude)

Programming an appropriate pacemaker output is one of the most critical programming steps. There are two

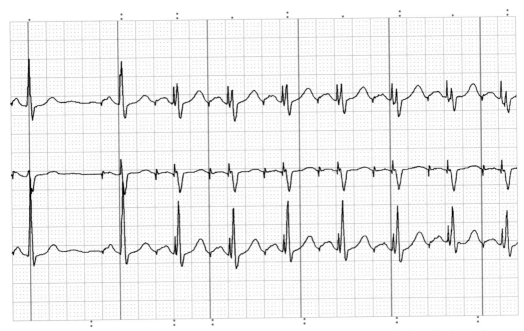

Fig. 8.14 Electrocardiographic tracing that begins with a rate of slightly less than 60 ppm. Criteria are met for the sudden bradycardia response algorithm and are followed by pacing at a rate of 100 ppm. This will continue for a predefined length of time.

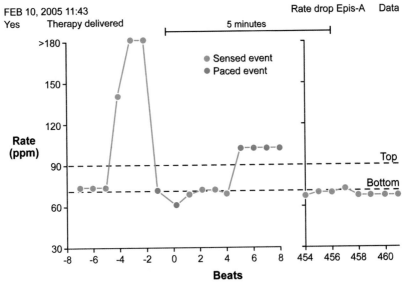

Fig. 8.15 Redrawn from a stored event from a patient with a pacemaker in place with Rate Drop Response (RDR™) programmed "on." The patient initially has a sudden rapid intrinsic rhythm per the pacemaker diagnostics. The intrinsic rate then drops precipitously and meets RDR criteria. The algorithm then results in pacing at a rate of 100 ppm. When the duration of the RDR pacing "times out," the stored event shows that the patient's rate returns to a rate of approximately 70 ppm.

goals in programming output: (i) ensure reliable capture with an adequate safety margin, preferably measured in voltage (as opposed to pulse duration); (ii) maximize pulse generator longevity to the extent this is consistent with the first goal. This requires getting the best safety margin at a pulse duration that provides minimal energy drain from the battery.

Adjustment of output is performed to extend pulse generator life by reducing output and battery drain or to manage increased or increasing stimulation thresholds. Pulse generators provide significant flexibility in pulse width (0.05–1.9 ms) and voltage amplitude (0.5–8.1 V) (these values vary between manufacturers and to some degree between models of a given manufacturer).

With good implantation technique and low-threshold lead designs, e.g., steroid-eluting leads, it is common to program the voltage output to values of ≤2.5 V (the nominal voltage for many pacemakers). (The voltage amplitude program is also affected by the programmed pulse width, see later.) By programming the output at an efficient but safe level, the projected battery life can be increased significantly. A decrease in output can also be used to eliminate extracardiac (diaphragmatic or pectoral muscle) stimulation.

In some patients, thresholds may increase after implantation. Although a transient and mild increase in thresholds is not uncommon in the first 4–6 weeks after implantation, higher outputs can be programmed until thresholds return to a stable level. Although this threshold evolution is largely avoided with steroid-eluting leads, it is reasonable to program higher outputs for the first 2–3 months post-implantation. We generally leave output parameters at nominal values until the patient returns for threshold measurement and then subsequently reprogram to lower outputs. If an auto-capture algorithm is being used that will check stimulation thresholds on a relatively frequent basis and respond automatically to a loss of capture, it may not be necessary to leave the initially programmed output parameters at higher values. Available auto-capture algorithms are summarized in Table 8.3.

High thresholds may be transient or permanent, and output programmability is useful in both situations. In patients with a transient threshold elevation, higher outputs can be used until thresholds return to a stable chronic level. In patients with chronically high thresholds, the pulse generator can be programmed to higher output to permit reliable pacing (albeit with reduced pulse generator longevity). Programming to higher outputs may be done to temporize until a solution is sought to achieve lower thresholds, or it may be the permanent solution, despite the additional battery drain, if there is some reason not to proceed with lead revision.

The output function (voltage or pulse width) that is reprogrammed to manage a rising threshold depends on the threshold value. Programming the pulse duration at or >1.0 ms (i.e., approaching rheobase, the

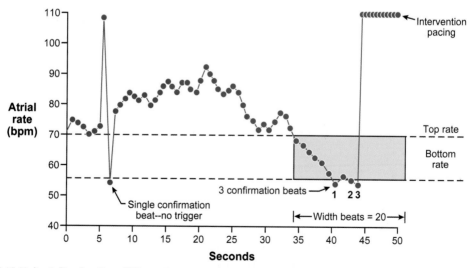

Fig. 8.16 Medtronic "Low Rate Detect." When pacing occurs at the programmed lower rate for the programmable consecutive number of detection beats, therapy is triggered. Low Rate Detect may be used as a backup to the method in Fig. 8.15 if the sudden drop in rate varies between slow and fast.

Table 8.3 Capture management algorithms.

Biotronik	**Atrial Capture Control (ACC)** looks for intrinsic activity as evidence of noncapture. ACC can be programmed "on" or to Automatic Threshold Monitoring (ATM). When programmed "on" the device may adjust pacing amplitude in the atrium. Unlike VCC, ACC does not evaluate atrial capture on a beat to beat basis. Once the threshold is determined and amplitude set it will not run another threshold until designated scheduled search
Ventricular Capture Control (VCC) measures the capture threshold and adjusts pacing amplitude to accommodate for changes, eliminating the need for a 2:1 safety margin and reducing battery consumption. VCC can be programmed "on," "off," or automatic threshold monitoring (ATM). When "off" user must program and determine threshold values and outputs. When "on" or ATM, the device performs two steps: signal quality check (SQC), capture threshold search (CTS). When "on," VCC also initiates continous capture control (CCC) which is a beat by beat assessment of ventricular capture on an ongoing basis and a back-up pulse in there is loss of capture
Boston Scientific	**Ventricular Automatic Capture** feature checks on a beat-to-beat basis for the evoked response. If there is an evoked response, beat-to-beat mode continues at an output of 0.5V above last measured threshold. If there is a loss of capture, the device delivers a backup safety pace at 1.5V greater than previously measured threshold (up to 4.5V). If there is a second loss of capture in two of four cardiac cycles, the device delivers another backup safety pace as described above. At this point, a confirmed loss of capture is declared and an Ambulatory Threshold Test is performed. Ambulatory Threshold Test is conducted every 21 hours or upon a confirmed loss of capture. The device performs an Ambulatory Threshold Test by starting at a voltage of 3.5V and stepping down in 0.2V decrements until reaching 1.0V and in 0.1V decrements thereafter. If the test is successfully completed, the device will return to beat-to-beat mode again pacing 0.5V above last measured threshold. If test cannot be successfully completed, i.e., no loss of capture detected (decremented to lowest output of 0.1V) or a measured threshold greater than 3.0V, the device will enter Retry mode. In Retry mode, the device will pace at twice the previous measured threshold (minimum of 3.5V and maximum of 5.0V)
Not available on atrial channel; not available on high-voltage devices
Medtronic	The Capture Management™ feature in Medtronic devices uses different capture verification methods for RV (evoked response), LV (LV pace induced RV sensing) and atrial (AV conduction [AVC] and atrial intrinsic suppression, i.e., atrial chamber reset [ACR]) chambers. These algorithms generally use sequences of three normal paces followed by a test pace, typically followed by a backup pace to avoid symptoms associated with these tests running while the patient is ambulatory
Capture Management generally operates by reducing pacing amplitude until capture is lost and then increase it again until capture is regained. Then, if programmed to adapt outputs rather than just monitor thresholds, output settings are adjusted above the measured thresholds according to the programmed safety margins. Capture Management nominally performs threshold measurements only once per day applying a programmable (nominal 2:1) voltage safety margin intended to cover circadian variations in threshold
Sorin Medical	No autothreshold algorithms on atrial lead
AutoThreshold – Three programmable values: (1) Off; (2) Auto; and (3) Monitor. In Monitor the system will do all the regular testing but not change the programmed amplitude value. In Auto the assessment is made and the amplitude value changed accordingly. Every 6 hours the device enters a Wait phase. At minimum this is a set of 8-V cycles where the output is put to 5V. The system then calibrates itself to differentiate between evoked potential and polarization. If the system successfully calibrates itself then a stepdown threshold is performed from 1.95V to 0.15V in 0.15-V increments. The last captured cycle is the threshold and the output is calculated with the minimum programmable output of 2.5V in the USA (1.5V OUS). The output determined will be in effect for 6 hours when the system performs the operation again. The only time there are backup pulses are during the calibration and threshold phases. There are no backup pulses during the 6-hour period
St. Jude Medical	Ventricular Autocapture™ (VAC) algorithm is beat to beat capture verification and provides a 5.0-V backup pulse with loss of capture. The VAC safety margin added is 0.25V. Atrial capture confirmation (ACap™ Confirm) is available in low- and high-voltage devices in addition to the VAC. CRT-D devices also have LV lead capture confirmation (LV Cap™ Confirm) and RV Cap™ Confirm algorithms in addition to the A Cap Confirm™ algorithm. A Cap™ Confirm, LV/RV Cap™ Confirm algorithms are not beat to beat capture verification, but rather a "threshold search" is performed every 8/24 hours and a safety margin is added which is algorithm specific

lowest voltage threshold at an infinitely long pulse duration) provides little additional safety margin and results in high current and energy drain.[15] If pulse duration testing defines a threshold >1.0 ms, increasing the output voltage while using a shorter pulse width is a better option.

Experts disagree about the optimal method to program the safety margin once the stimulation threshold has been established. Some devices will program or suggest programmable values after autothresholds are completed. Manual programming options that have been advocated include:
• Double the voltage amplitude
• Triple the pulse width
• Determine the capture threshold in microjoules and program the voltage amplitude and pulse width to achieve three times the threshold in microjoules. (This technique is rarely used with contemporary devices.)

At a given output voltage, if the pulse duration threshold is high, increasing the voltage is probably more useful. Otherwise, extending the pulse width even further may result in little gain, i.e., pulse duration beyond rheobase does not significantly alter capture threshold. Conversely, if pulse duration threshold is very low, i.e., in the range of 0.05–0.1 ms at a given output voltage, reducing the voltage and modestly prolonging the pulse duration may be considered. In general, programming at a pulse width close to the chronaxie (see Stimulation threshold in Chapter 1: Pacing and Defibrillation) minimizes battery drainage, and is preferred if an adequate safety margin can be found. Output programmability should not be a substitute for proper lead placement.

How much safety margin is enough, especially with contemporary leads? There is no universally agreed upon answer to this question. The safety margin in part depends on how often the threshold is checked and available options for intervening in the event of a threshold change. The frequency of threshold assessment ranges from the two extremes of with every beat with automatic algorithms to once a year with manual operator assessment.

In general, a larger safety margin is favored in patients who are pacemaker-dependent, placed on medications that may alter pacing thresholds, on dialysis, or who have metabolic abnormalities that may lead to wide swings in electrolytes and/or metabolic status. A larger safety margin is usually more important on the ventricular than the atrial lead so as to avoid asystole.

Determination of the stimulation threshold is a part of routine pacemaker follow-up. With autothreshold measurements, threshold assessment begins with selecting starting values for voltage and pulse width, and then observing the electrocardiogram and electrogram during output auto-decrement until capture is lost. The programmer for the specific device should provide clear directions on how to respond when capture is lost, e.g., move the programming head or release pressure from the programming screen (Fig. 8.17).

Despite the relative ease with which thresholds can be measured, it must be remembered that the risk of loss of capture includes not just asystole, but bradycardia-dependent tachyarrhythmias as well. Therefore, in pacemaker-dependent patients, equipment for external defibrillation should be available whenever thresholds are measured. Ideally, all thresholds should be measured on a temporary programming screen rather than a permanent screen, unless there is a specific reason to use a permanent screen. This is especially important when the device is near battery depletion, as programmability may be degraded.

Thresholds can also be determined by manually reprogramming the output to progressively smaller values until capture is lost. In the nonpacemaker-dependent patient, manual thresholds can be performed by first programming to the VVI mode and decreasing the rate until the patient's intrinsic rhythm is observed. The pacing rate is then increased until it exceeds the intrinsic ventricular rate. Thresholds can be performed by using a fixed pulse width and decrementing the voltage amplitude or by using a fixed voltage amplitude and decrementing the pulse width. We generally program the pulse width to 0.5 ms and decrement the voltage. The point at which capture is lost is noted, and the threshold defined as the last voltage amplitude at which capture was maintained. Another rapid method for checking thresholds in the nondependent patient uses simultaneous changes in rate and output variables. For example, with the pacemaker programmed to VVI at 40 ppm, if the intrinsic rate is 70, the next programming step could include VVI at 80 ppm, and very low output variables, e.g., voltage amplitude of 1.0 V and pulse width of 0.12 ms. If pacing is re-established, the stimulation threshold is ≤1.0 V, 0.12 ms. If capture is not re-established at 1.0 V and 0.12 ms, one of these two variables can be increased until capture occurs. Whether one increases pulse width or voltage amplitude for determination of stimulation threshold is in large part personal bias.

Other methods of assessing pacing safety margin have been available for years.[16,17] One manufacturer incorporates a Threshold Margin Test with magnet application.[16] With this technique, magnet application results in a rate of 100 ppm for three beats, followed by asynchronous pacing at the programmed rate. The first and second pacing artifacts at a rate of 100 ppm are

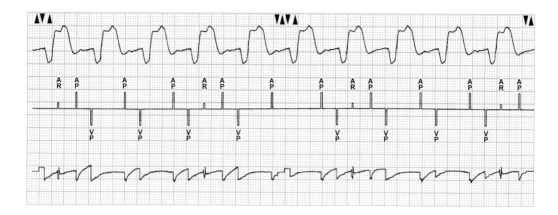

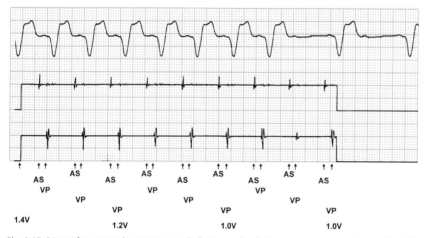

Fig. 8.17 Printout from pacemaker programmers displaying autothreshold testing. Ventricular voltage amplitude threshold test is performed with loss of ventricular capture at 1.0 V.

delivered at the programmed pulse duration. The third pacing artifact is delivered at 75% of the programmed pulse duration. Loss of capture on the third beat indicates a narrow margin of safety (Fig. 8.18).

Features that allow the pacemaker to automatically adjust output based on threshold changes conserve battery consumption, prolong device longevity, and protect patients from failure to capture due to increasing stimulation thresholds.[18–22] Automatic output adjustment and management is available in most devices and, as with any algorithm, operational features vary between manufacturers. The proprietary Auto-Capture™ system confirms capture on a beat-by-beat basis by monitoring the "evoked response" (ER) associated with the ventricular pacing output. The "evoked response" is deflection on the intracardiac electrogram that indicates that capture has occurred.[21,23] To detect the ER signal, a bipolar, low polarization pacing lead should be used. Each paced ventricular complex is assessed for capture by monitoring the ER signal. When no ER signal is detected, the AutoCapture system delivers a 5-V backup safety pulse within 80–100 ms. This backup safety pulse functions as the "safety margin." With two consecutive loss-of-capture events followed by backup safety pulses, the AutoCapture system automatically increases the output of the primary pacing pulse until capture is regained from the primary pacing pulse (Fig. 8.19). At the beginning of this increment, the first paced event is increased by 0.25 V. If capture is not confirmed with this paced event, the pulse amplitude continues to increase in 0.125-V steps* until

* In some devices with this feature the voltage increment may occur in 0.3-V steps.

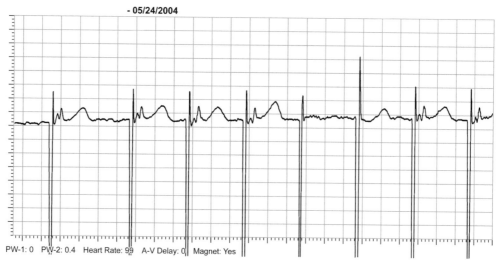

Fig. 8.18 Electrocardiographic tracings from a patient with a VVI Medtronic pacemaker programmed to a rate of 70 ppm. The pacemaker is capable of a Threshold Margin Test (TMT) during magnet application. With magnet application the rate goes to 100 ppm. The first pacing artifact fuses with the QRS and it is difficult to tell if there is a QRS complex present. However, there is a definite "T" wave that follows so by definition, "if there is repolarization there had to be depolarization." The second artifact results in definite capture. At the third pacemaker artifact there is failure to capture and a native QRS follows approximately 240 ms later. It is on the third output after magnet application when the pulse width is decreased to 80% of the programmed value.

capture is verified from the primary pacing pulse for two consecutive paced events. Once verification occurs, the pacemaker automatically initiates a threshold search. If capture for two consecutive events is not confirmed by the time the pacemaker output reaches 3.875 V, the pacemaker automatically reprograms to 4.5 V and 0.5 ms pulse width, or "high output mode" pacing.

Capture management algorithms vary a great deal between manufacturers. They may be responsible for some unusual electrocardiographic findings and, like any programmable feature, the provider needs to know and understand the nuances of the specific algorithm being employed (Fig. 8.20).

Several manufacturers have auto-capture management algorithms available for the atrial channel as well.

Because output adjustment is critical for both extremes, i.e., for maintaining an adequate safety margin and for prolonging battery longevity, automatic regulation of output has become a fairly standard feature and is used with increasing frequency.

Programming sensitivity

All pulse generators filter then sense the intracardiac electrogram delivered by the pacing leads. For atrial and ventricular sensing, the R and P waves must have a sufficient amplitude (millivolts) and slew rate (dV/dt) for proper sensing to occur. The programmed sensitivity is the smallest amplitude signal that the device recognizes (Figs 8.21 and 8.22). Events sensed on the atrial channel are defined as P waves, those sensed on the ventricular channel as R waves. For cardiac resynchronization therapy (CRT) devices there is also discrimination between sensing on the RV lead and sensing on the LV lead. Nominal ventricular sensitivity is usually in the range of 1.2–2.5 mV, and nominal atrial sensitivity is usually in the range of 0.5–1.2 mV. Although the amplitude of intracardiac R or P waves may be adequate at implantation, they may change over time due to metabolic or drug effects, myocardial damage, or lead dislodgment. Different intrinsic foci may not have different amplitudes on the sensing channels, so that extrasystoles may be undersensed despite normal sensing of normal rhythm, and vice versa.

Programming sensitivity to a smaller value increases the sensitivity of the amplifier, so that a smaller amplitude signal will be sensed as an event. (The terminology is confusing because the amplifier is made more sensitive as the number decreases, i.e., 1.25 mV is more sensitive than 2.5 mV.)

The sensing threshold should be determined during routine pacemaker follow-up and can be accomplished in multiple ways. Manual sensing thresholds can be obtained by programming the pacemaker to

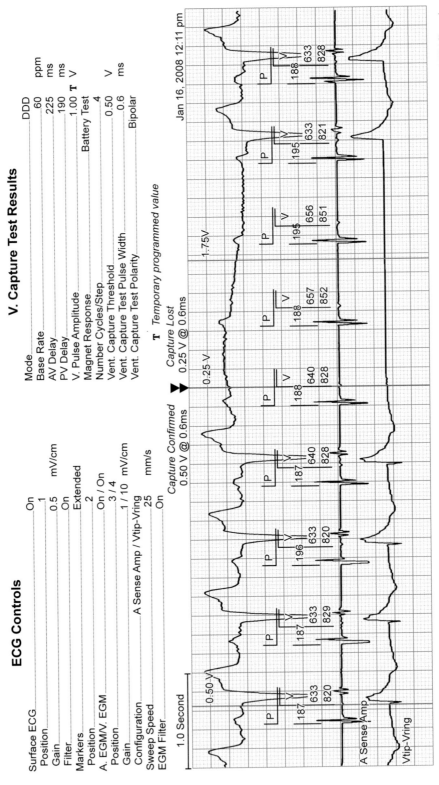

Fig. 8.19 Ventricular AutoCapture threshold test demonstrating loss of capture at 0.25V at 0.6 ms. Capture was confirmed at 0.25V at 0.6 ms. Following loss of capture the output returns to 1.75V. (From the collection of and with the permission of Paul A. Levine, MD, FHRS.)

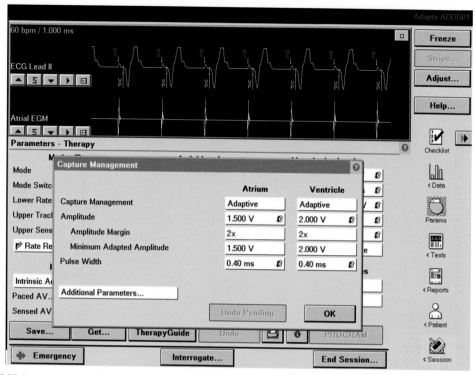

Fig. 8.20 Programmer screen showing options for a capture management algorithm.

progressively less sensitive values until there is failure to sense. (Sensing thresholds could also be determined by altering sensing values during programming to a triggered pacing mode, i.e., AAT or VVT.)

Automatic sensitivity adjustment is available in many pacemakers. Autosensing adjusts sensitivity on the basis of amplitude of the intrinsic waveform.[24,25] However, the method of dynamically altering sensitivity after paced or sensed events, available in implantable cardioverter-defibrillators (ICDs) for generations of devices, is now used in pacemakers; see Sensing sources). The purpose of automatic sensitivity is to prevent both oversensing and undersensing (Fig. 8.23). Although not as critical clinically as automatic output management, automatic sensing has merit and is used with increasing frequency. As noted early in this chapter, determination of sensing threshold via the programmer is often available.

The differential diagnoses for sensing abnormalities and approach to correcting such problems are discussed in Chapter 10: Troubleshooting.

Polarity programmability

Polarity programmability is available on most pacemakers with bipolar configuration. It allows program-

ming from unipolar to bipolar functions. (In some dual-chamber pacemakers, the polarities of the atrial and ventricular channels are independently programmable; in others, they are not.) This feature is helpful in patients who have myopotential or electromagnetic inhibition in the unipolar mode, but not in the bipolar mode. Unipolar and bipolar electrograms have different characteristics, and programming from one polarity to the other may eliminate the sensing of an unwanted electrogram or interfering signal. It is possible but improbable that sensing in one polarity configuration will be superior to that in the other (Fig. 8.23).

Polarity programmability may be helpful in a patient with a lead fracture or inner insulation failure. If the conductor to the ring electrode is fractured, reprogramming from bipolar to unipolar mode may restore effective pacing by using the intact conductor of the pacing lead and bypassing the damaged one (Fig. 8.24). This alternative should usually be considered a temporary measure, because whatever force resulted in fracture of one conductor may have damaged the other. In an increasing number of pulse generators, a change from bipolar to unipolar pacing configuration may be triggered automatically when a sudden change in

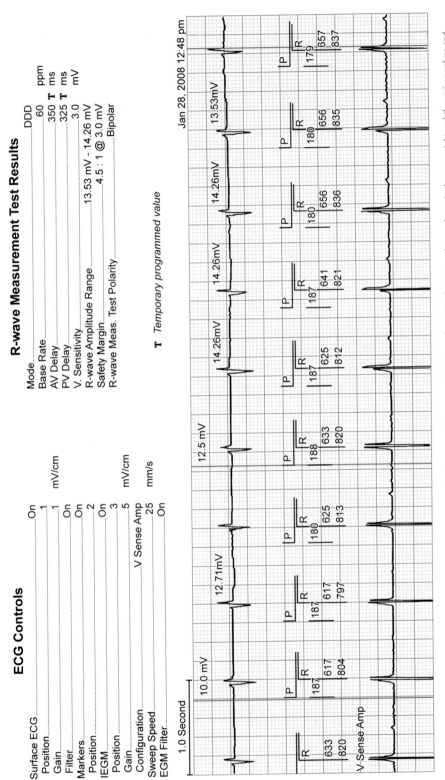

Fig. 8.21 R-wave amplitude test. It is displaying the Ventricular Sense Amplitude electrogram. The top tracing is the surface ECG. The test results are shown in the upper right and the various values and settings for the actual ECG and EGM recording are in the upper left. (From the collection of and with the permission of Paul A. Levine, MD, FHRS.)

A

ECG Controls

Surface ECG	On
Position	1
Gain	1 ____ mV/cm
Filter	On
Markers	On
Position	2
IEGM	On
Position	3
Gain	1 ____ mV/cm
Configuration	Atip-Aring
Sweep Speed	25 ____ mm/s
EGM Filter	On

A. Sense Test Results

Mode	DDD
Base Rate	30 **T** ppm
AV Delay	225 ms
PV Delay	200 ms
A. Sensitivity	0.3 mV
Magnet Response	Battery Test
Number Cycles/Step	4
P-Wave Amplitude	2.5 mV
Atrial Sense Test Polarity	Bipolar
Atrial Sense Safety Margin	8.3 : 1 @ 0.30mV

T *Temporary programmed value*

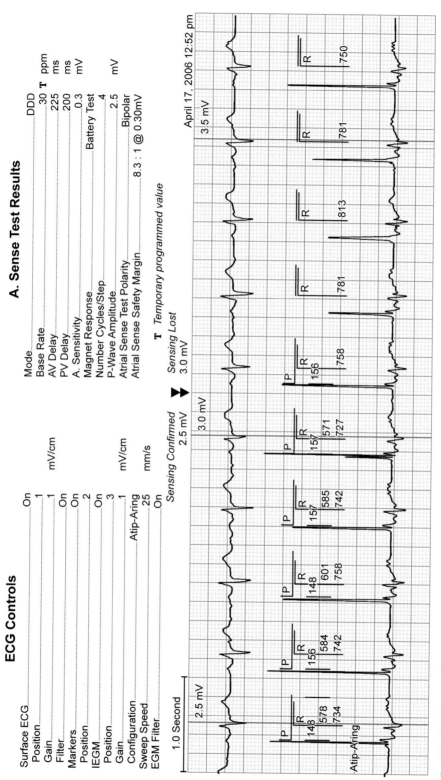

Fig. 8.22 (A) Trial sense test from a patient with a dual-chamber pulse generator. It is being run with the surface ECG, the event markers and the bipolar (Atip-Aring) electrogram being simultaneously displayed. Note the lack of P markers at the temporarily programmed sensitivity of 3.0 mV. Hence, the sensing threshold is the previous more sensitive setting at which there was consistent sensing for the number of cycles programmed for the test (4–10) and this value is shown in the data at the upper right. (B) Semiautomatic "Ventricular Sensing test." Under the central box with the new value, i.e., 9 mV, there is a display of the results the last time that this test was performed, at which time it was >12.5 mV. (From the collection of and with the permission of Paul A. Levine, MD, FHRS.)

(Continued)

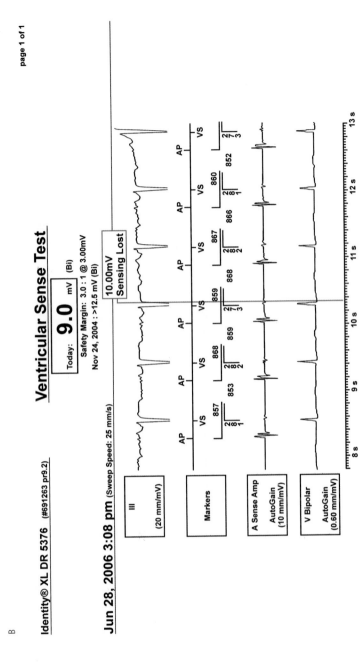

Fig. 8.22 (*Continued*)

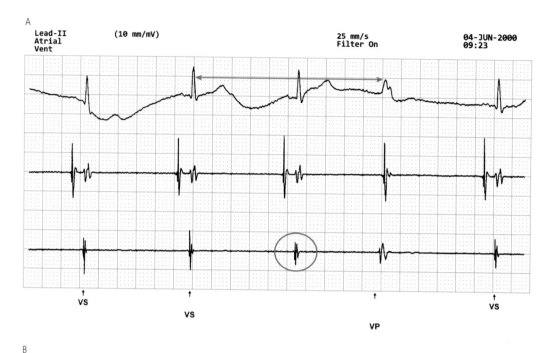

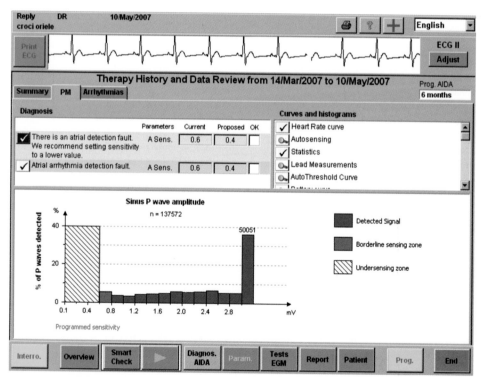

Fig. 8.23 (A) Electrocardiographic tracing from a patient with a dual-chamber pacemaker programmed to VVI mode at 30 ppm. (Top tracing, surface ECG; second tracing, atrial electrogram; third tracing, ventricular electrogram; marker channel at the bottom of the tracing.) Note that third QRS has no marker channel notation and is followed by a ventricular paced (VP) event. Measuring backward from the VP event by 2000 ms (30 ppm) it coincides with the prior ventricular sensed (VS) event. The measured R wave equaled 2 mV. When programmed to unipolar sensing configuration, the R wave measured 6 mV. Had an automatic sensitivity algorithm been programmed "on" this abnormality should be reprogrammed automatically avoiding any clinical sequelae. (B) Programmer screen displaying device diagnosis of atrial undersensing with sensing histogram. Based on this diagnosis the pulse generator proposes that atrial sensitivity be reprogrammed from 0.6 to 0.4 mV.

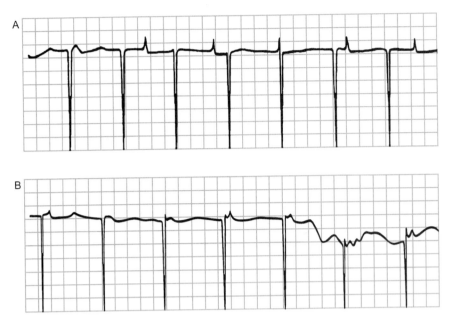

Fig. 8.24 Electrocardiographic tracings from a patient with a VVI pacemaker. (A) In the bipolar configuration, there is intermittent failure to capture. Capture is demonstrated only with the first two pacing stimuli. (B) Programmed to the unipolar configuration at the same pulse duration and voltage, the pacemaker demonstrates consistent capture. (From Hayes DL. Programmability. In: Furman S, Hayes DL, Holmes DR Jr, eds. A Practice of Cardiac Pacing, 3rd edn. Mount Kisco, NY: Futura Publishing Co., 1993:635–63, by permission of Mayo Foundation.)

impedance is detected during bipolar pacing, providing this programmable option is activated (Fig. 8.25).[26,27]

Refractory and blanking periods

Refractory and blanking periods are described in detail in Chapter 7: Timing Cycles. In brief, a refractory period can be defined as an interval during which a given sensing circuit does not respond to sensed events except to increment mode-switching counters. In contrast, events that occur during a blanking period are completely ignored, and not sensed at all.

Single-chamber pacemakers: Refractory period programming may be necessary in a variety of clinical circumstances. In the VVI mode, the ventricular refractory period (VRP) is the interval during which the ventricular sensing circuit does not respond to sensed events. The first portion of the VRP is usually a ventricular blanking period during which ventricular sensing is disabled after paced, sensed, and refractory sensed ventricular events. Depending on the pacemaker, the ventricular blanking period may be fixed, programmable, or dynamic. Refractory period programming in single-chamber pacing is not commonly required but can be advantageous in some situations.

Lengthening of the VRP may help prevent sensing of afterpotential depolarizations, T waves, or premature ventricular contractions. If the refractory period is too long, a closely coupled ventricular electrograms may be undersensed and a pacemaker stimulus could potentially fall on the T wave of the unsensed beat. In this circumstance, shortening the VRP would be appropriate.

When atrial pacing in the AAI mode, a refractory period that exceeds the intrinsic PR interval is desirable to avoid inhibition of atrial pacing as a result of far-field R-wave oversensing (Fig. 8.26).

Dual-chamber pacemakers: Refractory periods in dual-chamber, dual-sensing devices are more complex than single-chamber because the events and timing cycles in one channel affect those in the other. The refractory periods in the ventricular channel behave the same as during single-chamber sensing. The refractory periods in the atrial channel are quite different. After an atrial stimulus or a sensed atrial event, the initial portion of the atrioventricular interval (AVI) is the atrial blanking period. During this interval, atrial sensing does not take place. Depending on the pacemaker, the atrial blanking period is fixed, programmable, or dynamic, i.e., varying

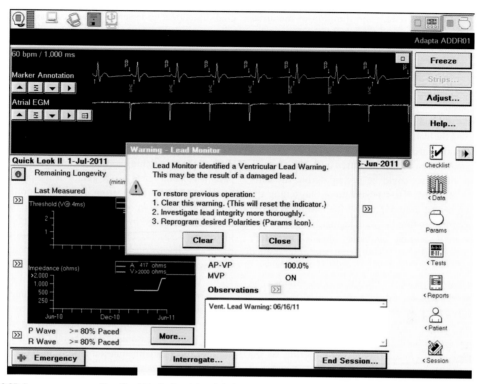

Fig. 8.25 Programmer screen with a "Lead Monitor" warning. If the lead monitor is programmed to adapt to a certain change in lead impedance, the pulse generator will reprogram from bipolar to unipolar pacing configuration.

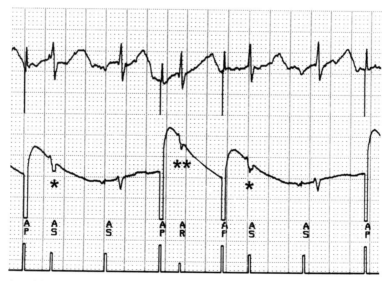

Fig. 8.26 Tracing obtained from a patient with a pacemaker programmed to the AAI mode. (Top, surface electrocardiogram; middle, atrial electrogram; bottom, marker channel.) Each atrial paced (AP) event is followed by an event that is labeled as an atrial sensed (AS) event. These events actually represent sensing of the QRS on the atrial sensing channel. The two events labeled with (*) fall outside the atrial refractory period and alter the timing cycle. The event labeled AR (**) occurs slightly earlier relative to the atrial pacing artifact that precedes it and falls in the atrial refractory period.

in relation to the strength and duration of the atrial event. (Blanking period programmability is summarized in Table 8.4.)

A ventricular blanking period is also initiated with a sensed or paced atrial event. The intent of this interval is to avoid sensing the electronic event of one channel in the opposite channel ("crosstalk"). The blanking period is usually programmable (Table 8.4). It may be desirable to prolong the blanking period to prevent crosstalk (Fig. 8.27). It may be necessary to shorten the blanking period if ventricular extrasystoles are sensed during this period, because the result could be pacing during the early portion of ventricular repolarization. Shortening the blanking period should diminish the likelihood of the QRS occurring within the blanking period.

The atrial sensing amplifier remains refractory for the remainder of the AVI plus the programmed PVARP.

The first portion of the PVARP disables atrial sensing after paced, sensed, and refractory sensed ventricular events, i.e., the post-ventricular atrial blanking period (PVAB). Once again, this interval may be fixed or programmable, depending on the pacemaker (Fig. 8.28).

Sensed events in the nonblanked portion of the TARP (TARP is composed of the AV interval and PVARP) are used for mode switching. Excessive atrial blanking may prevent mode switching, particularly at rapid ventricular rates. Minimal PVAB periods are preferred in patients at risk for 2:1 conduction of atrial flutter.

Programmable flexibility of the PVARP is especially important because of its role in preventing endless-loop tachycardia (ELT) (Fig. 8.29).[28,29] Because ELT can occur only when the PVARP is shorter than the retrograde (VA) conduction time, this is an especially important interval. However, not all patients have intact VA conduction and some have short retrograde conduction times. Algorithms to detect and interrupt ELT do so by automatically lengthening the PVARP or the AVI, or both periodically so that the retrograde P wave will fall into a refractory period and thus not be tracked (Fig. 8.30) (see Chapter 7: Timing Cycles).

Many pacemakers have a programmable "PVARP extension." If this feature is enabled, the PVARP is lengthened when a ventricular event is sensed that is categorized as a premature ventricular contraction (PVC). A PVC is defined as a ventricular event without an antecedent atrial event (i.e., two ventricular events in a row). Following a PVC, the PVARP is extended to prevent sensing retrograde atrial activation should it occur. PVARP extension may result in confusing electrocardiographic presentations. If the extended PVARP encompasses the subsequent atrial or ventricular event, the appearance of undersensing results. This is considered "functional undersensing," because it is a function of the extended PVARP (Fig. 8.31).

Mode switching

In a dual-chamber tracking mode it is important to avoid tracking paroxysmal atrial tachyarrhythmias. The device could be programmed to a nontracking mode, e.g. DDI, but function is then compromised when the patient is in a physiologic atrial rhythm and tracking is desired. Mode switching is available in all dual-chamber pacemakers and refers to the ability of the pacemaker to change automatically from a tracking mode to a nontracking mode in response to a rapid atrial rhythm that is characterized by the pacemaker as being pathologic (Fig. 8.32).[30–32] The nontracking mode to which the devices reverts during mode switching may be programmable and usually includes VVI, VVIR, DDI, and DDIR (Figs 8.33 and 8.34). The sensed atrial rate at which mode switching occurs is usually programmable. Mode switching is particularly useful for patients with known paroxysmal supraventricular rhythm disturbances but it is reasonable to program mode switch "on" for most patients unless it compromises or "locks out" some other desired programmable feature for the specific patient.

Many pacemakers provide extensive diagnostic data regarding events that meet mode-switch criteria. Depending on the mode-switching algorithm in use, inappropriate mode switching may occur although continued improvement of mode-switch algorithms has improved their accuracy. In many pacemakers, the appropriateness of mode switching can be verified by stored electrograms (Figs 8.35 and 8.36). There are multiple factors that may impact the appropriateness of mode switching, one main one being the mode-switching rate. Another factor is the presence of oversensed R waves on the atrial channel (i.e. far-field R-wave oversensing). No single rate is correct for all patients and the selection is simplified if the rate of the recurrent atrial tachyarrhythmia is known. It is tempting to set the detection rate significantly below the known tachyarrhythmia rate in an effort to detect all tachyarrhythmias. However, this may result in inappropriate mode switching, e.g., mode switching secondary to sinus tachycardia or atrial extrasystoles. Although no single value can be recommended for programming the detection rate, the caregiver is advised to review the patient's tachyarrhythmias, the nominally programmed value, and adjust appropriately. Some experts program the mode-switch rate to just above the anticipated maximum sinus rate. Also remember that the measured atrial rate is affected by blanking periods, particularly at high ventricular rates. Typically, mode

Table 8.4 Manufacturer-specific blanking characteristics.

	Atrial blanking after atrial event	Ventricular blanking after atrial pace	Ventricular blanking after ventricular event	Post-ventricular atrial blanking	Comments
Biotronik	Auto adjusts along with refractory period of AV delay	Programmable 30–70 ms in 5 ms increments, nominal 30	Programmable 100–220 ms in 10-ms increments, nominal is 100	Programmable 30–200 ms, nominal 100 ms after Vs, 150 ms after Vp	
Boston Scientific	NA	Programmable 30–200 ms Increment of 10 ms, nominal 40 ms	NA	Programmable 30–200 ms Increment of 10 ms, nominal 120 ms	
Medtronic	Nonprogrammable	Programmable	Nonprogrammable	Programmable	The nonprogrammable blanking periods are also sometimes referred to as "quiet-timer" blanking, as these variable length blanking intervals are enforced until the input stage of the sense amplifier is quiet enough, from a voltage standpoint, to turn it on again
Sorin	A-pacing = AV delay (during DDD mode or DDD operation of SafeR) A-pacing = 155 ms (during AAI operation of SafeR) A-sensing = 80 ms	A-pacing = true ventricular blanking of 30 ms but channel is committed or absolutely refractory for an additional 65 ms	V-pacing = 150 ms V-sensing = 100 ms	Programmable	
St. Jude	Defined as "Atrial Paced and Sensed Refractory" that is absolute refractory or blanked Atrial Paced Refractory is not programmable, except AAI/AAT modes Atrial Sense Refractory is programmable in single-chamber and dual-chamber modes	Programmable from 12 to 52 ms and Auto in which if a ventricular events falls in the first 12 ms of the V blanking period, another 12 ms will be added to the blanking period. This will continue until the V blanking period reaches 52 ms	Defined as "Ventricular Paced and Sensed Refractory" that is absolute refractory or blanked Ventricular Paced Refractory is programmable Ventricular Sensed Refractory is nonprogrammable	Programmable = 12–52 ms	

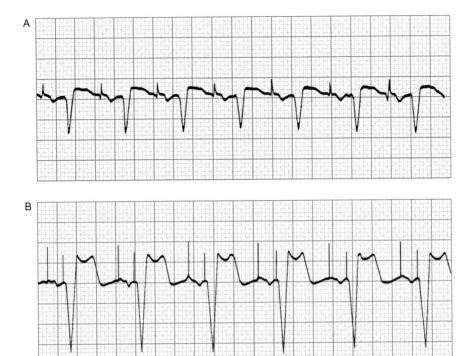

Fig. 8.27 (A) Electrocardiogram from a patient with a DDI pacemaker programmed to a rate of 86 ppm, atrioventricular (AV) interval of 165 ms and a blanking period of 13 ms. The interval from the atrial pacing stimulus to the intrinsic QRS complex is actually 220 ms. This abnormality occurs because the atrial output is sensed on the ventricular sensing circuit and inhibits ventricular output. AV nodal conduction is intact with a first-degree AV block. (B) When the blanking period is lengthened to 45 ms, crosstalk is prevented. A ventricular pacing stimulus occurs 165 ms after the atrial pacing stimulus, i.e., at the programmed AV interval. (From Hayes DL. Programmability. In: Furman S, Hayes DL, Holmes DR Jr, eds. Mount Kisco, NY: Futura Publishing Co., 1993:635–63, by permission of Mayo Foundation.)

switching is set to 175 bpm in the absence of known atrial tachyarrhythmia rates.

Programming rate-adaptive parameters

Parameters that determine rate adaptation in a sensor-driven pacemaker vary considerably depending on the sensor incorporated (Figs 8.37 and 8.38). Programming rate-adaptive parameters is discussed in Chapter 9: Rate-Adaptive Pacing.

Diagnostics – set-up and assessment

A variety of diagnostics are available on contemporary pacemakers, some of which have already been mentioned. Pacemakers are capable of detecting high atrial rate episodes, mode-switching events, high ventricular rate episodes, episodes that meet sudden bradycardia response criteria, etc.

During programming there will be an option to view "diagnostics." (This may be given a different name by some manufacturers.) As part of routine pacemaker evaluation, diagnostics are reviewed to see whether any events have been collected.

When programming a device for the first time, the diagnostic preferences must be selected (Fig. 8.39). Because there is a limitation to the number of events that can be stored in a pulse generator, it is usually not possible to select all of the available diagnostic categories. Category selection should be based on the patient's history. For many patients, selection of "high rate atrial episodes" is appropriate because it allows the caregiver to assess the events that trigger mode switching and the electrograms collected help to determine if the mode switching was appropriate (Figs 8.40–8.42).

Unexpected programming

There may be times when interrogation reveals something other than the expected programmed parameters. With contemporary devices, unexpected programming

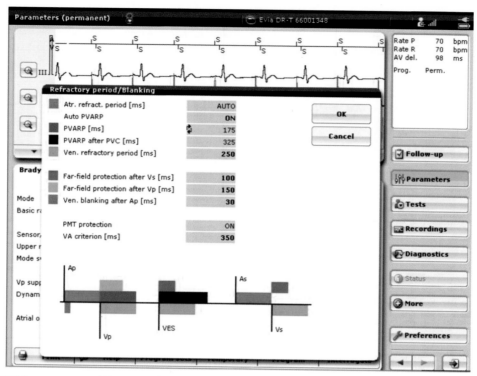

Fig. 8.28 Programmer screen which notes auto-PVARP to be "on." In addition, all of the refractory and blanking periods are listed and diagrammed. The diagram helps the clinician programming the device to better understand the interactions between the refractory and blanking periods and the difference in timing following a ventricular extrasystole (VES). After the VES, the PVARP is extended, dark blue.

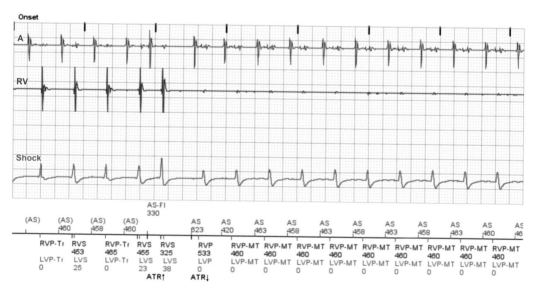

Fig. 8.29 Pacemaker mediated tachycardia from a CRT device; tracing from remote-monitoring. An atrial sense event (AS) occurs early and appears to alter timing that results in a sustained PMT. In this example the designation "MT" indicates the device is tracking at the maximum tracking rate allowed by the programmed settings.

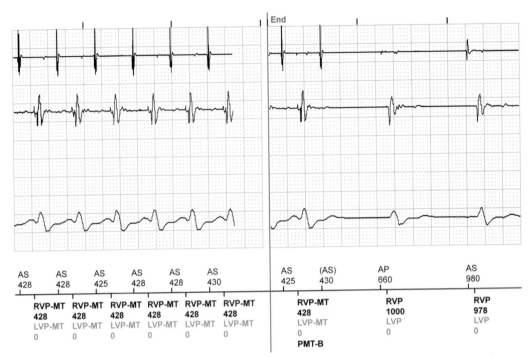

AS	AS	AS	AS	AS	AS	AS	(AS)	AP	AS
428	428	425	428	428	430	425	430	660	980
RVP-MT	RVP-MT	RVP-MT	RVP-MT	RVP-MT	RVP-MT	RVP-MT		RVP	RVP
428	428	428	428	428	428	428		1000	978
LVP-MT	LVP-MT	LVP-MT	LVP-MT	LVP-MT	LVP-MT	LVP-MT		LVP	LVP
0	0	0	0	0	0	0		0	0
						PMT-B			

Fig. 8.30 Stored episode demonstrating the end of a pacemaker mediated tachycardia (PMT). After meeting the criteria for this specific PMT termination algorithm the device extends the PVARP to 500 ms. As a result, the (AS) event falls in the refractory period. This ends the PMT and the paced rhythm resumes at 60 bpm, the programmed lower rate limit.

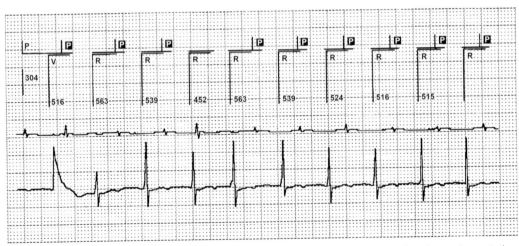

Fig. 8.31 Functional Undersensing. Tracing display: top, marker channel; middle, atrial electrogram; bottom, surface electrocardiogram. In the marker channel the first "P" indicates a sensed native atrial depolarization. All of the other "P" waves are displayed in a black square. This display is an indication for this manufacturer that the P wave is refractory, i.e., it is recognized but will not alter the timing cycle. Each of the refractory "P" waves is occurring in the PVARP. This is an example of functional atrial undersensing.

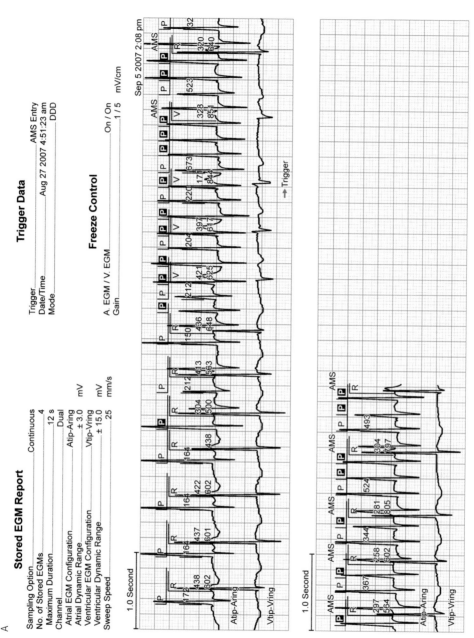

Fig. 8.32 (A) Mode-switch episode: top, marker channel; middle, atrial electrogram; bottom, ventricular electrogram. With the onset of a rapid atrial rhythm, many "p" waves fall in refractory, designated by the "shaded" P. The P waves that fall in the refractory period are counted for the purpose of determining whether a programmed atrial tachycardia detection rate has been achieved. Mode switch criteria are fulfilled where the notation "trigger" occurs, and AMS notes "automatic mode switching." (B) Diagnostic summary screen of mode-switch events. The example in (A) corresponds to the most recent entry on the summary screen. (From the collection of and with the permission of Paul A. Levine, MD, FHRS.)

(Continued)

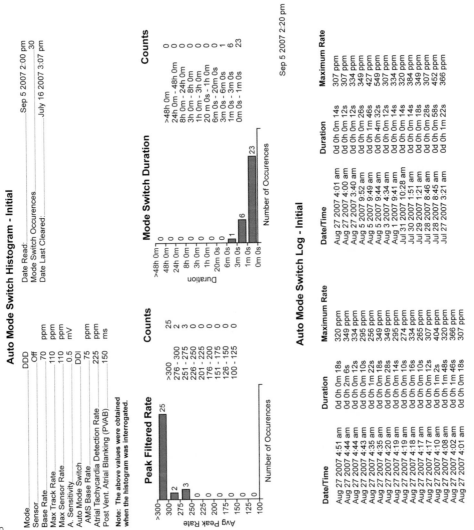

Fig. 8.32 (Continued)

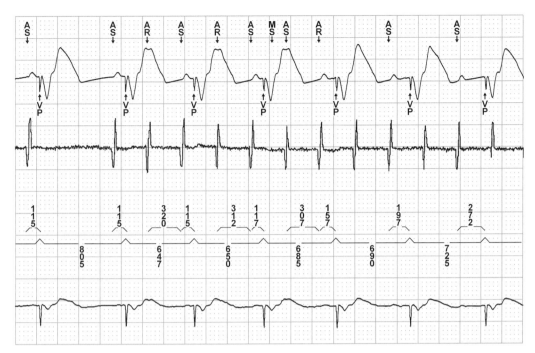

Fig. 8.33 Tracing from a patient that develops an atrial tachyarrhythmia resulting in mode-switching (MS). After the MS occurs there is continued atrial sensing (AS events) but the PV interval (AS to VP) varies and the ventricular pacing rate remains constant. This is characteristic timing for DDIR pacing mode.

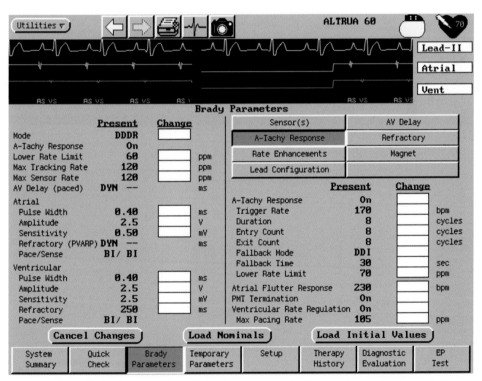

Fig. 8.34 Programmer screen from which the mode-switch algorithm is programmed in this pacemaker. Note that there are multiple programmable criteria for mode switching. In addition to turning it "on," criteria need to be set for the atrial tachycardia detection rate or "trigger rate," the number of cycles evaluated, the number of cycles to satisfy the criteria and mode switch and the number of cycles to return to the originally programmed mode, the mode and duration of time to lower the rate detected at the time the mode switch occurs back to the lower rate limit to be used during mode switching. In addition, an atrial flutter response can be activated.

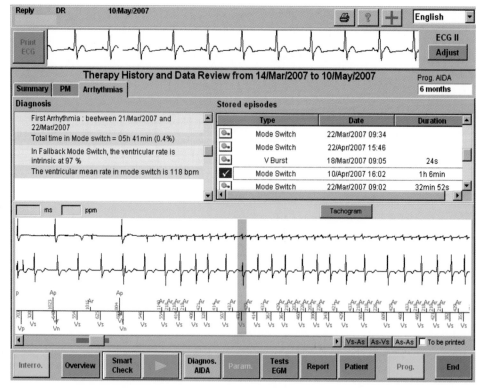

Fig. 8.35 Programmer screen displaying detection of an atrial tachyarrhythmia. The device notes the total time in mode-switch and mean ventricular rate during the event. The device provides the atrial and ventricular electrograms and marker channel.

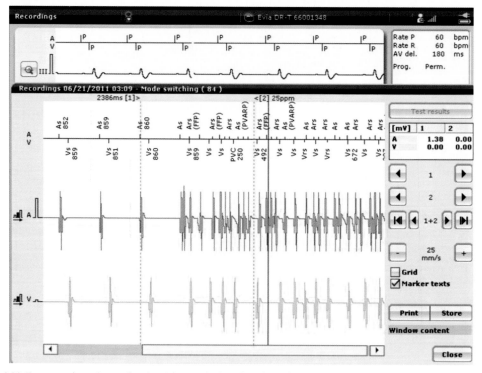

Fig. 8.36 Time-stamped stored event of mode switching. In the three-channel recording, the top channel is the marker channel; middle, atrial electrogram with an irregularly irregular rhythm consistent with atrial fibrillation; bottom, ventricular electrogram.

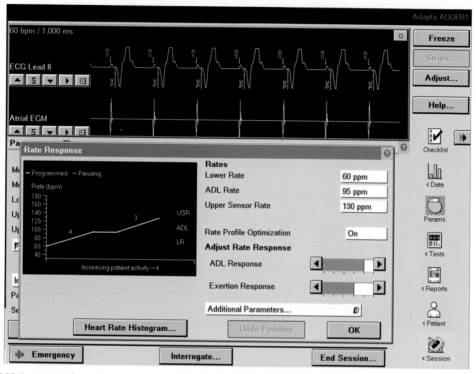

Fig. 8.37 Set-up screen for a rate-adaptive sensor, in this case an accelerometer. Programming options include the lower pacing rate and upper sensor-driven rate as well as the ADL, or activity of daily living, rate. In this device the ADL rate indicates the heart rate that would be desirable for the given patient with moderate activities. Rate profile optimization allows the pulse generator to adapt the ADL and exertional rate response levels one time each day. It does this by comparing the "sensor rate profiles" with a target rate profile.

probably occurs either because someone has reprogrammed the device and failed to document the changes or because the pacemaker has been exposed to electromagnetic interference.

Sources and management of electromagnetic interference are discussed in Chapter 12: Electromagnetic Interference.

Programming during routine follow-up

The importance of a systematic approach to programming during routine follow-up and troubleshooting cannot be overstated. Continued improvements in automaticity will undoubtedly further minimize the time required for programming,[17] but a defined approach to programming should be adopted to be certain that the pacemaker is thoroughly evaluated and to optimize pacemaker function. The following programming sequence for a rate-adaptive dual-chamber pacemaker (DDDR) is presented as a suggested approach. It is not critical that programming be performed in this specific sequence. (In fact, depending on the manufacturer of

the specific pacemaker, the way the programming screens are designed may favor another sequence that is more efficient.)

1 Interrogate the pacemaker and print out stored data
2 Assess magnet response
3 Determine underlying rhythm
4 Collect and review measured data
   • Lead impedance(s)
   • Intrinsic P and/or R-wave amplitude
   • Battery status and predicted longevity
5 Determine the atrial and/or ventricular stimulation thresholds.
6 Determine sensing thresholds.
7 Assess intrinsic AV conduction.
   • If AV conduction intact, consider algorithm to promote intrinsic ventricular conduction
8 Determine the appropriate upper rate limit by considering:
   • Physical activity
   • Subjective response to well-being during activity at current programmed values

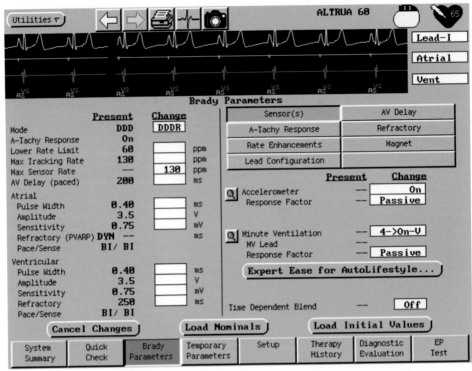

Fig. 8.38 Programming a dual-sensor pacemaker. At the time this screen shot was captured, both the accelerometer and minute ventilation sensors were "passive." When "passive" the sensor information is collected by the device but not used to actively alter the rate response. Behind the minute ventilation "drop-down" menu and partially obscured is an option for Expert Ease/Lifestyle. This option, if activated, assists the clinician by optimizing the behavior of the sensor based on the age of the patient. This feature will suggest programmed values for the lower rate limit, maximum sensor rate, and high rate response factor.

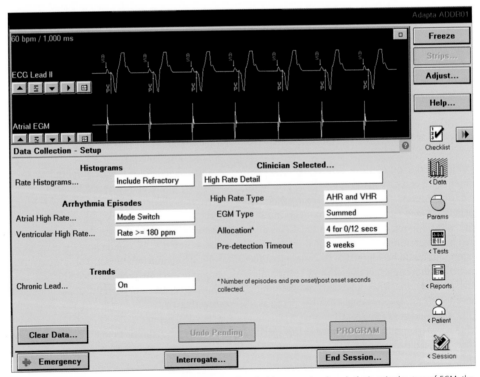

Fig. 8.39 Programmer screen to set up data collection. Options are given for histograms, trends, arrhythmia episodes, type of EGM, the number of episodes and amount of time, seconds, collected before and after the episode.

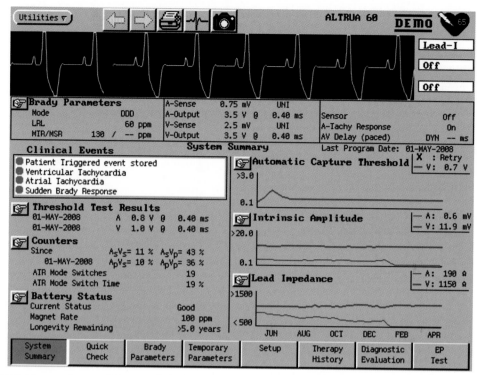

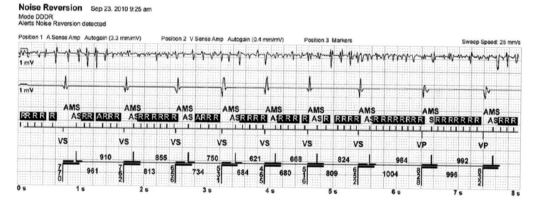

Fig. 8.40 A "summary" screen which notes multiple clinical events including: stored patient triggered event, ventricular tachycardia, atrial tachycardia and a sudden brady response.

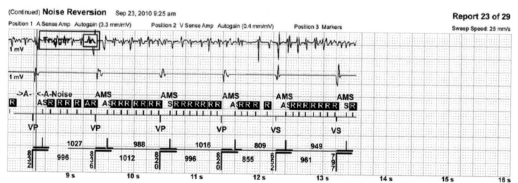

Fig. 8.41 Example of device detection of an atrial high rate episode that is labeled as 'noise reversion'. The patient was in atrial fibrillation and the device had appropriately mode-switched.

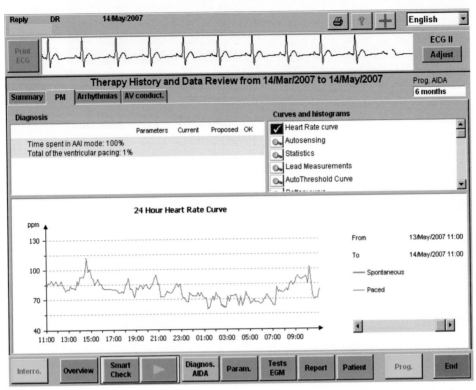

Fig. 8.42 A diagnostic screen displaying the 24-h heart rate trend. The device also reports how much time was spent in each pacing mode.

- Associated medical conditions.

9 Program AV delay variables, i.e., PAV/SAV, RAAVD.

10 Program rate-adaptive parameters:
- Assess exercise, either formally or informally (see Chapter 9: Rate-Adaptive Pacing).

11 Evaluate "other" parameters. For example, the need to:
- Activate the pacemaker-mediated tachycardia algorithm
- Turn on "mode-switching" algorithm
- Program PVARP extension "on."

12 Review "other" features available for the individual pacemaker, and program "on" desirable features (Fig. 8.43).

13 Review programmable telemetry options, and program as desired.

There are some pulse generators that will make programming suggestions based on details of the patient's history that have been entered in combination with collected data (Fig. 8.44) or not allow certain activities to occur based on measured data (Fig. 8.45). Additional discussion on management of routine follow-up is present in Chapter 13: Follow-up.

Defibrillator programming

ICDs incorporate many programmable parameters that enable device function to be tailored to an individual's cardiac disease. Many of the programmable features discussed in the pacemaker section of this chapter – pacing modes, programmable pacing output, mode switch, pacing rate-smoothing algorithms, and others – are currently available in defibrillators. However, in addition to providing sophisticated antibradycardia support, ICDs must be able to detect low-amplitude VF electrograms, to differentiate ventricular tachyarrhythmias from supraventricular tachycardias, and to deliver antitachycardia pacing (ATP) and high-energy shocks to treat tachyarrhythmias. These requirements necessitate additional programmable features. This section focuses on the operation and programming of these features and is divided into the following sections:
- ICD sensing
- ICD algorithms to detect tachyarrhythmias
- SVT-VT discriminators
- Ventricular therapies
- Atrial therapies
- Optimizing programming.

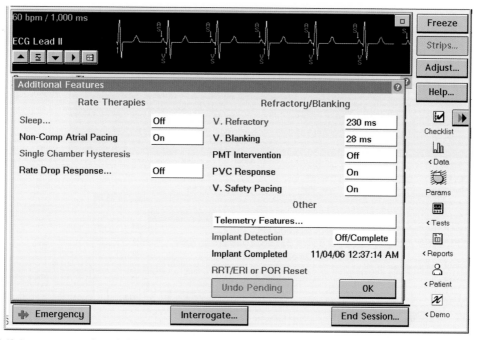

Fig. 8.43 Programmer screen from which "additional features" can be programmed. As noted in the programming sequence, the clinician should, at some point during the programming sequence, consider any parameters unique to the pulse generator that may benefit the patient.

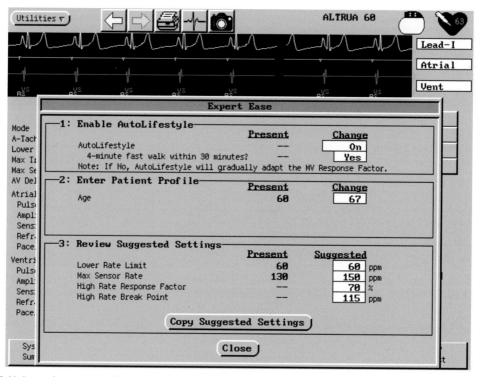

Fig. 8.44 Some pulse generators will make programming suggestions based on the patient's history. This screen demonstrates suggested programming changes for a rate-adaptive sensor.

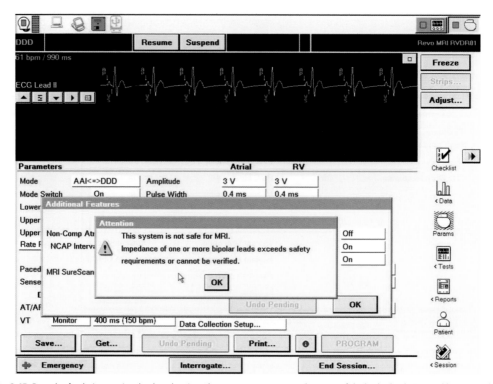

Fig. 8.45 Example of a device warning that based on impedance measurements on at least one of the leads, the device would not meet the safety criteria for magnetic resonance imaging (MRI).

Programming of resynchronization devices is covered in Cardiac resynchronization devices, below.

Implantable cardioverter-defibrillator sensing

"Sensing" is the process by which an ICD determines the timing of each atrial or ventricular electrical event from the electrogram. "Detection" occurs after analysis of a sequence of sensed events by the defibrillator to classify the rhythm and determine whether therapy should be delivered. "Oversensing" on the ventricular channel occurs when non-QRS potentials are greater than a reference threshold voltage and are considered sensed events; analogous oversensing occurs on the atrial channel. Oversensing may arise from intracardiac events (P or T waves) or extracardiac events (diaphragmatic signals, electromagnetic interference; Fig. 8.46) that lead the defibrillator to determine that cardiac events are present when in fact they are not. In contrast, undersensing occurs when the electrical signals of interest, whether QRS complexes or the electrograms of atrial fibrillation, do not reach the threshold voltage to be sensed as an event (Fig. 8.47). Because the number of sensed events is either too high (oversensing) or too low (undersensing), the rhythm may be misclassified by the ICD.

Determination of the intracardiac ventricular rate requires sensing each QRS complex once and avoiding detection of the subsequent T wave (which would result in double counting of a single event) while maintaining adequate sensitivity to detect fibrillatory electrograms of small amplitude.[33] Because the amplitude of VF may be small, ICDs must amplify ventricular electrograms 10 times more than those bradycardia pacemakers that used fixed gain sensing. The need to sense signals of markedly different amplitude has been addressed by a dynamic gain or sensitivity threshold. This effectively increases the sensitivity after each sensed or paced event until the next QRS occurs, at which point sensitivity is diminished (Fig. 8.48).[33,34] Consequently, oversensing of noncardiac signals is most likely to occur during slow heart rates, late in diastole, when sensitivity is greatest. This is particularly true after paced events, after which the attack rate (rate of increase in sensitivity or gain) is often greatest.

Generally, if the measured R wave during normal rhythm at implantation is at least 5 mV, spontaneous

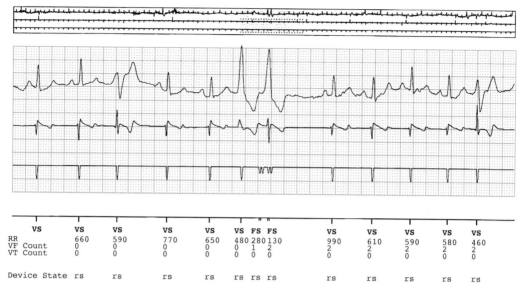

	VS	VS	VS	VS	VS	VS	FS	FS	VS	VS	VS	VS	VS
RR	660	590		770	650	480	280	130	990	610	590	580	460
VF Count	0	0		0	0	0	1	2	2	2	2	2	2
VT Count	0	0		0	0	0	0	0	0	0	0	0	0
Device State	rs	rs		rs	rs	rs rs rs			rs	rs	rs	rs	rs

Fig. 8.46 Oversensing. A recording from an implantable cardioverter-defibrillator is shown with surface electrocardiogram (top), electrogram (middle), and marker (bottom). Below are shown the markers again, annotated with cycle length and ventricular fibrillation (VF) and ventricular tachycardia (VT) counter values. During the ventricular couplet, the T wave exceeds the voltage threshold for sensing and is oversensed.

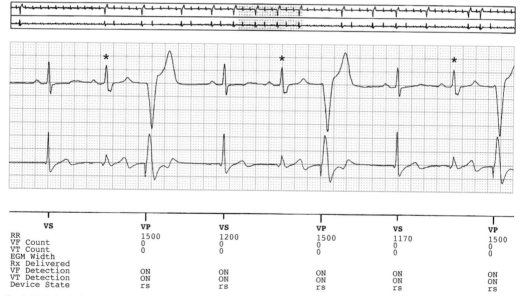

	VS	VP	VS	VP	VS	VP
RR		1500	1200	1500	1170	1500
VF Count		0	0	0	0	0
VT Count		0	0	0	0	0
EGM Width						
Rx Delivered						
VF Detection		ON	ON	ON	ON	ON
VT Detection		ON	ON	ON	ON	ON
Device State	rs	rs	rs	rs	rs	rs

Fig. 8.47 Undersensing. An implantable cardioverter-defibrillator recording is shown, as in the preceding figure. The QRS complexes marked with an asterisk have a right bundle branch block (RBBB) morphology due to intermittent bundle branch block and are not sensed. Note that the marked complexes appear smaller on the electrogram (bottom tracing) and are not sensed (no marker) and that a pacing pulse is inappropriately delivered shortly after the undersensed event (VP).

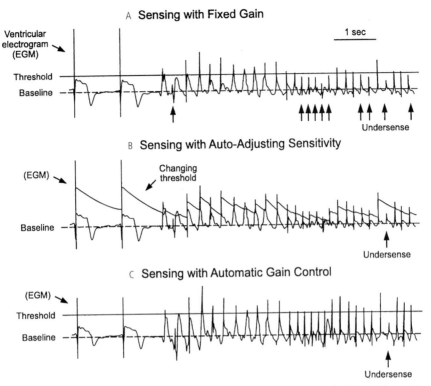

A Sensing with Fixed Gain

Ventricular
electrogram
(EGM)

1 sec

Threshold

Baseline

Undersense

B Sensing with Auto-Adjusting Sensitivity

(EGM)

Changing
threshold

Baseline

Undersense

C Sensing with Automatic Gain Control

(EGM)

Threshold

Baseline

Undersense

Fig. 8.48 Implantable cardioverter-defibrillator sensing systems. (A) Fixed gain (and sensitivity) requires that the sensed potential exceed a fixed threshold. Because of the highly variable amplitude during ventricular fibrillation, undersensing occurs (arrows). If the threshold is lowered, T-wave oversensing may occur (note that the threshold is just above the T-wave amplitude during sinus rhythm, first two complexes). (B) Autoadjusting sensitivity. The gain is fixed, but the threshold for sensing changes throughout the cardiac cycle. Undersensing is diminished. (C) Automatic gain control. The threshold for sensing is fixed, but the gain is adjusted throughout the cardiac cycle, so that very small electrograms are at a higher gain to increase the likelihood that they will exceed the sensing threshold. Undersensing is diminished. (Modified from Olson WH. Tachyarrhythmia sensing and detection. In: Singer I, ed. Implantable Cardioverter-Defibrillator. Armonk, NY: Futura Publishing Co., 1994:71–107, by permission of the publisher.)

VF is adequately sensed with nominal sensitivity settings (near 0.3 mV). In the absence of VF inductions during implant testing, an R wave >7 mV has been used.[22] During implant testing, it is useful to assess detection (see Implantable cardioverter-defibrillator detection, below) at the least sensitive setting (largest numerical value). This establishes a safety margin for sensing should a reduction in programmed sensitivity (increase in numerical value) be required in the future (e.g., due to oversensing). However, if intervening changes in medication or clinical status have occurred, induction of arrhythmia to reassess VF detection is recommended before sensitivity is reduced. During testing, assessment of sensing after a failed defibrillation shock is useful if VF sensing is borderline, as it tests the worst case scenario.

The manner in which dynamic sensing is applied differs among manufacturers. In the Boston Scientific devices, "sensitivity" is programmed to one of three values: "nominal," "most," and "least." A "fast" automatic gain control rapidly adjusts with each R wave, whereas a "slow" automatic gain control adjusts the overall dynamic range of the gain. Templates with unique attack rates for pacing, normal rate sensing, and tachycardia sensing are applied. In Medtronic devices, the concept is similar, except that slow automatic gain control does not occur. A sensitivity level is programmed by selection of the smallest signal that can be detected during the time in the cardiac cycle that sensitivity is maximum, nominally 0.3 mV in the ventricle (Fig. 8.49). St. Jude defibrillators offer programmable control over dynamic sensing function, in that the

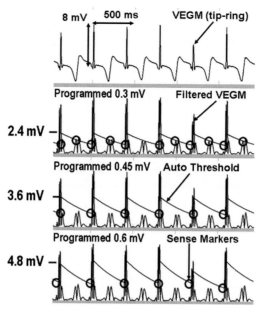

Fig. 8.49 Correction of T-wave oversensing with large R waves by adjusting programmed sensitivity. In Medtronic ICDs, the initial value of sensitivity is 8–10° – the programmed minimum sensitivity, depending on the model. Upper panel shows unfiltered true-bipolar ventricular electrogram. Second, third, and fourth panels show filtered electrogram with increasing sensitivity settings 0.3, 0.45, and 0.6 mV. The corresponding initial values of sensitivity are 2.4, 3.6, and 4.8 mV, respectively. The time constant for exponential decay of autoadjusting sensitivity is unchanged. Intermittent T-wave oversensing at a programmed sensitivity of 0.3 mV is corrected by decreasing sensitivity to 0.45 mV.

contour of the sensing envelope can be manipulated at multiple levels (Fig. 8.50).

Sensing sources

Implantable defibrillators record near-field signals between small, closely spaced electrodes to obtain sharp (high slew), discrete electrograms to determine the rate. Near-field signals may be obtained using true bipolar leads (sensing between dedicated tip and ring electrodes) or integrated bipolar leads (sensing between tip electrode and distal defibrillation coil; Fig. 8.51). In Medtronic ICDs from Secura™ on the near-field sensing source may be programmed true bipolar or integrated bipolar, to optimize sensing if R waves are small or T waves oversensed. Far-field signals recorded between widely spaced larger electrodes (defibrillation coil and pulse generator can) are used in morphology and noise detection algorithms, and during stored episode review to aid with electrogram interpretation. They integrate electrical information of a larger area and more closely approximate a surface ECG lead (Fig. 8.52).

For episode storage in single-chamber ICDs, near-field and far-field electrograms are stored to facilitate rhythm identification (nominal setting in Boston Sci-

entic, Medtronic, and Biotronik, programmable in St. Jude ICDs). In dual chamber ICDs, and atrial and ventricular near-field electrograms are selected, as near-field signals permit detection of lead noise, and the atrial electrogram facilitates rhythm identification. The exception is in patients with known 1:1 tachycardias, in whom storing the far-field electrogram is helpful. In ICDs that permit storage of three channels (latest generation Boston Scientific, St. Jude, and Biotonik ICDs), atrial and ventricular near-field channels and ventricular far-field channels are recorded.

Programming sensing

Nominal sensitivity settings permit VT/VF detection when the R wave exceeds 5 mV. Sensitivity is reprogrammed when testing indicates VF undersensing, or when T waves are oversensed. T waves that are prominent (Brugada syndrome) or delayed (long QT syndrome) increase the risk of T-wave oversensing. When T-wave oversensing occurs, programming options include decreasing sensitivity (Fig. 8.49), adjusting the sensing contour (in St. Jude Medical and Biotronik devices; Fig. 8.50), or modifying the filtering of the sensed signal to preferentially reduce T-wave amplitude (Biotronik, St. Jude Medical, Medtronic).

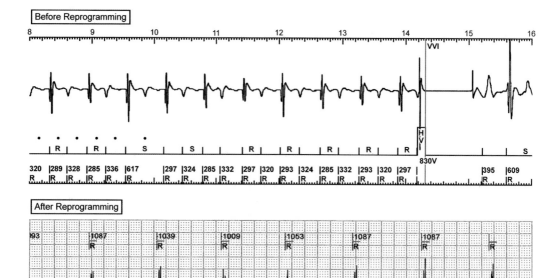

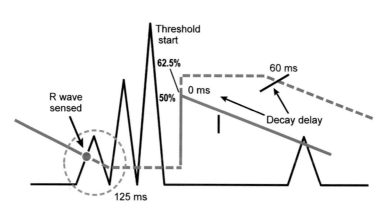

Fig. 8.50 Sensitivity adjustments in St. Jude defibrillators. Specific programmable features to correct T-wave oversensing. Upper panel: Upper strip in shows stored electrogram from a St. Jude ICD showing inappropriate shock for sinus tachycardia with T-wave oversensing. Lower strip is recorded from programmer after reprogramming decay delay from 0 to 220 ms. Lower panel: Diagram of programmable features to avoid and correct T-wave oversensing in St. Jude ICDs. Automatic sensitivity control begins to adjust sensing at the end of the 125-ms ventricular blanking period. Both the initial sensitivity (threshold start as percent of R-wave amplitude) and time delay before onset of linear decrease in sensing threshold (increase in sensitivity) are programmable parameters.

Medtronic Protecta™ devices use a T-wave discrimination algorithm (nominally "on") that compares the sensed electrogram with its derivative (which reduces T-wave amplitude) to identify T-wave oversensing and withhold shock. The approach to T-wave oversensing is discussed in Chapter 10: Troubleshooting, section on Ventricular oversensing: recognition and troubleshooting.

Implantable cardioverter-defibrillator detection

Before a tachycardia is shocked by an ICD, a sequence of steps transpire (Fig. 8.53):

1 The rate must exceed the VT cut-off
2 The tachycardia must last sufficiently long to trigger detection
3 If programmed "on" SVT-VT discriminators are applied

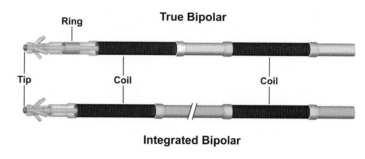

Fig. 8.51 True bipolar (top) and integrated bipolar (bottom) leads. True bipolar leads sense between a tip and dedicated ring electrode. Integrated bipolar leads sense between a tip and distal coil electrode. In some ICDs, a true biplar lead can be programmed to sense between tip and ring or tip and coil electrodes.

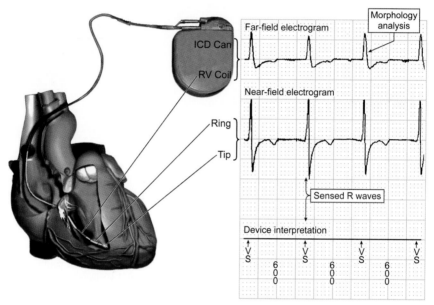

Fig. 8.52 ICD leads and electrograms. The left panel shows an ICD system including left-pectoral active can and RV lead. Right panel shows telemetered electrograms. The dual-coil lead uses true-bipolar sensing between tip and ring electrodes. Right panel shows telemetered high-voltage (shock), far-field (FF-VEGM) and sensing, near-field (NF-VEGM) electrograms with annotated markers. Arrows on marker channel denote timing of R waves sensed from true-bipolar electrogram. ICDs measure all timing intervals from this electrogram and display them on the marker channel, which also indicates the ICD's classification of each atrial and ventricular event by letter symbols. In this figure, VS indicates sensed ventricular events in the sinus rate zone and numbers indicate RR intervals. The stored near-field, rate-sensing electrogram is a wide-band (unfiltered) signal in Medtronic ICDs, but filtered in Boston Scientific and St. Jude ICDs. In St. Jude ICDs the filtered or unfiltered signal can be viewed.

4 If classified as VT/VF, ATP may be applied before or during capacitor charge

5 Following capacitor charge, reconfirmation determines whether arrhythmia is ongoing, and if so, a shock is delivered

6 Following a shock, redetection occurs. Redetection is programmable independent of initial detection.

Rate cut-off, duration, and zones

Initial detection of a ventricular arrhythmia is based on ventricular rate and arrhythmia duration. The rate criterion distinguishes between a tachyarrhythmia and a normal rhythm, and the duration requirement limits detection of nonsustained episodes. The rate at the time of detection is used to further classify the

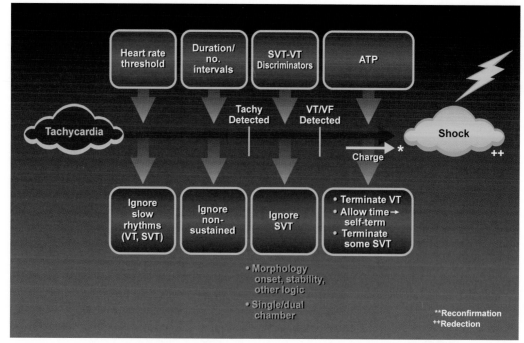

Fig. 8.53 Sequence of event leading to therapy. Each step provides an opportunity to prevent unnecessary shocks. A tachycardia must initial exceed the programmed heart rate threshold and duration threshold before a tachycardia is detected. Next, SVT-VT descriminators are applied. If these do not reject a tachycardia as SVT, VT/VF is detected. In the VF zone, ATP may delivered during the charge; in VT zones ATP is delivered as an independent therapy. Following charge completion, reconfirmation confirms ongoing tachycardia prior to shock delivery. After shock delivery, redetection determines whether VT/VF criteria remain satisfied.

rhythm into ventricular rate zones (Fig. 8.54). SVT-VT discriminators and therapies are independently programmable for each rate zone.[35] In programming detection and therapy zones, two general principles apply:

1 Detection of unstable (fast) VT and VF must be highly sensitive and therapies highly effective. The cost of this sensitivity is inappropriate treatment of rapid supraventricular tachycardias (SVTs)

2 Algorithms for rhythm discrimination and more than one sequence of ATP are programmed for slower (generally more hemodynamically stable) tachycardias to improve detection specificity and therapy tolerability. This improved specificity may come at the cost of some delay in detection and in the application of effective therapy.[36]

Arrhythmia detection begins with individual ventricular events and the inervals between them. After each sensed or paced event, the interval to the next sensed ventricular event determines the rate zone in which the next interval is classified (Fig. 8.55). A sequence of classified ventricular events is accumulated in VT and VF counters until criteria for arrhythmia

detection are met. The type of counting varies among manufacturers and between detection zones for one manufacturer (Medtronic). Because of highly variable electrogram amplitude during VF, some signal dropout may occur despite dynamic sensing. Therefore, to enhance sensitivity, initial detection, with St. Jude Medical devices as an exception, occurs when a certain percentage (usually 70–80%) of sensed events within a continuously rolling detection window fall within the VF zone (Fig. 8.56). In Boston Scientific defibrillators, X of Y counting is also used for detection in VT zones (Fig. 8.57).[36] Once the X of Y counter is satisfied, a programmable duration for which the arrhythmia must persist is required before therapy delivery.

In Medtronic defibrillators, X of Y counting is used for VF detection (Fig. 8.56), but consecutive interval counting is used for VT detection. Consecutive interval counting requires that a programmable number of consecutive intervals shorter (faster) than the VT cycle length be present for VT detection to occur; a single long (slow) interval resets the VT counter to zero (Fig. 8.58). This method increases specificity by avoiding detection of atrial fibrillation (AF) without

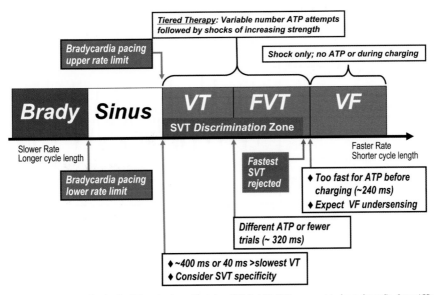

Fig. 8.54 ICD rate zones. See text for details. ATP, antitachycardia pacing; FVT, fast VT; SVT, supraventricular tachycardia. Some ICDs permit programming of an additional monitor-only zone.

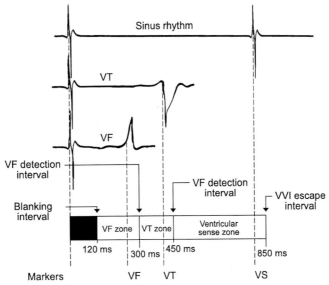

Fig. 8.55 Classification of each ventricular complex on the basis of cycle length. After each sensed or paced event, the time interval to the next sensed ventricular event determines its classification. If another ventricular event is sensed after the blanking period, but within the programmed ventricular fibrillation (VF) detection interval (typically 300–320 ms), the event is classified as a VF complex, regardless of the actual cause of the ventricular depolarization. A delay greater than the programmed VF interval but shorter than the maximum VT cycle length results in a ventricular tachycardia (VT) event. If the time between ventricular depolarizations exceeds the programmed length of the VT detection cycle, the event is sensed without classification as a tachyarrhythmia ("VS," for ventricular sensed event). If no event is sensed and the pacing rate interval is reached, a pacing impulse is generated. This example includes only two tachycardia zones (VF and VT). In most defibrillators, up to three tachycardia detection zones may be programmed to allow progressively more aggressive delivery of therapy for faster VTs. (From Olson WH. Tachyarrhythmia sensing and detection. In: Singer I. ed. Implantable Cardioverter-Defibrillator. Armonk, NY: Futura Publishing Co., 1994:71–107, by permission of the publisher.)

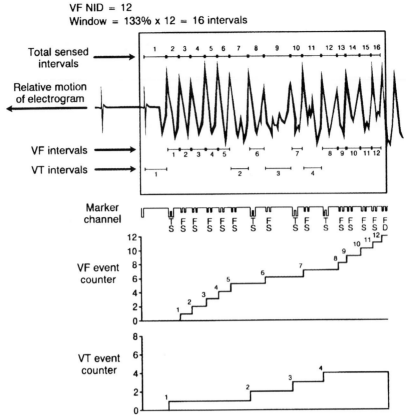

VF NID = 12
Window = 133% x 12 = 16 intervals

Fig. 8.56 Ventricular fibrillation (VF) detection (in a Medtronic implantable cardioverter-defibrillator). The box at the top shows the moving window during ventricular fibrillation (VF) detection. Twelve of the 16 intervals in the moving window must be shorter than the fibrillation detection interval for VF detection to occur. The marker channel demonstrates whether events are sensed as VF ("FS") or ventricular tachycardia (VT) ("TS"). The VF and VT counters below the markers show that VT counting is not reset by VF sensed events. The VF counter is never suddenly reset to zero under any circumstances, because, contrary to VT detection, a moving window is always used for VF detection. VF NID, number of intervals to detect ventricular fibrillation. (From Friedman PA, Stanton MS. The pacer-cardioverter-defibrillator: function and clinical experience. J Cardiovasc Electrophysiol 1995; 6:48–68, by permission of Futura Publishing Co.)

compromising VT sensitivity,[36] at the expense of non-detection of irregular VTs with a mean cycle length close to the VT cut-off rate. AF with a mean cycle length shorter than the tachycardia detection interval will be appropriately rejected if periodic intervals longer than the cut-off rate reset the tachycardia counter to zero. A third zone (Fast VT) may be added using either X of Y or consecutive interval counting.

For detection to occur in any zone in St. Jude defibrillators, a programmable number of intervals must be classified and counted in that zone. The classification of a sensed event depends on both the current interval and the average of the current interval and the previous three intervals (Table 8.5). The sinus counter is reset to zero whenever any interval is classified in a tachycardia zone. To prevent detection of bigeminy with average rates in a VT zone, a bigeminy detection algorithm withholds therapy if bigeminy is present.

The average ventricular tachyarrhythmia rate in patients with a secondary prevention indication is slower than the rate in primary-prevention patients (153 bpm vs. 200 bpm).[37,38] In patients with a primary-prevention indication, a VT rate cut-off of approximately 180 bpm with detection times of 7–9 s limits unnecessary shocks from slower and nonsustained arrhythmias.[39,40] For patients with known VT, a detection rate 30–60 ms longer (slower) than the slowest VT cycle length provides detection safety margin.[41,42] Patient-specific programming is discussed further in Optimizing programming, below.

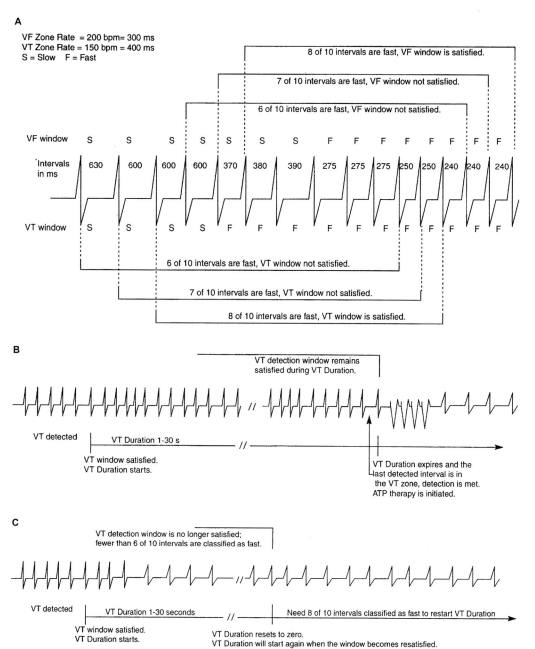

Fig. 8.57 Use of X of Y counting in multiple zones (in a Boston Scientific implantable cardioverter-defibrillator). (A) For each zone, the detection heart rate and tachycardia duration are programmed independently. Each zone has a detection window composed of the 10 most recent RR intervals. As each new interval is measured, it is defined as either fast – above the programmed rate threshold for the window – or slow. A window is satisfied when 8 of the 10 most recent RR intervals are fast and remains satisfied as long as 6 of 10 intervals in the moving window are fast. (B) Once a detection window is satisfied, a programmable duration timer is started, nominally 2.5 s for ventricular tachycardia (VT) and 1 s for ventricular fibrillation (VF). If after the duration timer expires the last detected interval is in the zone of the timer, detection is met and therapy is delivered (unless a detection enhancement is programmed; see text). When multiple zones are programmed "on," the higher zone takes priority over the lower zone. Up to three tachycardia zones (VT-1, VT, and VF) with independently programmable criteria and therapies may be used to enhance detection and specificity of therapy. (C) If the VT detection window does not remain satisfied until the end of the VT duration window, VT duration resets to zero, and timing will resume when the window becomes resatisfied. ATP, antitachycardia pacing. (Modified with permission from Boston Scientific ICD reference manual.)

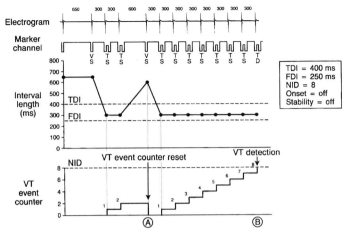

Fig. 8.58 Consecutive interval counting ventricular tachycardia (VT) detection (Medtronic). At the top is the ventricular electrogram with the individual intervals labeled in milliseconds. Beneath the electrograms are the corresponding markers for each sensed event. Next is a graph of the individual intervals, with dashed lines delineating the tachycardia detection interval (TDI) and fibrillation detection interval (FDI). At the bottom, the graph displays how each sensed event affects the VT event counter. The dashed line denotes the programmed number of intervals needed to detect VT (NID). In this figure, the third electrogram occurs at a cycle length of 300 ms, which is less than the programmed TDI of 400 ms; the VT counter increases to 1. Note that the marker channel displays a VT sense. At point "A," the VT counter is reset to zero by a sensed interval of 600 ms, which is longer than the TDI. At point "B," VT detection occurs, as the counter reaches the programmed NID of 8. Depending on the type of therapy programmed, antitachycardia pacing or charging of the capacitors would begin at this point. (From Friedman PA, Stanton MS. The pacer-cardioverter-defibrillator: function and clinical experience. J Cardiovasc Electrophysiol 1995; 6:48–68, by permission of Futura Publishing Co.)

Table 8.5 Classification of ventricular events in St. Jude defibrillators.

Interval average				
Current interval	Sinus	VT-1	VT-2	VF
Sinus	Sinus	Not binned	Not binned	Not binned
VT-1	Not binned	VT-1	VT-2	VF
VT-2	Not binned	VT-2	VT-2	VF
VF	Not binned	VF	VF	VF

Detection zone boundaries

Unanticipated ICD behavior may occur when arrhythmias straddle the rate detection zone boundaries. In older Boston Scientific, Medtronic (prior to Marquis™) and St. Jude (prior to Atlas 2™) devices, programming a VT zone with no therapies for use as a monitoring zone could accelerate therapy. This occurs because sensed events in the VT zone count towards detection in the adjacent faster zone (Fig. 8.59). Newer devices provide an independent monitor-only zone that avoids this limitation. In St. Jude ICDs, if VT is detected in the "monitor zone" SVT discriminators are disabled for all zones for that episode.

Committed and noncommitted shocks

The first defibrillators delivered committed shocks; once a tachyarrhythmia was detected and capacitor charging initiated, a shock was committed to follow, leading to treatment of nonsustained VT. Presently, the first shock is noncommitted in ICDs; after detection and capacitor charging, the pulse generator confirms (or "reconfirms") continuing tachyarrhythmia before delivery of a shock. If the arrhythmia has ended, the capacitors remain charged, but therapy is withheld and the device continues to monitor the rhythm (Fig. 8.60). Following the first shock, Medtronic devices are committed until the episode ends. In Boston Scientific devices shocks are committed following therapy diversion (i.e., two consecutive shocks cannot be diverted), whereas in in St. Jude Medical devices all shocks can be noncommitted.

Confirmation/reconfirmation is "trigger happy" so that even a few intervals shorter (faster) than the slowest VT interval (Boston Scientific) or 60 ms >VT interval (Medtronic before the Protecta series) result in shock delivery. Thus, a poorly timed, single premature ventricular complex or oversensed event during reconfirmation may lead to a shock (Fig. 8.61). Because the reconfrimation interval is linked to the VT interval in most ICDs, reconfirmation results in the first VF shock being committed when a long VT interval is

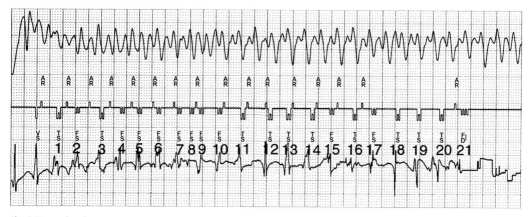

Fig. 8.59 Combined counter to avoid detection delay when a tachyarrhythmia straddles the ventricular tachycardia (VT) and ventricular fibrillation (VF) zones. In Medtronic ICDs, to avoid delayed detection when a tachyarrhythmia straddles the VT and VF zones, a combined counter that is incrementally activated by VT or VF events is used. When the sum of the VT and VF counters reaches a threshold (nominally 21), VF is detected unless eight or more of the preceding events were in the VT zone, in which case VT is detected. Events present in the VF zone (e.g., complex 17 and 15) result in detection as VF.

programmed. Reconfirmation has been modified in newer devices to minimize shock risk. In the Medtronic Protecta series, reconfirmation requires a cycle length within 60 ms of the detected tachycardia rate (as opposed to programmed VT rate) if the tachycardia is regular or a cycle length of the VF detection interval +60 ms in the VF zone. In new St. Jude Medical devices the reconfirmation rate is programmable to an operator-selected zone.

Redetection

Redetection is the process by which ICDs determine whether VT or VF detection criteria remain satisfied following therapy delivery (Fig. 8.53). Redetection nominally occurs more quickly than initial detection. While variable among manufacturers, during redetection SVT-VT discriminators are not applied, or are limited, in part because morphology-based detection enhancements are not reliable immediately following shock delivery due to transient shock-induced electrogram changes (see Morphology, below). In St. Jude ICDs, no SVT-VT discriminators are applied during redetection; in Medtronic devices, only stability is applied, and in Boston Scientific devices, Rhythm ID is modified so that functionally only stability (and V > A in dual chamber devices) is applied. Thus, sinus tachycardia following successful shock may lead to redetection, and rate-controlling medications (such as β-blockers) may prevent repetitive shocks.

When ATP during charge is programed on, reconfirmation determines whether VT is ongoing prior to shock delivery. Because reconfirmation after charge is not as specific as VT redetection, shocks are delivered after approximately 5% of successful ATP during charge sequences.[43,44]

SVT-VT discriminators

Inappropriate therapy delivered for nonventricular arrhythmias affects 8–40% of ICD recipients, has a deleterious effect on quality of life, can be associated with proarrhythmia, and leads to poor tolerance of life-saving ICD therapy.[45–48] Consequently, detection enhancements (SVT-VT discrimination algorithms) have been developed to improve the specificity of rhythm classification. When programmed "on," detection enhancements prevent delivery of therapy despite a tachycardia with rate and duration that meet detection if other rhythm characteristics indicate a supraventricular mechanism (Fig. 8.53). Because the overlap in heart rate between ventricular and supraventricular arrhythmias occurs predominantly in the "slower" tachycardia zones[49] and because the specificity of some discriminators decrease at faster rates, detection enhancements are most commonly applied only in VT zones <200 bpm, with the exception of some morphology algorithms, discussed below.[50,51]

There are two broad categories of single-chamber SVT-VT discriminators: morphology-based and interval-based enhancements. Morphology algorithms compare electrogram characteristics with a baseline template to distinguish SVT from VT. Interval-based algorithms assess R-R interval variability or abruptness of onset to discriminate AF and sinus tachycardia from VT. A summary of single-chamber detection enhancements and their operation is provided in Table 8.6. The general principles guiding optimal programming of single-chamber detection enhancements are as follows:

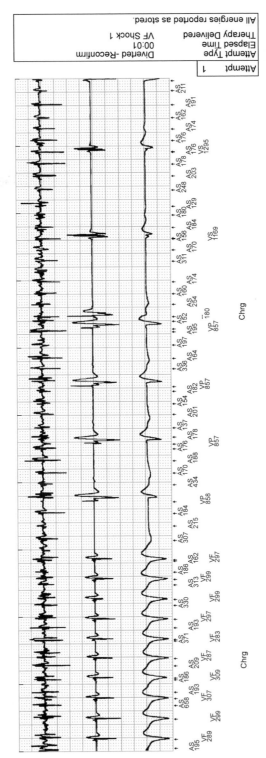

Fig. 8.60 Noncommitted shocks. Stored episode on a nonsustained ventricular tachycardia (VT) in a noncommitted device. From top to bottom are atrial electrogram, near-field ventricular electrogram, and far-field ventricular electrogram. Continuing atrial fibrillation is present. During capacitor charge, the VT terminates. Slow sensed events ("VS") after charge completion (at the second "Chrg" marker) indicate arrhythmia termination, so that the shock is withheld ("Diverted-Reconfirm" in the box at far right). Note that during the charge, pacing support ("VP") is provided.

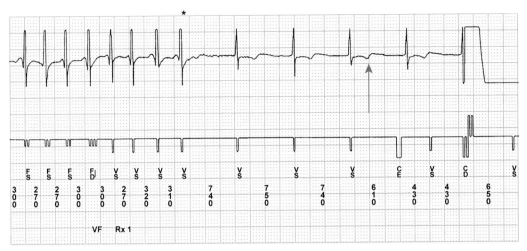

Fig. 8.61 T-wave oversensing during reconfirmation leads to a shock. Although the VT terminated (asterisk), immediately following charge end the T wave is oversensed (arrow), resulting in two short intervals and shock delivery.

Table 8.6 Single-chamber detection enhancements.

Detection enhancement	Function
Stability [inhibit therapy if ventricular rate is unstable (i.e., variable QRS intervals); or in some devices, accelerate therapy if unstable]	• Main use: differentiate atrial fibrillation (irregular, unstable intervals) from ventricular tachycardia (regular, stable intervals) • Strength: continuously assesses ongoing tachycardia, permitting detection even if initial misclassification occurs • Limitation: antiarrhythmic drugs may result in irregular intervals during VT leading to misclassification as SVT; atrial flutter with fixed conduction may be regular, leading to misclassification as VT • In Boston Scientific devices, can also be used to accelerate therapy (e.g., to avoid antitachycardia pacing in patient with known polymorphic ventricular tachycardia, which is irregular and unstable)
Onset (inhibit therapy if gradual onset)	• Main use: differentiate sinus tachycardia (gradual onset) from ventricular tachycardia (sudden onset) • Strength: one of limited number of approaches to distinguish sinus tachycardia from VT • Limitation: single assessment at arrhythmia onset does not permit "correction" if misclassification occurs due to ectopy (making ST onset appear abrupt) or VT onset below detection rate with gradual acceleration across ST-VT boundary (leading to misclassification of VT as ST)
Morphology discrimination (inhibit therapy if intracardiac morphology matches baseline rhythm morphology)	• Main use: differentiate ventricular from supraventricular arrhythmias irrespective of interval timing • Strength: continuously assesses ongoing tachycardia, permitting detection even if initial misclassification occurs; permits differentiation of regular flutter from VT. Most useful detection enhancement at very rapid rates (above 200 bpm) • Limitation: misclassifies aberrant SVT as VT; not useful immediately following shock due to shock-related distortion of the electrogram
Sustained rate duration (override inhibitor if fast rate persistent)	• Main use: limit the length of time inhibitor can withhold therapy during a high-ventricular-rate episode • Overrides therapy inhibitors after duration timer expires • Strength: prevents VT underdetection; particularly useful with algorithms that assess rhythm at single point in time (such as onset) • Limitation: degrades specificity by increasing the risk of shocking SVT Not routinely programmed on, and nominally "off" in many devices. • Many devices also have timers to limit the total duration of antitachycardia pacing therapies; after the programmed time elapses, the device delivers a shock, even if pacing therapies remain

1 Specificity enhancements are more liberally applied to slower (<200 bpm), hemodynamically tolerated VT zones, in which a modest delay in therapy is tolerable
2 Discrimination algorithms that continuously reassess the rhythm during tachycardia (such as "stability" or "morphology") are preferable to those that evaluate a tachycardia at a single point in time, and are generally used in patients with known AF
3 Discrimination algorithms that perform a single classification based on a limited number of ventricular events (such as "onset") are used judiciously and in conjunction with other detection enhancements.

The overall performance of discriminators is strongly influenced by the logic applied when several are programmed "on" simultaneously. Limited data suggest that analysis of ventricular electrogram morphology, alone or in combination with stability, provides the best single-chamber SVT-VT discrimination for the initial detection of VT.[52] Technical details vary among manufacturers, as do corresponding recommended program values, which are summarized in Tables 8.7 and 8.8.

SVT-VT discriminators may be explicitly linked to detection zones or programmed independently, depending on the manufacturer. In Boston Scientific ICDs, detection enhancements are programmed "on" for the entirety of one or both VT zones. In St. Jude ICDs, detection enhancements are programmable independently within the two VT zones (i.e., the cut-off rate

beyond which discriminators no longer apply need not match a VT or VF boundary), but they cannot overlap with the VF zone. Medtronic ICDs have a complex relationship between SVT-VT discriminators and detection zones. Onset and stability are only applied in the VT zones that use consecutive interval counting, and prevent detection by resetting detection counters (discussed below). PR Logic and Wavelet are applied only after detection (and thus for tachycardias in the VT zone, only applied if the tachycardia is not rejected by stability or onset when these are programmed "on"). Wavelet and PR Logic are applied up to an independently programmed SVT Limit that may overlap the VF zone. PR Logic is more specific in consecutive-interval VT zones than the VF zone, because it classifies irregular rhythms as AF in the VT zones; in Protecta devices the addition of Wavelet to PR Logic improves specificity in the VF or FVT via VF zones, for rates slower than the SVT Limit. Because 25% of SVTs are shocked due to rates for which SVT-VT discriminators are not applied, programming of SVT discriminators to sufficiently fast rates is essential (see Optimizing programming, below)

Single-chamber SVT-VT discriminators

Morphology: Morphology algorithms compare tachycardia electrograms with a patient-specific template recorded during normal rhythm. The operational

Table 8.7 Recommended programming of SVT-VT discriminators in single-chamber ICDs.

	Medtronic	Boston Scientific	St Jude
Stability*	40–50 ms, NID = 16	24–40 ms, duration 2.5 s[†]	80 ms
Onset	84–88%	9%[†]	100 ms
Morphology	3 of 8 electrograms ≥70% match	Rhythm ID "on"[†]	5 of 8 electrograms >60% match

*Less strict values are required for patients taking type I or III antiarrhythmic drugs.
[†]In devices with the Rhythm ID algorithm, stability and onset are not available.

Table 8.8 Recommended programming of SVT-VT discriminators in dual-chamber ICDs.

Medtronic PR Logic ™	Boston Scientific One Button Detection Enhancements™	Boston Scientific Rhythm ID™	St. Jude Rate Branch™
Afib/Aflutter: "on"	AFib rate threshold 200 beats/min	"on"	Rate branch "on"
Sinus Tach: "on"	Onset 9%		A = V branch: Morphology
Other 1:1 SVTs: "off"	Inhibit if unstable 10 ms		(sudden onset:passive to record response, but not
1:1 SVT boundary: 66%[†]	V rate > A rate "on"		use to classify)
	Sustained rate duration 3 min		A > V branch morphology combined with
			stability* using "ALL" logic

Note that these are generally useful settings, which may be customized for the individual patients.
*Stability at 80 ms with AV association of 60 ms.
†In devices in which this feature is programmable.

assumption is that supraventricular rhythms have the same morphology as the sinus rhythm template. Morphology has sensitivity for VT detection of 95–98% and a specificity of 72–85%.[46,52–55] Common elements present in all morphology algorithms include: (i) creation of a template by mathematically extracting electrogram features and storing them; (ii) recording electrograms during an unknown tachycardia; (iii) time aligning the template and tachycardia electrograms; (iv) classifying each tachycardia electrogram as a match or nonmatch based on its comparison with the template; (v) classifying the tachycardia as SVT or VT based on the number of electrograms that match the template. Various manufacturer's morphology algorithms differ in their electrogram source(s), methods of quantitative representation and alignment. Details of their function are shown in Figs 8.62–8.64.

Because morphology algorithms continually reassess a tachycardia, the risk of underdetection of significant arrhythmias while using them without override timers that override therapy inhibition is small.[46] In single-chamber ICDs, morphology algorithms are the only single-chamber discriminators that distinguish abrupt onset regular SVT (such as atrial flutter or atrioventricular nodal re-entrant tachycardia [AVNRT]) from VT.

Morphology algorithms have common failure modes (Table 8.9), some of which can be prevented with appropriate programming. An inaccurate template may be recorded because the electrogram has evolved (due to lead maturation or the development of bundle branch block) or because the template was recorded during an abnormal rhythm. Programming automatic template updates "on", and assessing templates at routine follow-up, minimizes the risk of misclassification due to an inaccurate template of the baseline rhythm. If automatic updates are not available, morphology should be disabled until a stable, chronic electrogram is present. Electrogram truncation occurs when the electrogram signal exceeds the dynamic range of the sensing amplifier, so that the maximum or minimum portions of the signal are clipped (Fig. 8.65). Variable truncation may result in mismatch of two signals that are otherwise identical. Truncation is eliminated by programming the amplitude scale so that the electrogram used for morphology analysis occupies 25–75% of the dynamic range. Alignment errors occur when similar electrograms are misaligned, leading to error in the calculated match score. Template and tachycardia electrograms are aligned by matching the morphology electrogram peak (Medtronic), onset (St. Jude), or near-field peak (Boston Scientific). Alignment errors may occur due to truncation (Medtronic), or due to rate-related, at times subtle, electrogram changes (St. Jude, Boston Scientific, or Medtronic). Avoiding truncation eliminates some

alignment errors. In dual-chamber ICDs, recording a template while atrial pacing at higher rates (e.g., 120 ppm) may prevent misalignment due to subtle electrogram changes (i.e., minor aberrancy). Pectoral myopotentials may distort the electrogram used for analysis leading to classification errors. In Medtronic ICDs, a different electrogram source can be selected. In St. Jude ICDs, near-field electrograms are used, so that pectoral myopotentials do not affect the morphology algorithm. Boston Scientific ICDs do use the far-field electrogram and lack a programmable adjustment to compensate for pectoral oversensing; limited early data suggest this problem is uncommon.[55,56] Rate-related aberrancy results in misclassification of SVT as VT due to tachycardia template mismatch.

In patients with known rate-related aberrancy, acquiring the template during rapid atrial pacing or disabling the morphology algorithm may prevent rhythm misclassification. In patients with pre-existing bundle branch block, the algorithm remains effective.[55] In patients with resynchronization systems, pacing is promoted, limiting template acquisition opportunities. In St. Jude CRT-D devices, morphology templates are not auto-acquired, so that updating should be manually performed at follow-up. Medtronic CRT-D systems will attempt to acquire templates, but will not alter bradycardia parameters to do so, whereas Boston Scientific devices will lower the pacing rate to 60 to update the template.

Stability: Stability differentiates AF (unstable, variable R-R intervals) from VT (stable, regular R-R intervals). When programmed "on," the stability algorithm withholds therapy despite ventricular rates in the tachycardia zone if the cycle length intervals are irregular (Figs 8.66 and 8.67). The rationale for this approach is that VTs have little variation in R-R intervals, in contrast to AF. In one study, the average stability (R-R variability) during VT episodes was 16 ± 15 ms, compared with 49 ± 15 ms during AF.[57] The stability enhancement prevents inappropriate detection of AF in up to 95% of AF episodes, with only a minimal decrease in VT sensitivity.[49,57,58] Atrial flutter may be regular and difficult to differentiate from VT in single-chamber devices; similarly, R-R intervals tend to regularize when AF is rapidly conducted (above approximately 170 bpm), limiting the utility of interval stability algorithms.[49,58] Antiarrhythmic medications may also affect the performance of the algorithm. Use of amiodarone or class IC antiarrhythmic drugs (e.g., flecainide or propafenone) may cause monomorphic VT to become irregular or polymorphic VT to slow, leading to rhythm misclassification.[59,60]

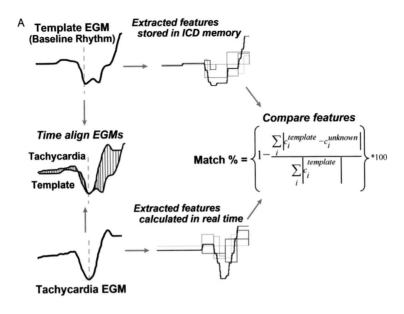

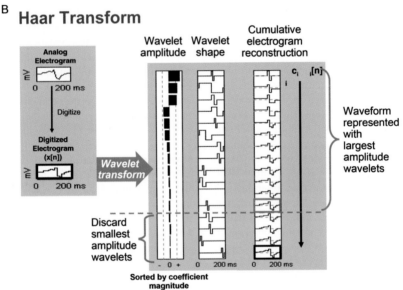

Fig. 8.62 Wavelet morphology algorithm (Medtronic). (A) A template is recorded during normal intrinsic rhythm (with rate <100), top left. The template is automatically updated (after confirmation that complexes are nonectopic) continuously, as needed. The electrogram source for the analysis is programmable (nominally RV coil to can). A mathematical transform is used to extract the electrogram features (top right figure). During tachycardia, the electrogram is recorded (bottom left figure), features are extracted in real time (bottom right panel), and the tachycardia and template electrograms are mathematically compared to derive a match score. Each complex is classified as SVT if the match score exceeds a programmable threshold value (nominally 70%). If ≥3 of eight complexes in a rolling window are SVT, the ongoing episode is classified as SVT. (B) The Haar transform is used to extract waveform characteristics and store them. (Reproduced with permission from Swerdlow CD, Brown ML, Lurie K, et al. Discrimination of ventricular tachycardia from a supraventricular tachycardia by a downloaded wavelet-transform morphology algorithm: a paradigm for development of implantable cardioverter defibrillator detection algorithms. J Cardiovasc Electrophysiol 2002; 13:432–41.)

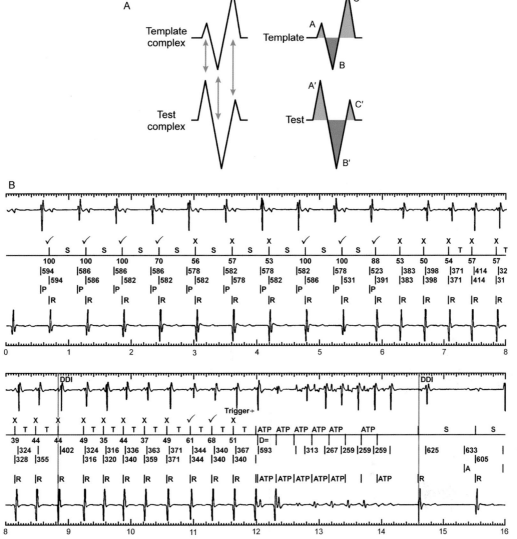

Fig. 8.63 (A) Morphology discrimination (St. Jude). An electrogram template is made during sinus rhythm, unique for each patient. During a tachyarrhythmia, each tachycardia complex ("test complex") is compared with the template. A morphology score is derived from the sum of the differences of aligned test complex and template. The % Match score is a function of the difference between the areas under the aligned complexes (i.e., [area A − area A″] + [area B − area B″] + [area C − area C″]). The % Match score required to consider a supraventricular complex is programmable. (B) Example of morphology discrimination and appropriate therapy for VT with 1 : 1 VA conduction. Bipolar atrial electrogram (RA), dual-chamber Marker Channel, and rate-sensing (RV) electrogram are shown. Asterisk denotes onset of VT during sinus tachycardia, identified by abrupt acceleration of ventricular rate and change in electrogram morphology without change in atrial rate. Morphology discriminator requires 5 of 8 match scores ≥60% to withhold therapy. During sinus tachycardia, scores exceed 60%. (Five are 100%, scores are labeled in the figure as "Match score.") During VT, most scores are <60%. Check marks above Marker Channel indicate that morphology algorithm classifies beats as supraventricular (labeled in the figure as "Match"). An "X" mark in the "match" row indicates a beat classified as VT morphology. "Trigger" in lower panel indicates detection of VT. "D" = at onset of ATP indicates that atrial rate = ventricular rate. "S" denotes intervals interval the "Sinus" zone longer than the VT detection interval of 400 ms. "T" denotes intervals in VT zone. DDI, mode switch. Time line is in section. Additional observations confirm the diagnosis of VT. The VT cycle length is moderately irregular. Changes in VV interval precede those in AA interval. Ventricular antitachycardia pacing (ATP) at right of lower panel results in transient VA block without acceleration of the atrial rate followed by 1 : 1 VA conduction. The near simultaneous atrial and ventricular activation during tachycardia is more typical of typical (antegrade, slow; retrograde, fast) AV nodal re-entrant tachycardia than VT, but the shortening of the AV interval at the onset of tachycardia is inconsistent with this diagnosis. Pacing-induced VA block without acceleration of the atrial rate is also unusual in AV nodal re-entry. (From Swerdlow CD, Friedman PA. Advanced ICD troubleshooting: Part 1. Pacing Clin Electrophysiol 2005; 28:1322–46, by permission of Blackwell Publishing.)

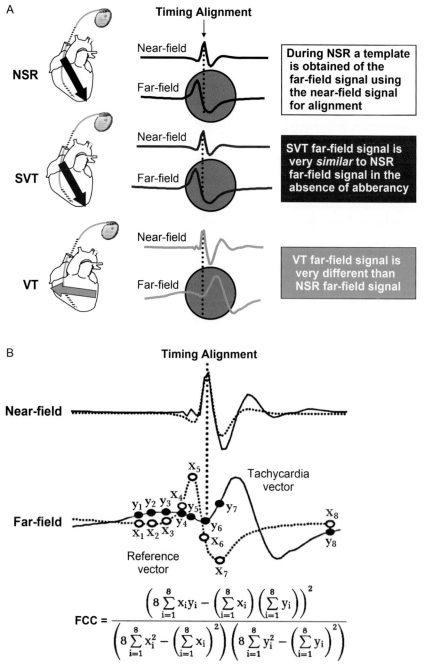

$$FCC = \frac{\left(8\sum_{i=1}^{8}x_iy_i - \left(\sum_{i=1}^{8}x_i\right)\left(\sum_{i=1}^{8}y_i\right)\right)^2}{\left(8\sum_{i=1}^{8}x_i^2 - \left(\sum_{i=1}^{8}x_i\right)^2\right)\left(8\sum_{i=1}^{8}y_i^2 - \left(\sum_{i=1}^{8}y_i\right)^2\right)}$$

Fig. 8.64 Vector Timing and Correlation (VTC) morphology algorithm (Boston Scientific). (A) Overview of algorithm function. (B) Comparison of tachycardia to template. The top panel depicts the local bipolar electrogram (labeled "near field") during normal rhythm (dotted line) and during tachycardia (solid line). The near-field electrogram generally has a greater slew (steeper rise) than the far-field signal, facilitating accurate alignment. It is used solely for aligning the far-field signals (bottom tracing). After alignment, the far-field template electrogram (dotted line) is compared with the far-field tachycardia electrogram (solid line) to classify the complex as supraventricular or ventricular by assessing eight points ("features") and calculating a feature correlation coefficient (FCC). If the FCC value of a tachycardia complex exceeds 94%, it is classified as supraventricular. If three or more out of 10 beats are classified as supraventricular, the ongoing tachycardia is classified as SVT. The values used by the algorithm are not programmable, the VTC is part of the Rhythm ID algorithm, which is programmed "on" or "off". In single-chamber programming Rhythm ID "on" activates VTC; in dual-chamber ICDs, programming Rhythm ID "on" activates VTC and interval-based dual-chamber algorithms together in an automatic, nonprogrammable manner. (Adapted from Lee MA, Corbisiero R, Nabert DR, et al. Clinical results of an advanced SVT detection enhancement algorithm. Pacing Clin Electrophysiol 2005; 28:1032–40, by permission of Blackwell Publishing.)

Table 8.9 Modes of morphology algorithm failure.

Type of morphology failure	Mechanism	Correction
Inaccurate template	Change in baseline electrogram due to lead maturation or intermittent bundle branch block, or recording of template during abnormal rhythm	Apply automatic template updates or use manual updates during known normal rhythm
Electrogram truncation (clipping)	Recorded electrogram signal exceeds sense amplifier range, altering its morphology	Adjust amplitude scale (Medtronic and SJM) so electrograms are 25–75% of dynamic range available
Alignment errors	Misalignment between tachycardia electrogram and template lead to miscalculation of "match" score	Eliminate clipping and/or change electrogram source (Medtronic), atrially pace at rapid rate to assess sensing (SJM)
Oversensing of pectoral myopotentials	Myopotentials distort the electrogram, altering its morphology	Change the electrogram source. Only affects algorithms utilizing far-field electrograms (Medtonic, Boston Scientific)
Rate related aberrancy	Morphology of electrograms change during SVT due to refractoriness (nonexcitability) of part of the conduction system	If reproducible, record template during rapid atrial pacing (while aberrancy present) and turn off autotemplate update; adjust match score to allow greater variability before defining VT; turn off morphology
SVT immediately following shocks	Shocks lead to transient distortion of morphology	Morphology is not used for redection

Source: adapted from Nof E, Glikson M, Luria D, Gard J, Friedman P. Beyond sudden death prevention: minimizing ICD shocks and morbidity, and optimizing efficacy. In Gussak I, Antzelevitch C, eds. Electrical Diseases of the Heart. Springer: 2011.

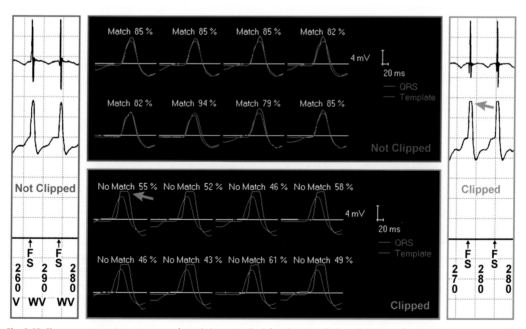

Fig. 8.65 Electrogram truncation as a source of morphology error. The left and top panels show electrograms from a patient in whom an SVT was appropriately rejected by a morphology algorithm. In the same patient, in the bottom and right panels, the gain of the far-field electrogram was too high for signal, so that the peak was clipped (note truncated signal at arrow). Because Medtronic ICDs use the electrogram peak for alignment, clipping of the signal can lead to misclassification by two mechanism: electrogram distortion and misalignment.

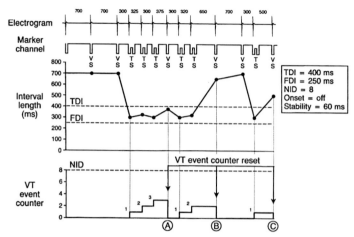

Fig. 8.66 Stability criterion (as implemented by Medtronic). Ventricular tachycardia (VT) counting commences with the first 300-ms interval. At point "A," the VT counter is reset to zero, since the cycle length of 375 ms, although less than the tachycardia detection interval (TDI), is >60 ms greater than the preceding interval, and the stability criterion is not met. Note that the marker channel registers a normal sensed event at that point even though the interval is less than the TDI. The stability criterion is not applied until after the VT counter reaches 3. At points "B" and "C," the VT counter is reset by intervals greater than the TDI. This pattern would be consistent with atrial fibrillation. FDI, fibrillation detection interval; NID, number of intervals needed to detect ventricular tachycardia. (From Friedman PA, Stanton MS. The pacer-cardioverter-defibrillator: function and clinical experience. J Cardiovasc Electrophysiol 1995; 6:48–68, by permission of Futura Publishing Co.)

Onset: Onset differentiates VT from sinus tachycardia based on the abruptness of arrhythmia onset (Fig. 8.68) The onset criterion rejects inappropriate detection of 64–98% of sinus tachycardias with heart rates in the VT zone, but results in underdetection of 0.5–5% of VTs.[49,57,58] Unlike stability, which continuously re-evaluates the rhythm diagnosis during tachycardia, onset is determined only once. Moreover, because ectopy preceding VT may mitigate the abruptness of arrhythmia onset, this enhancement is best limited to slow VT zones (heart rate <140–150 bpm), where the risk for overlap with sinus tachycardia is greatest, to avoid underdetection of faster VT.[61] In patients prone to sinus tachycardia and slow VTs, use of β-blockers and digitalis, which improve survival and reduce symptoms, respectively, may lower the risk of sinus tachycardia crossing the VT boundary. However, VT that begins slower than the VT detection rate and accelerates gradually across the sinus–VT rate boundary will always be misclassified as sinus tachycardia.

SVT-VT discriminator timers: Timers are available in ICDs to override detection enhancements and force therapy for ongoing tachycardia once the programmed duration expires. While designed to insure treatment of VT, available evidence indicates that they significantly increase the risk of shock with little or no safety benefit.[37] They are therefore generally programmed "off."

Dual-chamber SVT-VT discriminators

In addition to providing dual-chamber pacing functionality, dual-chamber defibrillators use atrial electrograms to enhance arrhythmia diagnosis.[62,63] Although manufacturers have adopted different approaches, the algorithms share many common principles:

• Comparison of atrial and ventricular rates. A ventricular rate that exceeds the atrial rate accurately identifies VT, eliminating the need for additional analysis.
• Identification of the presence of fibrillation in the atrium before applying stability algorithms.
• Identification of variation in PR intervals and presence of N:1 AV association to distinguish regular supraventricular rhythms such as sinus tachycardia and atrial flutter from VT.[64–66]

Overall, dual-chamber SVT-VT discriminators have a specificity of 60–95% for correctly identifying SVT episodes[62] and sensitivity over 98% for VT detection.[46] In the largest study comparing dual-chamber with single-chamber ICD detection, the odds of inappropriate SVT detection were decreased by half in the dual-chamber detection arm.[46] While the improved rhythm classification led to a reduction in inappropriate therapy, increased use of ATP was programmed in the single-chamber arm, so that shock rates did not differ in that study. Similarly, the DATAS study demonstrated a reduction by one-third in clinically significant adverse events with use of dual-chamber detection enhancements.[67] However, the use of dual-chamber ICDs is

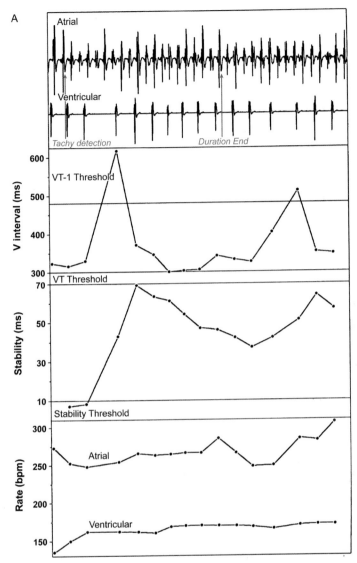

Fig. 8.67 The stability criterion (as implemented by Boston Scientific). (A) From top to bottom are the atrial and ventricular electrograms, ventricular interval, calculated stability, and atrial and ventricular rates. Atrial fibrillation with a rapid ventricular response is present. The ventricular interval drops below the ventricular tachycardia (VT) detection rate (475 ms in this example, shown as a line on the "V Interval" plot). Despite tachyarrhythmia detection and satisfaction of duration, therapy is withheld since the stability threshold (programmed to 30 ms in this example) is exceeded. (B) Stored episode with atrial electrogram (top tracing), and near-field ventricular electrogram (middle pacing), and far-field ventricular intervals. The sustained rate duration timer is fulfilled at 1 minute, rhythm is atrial fibrillation with a rapid ventricular response (note aberrancy can be seen in far-field electrogram in the 3rd–7th complexes) and the shock is inappropriate.

(Continued)

associated with an increased risk of lead dislodgment, and not all studies have shown benefit. Although expert opinion is divided, use of dual-chamber algorithms to improve SVT-VT rhythm classification is reasonable in patients in whom a VT zone with rates <200 bpm will be programmed, who are not in chronic atrial fibrilla-tion, and who do not have complete or high-grade AV block. This is discussed in more detail in Chapter 4: Choosing the Device Generator and Leads.

Comparison of atrial and ventricular rates: Because the ventricular rate exceeds the atrial rate in 80–90% of VTs

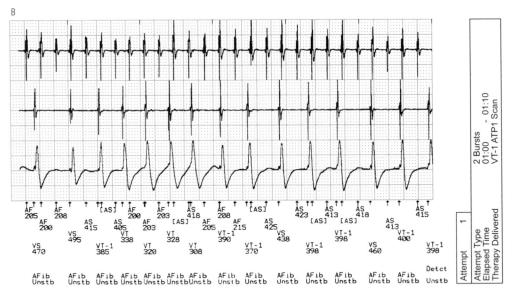

Fig. 8.67 (Continued)

in the VT zone of dual-chamber ICDs,[51,52] comparing atrial with ventricular rates is a simple and powerful SVT-VT discriminator if the atrial rate can be reliably measured. Algorithms that compare atrial and ventricular rates as their first step (Boston Scientific Rhythm ID™ and St. Jude) apply single-chamber discriminators to <10% of VTs, reducing the risk that they will misclassify VT as SVT.

Dual-chamber discrimination depends on accurate atrial sensing to classify arrhythmias reliably; the predominant cause of detection errors in dual-chamber ICDs has been atrial sensing errors.[68] Consistent far-field R-wave oversensing may misclassify VT as SVT because the atrial rate appears greater than the ventricular rate; intermittent far-field R-wave oversensing may misclassify SVT as VT in dual-chamber St. Jude and Medtronic ICDs if it is interpreted as AV dissociation. Atrial sensing function is optimized at implantation by lead placement at a site with a P wave of at least 1 mV and with absent or small far-field R waves (<25% of the atrial electrogram amplitude, in our experience). Selecting a lead with an interelectrode spacing of ≤10 mm minimizes far-field R waves because closely spaced electrodes create a smaller "antenna." Early observations with a lead with 1.1-mm interelectrode spacing support the concept that more closely spaced electrodes improve atrial sensing specificity, and early experimental work suggests totally intramyocardial electrodes may result in highly tissue-specific sensing.[69,70]

When P waves are not reliably sensed by an ICD, reprogramming sensitivity may result in acceptable function without surgical intervention. In most ICDs, atrial blanking after sensed ventricular event is programmable. Extending the blanking period and decreasing sensitivity may prevent far-field R-wave oversensing, but increases the risk of undersensing atrial fibrillation. The atrial sensing threshold start and decay delay are programmable to permit tailoring sensitivity programming, similar to the sensing function in the ventricle (Fig. 8.69). In Boston Scientific Vitality™ and newer ICDs, atrial blanking is programmable to a series of fixed values, or to SMARTSense™, in which after a short blanking period (15 ms), a period of reduced auto-adjusting sensitivity is present to minimize the risk of far-field R-wave oversensing, followed by full atrial sensitivity (Fig. 8.69). Figure 8.70 demonstrates far-field R-wave oversensing that is eliminated after prolonging the PVAB period. Older devices used fixed blanking periods following ventricular events, which could lead to underestimation of the atrial rate during atrial flutter and inappropriate therapy (due to the incorrect calculation that V > A rate).[70] To further minimize the risk of far-field R-wave oversensing, Medtronic ICDs analyze the pattern of activity sensed on the atrial lead to determine algorithmically whether sensed atrial events represent far-field R waves (Fig. 8.69). Intermittent far-field R-wave oversensing or frequent premature complexes disrupt the pattern, leading to algorithm error and tachycardia misclassification.

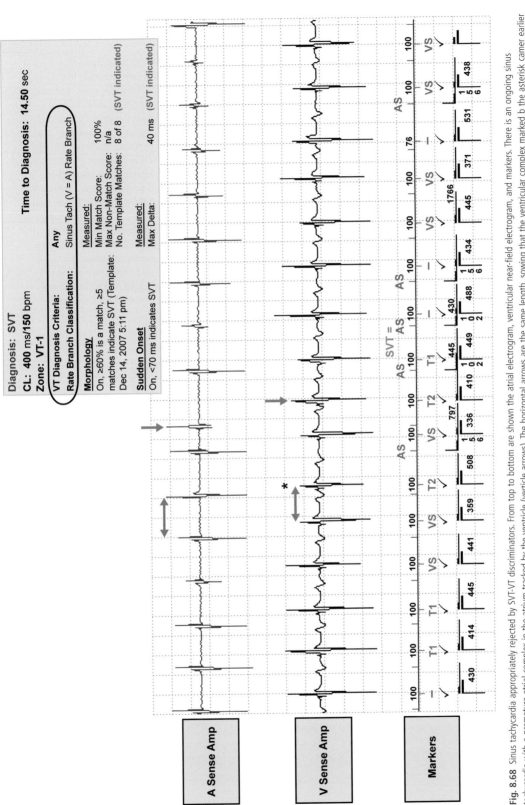

Diagnosis: SVT

CL: 400 ms/150 bpm   **Time to Diagnosis: 14.50 sec**

Zone: VT-1

VT Diagnosis Criteria: **Any**

Rate Branch Classification: **Sinus Tach (V = A) Rate Branch**

Morphology

On, ≥60% is a match, ≥5   Measured:

matches indicate SVT (Template: Min Match Score: 100%

Dec 14, 2007 5:11 pm)   Max Non-Match Score: n/a

                                  No. Template Matches: 8 of 8   (SVT indicated)

Sudden Onset   Measured:

On, <70 ms indicates SVT   Max Delta: 40 ms   (SVT indicated)

Fig. 8.68 Sinus tachycardia appropriately rejected by SVT-VT discriminators. From top to bottom are shown the atrial electrogram, ventricular near-field electrogram, and markers. There is an ongoing sinus tachycardia with a premature atrial complex in the atrium tracked by the ventricle (verticle arrows). The horizontal arrows are the same length, sowing that the ventricular complex marked b the asterisk came earlier than expected, making this a premature ventricular (or less likely, junctional) complex. Note that sudden onset criteria is on and is <70 ms, indicating a gradual onset and the presence of SVT. The morphology of the near-field electrograms also matches the baseline template (match score 100%, check marks at each complex below markers), also indicating SVT, so therapy is withheld. Note that the two algorithms (onset, morphology) are linked with "Any" logic, so that if any had indicated VT, therapy would have been delivered.

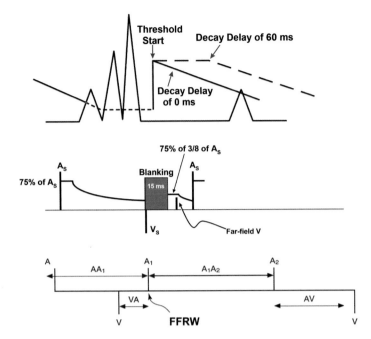

Fig. 8.69 Methods of prevention of far-field R-wave oversensing (FFRWO) on the atrial channel. Top panel: In St. Jude ICDs, sensing in the atrium following a sensed event is analogous to ventricular sensing. Threshold Start and Decay Delay are programmable. Middle panel: Boston Scientific ICDs use a short (15 ms) blanking period, followed by variable sensitivity designed to minimize FFRWO and permit sensing of atrial fibrillation. Bottom panel: Most Medtronic ICDs do not blank the atrial channel after sensed events, but instead, when there are two atrial events within a ventricular interval, look for a short–long pattern of A-A intervals to indicate FFRWO. After paced ventricular events, atrial sensitivity is transiently decreased. FFRW: far-field R wave oversensing.

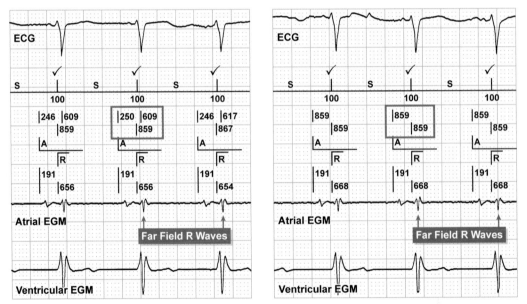

Fig. 8.70 Programming to eliminate far-field R-wave oversensing. In the left panel, far-field R waves are sensed on the atrial channel. Note in the boxed intervals the numbers "250" and "609." The time from the paced A to the oversensed R wave on the atrial channel is 250 ms. The ventricular signal is seen on the atrial electrogram. In the right panel, the ventricular signals are still seen on the atrial electrogram. However, due to reprogramming, they are no longer sensed on the atrial channel, and the AA interval (859 ms) happens to be the same as the VV interval. Note that sensing is sufficiently programmable to avoid sensing far-field R waves that have a larger amplitude than the atrial electrogram itself.

Decreasing the atrial sensitivity may eliminate intermittent far-field R-wave oversensing at the expense of increasing the risk of undersensing atrial fibrillation. In our experience, the risk of undersensing atrial fibrillation is low with atrial sensitivity as low as 0.45 mV. Far-field R-wave oversensing that occurs only after paced ventricular events does not increase the risk of inappropriate detection of SVT as VT. Elimination of far-field R-wave oversensing at implant and during follow-up results in effective dual-chamber SVT-VT discrimination.[46]

Manufacturer-specific dual-chamber SVT-VT discriminators are discussed below.

Enhanced onset and stability and Rhythm ID (Boston Scientific): The newest Boston Scientific dual-chamber defibrillators use either onset/stability or the morphology-based Rhythm ID detection enhancements. In dual-chamber ICDs the atrial lead permits the addition of two programmable features: V Rate > A Rate and AFib Rate Threshold. When V Rate > A Rate is "on" and true (defined as V rate > A rate by 10 bpm), therapy inhibitors (onset, stability, or both) are bypassed and therapy immediately delivered (Fig. 8.71). If false, therapy continues to be inhibited unless the tachycardia becomes stable (R-R intervals regularize) or V Rate > A Rate becomes true.

The AFib Rate Threshold increases specificity when used with stability by withholding therapy for unstable (irregular) ventricular rhythms only when the atrial lead confirms the presence of AF. An unstable (irregular) ventricular rhythm in the tachycardia zone that

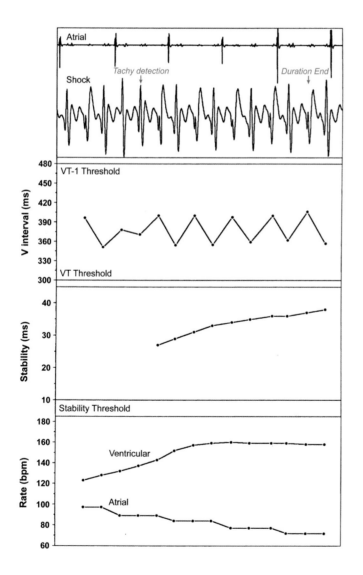

Fig. 8.71 Use of V Rate > A Rate (ventricular rate greater than atrial rate) to bypass therapy inhibitors. From top to bottom are the atrial and ventricular electrograms, the V intervals, the calculated stability, and the atrial and ventricular rates. The 10 most recent PP intervals and RR intervals are used to assess the rate in each chamber. An irregular ventricular tachycardia (VT) is present. The VT has a shorter interval (is faster) than the slow VT (VT-1) cut-off threshold. Thus, VT detection and duration are both satisfied (top box). Because the RR intervals are variable, the stability threshold is above the programmed value (in this case, 24 ms; not shown on graph). This inhibits therapy in a single-chamber device. However, because the ventricular rate is greater than the atrial rate, the stability inhibitor is bypassed and appropriate therapy delivered.

occurs in the absence of AF (as determined by the atrial lead), is classified as VT. Atrial undersensing increases the risk of treating AF as VT because an irregular rhythm will be treated as VT if the atrial rate is measured incorrectly to be below the AF rate threshold. If atrial lead sensing function is poor, programming the atrial lead from bipolar to "off" results in ventricular only SVT-VT discrimination, while still permitting atrial pacing for bradycardia support.

Rhythm ID™ integrates interval-based and morphology-based detection enhancements. Rhythm ID™ is programmed either "on" or "off," without additional operator programmable parameters. When programmed "on," if the ventricular exceeds the atrial rate (by 10 bpm), VT is declared and therapy is delivered (Fig. 8.72). Otherwise, the single-chamber morphology algorithm is applied (Fig. 8.64; see Morphology, above). A morphology match withholds therapy; a mismatch is further screened for rapidly conducted AF (defined as A rate > programmed mode switch rate and V rate unstable >20 ms) is performed. If AF is absent, therapy is delivered. During redetection, the morphology component of the algorithm is not included (Fig. 8.72B), because electrogram morphology may be distorted by the shock. The benefit of this algorithm is that it requires no custom programming; the limitation is that its errors cannot be corrected by troubleshooting. Early clinical results were impressive with 100% sensitivity for VT/VF, and 92% specificity for SVT.[71] However, the Rhythm ID Going Head to Head Trial (RIGHT), the first head-to-head comparison study between Boston Scientific Rhythm ID and Medtronic ICDs using the Wavelet (single-chamber) and PR Logic (dual-chamber) demonstrated equivalence of the two manufacturers algorithms with dual-chamber ICDs, but a greater number of inappropriate therapies with Rhythm ID in single chamber ICDs,[72] many inappropriate therapies were for slower VTs (<175 bpm), which are uncommon in primary prevention patients.[72] Starting with the Incepta device, additional programmability has been added. The Rhythm Match percent can be adjusted from the nominal value of 94% to individualize the algorithm's sensitivity and specificity, and beat by beat match scores is displayed.

PR Logic™ + Wavelet (Medtronic): Medtronic's PR Logic™ uses three programmable options that are independently programmed "on" or "off": AF/AT, sinus tachycardia, and other 1:1 SVT. The algorithm then analyzes the pattern of AA, VV, AV, and VA intervals hierarchically to classify the arrhythmia. An SVT limit criteria defines the fastest ventricular rate for which PR Logic is applied.[73,74] In its most current iteration, adaptive PR Logic (Entrust™ and newer), PR and RR intervals and expected variations are continuously analyzed; abrupt changes define VT. Wavelet (a morphology algorithm) has been added to PR Logic in the Protecta™ series ICDs, to increase the specificity of identifying AF in the VF zone (Fig. 8.73). Interval irregularity is not used as a descriminator by PR Logic in the VF zone because both AF and VF are irregular. If PR Logic classifies a tachycardia as VT/VF, therapy is not delivered unless confirmed by the Wavelet (morphology) algorithm. The combined algorithms are currently being further assessed.[75]

To avoid undersensing P waves, Medtronic ICDs nominally use no cross-chamber blanking in the atrium after sensed ventricular events and short (30 ms) atrial blanking after paced ventricular events. Consequently, far-field R waves are not uncommonly sensed on the atrial channel; true atrial events are differentiated from far-field R waves algorithmically (Fig. 8.74). As a practical matter, if far-field R-wave oversensing is consistently present or absent, the algorithm functions effectively. Intermittent far-field R-wave oversensing may lead to tachycardia misclassification. With poor atrial lead function, PR Logic can be turned off and Wavelet applied up to the SVT Limit (i.e. single-chamber morphology). In the first month post-implant, the other 1:1 SVTs is not programmed "on," because atrial lead dislodgment into the ventricle may result in misclassification of VT as SVT. Additionally, in the rare patient with AVNRT or orthodromic tachycardia (both typically 1:1 SVTs), ventricular ATP usually terminates the SVT, so that an intentional decision to deliver therapy may be appropriate. In consecutive interval counting VT zones, tachycardias rejected by single-chamber onset and stability are not assessed by PR Logic (see SVT-VT discriminators, above). Major clinical trials of PR Logic did not activate onset and stability; we routinely program these "off" in Medtronic dual-chamber ICDs, and favour PR Logic and Wavelet.

St. Jude Rate Branch™: St. Jude ICDs compare atrial and ventricular rates to sort a tachycardia into the A = V, A > V or V > A rate branch (Fig. 8.75). If V > A is true, the tachycardia is classified as VT and therapy delivered, eliminating up to 80% of tachycardias from further evaluation and possible algorithm error. In the other two rate branch arms, the individual detection enhancements (stability, morphology for A > V; onset, morphology for A = V) are individually programmed and combined using "any" or "all" logic (indicating how many of the SVT-VT discriminators must indicate VT for the episode to be classified as VT).[52] Based on the sensitivity and specificity of these combinations when applied to stored electrogram from spontaneous

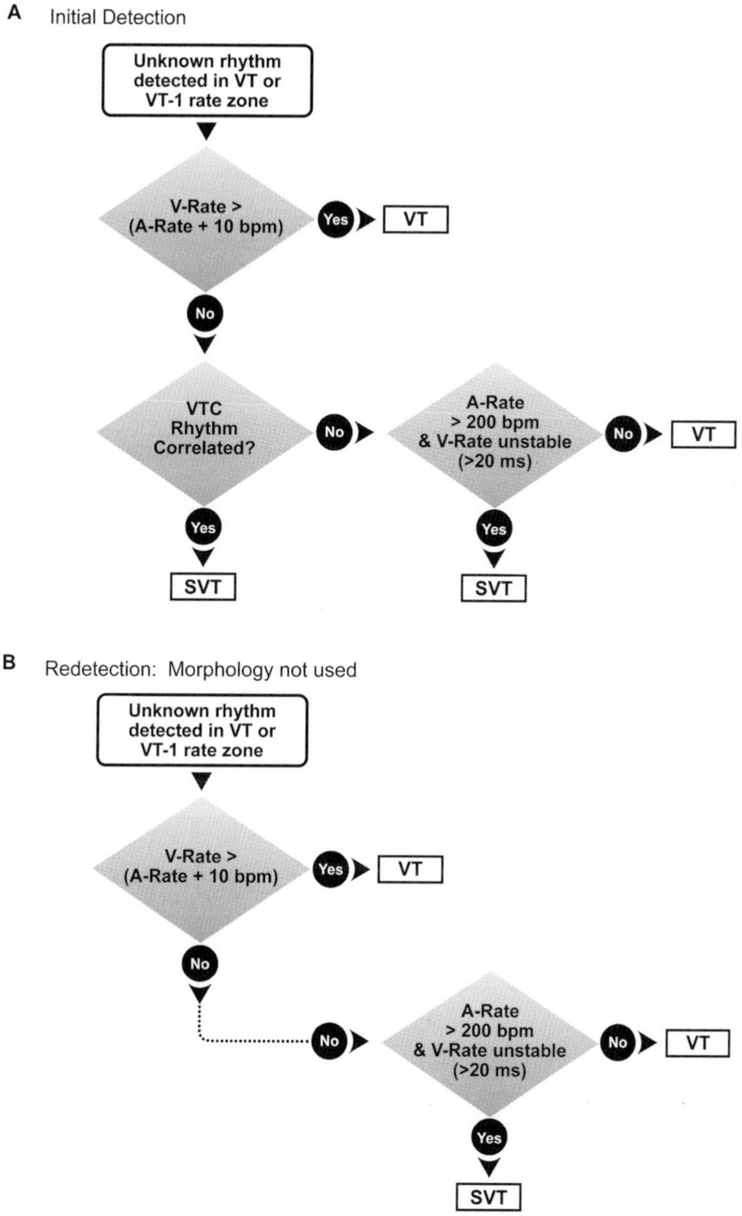

A   Initial Detection

```
┌─────────────────────┐
│   Unknown rhythm    │
│  detected in VT or  │
│   VT-1 rate zone    │
└─────────────────────┘
```

V-Rate > (A-Rate + 10 bpm) — **Yes** ▶ VT

No

VTC Rhythm Correlated? — **No** ▶ A-Rate > 200 bpm & V-Rate unstable (>20 ms) — **No** ▶ VT

Yes ↓ SVT   **Yes** ↓ SVT

B   Redetection: Morphology not used

```
┌─────────────────────┐
│   Unknown rhythm    │
│  detected in VT or  │
│   VT-1 rate zone    │
└─────────────────────┘
```

V-Rate > (A-Rate + 10 bpm) — **Yes** ▶ VT

No

········ **No** ▶ A-Rate > 200 bpm & V-Rate unstable (>20 ms) — **No** ▶ VT

Yes ↓ SVT

Fig. 8.72 (A) In the DR mode of Rhythm ID in a dual-chamber device, the first step is comparison of the atrial and ventricular rates. If the ventricular rate exceeds the atrial rate by at least 10 bpm, the rhythm is classified as VT for which therapy will be delivered. If V > A is not true, Vector Timing and Correlation is applied. If at least three of the last 10 beats are correlated, VTC classifies the rhythm as an SVT, for which therapy is inhibited. If VTC determines that the rhythm lacks sufficient correlation, atrial rate and ventricular rate stability are evaluated. If the atrial rate exceeds 200 bpm and the measured stability exceeds 20 ms, then the rhythm is classified as an SVT. Otherwise the rhythm is classified as a VT. (B) If Rhythm ID is enabled post-shock, the Vector Timing and Correlation portion of the algorithm is not used because there may be aberration of the signal morphology following shock delivery.

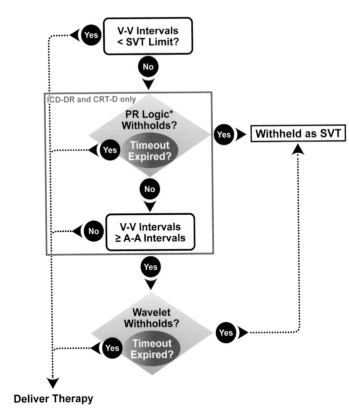

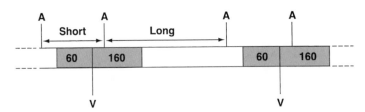

Fig. 8.73 Detection process in PR Logic (Medtronic). If the V-V intervals during tachycardia are shorter (faster) than the SVT limit, therapy is delivered. Otherwise, PR Logic, which assess the pattern and regularity of AA, VV, AV, and VA intervals, is applied. If it does not reject the tachycardia as SVT, and if the ventricular rate is not greater than the atrial rate , wavelet (morphology) is applied. Further details in text.

Fig. 8.74 Far-field R-wave oversensing. This subalgorithm determines whether sensed events on the atrial channel are due to atrial events or sensing of the far-field R wave. If each RR interval has exactly two atrial events and PP intervals alternate in a consistent manner, far-field R-wave oversensing can be diagnosed. The criteria must be met for 10 of the last 12 RR intervals to have atrial events rejected as far-field R waves. Further details in the text.

tachycardias in a clinical cohort, we use morphology in the A = V branch, and morphology or stability ("any" logic) in the A > V branch.[52,76] St. Jude dual-chamber ICDs also analyze AV association in conjunction with stability to test for N:1 flutters. We and others found a sensitivity of VT detection of 99% and specificity of SVT rejection up to 80% using optimal combinations and logic.[52,77] Detailed programming recommendations are summarized in Optimizing programming, below.

The Biotronic SMART® algorithm begins with rate branch sorting by assessing the V to A ratio. It then determines A and V stability, and association to classify tachycardias (Fig. 8.76).

Ventricular therapies

Antitachycardia pacing
ATP consists of short pacing sequences that terminate 80–95% of arrhythmia episodes without the need for

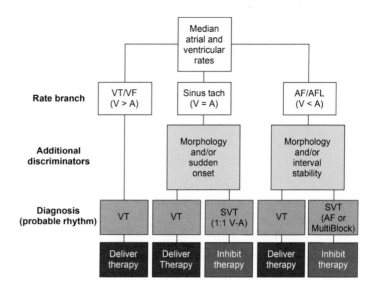

Fig. 8.75 Rate Branch™ Logic used in St. Jude Medical dual-chamber ICDs. See text for details.

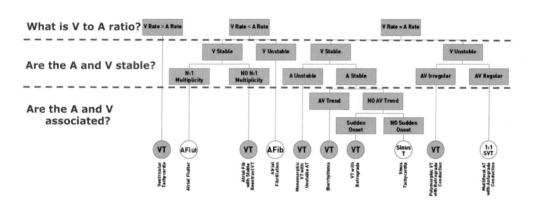

Fig. 8.76 Biotronik SMART® algorithm evaluates rate, onset, stability, and AV relationship on a beat-to-beat basis to discriminate SVT from VT.

shocks.[78–83] By pacing the ventricle at a rate greater than the tachycardia, the pacing impulses may enter the tachycardia circuit, to collide with the orthodromic tachycardia wavefront and extinguish re-entry (further discussed in Chapter 1: Pacing and Defibrillation).[84] ATP can be delivered as "bursts" (sequences of pacing pulses delivered at the same cycle length) or "ramps" (the cycle length shortens within the pulse train), or as a combination (Fig. 8.77). In 1–5% of patients, ATP may accelerate the arrhythmia,[77,78,85] which may lead to shock; the risk of syncope is <2%.[86] Due to the safety and efficacy of ATP, it is routinely applied, without the need for electrophysiologic testing.[87] ATP has been extensively studied. Key findings are as follow:

1 Burst more effectively terminates VT than ramp, and burst has a lower risk of acceleration.[88]

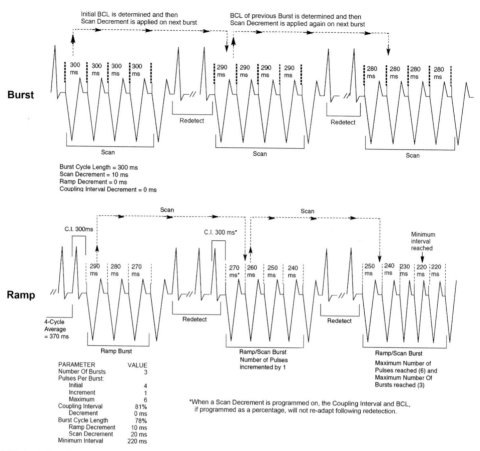

Fig. 8.77 Antitachycardia pacing. Top: in "burst" mode, a series of pacing pulses are given at the same cycle length. Subsequent bursts may have a shorter or an adaptive cycle, but the rate does not change within a burst. Bottom: in "ramp" mode, each pulse within a sequence comes at a progressively shorter interval. Terminology varies among manufacturers, with that of Boston Scientific shown in the figure. (Adapted with permission from Boston Scientific Manual.)

2 Within the commonly used clinical ranges of 69–88% of tachycardia cycle length, the ATP coupling interval and cycle length do not meaningfully affect efficacy.

3 The first ATP attempt is the most effective (up to 80%). ATP is limited to 1–2 sequences of eight pulses for fast VTs (heart rate >188 bpm); more are used to treat slow, relatively stable VTs.[86] Trial data show that 90% of fast VTs (up to 250 bpm) are terminated by two ATP bursts (eight pulses, 88% of VT cycle length), with a low risk of acceleration (4%) or syncope (2%).[39,86]

4 ATP is effective in CRT populations, with no difference between RV-delivered and biventricular-delivered ATP in the population as a whole. However, in patients with ischemic cardiomyopathy, biventricular ATP is more effective and may be less likely to accelerate the VT.[89] Efficacy is likely related to proximity to the re-entry circuit, facilitating impulse entry. We routinely program biventricular-delivered ATP when available.

Patient and arrhythmia characteristics affect ATP outcomes. ATP is less effective and more likely to accelerate VT as the ejection fraction decreases and the VT rate increases.[89–91] ATP is less effective when VT develops during sinus tachycardia.[92,93] Conversely, antiadrenergic medical therapy (β-blockers, antiarrhythmic drugs) augments ATP efficacy, in the case of membrane active drugs likely by slowing the VT rate. ATP is equally effective in ischemic and nonischemic cardiomyopathy.[85] Current generation ICDs deliver ATP therapy either before or during charge, and this feature is routinely programmed "on" with minimal or no effect on the timing of the first shock.[94]

In addition to terminating VT, ventricular ATP also reduces shocks for inappropriately detected SVT either by terminating SVT or delaying shock therapy, providing time for the SVT to terminate or slow. As ATP improves quality of life[86] and prevents appropriate and inappropriate shocks, it should be programmed "on" empirically in most patients, even if its efficacy has not been assessed.[44]

Defibrillation

The cumulative efficacy of ICD defibrillation shocks for VF termination exceeds 98%.[95,96] Current-generation defibrillators deliver up to 6–8 shocks per episode to ensure arrhythmia termination. Available maximal delivered shock energies range from approximately 25–36 J, enough to defibrillate most patients through an endocardial approach with biphasic waveforms and modern leads. The mean energy required for successful defibrillation at implant in current devices is approximately 10 J.[97–99] As discussed in Chapter 1: Pacing and Defibrillation, defibrillation threshold or margin testing is typically performed at implant to assess the energy requirements for defibrillation. Programming shock energy at 10 J above the defibrillation threshold results in a first-shock success rate of 87–93% during spontaneous VT/VF.[100] To maximize defibrillation success, all subsequent shocks are programmed to maximum output, and the polarity of the last shock in the sequence is reversed when this feature is available.

Some experts recommend programming a low first-shock strength when patient-specific implant testing indicates a low energy requirement for defibrillation (e.g., DFT + 10 J). Potential advantages of a lower first-shock energy include a reduced risk of syncope (due to faster charge time), battery preservation (particularly in the setting of frequent charges for VT storm or SVT), and reduction in post-shock myocardial depression.[100] Conversely, programming the first shock to maximal output may improve first-shock success, reducing the likelihood of repetitive shocks, may increase the odds of spontaneous termination due to the slightly longer charge time,[101] and a higher likelihood of cardioverting AF.

Low-energy cardioversion

Many monomorphic VTs are susceptible to low-energy shocks (1–5 J), even if they fail to respond to overdrive pacing. However, low-energy shocks are not pain-free, and they increase the risk that additional shocks will be necessary. Additionally, the vulnerable zone during ventricular tachycardia may extend from one cardiac cycle to the next R wave, so that a low-energy shock may induce VF. Thus, to prevent inducing VF, shocks to treat ventricular tachycardia should be programmed based on the defibrillation testing or at maximum output, not at low energies.

Interactions of antibradycardia pacing with tachycardia programming

The bradycardia and tachycardia functions of defibrillators can interact, putting constraints on programming options and device function. These vary among manufacturers, but common interactions exist:

• The maximum pacing rate must be 5–10 bpm slower than the slowest VT detection zone. This may become problematic in patients with slow VTs on antiarrhythmic medications who also have chronotropic insufficiency. The exception is in Sorin Medical devices, which permit the pacing upper rate limit to exceed the VT detection cut-off.

• Algorithms that promote pacing at more rapid rates impair VT detection. This results from the obligatory blanking and refractory periods following paced events, during which spontaneous ventricular activity is not detected. This phenomenon has been best characterized with the rate smoothing algorithm, but occurs with any high rate pacing.[102]

Most important interactions lead to programming lock-outs or parameter interaction warnings on the programmer, which should generally be heeded.[102]

In ICD recipients, bradycardia pacing may result in proarrhythmia, most commonly by algorithmically induced or permitted short–long–short R-R interval sequences. This is reviewed in Minimizing ICD proarrhythmia in Chapter 10: Troubleshooting.

Atrial defibrillators: detection and therapies

Implanted device therapy is infrequently used to maintain sinus rhythm because of the success of other strategies, including ablation.[103] A dedicated atrial defibrillator is no longer manufactured, although ventricular shocks will frequently cardiovert AF. Atrial pacing modestly reduces the risk of developing AF, and many devices offer atrial pacing algorithms to prevent or terminate AF.[104,105] Atrial termination and prevention therapies have been shown to reduce arrhythmia burden in subsets of ICD recipients using device-based arrhythmia detection (Fig. 8.78).[106] However, their ability to reduce the risk of clinically meaningful end-points

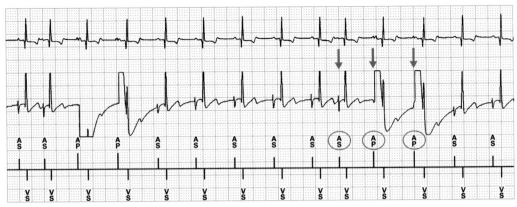

Fig. 8.78 Atrial rate stabilization is designed to prevent atrial fibrillation onset by eliminating pauses after premature atrial complexes (PACs). From top to bottom are shown the surface electrocardiogram, intracardiac electrogram, and markers. A PAC is present and sensed (first arrow, circled "AS" on marker channel). To prevent a long pause, two paced beats at gradually prolonging intervals are delivered (circled "AP" markers) until sinus rhythm returns ("AS" following the last "AP").

(symptoms, stroke, heart failure, etc.) has not been demonstrated.

When device therapy is used with a goal of maintaining sinus rhythm, the following general principles guide optimal programming:

1 Atrial pacing therapies should be used liberally. Even if efficacy is less than that of shocks, the main treatment goal is improvement in arrhythmia symptoms and quality of life.

2 Shock therapies are generally avoided. When used, they should be programmed to make the first shock work. In the clinically effective range, pain is more closely correlated with the number of shocks than with the shock strength.[107]

3 Patient preference is critical for effective programming. Some patients may prefer to self-administer therapies.

Atrial defibrillation is rarely offered because of the associated pain. However, several important safety rules must be considered when it is programmed: (i) ensure that detection of AF is reliable and that far-field R waves are not oversensed as AF; (ii) limit the duration of AF that receives cardioversion to 24 hours in patients who are not reliably anticoagulated; (iii) do not shock R-R intervals shorter than about 400–500 ms to prevent delivery of shocks into the vulnerable period of the preceding T wave; and (iv) use maximum or near-maximum strength shock to minimize the risk of shock-induced VF and maximize the probability of terminating AF. When device therapy is used to alleviate atrial fibrillation symptoms, it is most commonly in the

setting of an AV node ablation, the efficacy of which stems from the excellent control of the ventricular rate without pharmacologic therapy.[103]

Optimizing programming

Unnecessary shocks occur in roughly one-quarter of patients with ICDs.[108–110] Shocks may cause patients physical pain, psychologic trauma, and reduce their quality of life.[111] Shocks increase utilization of heathcare resources and are associated with increased mortality;[112–114] but it is not clear if they have a causal role in this increased mortality.

Optimal programming also minimizes ventricular pacing in nonresynchronization systems, as RV apical pacing introduces a left bundle branch block ECG pattern and dysynchrony leading to heart failure and AF in patients with ventricular dysfunction.[115–117]

Clinical trials have demonstrated that carefully selected empiric settings perform as well as clinician tailored individualized settings.[118,119] Population-specific parameters (e.g. routine programming in primary prevention) reduce all cause shocks by 50%.[119] In patients receiving an ICD for primary prevention of sudden death, the following programming principles are applied:

1 Use of a prolonged detection time (up to 9s) to avoid detection of self-terminating episodes

2 Use of VT rate cut-off at or above 180 bpm to prevent detection of slower rhythms that are often SVTs or well-tolerated VT (Fig. 8.79)

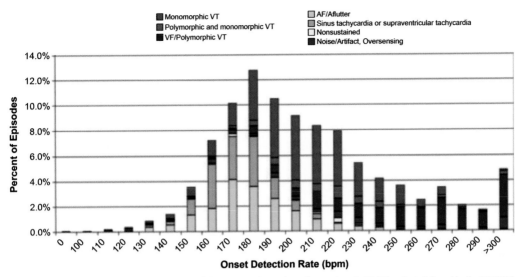

Fig. 8.79 Percentage of all shocks by rhythm type and detection rate in a cohort of approximately 15,000 patients followed by the LATITUDE remote monitoring system. (From Gilliam FR, Hayes DL, Boehmer JP, *et al*. Real world evaluation of dual-zone ICD and CRT-D programming compared to single-zone programming: the ALTITUDE REDUCES study. J Cardiovasc Electrophysiol 2011; 22:1023–9.)

3 Consistent application of SVT-VT discriminators to avoid treating SVT

4 Application of ATP even in fast detection zones.[3,9,21] Company-specific parameters used by the authors to achieve these aims are listed in Table 8.10.

In secondary prevention patients we program a VT zone 10–20 bpm slower than the slowest clinical arrhythmia, or 150–160 if the clinical VT rate is unknown. Therapy in the VT zone includes 2–4 ATP bursts (or more if hemodynamically stable VT is known to be present) of 81–88% burst cycle length, followed by maximum output shocks. The VF zone is programmed above 200–220 bpm. ATP before and during charge minimizes shock delivery. Use of multiple zones for detection rates <200 bpm is associated with fewer total shocks, fewer appropriate shocks, and fewer inappropriate shocks.[120] The programming strategies for specific patient populations is summarized in Table 8.11. Patient-independent general optimization programming is summarized in Table 8.12.

Cardiac resynchronization programming

In order for cardiac resynchronization to occur, a sufficient "dose" of therapy must be delivered. The "dose" is a function of the frequency of resynchronization pacing and of the effectiveness of each resynchronized beat. In order to be effective, the LV lead must capture the left ventricle. Programming outputs to ensure capture is discussed earlier in the chapter. The effectiveness of resynchronization is also modified by the programmed AV delay and the offset between RV and LV timing. The impact of these parameters, and their optimization, is reviewed in Chapter 2: Hemodynamics of Cardiac Pacing, and briefly discussed below. Lastly, optimized resynchronized pacing must be delivered nearly continuously (>92–98%)[121] in order to have a clinical impact. Events that disrupt ventricular tracking and permit intrinsic ventricular conduction, frequent PVCs, and rapidly conducted SVTs reduce the frequency of resynchronization. CRT devices incorporate algorithms designed to overcome these events in order to promote continuous resynchronization These are briefly discussed below, and in Chapter 13: Follow-up, and Troubleshooting cardiac resynchronization devices in Chapter 10: Troubleshooting.

Algorithms to promote continuous tracking

Tracking (ventricular pacing following a sensed atrial event) may not occur if the atrial event occurs during a refractory period or if intrinsic conduction is shorter than the programmed AV delay. Algorithms to address both scenarios exist. Because atrial complexes that

Table 8.10 Primary prevention ICD programming.

PG	Zone	Rate	Detect	Redetect	Therapy	Discriminators — Single-chamber	Discriminators — Dual-chamber and CRT-D
Med	VF	330 ms (182 bpm)	30/40 int	12/16 int	35J × 6, ATP during charge R-R>=230	Wavelet: ON SVT V. Limit: 300 ms <u>Other Enhancements</u> Stability: OFF Onset: OFF High rate timeout: OFF	<u>PR Logic</u> AF/Afi: ON (Protecta: Wavelet ON) Sinus Tach: ON Other 1:1 SVT: OFF SVT V. Limit: 300 ms <u>Other Enhancements</u> Stability: OFF Onset: OFF High rate timeout: OFF
	FVT via VF	240 ms (250 bpm)			ATP × 1, 35J × 5		
	Monitor	360 ms (167 bpm)	32 int		None		
BS	VF	200 bpm (300 ms)	7 s	1 s	Quick convert ATP ON, Shocks 41J × 8	<u>Enhancements (apply to VT and VT-1)</u> Rhythm ID VT Detection Enhancements ON Sustained rate duration OFF <u>SVT Discrimination</u> SVT discrimination: ventricle only SVT discrimination timeout: OFF SVT upper limit: 200 bpm / 300 ms Int Stab: 40 ms If 2 of 3 Sudden onset: ON 100 ms	<u>Enhancements (apply to VT and VT-1)</u> Rhythm ID VT Detection Enhancements ON Sustained rate duration OFF <u>SVT Discrimination</u> SVT discrimination: dual-chamber SVT discrimination timeout: OFF SVT upper limit: 200 bpm / 300 ms V < A Morph: ON Int stability: ON If All V = A Morph: ON Sudd onset: PASSIVE If Any
	VT	180 bpm (333 ms)	7 s	1 s	ATP1 Burst, Shocks 41J × 8		
	VT-1	160 bpm (375 ms)	9 s	1 s	ATP1&2 OFF, Shocks OFF		
SJM	VF	240 bpm / 250 ms	30 int	6 int	35J, 40J × 5, ATP while charging	<u>SVT Discrimination</u> Morph: ON Int Stab: 40 ms If 2 of 3 Sudden onset: ON 100 ms	<u>SVT Discrimination</u> SVT upper limit: 200 bpm / 300 ms V < A Morph: ON Int stability: ON If All V = A Morph: ON Sudd onset: PASSIVE If Any
	VT-2	181 bpm / 330 ms	30 int	6 int	ATP × 1, 40J × 4		
	VT-1	166 bpm / 360 ms	30 int		Monitor only		

ATP therapy	Rx
Burst	
Initial pulses	8
# of sequences	1
%RR	88%
Interval decrement	10
V-V Min inerval	200 ms
Chambers paced BiV Devices for ATP	
Medtronic	Program RV + LV
BS	Default BiV
SJM	Default RV only

Dependent patients: Turn all SVT discriminators OFF.

Chronic atrial fib with atrial port of BiV plugged: Use single chamber discriminators.

Acquiring morphology template:

1. Pace AAI > 100 bpm to see if bundle branch block aberrancy develops. If so, do not use morphology discriminators.

2. If no aberrancy with rapid pacing, manually acquire template at implant or at device check for Wavelet, Morphology, and Rhythm ID (Bos Sci will try to auto acquire template with lower rate of 60 bpm, Med will not alter brady params for auto collection, and SJM will not auto acquire with BiV)

Note: table updated periodically as new models emerge with different device functions. This table serves to depict programming concept of prolonged detection, consistent use of SVT-VT discriminators, and liberal application of ATP.

Acknowledgement: Brian Powell, MD, Marj Martin, RN, Tracy Webster, RN, Jim Ryan, RN

Table 8.11 Patient-specific optimized programming.

Disease state	Arrhythmia characteristic	Programming considerations	Rationale
Channelopathies	Rapid polymorphic VT/VF	Single detection zone for HR >200 bpm	• Clinical arrhythmia is rapid (so that a high cut-off rate is unlikely to underdetect significant arrhythmias; young patients can achieve rapid heart rates with exercise, increasing the risk of inappropriate detection of rhythms with HR <200 bpm
		Detection enhancements "off"*	• Enhancements are generally not effective in VF zone at rapid rates
		Avoid ATP	• Role in polymorphic VT/VF not established; possibility of proarrhythmia
	Frequent, nonsustained episodes	Prolong detection (to 30 of 40 beats or up to 7–9 s)	• Prevent inappropriate charging and shocks
	Long QT during sinus rhythm	Screen for T-wave oversensing and reprogram as necessary (see section Implantable cardioverter-defibrillator sensing)	• Avoid inappropriate shocks
Primary prevention (CAD or DCM)	Fast VT/VF is often monomorphic, HR >200	Use 2 detection zones, VT cut-off 180 bpm	• Minimize risk for inappropriate detections by not exposing detection algorithms to slower rates; two zones permits increased SVT-VT discriminator and ATP use in the lower HR zone
		ATP: use 1–2 sequences for HR <250	• Reduce risk of inappropriate and appropriate shock
Secondary Prevention (CAD, DCM)	Monomorphic VT with HR 120–200	Use 2–3 detection zones	• Permit increased detection enhancements and ATP for slower VT and tiered therapies
		Program detection enhancements "on;" use dual-chamber enhancements if available	• Decrease risk of inappropriate shock
	Fast VT/VF is often monomorphic, HR >200	Multiple sequence of ATP in slower zones; 1–2 sequences for 200 < HR < 250	• Terminate SVT and VT; reduce risk of appropriate and inappropriate shock
CHF	Bradycardias	Avoid RV pacing in non-CRT systems. Use RV pacing avoidance algorithms if available	• Chronic RV apical pacing desynchronizes the ventricles, increasing the risk of CHF
	VT/VF	Program as for primary and secondary prevention, above	
PAF	Atrial fibrillation and sinus bradycardia	Promote atrial pacing and minimize RV apical pacing	• Increased atrial pacing modestly reduces atrial fibrillation RV apical pacing increases risk of atrial fibrillation
		Atrial prevention and termination algorithms (if available)	• Atrial termination algorithms (ATP, HFB) reduce arrhythmia burden, but clinical significance is uncertain • May be particularly useful in patients with atrial flutter, incisional atrial re-entrant circuits • Avoid use in first month (possible lead dislodgment) • Avoid shocks for atrial arrhythmias

ATP, antitachycardia pacing; CHF, congestive heart failure; CRT, cardiac resynchronization therapy; HR, heart rate.
*While few data support use in this specific population, morphology up to 260 ms is nominally on in Medtronic Protecta™ series ICDs, and is reasonable to use in this population as well.

Table 8.12 Patient independent and general programming optimization.

	Programming	Rationale
Sensing	• Screen for far-field R-wave oversensing and program to eliminate it if present	Ensure appropriate detection enhancement operation
	• Screen for T-wave oversensing and program to eliminate it if present	Avoid double counting and inappropriate detection
Detection	• Use detection enhancements in all patients with intact AV nodal conduction and a VT zone with HR cut-off <200 bpm	Minimize the risk of inappropriate detection
	• Prolong number of intervals to detect or detection time in patients with frequent self-terminating arrhythmias (up to 30 out of 40 intervals or 7–9 s)	Prevent unnecessary capacitor charging and shocks
Bradycardia therapy	• Minimize RV pacing in all non-CRT systems	RV apical pacing promotes atrial fibrillation and congestive heart failure
	• Promote atrial pacing in patients with sinus node dysfunction	Reduce the risk of AF
Tachycardia therapy	• Program liberal ATP in VT zones <200 bpm and 1–2 ATP sequences in faster detection zones	Minimize the risk of inappropriate and appropriate shocks
	• Program first shock strength for VT or VF based on DFT or ULV testing or to maximum output. Program all subsequent shocks at maximum output	DFT or ULV based shock output not likely to transform VT to VF Maximum output shocks more likely to be effective and lower risk of repetitive shocks; longer charge time may allow spontaneous termination
Device function/ surveillance	• Check for device specific "recalls" at routine follow-up and reprogram accordingly	Some device "malfunction" can be corrected by specific manufacturer recommended programming. Example would include software errors (such as "latching") eliminated by turning off certain features
	• Enable patient alerts	These generate audible tones or vibratory alerts, advising the patient to seek care (see Chapter 13: Follow-up)
	• Enable remote monitoring	Automated monitoring generates web-based or other forms of physician notification when parameters (e.g., lead impedance) are out of range suggesting incipient malfunction (see Chapter 13: Follow-up)

AF, atrial fibrillation; ATP, antitachycardia pacing; AV, atrioventricular; CRT, cardiac resynchroniztion therapy; DFT, defibrillation threshold; HR, heart rate; RV, right ventricular; ULV, upper limit of vulnerability.

occur during the PVARP are not tracked, a premature atrial complex that falls in the PVARP and is intrinsically conducted to the ventricles may initiate a succession of nonresynchronized complexes. Algorithms such as Atrial Tracking Recovery™ (Medtronic) and Tracking Preference™ (Boston Scientific) shorten the PVARP to allow tracking of sequential atrial events that fall into the PVARP (Fig. 8.80). Negative AV Hysteresis algorithms (St. Jude), discussed in the pacing section above, shorten the AV interval following sensed ventricular events to promote ventricular stimulation.

Algorithms to manage premature ventricular complexes

PVCs may have detrimental effects in patients with heart failure by direct effects and by inhibiting resynchronization. Frequent PVCs themselves produce ventricular dyssynchrony that can lead to cardiomyopathy. Because they can occur early in the cardiac cycle, PVCs may inhibit ventricular pacing, limiting continuous CRT delivery. With algorithms such as Ventricular Sense Response™ (Medtronic), Biventricular Trigger (Boston Scientific), BiV with RVsense (Biotronik) a sensed ventricular event on either ventricular channel

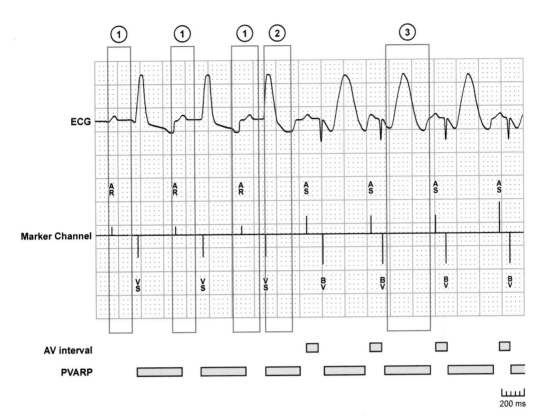

Fig. 8.80 Algorithm to promote continuous tracking (Atrial Tracking Recovery™, Medtronic, shown). The initial atrial complexes (labeled "1") occur during the PVARP and are not tracked. After eight AR–VS cycles, the algorithm shortens the PVARP to break the pattern (at "2"). The algorithmic intervention continues until AV tracking at programmed SAV resumes (at "3").

triggers an immediate ventricular pace, to promote resynchronization (Fig. 8.81). However, the value of these algorithms to achieve clinical resynchronization is not well established.

Algorithms to manage atrial fibrillation

Rapidly conducted AF frequently inhibits biventricular pacing. Algorithms such as Ventricular Rate Regulation™ (Boston Scientific) and Conducted AF Response™ (Medtronic) regularize the ventricular response AF by adjusting the pacing rate to minimize R-R interval variability and also increase the frequency of ventricular pacing (Fig. 8.82). The increased frequency of ventricular pacing has a minimal effect on the average heart rate. The latter issue is important, because inappropriately rapid pacing itself may depress ventricular systolic function. Resynchronization in patients with chronic AF typically also requires pharmacologic or nonpharmacologic rate control. We have a low threshold for offering AV node ablation to CRT recipients because it is associ-

ated with lower mortality, presumably because of near 100% resynchronization.[122]

Device-based optimization for cardiac resynchronization

Echo-based optimization assesses the effect of varying AV and VV intervals on Doppler-measured LV outflow or mitral inflow to define patient-specific best parameter settings. It is labor-intensive, and may require repetition over time.[123] This has led to great interest in device-based algorithms to identify AV and VV intervals that optimize hemodynamics (QuickOpt™, St. Jude Medical; SmartDelay™, Boston Scientific). The algorithms use intracardiac electrogram timing between leads and analysis of the atrial electrogram to derive optimal AV and VV intervals. However, the SMART-AV study found no difference at 6 months in clinical or echocardiographic end-points irrespective of whether the AV interval was echocardiograpahically optimized,

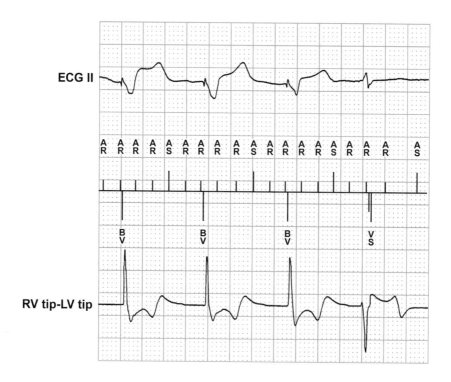

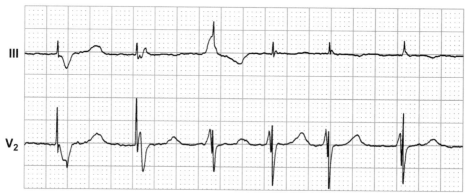

Fig. 8.81 Algorithm to promote resynchronization during ventricular ectopy. Top: surface ECG lead II, event markers, and the RV tip to LV tip electrogram are displayed during atrial fibrillation. The first three complexes represent biventricular pacing ("BV"). The last complex represents a conducted complex that was sensed ("VS"). The split marker associated with the "VS" indicates that a triggered pace pulse resulted. Bottom: hospital telemetry shows ventricular pacing occurring after the QRS onset due to the Medtronic Ventricular Sense Response™ algorithm, which introduces a triggered biventricular pacing pulse after each RV-sensed event. (From Swerdlow CD, Friedman PA. Advanced ICD troubleshooting: Part II. Pacing Clin Electrophysiol 2006; 29:70–96, by permission of Blackwell Publishing.)

algorithmically optimized by the device, or empirically set to 120 ms, and similar lack of benefit has been reported for other algorithms.[124,125] Thus, a reasonable strategy is proggramming an AV interval of 120 ms, with use of device algorithms in nonresponders. This is further discussed in Chapter 2: Hemodynamics of Cardiac Pacing.

Conclusions
Pacemakers and implantable defibrillators have undergone enormous technical advances since their early days. With the introduction of many new features, a large number of programmable parameters have been introduced to enable the caregiver to tailor device function to an individual's clinical arrhythmia. With a thor-

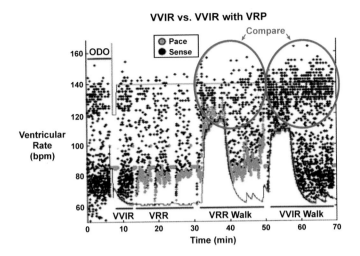

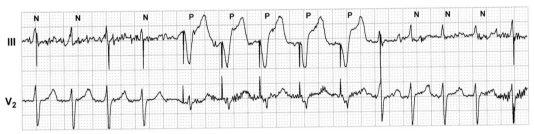

Fig. 8.82 Algorithms to manage atrial fibrillation. Top: example of a Holter graph in a patient at rest and during walking, showing the effect of a ventrical rate program (VRP) algorithm designed to regularize the ventricular rate during AF. With VRP "off" (VVIR only), there is a large variation in the cycle length of ventricular sensing beats during AF. During VVIR with VRP "on," there is a significant reduction in the variation in ventricular sensing beats with increasing ventricular pacing beats compared with VRP "off" at rest and during walking. (From Tse HF, Newman D, Ellenborgen KA, *et al.* Effects of ventricular rate regularization pacing on quality of life and symptoms in patients with atrial fibrillation (Atrial fibrillation symptoms mediated by pacing to mean rates [AF SYMPTOMS study]). Am J Cardiol 2004; 94:938–41). Bottom: hospital telemetry shows pacing during rapidly conducted atrial fibrillation due to an algorithm designed to maximize cardiac resynchronization pacing. This pacing, with the patient at rest, is distinct from rapid, rate-responsive pacing that is triggered by a sensor. (From Swerdlow CD, Friedman PA. Advanced ICD troubleshooting: Part II. Pacing Clin Electrophysiol 2006; 29:70–96, by permission of Blackwell Publishing.)

ough understanding of device operation function, it can indeed be optimized to provide life-prolonging therapy with minimal morbidity.

References

1 Chiu CC, Vicente KJ, Buffo-Sequeira I, Hamilton RM, McCrindle BW. Usability assessment of pacemaker programmers. Pacing Clin Electrophysiol 2004; 27:1388–98.

2 Bernstein AD, Daubert JC, Fletcher RD, *et al.* The revised NASPE/BPEG generic code for antibradycardia, adaptive-rate, and multisite pacing. North American Society of Pacing and Electrophysiology/British Pacing and Electrophysiology Group. Pacing Clin Electrophysiol 2002; 25:260–4.

3 Hayes DL, Von Feldt L, Higano ST. Standardized informal exercise testing for programming rate adaptive pacemakers. Pacing Clin Electrophysiol 1991; 14:1772–6.

4 Freedman RA, Hopper DL, Mah J, Hummel J, Wilkoff BL. Assessment of pacemaker chronotropic response: implementation of the Wilkoff mathematical model. Pacing Clin Electrophysiol 2001; 24:1748–54.

5 Page E, Defaye P, Bonnet JL, Durand C, Amblard A. Comparison of the cardiopulmonary response to exercise in recipients of dual sensor DDDR pacemakers versus a healthy control group. Pacing Clin Electrophysiol 2003; 26:239–43.

6 Sweeney MO, Bank AJ, Nsah E, *et al.* Extension and Managed Ventricular Pacing for Promoting Atrioventricular Conduction (SAVE PACe) Trial. Minimizing

ventricular pacing to reduce atrial fibrillation in sinus-node disease. N Engl J Med 2007; 357:1000–8.

7 Sweeney MO, Ellenbogen KA, Miller EH, Sherfesee L, Sheldon T, Whellan D. The Managed Ventricular pacing versus VVI 40 Pacing (MVP) Trial: clinical background, rationale, design, and implementation. J Cardiovasc Electrophysiol 2006; 17:1295–8.

8 Gillis AM, Purerfellner H, Israel CW, et al. Medtronic Enrhythm Clinical Study Investigators. Reducing unnecessary right ventricular pacing with the managed ventricular pacing mode in patients with sinus node disease and AV block. Pacing Clin Electrophysiol 2006; 29:697–705.

9 Sweeney MO, Ellenbogen KA, Tang AS, et al.; Managed Ventricular Pacing Versus VVI 40 Pacing Trial Investigators. Atrial pacing or ventricular backup-only pacing in implantable cardioverter-defibrillator patients. Heart Rhythm 2010; 7:1552–60.

10 Ogawa H, Ishikawa T, Matsushita K, et al. Effects of right atrial pacing preference in prevention of paroxysmal atrial fibrillation: Atrial Pacing Preference study (APP study). Circ J. 2008; 72:700–4.

11 Babu E, George G, Balachander J, Selvaraj R. Multiple inappropriate rate drop responses triggered by ventricular premature beats. Europace 2011; 13:1046.

12 Gammage MD. Rate-drop response programming. Pacing Clin Electrophysiol 1997; 20:841–3.

13 Johansen JB, Bexton RS, Simonsen EH, Markowitz T, Erickson MK. Clinical experience of a new rate drop response algorithm in the treatment of vasovagal and carotid sinus syncope. Europace 2000; 2:245–50.

14 http://manuals.medtronic.com/OrderManagement. In: Adapta/Versa/Sensia pacemaker reference guide. 2006: 5–33.

15 Hynes JK, Holmes DR Jr, Merideth J, Trusty JM. An evaluation of long-term stimulation thresholds by measurement of chronic strength duration curve. Pacing Clin Electrophysiol 1981; 4:376–9.

16 http://manuals.medtronic.com/OrderManagement. In: Adapta/Versa/Sensia pacemaker reference guide. 2006: 7–3.

17 St. Jude Medical Bradycardia Devices Supplemental Reference Manual. Vario Threshold Test. 2006: 16–35.

18 Ribeiro AL, Rincon LG, Oliveira BG, et al. Automatic adjustment of pacing output in the clinical setting. Am Heart J 2004; 147:127–31.

19 Sperzel J, Kennergren C, Biffi M, et al. Clinical performance of a ventricular automatic capture verification algorithm. Pacing Clin Electrophysiol 2005; 28:933–7.

20 Sperzel J, Nowak B, Himmrich E, et al. Acute performance evaluation of a new ventricular automatic capture algorithm. Europace 2006; 8:65–9.

21 Wood MA, Ellenbogen KA, Dinsmoor D, Hess M, Markowitz T. Influence of autothreshold sensing and sinus rate on mode switching algorithm behavior. Pacing Clin Electrophysiol 2000; 23:1473–8.

22 Swerdlow CD. Implantation of cardioverter defibrillators without induction of ventricular fibrillation. Circulation 2001; 103:2159–64.

23 Boriani G, Rusconi L, Biffi M, et al. Role of ventricular Autocapture function in increasing longevity of DDDR pacemakers: a prospective study. Europace 2006; 8:216–20.

24 Celiker A, Ceviz N, Kucukosmanoglu O. Long-term results of endocardial pacing with Autocapture threshold tracking pacemakers in children. Europace 2005; 7:569–75.

25 Castro A, Liebold A, Vincente J, Dungan T, Allen JC Jr. Evaluation of autosensing as an automatic means of maintaining a 2:1 sensing safety margin in an implanted pacemaker. Autosensing Investigation Team. Pacing Clin Electrophysiol 1996; 19:1708–13.

26 Felices Nieto A, Picon Intantes R, Diaz Ortuno F, Gimenez Raurell J, Herrera Rojas D, Lopez Cuervo JF. Loss of integrity of bipolar cardiac stimulation and its automatic correction. Report of 2 cases [in Spanish]. Rev Esp Cardiol 1994; 47:407–9.

27 Mauser JF, Huang SK, Risser T, et al. A unique pulse generator safety feature for bipolar lead fracture. Pacing Clin Electrophysiol 1993; 16:1368–72.

28 Barold SS. Termination of pacemaker endless loop tachycardia by an atrial extrasystole. Pacing Clin Electrophysiol 2001; 24:250–1.

29 Barold SS, Levine PA. Pacemaker repetitive nonreentrant ventriculoatrial synchronous rhythm: a review. J Interv Card Electrophysiol 2001; 5:45–58.

30 Lau CP, Leung SK, Tse HF, Barold SS. Automatic mode switching of implantable pacemakers: I. Principles of instrumentation, clinical, and hemodynamic considerations. Pacing Clin Electrophysiol 2002; 25:967–83.

31 Lau CP, Leung SK, Tse HF, Barold SS. Automatic mode switching of implantable pacemakers: II. Clinical performance of current algorithms and their programming. Pacing Clin Electrophysiol 2002; 25:1094–113.

32 Israel CW. Analysis of mode switching algorithms in dual chamber pacemakers. Pacing Clin Electrophysiol 2002; 25:380–93.

33 Friedman PA, Stanton MS. The pacer-cardioverter-defibrillator: function and clinical experience. J Cardiovasc Electrophysiol 1995; 6:48–68.

34 Brady PA, Friedman PA, Stanton MS. Effect of failed defibrillation shocks on electrogram amplitude in a nonintegrated transvenous defibrillation lead system. Am J Cardiol 1995; 76:580–4.

35 Glikson M, Friedman PA. The implantable cardioverter defibrillator. Lancet 2001; 357:1107–17.

36 Wood MA, Swerdlow C, Olson WH. Sensing and arrhythmia detection by implantable devices. In Ellenbogen KA, Kay GA, Wilkoff BL, eds. Clinical Cardiac Pacing and Defibrillation, 2nd edn. Philadelphia, PA: WB Saunders Company, 2000: 68–126.

37 Mansour F, Khairy P. Programming ICDs in the modern era beyond out-of-the box settings. Pacing Clin Electrophysiol 2011; 34:506–20.

38 Wilkoff BL, Hess M, Young J, Abraham WT. Differences in tachyarrhythmia detection and implantable cardioverter defibrillator therapy by primary or secondary pre-

vention indication in cardiac resynchronization therapy patients. J Cardiovasc Electrophysiol 2004; 15:1002–9.

39 Wilkoff BL, Williamson BD, Stern RS, et al. Strategic programming of detection and therapy parameters in implantable cardioverter-defibrillators reduces shocks in primary prevention patients: results from the PREPARE (Primary Prevention Parameters Evaluation) study. J Am Coll Cardiol 2008; 52:541–50.

40 Gasparini M, Menozzi C, Proclemer A, et al. A simplified biventricular defibrillator with fixed long detection intervals reduces implantable cardioverter defibrillator (ICD) interventions and heart failure hospitalizations in patients with non-ischaemic cardiomyopathy implanted for primary prevention: the RELEVANT [Role of long dEtection window programming in patients with LEft VentriculAr dysfunction, Non-ischemic eTiology in primary prevention treated with a biventricular ICD] study. Eur Heart J 2009; 30:2758–67.

41 Wilkoff BL, Ousdigian KT, Sterns LD, et al. A comparison of empiric to physician-tailored programming of implantable cardioverter-defibrillators: results from the prospective randomized multicenter EMPIRIC trial. J Am Coll Cardiol 2006; 48:330–9.

42 Dorian P, Philippon F, Thibault B, et al. Randomized controlled study of detection enhancements versus rate-only detection to prevent inappropriate therapy in a dual-chamber implantable cardioverter-defibrillator. Heart Rhythm 2004; 1:540–7.

43 Schoels W, Steinhaus D, Johnson WB, et al. Optimizing implantable cardioverter-defibrillator treatment of rapid ventricular tachycardia: antitachycardia pacing therapy during charging. Heart Rhythm 2007; 4:879–85.

44 Swerdlow CD, Shehata, M. Antitachycardia pacing in primary-prevention ICDs. J Cardiovasc Electrophysiol 2010; 21:1355–7.

45 Theuns DA, Klootwijk AP, Goedhat DM, Jordaens LJ. Prevention of inappropriate therapy in implantable cardioverter-defibrillators: results of a prospective, randomized study of tachyarrhythmia detection algorithms. J Am Coll Cardiol 2004; 44:2362–7.

46 Friedman PA, McClelland RL, Bamlet WR, et al. Dual-chamber versus single-chamber detection enhancements for implantable defibrillator rhythm diagnosis: the detect supraventricular tachycardia study. Circulation 2006; 113:2871–9.

47 Namerow PB, Firth BR, Heywood GM, Windle JR, Parides MK. Quality-of-life six months after CABG surgery in patients randomized to ICD versus no ICD therapy: findings from the CABG Patch Trial. Pacing Clin Electrophysiol 1999; 22:1305–13.

48 Pinski SL, Fahy GJ. The proarrhythmic potential of implantable cardioverter-defibrillators. Circulation 1995; 92:1651–64.

49 Swerdlow CD, Ahern T, Chen PS, et al. Underdetection of ventricular tachycardia by algorithms to enhance specificity in a tiered-therapy cardioverter-defibrillator. J Am Coll Cardiol 1994; 24:416–24.

50 Morgan JM, Sterns LD, Hanson JL, Ousdigian KT, Otterness MF, Wilkoff BL. A trial design for evaluation of empiric programming of implantable cardioverter defibrillators to improve patient management. Curr Control Trials Cardiovasc Med 2004; 5:12.

51 Wilkoff BL, Kuhlkamp V, Volosin K, et al. Critical analysis of dual-chamber implantable cardioverter-defibrillator arrhythmia detection: results and technical considerations. Circulation 2001; 103:381–6.

52 Glikson M, Swerdlow CD, Gurevitz OT, et al. Optimal combination of discriminators for differentiating ventricular from supraventricular tachycardia by dual-chamber defibrillators. J Cardiovasc Electrophysiol 2005; 16:732–9.

53 Boriani G, Occhetta E, Pistis G, et al. Combined use of morphology discrimination, sudden onset, and stability as discriminating algorithms in single chamber cardioverter defibrillators. Pacing Clin Electrophysiol 2002; 25:1357–66.

54 Klein GJ, Gillberg JM, Tang A, et al. Improving SVT discrimination in single-chamber ICDs: a new electrogram morphology-based algorithm. J Cardiovasc Electrophysiol 2006; 17:1310–9.

55 Lee MA, Corbisiero R, Nabert DR, et al. Clinical results of an advanced SVT detection enhancement algorithm. Pacing Clin Electrophysiol 2005; 28:1032–40.

56 Corbisiero R, Lee MA, Nabert DR, et al. Performance of a new single-chamber ICD algorithm: discrimination of supraventricular and ventricular tachycardia based on vector timing and correlation. Europace 2006; 8: 1057–61.

57 Brugada J, Mont L, Figueiredo M, Valentino M, Matas M, Navarro-Lopez F. Enhanced detection criteria in implantable defibrillators. J Cardiovasc Electrophysiol 1998; 9: 261–8.

58 Swerdlow CD, Chen PS, Kass RM, Allard JR, Peter CT. Discrimination of ventricular tachycardia from sinus tachycardia and atrial fibrillation in a tiered-therapy cardioverter-defibrillator. J Am Coll Cardiol 1994; 23: 1342–55.

59 Garcia-Alberola A, Yli-Mayry S, Block M, et al. RR interval variability in irregular monomorphic ventricular tachycardia and atrial fibrillation. Circulation 1996; 93: 295–300.

60 Swerdlow CD, Ahern T, Chen PS, et al. Underdetection of ventricular tachycardia by algorithms to enhance specificity in a tiered therapy cardioverter-defibrillator. J Am Coll Cardiol 1994; 24:416–24.

61 Schaumann A, von zur Muhlen F, Gonska BD, Kreuzer H. Enhanced detection criteria in implantable cardioverter-defibrillators to avoid inappropriate therapy. Am J Cardiol 1996; 78:42–50.

62 Lavergne T, Daubert JC, Chauvin M, et al. Preliminary clinical experience with the first dual chamber pacemaker defibrillator. Pacing Clin Electrophysiol 1997; 20:182–8.

63 Kühlkamp V, Dbrnberger V, Mewis C, Suchalla R, Bosch RF, Seipel L. Clinical experience with the new detection algorithms for atrial fibrillation of a defibrillator with dual chamber sensing and pacing. J Cardiovasc Electrophysiol 1999; 10:905–15.

64 Stadler RW. An adaptive interval-based algorithm for withholding ICD therapy during sinus tachycardia. Pacing Clin Electrophysiol 2003; 26:1189–201.

65 Li HG, Thakur RK, Yee R, Klein GJ. Ventriculoatrial conduction in patients with implantable cardioverter defibrillators: implications for tachycardia discrimination by dual chamber sensing. Pacing Clin Electrophysiol 1994; 17:2304–6.

66 Militianu A, Salacata A, Meissner MD, et al. Ventriculoatrial conduction capability and prevalence of 1:1 retrograde conduction during inducible sustained monomorphic ventricular tachycardia in 305 implantable cardioverter defibrillator recipients. Pacing Clin Electrophysiol 1997; 20:2378–84.

67 Almendral J, Arribas F, Quesada A, et al. Are dual chamber ICDs beneficial? The DATAS trial: a randomised trial focused on clinically significant adverse events. Presented at 15th Cardiostim, Nice, 16 June 2006.

68 Israel CW, Gronefeld G, Iscolo N, Stoppler C, Hohnloser SH. Discrimination between ventricular and supraventricular tachycardia by dual chamber cardioverter defibrillators: importance of the atrial sensing function. Pacing Clin Electrophysiol 2001; 24:183–90.

69 Asirvatham SJ, Bruce CJ, Danielsen A, et al. Intramyocardial pacing and sensing for the enhancement of cardiac stimulation and sensing specificity. Pacing Clin Electrophysiol 2007; 30:748–54.

70 de Voogt W, Van Hemel N, Willems A, et al. Far-field R-wave reduction with a novel lead design: experimental and human results. Pacing Clin Electrophysiol 2005; 28:782–8.

71 Kuhlkamp V, Dornberger V, Mewis C, et al. Clinical experience with the new detection algorithms for atrial fibrillation of a defibrillator with dual chamber sensing and pacing. J Cardiovasc Electrophysiol 1999; 10:905–15.

72 Gold MR, Ahmad S, Browne K, Berg KC, Thackeray L, Berger RD. Prospective comparison of discrimination algorithms to prevent inappropriate ICD therapy: primary results of the Rhythm ID Going Head to Head Trial (RIGHT). Heart Rhythm 2012; 9:370–7.

73 Olson WH. Dual chamber sensing and detection for implantable cardioverter-defibrillators. In: Singer I, Barold SS, Camm AJ, eds. Nonpharmacological Therapy of Arrhythmias for the 21st Century: The State of the Art. Armonk, NY: Futura Publishing Co., 1998: 385–421.

74 Gard JJ, Friedman PA. Strategies to reduce ICD shocks: the role of supraventricular tachycardia–ventricular tachycardia discriminators. Card Electrophysiol Clin 2011; 3:373–87.

75 Auricchio A, Meijer A, Kurita T, et al. Safety, efficacy, and performance of new discrimination algorithms to reduce inappropriate and unnecessary shocks: the PainFree SST clinical study design. Europace 2011; 13:1484–93.

76 Swerdlow CD, Friedman PA. Advanced ICD troubleshooting: Part I. Pacing Clin Electrophysiol 2005; 28:1322–46.

77 Boriani G, Biffi M, Dall'Acqua A, et al. Rhythm discrimination by rate branch and QRS morphology in dual chamber implantable cardioverter defibrillators. Pacing Clin Electrophysiol 2003; 26:466–70.

78 Hammill SC, Packer DL, Stanton MS, Fetter J. Termination and acceleration of ventricular tachycardia with autodecremental pacing, burst pacing, and cardioversion in patients with an implantable cardioverter defibrillator. Multicenter PCD Investigator Group. Pacing Clin Electrophysiol 1995; 18:3–10.

79 Bardy GH, Poole JE, Kudenchuk PJ, Dolack GL, Kelso D, Mitchell R. A prospective randomized repeat-crossover comparison of antitachycardia pacing with low-energy cardioversion. Circulation 1993; 87:1889–96.

80 Calkins H, el-Atassi R, Kalbfleisch S, Langberg J, Morady F. Comparison of fixed burst versus decremental burst pacing for termination of ventricular tachycardia. Pacing Clin Electrophysiol 1993; 16:26–32.

81 Wietholt D, Block M, Isbruch F, et al. Clinical experience with antitachycardia pacing and improved detection algorithms in a new implantable cardioverter-defibrillator. J Am Coll Cardiol 1993; 21:885–94.

82 Sweeney MO. Antitachycardia pacing for ventricular tachycardia using implantable cardioverter defibrillators: substrates, methods and clinical experience. Pacing Clin Electrophysiol 2004; 27:1292–305.

83 Wathen MS, Sweeney MO, DeGroot PJ, et al. Shock reduction using antitachycardia pacing for spontaneous rapid ventricular tachycardia in patients with coronary artery disease. Circulation 2001; 104:796–801.

84 Josephson ME. Clinical Cardiac Electrophysiology: Techniques and Interpretation, 2nd edn. Philadelphia, PA: Lea & Febiger, 1993: 417–615.

85 Sweeney MO. Antitachycardia pacing for ventricular tachycardia using implantable cardioverter defibrillators: substrates, methods and clinical experience. Pacing Clin Electrophysiol 2004; 27:1292–305.

86 Wathen MS, DeGroot PJ, Sweeney MO, et al. Prospective randomized multicenter trial of empirical antitachycardia pacing versus shocks for spontaneous rapid ventricular tachycardia in patients with implantable cardioverter-defibrillators: Pacing Fast Ventricular Tachycardia Reduces Shock Therapies (PainFREE Rx II) trial results. Circulation 2004; 110:2591–6.

87 Schaumann A, von zur Muhlen F, Herse B, Gonska BD, Kreuzer H. Empirical versus tested antitachycardia pacing in implantable cardioverter defibrillators: a prospective study including 200 patients. Circulation 1998; 97: 66–74.

88 Gulizia MM, Piraino L, Scherillo M, et al. A randomized study to compare ramp versus burst antitachycardia pacing therapies to treat fast ventricular tachyarrhythmias in patients with implantable cardioverter defibrillators: the PITAGORA ICD trial. Circ Arrhythm Electrophysiol 2009; 2:146–53.

89 Gasparini M, Anselme F, Clementy J, et al. BIVentricular versus right ventricular antitachycardia pacing to terminate ventricular tachyarrhythmias in patients receiving cardiac resynchronization therapy: the ADVANCE CRT-D Trial. Am Heart J 2010; 159:1116–23.

90 Ellenbogen KA, Levine JH, Berger RD, et al. Are implantable cardioverter defibrillator shocks a surrogate for sudden cardiac death in patients with nonischemic cardiomyopathy? Circulation 2006; 113:776–82.

91 Grimm W, Menz V, Hoffmann J, Maisch B. Failure of third-generation implantable cardioverter defibrillators to abort shock therapy for nonsustained ventricular tachycardia due to shortcomings of the VF confirmation algorithm. Pacing Clin Electrophysiol 1998; 21:722–7.

92 Mann DE, Kelly PA, Reiter MJ. Inappropriate shock therapy for nonsustained ventricular tachycardia in a dual chamber pacemaker defibrillator. Pacing Clin Electrophysiol 1998; 21:2005–6.

93 Kouakam C, Lauwerier B, Klug D, et al. Effect of elevated heart rate preceding the onset of ventricular tachycardia on antitachycardia pacing effectiveness in patients with implantable cardioverter defibrillators. Am J Cardiol 2003; 92:26–32.

94 Nof E, Glikson M, Luria D, Gard J, Friedman P. Beyond sudden death prevention: minimizing ICD shocks and morbidity, and optimizing efficacy. In Gussak I, Antzelevitch C, eds. Electrical Diseases of the Heart. Springer: (in press).

95 Pacifico A, Johnson JW, Stanton MS, et al. Comparison of results in two implantable defibrillators. Jewel 7219D Investigators. Am J Cardiol 1998; 82:875–80.

96 Hoffmann E, Steinbeck G. Experience with pectoral versus abdominal implantation of a small defibrillator: a multicenter comparison in 778 patients. European Jewel Investigators. Eur Heart J 1998; 19:1085–98.

97 Sticherling C, Klingenheben T, Cameron D, Hohnloser SH. Worldwide clinical experience with a down-sized active can implantable cardioverter defibrillator in 162 consecutive patients. Worldwide 7221 ICD Investigators. Pacing Clin Electrophysiol 1998; 21:1778–83.

98 Mehdirad AA, Love CJ, Stanton MS, Strickberger SA, Duncan JL, Kroll MW. Preliminary clinical results of a biphasic waveform and an RV lead system. Pacing Clin Electrophysiol 1999; 22:594–9.

99 Boriani G, Frabetti L, Biffi M, Sallusti L. Clinical experience with downsized lower energy output implantable cardioverter defibrillators. Ventak Mini II Clinical Investigators. Int J Cardiol 1998; 66:261–6.

100 Swerdlow CD, Russo AM, Degroot PJ. The dilemma of ICD implant testing. Pacing Clin Electrophysiol 2007; 30:675–700.

101 Wilkoff BL, Stern R, Williamson B, et al. Design of the Primary Prevention Parameters Evaluation (PREPARE) trial of implantable cardioverter defibrillators to reduce patient morbidity. Trials 2006; 7:18.

102 Glikson M, Beeman AL, Luria DM, et al. Impaired detection of ventricular tachyarrhythmias by a rate-smoothing algorithm in dualchamber implantable defibrillators: intradevice interactions. J Cardiovasc Electrophysiol 2002; 13:312–8.

103 Camm AJ, Kirchhof P, Lip GY, et al. Guidelines for the management of atrial fibrillation: the Task Force for the Management of Atrial Fibrillation of the European Society of Cardiology (ESC). Eur Heart J 2010; 31:2369–429.

104 Bruce GK, Friedman PA. Device-based therapies for atrial fibrillation. Curr Treat Options Cardiovasc Med 2005; 7:359–70.

105 Sweeney MO, Bank AJ, Nsah E, et al. Minimizing ventricular pacing to reduce atrial fibrillation in sinus-node disease. N Engl J Med 2007; 357:1000–8.

106 Friedman PA, Dijkman B, Warman EN, et al. Atrial therapies reduce atrial arrhythmia burden in defibrillator patients. Circulation 2001; 104:1023–8.

107 Jung J, Heisel A, Fries R, Kollner V. Tolerability of internal low-energy shock strengths currently needed for endocardial atrial cardioversion. Am J Cardiol 1997; 80:1489–90.

108 Wood MA, Stambler BS, Damiano RJ, Greenway P, Ellenbogen KA. Lessons learned from data logging in a multicenter clinical trial using a late-generation implantable cardioverter-defibrillator. J Am Coll Cardiol 1994; 24:1692–9.

109 Schmitt C, Montero M, Melichercik J. Significance of supraventricular tachyarrhythmias in patients with implanted pacing cardioverter defibrillators. Pacing Clin Electrophysiol 1994; 17:295–302.

110 Grimm W, Flores BF, Marchlinski FE. Electrocardiographically documented unnecessary, spontaneous shocks in 241 patients with implantable cardioverter defibrillators. Pacing Clin Electrophysiol 1992; 15:1667–73.

111 Ahmad M, Bloomstein L, Roelke M, Bernstein AD, Parsonnet V. Patients' attitudes toward implanted defibrillator shocks. Pacing Clin Electrophysiol 2000; 23:934–8.

112 Poole JE, Johnson GW, Hellkamp AS, et al. Prognostic importance of defibrillator shocks in patients with heart failure. N Engl J Med 2008; 359:1009–17.

113 Sweeney MO, Sherfesee L, DeGroot PJ, Wathen MS, Wilkoff BL. Differences in effects of electrical therapy type for ventricular arrhythmias on mortality in implantable cardioverter-defibrillator patients. Heart Rhythm 2010; 7:353–60.

114 Powell BD, Saxon LA, Boehmer JP. Survival after shock therapy in ICD and CRT-D recipients according to rhythm shocked: The Altitude Study Group. in 22nd Heart Rhythm Society Scientific Session Late-Breaking Abstract Session. 2011. San Francisco, CA.

115 Sharma AD, Rizo-Patron C, Hallstrom AP, et al. Percent right ventricular pacing predicts outcomes in the DAVID trial. Heart Rhythm 2005; 2:830–4.

116 Steinberg JS, Fischer A, Wang P, et al. The clinical implications of cumulative right ventricular pacing in the multicenter automatic defibrillator trial II. J Cardiovasc Electrophysiol 2005; 16:359–65.

117 Sweeney MO, Hellkamp AS, Ellenbogen KA, et al. Adverse effect of ventricular pacing on heart failure and atrial fibrillation among patients with normal baseline QRS duration in a clinical trial of pacemaker therapy for sinus node dysfunction. Circulation 2003; 107:2932–7.

118 Wilkoff BL, Ousdigian KT, Sterns LD, et al. A comparison of empiric to physician-tailored programming of

implantable cardioverter-defibrillators: results from the Prospective Randomized Multicenter EMPIRIC Trial. J Am Coll Cardiol 2006; 48:330–9.

119 Wilkoff BL, Williamson BD, Stern RS, *et al*. Strategic programming of detection and therapy parameters in implantable cardioverter-defibrillators reduces shocks in primary prevention patients: results from the PREPARE (Primary Prevention Parameters Evaluation) Study. J Am Coll Cardiol 2008; 52:541–50.

120 Gilliam FR, Hayes DL, Boehmer JP, *et al*. Real world evaluation of dual-zone ICD and CRT-D programming compared to single-zone programming: the ALTITUDE REDUCES study. J Cardiovasc Electrophysiol 2011; 22:1023–9.

121 Hayes DL, Boehmer JP, Day JD, *et al*. Cardiac resynchronization therapy and the relationship of percent biventricular pacing to symptoms and survival. Heart Rhythm 2011; 8:1469–75.

122 Dong K, Shen WK, Powell BD, *et al*. Atrioventricular nodal ablation predicts survival benefit in patients with atrial fibrillation receiving cardiac resynchronization therapy. Heart Rhythm 2010; 7:1240–5.

123 O'Donnell D, Nadurata V, Hamer A, Kertes P, Mohammed W. Bifocal right ventricular cardiac resynchronization therapies in patients with unsuccessful percutaneous lateral left ventricular venous access. Pacing Clin Electrophysiol 2005; 28:S27–S30.

124 Kamdar R, Frain E, Warburton F, *et al*. A prospective comparison of echocardiography and device algorithms for atrioventricular and interventricular interval optimization in cardiac resynchronization therapy. Europace 2010; 12:84–91.

125 Ellenbogen KA, Gold MR, Meyer TE, *et al*. Primary results from the SmartDelay determined AV optimization: a comparison to other AV delay methods used in cardiac resynchronization therapy (SMART-AV) trial: a randomized trial comparing empirical, echocardiography-guided, and algorithmic atrioventricular delay programming in cardiac resynchronization therapy. Circulation 2010; 122:2660–8.

9 Sensor Technology for Rate-Adaptive Pacing and Hemodynamic Optimization

David L. Hayes, Samuel J. Asirvatham, Paul A. Friedman
Mayo Clinic, Rochester, MN, USA

Indications for rate-adaptive pacing 408
Sensors available for rate-adaptive pacing 408
  Activity sensors 409
    Piezoelectric crystal (vibration sensor) 409
    Accelerometer (acceleration sensor) 410
  Minute ventilation sensors 411
  SonR sensor (previously called peak endocardial acceleration sensor) 411
  Right ventricular impedance-based sensor 412
  Stimulus-T or QT, sensing pacemaker 414
  Other sensors 414

Dual-sensor rate-adaptive pacing 415
Sensor applications for hemodynamic management 418
Programming 418
  Programmable parameters 420
Rate-adaptive pacing with cardiac resynchronization devices 424
  AV and V-V timing 424
Future of rate-adaptive sensors 425
References 425

Cardiac Pacing, Defibrillation and Resynchronization: A Clinical Approach, Third Edition.
David L. Hayes, Samuel J. Asirvatham, and Paul A. Friedman.
© 2013 Mayo Foundation for Medical Education and Research. Published 2013 by John Wiley & Sons, Ltd.

Rate-adaptive pacing has been a mainstay of bradycardia pacing programming for many years. The hemodynamic advantages of rate-adaptive modes, i.e., VVIR vs. VVI, AAIR vs. AAI, and DDDR vs. DDD, have been recognized since very early in the rate-adaptive pacing experience. Similarly, when dual-chamber rate-adaptive pacing was introduced, literature emerged demonstrating hemodynamic superiority of DDDR over DDD in the chronotropically incompetent patient. Rate-adaptive pacing may be similarly beneficial with cardiac resynchronization therapy (CRT) devices. Although there are other benefits of rate-adaptive pacing, correcting the chronotropic response remains the most important.

Indications for rate-adaptive pacing

The indications for rate-adaptive pacing are relatively straightforward (also reviewed in Chapter 2: Hemodynamics of Cardiac Pacing). VVIR pacing is indicated primarily for the patient with chronic atrial fibrillation and a slow ventricular response that requires bradycardia support. AAIR, not widely used, is appropriate for the patient with sinus node dysfunction and intact atrioventricular (AV) node conduction. Even though a significant number of patients require permanent pacing for sinus node dysfunction, many clinicians remain uncomfortable with a system that does not provide ventricular pacing support.

Chronotropic incompetence also remains the primary indication for DDDR pacing. However, pulse generators with the option of rate-adaptive pacing are reasonable to consider for any patient requiring dual-chamber pacing because of the clinical flexibility it may provide in the future. For example, should atrial fibrillation develop in a patient with a dual-chamber rate adaptive pacemaker, the pacemaker can be programmed to a single-chamber rate-adaptive mode, i.e., VVIR. In addition, if the patient has symptoms with traditional DDD upper rate response, i.e., symptomatic 2:1 AV block, optimal programming of sensor response in a DDDR pacemaker will minimize V-V cycle length variation.

Sensors available for rate-adaptive pacing

Sensors can also be classified as open-loop or closed-loop (Fig. 9.1). All commercially available sensors are open-loop sensors to some extent, in that the parameter being sensed requires input externally to optimize sensor response, and the sensor is unable to react appropriately to stimuli that do not affect the specific sensor. Conversely, a closed-loop system ideally does not require external input or manipulation because intrinsic feedback to the sensor self-regulates its response.

The ideal closed-loop sensor should closely mimic the normal sinus node and not require external input for programming. To mirror normal sinus node function, the sensor should have an anticipatory increase in heart rate prior to activity, increase the heart rate in proportion to the intensity of activity, gradually allow heart rate to return to normal after cessation of activity, and respond to nonphysical exertion (emotion). These characteristics of the ideal sensor are summarized in Table 9.1.

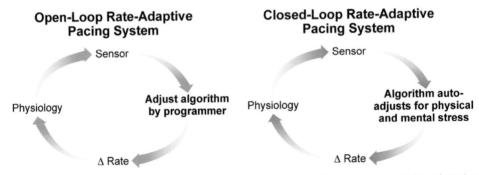

Fig. 9.1 Open-loop and closed-loop sensors. In the open-loop design, the parameter detected by the sensor is translated to a change in rate by use of an algorithm. Altering or optimizing the sensor requires input by the clinician. The rate change that results from the sensor activation does not have any negative feedback effect on the parameter that is being sensed. In the closed-loop design, the physiologic parameter, ideally both physical and mental, detected by the sensor is translated to a change in rate by use of an algorithm. However, the rate change resulting from sensor activation results in a change in the physiologic parameter in the opposite direction, i.e., a negative feedback loop. For a true closed-loop sensor, clinician input should not be necessary; that is, the ideal physiologic parameter that responds proportionally to all forms of stress should not need external input or manipulation by the clinician.

A variety of sensors appropriate for rate-adaptive pacing have been developed and clinically assessed; they are displayed in Fig. 9.2 as end-points of some physiologic response. Only a few of these sensors are clinically available. Others have previously been investigated and subsequently abandoned commercially. Even though some sensors may never have been clinically released as single-sensor rate-adaptive pacing systems, some iteration of the sensor technology may eventually be used for hemodynamic autoregulation in CRT or stand-alone implantable diagnostic devices.

Two varieties of sensors account for most rate-adaptive pacing systems worldwide. Activity sensing and minute ventilation have been the primary rate-adaptive pacing systems in the USA and have also been widely used throughout the world. Stimulus-T, or QT,

sensing pacemakers as well as an impedance-based sensor have been used less extensively but are currently in use. In some markets outside the USA another type of accelerometer is used that is incorporated into the tip of the pacing lead, originally known as "peak endocardial accelerating."

Activity sensors

Piezoelectric crystal (vibration sensor)

Activity-controlled pacing with vibration detection remains the most widely used form of rate adaptation because it is simple, easy to apply clinically, and rapid in onset of rate response (Fig. 9.3). The piezoelectric crystal is bonded to the inside wall of the pulse generator can. As the body moves and generates low-frequency vibrations that are transmitted to the torso, the piezoelectric crystal is slightly deformed. With the slight deformation the piezoelectric crystal produces a weak electrical current, which is then used as the basis of the algorithm to adjust the pacing rate.

The generated electrical currents from the piezoelectric crystal are "counted" based on the size of the output and whether it is large enough to cross a specified threshold. The number of outputs counted, i.e., the number that will meet criteria to alter the heart rate, is therefore a function of both the "size" of the signal (in turn dependent on the extent of movement) and the sensitivity to which the sensor threshold is programmed (Fig. 9.4).

Table 9.1 Characteristics of the ideal rate-adaptive sensor.

- *Proportional* to the level of metabolic demand
- *Speed of response* is appropriate to the onset and offset of metabolic demand
- *Sensitive* enough to detect both exercise and nonexercise (emotional) needs for rate increase
- *Specific* enough not to be influenced by signals not representing metabolic demand
- *Standard pacing lead* supports the rate-adaptive pacing system
- *Stability* of sensor in the long term
- *Easy* to program

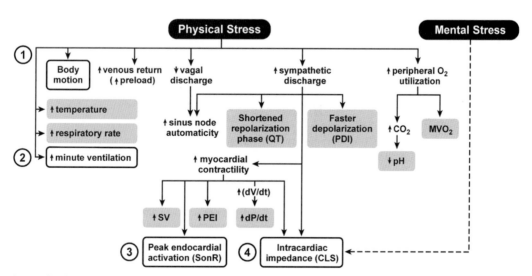

Fig. 9.2 Physiologic responses that have been investigated or clinically used for rate adaptation of permanent pacemakers. The boxed terms represent the end-points used for rate adaptation. PDI, paced depolarization integral; PEI, pre-ejection interval; MVO₂, myocardial oxygen consumption; SV, stroke volume.

Accelerometer (acceleration sensor)

The main difference between the piezoelectric crystal sensor and the accelerometer relates to the way in which the sensor is mounted within the pacemaker as well as the way in which the signal is utilized by the pacemaker. As opposed to being bonded to the inside of the pulse generator can, the accelerometer is suspended from the hybrid circuitry by a cantilever beam (Fig. 9.5). Movement that is perpendicular to the plane of the sensor generates an electrical signal that is then used to alter the pacing rate. Instead of counting signals above a certain threshold like a piezoelectric crystal, the accelerometer integrates the voltage that arises from the piezoelement. The pacemaker then differentially "weights" deflections of large amplitude, which allows a more proportional rate response to a given level of exertion to be achieved (Fig. 9.6).

The ability to respond to anterior/posterior motion allows accelerometer-based systems to respond more appropriately to specific activities, such as cycling. For example, the typical cyclist may not generate much vibratory sensation above the trunk level, which could result in a rate-adaptive pacemaker that incorporates a piezoelectric crystal having a limited response during the activity. Another advantage of the accelerometer is improved specificity of sensor response, i.e., it results in fewer inappropriate responses. For example, a vibration sensor will usually result in a greater rate increase when walking down stairs than walking up stairs because more vibration is generated walking down a flight of stairs.

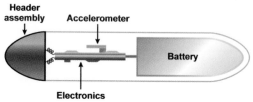

Fig. 9.5 Schematic drawing of how an activity sensor using an accelerometer is positioned within the pulse generator. The accelerometer is mounted on the hybrid circuitry of the pacemaker and is structurally insulated from the pacemaker can, i.e., independent of the mechanical forces of the surrounding tissue but dependent on patient motion. Signals can be processed by "peak counting" or acceleration integration. Acceleration integration achieved with the accelerometer allows all signals to be used to determine the level of rate response, because there is no amplitude threshold that must be exceeded.

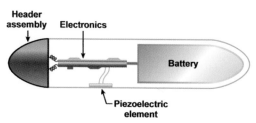

Fig. 9.3 Schematic drawing of how an activity sensor using a piezoelectric crystal is positioned within the pulse generator. The piezoelectric sensor was bonded to the inside surface of the pacemaker can and senses tissue vibration from mechanical forces transmitted by the surrounding tissues.

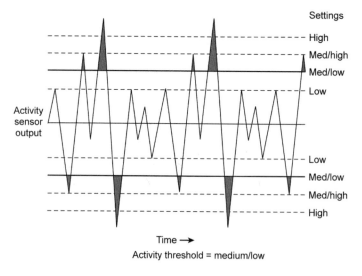

Fig. 9.4 Signals from a piezoelectric crystal. Various sized signals will be acted upon based on how the threshold of the sensor is programmed and whether a given signal or oscillation crosses the sensor threshold. (Redrawn from Medtronic, Adapta Technical Manual, pp. 2–15, with permission.)

Sensor

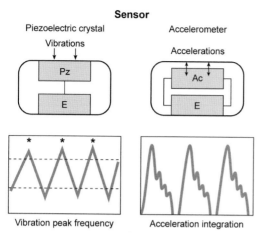

Fig. 9.6 Schematic comparison of how signals are processed in a piezoelectric crystal sensor vs. accelerometer-based sensor. The piezoelectric crystal will count any signal that crosses a given threshold. The accelerometer sensor integrates the voltages of the signals that come from the sensor element.

Rhythmic body motion such as that produced by walking or bicycle riding is typically in the range of 1–8 Hz. Non-exercise-related vibrations that arise from such sources as riding in a car or from nonspecific skeletal muscle noise are often >10 Hz. The accelerometer, which limits analysis of signals to the 1–10 Hz range, should be more specific in its response to activity.

There have been other variations of activity sensors but none has had the clinical success of the accelerometer.

Although accelerometers overcome some of the difficulties with piezoelectric crystal sensors, some problems remain. With prolonged duration activity, the amount of acceleration remains constant, but the physiologic demand for a higher heart rate increases. The extent of acceleration may be similar climbing uphill or moving downhill, but with considerably different requirement for increase in heart rate. Strenuous isometric exercise typically results in an increase in sinus rate, but will not be proportionately increased with accelerometer-based rate-adaptive pacing. In addition, neither vibration nor acceleration sensors will respond to non-movement-based exertion such as emotion or fever.

The overall experience with activity sensors has been very positive and even though accelerometer-based activity sensors now dominate the market and have theoretical and real advantages in some patients, the potential superiority of accelerometer-based technology is difficult to substantiate.[1]

Minute ventilation sensors

Minute volume (respiratory rate × tidal volume) has an excellent correlation with metabolic demand. There is a near-linear relationship between minute ventilation and heart rate below approximately 70% of VO_2max.[2] At higher workloads, minute ventilation increases more rapidly and this has to be taken into account in minute ventilation pacing algorithms to prevent an inappropriately high pacing rate.

For the purpose of rate-adaptive pacing minute volume measurement is accomplished as follows. Every 50 ms (20 Hz) the device will drive a current waveform between the pacemaker and the ring electrode (320 mA). The device then detects the resulting voltage between the lead tip and indifferent electrode on the header of the can (Fig. 9.7). When both current and voltage are known, transthoracic impedance can be measured between the ring electrode and the pacemaker can. Because transthoracic impedance varies with respiration and its amplitude varies with tidal volume, the impedance measurement can be used to determine respiratory rate and tidal volume, which in turn can be used to alter pacing rate.

Although the sensor has performed well clinically and the long-term reliability of the minute volume sensor has been excellent, the initial rate response of early minute volume sensors, i.e., at the onset of exercise, compared with an acceleration sensor, was often slower but subsequent generations of the sensor have improved the initial rate response. Inappropriate activation of a minute ventilation sensor is possible with coughing, abnormal breathing patterns, e.g., Cheyne–Stokes breathing, and at times by upper extremity movement. Inappropriate activation of a minute ventilation sensor may also occur when the patient is connected to some electrocardiogram (ECG) monitors that are also capable of documenting ventilatory frequency.[3]

SonR sensor (previously called peak endocardial acceleration sensor)

In healthy persons, the autonomic nervous system adjusts cardiac output to meet hemodynamic and metabolic requirements. Even in persons with chronotropic insufficiency, the autonomic nervous system controls the performance of the heart through changes in myocardial contractility.

SonR utilizes a microaccelerometer inside a hermetically sealed capsule incorporated in the tip of the pacing lead (Fig. 9.8). The microaccelerometer measures the amplitude of mechanical vibrations that are generated by the myocardium during the isovolumetric contraction phase of the cardiac cycle. The signal obtained is directly related to contractility of the myocardium and peak-to-peak values of the signal are

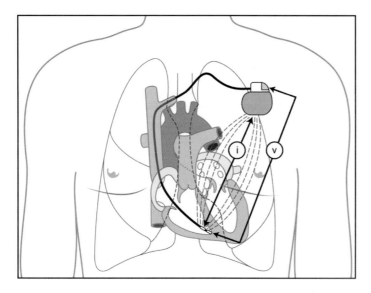

Fig. 9.7 The pacemaker sends a current (i) between the ring electrode and the pacemaker can. The sensor detects voltage (v) modulations between the tip electrode and the indifferent electrode on the pacemaker header that occur as a result of changes in transthoracic impedance.

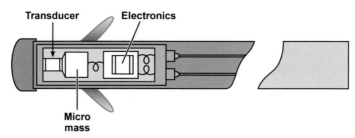

Fig. 9.8 Peak endocardial acceleration pacing system. The sensor is a microaccelerometer housed inside a rigid, perfectly hermetic capsule within the distal portion of the lead. An associated electronic circuit preprocesses the signal to ensure its correct transmission through the catheter. The rigidity of the capsule allegedly makes the sensor totally insensitive to ventricular pressures and to fibrosis on the lead tip, so that the sensor is sensitive only to the inertial forces generated by myocardial movement.

measured, i.e., peak endocardial acceleration (PEA) (Fig. 9.9). An algorithm calculates the pacing rate based on the variation of the peak endocardial signals against a dynamic reference value.[4]

Multiple studies have shown the sensor to be stable and reliable. In fact, as the lead becomes more fibrosed at the lead–myocardial interface there is even better transmission of myocardial signals, further improving sensor function.

Given the ability to detect early changes in contractility, the sensor has been investigated in patients with malignant vasodepressor syncope. Given the potential ability to react with a change in pacing rate prior to any systemic symptoms from a fall in heart rate or blood pressure (Fig. 9.10), SonR has been shown in small studies to have potential advantages in this group of patients.[5,6]

Although successful for rate adaptive pacing, the current application of this technology is for hemodynamics monitoring in CRT-D (see later).[7]

Right ventricular impedance-based sensor

Measuring intracardiac impedance can be used realtime as the basis for a rate-adaptive sensor. Multiple iterations of impedance based sensors have been tried.[8] Currently, one is commercially available.

Closed Loop Stimulation (CLS) translates myocardial contractility (inotropy) into rate variations mediated by the patients's own cardiovascular control system. It monitors and processes an intracardiac impedance signal associated with myocardial contraction dynamics on a beat-to-beat basis. The inotropic state of the heart is calculated through the use of subthreshold unipolar impedance measurements between the right ventricular

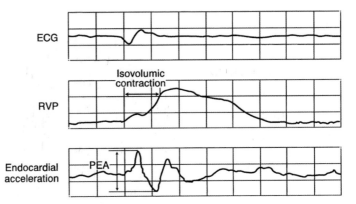

Fig. 9.9 Simultaneous electrocardiogram (ECG), right ventricular pressure (RVP) curve, and peak endocardial acceleration (PEA) waveform. The PEA is represented by the peak-to-peak value of the endocardial acceleration signal measured inside a time window containing the isovolumic contraction phase. (Reproduced with permission from Sorin Biomedica.)

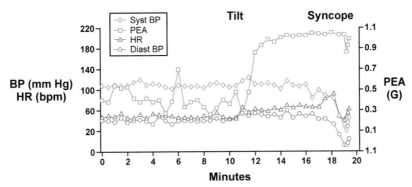

Fig. 9.10 Blood pressure (BP), heart rate (HR) and peak endocardial acceleration (PEA) measurements from a patient undergoing tilt testing for presumed neurocardiogenic syncope. The PEA increases dramatically at approximately 11 min. The patient subsequently has typical symptoms accompanied by a decrease in BP and HR approximately 7 min later. Reacting to the earlier increase in PEA has been shown in some patients to prevent or minimize the subsequent vasodepression. (Modified from Deharo JC, Peyre JP, Chalvidan T, *et al.* Continuous monitoring of an endocardial index of myocardial contractility during head-up tilt test. Am Heart J 2000; 139:1022–30, by permission of Futura Publishing Co.)

(RV) lead tip and the pacemaker can (Fig. 9.11). The impedance measurements correlate with dP/dt$_{max}$, which is a surrogate for ventricular contractility and in turn is a reflection of autonomic activity.[9,10] The impedance measured reflects changes in the proportion of blood and myocardium surrounding the electrode tip, which translates into ventricular contractility. As the myocardium reacts to changing demands, the impedance signal changes and the pacemaker drives the heart rate appropriately. Because CLS integrates directly into the cardiovascular control loop, it inherently benefits from the negative feedback system and cannot significantly overrespond or underrespond to physiologic variables, as long as the autonomic nervous system is intact. For

example, if CLS applies too much rate response to a particular stimulus, the autonomic nervous system will determine that the mean atrial blood pressure is too high for the given level of stress. The result is a decrease in contractility, which automatically reduces the CLS pacing rate. Therefore, the negative feedback provides CLS with normal physiologic control, allows optimal perfusion pressure, and maintains homeostasis. CLS differs from other sensors because its rate adaption is based on the principle of translating physiologic factors that influence cardiac demand into patient specific pacing rates. CLS has been US Food and Drug Administration (FDA) approved to respond to physiologic demands and acute mental stress.[11,12]

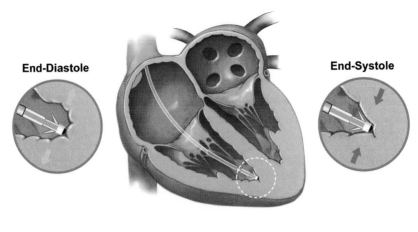

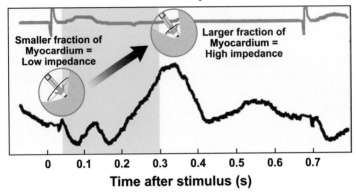

Fig. 9.11 Schematic representation of how changes in myocardial contractility are mapped to the time course of an impedance signal as a shift of the intracardiac impedance signal and used to derive a rate control parameter to assess the beat-by-beat changes in cardiac contraction. ms, milliseconds; a.u., arbitrary units for impedance. (Redrawn from Pieragnoli P, Colella A, Michellucci A, *et al.* A new algorithm for closed-loop stimulation: a feasibility study. Pacing Clin Electrophysiol 2003; 26:229–32, with permission.)

Changes in contraction dynamics result in changes in impedance. CLS can recognize these changes in impedance as predictors of syncope. The pacemaker reacts to such changes in the impedance curve with a proportional increase of the pacing rate in the range between the basic rate and the maximum sensor rate. As a therapy for neurocardiogenic syncope, CLS, with the resting rate control function turned off, interferes with any motion state as soon as the sympathetic system is activated causing an increase in contractility and can prevent an inadequate drop in the heart rate by accelerating the pacing rate.[13,14]

Stimulus-T or QT, sensing pacemaker
The interval from the onset of a paced QRS complex to the end of the T wave was used for rate-adaptive pacing for many years and although some devices with this sensor remain in service, it is no longer commercially available. Autonomic activity and heart rate affect this stimulus-T interval. Because of this relationship, measurement of the stimulus-T interval, a reflection of sympathetic activity, can be used for rate adaptation.

By definition, the "stimulus-T" sensor requires that a pacing stimulus be present and the "T" wave must be detectable. Given the preference to avoid right ventricular pacing when not necessary, the requirement for right ventricular pacing with this sensor was a significant disadvantage. In addition there were patients in which there was difficulty detecting and measuring the "stimulus-T" interval resulting in inappropriate sensor-driven rates.[15]

Other sensors
Several other rate-adaptive sensors have been used either investigationally or in commercially available pulse generators for a relatively brief period.

Temperature-sensing rate-adaptive pacemakers were available for a number of years, but never gained widespread acceptance, in part because a special pacing lead that incorporated a thermistor for temperature measurement was required. Also, because of the relatively slow response of central venous temperature, the sensor was somewhat slow to react and delivered a suboptimal rate response at low workloads.

The pre-ejection interval, the systolic interval from the onset of electrical ventricular depolarization to the onset of ventricular ejection, was used as a physiologic parameter for rate-adaptive pacing. For ventricular pacing, the pre-ejection interval is the interval between a RV pacing stimulus and the onset of contraction determined by an impedance catheter. The pre-ejection interval shortens as exercise workload increases, and this effect can be used as a signal to increase the pacing rate. An increase in heart rate does not appreciably affect the pre-ejection interval, i.e., no significant positive feedback occurs.

Stroke volume, also measured by an impedance catheter in the RV, has been used for rate-adaptive pacing by incorporation of a pacing algorithm that alters the pacing rate to keep the RV stroke volume relatively constant and within physiologic values.

Change in RV pressure, dP/dt, can be measured by a pressure transducer incorporated in the RV portion of the pacing lead. In clinical investigations and in follow-up, the sensor performed well but was never included in a market-approved device.

Mixed venous oxygen saturation, measured by hemoreflectance oximetry, varies with physical activity and changes rapidly with the onset of exercise (Fig. 9.12). For a rate-adaptive pacing system, the oximeter is incorporated within the pacing lead. There were early concerns about long-term stability and reliability of the sensor, but subsequent investigations suggest that it may be possible to design an O_2 saturation sensor that will have long-term stability and reliability.[16] This sensor also has potential advantages for hemodynamic management as well as management of comorbidities of the heart failure patient.

Paced depolarization integral, another sensor used many years ago, refers to the vector integral of the paced QRS, or ventricular depolarization gradient (VDG). During fixed-rate ventricular pacing, exercise and the effect of circulating catecholamines decrease the VDG. An increase in pacing rate increases the VDG. In a normal heart, therefore, the VDG should remain relatively unchanged during exercise and other forms of stress, representing a closed-loop rate-adaptive pacing system.

Dual-sensor rate-adaptive pacing

The overall performance of market-approved, single-sensor, rate-adaptive systems has been excellent. However, the perfect sensor would mimic the response of the normal sinus node at all levels of activity and during emotional stress and would be resistant to non-physiologic stimuli.

A multisensor rate-adaptive pacing system has the ability to improve specificity by having one sensor verify or cross-check the other. For example, with two operational sensors, if the first sensor indicated a rate response to a given stimulus, but the second sensor indicated that a rate increase was inappropriate, no rate increase would occur. Both sensors would have to indicate a rate increase before it would be allowed.

Because some sensors perform in a more physiologic manner at low levels of exercise and others perform in a more physiologic manner at high levels of exercise, a combination of two or more sensors has the potential

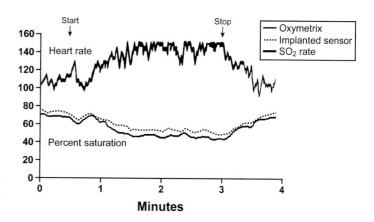

Fig. 9.12 Effect of exercise on right ventricular oxygen saturation measured by a permanently implanted rate-adaptive pacing system recording myocardial oxygen consumption in a canine. (Reproduced with permission from St. Jude Medical.)

to better simulate the normal sinus node response in some patients (Fig. 9.13).

Sensor programming must remain relatively simple even when more than one sensor is available. Although there should be options for choosing one sensor or both, if both sensors are used, the pacemaker must be capable of blending or mixing their responses (Fig. 9.14). At this time, the only dual-sensor that can simultaneously be programmed "on" is accelerometer and minute ventilation. A device with impedance based rate-adaptive pacing has an accelerometer as well. However, the accelerometer is used for sensor cross-checking only and the two sensors cannot be programmed "on" simultaneously. Dual-sensor technology is not an option in implantable cardioverter-defibrillators or CRT systems at this time.

There are relatively few investigations directly comparing single-sensor with dual-sensor systems. The Sensor and Quality of Life (SQL) study assessed the effect of single-sensor, minute ventilation or accelerometer, vs. dual-sensor programming on quality of life. Although pacing improved quality of life in this group of patients, neither single-sensor nor dual-sensor-driven pacing provided additional quality of life improvement.[17]

In the DUSISLOG study (Dual Sensor vs. Single Sensor comparison using patient activity LOGbook), patients were randomized to a single sensor, either minute ventilation or motion sensor and then reprogrammed after 3 months to the dual-sensor combination of minute ventilation and motion sensing. The investigators concluded that a single sensor achieved

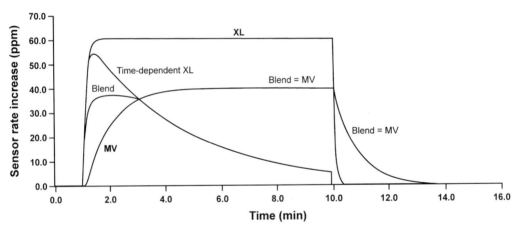

Fig. 9.13 Schematic representation of time-dependent interaction of two sensors. The diagram demonstrates sensor-indicated rates from rest to peak exercise for a minute ventilation sensor (MV) and an acceleration sensor (XL). The diagram depicts the potential superior outcome of blending the response of the two sensors. (Modified and reproduced with permission from Insignia Ultra Tech. Manual, p. 637.)

Fig. 9.14 Example from a patient in whom rate response was suboptimal with a single sensor. The pacemaker was capable of minute ventilation (MV) and acceleration sensing. The sequences were obtained with the patient completing a variety of tasks including: slow walk; brisk walk; walking to and riding up in an elevator; walking down stairs; walking up stairs. In each plot the dark line represents the actual heart rate achieved and the lighter line represents what the rate-adaptive sensors would have done had the patient been dependent on a sensor-indicated rate. (A) Pacemaker programmed so that minute ventilation is the primary sensor, i.e., acceleration programmed in such a way that it is effectively inactive. Note that the sensor-indicated rate is below the patient's actual rate at the onset of exercise, i.e., the MV sensor is relatively sluggish. Also note that the MV rate is lower than the patient's actual rate when coming down stairs and walking to and riding on an elevator. (B) Sensors programmed so that acceleration sensing is relatively "sensitive" and MV is programmed so that it is contributing little if anything to rate response. Acceleration sensing provides a rate similar to the patient's own rate during slow walk, but is suboptimal during brisk walk and walking down and up the stairs. Also note that the acceleration indicated rate is almost the same with walking up and down the stairs. (C) Example with both sensors programmed to complementary thresholds yields a rate response that very closely mimics the patient's own rate.

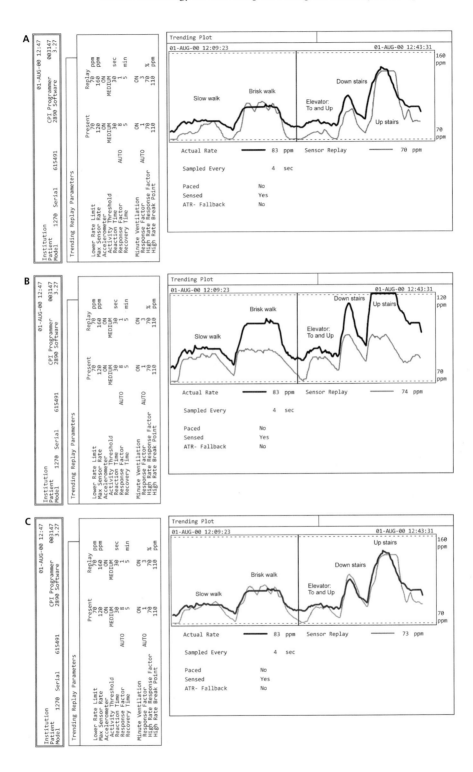

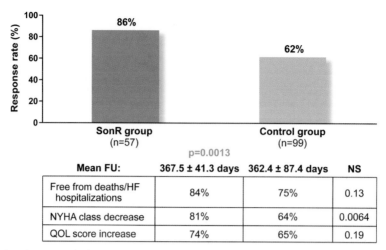

Mean FU:	367.5 ± 41.3 days	362.4 ± 87.4 days	NS
Free from deaths/HF hospitalizations	84%	75%	0.13
NYHA class decrease	81%	64%	0.0064
QOL score increase	74%	65%	0.19

Fig. 9.15 Results from the CLEAR study demonstrating that patients had better CRT performance when randomized to automatic optimization of the AV and V-V intervals. (Reproduced with permission of Sorin Biomedical, Paris, France.)

satisfactory rate adaptation for most patients. Dual-sensor programming provided additional clinical benefits in selected patients, specifically patients who were said to have "advanced atrial chronotropic disease."[18]

A more recent study of over 1000 patients with chronotropic incompetence demonstrated superiority of a blended sensor, i.e. minute ventilation and accelerometer, over accelerometer alone.[19]

There is no question that certain patients will benefit from dual-sensor technology, and when the sensors are carefully optimized they will benefit from the combination of sensors. It is also clear that sensor cross-checking prevents inappropriate false-positive rate response if complementary sensors are used.

Sensor applications for hemodynamic management

Given the increasing use of CRT devices and the prevalence of chronotropic incompetence in the heart failure population,[20] it was predictable that sensors implanted for rate-adaptive purposes would be investigated for their potential to aid in hemodynamic management in CRT patients.

Automatic determination of the AV interval by the PEA sensor in patients with AV block has been shown in several studies to be comparable to AV interval optimized by the accepted technique of Doppler echocardiography.[21,22]

In a relatively early study, the PEA sensor was assessed for its ability to reflect hemodynamic changes in patients with biventricular pacing and the PEA signals indicated improved hemodynamics with biventricular

and left ventricular pacing over right ventricular pacing.[23]

In the Clinical Evaluation of Advanced Resynchronization (CLEAR) trial SonR, to automatically program AV and interventricular (VV) delays in CRT, was compared with standard programming to determine if the sensor could dynamically optimize hemodynamic activity. The rate of responders, defined according to the primary end-point, was significantly better in the group automatically optimized using the sensor data but the benefit at 12 months was driven primarily by improvement in New York Heart Association (NYHA) functional class (Fig. 9.15).[24]

Monitoring and interpretation of activity and minute ventilation profiles have been used to predict when patients with CRT devices may be developing early cardiac decompensation. (Fig. 9.16).[25,26] Multivector impedance monitoring has also been shown to have potential for optimization of hemodynamics.[27] No doubt multiple other sensors will be incorporated for hemodynamic monitoring of multiple chronic disease states.

Programming

Contemporary rate-adaptive pacemakers, both single-sensor and dual-sensor systems, have an increasing degree of automaticity which assists in programming and optimization of sensor function. However, one basic tenet persists: every patient with a pacemaker programmed to a rate-adaptive pacing mode *must* be functionally assessed, in some way, to determine that the functional response to the sensor is appropriate. Despite

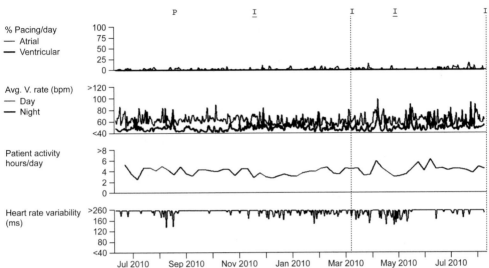

Device: **Secura DR D224DRG**
Serial Number: **PUG21...**

Initial Interrogation: Cardiac Compass Trends   **Page 3**

Fig. 9.16 Data from device interrogation depicting a trend of the patient's activity level. The level of activity is well maintained throughout the period represented. A decline of monitored activity as determined by the rate-adaptive sensor incorporated in the device may indicate early onset congestive heart failure.

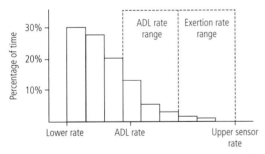

Fig. 9.17 Schematic of a rate profile demonstrating distribution of rates at rest and low level exertion, activities of daily living (ADL) and higher levels of exertion. (Reproduced with permission from Medtronic, Adapta Technical Manual, p. 27.)

autocalibration or autoprogramming of the sensor, there must be a clinical determination that the sensor response is appropriate, or, perhaps more importantly, that the sensor response is not inappropriate. At a minimum, sensor histograms should be assessed to determine if the patient's rate profile seems appropriate (Fig. 9.17). In many patients it is helpful to assess their rate response with exercise, either informal or formal.

Our approach is relatively simple. If the patient, regardless of age, performs at a very high functional aerobic capacity, a standard stress test that pushes the patient to a high level of exertion is reasonable to be certain that the sensor responds appropriately (Fig. 9.18). If formal treadmill exercise is performed and especially if a motion sensor is being evaluated, the patient should be encouraged to walk on the treadmill without holding on, i.e., allowing the arms to swing naturally at the sides. Gripping the treadmill tightly may blunt the response of the sensor.

Many device recipients do not routinely reach high levels of exertion and it is important to be certain that rate response is appropriate during an exertional range that corresponds to their activities of daily living. For these patients, casual exercise assessment is performed. If the patient is to be dismissed from the hospital in a rate-adaptive pacing mode, the assessment is performed in the hospital the morning after implantation. The rate response is reassessed in the outpatient clinic at approximately 3 months and subsequently depending on the sensor histogram profile (Fig. 9.19). Whether monitored by hospital telemetry or via the programmer in the outpatient device clinic, the patient is asked to walk at a casual pace in the corridor for approximately

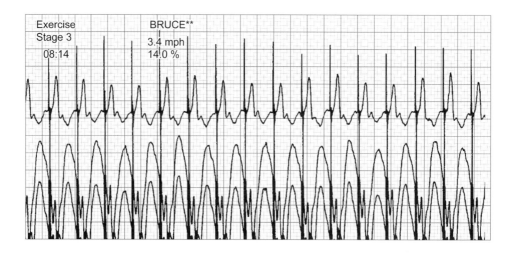

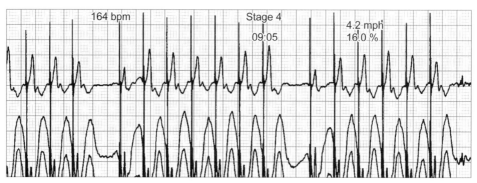

Fig. 9.18 Electrocardiographic tracings taken from a patient undergoing formal exercise assessment to observe and optimize sensor response. (A) 1:1 P-synchronous pacing at a rate of 175. (B) Pseudo-Wenckebach which correlated with the immediate onset of fatigue and inability to continue exercise.

2 min. The pacing rate achieved and the histogram are assessed during the walk or immediately afterward. Any patient capable of walking at a faster pace is asked to repeat the walk at a brisk pace.

Reassessment of sensor response should be considered if the patient has complaints of exertional fatigue (Fig. 9.20) or sudden changes in heart rate. Rate histograms can be invaluable in determining whether rate response is appropriate. For example, Fig. 9.20 displays a histogram in which the rates remain in the lowermost "bins," suggesting that the sensor is not programmed aggressively enough. Conversely, a histogram in which there is a significant amount of time at faster sensor-driven rates may suggest that the sensor is programmed too aggressively, especially if there are associated symptoms (Fig. 9.21).

If rate response is inadequate, whether determined by histograms or by exercise, determine whether the sensor needs to be programmed more sensitively and determine that the sensor is definitely programmed correctly. Terminology for sensor settings is not uniform among manufacturers; be certain that in an attempt to obtain more rate response, the sensor is not inadvertently being made even less sensitive.

Programmable parameters

There are elements of programming rate-adaptive parameters that are similar between devices. To program a specific sensor from a specific manufacturer optimally, you should consult the technical manual and/or contact the manufacturer if you have questions. The reader is also directed to a more extensive reference that goes into greater detail on each sensor.[28]

For most activity sensors it will be necessary to program a "threshold" for the sensor (Fig. 9.22). This can be defined as a programmable value for rate-

A Total Time Sampled: 0d, 0h, 1m, 57s
Sampling Rate: 1.6 seconds

Bin Number	Range (ppm)	Sample Counts
1	60 – 71	13
2	71 – 82	26
3	82 – 94	35
4	94 – 105	0
5	105 – 116	0
6	116 – 127	0
7	127 – 139	0
8	139 – 150	0
	Total:	74

B Total Time Sampled: 0d, 0h, 2m, 31s
Sampling Rate: 1.6 seconds

Bin Number	Range (ppm)	Sample Counts
1	60 – 71	14
2	71 – 82	3
3	82 – 94	1
4	94 – 105	3
5	105 – 116	57
6	116 – 127	8
7	127 – 139	9
8	139 – 150	0
	Total:	95

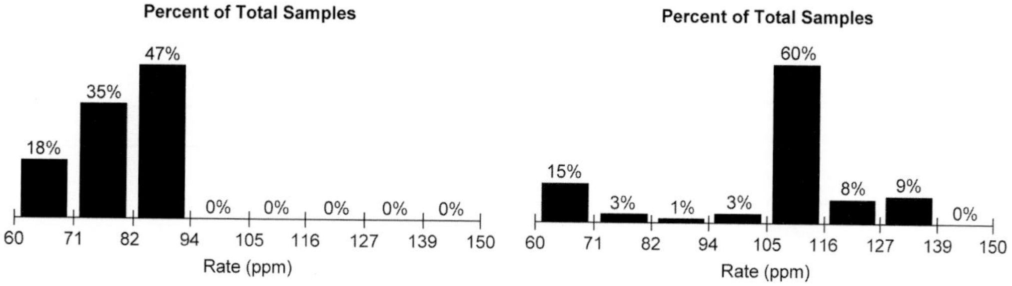

Percent of Total Samples

Fig. 9.19 Example from a patient that underwent an informal "hall walk" for approximately 2 minutes at a casual (left panel) and brisk (right panel) walk. The histograms would suggest that the sensor is programmed somewhat too aggressively because the patient achieved relatively rapid rates with the brisk walk. This simple assessment allows optimization for the individual patient.

ST. JUDE MEDICAL
© 1983-2007, St. Jude Medical, Inc.

Page 3a
Affinity® DR Model: 5330 Serial: 113110 PR 7.0
3650 Serial: 16081 (3330 v6. 1.0 PR18.1.8)

Sensor Indicated Rate Histogram

Mode............DDDR
Sensor............On
Base Rate............60 ppm
Max Sensor Rate............130 ppm
Threshold............Auto (–0.5)
  Measured Average Sensor............1.8
Slope............12
Reaction Time............Fast
Recovery Time............Medium

Date Read:............Aug 3, 2007 8:53 am
Total Time Sampled:............21d 17h 43m 8s
Date Last Cleared:............Jul 12, 2007 3:04 pm

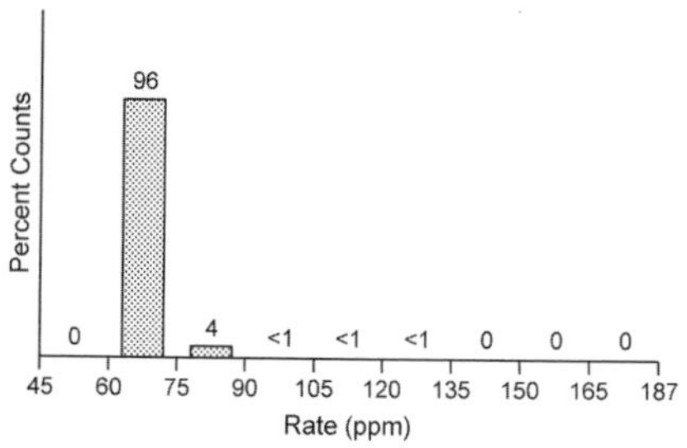

Note: The above values were obtained when the histogram was interrogated.

Bin Number	Range (ppm)	Time	Sample Counts
1	45 - < 60	0d 0h 0m 0s	0
2	60 - < 75	20d 20h 3m 36s	900,108
3	75 - < 90	0d 19h 56m 34s	35,897
4	90 - < 105	0d 1h 17m 20s	2,320
5	105 - < 120	0d 0h 18m 56s	568
6	120 - < 135	0d 0h 6m 42s	201
7	135 - < 150	0d 0h 0m 0s	0
8	150 - < 165	0d 0h 0m 0s	0
9	165 - 187	0d 0h 0m 0s	0
		Total:	939,094

Fig. 9.20 Sensor histogram in a patient where rate profile reflects inadequate chronotropic response. The base rate is programmed to 60 ppm and 96% of the heart rates captured in this histogram fall into the lowest rate bin of 60–75 ppm and only 4% fall into the next rate bin. (Courtesy of and copyrighted by St. Jude Medical.)

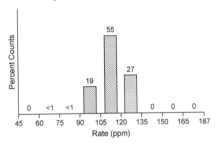

Page 1a
Integrity AFx™ DR Model: 5342 Serial: 279463 PR 6.6
3510P Serial: 15291 (3307 - 4.8.4m)

Sensor Indicated Rate Histogram

Mode...DDDR
Sensor...On
Base Rate...70 ppm
Max Sensor Rate..130 ppm
Threshold...1.0
    Measured Average Sensor.............................2.1
Slope...16
Reaction Time..Fast
Recovery Time   Medium

**Note: The above values were obtained
when the histogram was interrogated.**

Date Read:...Jun 6, 2005 15:40
Total Time Sampled: 0d 1h 32m 24s
Date Last Cleared: ....Jun 6, 2005 14:07

Bin Number	Range (ppm)	Time	Sample Counts
1	45 - < 60	0d 0h 0m 0s	0
2	60 - < 75	0d 0h 0m 4s	2
3	75 - < 90	0d 0h 0m 4s	2
4	90 - < 105	0d 0h 17m 14s	517
5	105 - < 120	0d 0h 50m 26s	1,513
6	120 - < 135	0d 0h 24m 36s	738
7	135 - < 150	0d 0h 0m 0s	0
8	150 - < 165	0d 0h 0m 0s	0
9	165 - 187	0d 0h 0m 0s	0
		Total:	2,772

Fig. 9.21 Sensor histogram in a patient in whom the rate profile is too aggressive and the patient's rate is primarily in the upper bins. (Courtesy of and copyrighted by St. Jude Medical.)

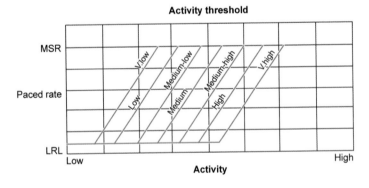

Fig. 9.22 Schematic diagram of the relationship between the "threshold" in an activity-sensing pacemaker and the rate response. (Reproduced with permission from Boston Scientific Ultra Insignia, p. 6.26.)

adaptive pacemakers that determine, in part, the level of activity necessary to activate the sensor. Programming the sensor threshold is not consistent across manufacturers (Fig. 9.23).

In addition, for most sensors it is necessary to program a rate-response value (Fig. 9.24). Although the terminology for the rate response factor will vary between manufacturers, the higher the rate response factor the steeper the sensor-indicated rate response (Fig. 9.25).

To define the rate at which the sensor-indicated rate increases and decreases, it is necessary to program a sensor acceleration or reaction time and deceleration

or recovery time (Fig. 9.26). These are programmable options for most sensors that determine how rapidly the pacing rate changes in response to increasing or decreasing stress.

Many rate-adaptive devices take "lifestyle" into consideration. That is, categorizing the patient by being very sedentary, moderately sedentary, minimally active, moderately active, very active, etc., assists the auto-rate adaptive programming in setting the appropriate ranges.[29]

It must be stressed that regardless of the sophistication of programmable options, the patient's sensor response must be assessed in some manner.

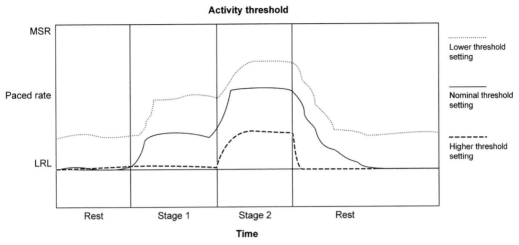

Fig. 9.23 Diagram of various activity thresholds demonstrating how different thresholds will affect the rate response during an exercise test. MSR, maximum sensor rate; LRL, lower rate limit. (Reproduced with permission from Boston Scientific Ultra Insignia, p. 6.26.)

Fig. 9.24 Diagrammatic representation of the effect of various rate response values. In this example, and terminology may vary between manufacturers, the greater the rate response value the steeper the sensor-indicated rate response. (Reproduced with permission from Boston Scientific Ultra Insignia, p. 6.24.)

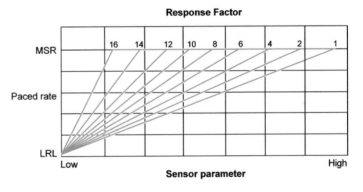

Fig. 9.25 Schematic depiction of the clinical effect of programming different rate response values. If too aggressive, the patient will achieve faster rates more quickly and perhaps faster than desirable. If not programmed aggressively enough, an appropriately fast rate response will not be achieved. (RRF = Rate Response Factor). (Reproduced from St. Jude Medical p. 8.5 courtesy of and copyrighted by St. Jude Medical.)

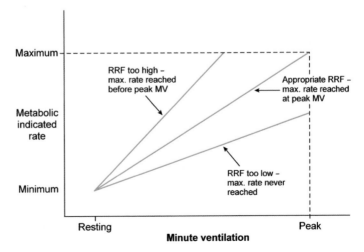

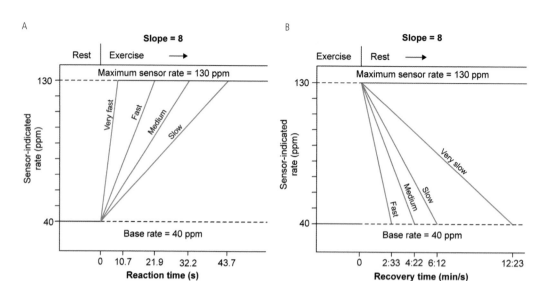

Fig. 9.26 Various example of programming (A) the reaction or acceleration times and (B) the recovery or deceleration times of a rate-adaptive sensor. (Reproduced from St. Jude Medical p. 8.5 courtesy of and copyrighted by St. Jude Medical.)

Rate-adaptive pacing with cardiac resynchronization devices

Patients with congestive heart failure (CHF) and who have had CRT devices implanted have specific requirements ideally aided with rate-adaptive pacing. Because of the underlying cardiomyopathy or from the use of negatively chronotropic drugs (β-blockers), chronotropic competence is often severely limited in patients with CHF. In some of these patients, however, even normal (predicted) increases in heart rate with activity may result in functional compromise (e.g. provocation of ischemia). Thus, careful evaluation and programming of rate-adaptive sensing is required in these patients.

To date, the literature is mixed whether rate-adaptive pacing should be activated in CRT devices. Conventional wisdom would suggest that those patients with intact sinus node function would be better served with their intrinsic atrial rate response. There is not consensus in the literature as to whether or not rate-adaptive pacing is hemodynamically or functionally superior for patients with CRT devices.[30,31]

AV and V-V timing

Interatrial conduction varies significantly in patients with CHF as a result of activity. In patients with standard dual-chamber pacemakers, this variation in interatrial conduction is of no significant physiologic consequence. With biventricular devices, however, optimization of the AV interval is greatly dependent on intra-atrial conduction. Optimal left atrial to left ven-

tricular contraction intervals may be quite different from right atrial to right ventricular conduction intervals, and optimal AV intervals with CRT devices need to factor in these differences. In present practice, the detailed programming of these intervals is of little value because intra-atrial conduction varies so significantly with exercise.

In the absence of automated hemodynamic based adjustment of the AV interval, it is unclear whether use of rate-adaptive AV intervals are beneficial in the CRT patient. In one study that assessed both rate-adaptive pacing "on and off" as well as rate-adaptive AV interval "on an off" did demonstrate a benefit from the use of both.[31] However, in another contemporary study the final recommendation was not to activate rate-adaptive AV delay in CRT patients.[32] Further studies are required.

Programming and offset between stimulation of the right and left ventricle is an option available in most presently implanted CRT devices. Because of increased capture latency and decreased intraventricular conduction time in the left ventricle compared with the right, often the left ventricular stimulus needs to be delivered earlier than the right ventricular stimulus to obtain optimal ventricular synchrony. Programming this optimization is typically done at rest (implant or followup), but both capture latency and intraventricular conduction time change significantly with exercise.

One study has been reported in which the SonR rate-adaptive sensor was used for dynamic optimization of V-V timing. The CLEAR trial was a prospective, multicenter, randomized, single-blind study in which 268 patients were randomized to automatic optimization of V-V and AV intervals by SonR or traditional clinical optimization techniques. The study demonstrated automatic optimization increased the responder rate to CRT by improving hemodynamic performance. Automatic interval optimization also has the potential of reducing time-consuming echocardiographic procedures associated with CRT optimization.[24]

Future of rate-adaptive sensors

Although rate-adaptive technology and the assessment of rate-adaptive sensors specifically for rate-adaptive pacing has been relatively stagnant for some time, the potential use of sensors in CRT systems has made sensor-technology much more dynamic in recent years.

The reassessment and application of older sensors for the purpose of hemodynamic monitoring in CRT systems as well as the development of new hemodynamic sensors will continue to drastically alter sensor technology in the near future. While new technology will primarily impact hemodynamic monitoring it will no doubt yield improvements in rate-adaptation as well.

References

1 Shukla HH, Flaker GC, Hellkamp AS, et al. Clinical and quality of life comparison of accelerometer, piezoelectric crystal, and blended sensors in DDDR-paced patients with sinus node dysfunction in the mode selection trial (MOST). Pacing Clin Electrophysiol 2005; 28:762–70.

2 Duru F, Cho Y, Wilkoff BL, et al. Rate responsive pacing using transthoracic impedance minute ventilation sensors: a multicenter study on calibration stability. Pacing Clin Electrophysiol 2002; 25:1679–84.

3 Southorn PA, Kamath GS, Vasdev GM, Hayes DL. Monitoring equipment induced tachycardia in patients with minute ventilation rate-responsive pacemakers. Br J Anaesth 2000; 84:508–9.

4 Greco EM, Ferrario M, Romano S. Clinical evaluation of peak endocardial acceleration as a sensor for rate responsive pacing. Pacing Clin Electrophysiol 2003; 26:812–8.

5 Deharo JC, Peyre JP, Ritter PH, Chalvidan T, Le Tallec L, Djiane P. Treatment of malignant primary vasodepressive neurocardiogenic syncope with a rate responsive pacemaker driven by heart contractility. Pacing Clin Electrophysiol 1998; 21:2688–90.

6 Deharo JC, Peyre JP, Chalvidan T, et al. Continuous monitoring of an endocardial index of myocardial contractility during head-up tilt test. Am Heart J 2000; 139:1022–30.

7 Donal E, Giorgis L, Cazeau S, et al. Endocardial acceleration (sonR) vs. ultrasound-derived time intervals in recipients of cardiac resynchronization therapy systems. Europace 2011; 13:402–8.

8 Kink A, Salo RW, Min M, Parve T, Rätsep I. Intracardiac electrical bioimpedance as a basis for controlling of pacing rate limits. Conf Proc IEEE Eng Med Biol Soc 2006; 1:6308–11.

9 Osswald S, Cron T, Grädel C, et al. Closed-loop stimulation using intracardiac impedance as a sensor principle: correlation of right ventricular dP/dtmax and intracardiac impedance during dobutamine stress test. Pacing Clin Electrophysiol 2000; 23:1502–8.

10 Coenen M, Malinowski K, Spitzer W, et al. Closed loop stimulation and accelerometer-based rate adaptation: results of the PROVIDE study. Europace 2008; 10:327–33.

11 Chandiramani S, Cohorn LC, Chandiramani S. Heart rate changes during acute mental stress with closed loop stimulation: report on two single-blinded, pacemaker studies. Pacing Clin Electrophysiol 2007; 30:976–84.

12 Wiegand U, Nuernberg M, Maier SK, et al. The COGNITION study rationale and design: influence of closed loop stimulation on cognitive performance in pacemaker patients. Pacing Clin Electrophysiol 2008; 31:709–13.

13 Occhetta E, Bortnik M, Audoglio R, Vassanelli C; INVASY Study Investigators. Closed loop stimulation in prevention of vasovagal syncope. Inotropy Controlled Pacing in Vasovagal Syncope (INVASY): a multicentre randomized, single blind, controlled study. Europace 2004; 6:538–47.

14 Kanjwal K, Karabin B, Kanjwal Y, Grubb BP. Preliminary observations on the use of closed-loop cardiac pacing in patients with refractory neurocardiogenic syncope. J Interv Card Electrophysiol 2010; 27:69–73.

15 Ruiter JH, Barrett MJ, Weteling L, Jansen R. Malfunction of the automatic slope adjustment of the QT sensor in patients with normal QT intervals. Pacing Clin Electrophysiol 2004; 27:405–7.

16 Kjellstrom B, Linde C, Bennett T, Ohlsson A, Ryden L. Six years follow-up of an implanted SvO(2) sensor in the right ventricle. Eur J Heart Fail 2004; 6:627–34.

17 van Hemel NM, Holwerda KJ, Slegers PC, et al. Sensor and Quality of Life (SQL). The contribution of rate adaptive pacing with single or dual sensors to health-related quality of life. Europace 2007; 9:233–8.

18 Padeletti L, Pieragnoli P, Di Biase L, et al. Is a dual-sensor pacemaker appropriate in patients with sino-atrial disease? Results from the DUSISLOG study. Pacing Clin Electrophysiol 2006; 29:34–40.

19 Coman J, Freedman R, Koplan BA, et al.; LIFE Study Results. A blended sensor restores chronotropic response more favorably than an accelerometer alone in pacemaker patients: the LIFE study results. Pacing Clin Electrophysiol 2008; 31:1433–42.

20 Brubaker PH, Kitzman DW. Prevalence and management of chronotropic incompetence in heart failure. Curr Cardiol Rep 2007; 9:229–35.

21 Leung SK, Lau CP, Lam CT, et al. Automatic optimization of resting and exercise atrioventricular interval using a peak endocardial acceleration sensor: validation with Doppler echocardiography and direct cardiac output measurements. Pacing Clin Electrophysiol 2000; 23:1762–6.

22 Dupuis JM, Kobeissi A, Vitali L, et al. Programming optimal atrioventricular delay in dual chamber pacing using peak endocardial acceleration: comparison with a standard echocardiographic procedure. Pacing Clin Electrophysiol 2003; 26:210–3.

23 Bordachar P, Garrigue S, Reuter S, *et al.* Hemodynamic assessment of right, left, and biventricular pacing by peak endocardial acceleration and echocardiography in patients with end-stage heart failure. Pacing Clin Electrophysiol 2000; 23:1726–30.

24 Ritter P, Delnoy PP Padeletti L, *et al.* A randomized pilot study of optimization of cardiac resynchronization therapy in sinus rhythm patients using a peak endocardial acceleration sensor vs. standard methods. Europace 2012; 14: 1324–33.

25 Page E, Cazeau S, Ritter P, Galley D, Casset C. Physiological approach to monitor patients in congestive heart failure: application of a new implantable device-based system to monitor daily life activity and ventilation. Europace 2007; 9:687–93.

26 Fung JW, Yu CM. Implantable cardiac resynchronization therapy devices to monitor heart failure clinical status. Curr Heart Fail Rep 2007; 4:48–52.

27 Khoury DS, Naware M, Siou J, *et al.* Ambulatory monitoring of congestive heart failure by multiple bioelectric impedance vectors. J Am Coll Cardiol 2009; 53:1075–81.

28 Ellenbogen KA, Wilkoff BL, Kay GN, Lau CP. Clinical Cardiac Pacing, Defibrillation and Resynchronization Therapy, 4th edn. Philadelphia: Saunders/Elsevier, 2011.

29 Schuster P, Faerestrand S, Ohm OJ, Schouten V. Proportionality of rate response to metabolic workload provided by a rate adaptive pacemaker with automatic rate profile optimization. Europace 2005; 7:54–9.

30 Van Thielen G, Paelinck BP, Beckers P, Vrints CJ, Conraads VM. Rate response and cardiac resynchronisation therapy in chronic heart failure: higher cardiac output does not acutely improve exercise performance: a pilot trial. Eur J Cardiovasc Prev Rehabil 2008; 15:197–202.

31 Tse HF, Siu CW, Lee KL, *et al.* The incremental benefit of rate-adaptive pacing on exercise performance during cardiac resynchronization therapy. J Am Coll Cardiol 2005; 46:2292–7.

32 Melzer C, Bondke H, Körber T, Nienaber CA, Baumann G, Ismer B. Should we use the rate-adaptive AV delay in cardiac resynchronization therapy-pacing? Europace 2008; 10:53–8.

10 Troubleshooting: Interpreting Diagnostic Information to Ensure Appropriate Function

Charles D. Swerdlow[1], Paul A. Friedman[2], Samuel J. Asirvatham[2], David L. Hayes[2]

[1]Cedars-Sinai Heart Center at Cedars-Sinai Medical Center; David Geffen School of Medicine, University of California, Los Angeles, CA, USA
[2]Mayo Clinic, Rochester, MN, USA

Pacemaker troubleshooting 428
Clinical assessment 428
Identifying the pulse generator 429
Electrocardiographic interpretation 430
Lead integrity 430
Pulse generators 432
Clinical troubleshooting 432
  Pacing and sensing threshold evaluation 432
  Assessing the pacing rate 435
Diagnostic features 439
Unexpected device failure 439
Operative evaluation of pacing systems 440
Focused troubleshooting 440
Failure to capture 441
Pseudo-malfunctions 452
Failure to pace (no output) 454
Undersensing 458
Alteration in programmed pacing rate 462
New symptoms after pacemaker implantation 464
ICD troubleshooting 472
Diagnostic tools for ICD troubleshooting 472
  History, physical, and basic laboratory data 472
    Device-focused history and physical 472
    Findings pertinent to presentation with
      shocks 472
    Patient activity 472
    Symptoms 472
    Shocks patterns 473
    Phantom shocks 473
  Radiography 473
  ICD Diagnostics 473
  Analysis of ICD electrograms and marker
    channels 473
    Electrogram sources 473
    Stored and real-time electrograms 476
Evaluating appropriateness of delivered therapy 476

Ventricular oversensing: recognition and
  troubleshooting 476
  Intracardiac signals 476
  Extracardiac signals 485
Distinguishing VT from SVT in ICD stored
  electrograms and episode data 488
  Analysis of dual-chamber electrograms 488
  Analysis of single-chamber, ventricular
    electrograms 489
Troubleshooting errors in SVT-VT discrimination 495
  Ventricular rate in SVT compared with the VT/
    VF rate boundary 498
  Ventricular rate in SVT compared with the
    fastest rate at which SVT-VT discriminators
    apply 498
  Failure of SVT-VT discriminators 499
  Troubleshooting errors in SVT-VT discrimination
    due to atrial sensing problems 501
Determining if shocks for VT are necessary 506
  Minimizing ICD proarrhythmia 506
  Minimizing therapy for self-terminating VT/VF 507
  Optimizing ATP 507
  Miscellaneous factors 507
Approach to the patient with frequent shocks 510
  Emergency management 510
  VT storm 510
Unsuccessful shocks 511
  Determining that shocks are truly ineffective 511
  Patient-related factors 512
  ICD system-related factors 512
Failure to deliver or delayed therapy: underdetection
  and undersensing 515
  Problems corrected by ICD programming 515
    ICD inactivation 515
    VT slower than the programmed detection
      interval 515
    SVT-VT discriminators 515

Cardiac Pacing, Defibrillation and Resynchronization: A Clinical Approach, Third Edition.
David L. Hayes, Samuel J. Asirvatham, and Paul A. Friedman.
© 2013 Mayo Foundation for Medical Education and Research. Published 2013 by John Wiley & Sons, Ltd.

Oversensing of stimuli delivered by other
implanted electronic devices 517
Intra-device interactions due to cross-chamber
blanking periods 518
Problems that may require system revision 519
Undersensing of VF 519
Troubleshooting ICD lead failure 521
Differential diagnosis of pace-sense lead
fractures 521
Noise oversensing with a normal
impedance 522
High impedance with or without
oversensing 522
Discriminating fractures from connection
problems 525
Discriminating fractures from functioning leads
with high impedance 529
Approach to the patient with a suspected
pace-sense lead fracture 529
Other ICD lead failures 531

High-voltage conductor failures 531
Outer insulation failures 532
Lead failure diagnostics 533
Lead Integrity Alert™ 533
Lead Noise Algorithm™ 533
**Troubleshooting cardiac resynchronization
devices 533**
Failure to respond to resynchronization pacing 533
Resynchronization <90–95% of R-R intervals 534
Ventricular sensing of conducted sinus or
atrial-paced rhythm 534
Ventricular sensing of conducted AF 537
Resynchronization ≥90–95% of RR intervals 541
Troubleshooting other problems in CRT systems 542
Phrenic nerve stimulation 542
CRT proarrhythmia 543
Ventricular sensing problems 543
References 546

Pacemaker troubleshooting

Pacemaker diagnostics and automaticity have become increasingly more sophisticated. Knowledge of the device capabilities and the clinical situation of the patient is key to successful troubleshooting. Whether a patient has a clinical episode that suggests system malfunction or is having routine follow-up, device evaluation should be performed in an orderly fashion so that potential malfunction is not overlooked. Some instances of device "malfunction" are not malfunctions at all, but rather are the result of an inappropriately programmed device functioning as programmed or unrecognized appropriate function, i.e., pseudo-malfunction. In some instances, early component failure is intermittent, and even meticulous evaluation of the system may not initially reveal a problem.

Successful troubleshooting requires a systematic approach (Table 10.1). Noninvasive evaluation should be exhausted first and involve careful evaluation of any symptoms; the pacing indication; available electrocardiographic tracings; the function and radiographic appearance of the lead system; and stored information obtained by telemetry from the pulse generator. Noninvasive diagnosis and correction of any malfunction are always preferable to operative management. Before invasive troubleshooting, one should take advantage of every possible source of assistance, including careful review of the technical manual and contacting the manufacturer for help. If noninvasive evaluation is unrewarding, operative assessment may be necessary.

In order to adopt a systematic approach to troubleshooting, an understanding of the common problems encountered in a device clinic and their causes is necessary.

The most common problems encountered in pacemaker management include:

- Failure to sense
- Failure to capture
- Failure to output
- Change in magnet rate
- Recurrent preimplant symptoms
- Palpitations/tachyarrhythmias
- Hemodynamic compromise
- Device advisory or recall.

Clinical assessment

Knowing the patient and taking a careful history are very important in evaluating any pacing system, especially if malfunction is suspected. Clinical assessment should include the following information: the original indication for pacing, whether or not the patient is pacemaker-dependent, activity immediately preceding the clinical event, symptoms experienced by the patient during the event, observations made by witnesses, and

Table 10.1 Troubleshooting steps.

Clinical assessment
   Indication for pacing
   Focused history and physical examination
   Review of operative report
Electrocardiography
   Rate
   Pacing and sensing
   QRS axis
   Magnet response
Chest radiograph
   Device type and location
   Proper contact between lead pins and setscrews
   Lead integrity
   Lead position
Pacemaker interrogation
   Sensing threshold(s)
   Pacing threshold(s)
   Lead impedance
   Battery status
   Special features
   Histograms
   Trend data
   Counters
Programming
Review technical manual for other "clues" to perceived
   malfunction
Contact the manufacturer for assistance
Operative assessment
   Appearance of pocket
   Assessment of lead connection(s)
   Visual inspection of lead(s)
   Electrical assessment of lead(s)
   Patency of venous system

Table 10.2 Toll-free, 24-h telephone numbers of manufacturers.*

Biotronik	1-800-547-0394
Boston Scientific	1-800-CARDIAC
Sorin/ELA	1-800-352-6466
Medtronic	1-800-328-2518
St. Jude Medical	1-800-722-3774

*As of January 2012.

Many devices store information on lead models, acute threshold data, clinical information (e.g., medication regimen), name of institution where the device was implanted, and name of the implanting physician in their memory, for retrieval upon interrogation. All manufacturers have toll-free numbers that may be used to obtain implant information (generally kept by the manufacturer of the pulse generator), such as device model and lead models (Table 10.2). The manufacturers can also provide technical information about device and lead performance and assist with electrocardiographic interpretation and troubleshooting. (If calling for implant information ask for "patient registration" and if calling for troubleshooting assistance ask for "brady technical support".)

It is also very useful (but sometimes difficult) to obtain the chest radiograph taken immediately after implantation for comparison with current radiographs (see Chapter 11: Radiography of Implantable Devices).

Identifying the pulse generator

The first step in troubleshooting is pacemaker interrogation. However, interrogation requires knowing the pulse generator manufacturer, because pulse generators only communicate with programmers made by the same manufacturer. Methods to identify the manufacturer include review of the pacing system identification card that all patients should carry, review of medical records that identify the pacemaker manufacturer, or radiographic identification.

With a high-quality posteroanterior chest X-ray, it may be possible to see a radiographic code that will identify the manufacturer (Chapter 11, Fig. 11.3). Alternatively, interrogation with available programmers can be attempted. No adverse consequences should occur from attempting to interrogate the device with a noncompatible programmer. In the event that interrogation by multiple programmers is unsuccessful or not possible, i.e., programmers from multiple manufacturers not available, calls can be made to "patient registration" for each of the device manufacturers. You will

duration of the event. Symptoms of pacing system malfunction may be subtle and include fatigue, weakness, confusion, neck pulsations, or activity intolerance. Some types of pacing system malfunctions may occur totally without symptoms. For example, intermittent failure to capture in the nonpacemaker-dependent patient or undersensing may not be associated with any symptoms and may be discovered only at the time of routine evaluation. During routine follow-up, the patient should be asked about symptoms potentially related to pacemaker complications, such as recurrence of preimplant symptoms, syncope, near-syncope, palpitations, and any perception of a slow, fast, or irregular pulse. It is important to obtain information from the operative report if possible, including device model, lead models, acute intraoperative pacing and sensing thresholds, and impedance values, and any difficulties encountered during implantation.

need to provide the patient's name and possibly the date of birth. If the manufacturer's products were implanted and appropriately registered, the information should be on record. If the appropriate programmer is not immediately available, the company should be contacted at the number given in Table 10.2 and assistance requested.

Electrocardiographic interpretation and troubleshooting is made significantly easier once the pulse generator is identified, programmer acquired, and interrogation completed.

Electrocardiographic interpretation

If presented with a paced electrocardiogram and no other information, it is reasonable to approach interpretation with several specific questions:
• Is pacing occurring in the atrium, the ventricle, or both?
• Is sensing occurring in the atrium, the ventricle, or both?
• Based on the first two questions, is it possible to identify the pacing mode or at least narrow the possible options?
• What are the lower and (if applicable) upper rate limits?
• What other measurable intervals are present? For example, what is the atrioventricular (AV) interval; more specifically, what are the AV, PV, or AR intervals?
• Is there any evidence that the programmed rate, if identifiable, has been violated?
• On the electrocardiographic tracing available is there evidence of normal sensing and capture?

Only after extracting as much information regarding what is believed to be "normal" operation should attention be turned to any possible abnormality.

Lead integrity

The lead system is the most vulnerable component of the pacing system and the most frequent site of system failure other than expected battery failure (depletion). Lead technology continues to improve, and many manufacturers now have lead performance data that can be accessed through their published product performance reports.

Insight regarding etiology of transvenous lead failure, presenting signs of failure, and time distribution of failure can be gained from data from a multicenter registry of recognized lead and pulse generator problems.[1] It should be emphasized that this registry includes only leads and pulse generators that have been removed from service; it is not a prospective registry of all implants. Insulation defects are the most common cause of failure, followed by conductor and fixation failure, although there is variability depending on lead construction. From registry data, when the distribution of lead failure by number of years in service was analyzed, the median time to failure for all leads was 7.2 ± 5.2 years, with a "failure" peak in the first year followed by a second peak at approximately year 9. The adverse clinical events (most commonly syncope) and their relationship to the mechanism of failure are shown in Fig. 10.1.

If there is concern or evidence of lead failure, it may be helpful to look at product performance data available from the manufacturer. Most manufacturers

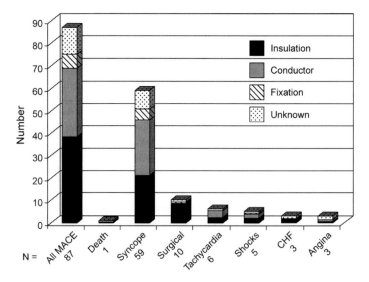

Fig. 10.1 Major adverse clinical events (MACE); and their relationship to the causes of; transvenous lead failure. (From Hauser RG, Hayes DL, Kallinen LM, *et al.* Clinical experience with pacemaker pulse generators and transvenous leads: an 8-year prospective multicenter study. Heart Rhythm 2007; 4:154–60, by permission of Elsevier.)

make product performance information available on a regular basis. Another valuable source, albeit somewhat to difficult to navigate, is the Food and Drug Administration (FDA) website, specifically the MAUDE database (http://www.accessdata.fda.gov/scripts/cdrh/cfdocs/cfMAUDE/search.cfm).

The chest radiograph is a valuable component in lead evaluation (see Chapter 11: Radiography of Implantable Devices). The lead should be inspected in its entirety, from the contact of the pin with the setscrew to the position of the lead within its cardiac chamber. Unfortunately, deterioration of the lead insulation is rarely visible on the chest radiograph, and fractures of the coil are not always obvious. A frequent site of lead damage if a subclavian implant approach has been utilized is the region between the first rib and the clavicle; this site should be carefully inspected for coil fracture (subclavian crush syndrome). The risk of subclavian crush becomes higher if multiple leads are in place. If an older chest radiograph is available for comparison, the presence of gross lead dislodgment can be determined. This presentation is becoming less common because subclavian approach is now less frequently used.

Abandoned leads in contact with the electrode of an active lead may cause an artifact, which can be interpreted by the pacemaker as a cardiac event and cause inappropriate inhibition. Although findings on the chest radiograph suggestive of lead fracture, dislodgment, or poor connection between the lead pin and generator setscrew are helpful in identifying lead problems, absence of such findings does not exclude lead failure. (For detailed information on the radiographic appearance of pacing systems, see Chapter 11: Radiography of Implantable Devices)

Lead evaluation should also include the measured lead impedance. For currently available leads, an impedance >2000 Ω indicates a conductor fracture or loose setscrew, and low impedance (<200 Ω indicates an insulation defect. (Note: expected impedance is a function of lead design, so that for some leads values >1500 Ω are abnormal. A call to the manufacturer is helpful in determining an acceptable impedance range for a given lead model.) Most contemporary pacemakers periodically measure and store impedance values, and creates plots or tables summarizing periodic values, facilitating detection of changes in lead function (Fig. 10.2). Even if a measured value is within the "normal" range for that particular lead, a notable change in impedance from previous values should raise suspicion. Most pulse generators have the ability to respond to a sudden change in impedance by automatically reprogramming the

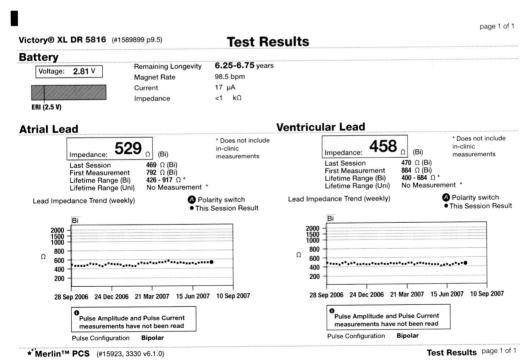

Fig. 10.2 Telemetry printout noting atrial and ventricular; lead impedances but also a "trend" of impedance; values for both leads. In this example the trend displays information for approximately 11 months and impedance values are stable for both leads.

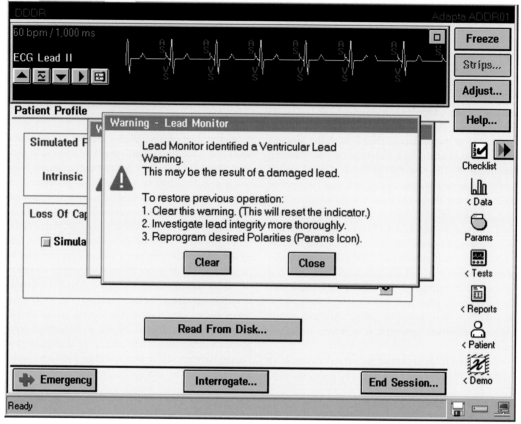

Fig. 10.3 A programmer "screen" with a warning that the lead monitor identified a ventricular lead warning. Such a warning may be a sudden change in lead impedance resulting in automatic switch from bipolar to unipolar pacing configuration.

pacemaker from bipolar to unipolar pacing and sensing configuration (Fig. 10.3).

Pulse generators

Multicenter registry data provide insight into pulse generator failure mechanisms and associated adverse clinical events. The single most common reason for pulse generator removal from service was expected battery depletion, accounting for 92% of removals. Other reasons included medical advisory or recall (4%), electronic failure (2%), connector failure (1%), and unknown cause of failure (1%).[1] The impact of rate responsiveness on observed battery longevity is shown in Fig. 10.4. Figure 10.5 demonstrates major adverse clinical events and their relationship to pulse generator removal.

Clinical troubleshooting

The number of programmable features available in pacemakers continues to increase. Although these options permit individualizing optimal pacing therapy for patients, they can make troubleshooting a complex endeavor. A detailed understanding of the correct function of these devices is necessary to provide comprehensive evaluation; technical manuals and expert representatives from the manufacturer provide important assistance.

Pacing and sensing threshold evaluation

An initial step in troubleshooting is to determine the patient's native rhythm. This may require turning down the rate of the pacemaker or programming it to a non-tracking ventricular mode, or both. The presence, type, and time to appearance of a spontaneous rhythm after the pacing rate is lowered should be noted. If the patient is found to have no underlying rhythm (usually defined as absence of a native rhythm with the pacemaker programmed to 30 bpm), care should be taken to ensure that the patient does not become asystolic for

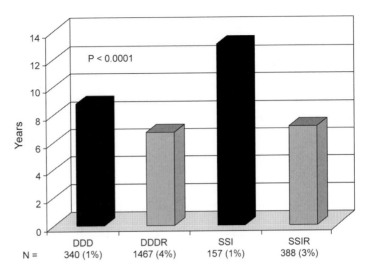

Fig. 10.4 Observed pulse generator battery longevity assessed by those with vs. those without the capability of rate-responsiveness. The percentages along the abscissa represent the proportion of pulse generators that failed in ≤3 years, the definition of premature battery failure in this registry. (From Hauser RG, Hayes DL, Kallinen LM, et al. Clinical experience with pacemaker pulse generators and transvenous leads: an 8-year prospective multicenter study. Heart Rhythm 2007; 4:154–60, by permission of Elsevier.)

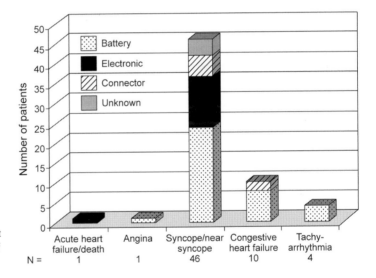

Fig. 10.5 Major adverse clinical events and their relationship to the causes of pulse generator failure. (From Hauser RG, Hayes DL, Kallinen LM, et al. Clinical experience with pacemaker pulse generators and transvenous leads: an 8-year prospective multicenter study. Heart Rhythm 2007; 4:154–60, by permission of Elsevier.)

any significant length of time during the troubleshooting session.

Pacing thresholds should then be evaluated. Most devices allow automated evaluation of pacing thresholds; the output is incrementally decreased until loss of capture occurs, and termination of the test results in immediate pacing at pretest values (Fig. 10.6). Pacing thresholds can always be obtained manually. In pacemaker-dependent patients, threshold testing should be performed in the safest possible manner which is usually a mechanism that results in the pacemaker reverting to the permanently programmed output when

loss of capture noted. The operator should be familiar with the programmer emergency pacing feature should it become necessary to restore nominal pacing outputs quickly. After determination of the pacing threshold(s), the chronically programmed output parameters, i.e., voltage amplitude and pulse width, should be reassessed to be certain that the patient has an adequate safety margin. There are several ways to program output parameters to ensure an adequate safety margin. These are described in detail in Chapter 8: Programming. During the evaluation of pacing thresholds, the presence or absence of ventriculoatrial conduction should be

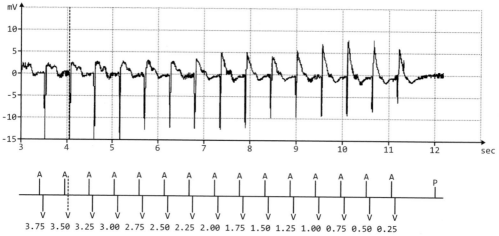

Amplitude V thresh.   3.5 V   Adjust the threshold ⬅ ➡

A

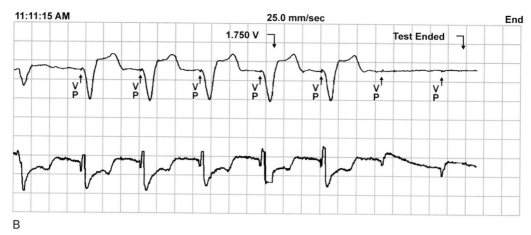

B

Fig. 10.6 Two examples of autothreshold determination by the programmer. Autothreshold determination allows ventricular thresholds to be determined in the pacemakerdependent patient, with minimal risk of clinically significant asystole. (A) Ventricular capture is maintained to the lowest value of 0.25 V. (B) Ventricular capture is lost at 1.75 V.

noted, and the patient should be questioned about symptoms of pacemaker syndrome, especially if it is suspected on the basis of the clinical findings.

Threshold values should be compared with those at implantation if possible. The development of exit block, some medications, severe electrolyte or meta-

bolic abnormalities, lead dislodgment, and occurrence of new myocardial infarction may affect pacing thresholds (Table 10.3).

Many devices offer automated periodic assessment of pacing threshold in the ventricle, with adjustment of the pacing output to maintain capture with a safety margin that minimizes battery depletion (Fig. 10.7).[2,3] In these devices, the output on the ventricular channel may be different at the time of interrogation from that initially programmed because of self-adjustment of the device. Additionally, electrocardiographic monitoring during a periodic threshold check may give the appearance of device malfunction due to variations in pacing outputs during the self-diagnostic test.

The sensing threshold in each chamber should be assessed. Some devices automatically measure the native atrial and ventricular electrograms,[4] whereas in older devices the value may require manual measure-

ment. The measured sensitivity should be compared with the programmed value to ensure that the chronically programmed sensitivity value is adequate.

Assessing the pacing rate

An understanding of basic pacemaker timing cycles is mandatory (explained in detail in Chapter 7: Timing Cycles). Many abnormal-appearing electrocardiograms actually represent normal device function when it is understood how the device is programmed.

To know whether the pacing rate is appropriate, it is first necessary to determine the pacing mode and programmed lower and (if applicable) upper rate limits. Under certain circumstances, the rate may be outside programmed values. The upper rate limit may be overridden by the spontaneous sinus rhythm, atrial or ventricular tachyarrhythmias, or, in very rare instances, runaway pacemaker (see later).

Several optional features allow intrinsic rates below the programmed lower rate limit to occur without pacing under specific circumstances. Some devices have a nocturnal or sleep function. During sleep time, the pacemaker allows programming of the lower rate limit to a rate generally 10 or 15 ppm less than that during wake time, replicating the natural circadian sleep–wake cycle. If it is not known that a "sleep rate" is programmed "on," confusion may arise when the patient's paced rate decreases at the programmed time.

Hysteresis allows the intrinsic heart rate to decrease to a rate below the lower rate limit before pacing begins

Table 10.3 Effect of drugs on pacing thresholds.

Increase in threshold
Bretylium
Encainide*
Flecainide
Moricizine*
Procainamide†
Propafenone
Sotalol
Decrease in threshold
Atropine
Epinephrine
Isoproterenol
Corticosteroids

*Off market in the USA.
†At supratherapeutic levels.

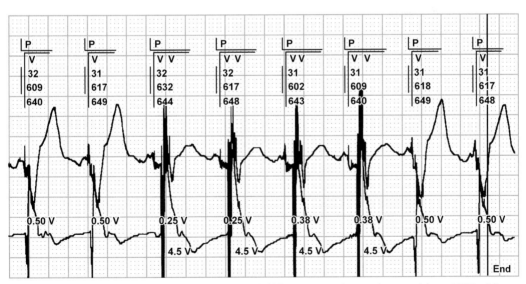

Fig. 10.7 Electrocardiographic tracing demonstrating automatic threshold determination. In this example, capture is lost at 0.25V and the output is automatically increased to 0.38V, which fails to capture, and the device again increases output to 0.5V, and confirms capture for two consecutive beats. If one is not familiar with this specific function, it may suggest malfunction.

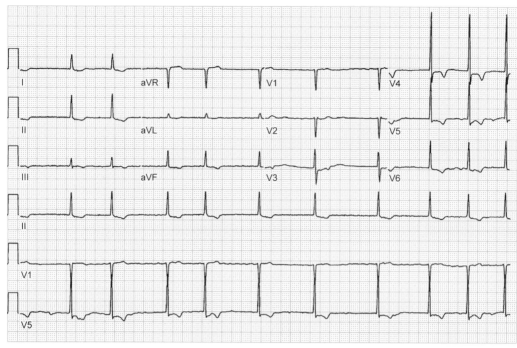

Fig. 10.8 A portion of a 12-lead ECG from a patient with a VVI pacemaker programmed to a pacing rate of 60 ppm, i.e., VV interval of 1000 ms. However, an interval of approximately 1240 ms is explained by a programmed hysteresis rate of 40 ppm, i.e., 1500 ms. This means that if an intrinsic QRS complex is present, the pacemaker will wait for 1500 ms to "time-out" before delivering the fi rst paced artifact. Once pacing has occurred, pacing will continue at the programmed lower rate, i.e., intervals of 1000 ms, unless intrinsic ventricular depolarization occurs and again initiates the hysteresis interval.

at the programmed lower rate (Fig. 10.8). However, if the intrinsic rate slows below the hysteresis rate, then pacing will commence at the lower rate limit (which by definition is faster than the hysteresis escape rate). Thus, hysteresis permits intrinsic rhythms slower than the programmed lower rate limit, but will not result in pacing at rates below the lower rate limit, distinguishing it from "sleep rate" function. Although useful in patients whose intrinsic rate approximates that of the programmed lower rate limit to promote native conduction, hysteresis has been a source of confusion for many years. Unless it is realized that hysteresis is programmed "on" and the mechanism of this feature is understood, electrocardiographic tracings are often misinterpreted as "oversensing," because the cycle length is intermittently longer than the recognized programmed lower rate limit.

Multiple parameters affecting the AV intervals are programmable. Independently programmable paced and sensed AV intervals allow for more consistent mechanical AV activation in patients with interatrial and intra-atrial conduction delay, but can cause confu-

sion when electrocardiographic tracings are interpreted. This effect may also cause minor variations in the paced lower and upper rates. Rate-adaptive AV delay is available in most dual-chamber pacemakers. Because the rate-adaptive AV interval affects the total atrial refractory period and therefore the achievable upper rate limit, confusion may arise (see Chapter 7: Timing Cycles).

Another classic source of confusion during assessment of pacing rates and alterations in cycle length is rate smoothing. Rate smoothing avoids abrupt changes in pacing rate, such as those that can occur during a sudden transition to pseudo-Wenckebach or 2:1 upper rate behavior, and may eliminate symptoms associated with sensed dysrhythmic events. Rate smoothing controls sudden changes in pacing rate by monitoring the interval between ventricular events (both paced and sensed) and storing the most recent RR interval in memory (Fig. 10.9). On the basis of this RR interval and the programmed rate-smoothing percentage, the pulse generator sets up two rate-control windows for the next cycle – one for the atrium and one for the

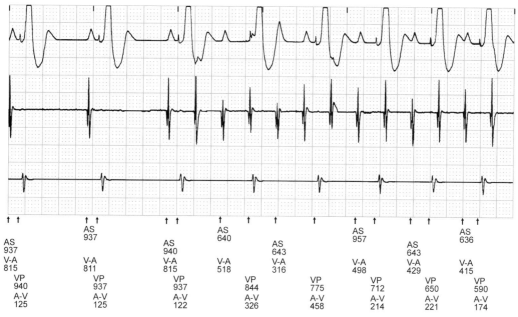

	AS 937		AS 640		AS 957		AS 636
AS 937		AS 940		AS 643		AS 643	
V-A 815	V-A 811	V-A 815	V-A 518	V-A 316	V-A 498	V-A 429	V-A 415
VP 940	VP 937	VP 937	VP 844	VP 775	VP 712	VP 650	VP 590
A-V 125	A-V 125	A-V 122	A-V 326	A-V 458	A-V 214	A-V 221	A-V 174

Fig. 10.9 Rate smoothing can confound electrocardiographic interpretation if one is not familiar with it or aware that it is programmed "on." In this tracing, normal sinus rhythm is replaced by an atrial tachyarrhythmia. Rather than an abrupt increase in the paced ventricular rate in response to the atrial tachyarrhythmia, there is gradual shortening of the VV cycle length. The cycle length is regulated by rate smoothing and is allowed to change by the programmed smoothing factor; in this example, the smoothing factor is 9%. AS, atrial sensing; V-A, interval from ventricular sensed or paced event to atrial paced event; VP, ventricular pacing.

ventricle. For example, if the monitored VV interval is 800 ms and 6% rate smoothing is programmed, the algorithm allows the upcoming ventricular rate of the cycle to increase or decrease a maximum of 6%, or ±48 ms (752–848 ms). Rate stabilization algorithms function in an analogous manner to prevent long pauses, and similarly can result in "unexpected" pacing on the surface ECG.

Other algorithms also result in "unexpected" atrial pacing or intrinsic conduction. For example, atrial fibrillation (AF) suppression algorithms may maintain atrial pacing at a rate slightly faster than the intrinsic rate, and periodically extends the cycle length to reassess the intrinsic rate.[5] Once intrinsic conduction is seen, the rate is again increased to maintain atrial pacing. Thus, surface electrocardiography reveals predominantly paced atrial rhythms with spontaneously slow, up to two conducted intrinsic beats, and then more rapid atrial pacing. Ventricular avoidance pacing algorithms may also result in tracings with predominantly paced atrial rhythms with what may appear to be inappropriate lack of ventricular pacing artifacts.[6]

Most manufacturers have some variation of rate drop response or sudden brady response, designed primarily for patients with neurocardiogenic syncope. This type of feature is triggered when the native heart rate decreases through a programmed rate-drop window, after which the device paces at a faster programmed rate (generally 90–100 ppm) until spontaneous rhythm is detected. Other devices offer some type of search hysteresis, in which the device paces for a programmed number of cycles at an accelerated rate (usually 90–100 pulses/min) when the native rate drops below the lower rate limit. Search hysteresis can lead to misinterpretation of the electrocardiogram if the feature is not well understood or if the healthcare professional interpreting the electrocardiogram is unaware that the feature is programmed "on" (Fig. 10.10).

Rate-adaptive sensors can also cause confusion. Sensors based on physiologic stimuli, such as thoracic impedance or intracardiac impedance measurements, may increase the pacing rate even when the patient is not physically active (as with activity-based sensors). The sensor-driven rates may therefore cause confusion because the paced rates may seem inappropriate for a given activity (Fig. 10.11). Patients may experience symptoms of fatigue or effort intolerance if the sensor is not programmed aggressively enough and symptoms

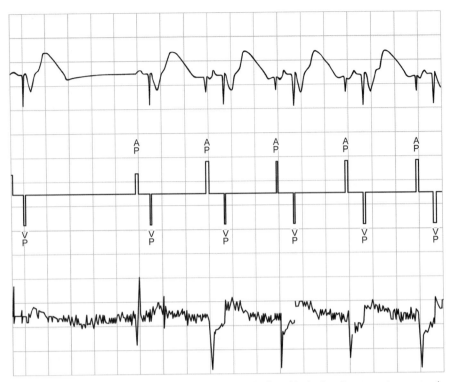

Fig. 10.10 Sudden onset of pacing at a rate of 100 ppm. This occurs as a result of a sudden bradycardia response, i.e., a pacemaker feature that will pace at a faster rate for a programmed period of time when there is a drop in heart rate that meets preset criteria of the algorithm. The purpose of this feature is to better support the patient's blood pressure when neurocardiogenic responses result in cardio-inhibition, which is often accompanied by vasodepression.

Sensor Indicated Rate Histogram

Sensor	On	Date Read	9 Jan 2000 12:22
Base Rate	90 ppm	Total Time Sampled	0d 0h 1m 26s
Max Sensor Rate	110 ppm	Sampling Rate	16 s
Slope	11		
Threshold	2.0		
Measured Average Sensor	2.1		
Reaction Time	Fast		
Recovery Time	Medium		

Note: The above values were obtained when the histogram was interrogated.

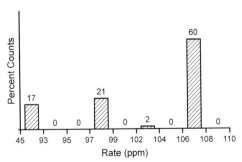

Bin Number	Range (ppm)	Time	Sample Counts
1	45 - 93	0d 0h 0m 14s	9
2	93 - 95	0d 0h 0m 0s	0
3	95 - 97	0d 0h 0m 0s	0
4	97 - 99	0d 0h 0m 17s	11
5	99 - 102	0d 0h 0m 0s	0
6	102 - 104	0d 0h 0m 1s	1
7	104 - 106	0d 0h 0m 0s	0
8	106 - 108	0d 0h 0m 52s	32
9	108 - 110	0d 0h 0m 0s	0
		Total:	53

Note: Sensor Param. changed since histogram was cleared.

Fig. 10.11 Inappropriate sensor response is determined from the "Sensor Indicated Rate Histogram." During a casual walk of 1 min 26 s, the patient's heart rate varied from the lowest rate bin to a point near the maximum sensor rate of 110. Sixty percent of the counts were in the 106–108 ppm rate bin. The patient complained of dyspnea during the casual walk. With reprogramming to less aggressive rate-adaptive parameters, the walk was well tolerated.

of palpitations or tachycardia if it is programmed too aggressively (see Chapter 9: Rate-Adaptive Pacing).

Diagnostic features

Most contemporary devices offer sophisticated diagnostic options that can help troubleshoot potential causes of clinical events and aid in optimal programming and detection of potential problems before symptoms develop.[7–9] Such diagnostic features include the number of mode-switching events, number of high-rate atrial events, number of ventricular high-rate episodes, number of ectopic events, percentage of time paced and sensed in all chambers, electrograms, and trending of such values as lead impedance.

Pacemakers provide diagnostic interpretation channels. An electrocardiographic recorder from the programmer is applied to the patient, and telemetry is established with the pacemaker. The marker channel offers real-time, simultaneous electrocardiographic signals and markers denoting paced and sensed events as well as refractory events occurring in each channel. This feature is especially helpful in attempting to determine whether the device is undersensing or oversensing, or if "functional" sensing abnormalities exist (Fig. 10.12).

In nonpacemaker-dependent patients who have experienced a clinical event suggesting possible pacing system failure which is not identified by a thorough noninvasive evaluation, Holter monitoring or an event recorder may be considered (Fig. 10.13).

Battery voltage should always be assessed during troubleshooting. Battery depletion, although expected, is still the most common cause of pacemaker failure.[1] Some devices provide a measured numerical battery voltage, which should generally be above 2.4 V in lithium-based batteries, and others give a "gas gauge" representation of battery status. Another way to grossly assess battery voltage is to note the magnet rate. All pacemakers have a characteristic magnet rate that changes predictably as the battery voltage decreases. Unfortunately, each manufacturer uses a different magnet rate, necessitating knowledge of or access to that information to ascertain battery status. Assessment of the magnet rate is a key component in transtelephonic pacemaker monitoring. As the battery approaches depletion, most devices reset to a backup mode. Backup mode is usually fixed-rate ventricular pacing at maximal output. Most devices also lose telemetry function and programmability when the battery nears imminent failure.

Unexpected device failure

Contemporary pacemakers and implantable cardioverter-defibrillators (ICDs) have achieved an extraordinary level of reliability. However, rare random component failures occur.[1]

If a component malfunction is suspected, the manufacturer should be asked whether similar problems have been reported. Physicians should report adverse device events via the FDA's MedWatch program using a simple

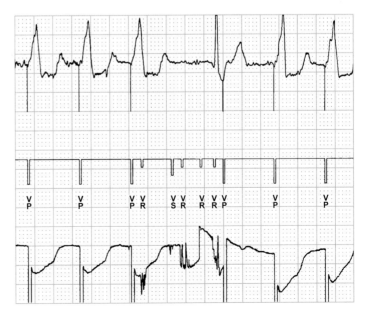

Fig. 10.12 Programmer-derived tracing with: top, surface ECG; middle, marker channel; bottom, ventricular electrogram. On the surface ECG there is a VV interval that is longer than any other interval present on the tracing. On the marker channel the pause correlates with multiple ventricular sensed events (VS) and ventricular events that occur in a refractory period (VR). This represents oversensing that was caused by a conductor coil fracture. Although oversensing would be suspected based on the surface tracing alone, the marker channels confirm oversensing and provide diagnostic information as to the mechanism. The sharp, saturated electrograms are consistent with "make-break" contact noise from a fracture site.

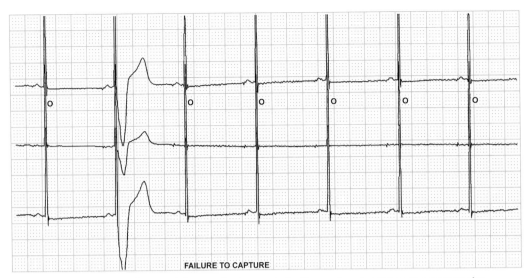

FAILURE TO CAPTURE

Fig. 10.13 Three-channel tracing from an ambulatory monitor that was obtained because the patient had recurrent symptoms after pacemaker implantation. The tracing demonstrates failure to capture and the pacemaker malfunction correlated with symptoms. The patient was found to have developed excessively high pacing thresholds on epicardial pacing leads.

online form (https://www.accessdata.fda.gov/scripts/medwatch/). Other sources of information also exist. There is no comprehensive, mandatory database of pacemaker pulse generator and lead usage and function at present in the USA.

Operative evaluation of pacing systems

Sometimes the status of a pacing system is impossible to determine noninvasively. If intermittent system failure is strongly suspected clinically and comprehensive noninvasive evaluation has been unrevealing, operative assessment may be required.

Invasive troubleshooting should begin with pulse generator manipulation in the open pocket while the electrocardiogram is observed for abnormalities in pacing or sensing. After delivery of the generator from the pocket, the connection between the pins and the setscrews should be inspected. The lead or leads should then be disconnected from the pulse generator, and thresholds, current, and impedance should be directly measured by the pacing system analyzer before any further manipulation of the leads. Normally, only minor variation exists between the values obtained by telemetry and those obtained by direct measurement; gross differences suggest lead abnormalities. One of the most important measurements obtained at the time of intraoperative troubleshooting is lead impedance. After the electrical integrity of the lead is assessed, the leads should be carefully dissected away from any fibrous tissue and visually inspected. Any obvious breaks in the insulation or fractures in the coil should be noted, especially in the area under any anchoring or purse-string sutures. Blood in the lead is *de facto* evidence of a breach in the insulation. Unfortunately, only that portion of the lead that is extravascular can be visually inspected. Any breach of lead integrity would likely warrant lead replacement. Attempting lead repair is rarely, if ever, the best approach.

However, one is sometimes left with a clinical situation strongly suggestive of pacing system malfunction and no obvious point of failure. In that case, careful consideration could be given to empirically placing a new lead, especially the ventricular lead in a pacemaker-dependent patient. However, empiric replacement of any portion of the pacing system should be considered only as a last resort.

Focused troubleshooting

Now that the broader troubleshooting issues have been discussed, we focus on specific, presenting clinical problems. Most problems can be categorized by electrocardiographic abnormalities:
• Failure to capture
• Failure to output
• Undersensing
• Alteration of pacing rate.
Or by patient symptoms:
• Syncope or near-syncope
• Palpitations
• Fatigue.

Each category is discussed after a differential diagnosis has been provided. Some problems occur more commonly early after implantation (i.e., within the first few weeks post-implant), some much later, and others completely independent of time. An attempt is made to classify each abnormality by whether it is most likely to occur early, late, or at any time after implantation.

Failure to capture

The differential for failure to capture and the most likely time of appearance for the abnormality are as follows:

- Lead dislodgment   Early
- Damage at the   At any time
  electrode–myocardial
  interface
- Exit block   After the first 4–6 weeks
- Perforation   Acute (usually manifest
                                                   within 48 h)
- Lead fracture   Usually late
- Lead insulation failure   Usually late
- Loose setscrew (Fig.   Usually early
  10.14)
- Battery failure (Fig.   Usually late
  10.15)
- Circuit failure   At any time
- Air in pocket (unipolar)   Acute
- Pseudo-malfunction   At any time
- Metabolic or drug effect   At any time

A clinical approach to assessment of the most common causes of failure to capture is detailed in Table 10.4.

Lead dislodgment usually occurs within the first few weeks after implantation. It may be microdislodgment or macrodislodgment. Macrodislodgment implies that the problem is radiographically evident. Microdislodgment implies that the clinical situation is consistent with dislodgment, but that there is no radiographic evidence that the lead has moved (see Chapter 6: Implant-Related Complications).

With lead dislodgment, failure to capture may be intermittent or persistent. It is often, but not always, accompanied by sensing abnormalities (Fig. 10.16). If macrodislodgment is confirmed, the lead should be repositioned. The diagnosis of microdislodgment should be entertained and the lead repositioned only if other causes of failure to capture have been excluded.

In Fig. 10.17, atrial lead dislodgment leads to cross-stimulation. Cross-stimulation is defined as stimulation of a cardiac chamber different from the one to which the stimulus is directed. This may result from atrial lead dislodgment into the ventricle or from atrial lead stimulation near the tricuspid valve or in the coronary sinus. Cross-stimulation as a reversal of lead connection may also occur but is uncommonly reported (Fig. 10.18).

Elevated thresholds may be due to a variety of causes, including lead dislodgment, perforation, loss of lead integrity (e.g., fracture or insulation defect), damage at the electrode–myocardium interface and metabolic, electrolyte, or drug changes (Fig. 10.13). Although the etiology of the elevated pacing threshold must be determined and managed, as a temporary measure an attempt should be made to re-establish capture by increasing output parameters.

Damage at the electrode–myocardial interface may occur from several causes. Myocardial infarction, an infiltrative cardiomyopathic process, or localized damage secondary to cardioversion or defibrillation could damage the myocardium at the site of the electrode.[10] With an infiltrative process, the alteration in pacing or sensing threshold may be permanent. Following myocardial infarction, cardioversion, or defibrillation, the changes may be transient or permanent.

Altered pacing-sensing thresholds after cardioversion-defibrillation occur if the electrical current is transmitted through the lead and results in a circumscribed burn at the electrode–myocardial interface (Fig. 10.19). The threshold alteration is usually transient, minutes or hours. The potential risk may be minimized, but not completely eliminated, by maximizing the distance between the cardioversion pads and the implanted device.

Exit block, by definition, is manifested as increased thresholds. Exit block is defined as chronically elevated thresholds, presumably due to excessive fibrosis or some other problem at the electrode–myocardial interface. True exit block is uncommon, and the cause is not well understood. Steroid-eluting leads generally, but not always, prevent exit block. The diagnostic problem is trying to differentiate exit block from microdislodgment. If microdislodgment is the presumed diagnosis, the lead is repositioned and thresholds improve and are maintained long term, microdislodgment is confirmed as the correct diagnosis. If exit block is the real problem, the thresholds will rise again. If this occurs with steroid-eluting leads, the only option is to program the pacing output to levels that allow consistent pacing and maintain an adequate safety margin. Most contemporary pacemakers can be programmed to maximum outputs of approximately 7.5 V and 1.5 ms. If capture cannot be maintained at these levels, therapeutic options are limited. Repositioning the ventricular lead or placing a new lead in an alternative ventricular site may be successful. Alternatively, coronary sinus pacing may be considered with long-term outcomes of coronary sinus pacing becoming more predictable.[11] Epicardial pacing could also be considered even though epicardial

ECG Controls

Surface ECG	On
Position	1
Gain	0.5 mV/div
Filter	Off
Markers	On
Position	2
IEGM	On
Position	2
Gain	2.5 mV/div
Configuration	V IEGM Uni
Sweep Speed	25 mm/s

Programmed Parameters

Mode	DDD
Base Rate	60 ppm
A-V Delay	175 ms
P-V Delay	150 ms
Magnet Response	Temporary Off
Temporary 30	Off

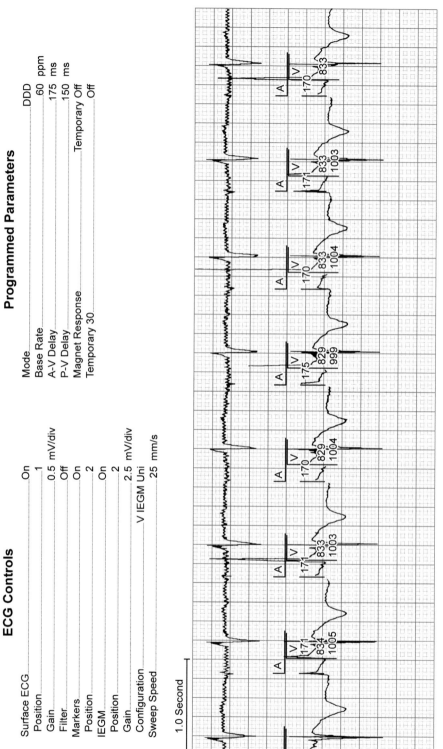

Fig. 10.14 Surface ECG (top) and unipolar ventricular electrogram (bottom) from a patient who presented with ventricular failure to output at a routine followup. No ventricular pacing artifacts could be seen on the surface ECG when programmed to DDD or DOO mode. This tracing, obtained in a DDD mode, demonstrates that the pacemaker is delivering atrial and ventricular outputs. However, failure of the ventricular pacing output to be seen on the surface ECG suggests that the circuit is interrupted. In this case the chest X-ray demonstrated a connector pin that was not fully engaged in the connector block.

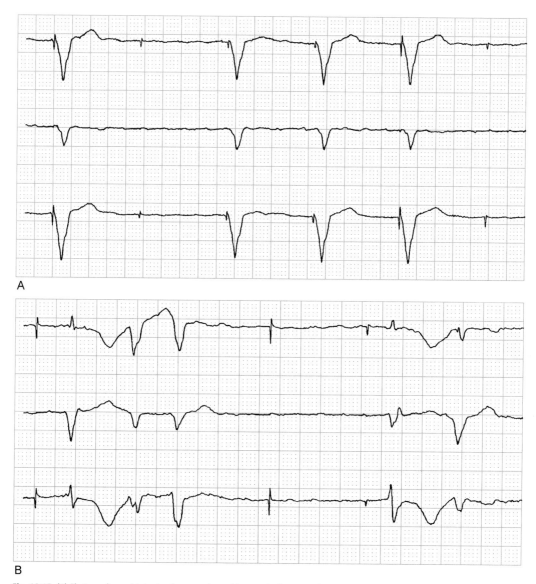

Fig. 10.15 (A) Electrocardiographic tracing from a patient with a ventricular pacemaker and recurrent near-syncope. The patient had not had her pacemaker checked in several years. The electrocardiogram reveals intermittent failure to capture, and troubleshooting results were consistent with nearly total battery depletion. (B) The patient was admitted to the hospital, and a subsequent tracing demonstrated complete failure to capture and ventricular rhythm disturbances secondary to the bradycardia. At the time of pulse generator replacement, lead function was normal.

thresholds are characteristically higher than endocardial thresholds, which may not be the case in the patient with exit block on a transvenous lead. Again, long-term outcome cannot be predicted and only long-term observation will determine success.

The use of systemic steroids to treat high outputs may be contemplated. Large doses of systemic steroids usually result in a decrement in pacing thresholds. However, when administration is discontinued, the thresholds generally increase again. Long-term use of steroids is obviously not desirable because of the systemic side effects.

Perforation may also cause elevated thresholds and is discussed in Chapter 6: Implant-Related Complications.

Metabolic and drug alterations may also affect thresholds and result in failure to capture.[12–20] Drugs that may affect pacing thresholds are listed in Table 10.3. Two

Table 10.4 Failure to capture.

Determine pacing threshold
Able to obtain consistent capture at higher output – yes or no

Check impedance
If low – recheck in unipolar configuration
- If impedance normal in unipolar configuration suggests loss of integrity of the outer insulation
If high – recheck in unipolar configuration
- If impedance normal in unipolar configuration suggests defect in the outer conductor coil
- Obtain chest X-ray and inspect carefully for conductor coil fracture and connection at the connector block
If normal – obtain chest X-ray to look for dislodgment
- Gross dislodgment – reposition
- No definite evidence of dislodgment, consider other causes for a rise in threshold
  - Damage at the electrode–myocardial interface
  - Drugs that may raise pacing thresholds
  - Exit block (assumes lead is not acutely placed)

comments should be made about drug therapy. Class IC antiarrhythmic agents are the most likely drugs to affect pacing thresholds. If a pacemaker-dependent patient is placed on a Class IC agent, administration should be done cautiously and the patient's course followed carefully. This class of drugs may also affect sensing thresholds (Fig. 10.20).[13–15,21]

A common misconception is that amiodarone will frequently result in an increase in pacing thresholds. Amiodarone can raise pacing thresholds secondary to drug-induced hypothyroidism.[17] In the euthyroid patient, amiodarone rarely if ever causes elevated pacing thresholds.

Most severe metabolic disturbances can affect pacing and sensing thresholds.[22–25] Hyperkalemia is the most commonly encountered metabolic disturbance to do so. The most frequent clinical scenario is in the pacemaker patient who is undergoing dialysis. Although programming output or sensing variables may help in

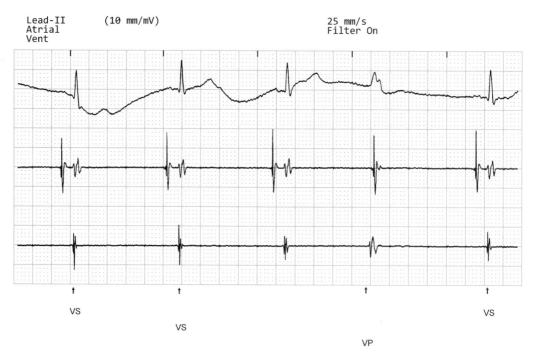

Fig. 10.16 Tracing from a patient with the pulse generator programmed to VVI at a rate of 30 ppm. The surface tracing, top, reveals a single paced beat and corresponds to a ventricular pace (VP) marker. (The second tracing from the top represents the atrial electrogram and the bottom tracing represents the ventricular electrogram.) It is important to take advantage of all of the information offered by the pacemaker, but it is just as important to take advantage of information "not provided" by the pulse generator. In this example, all of the ventricular events are labeled on the marker channel with the exception of the third ventricular event. This is because the event was not sensed and therefore not labeled as a VS event. The interval from the paced event backward to the second event equals approximately 2000 ms or 30 ppm.

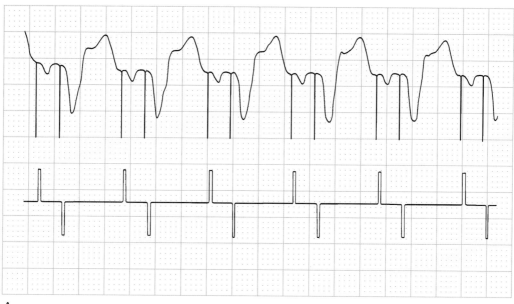

A

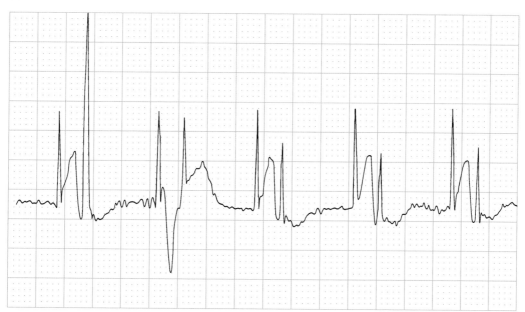

B

Fig. 10.17 (A) Electrocardiographic tracing shortly after the implantation of a dual-chamber pacemaker. The tracing confirms atrial and ventricular capture. (B) Electrocardiographic tracing from the same patient at a 4-week follow-up examination. The atrial pacing artifact results in ventricular stimulation, and the ventricular artifact occurs at the same atrioventricular interval but falls after the ventricular depolarization. Chest radiography confirmed that the atrial lead had dislodged into the ventricular lead. Because the intrinsic deflection of the ventricular depolarization was consistently falling within the blanking period, the atrioventricular interval was not disturbed.

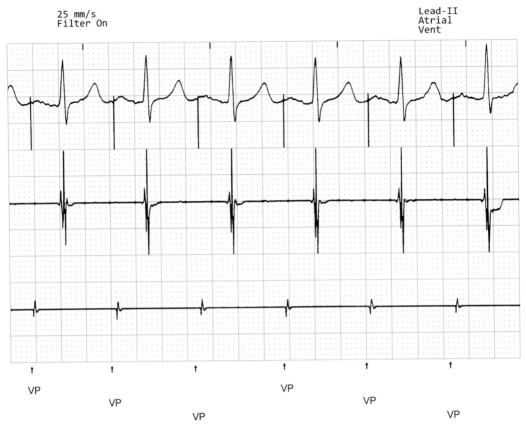

Fig. 10.18 Telemetry from a dualchamber pacemaker; top channel is surface ECG; second channel atrial electrogram; third channel ventricular electrogram and bottom channel is of "markers." The pacemaker is programmed to the VVI mode during this tracing, but there is consistent atrial pacing and the ventricular EGM channel actually displays the atrial electrogram. The ventricular lead had been connected to the atrial port of the dual-chamber pacemaker and the atrial lead connected to the ventricular port.

the short term, the definitive treatment is to lower the potassium levels and avoid subsequent episodes of hyperkalemia.

Older studies have documented sensing and pacing threshold variations with such everyday activities as sleeping and eating.[15–17] Although well documented, the threshold variations are minimal. In addition, with the low achievable pacing thresholds and outstanding sensing thresholds achievable with contemporary pacing systems as well as a broad range of programming options, the issue is rarely clinically significant.

Loose setscrew can cause failure to capture. Although this is usually detected in the early post-implantation period, a setscrew that has not been effectively tightened may not work loose for months. The clinical presentation of a loose setscrew depends on the degree of contact between the connector pin and the header. If the header and pin are completely disconnected, complete failure to output occurs because of the circuit interruption. If failure of contact is intermittent, failure to output is also intermittent (Fig. 10.14). Although this is the most common presentation, minimal contact between pin and header may allow transmission of a pacing artifact but inadequate energy is transmitted to result in capture. Intermittent contact may also lead to oversensing with consequent inhibition of pacing.

Conductor coil fracture may produce failure to capture, failure to output, and sensing abnormalities (Fig. 10.21). Although this could theoretically happen at any time, it is most often a "late" or chronic complication. In complete fracture, the electrocardiographic findings are persistent. In "make-or-break" fracture, the electrocardiographic abnormalities are intermittent. If the fracture is complete, i.e., the circuit is interrupted, failure to output occurs. If the break is incomplete, i.e., only a portion of the output pulse is transmitted to the

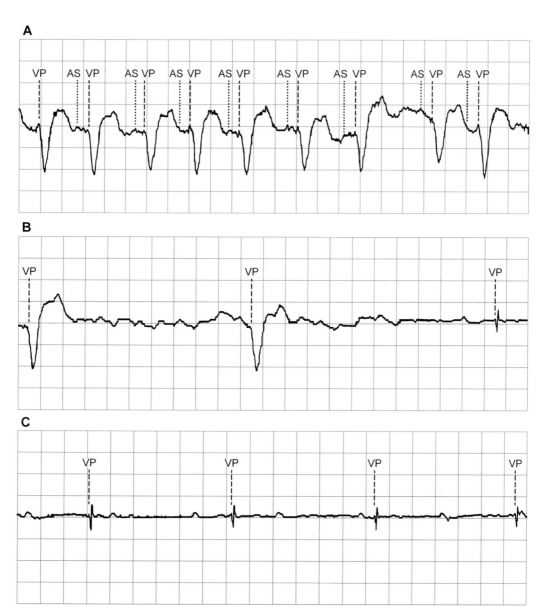

Fig. 10.19 (A) Baseline electrocardiographic tracing from a patient with a dual-chamber pacemaker with underlying atrial fibrillation. (The "marker" notations have been added to facilitate interpretation of the tracing.) The atrial fibrillation is being tracked by the ventricular channel, resulting in an irregular paced ventricular rhythm. (B) The pacemaker has been programmed to a VVI mode at a rate of 30 bpm and the patient has been cardioverted using the precautions discussed in the text. However, despite all precautions being taken, the pacemaker is not functioning as programmed with apparent paced rates that are less than the programmed 30 bpm and failure to capture with the third pacing artifact. Also notes atrial fibrillation persists at this point. (C) Tracing obtained shortly after the one shown in panel B now demonstrates an underlying sinus rhythm. However, there is complete failure to capture. An emergency temporary pacing wire was placed but within a very short period of time the ventricular pacing threshold improved and ventricular capture was consistent via the permanent pacemaker and the temporary wire removed. However, no atrial functions could be restored on the pacemaker consistent with permanent damage to the pacemaker during the cardioversion. The pulse generator was replaced and chronic pacing and sensing thresholds on both leads were acceptable.

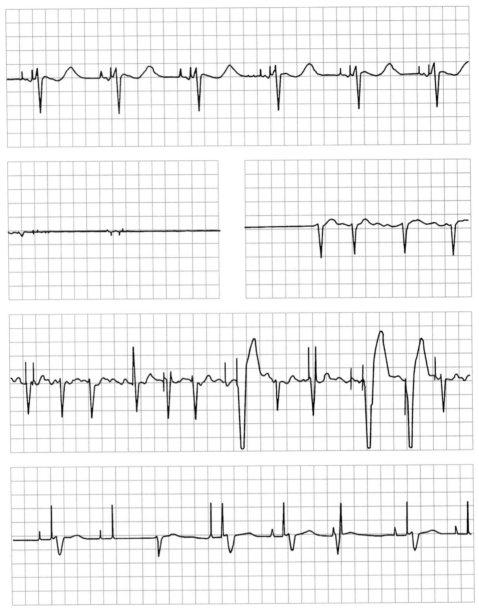

Fig. 10.20 Series of electrocardiographic tracings from a patient who received a dual-chamber pacemaker for tachycardia-bradycardia syndrome. The top tracing, obtained on day 1 post-implant, reveals dual-chamber pacing with atrial capture and ventricular fusion or pseudo-fusion. (Without an intrinsic ventricular event, it is impossible to state with certainty whether any degree of fusion exists.) The second tracing, obtained on day 5 post-implant, demonstrates a flat line that suggests an artifact. In fact, a monitoring electrode had fallen off, resulting in 21 s of artifactual recording. The third tracing, obtained on day 6 post-implant, reveals intermittent ventricular failure to sense and capture. The underlying rhythm appears to be atrial fibrillation. The bottom tracing, obtained on day 7 post-implant, suggests intermittent failure to capture and sense in both chambers. Administration of propafenone had been started for treatment of tachyarrhythmias. The drug resulted in significant elevation of both pacing and sensing thresholds.

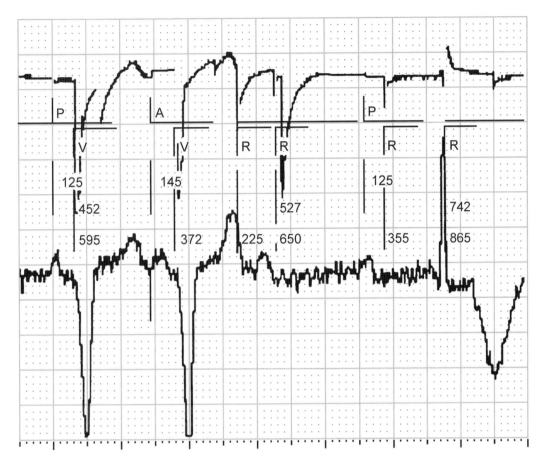

Fig. 10.21 Electrocardiographic tracing obtained by the programmer in a patient with a ventricular lead fracture. The electrogram identifi es intrinsic ventricular events (R) where none occur, because escaping current is sensed by the pacemaker and identified as a ventricular event. There is evidence of failure to capture, identified by a paced ventricular output (V) without a corresponding paced ventricular event on the surface electrocardiogram (lower tracing). Also, there is functional atrial undersensing, i.e., intrinsic P waves are not sensed because the post-ventricular atrial refractory period (PVARP) has been extended. The electrogram (upper tracing) is erratic because of the lead fracture. P, intrinsic atrial event; A, paced atrial event.

heart, failure to capture is seen. Often, both manifestations are present. Escaping current at the "break" may also cause sensing abnormalities.

Although programming a bipolar lead to a unipolar pacing and sensing configuration may restore normal pacing, this "fix" should be considered temporary (Fig. 10.22). Whatever mechanism fractured the outer coil of a coaxial lead could eventually affect the inner coil also.

Insulation break also can produce a variety of clinical manifestations and is most often a "late" complication. Insulation defects may involve the outer insulation or, in a bipolar lead, the insulation between conductors. Sensing abnormalities are the most common electro

cardiographic manifestation.[1] These can be diagnosed as a reduction in bipolar lead impedance with normal uinpolar impedance in leads at risk for this failure mode. Failure to capture and failure to output, intermittent or persistent, may also be seen (Figs 10.23 and 10.24).

As with conductor coil fracture, programming a bipolar lead to unipolar pacing and sensing configuration may restore normal pacing and sensing. If the insulation defect is in a ventricular lead in a pacemaker-dependent patient, even if programming to a unipolar configuration restores normal function, this should be considered a temporary solution and the lead should be replaced.

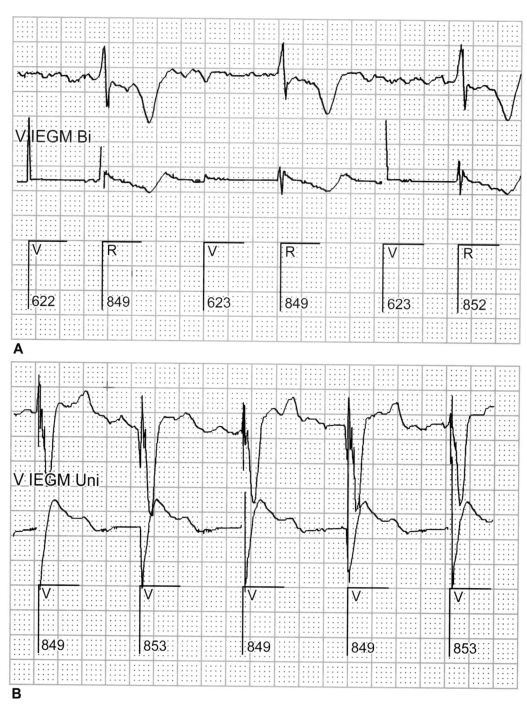

Fig. 10.22 (A) Programmer-derived surface electrocardiogram, ventricular bipolar intracardiac electrogram, and markers demonstrating VVI pacing at 70 ppm with failure to capture. Telemetered ventricular impedance was >9999 Ω. (B) Reprogrammed to the unipolar pacing configuration at the same output settings, ventricular capture is now consistent and the lead impedance is within normal range.

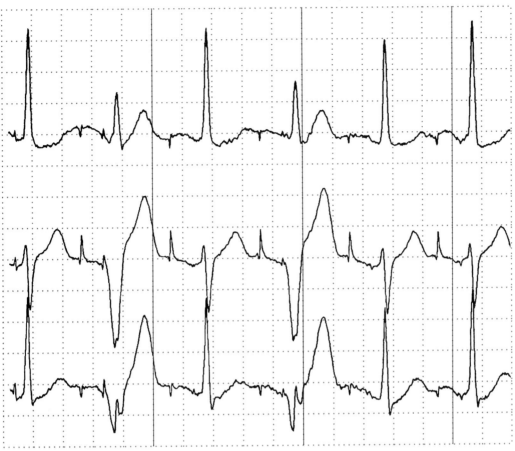

Fig. 10.23 Electrocardiographic tracing obtained from a patient with an older ventricular polyurethane pacing lead on advisory. There is intermittent ventricular failure to capture. The finding is relatively subtle. The second and fourth ventricular events are paced. The other ventricular events are intrinsic. The ventricular pacing artifact precedes the intrinsic ventricular events, but fails to capture. Interrogation revealed a lead impedance of <250 Ω.

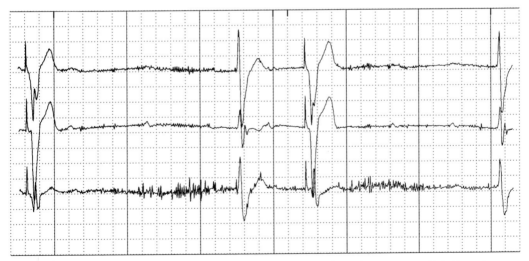

Fig. 10.24 Electrocardiographic tracing obtained from a patient with a pacing lead on advisory due to an unacceptable incidence of insulation failure. In this example, there are two pauses. The intervals are not exact multiples of the paced VV cycle (the distance from the second to third ventricular event). Without marker channel or intracardiac electrograms, it is not possible to say whether this is an example of oversensing or whether there is an undetected paced ventricular artifact with failure to capture. However, with the lead advisory, the possibility of a defective lead is difficult to ignore.

Battery depletion is an expected late occurrence.[1] Fortunately, battery depletion is almost always a predictable phenomenon, one that is readily detected as part of a regular follow-up program.[26] Some pulse generators have had battery depletion patterns that were unpredictable or earlier than projected. If a pulse generator is known to have unpredictable or sudden battery failure, the device should be prophylactically replaced, following guidelines provided by the manufacturer.

Air in the pocket is a complication that is rarely seen but may result in a pacing failure if the pacemaker is functioning in a unipolar pacing configuration. Because a pacemaker in the unipolar pacing configuration must make tissue contact to complete the circuit, air can insulate the pacemaker and prevent tissue contact. Historically, this was of greater potential when one side of the pacemaker was coated and the coated side was placed next to the underlying muscle. This meant that contact had to be maintained with the anterior portion of the pulse generator. This is no longer the case and any surface of the device programmed to the unipolar configuration that is in contact with tissue should maintain normal function. Therefore, even if there was air or fluid anterior to the pulse generator that prevented tissue contact, it would still be maintained on the posterior surface.

Circuit or component failure is rare. Contemporary pacemakers have achieved an extraordinary level of reliability. If a circuit or component failure occurs, the clinical manifestation is usually not predictable and almost any electrocardiographic abnormality is possible.[26]

Pseudo-malfunctions

Several pseudo-malfunctions may suggest failure to capture. Functional failure to capture occurs if a pacing artifact is delivered when the ventricle is functionally refractory. For example, during magnet application and asynchronous pacing, a pacing artifact that occurs early after an intrinsic event will not capture the myocardium (Fig. 10.25).

Isoelectric atrial or ventricular depolarization may suggest failure to capture; i.e., a pacing artifact is recorded but there is minimal, if any, electrocardiographic evidence of depolarization (Fig. 10.26).[22] Confirmation can be obtained by a multichannel recording (Fig. 10.27).

Electrical artifact, i.e., nonpacemaker output artifact, may be misinterpreted as being pacemaker artifact and therefore may suggest failure to capture. Electrical artifact can present in many ways. If there is very regular and very rapid artifact present, one should be suspicious of 60-cycle interference. The first question to ask

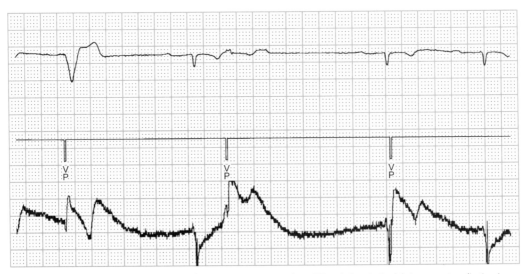

Fig. 10.25 Single-lead electrocardiographic tracing from a patient programmed to a VVI mode but obtained during magnet application, i.e. VOO. The first ventricular paced event (VP) results in ventricular capture. The second VP occurs approximately 360 ms after an intrinsic ventricular event. The myocardium is refractory from the intrinsic depolarization which results in "functional" failure to capture. The third VP appears to occur simultaneously with an intrinsic beat but there is no alteration in intrinsic QRS morphology, i.e. pseudo-fusion beat results.

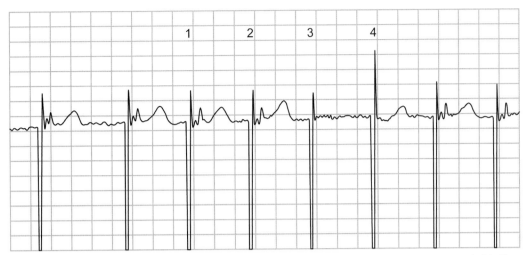

Fig. 10.26 Transtelephonic tracing with magnet application. The first magnet beat is labeled "1." There is failure to capture on the "third" magnet evoked pacing artifact. On the beat that follows, 4, it is difficult to separate a paced QRS from the pacing artifact. Given the accepted variation of pacemaker artifact size when a digital recording system is used, it would be possible to assume that the artifact was a larger variation of the artifact seen in beat 3 and that there was again failure to capture. However, the artifact labeled "4" is followed by a definite T wave. If there is repolarization there had to be depolarization. Therefore, capture was normal with the artifact labeled "4."

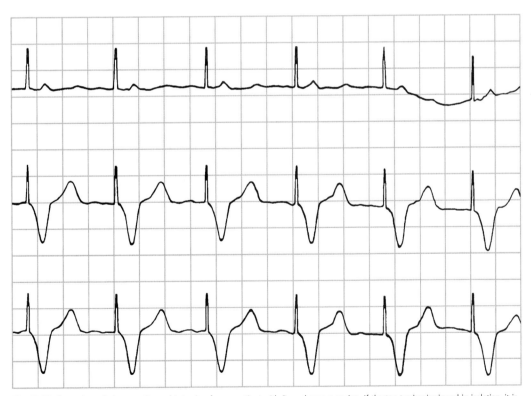

Fig. 10.27 Three-channel electrocardiographic tracing from a patient with P-synchronous pacing. If the top tracing is viewed in isolation, it is difficult to tell which chamber is paced and if there is capture. However, a clue in the top recording is that there appears to be ventricular repolarization, i.e., a T wave; therefore, there must have been depolarization, even if the QRS is difficult to identify.

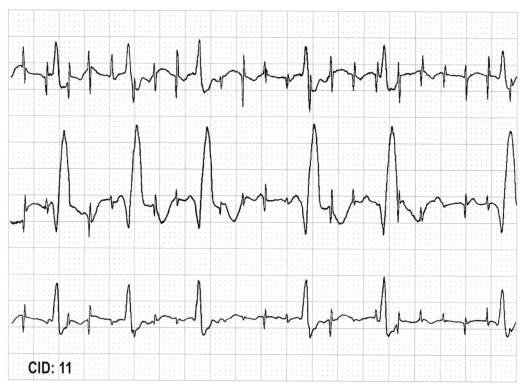

CID: 11

Fig. 10.28 Artifact noted in this tracing obtained during a medical procedure. The patient was asymptomatic. There was a source of 60-cycle interference in the procedure room. When this equipment was turned off, the electrical artifact stopped.

is whether the patient is symptomatic. If not, then before reacting to the electrocardiographic finding, look for and disable any possible source of electrical interference (Fig. 10.28).

Failure to pace (no output)
- Battery failure
- Circuit failure
- Lead fracture
- Insulation failure
- Oversensing
- Loose setscrew
- Crosstalk
- Unipolar lead with pulse generator programmed to bipolar configuration
- Pseudo-malfunction:
  - Ventricular pacing avoidance algorithm
  - Small bipolar pacing artifacts
  - Sleep function (reduction in rate under specific circumstances)
  - Isoelectric intrinsic rhythm.

A clinical approach to assessment of the most common causes of failure to output is detailed in Table 10.5.

Battery failure (Fig. 10.15), circuit or component failure, lead fracture, insulation defect, and loose setscrew have all been discussed as potential causes of failure to output.

The most common cause of failure to output is oversensing. Oversensing implies that something is sensed other than an intrinsic atrial or ventricular depolarization, and therefore the timing cycle is reset and the pacing output inhibited (Fig. 10.29). As previously noted, oversensing may be a manifestation of lead failure, either conductor coil fracture or insulation defect (Fig. 10.24).

Crosstalk occurs when an atrial pacing output is sensed on the ventricular sensing channel, inhibiting ventricular output (Figs 10.30–10.32). Mechanisms that contribute to crosstalk include high atrial output, ventricular sensitivity programmed to a very sensitive value, and positioning of atrial and ventricular leads in close proximity.

In an effort to prevent crosstalk, pacemakers incorporate a post-atrial ventricular blanking period (see Chapter 7: Timing Cycles). The blanking period is the initial portion of the AV interval. During this period, decay of the atrial pacing output is maximal and the

Table 10.5 Failure to pace (output).

Assess multichannel electrocardiogram to determine whether pacing artifacts may be visible in one lead but not another – if artifacts are indeed present, no further evaluation needed

Reprogram the pulse generator to high output settings and to a pacing rate that is unequivocally faster than the patient's underlying rhythm

Obtain telemetry with markers

- If telemetry verifies that the pacemaker is delivering an output at the programmed rate, the pacing circuit has been interrupted and should be carefully evaluated for circuit interruption:
  - Perform pocket manipulation while monitoring the patient; ability to see intermittent output would suggest a loose connection in the connector block
  - Check lead impedance; if there is circuit interruption the lead impedance will be very high
  - Carefully inspect connector block radiographically
  - Carefully inspect the entire length of the lead radiographically

Invasive troubleshooting will probably be necessary at this point

- If no output is seen on telemetry, is there telemetric evidence of other sensed events that may be inhibiting output? If there is evidence of sensed events that do not correlate with any intrinsic cardiac activity:
  - Reassess the lead carefully looking for an intermittent loss of integrity, either insulation or conductor coil, that could be the source of leaking current sensed as activity and inhibiting output
  - Look for any sources of electromagnetic interference. Remove any potential sources from the environment and recheck telemetry

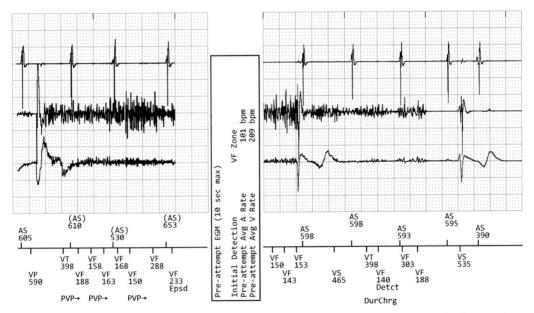

Fig. 10.29 Electrocardiographic tracing from ICD interrogation. Upper tracing, atrial electrogram; middle tracing, ventricular electrogram; lower tracing, surface electrocardiogram; marker channel at the bottom of the figure. There is significant artifact/noise on the ventricular EGM resulting in inhibition of ventricular pacing because the noise is oversensed as ventricular activity and classified as ventricular tachyarrhythmia, i.e., VT, VF.

atrial output has the greatest potential for being sensed on the ventricular channel. If something is sensed immediately after the blanking period, it is not possible to distinguish between crosstalk and an intrinsic event. As a safety measure, dual-chamber pacemakers deliver a ventricular pacing artifact at a foreshortened AV interval if something is sensed in the interval after the blanking period. This portion of the AV interval has been dubbed the crosstalk sensing window. If something is sensed in the crosstalk sensing window, ventricular safety pacing results in effective ventricular capture at a short AV interval, usually 100–110 ms, and

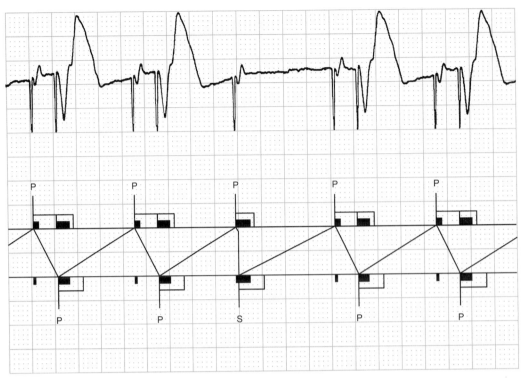

Fig. 10.30 Electrocardiographic example of "crosstalk." Although crosstalk appears to be the most likely cause of ventricular failure to output when the surface electrocardiogram is assessed, it is confirmed by the telemetered "ladder diagram." The ladder diagram, a type of diagnostic channel that is not commonly seen with contemporary devices, confirms that the atrial output was detected almost simultaneously on the ventricular sensing channel and that ventricular output was inhibited. P, paced; S, sensed.

prevents ventricular asystole (Fig. 10.33). If an intrinsic ventricular event is sensed in the crosstalk sensing window, e.g., a premature ventricular contraction, the ventricular safety pacing artifact is delivered within the intrinsic event or shortly after and not during ventricular repolarization (T wave). The ventricle would be refractory and the pacing artifact would not depolarize the ventricle, i.e., functional failure to capture.

When ventricular events are sensed on the atrial sensing channel and reset the timing cycle, the most appropriate description for this abnormality is far-field sensing (Fig. 10.34). The longer intervals are equal to the AR or AV interval plus the programmed AA interval; e.g., if the AR interval is 200 ms and the programmed lower rate limit is 60 ppm, or 1000 ms, the interval lengthened as a result of far-field sensing is 200 plus 1000, or 1200 ms. This effect can usually be eliminated by lengthening the atrial refractory period so that the intrinsic ventricular event is ignored or by programming the atrial channel to a less sensitive value (Fig. 10.35). The former may reduce the upper rate limit of the pacemaker, whereas the latter may result in failure to mode switch during AF.

Oversensing can be caused by many things, which can be classified as:
- Biologic sources of interference, e.g., retrograde P wave, T-wave myopotentials
- Paced ventricular afterdepolarization, i.e., sensing the "decay" of the ventricular pacing output
- Nonbiologic sources of electromagnetic interference (see Chapter 12: Electromagnetic Interference).

If myopotential inhibition is suspected, a series of maneuvers should be performed in an effort to document the cause (Fig. 10.36). In our pacemaker clinic, a series of isometric maneuvers is accomplished while the electrocardiogram is monitored:
- Hands clasped, pulling against each other
- Palms of hands together, pushing against each other
- Reaching with right arm across left shoulder
- Reaching with left arm across right shoulder
- Pocket manipulation (although not specifically to bring out myopotential inhibition, but instead to assess

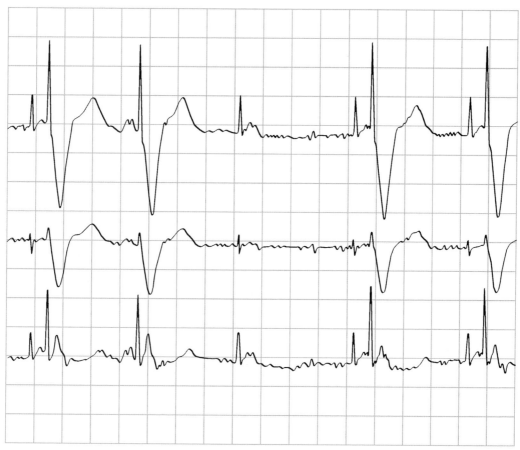

Fig. 10.31 Three-channel tracing from an ambulatory monitor. The tracing begins with AV sequential pacing with a short AV interval, approximately 100 ms, which probably represents ventricular safety pacing, although this cannot be proven without more diagnostic information and programming information. This is followed by an intrinsic atrial depolarization with ventricular tracking. The next event is an atrial paced event without a subsequent ventricular event, i.e., ventricular output inhibition. This is again followed by two cycles of AV sequential pacing, again with a relatively short AV interval. The paced AA interval is consistent between the final two intervals on the tracing. The ventricular failure to output could represent some event that was oversensed on the ventricular sensing channel. However, the consistency of the AA interval and the lack of any artifact on any of the three channels would suggest that oversensing of external noise or an isoelectric event is less likely and crosstalk more likely. If the other AV intervals reflect safety pacing then it is possible that whatever is being sensed as crosstalk during these cycles is instead being sensed beyond the crosstalk sensing window and inhibiting output.

for integrity of the lead or leads and integrity of the lead–connector block connection, this procedure is carried out in concert with the other maneuvers).

If maneuvers induce myopotential inhibition, the programmed sensitivity is made less sensitive and the maneuvers are repeated in an effort to find a sensitivity value at which significant myopotential inhibition no longer occurs but sensing of intracardiac events is still intact (Fig. 10.37).

When an interval longer than the programmed lower rate is observed, the point of sensing can be determined by measuring backward from the pacing artifact that terminates the longer interval (Fig. 10.38). For example, if a VVI pacemaker is programmed to 60 ppm, 1000 ms, and an interval of 1500 ms is observed, measuring back 1000 ms from the pacing artifact that ends the 1500-ms interval marks the point of sensing, i.e., the point at which the timing cycle is reset.

An incompatible lead-header combination is a clinical possibility, but is rarely seen. Lead design and compatibility are discussed in Chapter 4: Choosing the Device Generator and Leads. Any incompatibility of the

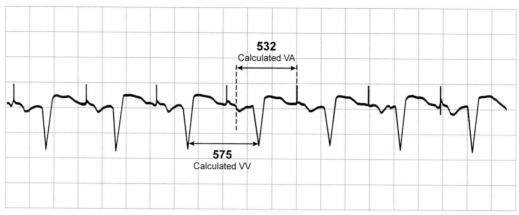

Fig. 10.32 Single-lead tracing from a patient with a dualchamber pacemaker programmed to the DDI mode and a rate of 86 ppm, AVI 165 ms and a ventricular blanking period of 13 ms. The tracing demonstrates a ventricular rate of approximately 104 ppm, RR interval = 575 ms. If the programmed rate is supposed to be 697 ms (86 ppm), the VA interval should be 697 ms − 165 ms (programmed AVI) = 532 ms. However, the effective rate is at a cycle length of 575 ms. 575 ms − the calculated VA interval of 532 ms = AVI of 43 ms. This means that there was sensing of ventricular activity at 43 ms after the atrial output which terminated the AVI and initiated the VA interval. This occurred because there was consistent sensing of the atrial output on the ventricular sensing channel, i.e., crosstalk, but the tracing appears relatively normal because the patient has consistent, albeit prolonged, AV conduction. The abnormality is only clear once the programmed parameters are known.

lead and header should be readily apparent at the time they are connected. To be certain that an adequate connection has been established at the time of implantation if pacing output is not observed, a magnet should be applied to confirm output and capture and/or device interrogation should be performed and thresholds documented via the programmer.

With international standard 1 (IS-1) lead-header designs, unipolar and bipolar leads are of the same dimensions. If a unipolar IS-1 lead is connected to a bipolar pacemaker that is programmed to a bipolar configuration, no pacing will occur. Most contemporary pacemakers detect the incompatibility and prevent the programming combination, allowing the pacemaker to be programmed only to a unipolar configuration.

Pseudo-malfunctions may also suggest failure to output. Small bipolar pacing artifacts may not be visible on the electrocardiogram and raise the question of failure to output or of oversensing.

Digital recording systems may also give the appearance of failure to output.[21] Digital recording systems, the type of electrocardiographic recording system used by most hospitals and offices today, artificially create the pacing artifact (Fig. 10.39). As a function of the system, pacing artifacts may not always be seen. Clues to this abnormality is that the ventricular depolarizations with and without pacing artifacts are of the same morphology. In Fig. 10.40 this pseudo-malfunction is associated with true failure to capture in a patient

with exit block. In this situation, another clue is that all the pauses are a multiple of the programmed lower rate.

Ventricular avoidance pacing algorithms are designed to allow the patient's intrinsic ventricular conduction to dominate and minimize ventricular pacing. Multiple algorithms are available to achieve this outcome (see Chapter 8: Programming). With some algorithms the ventricular output may be inhibited in an attempt to allow intrinsic conduction to occur. This may give the appearance of intermittent failure to output and may be misinterpreted as pacemaker malfunction if the programmed settings are not known (Figs 10.41 and 10.42).

Although not a pseudo-malfunction, a possible error of interpretation may be due to failure to recognize a near-isoelectric P or R wave on a surface ECG lead. If an event is truly isoelectric, an intracardiac electrogram or a diagnostic interpretation channel is necessary to make the diagnosis. Figures 10.43–10.45 show examples of near-isoelectric events. A basic tenet to remember in troubleshooting is that even without a recognizable depolarization, a subsequent repolarization, i.e., a T wave, affirms a preceding depolarization.

Undersensing
• Change in intrinsic complex, e.g., bundle branch block, ventricular fibrillation, ventricular tachycardia, AF
• Myocardial infarction

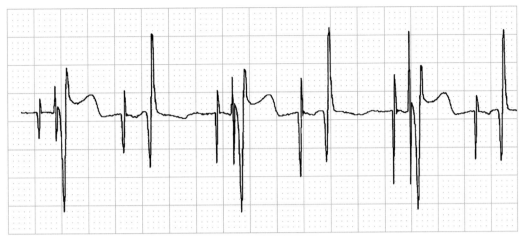

A

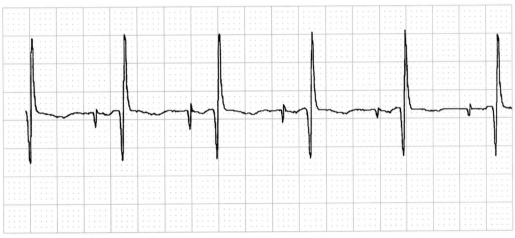

B

Fig. 10.33 (A) Electrocardiographic tracing from a pediatric patient with a dual-chamber pacemaker after surgical correction of a congenital cardiac anomaly. The atrial lead was programmed to excessively high outputs. Every other ventricular event is paced at an abbreviated atrioventricular interval consistent with ventricular safety pacing. We were unable to explain the bigeminal occurrence of the safety pacing. (B) Tracing obtained after reprogramming of the atrial output to values that allowed for an adequate safety margin but no longer resulted in ventricular safety pacing.

• Lead dislodgment or poor positioning (Figs 10.46–10.48)
• Lead insulation failure
• Magnet application
• Battery depletion
• Pulse generator component failure or header abnormality (Fig. 10.49)
• Metabolic or drug effect
• Functional undersensing.

A clinical approach to assessment of the most common causes of undersensing is detailed in Table 10.6.

Any event that results in an intrinsic complex that differs from the intrinsic complex that was present and measured at the time of pacemaker implantation may cause undersensing. For example, a premature ventricular contraction, which may actually appear larger than the normally conducted ventricular event on the surface electrocardiogram, may not be sensed (Fig. 10.50). Making the ventricular sensing channel more sensitive may allow normal sensing of premature ventricular contractions. However, if the undersensing is only intermittent, the premature ventricular

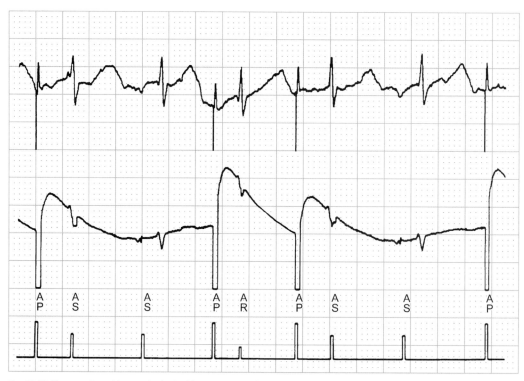

Fig. 10.34 Electrocardiographic example obtained from a patient with an AAI pacemaker. The programmed AA cycle length is 95 ppm, 630 ms. However, some AR intervals are >630 ms. This occurs because there is far-field sensing; i.e., the ventricular event is sensed on the atrial sensing channel and resets the timing cycle. This is verified on the simultaneous marker channel. Three ventricular events – first, third, and fourth – are sensed as atrial events. AP, atrial paced event; AR, atrial event occurring in the refractory period; AS, atrial sensed event.

contractions occur rarely, and the normally conducted beats are appropriately sensed, it may not be necessary to take any additional action.

Undersensing in either chamber is theoretically troublesome because of the potential for competitive pacing. Specifically, the concern is one of pacing in a vulnerable portion of the cardiac cycle, i.e., during repolarization. Pacing on a T wave could initiate ventricular fibrillation or ventricular tachycardia, and pacing during atrial repolarization could initiate AF. Both have been documented, but both are uncommon. This conclusion is supported by the fact that although magnet application results in competitive pacing, as a routine part of transtelephonic follow-up it is rarely identified as inducing a tachyarrhythmia.

As noted above, any event that damages the myocardium at the electrode–myocardial interface could alter sensing thresholds. Undersensing may be a manifestation of conductor coil fracture and insulation break. In fact, sensing abnormalities are the most common elec-trocardiographic manifestation of loss of insulation integrity.

Also noted previously, metabolic disturbances and drugs can affect sensing thresholds. Class IC antiarrhythmic agents are the most likely to alter sensing thresholds, and hyperkalemia is the most common metabolic disturbance to result in undersensing.

Sensing may not be reliable when pacemaker battery reaches a very low voltage level.

As noted below, the first programming step used to correct undersensing is often to make the sensing channel more sensitive, i.e., a smaller number, although uncommon exceptions occur.

Functional undersensing occurs when an intrinsic event falls within a blanking period or refractory period and is not sensed as a function of the pacemaker programming. This can cause confusion in electrocardiographic interpretation unless electrograms or a marker channel is available. Figure 10.21 demonstrates functional undersensing as a result of extension of the

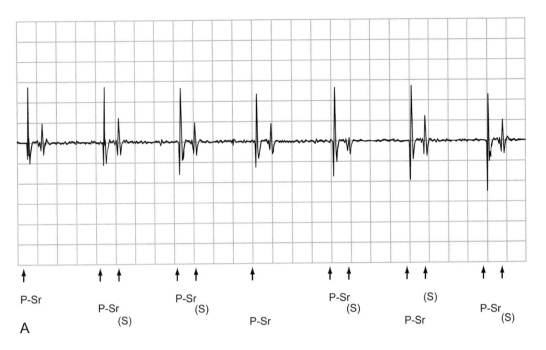

A

Arrhythmia Logbook- Arrhythmia Log						
Episode	Date/Time		Type	Onset (bpm)	Max (bpm)	Duration (HH:MM:SS)
20472	02-JUN-2004	13:12	Tach	320	320	--------
20471	02-JUN-2004	11:49	Tach	280	290	--------
20470	29-MAY-2004	18:21	Tach	280	290	--------
20469	28-MAY-2004	19:30	Tach	290	290	--------
20468	28-MAY-2004	19:29	Tach	290	290	--------
20467	28-MAY-2004	19:27	Tach	290	290	--------
20466	28-MAY-2004	18:36	Tach	300	300	--------
20465	28-MAY-2004	15:47	Tach	300	300	--------
20464	27-MAY-2004	12:05	Tach	300	300	--------
20463	27-MAY-2004	10:16	Tach	290	300	--------
20462	26-MAY-2004	11:11	Tach	290	290	--------
20461	23-MAY-2004	17:56	Tach	300	300	--------
20460	23-MAY-2004	17:55	Tach	290	290	--------
20459	22-MAY-2004	13:21	Tach	300	300	--------
20458	22-MAY-2004	13:20	Tach	290	290	--------
20457	19-MAY-2004	12:54	Tach	290	300	--------
20456	17-MAY-2004	19:00	Tach	290	290	--------
20455	07-MAY-2004	15:46	Tach	300	300	--------
20454	05-MAY-2004	15:59	Tach	290	300	--------
20453	05-MAY-2004	13:39	Tach	300	320	--------
20452	05-MAY-2004	13:37	Tach	290	300	--------
20451	05-MAY-2004	13:33	Tach	300	300	--------
20450	05-MAY-2004	13:31	Tach	300	300	--------
20449	05-MAY-2004	13:15	Tach	300	320	--------
20448	05-MAY-2004	12:34	Tach	300	300	--------
20447	05-MAY-2004	12:32	Tach	290	290	--------
20446	05-MAY-2004	12:30	Tach	290	300	--------
20445	05-MAY-2004	12:27	Tach	290	300	--------
20444	05-MAY-2004	12:23	Tach	290	300	--------
20443	05-MAY-2004	12:21	Tach	290	300	--------
20442	05-MAY-2004	11:37	Tach	300	320	--------
20441	05-MAY-2004	11:07	Tach	280	290	--------
20440	05-MAY-2004	11:02	Tach	300	300	--------
20439	05-MAY-2004	10:53	Tach	290	300	--------
20438	05-MAY-2004	10:45	Tach	290	300	--------
20437	05-MAY-2004	10:36	Tach	300	300	--------
20436	05-MAY-2004	10:29	Tach	280	300	--------
20435	05-MAY-2004	09:42	Tach	290	290	--------
20434	05-MAY-2004	09:30	Tach	290	290	--------
20433	05-MAY-2004	09:04	Tach	250	260	--------

B

Fig. 10.35 Refractory. (A) Programmer-derived tracing that demonstrates sensor-driven atrial pacing (P-Sr) and intermittent sensed (S) events that follow the sensor-driven atrial event. The pacemaker was programmed AAIR at a rate of 75 ppm; atrial refractory period of 280 ms. (B) The arrhythmia logbook had recorded very frequent atrial tachycardias. Although this represents far-field sensing, the far-field events fall within the programmed ARP and therefore do not alter the pacing rate. However, for purposes of tachycardia detection they are counted and the double counting results in the arrhythmia logbook recording this as a tachycardia.

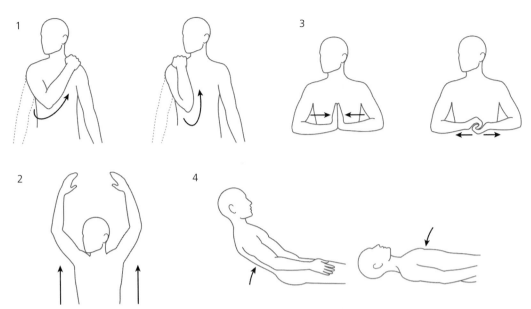

Fig. 10.36 Cartoon depictions of various maneuvers used to provoke interference during troubleshooting a permanent pacemaker. These include: 1. Hands clasped, pulling against each other. 2. Palms of hands together, pushing against each other. 3. Reaching with right arm across left shoulder. 4. Reaching with left arm across right shoulder.

post-ventricular atrial refractory period (PVARP). Because the PVARP is extended in consecutive cycles, the P waves are consecutively within this period and therefore not tracked. The appearance is of true undersensing, but function is normal.

When undersensing occurs (Fig. 10.51), the approach should be as follows:
- Determine the cause of the undersensing
- Assess the amplitude of the undersensed event and compare the measured signal amplitude with the programmed sensitivity
- If possible, correct whatever change has resulted in undersensing
- If the cause of the undersensing cannot be corrected or if immediate resolution is required, reprogram the sensitivity to a more sensitive value.

Alteration in programmed pacing rate
- Circuit failure
- Battery failure
- Magnet application
- Hysteresis
- Crosstalk
- Undocumented reprogramming
- Oversensing
- Runaway pacemaker

- Malfunction of electrocardiographic recording equipment; alteration in paper speed.

Undocumented reprogramming is probably the most common cause of an alteration in the programmed pacing rate; i.e., another healthcare professional has reprogrammed the pacing rate and failed to document the change. To avoid this, a system should be in place whereby any reprogramming requires that the pacemaker be interrogated, the programmed values stored and the programming change recorded in the patient's medical record.

Hysteresis, crosstalk, far-field sensing, and oversensing alter pacing rate, as previously described. If hysteresis is the cause of the altered rate, obviously no action need be taken, because the hysteresis is presumably desirable. If oversensing of any type is causing the altered pacing rate, steps should be taken to correct or remove the source that is being oversensed (see earlier).

Circuit or component failure could alter the programmed rate in an unpredictable fashion. Runaway pacemaker is a manifestation of a component failure or a software-based programming error that results in pacing at dangerously fast rates, in excess of 1000 ppm. It is most likely to occur if a pacemaker is in the field of therapeutic radiation.[23,24] Therapeutic radiation can cause failure of the complementary oxide semiconduc-

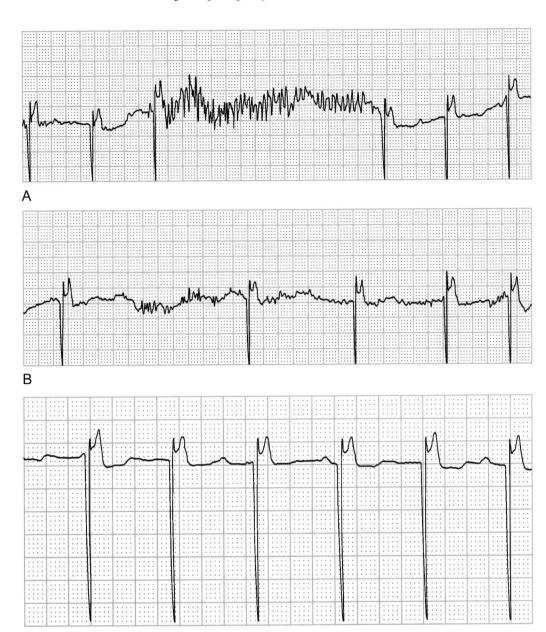

Fig. 10.37 Series of electrocardiographic tracings obtained during provocative maneuvers to induce myopotential inhibition in a patient with a pacemaker programmed to the VVI mode. There is significant inhibition at programming to 1 mV (A) sensitivity. Inhibition decreases at 2.0 mV (B) and is absent at 4.0 mV (C).

tor. The failure is unpredictable by both time of exposure and total radiation. Runaway pacemaker constitutes an emergency. If the patient is hemodynamically compromised, the pacemaker must be urgently disconnected. If time allows, the pacing lead can be properly released from the pacemaker. If hemodynamic failure does not allow the extra time required to properly release the lead, the lead should be transected and temporary pacing should be available if necessary.

Confusion may arise if there is malfunction of the electrocardiographic recording equipment; e.g., the paper sticks or the speed is not constant. This defect

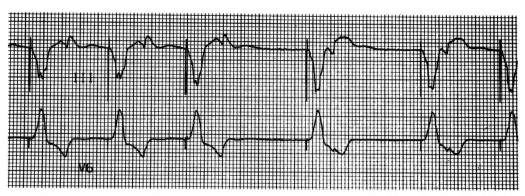

Fig. 10.38 Electrocardiographic tracing from a patient with a VVI pacemaker. The programmed rate of the pacemaker is 70 ppm, 857 ms, but there are longer intervals. Measuring 857 ms backward from the ventricular pacing artifact that ends the longer intervals determines that the point of sensing is either a retrograde P wave or a T wave. Without electrograms or a diagnostic interpretation channel, one cannot be certain which event was oversensed. (From Hayes DL, Zipes DP. Cardiac pacemakers and cardioverter-defibrillators. In Braunwald E, Zipes DP, Libby P, eds. Heart Disease: A Textbook of Cardiovascular Medicine, 6th edn. Philadelphia: WB Saunders Co., by permission of the publisher.)

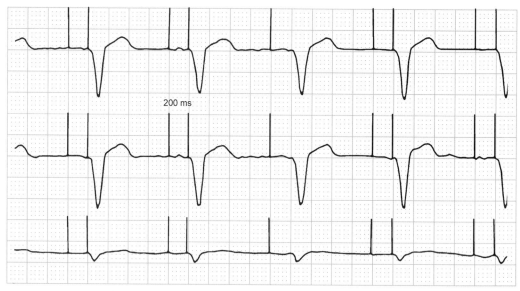

Fig. 10.39 Part of a 12-lead ECG from a patient with a dualchamber pacemaker. The paced QRS morphology is the same for all beats in each of the three channels depicted. However, there is no discernible pacing artifact preceding the third QRS complex. This complex is indeed paced, the patient is completely pacemaker-dependent, but due to the digital recording system, the pacemaker artifacts are not always reliably seen. This may be a source of confusion when interpreting the paced electrocardiogram.

can give the appearance that the pacing rate is different from the programmed rate or erratic. The clinical approach to an alteration in pacing rate depends entirely on the cause.

New symptoms after pacemaker implantation

As initially discussed, some of the most frequently encountered new complaints after pacemaker place-ment are recurrent syncope or presyncope, fatigue, and palpitations. Several pacemaker-specific causes should be considered in the paced patient complaining of these symptoms.

- Pacemaker syndrome
- Failure to capture
- Reversion to backup mode
- Inappropriate programmed rate or sensor

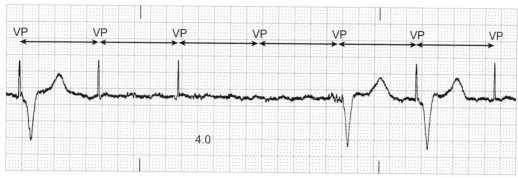

Fig. 10.40 Electrocardiographic tracing from a patient with a pacemaker programmed to the VVIR pacing mode. The lower rate of the pacemaker is programmed to 60 ppm. The tracing was obtained urgently in the emergency department and demonstrates intermittent failure to capture and a long pause without evidence of pacing artifacts, a suggestion of oversensing (pacemaker telemetry was not available at the time). Careful inspection of the second ventricular depolarization reveals the lack of a pacing artifact. This patient was pacemaker-dependent, and all ventricular activity was paced. Pacing artifacts occur during the interval that appears to be a pause without any pacing activity. This finding was proven by intracardiac electrograms. It can also be suspected from the surface electrocardiogram, because the pause is an even multiple of the programmed lower rate interval. If this were oversensing, a pause that was an exact multiple of the pacing rate would be unlikely. The inability to detect pacing artifacts is not uncommon with digital recording systems.

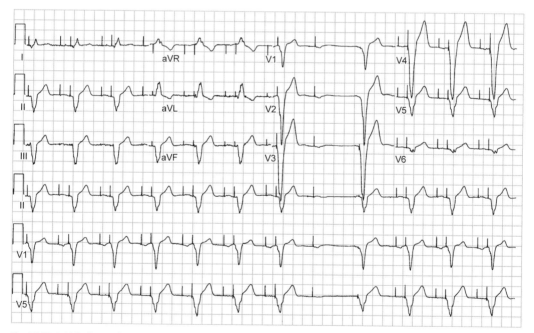

Fig. 10.41 A 12-lead ECG where there is a single episode of ventricular failure to output after a paced atrial event. This is an example of Managed Ventricular Pacing (MVP), a ventricular pacing avoidance algorithm. The pacemaker performs periodic one-cycle checks for AV conduction and the opportunity to resume AAIR or AAI therapy.

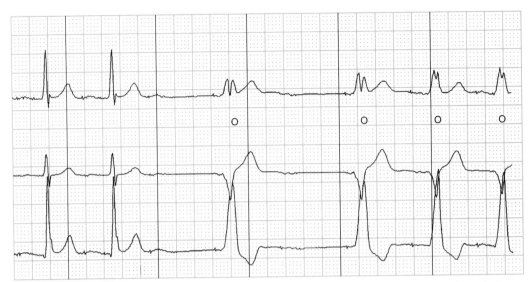

Fig. 10.42 Three-channel recording from an ambulatory monitor. The tracing begins with atrial pacing and intrinsic ventricular conduction with a narrow-complex QRS. This is followed by atrial pacing and capture and no subsequent ventricular pacing output. The next event seen is an atrial pacing artifact that occurs immediately before a wide-complex QRS escape. (The atrial artifact gives the appearance of a pseudo-pseudo-fusion event.) The initial wide-complex event is followed by another atrial pacing artifact and yet another which is immediately followed by another wide-QRS escape complex. The last two RR cycles occur at a shorter cycle length and there is presumed AV nodal conduction from the atrial paced artifacts, but with a continued wide QRS morphology. This is an example of managed ventricular pacing (MVP), one of the ventricular pacing avoidance algorithms. With this algorithm, if two of the four most recent nonrefractory A-A intervals are missing a ventricular event, the pacemaker will identify this as a persistent loss of AV conduction and switch to the DDDR or DDD mode. However, in this example, there are only single A-A intervals missing a ventricular event, so the switch to DDD mode does not occur. This is normal function.

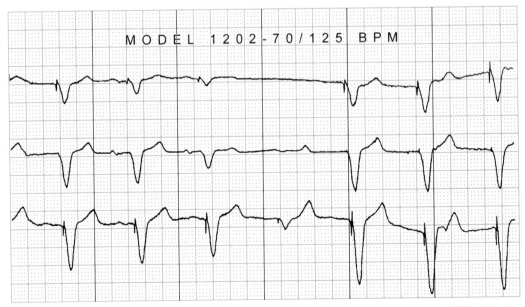

Fig. 10.43 Three-channel recording from a patient with a DDD pacemaker. The top tracing would suggest oversensing with failure to output unless the other ECG leads were available for comparison. The tracing also demonstrates varying degrees of fusion beats. (Tracing courtesy of Dr. Seymour Furman.)

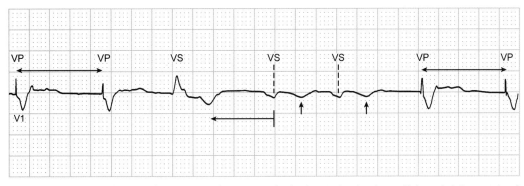

Fig. 10.44 Electrocardiographic tracing from a patient with a VVI pacemaker. (Marker notations have been added to assist in interpretation of the tracing.) After the third ventricular event which is an intrinsic event (VS), there appears to be some baseline activity but no clear-cut cardiac activity. However, measuring backward from the subsequent paced ventricular event by the interval equal to the programmed pacing rate appears to indicate that the activity in the baseline is two intrinsic ventricular events and T waves.

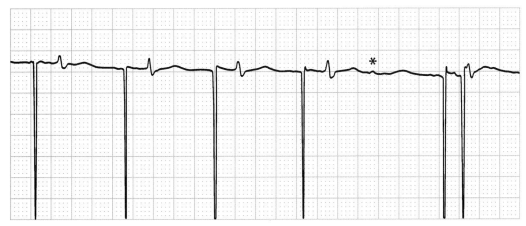

Fig. 10.45 Transtelephonic tracing from a patient with a dual-chamber pacemaker. Measuring back from the final ventricular paced event by an interval equal to the AA interval shows that a small-amplitude complex representing an intrinsic ventricular event is present, noted by (*). (The AA interval is used for measurement because only one paced ventricular event occurs. If there is no alteration of the AV or AR interval, the AA interval should generally be equivalent to the VV interval.)

- Symptomatic upper rate response
- Primary myocardial abnormality or ventricular rhythm disturbance.

Pacemaker syndrome should be suspected if the paced patient complains of general malaise and fatigue. This diagnosis is discussed in Chapter 2: Hemodynamics of Cardiac Pacing. Symptoms include the following:

- General malaise and fatigue
- Chest discomfort
- Cough
- Symptomatic cannon A waves
- Presyncope or syncope
- Confusion
- Dyspnea on exertion.

As part of the troubleshooting process, blood pressure readings should be obtained with and without pacing if the patient is not pacemaker dependent. Blood pressure differences may be even more dramatic if paced and nonpaced pressures are checked in the supine and upright positions. It must be remembered that pacemaker syndrome can occur with any pacing mode if AV synchrony is uncoupled.

Failure to capture or output may result in relative bradycardia and symptoms compatible with low cardiac output. Failure to restore rate response adequately, i.e.,

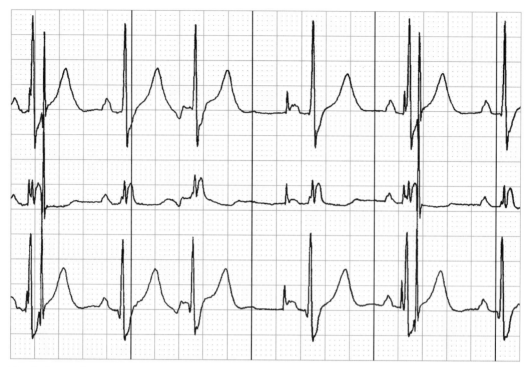

Fig. 10.46 Tracing from an ambulatory monitor shows intermittent atrial failure to sense. This is best seen at the fifth ventricular complex. A P wave precedes the intrinsic ventricular event, but this is not sensed, and an atrial pacing artifact occurs immediately before the intrinsic ventricular complex. The ventricular complex is sensed in the crosstalk sensing window. As a result, the ventricular pacing artifact is delivered early after the intrinsic ventricular event, i.e., ventricular safety pacing.

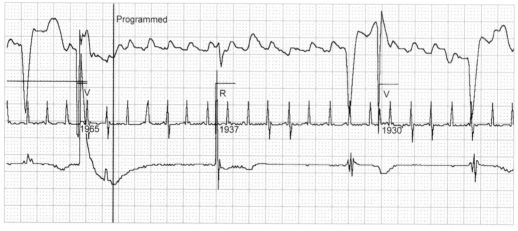

Fig. 10.47 Telemetry with surface electrocardiogram, top; atrial electrogram, middle; and ventricular electrogram, bottom. Markers are present on the ventricular channel. There are six ventricular events but only three with "marker" annotation. The first ventricular event is not sensed and not annotated. The second ventricular event is labeled as a paced ventricular (V) event; the third is an intrinsic ventricular event (R); the fourth is not sensed and is followed approximately 360 ms later by a paced ventricular event (V); and the final event is not sensed.

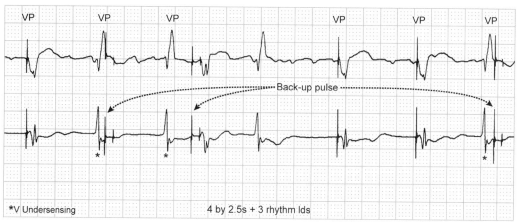

Fig. 10.48 Two-channel rhythm strip from a patient with a pacemaker programmed to the VVI mode with AutoCapture. There is intermittent ventricular undersensing. The (*) note ventricular events that are not sensed and followed by a pacing artifact. Because there is failure to capture, albeit functional failure to capture, the AutoCapture mechanism follows this with a second pacing artifact delivered at higher output. On one occasion the second output is distant enough from the intrinsic ventricular depolarization that the myocardium is no longer refractory and paced depolarization occurs. On the others (arrowhead) there is functional failure to capture on the second output because the myocardium is still refractory.

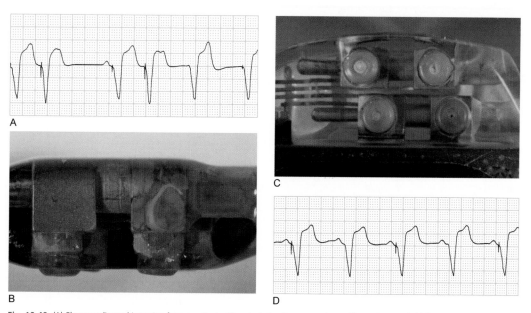

Fig. 10.49 (A) Electrocardiographic tracing from a patient with a dual-chamber pacemaker and intermittent atrial failure to sense. Despite reprogramming, the intermittent atrial undersensing persisted. (B) Side view of pulse generator and (C) top view. At the time of pulse generator replacement, inspection revealed an area of corrosion at the site of one of the atrial grommets. (D) After pulse generator replacement, no further atrial undersensing was noted. Normal P-wave tracking is noted in this tracing.

persistent chronotropic incompetence, may also be accompanied by symptoms compatible with low cardiac output.

Exposure of the pacemaker to electromagnetic interference could potentially cause reversion to a backup mode. Because most backup pacing modes are non-rate-responsive and often single-chamber, patients may experience symptoms of pacemaker syndrome or

general fatigue, effort intolerance from lack of chronotropic support and loss of AV synchrony.

Palpitations are also frequently reported by paced patients. These may be due to the following:
• Intrinsic tachyarrhythmia
• Ventricular tracking of an atrial tachyarrhythmia
• Pacemaker-mediated tachycardia
• Excessive rate response from a sensor-driven pacemaker
• Search hysteresis.

Before mode switching was available, ventricular tracking of atrial tachyarrhythmias was a frequent source of palpitations. Without mode switching, treatment often required programming the pacemaker to a nontracking mode.

Pacemaker-mediated tachycardia (PMT) may occur when AV synchrony is uncoupled and a ventricular event results in retrograde atrial activation. The retrograde atrial event is sensed on the atrial sensing channel of the pacemaker and initiates the AV interval (AVI). When the AVI times out, a ventricular pacing artifact is delivered. If retrograde conduction is sustained, the patient will have a sudden increase in their paced rate, usually to a rate at or near the programmed maximum tracking rate. The tachyarrhythmia will persist until retrograde atrial activation ends, the retrograde atrial

Table 10.6 Failure to sense.

• Check sensing threshold; automatic sensing threshold or manual
• If possible, reprogram sensitivity to a value more sensitive than the measured value
• If unable to program to a sensitivity value that will allow consistent sensing and/or if there is concern that the sensitivity value necessary is so sensitive that oversensing may be a concern, recheck in the unipolar sensing configuration
  • If unipolar sensing thresholds are improved, be suspicious of a loss of lead integrity, especially an insulation defect
  • Check impedance value
• Depending on whether the sensing abnormality is early or late after implant, work through the differential diagnoses

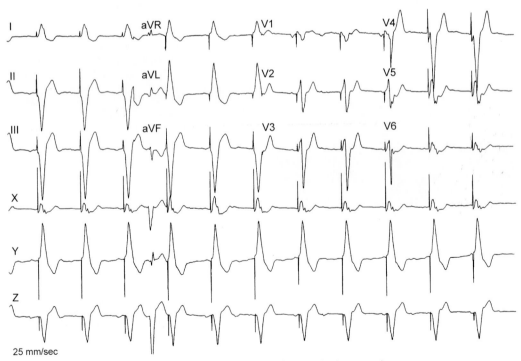

25 mm/sec

Fig. 10.50 Electrocardiographic tracing in which a single premature ventricular contraction is not sensed.

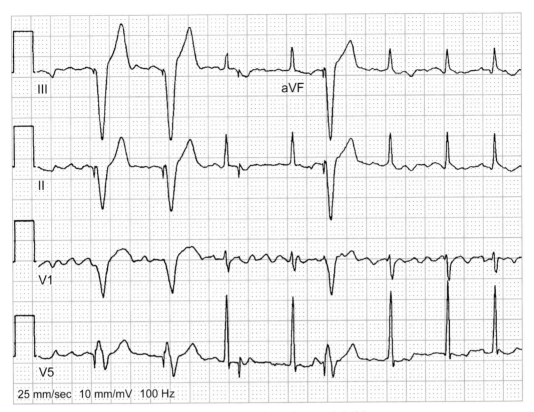

Fig. 10.51 Electrocardiographic tracing demonstrating VVI pacing with intermittent ventricular failure to sense.

event falls in the post-ventricular refractory period and is not sensed or a PMT termination algorithm is invoked (see Chapter 8: Programming). PMT is most commonly initiated by a premature ventricular event or atrial failure to capture.

A rate-adaptive sensor programmed too aggressively as well as search hysteresis can also cause symptoms (see earlier) as a result of relatively sudden rate alteration. Occasionally, patients who are paced after being chronotropically incompetent for a long period of time may have poor tolerance of the new rate response. Although paced rates may be appropriate, patients may have a sensation of relative tachycardia and complain of palpitations. This may require reprogramming the pacemaker to a less aggressive rate response and allowing the patient to adjust slowly to faster rates. The rate response can then be reprogrammed as tolerated.

As discussed in Chapter 8: Programming, an inappropriately programmed rate-adaptive sensor may result in suboptimal cardiac output, which can be corrected by optimization of sensor settings.

Patients who have abrupt 2:1 AV block at the upper rate limit may have symptoms from the sudden change in ventricular rate. Although this is much less common at present given the fact that most patients are programmed to a rate-adaptive mode, 2:1 AV block upper rate response may lead to symptoms, and caregivers need to understand the phenomenon. A sudden decrease in heart rate obviously affects cardiac output (cardiac output = heart rate × stroke volume). If this upper rate behavior is recognized as the cause of the patient's symptoms, reprogramming the pacemaker may alleviate the problem. Programming changes include the following:
- Shortening the total atrial refractory period to allow a higher achievable upper rate limit
- Shortening the PVARP
- Programming "on" rate-adaptive PVARP
- Programming "on" rate-adaptive AV delay
- Programming "on" or optimizing sensor-driven pacing, or both
- Programming "on" another feature, such as rate smoothing or fallback, to minimize sudden changes in cycle length.

Primary cardiac abnormalities may also result in suboptimal cardiac output. Development of a primary cardiomyopathic process, left ventricular dysfunction due to ischemic disease or tachyarrhythmias may be manifested by symptoms compatible with low cardiac output.

The number and versatility of current pulse generators and lead systems available challenge the caregiver to understand all the various devices and their features when assessing a system for potential malfunction. A thorough understanding of pacemaker timing cycles and electrocardiography (Chapter 7: Timing Cycles), pacemaker radiography (Chapter 11: Radiography of Implantable Devices), and programming (Chapter 8: Programming) is critical for successful troubleshooting. An understanding of the clinical situation, a systematic approach to troubleshooting, assessment of pacing system integrity, and judicious use of manufacturers' technical support teams can help distinguish between malfunction and apparent malfunction.

ICD troubleshooting

ICDs are susceptible to all types of troubles that pacemakers can experience, as well as troubles specific to high-voltage, antitachycardia devices. These troubles can be minimized by attention to intraoperative technique (Chapter 5: Implanting and Extracting Cardiac Devices), thoughtful perioperative programming (Chapter 8: Programming), and analysis of in-office or remote follow-up data (Chapter 13: Follow-up). The primary ICD-specific problems that require troubleshooting include shocks, ineffective antitachycardia therapy, and failure to deliver antitachycardia therapy. This section reviews the diagnostic tools of ICD troubleshooting and addresses these three specific problems, emphasizing the response to shocks, the most common troubleshooting problem. Additionally, we consider the differential diagnosis of ICD lead failures presenting with abnormal lead diagnostics and/or inappropriate shocks.

Diagnostic tools for ICD troubleshooting

History, physical, and basic laboratory data
Device-focused history and physical: Key elements include the following:

1 The initial indication for ICD therapy (primary prevention, secondary prevention, or cardiac resynchronization) because secondary prevention patients have a higher rate of true VT/VF than primary prevention patients.[27]

2 The causes of previous shocks may provide a clue to the cause of present shocks.

3 Similarly, a history of other arrhythmias may be helpful: rapidly-conducted SVT or AF raises this pos-

sibility as a precipitant of ICD shocks. In contrast, therapy for SVT does not occur in patients with permanent, complete AV block.

4 Cardiac drug initiation and withdrawal may provide clues to presenting symptoms including arrhythmias and nonarrhythmic syncope. Key points related to antiarrhythmic drugs are summarized in Chapter 1: Pacing and Defibrillation (see Drugs and defibrillators). Drugs associated with hypokalemia (e.g. diuretics) may be proarrhythmic. Those associated with hyperkalemia (e.g. aldosterone antagonists, angiotensin converting enzyme inhibitors, angiotensin receptor blockers) may contribute to undersensing during VT/VF or elevation in pacing threshold. Drug-induced orthostatic syncope (e.g., nitrates, diuretics, angiotensin converting enzyme inhibitors, angiotensin receptor blockers) should be considered in patients who present with syncope and have nominal ICD interrogations. Blocker withdrawal or dose reduction may cause an increase in maximum sinus rate or ventricular rate of conducted atrial arrhythmias.

5 Other implanted electronic devices including pacemakers, neurostimulators, ventricular assist devices, and devices for nonexcitatory cardiac stimulation may result in device–device interactions.

6 History and ECG may indicate exacerbation of ischemia as a cause of VT/VF.

7 History and physical may also suggest exacerbation of heart failure as a precipitating cause.

8 Audible tones or vibrations[28] from the ICD represent a patient alert caused by a detected arrhythmia or abnormal diagnostic. In Medtronic ICDs, alerts that sound every 4 hours indicate impedance or oversensing findings suggestive of a lead or connector problem.

Findings pertinent to presentation with shocks: These include patient activity at the time of shock, symptoms preceding the shock, and spatial or temporal patterns of shocks.

Patient activity: Multiple shocks during vigorous exercise suggest inappropriate therapy for sinus tachycardia or rapidly conducted AF if the integrity of lead system is verified. Stretching may provoke oversensing due to a lead insulation defect or conductor fracture. Pectoral muscle exercise may result in oversensing if an insulation defect is present in the pocket. Deep breathing, straining, or sitting up provoke in oversensing of diaphragmatic myopotentials.

Symptoms: Rapid palpitations preceding a shock suggest that the shock was delivered in response to a true arrhythmia (either SVT or VT), but does not exclude oversensing. The patient may experience palpitations due to ATP delivered in response to oversensing.

Preceding syncope occurs in only a minority of shocks.[29] It may be caused by true VT/VF resulting in hemodynamic collapse; but, in pacemaker-dependent patients, oversensing may cause inhibition of pacing and profound bradycardia while the ICD is detecting VF and charging. However, because most VT/VF episodes are not preceded by symptoms,[30] absence of symptoms does not indicate absence of VT/VF.

Shocks patterns: Recurrence of shocks in the same physical environmental may indicate inappropriate shocks due to external electromagnetic interference (EMI). In most studies, the first shock success rate for termination of true VT/VF is 80–90%.[31] Thus most clinical episodes of true VT/VF are terminated by one or two shocks. In contrast, repetitive shocks within seconds suggests inappropriate shocks in response to sensed events that are not terminated by the shock (e.g. sinus tachycardia, or oversensing of rapid physiologic or nonphysiologic signals). In previous reports, shocks for causes other than VT/VF occurred in clusters of 4.0 ± 2.0 per episode, compared with 1.6 ± 0.9 shocks per episode for true VT/VF.[32,33]

Phantom shocks: Some patients report experiencing "shocks" in the absence of shock delivery by the ICD.[34] This may occur either in patients with previous ICD shocks as a symptom of anxiety or in patients who have never experienced an actual ICD shock as "little shock."

Radiography

System radiography is discussed in Chapter 11: Radiography of Implantable Devices, and briefly in Chapter 13: Follow-up. It is particularly helpful in identifying lead positions, lead dislodgments, the relationship between defibrillation shock vectors and the mass of LV myocardium, specific lead and connection failure modes. Intraoperative radiography and cine fluoroscopy may be useful adjuncts in specific troubleshooting problems, as discussed below.

ICD Diagnostics

ICDs include all diagnostics present in pacemakers, including indicators of battery status, automatic measurement of P and R waves, and automated measurement of pacing impedance. They store the programmed parameters described in Chapter 8: Programming, which are vital to interpreting ICD function. In addition, they include ICD-specific diagnostics. The most commonly used diagnostics relate to classification of device-detected arrhythmia episodes, the high-voltage system, and specific metrics of oversensing common in ICDs. In addition to electrograms (EGMs), ICDs store specific data relating to device-detected arrhythmia

episodes that satisfy the rate and duration criteria for VT/VF detection (or monitor zones), including the specific criteria used to classify the rhythm as VT or SVT and the ICD's interpretation of the success or failure of delivered therapy. Some dual-chamber and cardiac resynchronization ICDs also store data regarding the duration and ventricular rate of AF episodes that do not satisfy ventricular rate criteria. Diagnostics specific to the high-voltage system include shock lead impedance, charge time for the high-voltage capacitors, and measured delivered energy for each delivered shock therapy. These are discussed in relation to diagnosis of high-voltage lead problems (see High-voltage conductor failures, below) and evaluating ineffective therapy (see ICD system-related factors, below). Some ICDs include specific oversensing diagnostics intended to facilitate diagnosis of T-wave oversensing or lead and connection problems. ICDs also diagnostics also indicate the cause of any auditory or vibratory patient alert.

Analysis of ICD electrograms and marker channels

Electrogram sources Analysis of ICD electrograms and marker channels is the cornerstone of troubleshooting the response to sensed events and detected tachycardias. ICDs store two or more electrograms recorded between various implanted electrodes. Typically, one or more source electrograms are programmable (Fig. 10.52). Two primary electrograms are available in most modern ICDs: the ventricular sensing (near-field) electrogram recorded between lead tip electrode and the adjacent ring or coil and the shocking electrogram recorded between or among two or three high-voltage electrodes. Other useful electrograms available in some ICDs include the leadless ECG recorded between the can and SVC coil on dual-coil defibrillation leads,[35] the atrial bipolar sensing electrogram in dual-chamber or cardiac resynchronization ICDs, and the LV electrogram in cardiac resynchronization ICDs.

The ICD determines the timing of each atrial and ventricular sensed event from the corresponding sensing channel. The timing of these events as sensed by the ICD's circuitry is displayed on the corresponding marker channel. In addition to displaying the interval between sensed events, the marker channel provides information about the timing of sensed events in relation to programmed detection intervals and intervals of the pacemaker timing cycle. ICD detection algorithms make most decisions by analysis of the atrial and ventricular intervals displayed on the marker channel. The most common analysis performed on the far-field channel is analysis of ventricular electrogram morphology. The closely spaced, near-field electrogram usually provides a sharp, short, local signal for timing that does

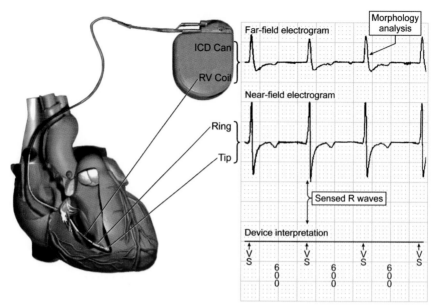

Fig. 10.52 ICD leads and electrograms. The left panel shows an ICD system including left-pectoral active can and RV lead. Right panel shows telemetered electrograms. The dual-coil lead uses true-bipolar sensing between tip and ring electrodes. Right panel shows telemetered high-voltage (shock), far-field (FF-VEGM) and sensing, near-field (NF-VEGM) electrograms with annotated markers. Arrows on marker channel denote timing of R waves sensed from true-bipolar electrogram. ICDs measure all timing intervals from this electrogram and display them on the marker channel, which also indicates the ICD's classification of each atrial and ventricular event by letter symbols. In this figure, VS indicates sensed ventricular events in the sinus rate zone and numbers indicate RR intervals. The stored near-field, rate-sensing electrogram is a wide-band (unfiltered) signal in Medtronic ICDs, but filtered in Boston Scientific and St. Jude ICDs. (From Friedman PA, Swerdlow CD, Hayes DL. Troubleshooting. In: Hayes DL, Friedman PA, eds. Cardiac Pacing and Defibrillation: A Clinical Approach, 2nd edn. West Sussex, UK: Wiley-Blackwell, 2008: 401–516, by permission of Friedman, Swerdlow, and Hayes.)

not exceed the short ventricular blanking period. However, its small field of view limits information about global ventricular electrogram morphology. A modeling study reported that the fraction of ventricular myocardium recorded by the true-bipolar, integrated-bipolar, and far-field electrograms as 3–7%, 20–35%, and 50–70%, respectively.[36] An important limitation of near-field signals is that electrogram morphology in VT may be indistinguishable from that during sinus rhythm in at least 5–10% of VTs (Fig. 10.53).[37,38]

Far-field electrograms usually are recorded between widely spaced shocking electrodes. They have two roles in troubleshooting. In analysis of true tachycardias, they are useful for comparing the morphology of tachycardia ventricular electrograms with that stored or real-time sinus templates to determine if the rhythm is VT or SVT. In analysis of ventricular sensing problems, the far-field electrogram is used as a check on the sensing electrogram. Ventricular sensed events that occur on the sensing channel but not far-field channel indicate oversensing. True intracardiac electrograms that are

not associated with events on the marker channel indicate undersensing, except for events that time in true ventricular blanking periods or rare marker-telemetry problems. Far-field electrograms recorded between one sensing and one shocking electrode (e.g., RV ring to can or LV tip to can) have the appearance of typical unipolar electrograms.

Atrial electrograms in dual or cardiac resynchronization ICDs are used to distinguish VT from SVT, identify primary atrial arrhythmias such as AF, and analyze atrial sensing problems. The leadless ECG can be helpful in identifying atrial activation from a single-chamber ECG.[35] Floating bipolar atrial electrograms on one model of "VDD" ventricular ICD lead can also be used for analysis of atrial electrograms.[39,40]

In troubleshooting, each electrogram must be interpreted in the context of applied filter settings, especially for ventricular sensing electrograms. Manufacturers may display only wide-band (unfiltered) signals, only narrow-band (filtered) signals, or both (Fig. 10.54). Filtered signals permit direct visualization of the actual signal that is compared with the sensing threshold to

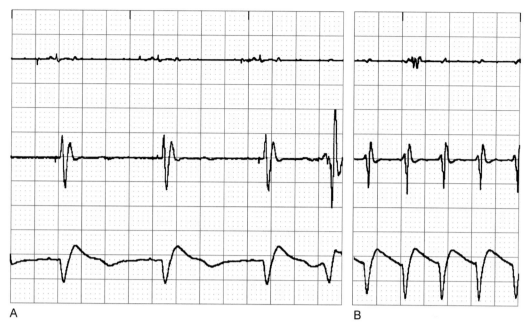

A   B

Fig. 10.53 Difficulty in distinguishing between supraventricular rhythm (or at times paced rhythm) and ventricular tachycardia (VT) seen only by near-field electrograms. Top to bottom are shown the atrial, rate (near-field), and shock (far-field) electrograms. (A) Recording before arrhythmia onset. (B) Tracing during VT; note that the ventricular rate (bottom two tracings) is greater than the atrial rate (top tracing). The amplitude and morphology of the near-field (middle) tracings are similar in (A) and (B), with only minor differences in the electrogram onset, despite VT in (B). In contrast, the morphologic differences are more evident on the far-field (bottom) tracing. The morphologic difference between supraventricular tachycardia and VT may be subtle when only near-field electrograms are available and, in contrast to this example, the differences are usually best seen in the terminal portion of the electrogram. (From Friedman PA, Swerdlow CD, Hayes DL. Troubleshooting. In: Hayes DL, Friedman PA, eds. Cardiac Pacing and Defibrillation: A Clinical Approach, 2nd edn. West Sussex, UK: Wiley-Blackwell, 2008: 401–516, by permission of Friedman, Swerdlow, and Hayes.)

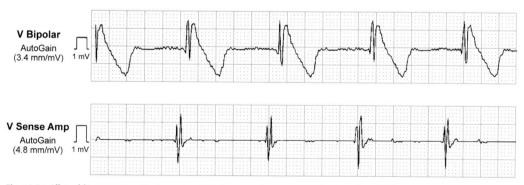

V Bipolar
AutoGain
(3.4 mm/mV)   1 mV

V Sense Amp
AutoGain
(4.8 mm/mV)   1 mV

Fig. 10.54 Effect of filtering on true-bipolar sensing EGM. Upper panel shows low-amplitude unfiltered EGM. Lower panel shows that filtered EGM markedly reduces T-wave amplitude and alters morphology of R wave. The change in scale indicates that the R-wave amplitude is reduced by filtering.

determine if a signal is sensed. Typically, filtering alters signal amplitude. The filtered R wave usually has a lower amplitude than the unfiltered R wave, but occasionally the filtered R wave is larger. When filter settings are programmable (St. Jude Unify/Fortify ICD family), displaying the filtered R wave permits assessing the effect of filtering on R and T-wave amplitude.

Stored and real-time electrograms Stored electrograms and their corresponding interval and episode data are the primary source data for diagnosing the mechanism of tachycardias that ICDs detect, regardless of whether therapy is delivered or withheld or whether therapy is delivered in response to oversensing or true a true tachycardia. They are also essential to assessing the response to delivered therapy.

Real-time electrograms provide complementary information in specific situations. Comparison of ventricular electrograms recorded in real time when the patient's conducted rhythm is known may assist in identifying the electrogram during a stored episode as ventricular or supraventricular in origin: the morphology of stored SVT episodes resembles that of the usual supraventricular rhythm in the absence of aberrancy or post-shock distortion (Fig. 10.55).[30,37] Rapid atrial pacing can provoke rate-related aberrancy. Assessment of VA conduction during ventricular pacing provides supportive information related to the likelihood that a 1:1 tachycardia is VT. Real-time electrograms are particularly useful in troubleshooting reproducible oversensing events, including those provoked by various maneuvers such as lead or connector problems in the pocket that may be identified by pocket manipulation. Pectoral or diaphragmatic myopotentials can be provoked by pectoral muscle exercise and straining, respectively. If a patient describes a stereotypical maneuver that reproduced the event (e.g., reaching or coughing), repeating the maneuver during electrogram recording may be diagnostic (Fig. 10.56). Some ICDs provide real-time telemetry of more electrograms than they can store. When multiple electrogram sources are available, recording each of the possible electrograms often permits isolating the problem to a specific electrode. This is particularly helpful in Medtronic ICDs that permit programming ventricular sensing to either true-bipolar or integrated-bipolar vectors. In these ICDs, oversensing problems isolated to the connection of the ring to the header may be resolved noninvasively (Fig. 10.57).

Evaluating appropriateness of delivered therapy

ICDs may deliver therapy either in response to a tachyarrhythmia (SVT or VT) or oversensing of nonar-

rhythmic electrical signals. Figure 10.58 summarizes our approach:

1 Determine if therapy was delivered in response to oversensing or a true tachycardia
2 If oversensing occurred, determine its cause and correct its cause
3 If a tachycardia occurred, determine if it was VT or SVT
4 If VT occurred, determine if: (a) it could have been prevented, (b) therapy was necessary, and (c) if ATP should have been delivered instead of a shock.

Ventricular oversensing: recognition and troubleshooting

Oversensing is defined as sensing of signals other than local depolarization at the sensing electrodes. The oversensed signals may originate from physiologic or nonphysiologic sources. In ICD patients who require ventricular bradycardia pacing, oversensing may manifest identically to oversensing in pacemakers: ventricular oversensing may present as failure to deliver an expected ventricular pacing stimulus. In dual-chamber ICDs, atrial oversensing presents as inappropriate mode-switching or tracking of nonphysiologic signals. However, in ICDs oversensing most commonly manifests as inappropriate detection of VT or VF, and this section focuses on that presentation.

Oversensing often results in characteristic patterns of stored EGMs and associated markers (Fig. 10.59).[41,42] Ventricular oversensing of physiologic, intracardiac signals results in exactly two ventricular events for each cardiac cycle (such as a ventricular electrogram and its T wave). In contrast, oversensing of intracardiac, nonphysiologic signals results in a sensing electrogram comprised of the superposition the true cardiac signal and an independent, unrelated signal. Often, extracardiac signals are rapid (e.g., external electromagnetic interference, myopotentials), replacing the isoelectric baseline with high-frequency signals that have no relationship to the cardiac cycle.[41–44] Some authors refer to all such signals as "noise." We prefer to restrict the term noise to signals originating from lead failures or connection problems that usually require system revision.

Intracardiac signals *T-wave oversensing:* T-wave oversensing is the most common, clinically significant cause of intracardiac oversensing. It presents as alternating high-frequency (local electrogram) and low-frequency (T wave) morphologies on the sensing electrogram.[41] Device detected R-R intervals must be consistent with successive R-T and T-R intervals. ICD-measured R-R intervals during T-wave oversensing may alternate, but the magnitude of alternation often is small, especially

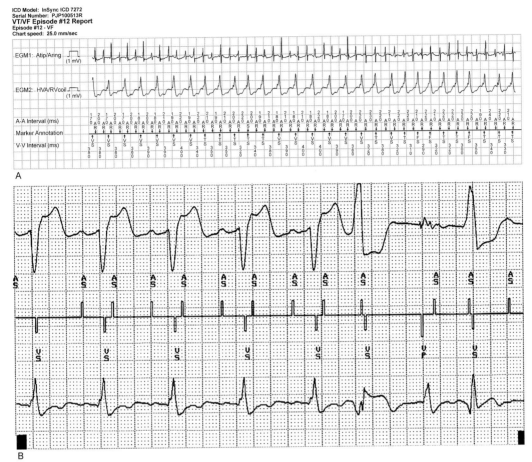

ICD Model: InSync ICD 7272
Serial Number: PJP100513R
VT/VF Episode #12 Report
Episode #12 - VF
Chart speed: 25.0 mm/sec

Fig. 10.55 Use of real-time telemetry to assess baseline electrogram morphology during sinus rhythm. (A) Stored electrograms from an episode of wide-complex tachycardia. From top to bottom are the atrial electrograms, far-field (can to right ventricular [RV] coil) electrogram, and marker channels. Atrial electrograms show continuing atrial flutter, whereas ventricular electrograms show a regular wide-complex tachycardia, which could represent conducted atrial flutter or concomitant ventricular tachycardia. (B) Real-time recordings during sinus rhythm showing (top to bottom) surface electrocardiogram marker channels, and far-field (can to RV coil) electrogram. Note the similarity between the far-field electrogram during sinus rhythm and the electrogram morphology during the episode in (A), indicating that the tachycardia was rapidly conducted atrial flutter. Also incidentally noted in (B) is far-field R-wave oversensing (sensing of the QRS on the atrial channel), seen as an "AS" marker immediately following the "VS" marker. The PR Logic detection algorithm can take far-field R-wave oversensing into consideration if it is consistently present. (From Friedman PA, Swerdlow CD, Hayes DL. Troubleshooting. In: Hayes DL, Friedman PA, eds. Cardiac Pacing and Defibrillation: A Clinical Approach, 2nd edn. West Sussex, UK: Wiley-Blackwell, 2008: 401–516 by permission of Friedman, Swerdlow, and Hayes.)

during tachycardia or if the QT interval is prolonged; such alternation is not required for the diagnosis. Similarly, alternation of electrogram amplitude without alternation in morphology suggests true tachycardia, typical of T-wave oversensing (Fig. 10.60). A simultaneous, stored far-field electrogram or real-time ECG confirms that alternate low-frequency electrograms represent T waves. Alternatively, in dual-chamber ICDs,

T-wave oversensing can be identified in sinus rhythm by the fixed relationship of the preceding atrial electrogram to the high-frequency ventricular electrogram.

T-wave oversensing may be divided into oversensing of paced T waves and oversensing of spontaneous T waves. Post-pacing T-wave oversensing can inhibit bradycardia pacing[45,46] or cause ATP to be delivered at a longer-than-programmed cycle length.[19] It does not

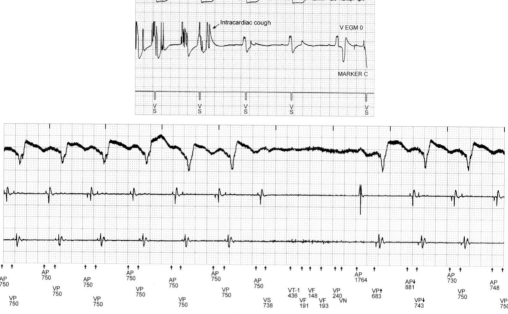

Fig. 10.56 Provocative maneuvers during real-time telemetry to diagnose system malfunction. (Top) Cough during real-time telemetry. From top to bottom are the surface electrocardiogram (ECG), far-field ventricular electrogram, and marker channel. During the cough, electrical noise is seen on the far-field electrogram (recorded between the coil and the device can) while the surface ECG displays continuing normal sinus rhythm, confirming that the electrical noise is noncardiac. The marker channel shows appropriate QRS sensing (one sensed event for each QRS), indicating that the fracture involves the shocking coil but spares the conductors to the tip or ring used for sensing. (Bottom) Oversensing of diaphragmatic myopotentials during deep inspiration. The patient has marked underlying sinus bradycardia and high-grade atrioventricular block. From top to bottom are shown the surface ECG, atrial electrogram, ventricular electrogram, and markers. With deep inspiration, diaphragmatic myopotentials are sensed as ventricular tachycardia (VT) and ventricular fibrillation (VF) events (beginning at marker VT-1 436). During VT/VF detection, pacing is suspended, resulting in a pause. This patient had received a shock during deep breathing exercises. Reprogramming from "nominal" to "least" sensitivity eliminated the problem. Assessment of adequate ventricular fibrillation detection should be performed when sensitivity is diminished. (From Friedman PA, Swerdlow CD, Hayes DL. Troubleshooting. In: Hayes DL, Friedman PA, eds. Cardiac Pacing and Defibrillation: A Clinical Approach, 2nd edn. West Sussex, UK: Wiley-Blackwell, 2008: 401–516, by permission of Friedman, Swerdlow, and Hayes.)

typically cause inappropriate detection of VT, but may increment VT or VF counters and thereby increase the likelihood that nonsustained VT will be detected. It is corrected by increasing the post-pacing ventricular blanking period.

Oversensing of spontaneous T waves during baseline rhythm or SVT may cause inappropriate detection of either VT or VF, depending on the sensed R-T and T-R interval and the programmed VF detection interval. T-wave oversensing that occurs during monomorphic VT may result inappropriate detection of VF, and delivery of a shock instead of ATP. There are conflicting reports regarding the effect of the sensing vector (true-bipolar or integrated-bipolar) on T-wave oversens-

ing;[47,48] uncontrolled variables may be responsible. The likelihood of T-wave oversensing probably differs in different ICDs from different manufacturers depending on the method of autoadjusting sensitivity and bandwidth of the ventricular sensing amplifier. For example, T-wave oversensing has been a vexing problem for Medtronic and older St. Jude ICDs, with bandwidths of 14–40 Hz and 12–60 Hz, respectively. However, the bandwidth of Boston Scientific ICDs is 21–85 Hz. In a recent study, T-wave oversensing accounted for only 1.5% of all oversensing episodes.[49] St. Jude Medical claims that an enhanced sensing filter in the Unify™/Fortify™ family reduces T-wave oversensing in bench testing. The potential risk of such filtering is underdetection

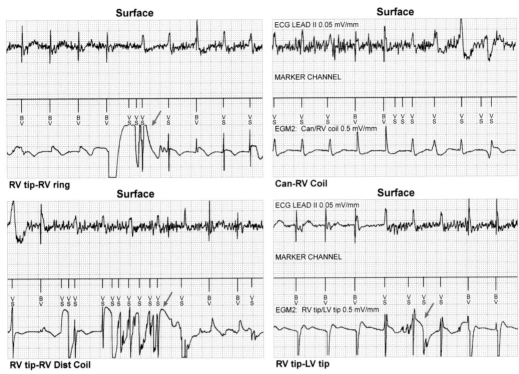

Fig. 10.57 Using multiple real-time electrogram channels to diagnose the source of malfunction in a patient who received a shock while shaking his cardiologist's hand the day after a CRT-D (resynchronization ICD) implant. In all four panels, the top tracing is the surface ECG (which contains artifact due to hand-shaking during recording in effort to reproduce malfunction); the second row depicts the marker channels, which show device interpretation of events; the bottom row shows the device electrogram (RV tip to RV ring from the true-bipolar lead is top left; RV tip to RV distal coil bottom left; can to RV coil top right; RV tip to LV tip bottom right). Note that in all of the panels there are more "VS" markers than surface QRS complexes, consistent with oversensing of noise. "VS" is seen (as opposed to "TS" or "FS") because detection is turned off for troubleshooting. The noise is seen in all of the electrograms (arrows) except the can to RV coil electrogram (top right). The can to RV coil tracing is the only one in which the RV tip is not part of the circuit. This suggests the problem lay in the conductor or connection to the RV tip. At reoperation, a loose setscrew was found in the RV-tip port of the header. (From Friedman PA, Swerdlow CD, Hayes DL. Troubleshooting. In: Hayes DL, Friedman PA, eds. Cardiac Pacing and Defibrillation: A Clinical Approach, 2nd edn. West Sussex, UK: Wiley-Blackwell, 2008: 401–516, by permission of Friedman, Swerdlow, and Hayes.)

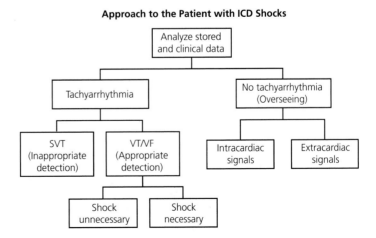

Fig. 10.58 Approach to the patient with ICD shocks.

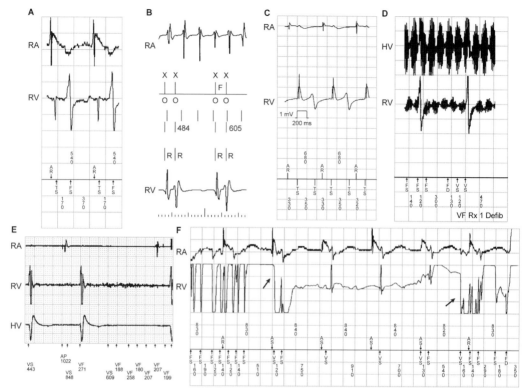

Fig. 10.59 Types of oversensing resulting in inappropriate detection of VT/VF. (A–C) Oversensing of physiologic, intracardiac signals. (A) P-wave oversensing in sinus rhythm from integrated bipolar lead with distal coil near the tricuspid valve. (B) R-wave double counting during conducted AF in a biventricular sensing ICD. (C) T-wave oversensing in patient with low-amplitude R wave (note mV calibration marker). (D) Electromagnetic interference from a power drill has higher amplitude on widely spaced high-voltage electrogram than on closely spaced true bipolar sensing electrogram. (E) Diaphragmatic myopotential oversensing in a patient with an integrated bipolar lead at the RV apex. Note that noise level is constant, but oversensing does not occur until automatic gain control increases the gain sufficiently, about 600 ms after the sensed R waves. (F) Lead fracture noise results in intermittent saturation of amplifier range denoted by arrow. RA, right atrium; RV, right ventricular sensing electrogram; HV, high-voltage electrogram. (From Friedman PA, Swerdlow CD, Hayes DL. Troubleshooting. In: Hayes DL, Friedman PA, eds. Cardiac Pacing and Defibrillation: A Clinical Approach, 2nd edn. West Sussex, UK: Wiley-Blackwell, 2008: 401–516, by permission of Friedman, Swerdlow, and Hayes.)

of VF (see later). New Medtronic ICDs (Protecta™ family) reduce T-wave oversensing using an algorithm that withholds ICD therapy when T-wave oversensing is identified as the source of device-detected tachycardia based on lower frequency content of the oversensed T waves. In bench testing, the algorithm markedly reduced inappropriate ICD therapies without compromising sensing and detection of VF.[50]

Once T-wave oversensing occurs, the clinical approach depends on whether it happens in the setting of adequate R waves (≥3 mV) with varying T-wave amplitude or small R waves (<3 mV) with constant or increasing T-wave amplitudes (Fig. 10.60).[51] T-wave oversensing often occurs in the setting of low-amplitude

R waves because the sensing threshold decays from a fraction of the low-amplitude preceding R wave.[52] To compound the problem, patients with low-amplitude R waves may require lower minimum sensing thresholds to ensure reliable sensing of VF. T-wave oversensing in this setting may be a warning that detection of VF may be unreliable. Testing of VF detection should be considered. The ventricular lead may need to be revised or a separate pace and/or sense lead added to ensure reliable sensing in VF.

Troubleshooting is challenging because T-wave oversensing is often transient and unpredictable.[51,53] Unpredictable variations in amplitude of the filtered and rectified R-wave may be responsible (Fig. 10.61).[54] For

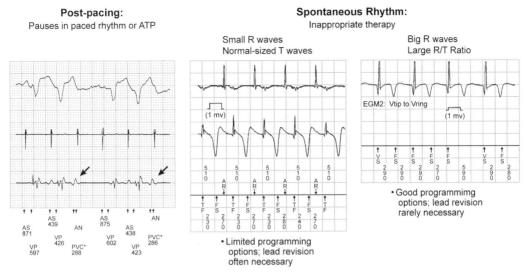

Fig. 10.60 Classification of T-wave oversensing. During pacing (left panel) T-wave oversensing may cause a pause. From top to bottom in the left panel are shown the surface ECG, atrial electrogram, ventricular electrogram, and marker annotations. The oversensed T wave is indicated with an arrow on the ventricular electrogram. The middle panel shows T-wave oversensing with a very small R-wave to T-wave ratio, in this case due to small R waves and normal sized T waves. From top to bottom are atrial electrogram, near-field ventricular electrogram, and markers. Reprogramming options are limited in this situation, and lead revision is often necessary. It is important that the near-field ventricular electrogram be reviewed (as opposed to far-field), as this represents the signal the ICD uses for rate detection. The right panel shows T-wave oversensing in the setting of a large R/T ratio; this is typically corrected with device reprogramming. From top to bottom are the ventricular near-field electrogram and markers. (From Friedman PA, Swerdlow CD, Hayes DL. Troubleshooting. In: Hayes DL, Friedman PA, eds. Cardiac Pacing and Defibrillation: A Clinical Approach, 2nd edn. West Sussex, UK: Wiley-Blackwell, 2008: 401–516, by permission of Friedman, Swerdlow, and Hayes.)

large R waves, unpredictable changes in T-wave amplitude complicate troubleshooting.

Specific programming features may be used to reduce T-wave oversensing, provided that sensing of VF is reliable. Because most may compromise sensing during VF, usually they are implemented reactively after T-wave oversensing has occurred rather than proactively at implant.

1 The simplest is to reduce ventricular sensitivity to a less sensitive (higher) value.

2 St. Jude ICDs provide a programmable "Threshold Start" and "Decay Delay," which are designed to reduce over-sensing of spontaneous T waves. Models of the Unify™ and Fortify™ families also provide an enhanced sensing filter designed to minimize T-wave oversensing.

3 The apparent alternation of ventricular EGM morphologies caused by T-wave oversensing may be exploited to prevent inappropriate detection of VT. The SVT-VT morphology discriminator may be programmed "on" to classify alternate EGMs as "sinus" and thereby withhold inappropriate detection.

4 As a temporary measure, T-wave oversensing may be reduced by forcing short-term ventricular pacing, altering the sequence of repolarization, and thus reducing T-wave amplitude. The reliability of these approaches is not established.

5 Some Medtronic ICDs (Secura™ /Consulta™ and Protecta™ familes) permit sensing from either the true-bipolar EGM or the integrated-bipolar EGM when a true-bipolar lead is connected. Integrated-bipolar sensing may prevent T-wave oversensing, especially when true bipolar R-waves are small compared with the integrated bipolar R-waves (Fig. 10.61).

6 Medtronic ICDs of the Protecta™ family include an algorithm that classifies oversensing T waves as T waves rather than R waves (Fig. 10.62).[55]

R-wave double-counting: R-wave double-counting occurs if the duration of the sensed EGM exceeds the short ventricular blanking period in ICDs. Presently, it is rare, but probably more common with integrated-bipolar than true-bipolar leads.[56] It may be a specific problem for Biotronik ICDs attached to other manufacturers

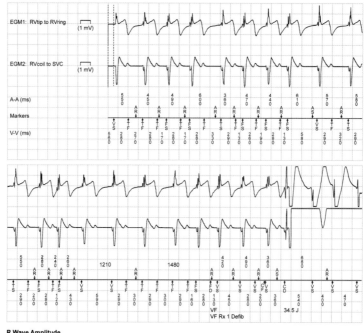

R Wave Amplitude

At implant	6.0 mV	Highest	6.0 mV
Last	3.3 mV	Lowest	1.7 mV

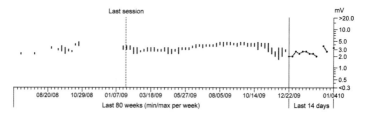

Sensing Simulation (0.3 mV sensitivity)

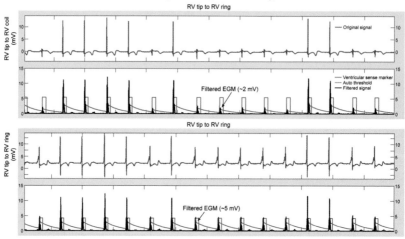

Fig. 10.61 T-wave oversensing due to low and varying R wave amplitude corrected by altering sensing vector. (A) Panels show unfiltered RV true-bipolar sensing EGM, high-voltage EGM, and dual-chamber markers. The Fast VT detection interval is 310 ms, and the VF detection interval is 240 ms. The calibration marker shows that the unfiltered R wave amplitude on the sensing EGM is 2.5–3.5 mV. The panels are not continuous. T-wave oversensing results in R-T intervals in the Fast VT zone (TF marker) and T-R intervals in the VF zone (FS marker). (B) R-wave amplitude trend. It shows that amplitudes decreased from 6.0 mV at implant to a range of about 1.7–3.5 mV in last month. (C) The panel shows simultaneous EGMs from a Holter monitor in the same patient that records telemetered ICD EGMs. It was recorded 1 week after T-wave oversensing. In the upper panel, the top tracing shows the unfiltered true-bipolar signal in blue. The bottom tracing shows the filtered signal in black. The pink curve shows the auto-adjusting sensitivity threshold. Red rectangles show post-sensing 120 ms blanking period. The R wave amplitude shows great a beat-to-beat variation. The safety margin for T-wave oversensing is the voltage (vertical distance) between the pink sensing threshold and black EGM amplitude of the T wave. Although T-wave oversensing did not occur because the filtered T waves remain below the sensing threshold, the safety margin is low when the R wave is small. The lower panel shows corresponding filtered and unfiltered EGMs for the integrated-bipolar signal. R wave amplitude varies much less beat-to-beat, and the safety margin for T-wave oversensing is greater.

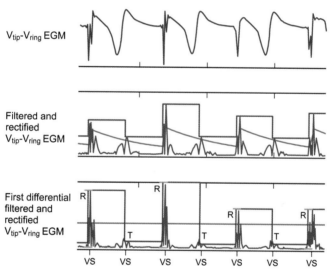

Fig. 10.62 Algorithm to reject T-wave oversensing. Upper tracing: V_{tip}-V_{ring} EGM with large T waves and T-wave oversensing. Middle tracing: signal after standard sense amplifier filtering and rectification (purple line), automatic adjusting sensing threshold (red), and peak amplitude at each sensed event (blue; the peak amplitude for each sensed event is held until the next sensed event). Bottom tracing: first derivative of the filtered and rectified EGM (purple line) its peak amplitude at each sensed event (blue), and adaptive threshold used to separate possible R and T waves (red horizontal line). The algorithm recognizes oversensed T waves with lower frequency content than the preceding sensed R waves by automatically comparing signal amplitudes in the filtered/rectified sensing EGM and its first derivative (which further attenuates low-frequency signals) to identify patterns of alternating signal frequency content. Using an analysis window of six sensed events, the algorithm first automatically identifies possible R and T waves based on comparing peak amplitudes and patterns of the first derivative of the filtered/rectified sensing EGM. For each analysis window, the adaptive threshold is set to a fraction of the three largest first differential EGM peak amplitudes. The algorithm assumes that possible R waves are above threshold and possible T waves are below threshold. An alternating RT pattern with 3Rs and 3Ts or 4Rs and 2Ts in the six sensed events analysis window is required. RT pairs are confirmed when the R-wave/T-wave (R/T) ratio in the filtered/rectified sensing EGM is less than the R/T ratio measured in the first differential filtered/rectified EGM. This approach does not increase the risk of undersensing because the operation of the standard ICD sensing channel is not modified. It does not prevent oversensing of T waves, but rather allows the ICD to withhold therapy when T-wave oversensing pattern is recognized. Testing on more than 1000 VT/VF episodes showed no loss in sensitivity to true VT/VF. VS, Ventricular sensed event. (Reproduced with permission from Cao J, Gillberg JM, Swerdlow CD. A fully automatic, implantable cardioverter-defibrillator algorithm to prevent inappropriate detection of ventricular tachycardia or fibrillation due to t-wave oversensing in spontaneous rhythm. Heart Rhythm 2012; 9:522–530.)

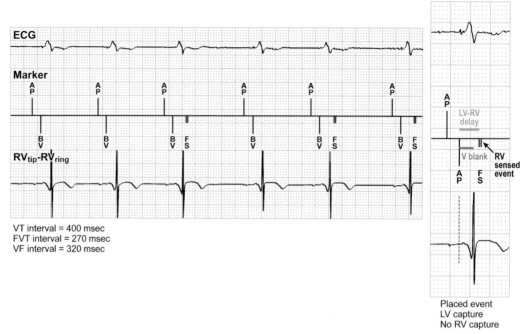

Fig. 10.63 Intermittent R-wave double-counting as a result of loss of RV capture in a cardiac resynchronization ICD patient with left bundle branch block. Left main panel shows surface ECG, atrial and ventricular marker channels, and true bipolar right ventricular (RV) EGM. The third, fifth, and sixth R waves are double-counted, as shown in insert on right. Simultaneous biventricular pacing activates the left ventricle (LV). After the LV-RV conduction delay, the wavefront arrives at the RV sensing bipole, corresponding to a sensed in interval in the ventricular fibrillation (VF) zone (VS) and incrementing the VF counter. This condition alone will not result in VF being detected even if all beats are oversensed, but transient nonsustained ventricular tachycardia (VT) in the VF zone could result in inappropriate detection of VF, because the baseline VF counter may be as high as 50% of its maximum value.

integrated-bipolar leads.[57] R-wave double-counting results in alternation of ventricular cycle lengths that produces a characteristic "railroad track" pattern on a plot of stored of ventricular intervals. Because the second component of the R wave is sensed as soon as the blanking period terminates, the double-counted RV-RV or RV-LV interval measures within 20 ms of the ventricular blanking period and is always classified in the VF zone (Fig. 10.63). Inappropriate detection of VF may occur despite a true ventricular rate below the VT detection interval.

Consistent R-wave double-counting may occur as a result of local ventricular delays in the baseline state in native rhythm or conduction delays caused by use-dependent effects of sodium channel blocking antiarrhythmic drugs or hyperkalemia. It may also occur with loss of RV capture in cardiac resynchronization ICDs. The ICD counts both the paced ventricular event and the conducted wavefront arriving at the RV bipole as a result of LV capture, if the interventricular conduction delay exceeded the ventricular blanking period. R-wave double-counting was a common problem in early cardiac resynchronization ICDs that used Y-adapted or extended bipolar sensing between RV and LV electrodes.[43] The composite ventricular EGM included deflections from the RV and the LV, both of which could be counted as separate R waves. For this reason, all current CRT devices sense only using a right ventricular bipole for tachyarrhythmia detection. Occasional R-wave double-counting may occur during premature ventricular complexes (PVCs).

Most consistent R-wave double-counting now results from transient or reversible events such as hyperkalemia, drug effects, or lead failure in cardiac resynchronization ICDs; and most intermittent R-wave double-counting is not clinically significant. Some ICDs permit programming to increase the ventricular blanking period from the nominal value (120–125 ms) to higher values, up to 170 ms. Occasionally, reducing ventricular sensitivity

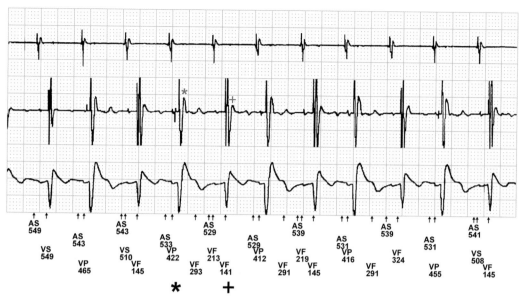

Fig. 10.64 Oversensing of P and T waves related to dynamic gain in a Ventak series implantable cardioverter-defibrillator. Note that oversensing occurs after ventricular pacing, because dynamic gain for sensing is increased rapidly following paced events. From top to bottom are the atrial, near-field ventricular (rate), and far-field ventricular (shock) electrograms. After a paced event (VP 422, asterisk), the T and P waves are both oversensed on the ventricular channel. Because of the short time between the pacing pulse and the T wave, these are detected as fibrillation-sensed events (VF 293 and VF 213). The next QRS complex is also sensed as a ventricular fibrillation event (VF 141) and is not paced. The absence of pacing (and its effect on dynamic sensing gain) prevents ventricular oversensing of the atrial event, and it is followed by a paced ventricular event after elapse of the atrioventricular interval (VP 412). This ventricular paced event, in turn, leads to repetition of the oversensing of the T wave at VF 291, the P wave at VF 219, and so on. (From Friedman PA, Swerdlow CD, Hayes DL. Troubleshooting. In: Hayes DL, Friedman PA, eds. Cardiac Pacing and Defibrillation: A Clinical Approach, 2nd edn. West Sussex, UK: Wiley-Blackwell, 2008: 401–516, by permission of Friedman, Swerdlow, and Hayes.)

can avoid R-wave double-counting; but ventricular sensitivity should not be reduced unless reliable sensing of VF is confirmed at the reduced level of sensitivity.

P-wave oversensing: P-wave oversensing may occur if the distal coil of an integrated bipolar lead is close to the tricuspid valve and the sensed P-R interval exceeds the cross-chamber ventricular blanking period (Fig. 10.64). It is rare in adults with ventricular sensing electrodes near the RV apex, but it may occur in children or in adults if the RV electrode is positioned in the proximal septum or inflow region of the RV. P-wave oversensing on a true-bipolar sensing lead early after implant usually indicates dislodgement to the atrium. If P-wave oversensing occurs during a 1 : 1 rhythm, the device-detected RR pattern is similar to that of R-wave double-counting, provided that the sensed P-R or R-P interval is short. However, oversensing of atrial activation as R waves during AF or atrial flutter can cause inappropriate detection of VF independent of the ventricular rate.

Consistent oversensing of spontaneous P waves often requires lead revision. One mitigation strategy is to force atrial pacing using DDDR or Dynamic Overdrive modes. This shortens the ventricular cycle length (preventing ventricular sensitivity from reaching its minimum value) and introduces cross-chamber ventricular blanking after each atrial event (reducing the likelihood of oversensing P waves).

Extracardiac signals *External electromagnetic interference:* External electromagnetic interference[41–44] is reviewed in Chapter 12: Electromagnetic Interference. It results in greater signal amplitude on the high-voltage electrogram recorded from widely-spaced electrodes than on the sensing electrogram recorded from closely spaced electrodes. The source signal recorded on the far-field electrogram usually is continuous, but oversensing oversensing may be intermittent due to automatic adjustment of sensitivity. Clinical conditions may suggest a specific identifiable cause (see Chapter 12: Electromagnetic Interference). Some manufacturers

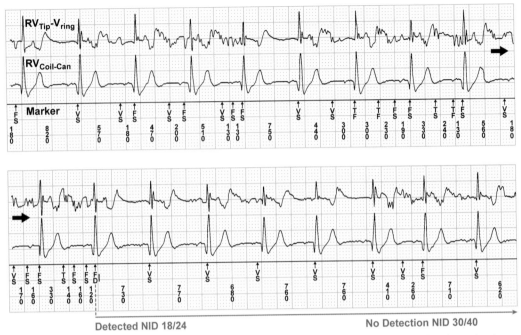

Fig. 10.65 Stored electrogram shows intermittent oversensing caused by lead fracture. Pace-sense (V_{tip}-V_{ring}), high-voltage ($RV_{coil-can}$), and marker channels are shown; VS, TS, and FS, intervals in sinus, ventricular tachycardia (VT), and ventricular fibrillation (VF) zones, respectively; FD, detection of VF. Upper and lower panels are continuous. Pace-sense channel shows intermittent, high-frequency, oversensing of nonphysiologic noise characteristic of lead fracture or header-connector problem. At the programmed number of intervals to detect VF (NID) 18/24, inappropriate detection of VF occurs near left of the bottom panel, resulting in an inappropriate shock (not shown). Coincident with detection of VF, oversensing decreases greatly. VF would not have been detected at higher values of NID. VS, Ventricular sensed event; VP, ventricular paced event; FS, ventricular interval in VF zone. (Reproduced with permission from Swerdlow CD, Gillberg, JM, Khairy P. Sensing and detection. In: Ellengogen KA, Kay GN, Lau C, Wilkoff BL, eds. Clinical Cardiac Pacing, Defibrillation, and Resynchronization Therapy. 4th edn. Philadelphia, PA: Saunders Company, 2011, 56–126.)

(St. Jude, Sorin, Boston Scientific) have specific ICD algorithms to reduce or prevent inappropriate detection of VF in the presence of EMI, but they have not been validated in peer-reviewed publications.

Lead and connection problems: Identifying oversensing of this type is critical because it indicates failure of the integrity of the ICD system and usually requires system revision. The primary mechanisms include connection (header, adapter, or setscrew) problems and lead insulation failure or conductor fracture. The characteristic presentation is of intermittent "noise." Lead and connector noise has four typical characteristics (Fig. 10.65):
1 High-frequency components typically result in intervals within 20 ms of the ventricular blanking period (130–150 ms) and many intervals below 200 ms.
2 Substantial variability in amplitude or frequency occurs.
3 High-amplitude signals saturate the amplifier.

4 The noise signal is limited to the sensing electrogram unless the problem relates to the RV coil in an integrated bipolar lead or to both sensing and high-voltage conductors or connectors.

Because noise always results in extremely rapid oversensing, inappropriate detection always occurs in the VF zone. Lead or connection problems often present with abnormalities of pacing impedance, with or without noise oversensing. For differential diagnosis and management of presentations associated with noise oversensing alone, impedance abnormalities alone, or both, see Differential diagnosis of pace-sense lead fractures, below.

Myopotential oversensing: Diaphragmatic myopotentials are most prominent on the sensing electrogram. Oversensing usually occurs after long diastolic intervals or after ventricular paced events when amplifier sensitivity or gain is maximal. It often ends with a sensed R wave,

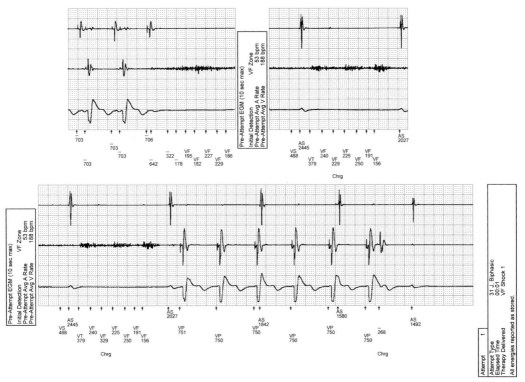

Fig. 10.66 Oversensing of diaphragmatic myopotentials leading to inappropriate detection of ventricular fibrillation (VF), transient asystole, and shock delivery. The patient was performing deep breathing exercises when she felt dizzy and received a shock. These are stored episode data from the patient whose real-time telemetry findings are shown in Fig. 10.56B. (B) From top to bottom are the atrial, ventricular near-field (rate) and ventricular far-field (shock) electrograms. (A) Diaphragmatic myopotential oversensing leads to inappropriate detection of VF. Pacing is withheld during ventricular tachycardia (VT)/VF detection, leading to asystole (note that QRS complexes are absent on the far-field electrogram [bottom tracing], but noise is present on the near-field electrogram [middle tracing]). (B) Oversensing resolves and pacing resumes (at VP 751), presumably because the patient stopped the deep breathing exercises after the dizzy spell. During reconfirmation (at the second "Chrg" marker), pacing is withheld to determine whether VT or VF is still present. As this patient has high-grade atrioventricular block, asystole recurs and is shocked by the algorithm, which inappropriately assumes that asystole represents fine VF. Newer versions of this algorithm do not shock for asystole, but rather provide pacing support. (From Friedman PA, Swerdlow CD, Hayes DL. Troubleshooting. In: Hayes DL, Friedman PA, eds. Cardiac Pacing and Defibrillation: A Clinical Approach, 2nd edn. West Sussex, UK: Wiley-Blackwell, 2008: 401–516, by permission of Friedman, Swerdlow, and Hayes.)

which abruptly reduces sensitivity. In pacemaker-dependent patients, diaphragmatic oversensing causes inhibition of pacing, resulting in persistent oversensing and inappropriate detection of VF (Fig. 10.66). Clinically, this may manifest as syncope due to inhibition of pacing followed by an inappropriate shock. This is an exception to the clinical rule that antecedent syncope usually indicates an appropriate shock. A short time constant for automatic adjustment of sensitivity increases the probability of this type of oversensing. It is most common in male patients who have integrated bipolar leads in the RV apex.[48,58] Oversensing of diaphragmatic myopotentials may be corrected by reducing ventricular sensitivity, provided that VF sensing and

detection are reliable at the reduced level of sensitivity. In pacemaker-dependent patients it may also be reduced by pacing at a faster rate. Noise rejection algorithms may be effective in preventing oversensing due to diaphragmatic myopotentials. Occasionally, correction requires insertion of a new rate-sensing lead away from the diaphragm.

Pectoral myopotentials are more prominent on a far-field electrogram that includes the ICD can rather than the near-field EGM. Because ICDs do not use this EGM for rate-counting, oversensing of pectoral myopotentials does not cause inappropriate detection during normal intrinsic rates if the ventricular lead is intact, but pectoral myopotentials may lead to misclassification during exercise-induced sinus tachycardia by SVT-VT discriminators that use far-field electrogram morphology (Medtronic, Boston Scientific). As in pacemakers, pectoral myopotential oversensing may be suspected if symptoms occur during arm motion and can often be demonstrated in the clinic by having the patient forcefully press his or her hands together while the intracardiac EGM is monitored.

Distinguishing VT from SVT in ICD stored electrograms and episode data

If therapy is delivered in response to a true tachycardia, the caregiver must distinguish VT from SVT. This process is distinct from and independent of the SVT-VT discrimination by ICD algorithms as reviewed in Chapter 8: Programming (see SVT-VT discriminators).

Our approach is summarized in Fig. 10.67. Analysis of dual-chamber electrograms is more accurate than analysis of single-chamber electrograms, providing atrial sensing is reliable.[59,60]

Analysis of dual-chamber electrograms Analysis of atrial and ventricular rates and AV relationships comprise the foundations of dual-chamber rhythm analysis. In single-chamber ICDs a leadless ECG between can and SVC coil may be used to determine the AV relationship during tachycardia, providing atrial and ventricular electrograms can be distinguished reliably. If the ventricular rate is faster than the atrial rate, the diagnosis is VT. Interpretive issues arise for tachycardias in which the atrial rate is equal to or more than the ventricular rate.

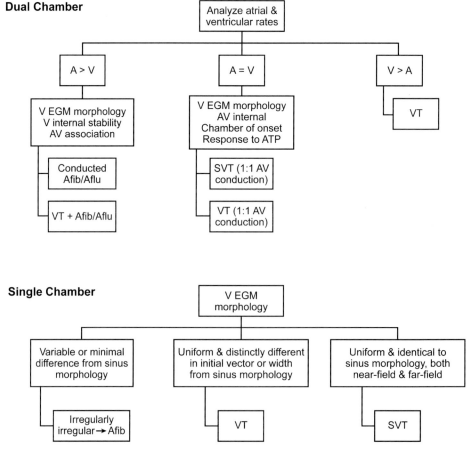

Fig. 10.67 Method for analysis of stored electrograms in dual-chamber ICDs (upper panel) and single-chamber ICDs (lower panel). ATP, antitachycardia pacing; AFib, atrial fibrillation; AFlu, atrial flutter. See text for details. (Modified from Swerdlow C, Friedman P. Advanced ICD troubleshooting: Part I. Pacing Clin Electrophysiol 2005; 28:1322–46, Blackwell Publishing, with permission.)

Tachycardias with 1:1 AV relationship: Most tachycardias with 1:1 AV relationship are SVT, primarily sinus tachycardia, or atrial tachycardia. In early studies, VT with 1:1 VA conduction accounted for less than 10% of VTs detected by ICDs in early studies,[61] but more than 20% in more recent studies such as EMPIRC. The principal differentiating features between SVT and VT with 1:1 AV relationship include morphology of the ventricular electrogram, chamber of onset, and response to ventricular ATP. Atrial tachycardia usually begins with a short P-P interval (i.e., a premature atrial complex) followed by a short R-R interval. Each conducted R-R interval is determined by the preceding P-P interval (Fig. 10.68). In contrast, VT begins with a short R-R interval (Fig. 10.69). A few beats of AV dissociation may occur until 1:1 ventriculoatrial conduction stabilizes. In sinus tachycardia, the atrial rhythm accelerates gradually with an approximately stable PR interval. Atrial electrogram morphology in sinus tachycardia may differ from the morphology of abnormal atrial electrograms (atrial tachycardia or retrograde electrograms in VT or reciprocating tachycardias), but these differences may be subtle, and their absence should not be considered as confirmatory of sinus P waves. The response to ATP may provide additional evidence (Fig. 10.70; see further discussion below).

Tachycardias with atrial rate higher than ventricular rate: Rapidly conducted AF or atrial flutter may be difficult to distinguish from VT during these atrial arrhythmias (Figs 10.71 and 10.72). Most VT during paroxysmal AF is fast enough to be classified in the VF or FVT zone.[62] The single-chamber criteria of abnormal ventricular morphology and regular ventricular rate (stability) are most helpful for diagnosing VT during AF. Conducted atrial flutter may be diagnosed in the presence of abnormal ventricular morphology if consistent 2:1 AV association or Mobitz 1 AV block is present. In contrast, VT during atrial flutter is diagnosed based on abnormal ventricular electrogram morphology and AV dissociation (Fig. 10.71).

Analysis of single-chamber, ventricular electrograms

The morphology, abruptness of onset, and regularity of ventricular electrograms form the foundation of single-chamber SVT-VT discrimination.

Morphology: Analysis of ventricular electrogram morphology is the most powerful tool for distinguishing VT from SVT on single-chamber recordings. Morphology analysis is best performed on far-field electrograms, preferably multiple electrograms. Morphology analysis is less accurate when performed on a single, near-field electrogram (Fig. 10.53). We and others are unable to discriminate VT from SVT reliably using near-field electrograms in at least 10% of VTs.[37,63] It is also less accurate if the electrogram is recorded at such high gain that the peak is truncated so that the entire electrogram cannot be analyzed. Whenever possible, a real-time, reference electrogram of conducted baseline rhythm should be recorded to compare morphology with that of the stored electrogram (Figs 10.55 and 10.73).

The rhythm is classified as SVT if electrogram morphology is uniform and identical to the sinus and/or baseline morphology. It is classified as VT if morphology is uniform and distinctly different from the sinus morphology. However, rate-related bundle branch block and more subtle forms of rate-related aberrancy may distort conducted beats, and there are no validated criteria for distinguishing aberrantly-conducted beats from VT or for determining precisely how much difference in electrogram morphology is sufficient to distinguish VT from SVT. A preliminary report indicates that specific electrogram features on the far-field electrogram correlate strongly with VT.[64] These include marked alteration of the electrogram onset (new Q waves, QS pattern, or pseudo-delta wave), marked increase in S-wave amplitude, or marked change in electrogram duration. In contrast, changes in amplitude only or low-amplitude terminal variations in the electrogram do not correlate with VT. During rapidly conducted AF, R-R intervals frequently demonstrate subtle beat-to-beat variation in morphology, the intracardiac correlate of rate-related aberrancy. In contrast, electrograms during VT tend to be uniform.

The vector of the far-field electrogram may also be helpful. For example, the far-field, coil–can electrogram in Medtronic, Boston Scientific, and St. Jude ICDs is recorded with the coil negative and can positive. In conducted SVT, the apex of ventricles is activated before the base, and the dominant component of this electrogram is almost always positive. A change from primarily positive to negative initial component of the far-field electrogram correlates strongly with VT, but the absence does not confirm SVT.[65] After shocks, electrogram morphology cannot be used to discriminate VT from SVT until post-shock distortion due to lead polarization and local muscle injury resolves (Fig. 10.73).

Regularity of the ventricular rhythm: Typically, the ventricular rhythm is irregularly irregular in conducted AF and more regular in monomorphic VT. However, in conducted AF beat-to-beat cycle length variability decreases as the ventricular rate increases. At ventricular rates above about 170/min, conducted AF may have periods in which variability is as low as 20 ms between

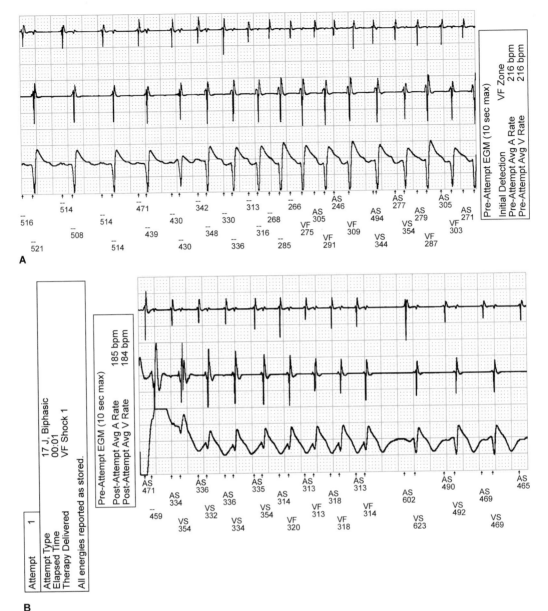

Fig. 10.68 Use of stored episode data for diagnosis of arrhythmia. All tracings are from the same patient. From top to bottom are atrial, rate (near-field) and shock (far-field) electrograms. (A) Episode of atrial tachycardia. Beginning with the fifth atrial complex (cycle length, 430), the atrial rate accelerates and is conducted rapidly to the ventricles. The changes in AA intervals precede the changes in VV intervals, as expected in atrial tachycardia (AA 430 leads to VV 430, AA 342 leads to VV 348, AA 330 leads to VV 336, and so on). Also, the far-field morphology is unchanged, consistent with supraventricular tachycardia. The atrial tachycardia is detected as ventricular fibrillation (VF), leading to a shock. (B) After the shock, nine atrial tachycardia complexes are conducted with a wide QRS (most likely a result of the shock) and are followed by resumption of sinus rhythm. Despite the wide QRS complex, the fact that the AA intervals "drive" the VV intervals confirms a supraventricular rhythm. (C) Subsequent development of ventricular tachycardia (VT). The tachycardia begins with a ventricular complex (with cycle length 285). The ventricular rate is greater than the atrial rate, and the morphology of both near-field and far-field electrograms is different from the sinus morphology (as seen in the first four ventricular complexes). (D) After a successful shock (the first four complexes are sinus tachycardia with aberrant QRS, as seen in B), VT recurs. The tachycardia begins with a ventricular complex (VF 281), has a ventricular rate exceeding the atrial rate, and has a morphology that is different from the aberrantly conducted sinus tachycardia, all consistent with the diagnosis of VT. This example demonstrates how the initiation of VT during an aberrant supraventricular rhythm can be diagnosed. (From Friedman PA, Swerdlow CD, Hayes DL. Troubleshooting. In: Hayes DL, Friedman PA, eds. Cardiac Pacing and Defibrillation: A Clinical Approach, 2nd edn. West Sussex, UK: Wiley-Blackwell, 2008: 401–516, by permission of Friedman, Swerdlow, and Hayes.)

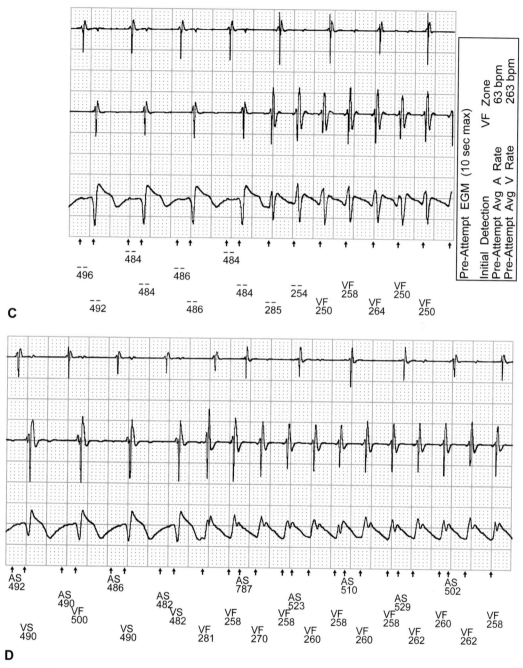

Fig. 10.68 (*Continued*)

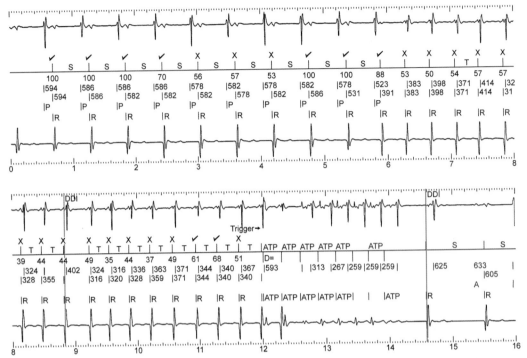

Fig. 10.69 Appropriate therapy for VT with 1:1 VA conduction. Bipolar atrial electrogram (RA), dual-chamber marker channel and rate-sensing (RV) electrogram are shown. Onset of VT during sinus tachycardia is identified by abrupt acceleration of ventricular rate and change in electrogram morphology without change in atrial rate. Morphology discriminator requires five of eight match scores 60% to withhold therapy. During sinus tachycardia, scores exceed 60%. (Five are 100%.) During VT, most scores are <60%. Check marks above marker channel indicate that morphology algorithm classifies beats as supraventricular. "X" marks indicate beats classified as VT morphology. The VT cycle length is moderately irregular. Changes in VV interval precede those in AA interval. Ventricular antitachycardia pacing (ATP) at right of lower panel results in transient VA block without acceleration of the atrial rate followed by 1:1 VA conduction. The near-simultaneous atrial and ventricular activation during tachycardia is more typical of typical (antegrade, slow; retrograde, fast) AV nodal re-entrant tachycardia than VT, but the shortening of the AV interval at the onset of tachycardia is inconsistent with this diagnosis. Pacing-induced VA block without acceleration of the atrial rate is also unusual in AV nodal re-entry. "Trigger" in lower panel indicates detection of VT. "D =" at onset of ATP indicates that atrial rate = ventricular rate. "S" denotes intervals interval the "Sinus" zone longer than the VT detection interval of 400 ms. "T" denotes intervals in VT zone. DDI, mode switch. Time line is in section. (From Swerdlow C, Friedman P. Advanced ICD troubleshooting: Part I. Pacing Clin Electrophysiol 2005; 28:1322–46, Blackwell Publishing, by permission.)

successive cycle lengths or 30–40 ms over a few cycle lengths, a range that is common in VT.[66,67] Inappropriate detection of rapidly conducted AF requires only that the detection algorithm's interval-stability criterion be met for the short duration of detection at any time during the conducted arrhythmia.

In patients with paroxysmal AF, VT may be detected inappropriately during ongoing AF. When interval stability criteria are active, inappropriate detection occurs during a period of increased regularity in conducted intervals. Thus, prior to detection the ventricular rate is usually fast and more irregular. In contrast, VT

during AF usually begins with an abrupt acceleration to a rapid ventricular rate. The exception to this rule is regularization of the atrial rhythm resulting in 1:1 conduction of atrial flutter and/or tachycardia (Fig. 10.74). An additional interpretive difficulty is that amiodarone or type IC antiarrhythmic drugs may cause monomorphic VT to become markedly irregular or polymorphic VT to slow, causing irregular intervals during true VT in the VT rate zone.[68,69]

Onset: Sinus tachycardia accelerates gradually and is always detected at the sinus–VT rate boundary

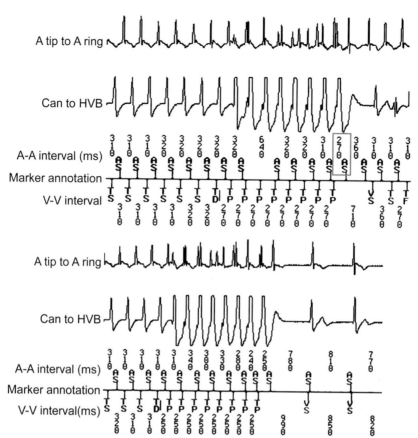

Fig. 10.70 Effect of ventricular antitachycardia pacing on SVT with 1:1 AV relationship. Atrial electrogram (A tip to A ring), high-voltage ventricular electrogram (can to HVB), and dual-chamber marker channel are shown. Upper panel: burst ventricular antitachycardia pacing at cycle length 270 ms is applied to SVT with cycle length 310–320 ms. The atrial interval after the last paced beat is accelerated to the pacing rate, probably indicating entrainment of the atrium. The AAV response at termination of pacing is diagnostic of atrial tachycardia. Lower panel: burst ventricular pacing at cycle length 250 ms accelerates the last two atrial intervals to the pacing cycle length and terminates tachycardia. This response does not distinguish between VT and SVT. (From Swerdlow C, Friedman P. Advanced ICD troubleshooting: Part I. Pacing Clin Electrophysiol 2005; 28:1322–46, Blackwell Publishing, by permission.)

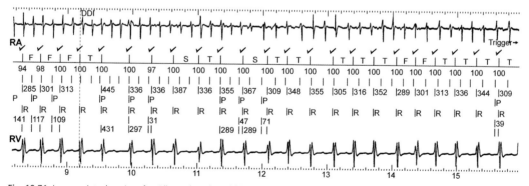

Fig. 10.71 Inappropriate detection of rapidly conducted atrial fibrillation. Stability and morphology algorithms are combined with "any" in this St. Jude ICD so that VT is diagnosed if either discriminator classifies rhythm as VT. Stability algorithm incorrectly classifies rhythm because ventricular cycle lengths regularize. Morphology algorithm correctly classifies rhythm as SVT. The rhythm would have been classified correctly if the morphology discriminator alone had been programmed. "F" markers indicate ventricular intervals in VF (Fib) zone. Other abbreviations as in Fig. 10.76. (From Swerdlow C, Friedman P. Advanced ICD troubleshooting: Part I. Pacing Clin Electrophysiol 2005; 28:1322–46, Blackwell Publishing, by permission.)

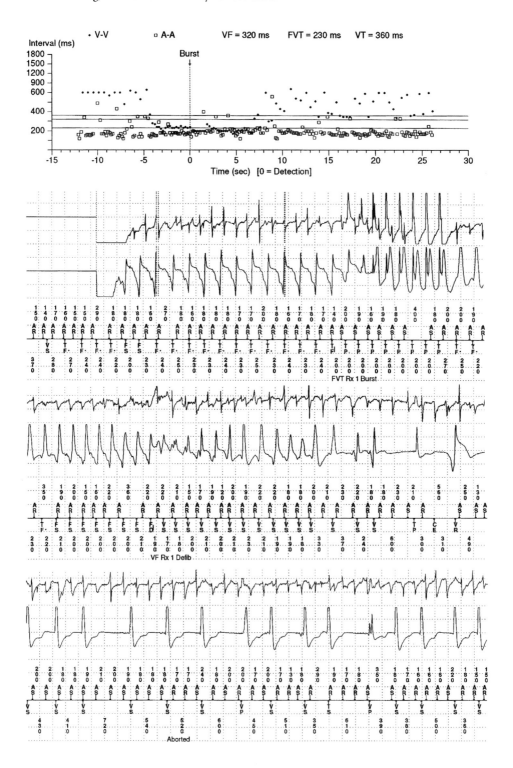

Fig. 10.72 VT during paroxysmal atrial fibrillation. Interval plot (upper panel) and continuous stored electrogram are shown. VT at cycle length 230 ms is diagnosed by AV dissociation and rate as "Fast VT." Change in morphology is clear on ventricular electrogram, but is not used for diagnosis. Antitachycardia pacing is delivered toward the right side of the first electrogram panel. It changes the morphology of VT, which becomes polymorphic and terminates toward the right side of the middle electrogram panel (type II break). VF is detected during this delayed termination ("VF Defib Rx 1" in middle of middle panel), but shock is aborted (Aborted) in middle of bottom panel. Dual-chamber interval plot at top shows onset of VT during atrial fibrillation, persistence of VT after antitachycardia pacing and subsequent termination. Most VT that occurs during paroxysmal atrial fibrillation is rapid and has cycle lengths classified in the VF zone using traditional programming. Antitachycardia pacing therapy for "fast" VT reduces inappropriate shocks. Ventricular intervals are classified as TS (fast VT), VS (ventricular sensed – sinus zone or during capacitor charging), FS (VF zone), TP (antitachycardia pacing), and VR (ventricular refractory) period after end of capacitor charging (CE). (From Swerdlow C, Friedman P. Advanced ICD troubleshooting: Part I. Pacing Clin Electrophysiol 2005; 28:1322–46, Blackwell Publishing, by permission.)

←——

(Fig. 10.73). In contrast, the onset of VT or paroxysmal SVT (including AF) is abrupt unless it originates during sinus tachycardia or SVT. However, if VT starts abruptly with an initial rate below the programmed VT detection rate, the beginning of the stored electrogram does not record the onset of the arrhythmia. Rather, it records the VT as it accelerates across the programmed, sinus–VT rate boundary. In Medtronic ICDs, stored (flashback) intervals preceding the stored electrogram may permit correct diagnosis of an abrupt-onset arrhythmia at a rate slower than the VT detection rate (Fig. 10.75). In the absence of flashback intervals, the few seconds of stored electrograms prior to initial detection are insufficient to determine categorically that an arrhythmia accelerated gradually.

Temporal relation between near-field and far-field electrograms: During conducted rhythms, the RV apical electrogram usually is recorded within 20 ms of QRS onset in the absence of right bundle branch block. If the RV sensing electrode is close the RV apex, it is usually activated early in SVT. Late activation suggests VT. In one study, the delay in onset of the near-field sensing electrogram relative to the far-field electrogram was 22 ± 14 ms in sinus rhythm, 17 ± 14 ms in SVT, and 83 ± 41 ms in VT (Fig. 10.76).[70]

Response to therapy: When atrial rate exceeds ventricular rate, abrupt termination of a regular tachycardia by ventricular ATP pacing without alteration of the atrial rhythm is essentially diagnostic of VT. However, during AF, retrograde concealed conduction from ventricular ATP may result in post-pacing pauses and/or slowing of antegrade conduction that must be distinguished from true termination of VT. In contrast, termination of tachycardias with 1 : 1 AV association by ATP is not helpful because ventricular ATP terminates >50% of inappropriately detected 1 : 1 SVTs.[70] However, the atrial response to ATP may be diagnostic. In ICD

patients, the vast majority of 1 : 1 SVTs treated by ventricular ATP are atrial tachycardias. They are terminated by ventricular ATP only if the atrial rate accelerates during pacing. Thus, atrial tachycardia can be excluded if a 1 : 1 tachycardia terminates while high-grade VA block occurs at the onset of ATP and the atrial rate slows during ATP. The differential diagnosis then is VT or AV nodal re-entrant tachycardia. The response to unsuccessful ATP may also be helpful. If the atrial cycle length is unchanged by ventricular ATP (tachycardia in the atrium does not depend on retrograde conduction, so that the ventricle is dissociated from the atrium), the diagnosis is SVT. If the atrial rate accelerates to the ventricular rate during ventricular ATP, the response at the end of unsuccessful pacing therapy may be helpful. A VAA response is one in which following the termination of ventricular pacing, two sensed atrial events occur before the next sensed ventricular event (V_PAA). It is diagnostic of atrial tachycardia (Fig. 10.70).[71] A VAV (V_PAV_S) response may occur in VT, AV nodal re-entrant SVT and AV re-entrant SVT. A VVA (V_PV_SA) response is diagnostic of VT.

If multiple arrhythmias occur with similar electrogram morphology and ventricular rate, one episode may permit definitive diagnosis for all episodes. In tachycardias with 1 : 1 AV association, transient AV block permits the diagnosis of SVT; transient VA block permits the diagnosis of VT. A regular tachycardia during paroxysmal AF may be identified as VT if a tachycardia with the same rate and morphology occurred during sinus rhythm.

Troubleshooting errors in SVT-VT discrimination

In this section, we consider how to determine why SVT was detected inappropriately and what types of solutions may be applied. We address details of programming solutions in Chapter 8: Programming. Tables 8.7 and 8.8 in Chapter 8 summarize our approach.

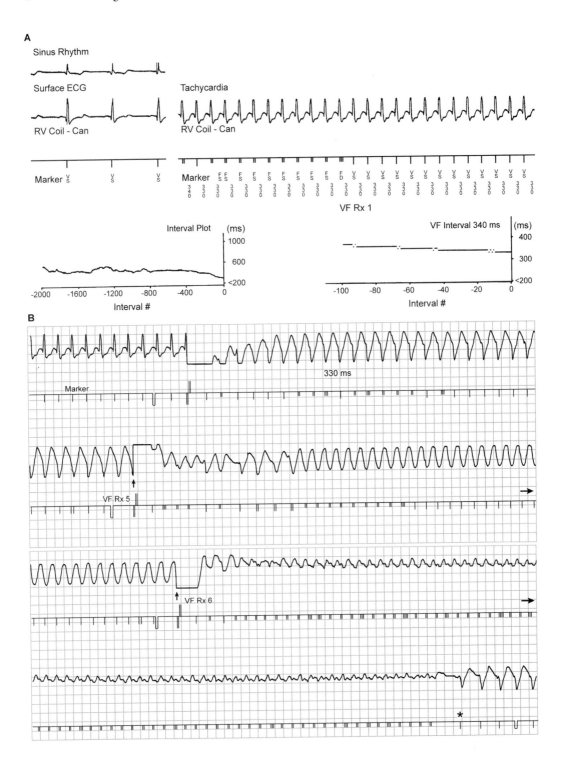

Fig. 10.73 Proarrhythmia caused by inappropriate shock for sinus tachycardia during rate-only detection. (A) The top left tracing shows electrograms recorded from high-voltage leads (HVA-HVB) during sinus rhythm. The top right tracing shows the initial stored electrogram from the treated tachycardia. The electrograms in these two panels are essentially identical, indicating that treated arrhythmia is SVT. The electrogram during tachycardia is clipped at the maximum amplitude of +8 mV. The lower panels are "flashback interval" plots of the RR-interval cycle lengths prior to rate-only detection of VF, which occurs at the right side of each panel. The interval number prior to detection is plotted on the abscissa, and the corresponding interval is plotted on the ordinate. The lower left panel shows 2000 RR intervals prior to detection. A tachycardia is present throughout. Shortly after the 400th interval, the rhythm accelerates gradually in a manner typical of sinus tachycardia and decreases below the programmed VF detection interval of 340 ms. The lower right panel shows this gradual acceleration on an expanded scale during the last 100 intervals prior to detection. Cycle-length measurements are truncated to the nearest 10 ms. (B) Stored electrogram during therapy of the tachycardia detected in (A). The first VF shock (VF Rx 1) results in widening of the electrogram without change in the cycle length of 330 ms. This is probably due to shock-induced right bundle branch block, which was documented in this patient at electrophysiologic testing. The tracing is discontinuous at the end of the first line and continuous thereafter. Shocks 2, 3, and 4 resulted in no change in rate or electrogram morphology. On the second line, the fifth VF shock (VF Rx 5) induces VT with cycle length 280 ms, despite appropriate synchronization to the nadir of the R wave. The sixth VF shock (VF Rx 6) accelerates the VT to cycle length 210 ms. This rhythm terminates spontaneously 21 s later, and sinus tachycardia with a wide electrogram resumes (asterisk). No additional shocks were delivered during these 21 s, because the maximum number of therapies per zone is six in this ICD. The patient reported that during exertion he experienced multiple shocks followed by syncope. The programmed shock strength was 24 J for the first shock and 34 J for subsequent shocks. (From Swerdlow C. Optimal programming of sensing and detection in single chamber ventricular ICDs. Card Electrophysiol Rev 2001; 5:85–90, Springer, by permission.)

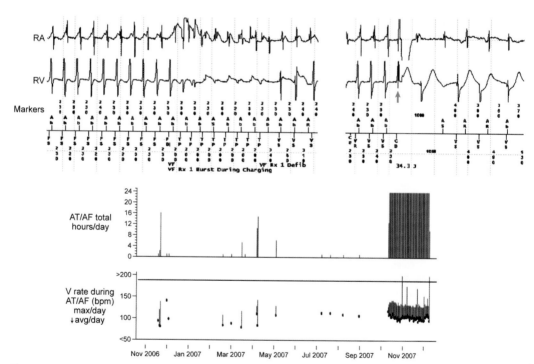

Fig. 10.74 Therapy for 1:1 conduction of atrial flutter. Upper panel shows atrial and far-field ventricular EGM combined with dual-chamber markers. The left side of the panel shows ATP during charging (TP). The atrial cycle length does not change during ATP, excluding VT with 1:1 VA conduction. The right side shows inappropriate shock after charging period (not shown), terminating the atrial arrhythmia (CD on marker channel, red arrow). The lower panel displays diagnostics for the total hourly atrial fibrillation (AF) burden in each day and the maximum ventricular rate in AF/atrial flutter. When the patient received this shock in December 2007, he had been in asymptomatic AF/atrial flutter for approximately 6 weeks without anticoagulation. He was thus at risk for a thromboembolic event with cardioversion, although one did not occur. The plot of ventricular (V) rate during atrial tachycardia (AT)/AF shows that his ventricular rate approached the single zone detection interval of 188 bpm on several days before exceeding it on the day of the shock. Remote monitoring would likely have identified new onset atrial arrhythmia with rapid ventricular rate, permitted early cardioversion, anticoagulation, and pharmacologic or ablative preventive therapy.

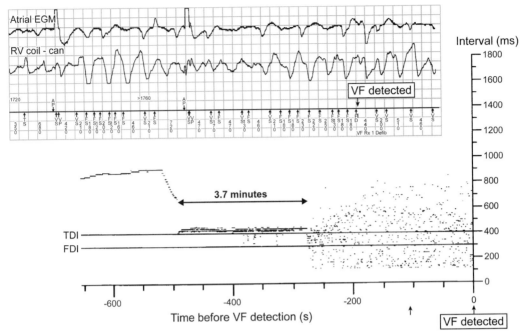

Fig. 10.75 Underdetection of VT and undersensing of VF. The lower panel is a "flashback interval" plot of RR-interval cycle lengths prior to detection of VF, which occurs at the right side of each panel. The interval number prior to detection is plotted on the abscissa, and the corresponding interval is plotted on the ordinate. Horizontal lines indicate the VT detection interval (TDI) of 400 ms and VF detection interval (FDI) of 320 ms. Shortly after the 500th interval preceding detection, regular tachycardia begins abruptly. The constant cycle length indicates reliable sensing. This VT is not detected despite reliable sensing because the cycle length is more than the programmed TDI. VT persists for 3.7 min until approximately interval 280 prior to detection, when sensed intervals become highly variable. This indicates degeneration of the rhythm to VF with undersensing that delays detection. During VT and VF, atrial flashback intervals (not shown) indicated lower rate limit bradycardia pacing at 40 bpm (1500 ms). The upper panel shows stored atrial and far-field ventricular electrograms immediately prior to detection with atrial and ventricular marker channels. Specific undersensed electrograms cannot be identified because the rate sensing electrogram was not recorded. However, long-sensed RR intervals ending with VS markers indicate undersensing and correspond to long interval in upper panel. "VF Therapy 1 Defib" at lower right (arrow) denotes detection of VF. (From Swerdlow C, Friedman P. Advanced ICD troubleshooting: Part I. Pacing Clin Electrophysiol 2005; 28:1322–46, Blackwell Publishing, by permission.)

Ventricular rate in SVT compared with the VT/VF rate boundary Inappropriate detection of SVT as VT or VF requires that SVT exceed the corresponding rate boundary (VT or VF) for a sufficient duration to satisfy the programmed detection criterion. From the perspective of ICD programming, the simplest solution is to prevent conduction of SVT in the VT/VF rate zones either with drugs or ablation to prevent SVT/AF or to slow the ventricular rate when AF occurs.

An alternative, and complementary, solution is to shorten (increase the heart rate of) the VT or VF detection interval, but this may increase the risk of not detecting VT. Several studies directly or indirectly confirm that shorter detection intervals reduce inappropriate therapy of SVT. These include the EMPIRIC[72] and PREPARE[73] studies; see Chapter 8: Programming

(see Optimizing programming). In EMPIRIC, SVT-VT discriminators reduced the fraction of SVT episodes that received inappropriate therapy after satisfying rate and duration criteria for VT, but they did not reduce the absolute incidence of inappropriate therapies for SVT because patients who did not have SVT-VT discriminators programmed had shorter VT detection intervals than those who had SVT-VT discriminators programmed (mean 360 vs. 400 ms). The shorter (faster) VT detection intervals meant that their devices were exposed to fewer tachycardias.

Ventricular rate in SVT compared with the fastest rate at which SVT-VT discriminators apply When SVT-VT discriminators are programmed, approximately 25% of inappropriate therapy is caused by

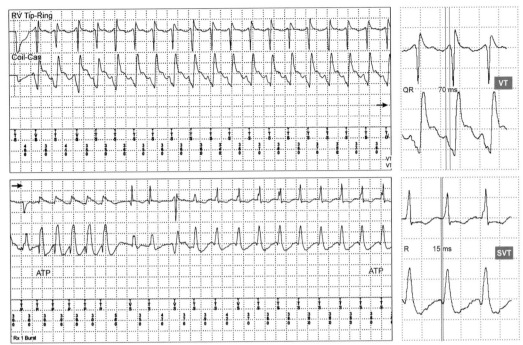

Fig. 10.76 Morphology analysis of single-chamber EGMs. The left panel shows continuous recordings of the true-bipolar (near-field, upper EGM) and high-voltage (far-field, lower) EGM. ATP delivered at beginning of lower left panel shows conversion of regular tachycardia with one morphology at cycle length 360 ms to a regular tachycardia with different morphology at cycle length 380 ms, still below the VT detection interval of 400 ms. The right panel enlarges three complexes for analysis. The initial component of the far-field EGM is directed inferiorly in the first tachycardia, highly correlated with VT, because conducted EGMs originate at the insertion of the His–Purkinje system near the apex, not the base. It is directed superiorly after ATP, consistent with either VT or SVT. In the first tachycardia, the near-field EGM begins 70 ms after the far-field EGM, indicating that the RV apex is activated late, typical of VT or LBBB during SVT. In the second tachycardia, the RV EGM begins 15 ms after the far-field EGM. Early activation of the RV apex via the right bundle is characteristic of SVT. Thus, the diagnosis is VT terminated to SVT. The morphology of the EGM in the second tachycardia was identical to a real-time EGM recorded in sinus rhythm.

SVT with ventricular cycle lengths shorter than the minimum cycle length to which SVT discriminators apply.[74–76] In most cases, SVT-VT discriminators do not withhold inappropriate therapy for SVT if the majority of ventricular intervals (typically 70–80%) are shorter than the SVT limit. Therefore, rapidly conducted AF may be classified as VT even if the mean cycle length is 20–40 ms longer than the SVT limit. Programming a sufficiently short, minimum cycle length for SVT-VT discrimination is essential to reliable rejection of SVT.

The principal reason that the SVT limit cycle length is programmed slower than optimal for SVT-VT discrimination is concern that, if the algorithm incorrectly misclassifies VT as SVT, the patient may collapse or die. This problem may be reduced by optimal use of β-blockers or other drugs to reduce ventricular rate during rapidly conducted AF. Increasing the duration for detection of VT/VF may also reduce inappropriate detection of AF, because rapid conduction during AF may be transient. Finally, high-rate time out features may reduce the risk of inappropriately withholding therapy from true VT, but they ensure inappropriate treatment of all SVTs that satisfy the high-rate criterion for the duration of the time-out period (Chapter 8: Programming, see SVT-VT discriminator timers) for details.

Failure of SVT-VT discriminators If SVT is detected inappropriately and the ventricular rate is in the zone of SVT-VT discrimination, either the discriminator(s) failed or discrimination did not apply for a specific reason. For example, many discriminators apply only to initial detection of VT, but not redetection (Chapter

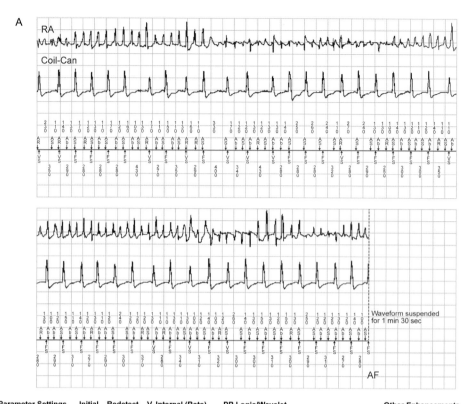

Parameter Settings	Initial	Redetect	V. Internal (Rate)	PR Logic/Wavelet		Other Enhancements	
VF On	30/40	12/16	320 ms (188 bpm)	AF/Afl	On	Stability	Off
FVT Off				Sinus Tach	On	Onset	Off
VT Off	16	12		Other 1:1 SVTs	Off	High Rate Tmeout	
Monitor Monitor	32		370 ms (162 bpm)	Wavelet	On, Match = 70%	VF Zone Only	Off
				Template	14-Jan-2010, Auto = On	T Wave	On
				SVT V. Limit	260 ms	RV Lead Noise	On + Timeout
						RV Lead Noise	0.75 min

Fig. 10.77 Rapidly conducted AF is rejected for the wrong reason. **(A)** Atrial and far-field ventricular EGMs are shown with marker channel during rapidly conducted AF in the VF zone of the ICD. Programmed values for this Medtronic ICD are also shown. (B) The upper panel shows that Wavelet morphology analysis would have classified the rhythm as SVT (≥3 of 8 intervals with match score ≥70%). The lower panel shows the episode summary. It indicates that the Wavelet morphology feature was not applied because therapy was withheld by "other criteria." In this case extremely rapid atrial activations at 100–160 ms resulted in incorrect diagnosis of AV association. The rule for AV association in this ICD (PR Logic™) classifies beats as dissociated if either PR average – PR current >40 ms or there is no P wave in the current RR interval. If 4 of the last 8 beats are dissociated, the rhythm is classified as dissociated. Extremely rapid atrial activation ensured the interval between the ventricular EGM and preceding P wave was classified as a stable AV interval. Although the rhythm was classified correctly, similarly rapid atrial activation during VT could result in misclassification, preventing application of the Wavelet morphology algorithm.

8: Programming, see Committed and noncommitted shocks).

Failure of SVT-VT discrimination may be diagnosed using the text episode summary that provides numerical data regarding the measured values of specific discriminators such as onset, stability, and morphology during the episode in comparison with the programmed values for withholding the diagnosis of VT. Even if the rhythm is classified correctly as SVT, these summaries should be inspected. Sometimes SVT is diagnosed correctly, but for the wrong reason (Fig. 10.77). Other times, SVT may be rejected, but with an insufficient safety margin (Fig. 10.78). In some ICDs, the marker channel also indicates the criteria used to classify the rhythm as SVT or VT (Fig. 10.71), especially status of dual-chamber discriminators and match scores for morphology algorithms. (See Chapter 8: Programming, SVT-VT discriminators section for solu-

B

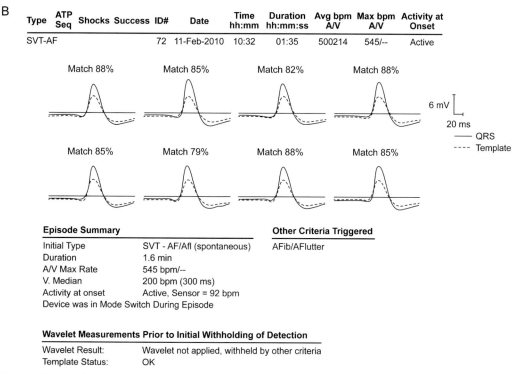

Type	ATP Seq	Shocks	Success	ID#	Date	Time hh:mm	Duration hh:mm:ss	Avg bpm A/V	Max bpm A/V	Activity at Onset
SVT-AF				72	11-Feb-2010	10:32	01:35	500214	545/--	Active

Match 88%   Match 85%   Match 82%   Match 88%

6 mV

20 ms

—— QRS

---- Template

Match 85%   Match 79%   Match 88%   Match 85%

Episode Summary

Initial Type	SVT - AF/Afl (spontaneous)
Duration	1.6 min
A/V Max Rate	545 bpm/--
V. Median	200 bpm (300 ms)
Activity at onset	Active, Sensor = 92 bpm
Device was in Mode Switch During Episode	

Other Criteria Triggered

AFib/AFlutter

Wavelet Measurements Prior to Initial Withholding of Detection

Wavelet Result:	Wavelet not applied, withheld by other criteria
Template Status:	OK

Fig. 10.77 *(Continued)*

tions to SVT-VT discrimination failures for specific single and dual-chamber discriminators including morphology algorithms.)

Troubleshooting errors in SVT-VT discrimination due to atrial sensing problems Accurate sensing of atrial EGMs is essential for discrimination between VT/VF and rapidly conducted SVTs by dual-chamber algorithms that compare atrial and ventricular intervals or rate. Atrial lead dislodgment, oversensing of far-field R waves, or undersensing due to low-amplitude atrial EGMs or atrial blanking periods can cause inaccurate identification of atrial EGMs. Atrial undersensing results in misclassification of conducted AF as VT due to ventricular rate greater than measured atrial rate. Atrial oversensing may result in either misclassification of VT as SVT or of SVT as VT.

Far-field R-wave oversensing: The most important steps to prevent oversensing of far-field R waves occur at implant: use an atrial lead with short (≤10 mm) interelectrode distance and position the atrial lead on the lateral wall or some other location with a small far-field R wave. The relative size of the atrial and far-field

ventricular electrograms at implant predict the likelihood of far-field R-wave oversensing. If the atrial electrogram is four times the size of the far-field R-wave the problem is rare; if the ratio is 2:1 it is often manageable.

The simplest and preferred method for reducing oversensing of far-field R waves after sensed ventricular events is to decrease atrial sensitivity, if this can be done without undersensing of true atrial electrograms during sinus rhythm and AF. Atrial sensitivity can be reduced to 0.45 mV with a low risk of undersensing AF. Less sensitive values should be programmed only if the likelihood of rapidly conducted AF is low. Far-field R wave oversensing that occurs only after paced ventricular events (when auto-adjusting atrial sensitivity is maximal) does not cause inappropriate detection of SVT as VT, but it may cause inappropriate mode switching and can contribute to inappropriate detection of AF or atrial flutter.

Post-ventricular atrial blanking: To prevent oversensing of far-field R waves, older dual-chamber ICDs had fixed post-ventricular atrial blanking (PVAB) periods, similar to those in pacemakers. With a fixed blanking period,

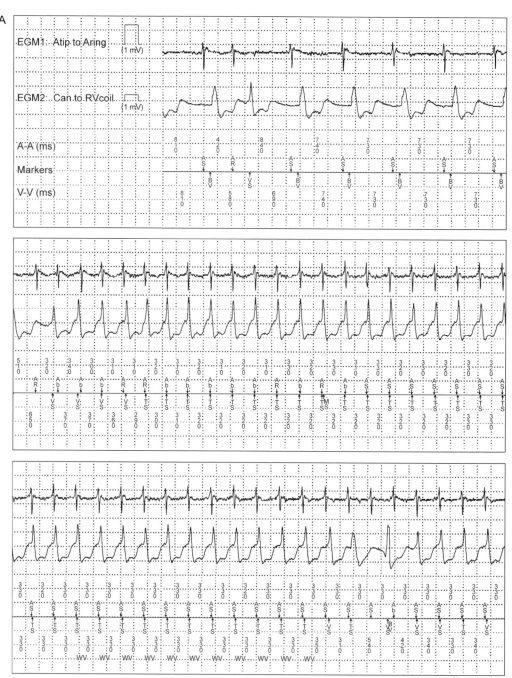

Fig. 10.78 Appropriate rejection of SVT with insufficient safety margin in a cardiac resynchronization ICD. (**A**) Rejection of abrupt onset 1:1 SVT by morphology, where onset and stability would have failed. Atrial and coil-CAN (far-field) ventricular EGM are shown. BV, biventricular pacing; TS, intervals in VT zone; WV, rhythm classified as SVT by Medtronic Wavelet morphology algorithm after number of intervals to detect VT has been satisfied. (B) Upper panel shows interval plot with abrupt onset of 1:1 tachycardia. Middle panel shows beat-to-beat morphology match between template (dotted line) and SVT (solid line). Match scores are listed in lower panel. Although 5 of 8 values meet or exceed the threshold of 70%, 3 of them are at the boundary of 70%. In this case, the first step is to evaluate the template match in sinus rhythm. Because this is a cardiac resynchronization ICD, the template is not updated regularly. If the match is poor, it should be updated. If the match is good, lowering the programmed SVT threshold slightly may prevent future misclassification of SVT as VT, but may slightly increase the risk of misclassifying VT as SVT. Other considerations include increasing beta blockers or catheter ablation, providing the LV lead is chronic.

B

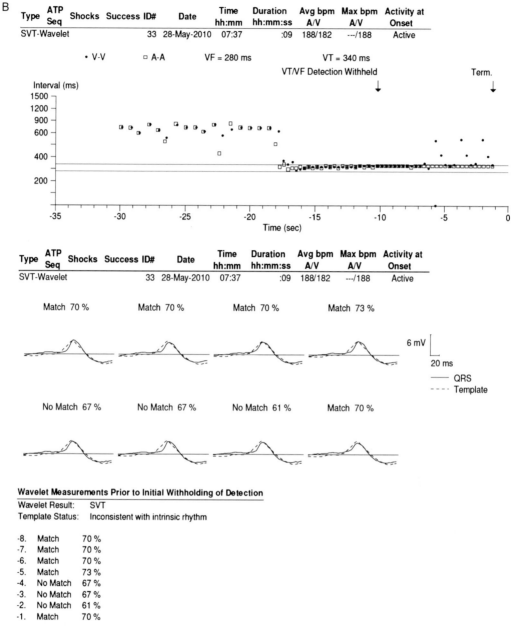

Type	ATP Seq	Shocks	Success	ID#	Date	Time hh:mm	Duration hh:mm:ss	Avg bpm A/V	Max bpm A/V	Activity at Onset
SVT-Wavelet				33	28-May-2010	07:37	:09	188/182	---/188	Active

• V-V   □ A-A   VF = 280 ms   VT = 340 ms

VT/VF Detection Withheld

Term.

Type	ATP Seq	Shocks	Success	ID#	Date	Time hh:mm	Duration hh:mm:ss	Avg bpm A/V	Max bpm A/V	Activity at Onset
SVT-Wavelet				33	28-May-2010	07:37	:09	188/182	---/188	Active

Match 70 %   Match 70 %   Match 70 %   Match 73 %

6 mV

20 ms

—— QRS
- - - - Template

No Match 67 %   No Match 67 %   No Match 61 %   Match 70 %

Wavelet Measurements Prior to Initial Withholding of Detection

Wavelet Result: SVT
Template Status: Inconsistent with intrinsic rhythm

-8.	Match	70 %
-7.	Match	70 %
-6.	Match	70 %
-5.	Match	73 %
-4.	No Match	67 %
-3.	No Match	67 %
-2.	No Match	61 %
-1.	Match	70 %

Fig. 10.78 (Continued)

the blanked proportion of the cardiac cycle increases with the ventricular rate. Atrial undersensing caused by PVAB causes underestimation of the atrial rate, resulting in inappropriate detection of VT (Fig. 10.79).[77] However, without PVAB, atrial oversensing of far-field R waves could cause overestimation of the atrial rate during tachycardias with a 1:1 AV relationship.[75] This may result in either inappropriate rejection of VT as

SVT, if far-field R waves are counted consistently as atrial EGMs, or inappropriate detection of SVT as VT, if they are counted inconsistently.[78]

Medtronic ICDs, which have short, nominal PVABs, reject far-field R waves algorithmically by identifying a pattern of atrial and ventricular events that fulfill specific criteria (Fig. 10.80). Intermittent sensing of far-field R waves or frequent premature atrial sensed events

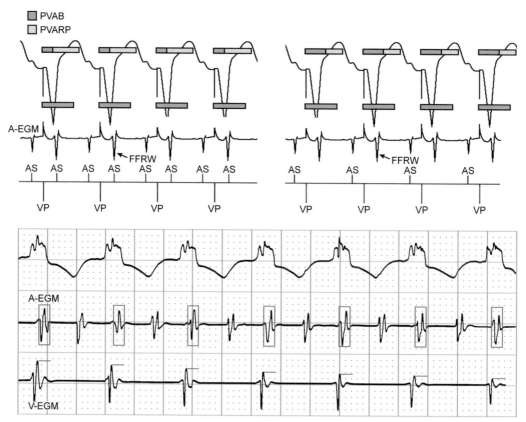

Fig. 10.79 Effect of post-ventricular atrial blanking. Upper panel shows ECG, atrial electrogram, and marker channel during atrial sensed-ventricular paced rhythm. First segment of lower horizontal bar denotes postventricular atrial blanking period (PVAB). Second segment denotes post-ventricular atrial refractory period (PVARP). FFRW denotes far-field R wave on atrial channel. With a short post-ventricular atrial blanking period (left), far-field R waves are oversensed. Longer post-ventricular atrial blanking period (right) prevents oversensing of far-field R waves. Lower horizontal line bar denotes post-pacing ventricular blanking period. Lower panel shows ECG, atrial, and ventricular electrograms from atrial flutter with 2:1 AV conduction. Horizontal bars on ventricular channel denote postventricular atrial blanking, which results in atrial undersensing of alternate atrial flutter electrograms (in boxes). Resultant incorrect calculation of atrial rate causes inappropriate shock (arrow) for atrial flutter because the ICD interprets the ventricular rate to be more than the atrial rate. (From Swerdlow C, Friedman P. Advanced ICD troubleshooting: Part I. Pacing Clin Electrophysiol 2005; 28:1322–46, Blackwell Publishing, by permission.)

disrupt this pattern, so that the algorithm is unable to identify far-field R waves. During sinus tachycardia, the algorithm then identifies a regular ventricular rhythm with dissociated sensed atrial events faster than the ventricular rate, resulting in misclassification as VT during atrial arrhythmia. Thus, whenever possible, far-field R waves should be rejected by other methods.

Medtronic ICDs (starting with the Entrust family) and Boston Scientific ICDs (starting with Vitality family) may use a brief PVAB or a period of reduced, automatically adjusting sensitivity (or both) to reject far-field R waves without preventing detection of AF. St. Jude ICDs, and Medtronic ICDs starting with the Entrust family, provide programmable atrial blanking after sensed ventricular events to individualize the tradeoff between oversensing of far-field R waves and undersensing of atrial EGMs in AF. St. Jude ICDs also provide programmable atrial sensing Threshold Start and Decay Delay, corresponding to the same features in the ventricular channel.

Atrial undersensing in AF: Atrial undersensing during rapidly conducted AF may be caused either by atrial blanking periods, as noted above, or by low amplitude electrograms. In either case, the result is incorrect

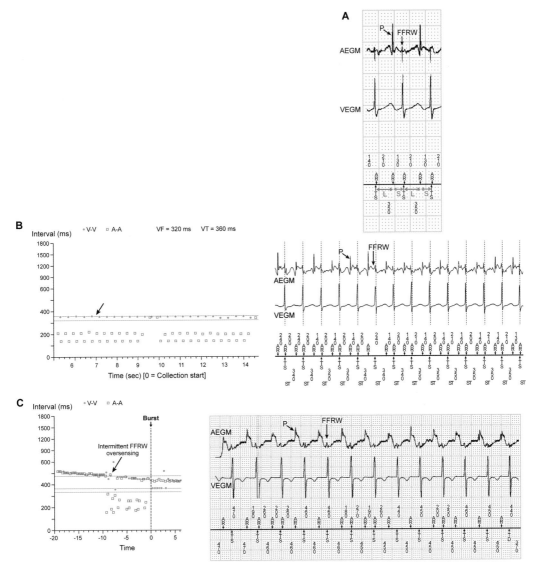

Fig. 10.80 Algorithmic rejection of far-field R waves (FFRW) by pattern analysis. ICDs with minimum cross-chamber blanking (Medtronic) reject FFRWs by the timing pattern of atrial and ventricular intervals. Atrial events are classified as FFRWs if all the following criteria are met: (1) there are exactly two atrial events for each V-V interval; (2) timing of one P wave is consistent with a FFRW (R-P interval <160 ms); (3) there is a stable interval between the FFRW and the ventricular electrogram (VEGM); (4) there is a short–long pattern of P-P intervals (to distinguish FFRW oversensing from atrial flutter); and (5) the pattern occurs frequently (4 of 12 intervals). (A) Atrial electrogram (AEGM), VEGM, and dual-chamber event markers are shown. All five criteria for FFRWs are fulfilled. Horizontal double-ended arrows below event markers denote alternation of long (L) and short (S) atrial intervals; AR, atrial refractory event; P, P wave; TS, ventricular event in ventricular tachycardia zone. (B) Interval plot (left) and stored EGM (right) from episode of sinus tachycardia with consistent FFRW oversensing that is classified correctly. On the interval plot, open squares denote A-A interval and closed circles denote V-V interval. Horizontal lines denote ventricular tachycardia (VT) and ventricular fibrillation (VF) detection intervals of 400 and 320 ms, respectively. Alternating A-A intervals whose sum equals that of the VV intervals produce a characteristic "railroad track" appearance (arrow). The algorithm rejects FFRWs despite the fact that FFRW oversensing does not occur for one V-V interval between seconds 9 and 10. (C) Interval plot (left) and stored EGM (right) from episode of sinus tachycardia with inconsistent FFRW oversensing that was detected inappropriately as VT. Intermittent oversensing of FFRWs occurs as sinus tachycardia accelerates gradually across the VT detection interval of 480 ms (arrow), resulting in inappropriate therapy ("Burst" antitachycardia pacing marker on interval plot, VT marker on EGM event markers). (From Swerdlow CD, GIllberg JG, Olson WH. Sensing and detection. In: Ellenbogen KA, Kay GN, Lau C, Wilkoff BL, eds. Cardiac Pacing and Defibrillation: A Clinical Approach, 3rd edn. Philadelphia, PA: Saunders Company, 2007: 75–160, by permission of Swerdlow, Gillberg, and Olson.)

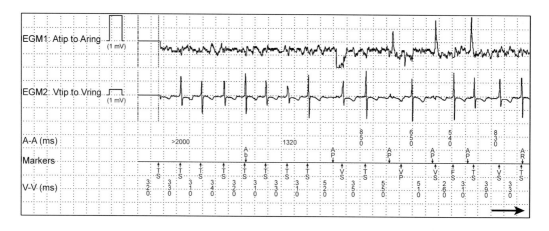

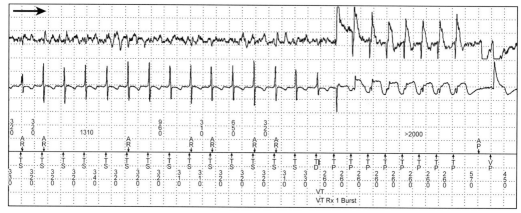

Fig. 10.81 Inappropriate therapy of rapidly-conducted AF due to atrial undersensing. Atrial and true-bipolar RV sensing EGMs are shown with dual-chamber marker channel. The calibration marker shows that the atrial EGMs have low amplitude (mostly less than 0.3 mV). Marker channel shows few atrial sensed events, indicating atrial undersensing.

classification of a tachycardia with ventricular rate greater than atrial rate, usually resulting in a diagnosis of VT. Floating atrial electrodes on ventricular ventricular ICD leads may be particularly prone to this type of undersensing, as well as far-field R-wave oversensing because of the high gain amplification required to identify atrial electrograms with this lead (Fig. 10.81).[40]

Determining if shocks for VT are necessary

If a shock has been delivered in response to true VT, it is important to consider whether the shock was necessary or preventable. Troubleshooting to reduce shocks for VT includes minimizing ICD proarrhythmia, minimizing treatment of self-terminating VT, ensuring optimal delivery of ATP, and other factors.

Minimizing ICD proarrhythmia

Excluding lead dislodgments, the most common causes of ICD proarrhythmia is bradycardia pacing in patients with inducible VT. Proposed mechanisms include short–long–short sequences that are either pacing facilitated or pacing permitted,[79] atrial preference pacing,[80] and noncompetitive atrial pacing.[81] Rate-smoothing algorithms that aimed reduce short–long–short sequences have not shown consistent benefit.[82] Surprisingly, even VVI pacing at 40 bpm may be proarrhythmic (Fig. 10.82).[83] Occasionally, pacing-facilitated short–long–short VT can be due to Wenckebach upper rate response.[83] In this case, the upper tracking rates can be increased, and PVARP reduced.[79] When the paced QRS morphology and VT morphology are similar shortly after ICD implant, mechanical irritation from the ventricular lead should be considered.

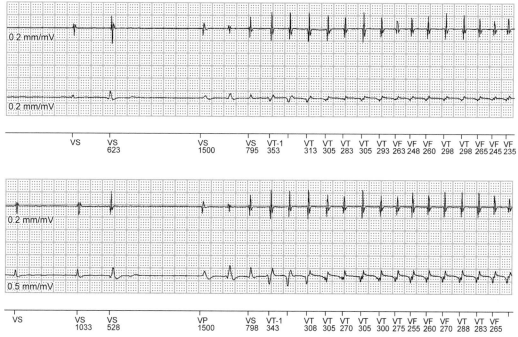

Fig. 10.82 Proarrhythmia from bradycardia pacing. Upper and lower panels show stored EGMs from distinct episodes of rapid VT. In each panel, integrated-bipolar sensing EGM, shock EGM, and single-chamber marker channel is shown. Each episode begins with a post-PVC pause terminated by ventricular (VVI) pacing (VP) at 40 bpm (1500 ms). This patient had these two episodes of VT in the first 10 days after implant of a primary prevention ICD. After programming the ICD to OVO (no pacing) mode, the patient has had no further episodes of VT in 20 months of follow-up.

Minimizing therapy for self-terminating VT/VF

Optimizing duration for detection of VT/VF is discussed in Chapter 8: Programming. Data from the REL-EVANT study show that about 90% of VT episodes will terminate between 12 and 30 beats.[84] The PREPARE[73] and RELEVANT[84] studies demonstrate the safety of increasing detection durations, providing consecutive-interval counting is not used (see Chapter 8: Programming for details).

Optimizing ATP

Optimal initial programming of ATP is discussed in Chapter 8: Programming (see Optimizing programming). Analysis of the return cycle after unsuccessful ATP may permit tuning ATP if it is unsuccessful. If the VT is not reset, propagated wavefronts from ATP stimuli have not reached the re-entry circuit; adding stimuli may improve efficacy by peeling back refractoriness between the pacing site and re-entry circuit. If the circuit is reset, ATP pulses traverse the circuit orthodromically without causing bidirectional block; addition of a premature stimulus at the end of the pacing train

("burst +" mode) may achieve sufficient prematurity to induce block in the circuit.

ICDs misclassify effective ATP as ineffective if VT/VF recurs before the ICD identifies episode termination and reclassifies the post-therapy rhythm as sinus (Fig. 10.83). The ICD then escalates therapy to shocks rather than starting a new initial detection sequence. This may also occur if SVT begins after successful ATP but before ICD-defined episode termination because of frequent premature beats or nonsustained tachycardia. Decreasing the duration for redetection of sinus rhythm in St. Jude ICDs may correct this classification error.

Miscellaneous factors

Inappropriate redetection of SVT as VT after appropriate therapy is a vexing problem (Fig. 10.84). This may be prevented by use of SVT-VT discrimination in redetection, when this feature is available (Fig. 10.85). If therapy is delivered for nonsustained VT or SVT after ATP or shocks, increasing the duration for redetection may prevent inappropriate redetection of delayed

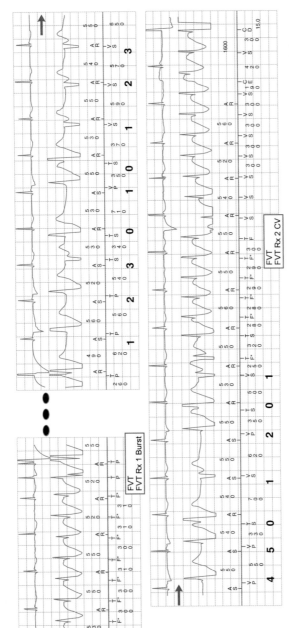

Fig. 10.83 Failure to identify post-therapy sinus rhythm because of rapid reinitiation of ventricular tachycardia (VT) after successful therapy. Atrial EGM, ventricular true bipolar EGM, and EGM markers classify the rhythm as sinus (eight consecutive intervals). Therefore, VT is inappropriately redetected instead of being detected de novo for the second time. This results in delivery of the second programmed Fast VT (FVT) therapy, cardioversion, rather than repeat delivery of the previously successful antitachycardia pacing (ATP) stimulus, which is both painless and more energy efficient. Redetection marker (FV Rx 2 CV) indicates onset of capacitor charging for the second VT therapy. Shock is not shown. Large numbers below right side of upper panel and left side of lower panel show value of sinus rhythm counter, which increments for each interval in the sinus zone (VS) and is reset to zero by premature ventricular complexes (PVCs) with a coupling interval of less than the VT detection interval of 400 ms (TS). VS markers indicate unclassified ventricular intervals during capacitor charging. AS, Atrial sensed event; AR, atrial intervals in pacing refractory period. (From Swerdlow CD, Gillberg JG, Olson WH. Sensing and Detection. In: Ellenbogen KA, Kay GN, Lau C, Wilkoff BL, eds. Cardiac Pacing and Defibrillation: A Clinical Approach, 3rd edn. Philadelphia, PA: Saunders Company, 2007: 75–160, by permission of Swerdlow, Gillberg, and Olson.)

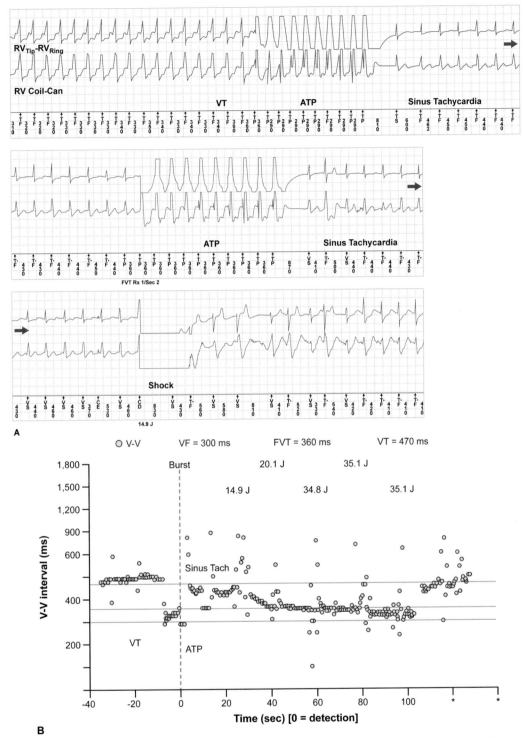

Fig. 10.84 Redetection. Inappropriate therapy of sinus tachycardia after appropriate therapy for ventricular tachycardia (VT) in a single-chamber ICD. Ventricular sensing and high-voltage leads are shown with event markers. (A) Continuous stored EGM strips after detection of VT. The top strip shows successful antitachycardia pacing (ATP) of VT followed by sinus tachycardia in the Fast VT (FVT) zone (TF on event markers). The second strip shows the first inappropriate sequence of ATP. The third strip shows the first of five shocks delivered after ATP. (B) Interval plot shows the entire episode. No US ICD manufacturer provides for VT-supraventricular tachycardia (SVT) discrimination after ATP. RV, Right ventricular; VF, ventricular fibrillation. (From Swerdlow CD, Friedman PA. Advanced ICD troubleshooting. Part II. Pacing Clin Electrophysiol 2006; 29:70–96.)

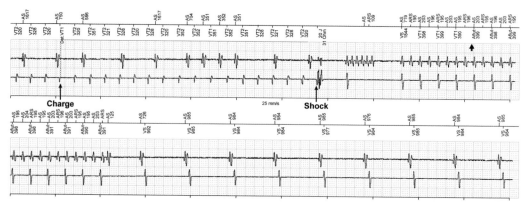

Fig. 10.85 SVT-VT discriminators in redetection. Dual-chamber EGM markers, atrial EGM, and true bipolar EGM are shown in this continuous strip from a Biotronik Lexos ICD, Model 347000. Rhythm at beginning of upper panel is VT with ventricular-atrial (VA) dissociation. Vertical dotted line indicates detection and start of capacitor charging ("Charge"). Black horizontal line indicates period of capacitor charging followed by successful shock. Post-shock nonsustained atrial flutter begins toward right side of upper panel, continues into lower panel, and shows transient atrial flutter followed by conversion to sinus rhythm. Ventricular rhythm is classified by the lower row of markers as VT2 (faster VT zone) before shock, VT1 (slower VT zone) for the first four ventricular EGMs of atrial flutter, and conducted atrial flutter ("Aflut") beginning at the fifth conducted ventricular EGM during atrial flutter (arrowhead). Without SVT-VT discrimination in redetection, VT would have been redetected after 10 intervals. (From Friedman PA, Swerdlow CD, Hayes DL. Troubleshooting. In: Hayes DL, Friedman PA, eds. Cardiac Pacing and Defibrillation: A Clinical Approach, 2nd edn. West Sussex, UK: Wiley-Blackwell, 2008: 401–516, by permission of Friedman, Swerdlow, and Hayes.)

termination of VT (type II break) or post-shock non-sustained VT or shock-induced atrial arrhythmia.

Use of sufficiently strong first shocks minimizes the number of shocks delivered for each true VT/VF episode and has the greatest likelihood of terminating rapidly conducted AF.

Approach to the patient with frequent shocks

Frequent or repetitive shocks constitute an emergency, both because of underlying medical conditions that my precipitate an exacerbation of true arrhythmias, and because repetitive shocks may cause post-traumatic stress disorder.[84,85]

Emergency management

In addition to standard emergency department care, the appropriate programmer should be applied immediately to interrogate the ICD and determine the cause of shocks. Usually, it is preferable to disable automatic ICD shocks while the physician is determining the cause of shocks after applying self-adhesive electrodes from an external defibrillator.

If a programmer is not available immediately, a magnet should be applied to the ICD and left in place after external defibrillator electrodes are applied. The magnet disables detection of VT and VF without altering programmed pacing parameters. In most ICDs,

detection of VT/VF is reactivated as soon as the magnet is withdrawn. However, some Boston Scientific ICDs remain inactivated if a magnet is applied for more than 30 s. If shocks are caused by a lead problem, either defibrillation or bradycardia/ATP may be unreliable. Thus, continuous ECG monitoring with a backup external defibrillator must continue until interrogation appropriate ICD function assured both with respect to lead integrity and arrhythmia detection.

If shocks occur before a programmer or magnet is applied, ECG monitoring permits determination as to whether the shocks are delivered in response to a true tachycardia (VT/VF or SVT) or during baseline rhythm (oversensing). If not, interrogation will determine the cause of shocks. Once this determination is made, appropriate interventions for SVT and most oversensing problems are straightforward; the condition that represents the greatest risk is VT storm.

VT storm

VT storm is defined as three independent episodes of VT (or VF) requiring ICD therapy or external intervention within 24 hours.[86] Most ICD patients with VT storm present with frequent shocks, and most frequent shocks for VT/VF constitute VT storm, but the two terms are not synonymous: VT storm can present without shocks as frequent episodes of VT terminated

Table 10.7 Potential causes of recurrent ventricular tachyarrhythmias.

Progressive heart disease, ventricular dysfunction
Thyroid dysfunction (particularly hyperthyroidism in patients receiving amiodarone)
Electrolyte abnormalities (consider in patients who are taking diuretics or who have acute gastrointestinal illness); particularly hypokalemia, hypomagnesemia
Ischemia (favored by polymorphic ventricular tachycardia and ventricular fibrillation)
Noncompliance with medications or with diet
Drug effects (proarrhythmia, change in dose, noncompliance, drug interactions)

by ATP. More commonly, a patient presents with a few shocks, but ICD interrogation reveals many more true VT episodes terminated by ATP. Conversely, repetitive shocks may indicate multiple failed cardioversions/ defibrillations for a single episode of VT/VF or shocks delivered in response to multiple self-terminating episodes of VT. The solution to the latter usually includes prolonging duration for detection of VT/VF and/or prescribing an antiarrhythmic drug to reduce the frequency of VT/VF. The approach to unsuccessful defibrillation is discussed below (see Unsuccessful shocks).

True VT storm comprises recurring episodes after successful termination by shocks or ATP, and it represents a true medical emergency. The acute approach includes the following:

1 *Identification and treatment of precipitating medical or device-related causes.* Medical causes include acute ischemia, exacerbation of heart failure, metabolic abnormalities, and drug effects (Table 10.7). Diagnosis of acute coronary syndromes during VT storm is difficult because multiple shocks can cause changes in repolarization and elevations of troponin I.

2 *Appropriate ICD programming.* We have excluded shocks delivered for self-terminating VT from the definition of VT storm. However, most shocks are delivered after unsuccessful ATP, and, unlike shocks which require charging and confirmation periods after detection of VT, ATP is delivered immediately after detection duration is met. Thus, prolonging duration for initial detection is desirable unless ATP is uniformly successful. Increasing the duration required for redetection of VT or VF may permit the ICD to recognize true termination of VT. Usually, multiple trials of ATP should be programmed if VT is tolerated hemodynamically, and ATP settings should be optimized as discussed in Chapter 8: Programming (see Antitachycardia pacing). Occasionally, VT storm may be triggered by pacing-induced proarrhythmia. Rarely, this occurs shortly after

initiation of resynchronization pacing.[87] Reprogramming bradycardia or resynchronization pacing may relieve the problem acutely. If frequent ICD shocks continue to be required after acute interventions, the programmed first-shock strength may be reduced temporarily to conserve ICD battery. VT storm is the only clinical context in which we consider use of low-energy shocks for VT in adults.

3 *Drugs.* Reports of drug administration in VT storm are limited.[88–91] The only approach supported by controlled data includes administration of maximally tolerated doses of β-blockers.[90] Intravenous amiodarone probably is the most commonly administered antiarrhythmic drug, unless thyrotoxicosis is suspected.[92]

4 *Neuraxial modulation.* Increasingly, neuraxial modulation is recognized as an effective acute therapy, including sedation, general anesthesia with propofol, and thoracic epidural anesthesia.[61] Limited data support the long-term efficacy of surgical left cardiac sympathetic denervation.[61]

5 *Catheter ablation.* Unless precluded by comorbidities, ablation often has a major role in long-term therapy to prevent recurrence of VT storm.[93–95]

Unsuccessful shocks

The approach to ineffective ATP is considered in Optimizing ATP section, above. Here we consider the approach to ineffective shocks. Because the outcome of defibrillation is probabilistic, occasional shocks fail to terminate VF; but failure of two maximum-output shocks is rare if the safety margin is adequate.[31,42,96]

Determining that shocks are truly ineffective

Review of stored electrograms permits distinguishing failed cardioversion or defibrillation from other reasons that an ICD may classify shocks delivered for VT/VF as unsuccessful. First, the caregiver must assess the level of certainty that the first shock was delivered for VT rather than SVT, especially in single-chamber ICDs. Failure of multiple high-output shocks to terminate a regular tachycardia suggests sinus tachycardia because monomorphic VT and nonsinus SVT usually are terminated by one or two shocks. If the diagnosis of VT is confirmed before the first shock, the post-shock rhythm should be inspected. ICDs misclassify effective therapy as ineffective if VT/VF recurs before the ICD recognizes that the VT/VF episode has terminated. Decreasing the duration for redetection of sinus rhythm (St. Jude) may correct this classification error. ICDs also misclassify effective therapy as ineffective if the post-shock rhythm is SVT in the VT rate zone (e.g., catecholamine-induced sinus tachycardia or shock-induced AF). Post-shock changes in ventricular electrogram morphology may make accurate discrimination between VT and SVT challenging, especially in single-chamber ICDs.

Prolonged episodes of VT/VF caused by delayed detection and/or prolonged charge times may increase the shock strength required, resulting in true failure of cardioversion or defibrillation. When this occurs, the clinical approach should include shortening the detection time. Occasionally, a prolonged episode of VT slower than the VT detection interval degenerates to VF due to secondary ischemic or metabolic effects. In this case, the goal is to program therapy for the initial, slower VT.

Shocks from chronic ICD systems that defibrillated reliably at implantation may fail to terminate true VT or VF because of patient-related or ICD system-related reasons. In chronically implanted systems, most patient-related causes of unsuccessful shocks can be reversed, but most system-related causes require operative intervention (Table 10.8).

Patient-related factors

Patient-related factors that raise defibrillation thresholds (DFTs) reversibly at the cellular level include hyperkalemia, antiarrhythmic drugs, and ischemia. Pleural or pericardial effusions create parallel intrathoracic current paths that shunt current away from the heart. Progressive cardiac enlargement or interval infarction may also raise DFT and are less easily reversed. DFTs may increase after administration of antiarrhythmic drugs, especially amiodarone.[27,28,97,98] Usually, noninvasive device testing should be performed to confirm reliable defibrillation after the cause has been reversed.

A few patient-related causes that would otherwise require operative revision may be resolved by programming shock pathway and waveform parameters. For ICDs with fixed-tilt waveforms, waveform duration depends on output capacitance and pathway resistance.[99] ICDs with programmable waveform duration or tilt (St. Jude) permit optimization of waveform parameters independent of pathway resistance. Shortening the entire waveform may reduce DFT.[100] Waveform optimization (available in St. Jude ICDs) may result in acceptable defibrillation safety margins without system hardware revision.[101] Migration of an active-can pulse generator low on the chest wall can increase DFT by altering the shock vector. This may be resolved by excluding the pulse generator from the shock circuit.

ICD system-related factors

These factors are summarized in Table 10.8.[102] Figures 10.86 and 10.87 provide illustrative examples.

Isolated failure of high-voltage leads may prevent delivery of effective therapy despite appropriate detection. Low-voltage impedance testing of high-voltage

Table 10.8 Causes of failed defibrillation shocks.

Device-related
- Battery depletion
- Component failure
- Crumpling of epicardial patch
- Dislodgment of transvenous lead

Medical or biologic
- Evolution of defibrillation threshold over time (especially if threshold at implantation exceeded 15 J)
- Pneumothorax
- Myocardial infarction
- Drug proarrhythmia or alteration of defibrillation threshold
- Electrolyte abnormalities
- Probalistic nature of defibrillation (if fewer than two shocks fail)

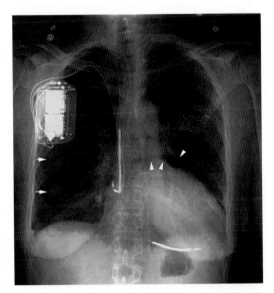

Fig. 10.86 Pneumothorax, as seen in this chest radiograph (arrows), can result in ineffective defibrillation. Also present is a pneumopericardium (arrowheads). (Friedman PA, Swerdlow CD, Hayes DL. Troubleshooting. In: Hayes DL, Friedman PA, eds. Cardiac Pacing and Defibrillation: A Clinical Approach, 2nd edn. West Sussex, UK: Wiley-Blackwell, 2008: 401–516, by permission of Friedman, Swerdlow, and Hayes.)

leads permit detection of shocking lead fractures before they manifest clinically. These fractures occurred commonly epicardial systems, in which the leads for sensing and for shocking are mechanically distinct.[32,103] Isolated high-voltage fractures of transvenous leads are less common, and precise data on the range of acceptable high-voltage lead impedances are limited.[104] Use of

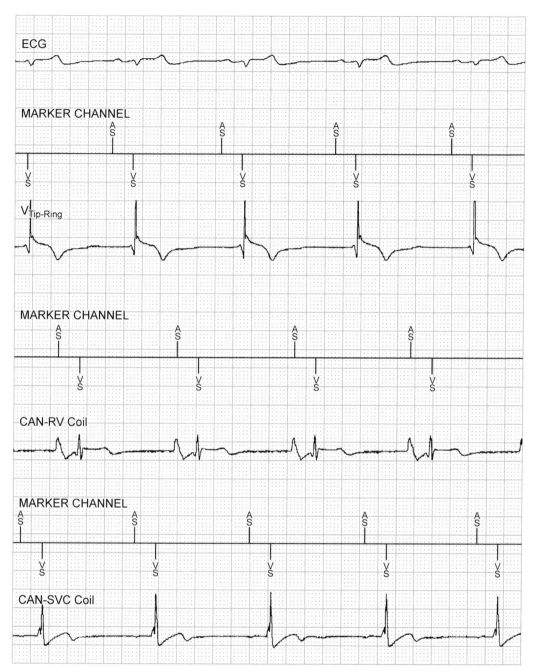

Fig. 10.87 Reversed high-voltage connections at ICD implant. From top to bottom, panels show recordings in sinus rhythm: surface ECG lead II, true-bipolar sensing EGM, CAN-RV coil EGM, and CAN-SVC coil EGM. The large P wave on the cab-RV coil EGM and absence of one on the CAN-SVC coil EGM indicates reversed high-voltage connections. These will not be identified if only the sensing EGM is evaluated before shock testing.

A

Treated VT/VF Episode #100

Episode #100: 25-Nov-2009 04:46:15

Episode Summary		Initial VT/VF Detection Withheld By
Initial Type	VF (spontaneous)	None
Duration	47 min	
V. Max Rate	400 bpm	
V. Median	375 bpm (160 ms)	
Activity at onset	Rest, Sensor = 60 bpm	
Last Therapy	VF Rx6: Defib, Unsuccessful	

Therapies	Delivered	Charge	Ohms	Energy
VF Rx 1 Defib	0.0 J	4.49 sec	<20 ohms	0.0 - 25 J
VF Rx 2 Defib	0.0 J	2.90 sec	<20 ohms	20 - 35 J
VF Rx 3 Defib	0.0 J	1.26 sec	<20 ohms	28 - 35 J
VF Rx 4 Defib	0.0 J	0.92 sec	<20 ohms	30 - 35 J
VF Rx 5 Defib	0.0 J	0.74 sec	<20 ohms	31 - 35 J

B

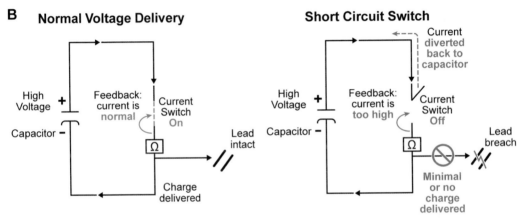

Normal Voltage Delivery   Short Circuit Switch

Fig. 10.88 Aborted shock due to lead-can abrasion. (A) Treated VT/VF summary: Note that the delivered energy is 0.0 J, the charge times are very short, and impedance abnormally low. This occurs when a short-circuit is present and short-circuit protection has been triggered. In the schematic, normal current flow is on the left, and a short-circuit is shown on the right. If currents are too high, a switch is tripped to cut off current flow to prevent circuit damage. The delivery energy prior to shutoff is typically <3 J, consistent with the 0.0–0.3 J energy delivery seen in the device report. Note that in the "Energy" column in the VT/VF report, the starting energy after a short-circuit protection is a few joules below the desired shock energy, because only a small amount of energy has been drained from the capacitor. (B) Normal shock energy delivery (left) and aborted shock energy delivery (right). (From Friedman PA, Rott MA, Wokhlu A, Asirvatham SJ, Hayes DL, eds. A Case-Based Approach to Pacemakers, ICDs, and Cardiac Resynchronization, Vol. 2, Advanced Questions for Examination Review and Clinical Practice. Minneapolis, MN: Mayo Foundation for Medical Education and Research Cardiotext Publishing, 2011: 62–5, Figs 55.5, 55.7.)

single coil systems and programming to exclude electrodes from the defibrillation circuit may increase the high-voltage impedance outside of the nominal range in the absence of malfunction. Low-voltage lead integrity measurements do not identify high-voltage insulation failures due to lead-can abrasions. The dielectric of the insulation coating remains intact during the test pulses but breaks down during high-voltage pulses, resulting in aborted shocks (Fig. 10.88). High-voltage connection problems (e.g., an incompletely inserted lead pin) can also result in failure to deliver a shock. Such connection problems may be detected by low-voltage impedance tests. We are not aware of published data regarding the clinical spectrum of high-voltage connection problems.

Pulse generator failures are a rare cause of failure to deliver therapy. They may be random or systematic. The root causes of systematic failures include internal battery shorting,[105] and electrical overstress failures of high-voltage components.[106] Electrical overstress failure is a term applied to semiconductor failure caused by application of extreme voltages or currents for a sufficient duration to cause a transistor to fail catastrophically.[106] These failures may occur in the sealed components of the pulse generator or header.

Failure to deliver or delayed therapy: underdetection and undersensing

Underdetection and undersensing or may be caused by ICD system performance, programmed values, or a combination of the two, resulting in failure to delivery therapy or delay in therapy. Usually, underdetection is caused by programming issues (including human error) and undersensing is caused by ICD system or patient issues.

Problems corrected by ICD programming

ICD inactivation An ICD may be inactivated by programming (e.g., preceding surgery to avoid oversensing of electrocautery) or, in some Boston Scientific models, by prolonged contact with an external magnet. One study reported an unexplained 11% annual incidence of transient suspension of detection.[107] ICD inactivation usually occurs in hospitals. Devices inactivated for surgical interventions must be reactivated before the patient leaves a monitored hospital bed.[108] Boston Scientific ICDs offer a "Change Tachy Mode with Magnet" feature that permits inactivation by holding a magnet over it for at least 30 s. Initially, tones synchronous with R waves are emitted (if the ICD is in the monitor plus therapy mode); tones become continuous when inactivation occurs. Because environmental magnets (e.g., stereo speakers, motors) have in rare instances inactivated these ICDs, we routinely program this feature "off" to prevent environmental magnets from inactivating these ICDs. This problem is addressed in Medtronic ICDs with an audible patient alert that sounds if programmed detection or therapy is "off" for longer than 6 hours.

VT slower than the programmed detection interval In most ICD patients, VT with cycle lengths >400–450 ms are tolerated well, but repeated inappropriate therapies are not. SVT-VT discrimination algorithms (except those in Sorin models[42,96,109]) deliver fewer inappropriate therapies if the VT detection interval is programmed to a shorter (faster) cycle length, because fewer SVTs are evaluated. Nevertheless, slow VT can be life-threatening in patients with severe LV dysfunction or ischemia;[110] thus, treating slower VT is important some patients with advanced heart failure (Fig. 10.89). The VT detection interval should be increased if antiarrhythmic drug therapy is initiated, particularly with amiodarone or a sodium-channel blocking (type 1A or 1C) drug.[111,112] Some experts advise measuring the cycle length of induced VT at electrophysiologic testing after beginning drug therapy.[112] However, spontaneous VT may be slower than induced VT.[113]

SVT-VT discriminators SVT-VT discriminators may prevent or delay therapy if they misclassify VT or VF as SVT.[63,69,114,115] Discriminators that re-evaluate the rhythm diagnosis during an ongoing tachycardia (e.g., stability, most dual-chamber algorithms) reduce the risk of underdetection of VT compared with those that withhold therapy if the rhythm is not classified correctly by the initial evaluation (e.g., onset, chamber of origin algorithms). The minimum cycle length for SVT-VT discrimination should be set to prevent clinically significant delay in detection of hemodynamically unstable VT.

Single-chamber discriminators: The sensitivity of discriminators for detection of VT is best determined from analysis of dual-chamber electrograms; physician analysis of single-chamber electrograms overestimates sensitivity.[60] Although spontaneous VT often begins with irregular R-R intervals, stability algorithms classify it as VT as soon as R-R intervals regularize, even transiently. Thus they rarely prevent detection of monomorphic VT (approximately 0.5%). Morphology discriminators also re-evaluate rhythm diagnosis during ongoing tachycardias. However, if they misclassify monomorphic VT initially, the error usually persists and prevents detection for the duration of the tachycardia. The St. Jude morphology algorithm, which analyzes only the near-field electrogram, continuously misclassifies at least 5–10% of monomorphic VTs as SVT, but when it is restricted to the V = A and V < A rate branches, only 1–2% of VTs are misclassified.[61] The Medtronic morphology algorithm, which analyzes high-voltage electrograms, was reported to misclassify 1–2% of VTs as SVTs based on single-chamber data,[115] but the true error rate is likely higher. Limited data regarding the Boston Scientific Guidant algorithm report no episodes of VT misclassified as SVT.[117,118] Direct comparison of these three algorithms showed that the Medtronic, Boston Scientific, and St. Jude algorithms correctly clas-

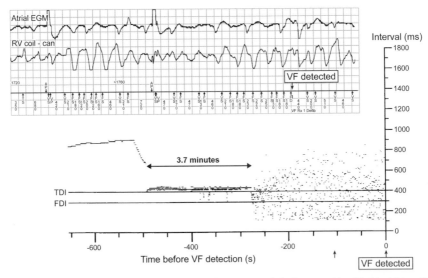

Fig. 10.89 Ventricular tachycardia (VT) slower than the programmed detection interval. The lower panel is a "Flashback Interval" plot of R-R interval cycle lengths before detection of ventricular fibrillation (VF), which occurs at the right side of each panel. The interval number before detection is plotted on the abscissa, and the corresponding interval is plotted on the ordinate. Horizontal lines indicate the VT detection interval (TDI) of 400 ms and the VF detection interval (FDI) of 320 ms. Shortly after the 500th interval preceding detection, regular tachycardia begins abruptly. The constant cycle length indicates reliable ventricular sensing. Atrial flashback intervals (not shown) demonstrated atrioventricular (AV) dissociation. This VT is not detected despite reliable sensing, because the cycle length is greater than the programmed TDI. VT persists for 3.7 minutes until approximately interval 280 before detection, when sensed intervals become highly variable. This indicates degeneration of the rhythm to VF with undersensing that delays detection. During VT and VF, atrial flashback intervals (not shown) indicated lower rate limit bradycardia pacing at 40 bpm (1500 ms). The upper panel shows stored atrial and far-field ventricular EGMs immediately before detection with atrial and ventricular channel showing event markers. Specific undersensed EGMs cannot be identified because the rate-sensing EGM was not recorded. However, long sensed R-R intervals ending with ventricular sense (VS) markers indicate undersensing and correspond to long intervals in the upper panel. "VF Rx 1 Defib" at lower right (arrow) denotes "VF detected." AP, Atrial paced event; FD, VF detected; FS, intervals in VF zone. (From Swerdlow C, Friedman P. Advanced ICD troubleshooting. Part I. Pacing Clin Electrophysiol 2005; 28:1322–46.)

sified 92%, 70%, and 46% of rapidly conducted atrial arrhythmias, respectively.[119] In contrast, the onset discriminator uniformly misclassifies VT if it either accelerates gradually across the sinus–VT zone boundary or occurs during SVT with cycle length in the VT zone.

Dual-chamber discriminators: Discriminators that withhold VT therapy for 1:1 arrhythmias run the risk of withholding therapy if the atrial lead dislodges to the ventricle and the ventricular electrogram is recorded on both channels. These should not be programmed until the atrial lead is stable (Medtronic 1:1 SVT rule and St. Jude 1:1 Rate Branch without additional discriminators).

VT with 1:1 VA conduction was difficult diagnosis for early dual-chamber algorithms using only onset and predetermined AV-VA patterns. Algorithms that identified dynamic changes in AV-VA relationships (Fig.

10.90) or chamber of origin (Fig. 10.91) improved performance. Boston Scientific's Rhythm ID® and St. Jude's Branch® misclassify SVT only if a morphology match occurs.[120,121] The present version of Medtronic's PR Logic® misclassifies SVT only if both a morphology match occurs and other rules do not classify the rhythm as SVT. Single-chamber stability may be programmed in Medtronic dual-chamber ICDs to reject AF during redetection. In this case, stability is applied before the dual-chamber algorithm. Because stability responds to irregular rhythms by resetting the VT counter to zero, rhythms rejected by stability are not evaluated by the dual-chamber algorithm. Thus, stability may delay detection of VT even if the ventricular rate is greater than the atrial rate.

Sustained-duration override features deliver therapy if an arrhythmia satisfies the ventricular rate criterion for a long programmed duration even if discriminators

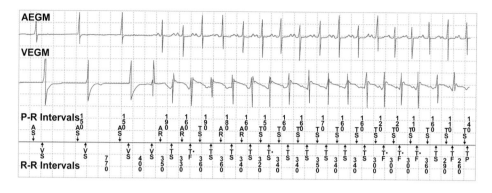

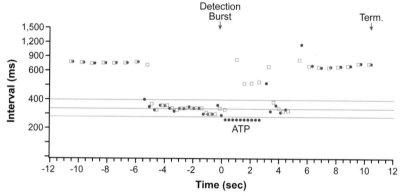

Fig. 10.90 Appropriate detection of ventricular tachycardia (VT) with 1:1 ventricular-atrial (VA) conduction by abrupt change in P-R pattern and ventricular rate. Upper panel: dual-chamber stored EGMs and dual-chamber EGM markers. Note that upper numerical values indicate P-R interval, not P-P interval. Lower panel: interval plot. VT starts in the ventricle with a premature ventricular complex, followed by abrupt change in ventricular rate, ventricular EGM morphology, and the PR-RR relationship (Medtronic PR Logic). Fast VT (FVT) detection at right of EGM is followed by burst antitachycardia pacing (VT Rx 1 Burst), designated by ATP on interval plot. This results in abrupt termination of VT. Note that older versions of this algorithm, which discriminated VT from SVT based only on the PR-RP percentage, may have classified this long-RP tachycardia incorrectly as SVT. AEGM, Atrial electrogram; TF, interval in FVT zone; TS, interval in VT zone; VEGM, ventricular (true bipolar) electrogram;VS, ventricular sensed event. (From Swerdlow CD, Gillberg JG, Olson WH. Sensing and detection. In: Ellenbogen KA, Kay GN, Lau C, Wilkoff BL, eds. Cardiac Pacing and Defibrillation: A Clinical Approach, 3rd edn. Philadelphia, PA: Saunders Company, 2007: 75–160, by permission of Swerdlow, Gillberg, and Olson.)

indicate SVT. These include Sustained Rate Duration (Boston Scientific), Extended High Rate (St. Jude), Maximum Time to Diagnosis (St. Jude), or High Rate Timeout (Medtronic). The premise is that VT will continue to satisfy the rate criterion for the programmed duration while the ventricular rate during transient sinus tachycardia or AF will decrease below the VT rate boundary. The limitation is delivery of inappropriate therapy when SVT exceeds the programmed duration. The incidence of inappropriate detection of SVT is approximately 10% at 1 min and 3% at 3 min.[114,116] Additionally, the SVT limit should be set to prevent clinically significant delay in detection of hemodynam-ically unstable VT. Medtronic ICDs beginning with the Protecta™ family include a zone-specific High Rate Timeout feature which may be activated only in the VF zone.

Sometimes, discriminators my correctly withhold therapy for SVT, but for the wrong reasons. Inspection of the text episode summary may identify such concerns (Fig. 10.77).

Oversensing of stimuli delivered by other implanted electronic devices Interactions between ICDs and separate pacemakers became rare after ICDs incorporated dual-chamber bradycardia pacing. These interactions

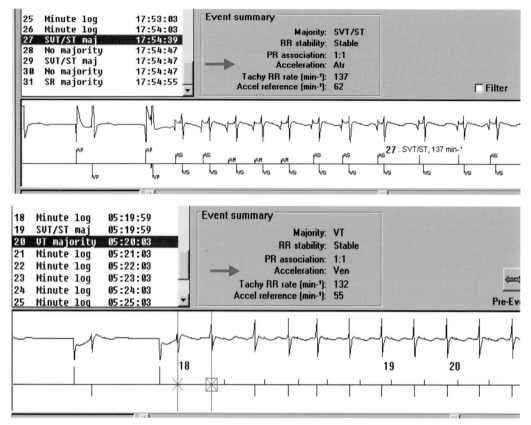

Fig. 10.91 Classification of 1:1 tachycardias by chamber of origin. The Sorin Parad algorithm classifies 1:1 tachycardias by chamber of onset. Stored ventricular EGM is shown with dual-chamber event markers (top, atrial; bottom, ventricular). Event log and Event summary are shown above each stored EGM. Upper panel: supraventricular tachycardia (SVT) is diagnosed by atrial onset. Lower panel: ventricular tachycardia (VT) is diagnosed by ventricular onset. (From Swerdlow CD, Gillberg JG, Olson WH. Sensing and detection. In: Ellenbogen KA, Kay GN, Lau C, Wilkoff BL, eds. Cardiac Pacing and Defibrillation: A Clinical Approach, 3rd edn. Philadelphia, PA: Saunders Company, 2007: 75–160, by permission of Swerdlow, Gillberg, and Olson.)

have been reviewed.[122–124] The principal interaction that may delay or prevent ICD therapy is oversensing of high-amplitude pacemaker stimulus artifacts. If this occurs during VF, automatic adjustment of sensing threshold may cause repetitive undersensing of VF electrograms. This is of greatest concern if an ICD shock initiates a rest of the pacemaker to unipolar pacing with maximum output. Other electronic devices such as transcutaneous electrical nerve stimulation (TENS) units may emit pulses that can be oversensed and tracked by the ICD, preventing sensing of low amplitude VF electrograms. Pacemaker–ICD interactions that can be avoided if proper testing is performed.[125]

Intra-device interactions due to cross-chamber blanking periods Under most conditions, ICDs apply only the minimum cross-chamber ventricular blanking required to prevent crosstalk resulting from an atrial pacing stimulus. During high-rate atrial or dual-chamber pacing, ventricular sensing may be restricted to short periods of the cardiac cycle because of the combined effects of ventricular blanking after ventricular events and cross-chamber ventricular blanking after atrial pacing. If a sufficient fraction of the cardiac cycle is blanked, systematic undersensing of VT or VF may occur. When pacing and blanking events occur at intervals that are multiples of a VT cycle length, ventricular complexes may be repeatedly undersensed, delaying or preventing detection.[126–128]

This occurs most commonly with the Rate Smoothing algorithm.[126–128] This algorithm is intended to prevent VT/VF initiated by sudden changes in

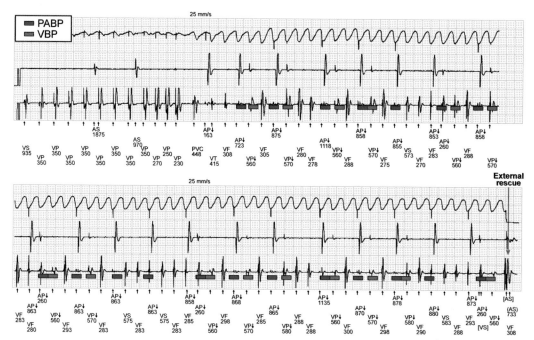

Fig. 10.92 Failure to detect VT due to an intradevice interaction. The rate-smoothing algorithm introduced atrial and ventricular pacing complexes with associated blanking periods that prevented detection of VT during post-implant testing. An external rescue shock was required. Shown from top to bottom are surface ECG, atrial electrogram, ventricular electrogram, and event markers. At top, VT is induced by programmed electrical stimulation with drive cycle length 350 ms and premature stimuli at 270, 250, and 230 ms (intervals labeled next to event markers). The first sensed ventricular event occurs 448 ms after the pacing drive ("PVC 448"). The rate smoothing algorithm drives pacing to prevent a pause after the "premature ventricular complex" (PVC), labeled AP↓1638. A ventricular-paced event does not follow the first AP↓ because a ventricular event is sensed (VT 415). Subsequent rate smoothing generated atrial and ventricular pacing pulses (indicated by AP↓ and VP↓ markers, respectively). The resultant post-pacing blanking periods are shown in the figure as horizontal bars. PAB denotes cross chamber (post-atrial-pace) ventricular blanking period. VBP denotes same-chamber (post-ventricular pace) blanking period. Together, they prevent approximately four of every six VT complexes from being sensed. Since the VT counter must accumulate eight out of 10 consecutive complexes in the VT zone for detection of VT to occur, VT is not detected. (From Friedman PA, Swerdlow CD, Hayes DL. Troubleshooting. In: Hayes DL, Friedman PA, eds. Cardiac Pacing and Defibrillation: A Clinical Approach, 2nd edn. West Sussex, UK: Wiley-Blackwell, 2008: 401–516, by permission of Friedman, Swerdlow, and Hayes.)

ventricular rate.[129] It prevents sudden changes in ventricular rate by pacing both the atrium and the ventricle at intervals based on the preceding (baseline) R-R interval. As an unintended consequence, it may prevent sensing of VT/VF in some patients, because it introduces repetitive post-pacing blanking periods (Fig. 10.92). The algorithm applies rate smoothing to baseline intervals independent of their cycle length, including intervals in the VT or VF zones. Intra-device interactions that result in delayed or absent detection of VT/VF are most common and most dangerous when VT is fast. The parameter interrelationships that result in delayed or absent detection of VT/VF are complex and difficult to predict, but they usually elicit a programmer warning. Generally, aggressive rate

smoothing (a small allowable percentage change in R-R intervals), a high upper pacing rate, and a long and fixed AV interval favor undersensing and should be avoided. If rate smoothing is required, the AV delay should be dynamic, the upper rates should be 125 bpm or less, and parameter combinations that result in warnings should be avoided. This programming reduces, but does not eliminate, the risk of undersensing when Rate Smoothing is used.[126–128,130]

Problems that may require system revision

Undersensing of VF Undersensing of VF is rare in modern ICDs. It occurs due to combinations of

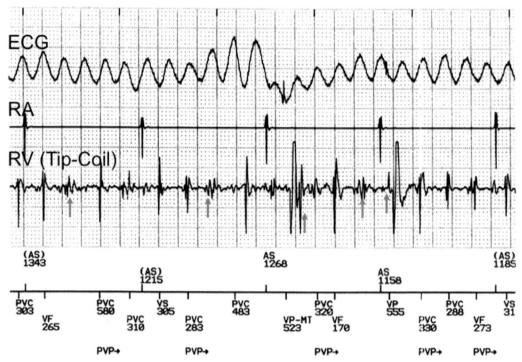

Fig. 10.93 Undersensing of ventricular fibrillation (VF) despite normal R wave in sinus rhythm (18.5 mV). Programmer strip recorded at implantation testing of a Boston Scientific Prizm ICD shows electrocardiogram (ECG), right atrial (RA) EGM, and integrated bipolar right ventricular (RV) sensing EGM (Tip-Coil) during implantation testing. The VF EGMs have highly variable amplitudes, resulting in undersensing of low-amplitude EGMs immediately after high-amplitude ones (arrows). Intermittent ventricular pacing (VP) introduces postpacing blanking periods. Slow Automatic Gain Control may contribute to this type of undersensing. AS, atrial sensed event; PVC, premature ventricular complex; PVP→, extension of post-ventricular atrial refractory period (PVARP); VP, ventricular paced event. (Modified from Dekker LR, Schrama TA, Steinmetz FH, *et al.* Undersensing of VF in a patient with optimal R wave sensing during sinus rhythm. Pacing Clin Electrophysiol 2004; 27:833–4.)

programming (sensitivity, rate, or duration), low-amplitude EGMs, rapidly varying EGM amplitude, drug effects, and post-shock tissue changes. Presently, the most common causes of VF undersensing are drug or hyperkalemic effects that slow VF into the VT zone, ischemia, and rapidly varying EGM amplitude.[42,131] ICDs that adjust the dynamic sensing floor based on the amplitude of the sensed R wave (Boston Scientific) may be the most vulnerable to rapidly varying EGM amplitude (Fig. 10.93). ICD features that reduce sensitivity to prevent T-wave oversensing may also result in undersensing of VF (Fig. 10.94).[54] Prolonged ischemia from sustained VT slower than the VT detection interval may cause deterioration of signal quality, resulting in undersensing of VF. Lead, connector, or generator problems may also manifest as undersensing.

The value of assessing the baseline-rhythm R wave in predicting the reliability of sensing VF is uncertain in present ICDs. Overall, the statistical correlation between R-wave amplitude in VF and baseline rhythm is weak.[132,133] Two studies report that sensing of VF is

adequate with nominal sensitivities near 0.3 mV if the baseline R wave is sufficiently large (≥5 mV or ≥7 mV[134]). Reliable sensing of VF cannot be predicted from baseline EGMs if the baseline ventricular rhythm is paced; sensitivity is programmed to a less sensitive value than nominal (e.g., to avoid T-wave oversensing); or patients have other implanted electronic devices. However, clinically significant undersensing of VF or polymorphic VT may occur despite adequate sinus rhythm R waves.[54,131] In these instances, undersensing occurs because automatic adjustment of sensitivity responds too slowly to variations in R-wave amplitude, rather than because low-amplitude R waves are undersensed consistently. The reproducibility of this phenomenon is unknown, as is the extent to which it can be predicted at implantation. Therefore, it is uncertain whether reasonable testing at implantation can detect this infrequent cause of undersensing. Further, with true-bipolar sensing and present digital sensing amplifiers, clinically significant undersensing of VF is rare at implant and unrelated to sinus rhythm R-wave amplitude, even

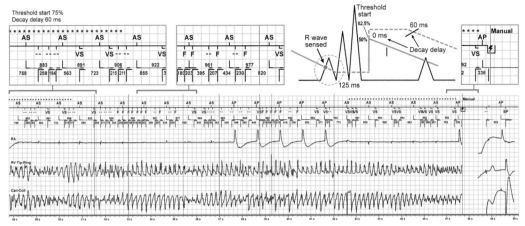

Fig. 10.94 Undersensing resulting in failure to detect VF due to features to prevent T-wave oversensing. The continuous real-time EGM in lower panel shows atrial, true-bipolar sensing, and high-voltage EGMs during implant testing in a St. Jude ICD. The programmed number of intervals to detect VF is 12. External shock at right was delivered at 48 s. Upper panels enlarge the dual-chamber marker channel, showing multiple long ventricular intervals up to 820 ms during VF. These long intervals prevented the interval + interval average counting method from detecting VF. Insert at top right shows the increased Decay Delay of 60 ms (nominal 0 ms) and Threshold Start set at 75% of the preceding EGM amplitude (nominal 50% in this model).

Fig. 10.95 Multilumen lead body design (left) and coaxial lead body design (right). Coaxial design has a higher risk of lead failure, and is no longer used for ICD leads. Failure may result from degradation of the internal insulation separating the conductors. Further details in the text. (From Friedman PA, Swerdlow CD, Hayes DL. Troubleshooting. In: Hayes DL, Friedman PA, eds. Cardiac Pacing and Defibrillation: A Clinical Approach, 2nd edn. West Sussex, UK: Wiley-Blackwell, 2008: 401–516, by permission of Friedman, Swerdlow, and Hayes.)

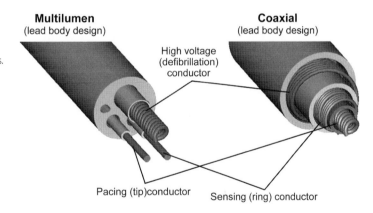

below 3 mV.[135] Undersensing of spontaneous VT/VF in the VF zone is similarly rare. However, rare instances of VF undersensing due to consistent, extremely low-amplitude R waves (e.g. 1 mV) is an indication for lead revision (or reprogramming the sensing vector in Medtronic ICDs).

Troubleshooting ICD lead failure
Leads have been and continue to be the weakest link in ICD systems. The radiography of lead failure is reviewed in Chapter 11: Radiography of Implantable Devices. The vast majority of presently functioning ICD leads have multilumen construction (Fig. 10.95). Lead fail-

ures may involve either the high-voltage or pace-sense components. Of these, pace-sense failures both are more common and present the greatest diagnostic challenges; the majority of these failures are fractures.

Differential diagnosis of pace-sense lead fractures
Historically, ICDs monitored for pace-sense fractures using the same automated measurements of pacing impedance developed for pacemakers. ICD pace-sense lead fractures may present as they do in pacemaker systems with failure to capture or failure to pace due to oversensing. However, despite daily automated measurements of pacing impedance, ICD pace-sense

Table 10.9 Differential diagnosis of lead fracture.

EGM	Z	Condition
Noise	Normal	Fracture
Noise	High	Fracture
		Connection problem
Normal	High	Fracture
		Connection problem
		Normally functioning lead

EGM, electrogram; Z, impedance.

fractures present most commonly as inappropriate shocks caused by oversensing of rapid, nonphysiologic potentials (noise) (see Section Extracardiac signals, above).[136–138]

Monitoring of both rapid oversensing and impedance enhances early detection of lead fractures compared to monitoring of impedance alone.[139] However, conditions other than lead fracture can cause both high impedance and oversensing;[140,141] and overdiagnosis of lead fracture results in unnecessary lead replacements, with corresponding morbidity.[142]

Table 10.9 summarizes the differential diagnosis for patients who present with noise oversensing alone, high pace-sense impedance alone, or both. For the distinguishing characteristics of noise oversensing see Ventricular oversensing: recognition and troubleshooting (see earlier) and Fig. 10.65:

1　High-frequency components
2　Highly variable signals
3　Amplifier saturation, and
4　Normal high-voltage electrogram.

However, noise may have atypical signal characteristics (Fig. 10.96). Limited data suggest that noise related to lead fractures may be exacerbated by pacing, especially high-output pacing (Fig. 10.97).[143]

Noise oversensing with a normal impedance In our experience, noise oversensing with a normal impedance is diagnostic of lead failure if it presents more than 30 days postoperatively. Other specific conditions can result in extremely short sensed R-R intervals with normal impedance (Fig. 10.98). This paragraph focuses on distinguishing noise oversensing from other causes of extremely rapid sensed events. Header seal-plug problems shortly after implant or generator change[144] present with uniform, medium frequency signals that may have widely varying cycle lengths corresponding to the intervals between identical air bubbles escaping from the seal plug (Fig. 10.99), device–device interac-

tions and lead–lead mechanical interactions (chatter)[56] can be suspected based on the patient's history or a radiograph showing other devices or retained leads. Sometimes lead–lead interactions are the first indicator of a lead dislodgment. Unusual cases of true VF[56] may have cardiac cycle lengths within 20 ms of the ventricular blanking period. Recording a far-field ventricular electrogram facilitates the diagnosis of VF. Diaphragmatic myopotentials (see Extracardiac signals, above; Fig. 10.56) have been misdiagnosed as lead noise. Although they have high frequency, they are low-amplitude, relatively uniform signals that cause oversensing only when sensitivity is maximal, either after long diastoles or paced beats. They usually occur with integrated bipolar leads placed at the RV apex.

In ICDs, extremely short R-R intervals near the ventricular blanking period do not represent successive cardiac depolarizations except occasionally during VF. Medtronic ICDs count these very short intervals as a measure of nonphysiologic oversensing to provide early warning of lead fracture; they store this count as the Sensing Integrity Counter. A high or rapidly increasing Sensing Integrity Count (total >300 or 10 per day for 3 consecutive days) is a sensitive indicator of pace-sense lead fracture,[58,145,146] but in isolation it is nonspecific. The specificity of a high sensing integrity count for lead/connector problems is approximately 20%.[53] The most common cause of isolated, extremely short R-R intervals is a combination of an oversensed physiologic event and appropriately sensed R-waves. In P-wave oversensing, the nonphysiologic short interval is the PR interval. In R-wave double-counting, it is the interval between initial and terminal deflections of a true ventricular EGM. In T-wave oversensing, the interval is bounded by an oversensed T-wave and a PVC (Fig. 10.100).[56] However, these nonphysiologic combinations of physiologic signals rarely result in repetitive oversensing, which is common in lead or connector problems. Repetitive, transient oversensing may be identified by stored nonsustained tachycardias. The combination of isolated extremely-short R-R intervals and repetitive rapid oversensing (defined as at least two nonsustained tachycardias with duration ≥5 intervals and mean cycle length ≤220 ms) has a positive predictive value for lead or connector problems of approximately 80%,[53,56] even with a normal pace-sense impedance. This observation forms the basis for use of the combination of a high sensing integrity count and two rapid nonsustained tachycardias to trigger the Medtronic Lead Integrity Algorithm® (see Lead failure diagnostics, below).[53]

High impedance with or without oversensing The differential diagnosis of high impedance includes lead

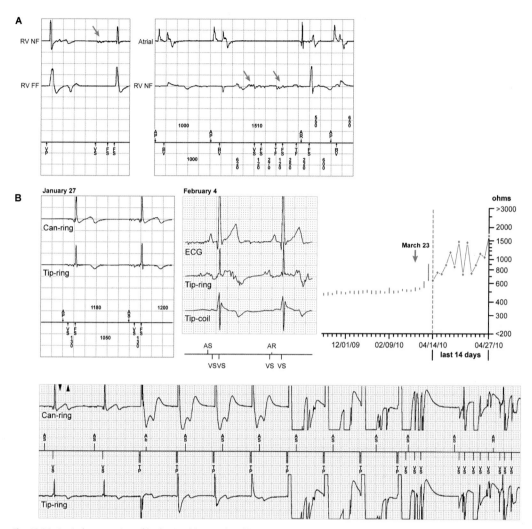

Fig. 10.96 Atypical presentations of lead noise. (A) Examples of low amplitude lead noise that might be confused with diaphragmatic myopotentials. Usually, lead noise is intermittent and variable. Diaphragmatic myopotentials vary with respiration. (B) Cyclical lead noise preceding pacing-induced exacerbation of noise and impedance rise. Left upper panel displays stored EGM triggered by nonphysiologically short R-R interval. It shows presystolic oversensing of low-amplitude signal. In this single-chamber, primary-prevention ICD, the differential diagnosis includes P-wave oversensing and diaphragmatic myopotential oversensing. Both are rare with true-bipolar sensing. The patient was seen in clinic on February 4. Real time EGMs show oversensing of noncardiac signals preceding P waves, excluding P-wave oversensing. Deep respirations did not reproduce oversensing. High output pacing did not initiate oversensing. The patient was followed with weekly remote monitoring transmissions and seen in clinic on alternate weeks. On March 23, high output pacing (TP) produced post-pacing noise on both EGMs involving the ring electrode (bottom panel) characteristic of lead fracture. However, only single oversensed events had occurred spontaneously. Detection of VF was disabled. Approximately 3 weeks later, intermittent impedance changes occurred. Intraoperative unipolar recordings and returned-product analysis of the extracted lead confirmed a fracture of the cable to the ring electrode.

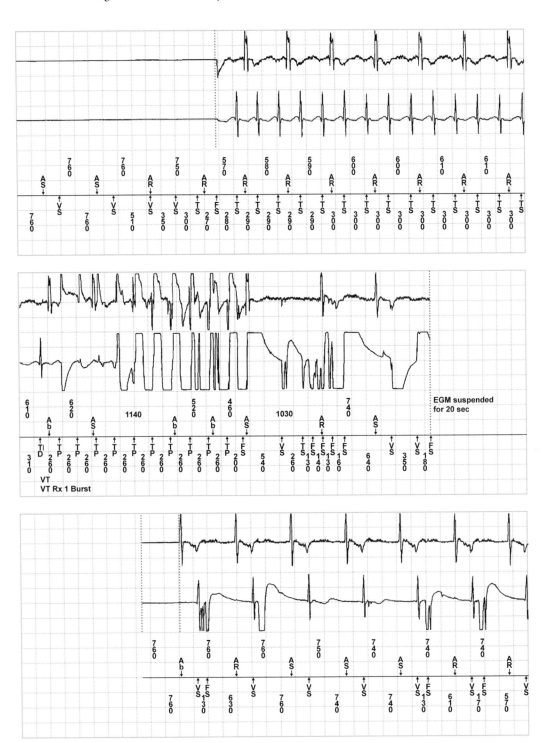

Fig. 10.97 ATP initiates lead noise. Atrial, true-bipolar RV EGM, and dual-chamber marker channel show the onset of VT in upper panel and termination of VT by ATP in the middle panel. High output ATP initiates lead noise resulting in oversensing that prevented the ICD from recognizing termination of VT for 20 s. In the lower panel, noise continued immediately following sensed ventricular EGMs. The reason for the temporal correlation of noise signals with spontaneous EGMs is unknown.

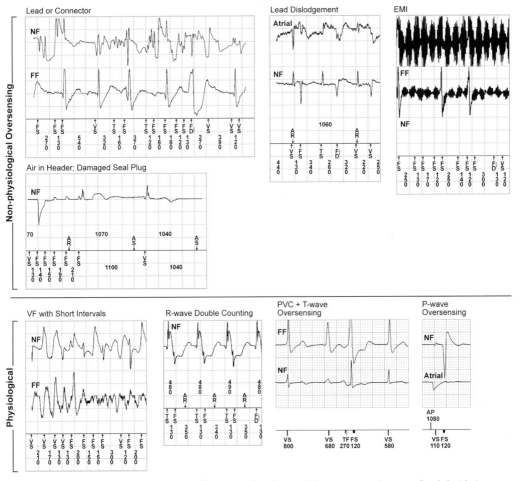

Fig. 10.98 Recordings show characteristic EGMs for different types of rapid nonphysiologic oversensing (upper panel) and physiologic oversensing (lower panel). (Reprinted with permission from Gunderson BD, Swerdlow CD, Wilcox JM, Hayman JE, Ousdigian KT, Ellenbogen KA. Causes of ventricular oversensing in implantable cardioverter defibrillators: Implications for diagnosis of lead fracture. Heart Rhythm 2010; 7:626–633.)

fractures, connection problems between the lead and ICD,[144,147–149] and normally functioning leads. All three may present as high impedance without oversensing, but only fractures and connection problems present with oversensing, and only fractures require lead replacement. Despite considerable effort, we have failed to identify characteristics of noise oversensing that separate lead fractures from connection problems (Fig. 10.101). However, analysis of characteristics of impedance trends and the relationship between these characteristics and noise oversensing can discriminate fractures from connection problems that were misdiagnosed as fractures.[141]

Discriminating fractures from connection problems
Connection problems may include loose setscrews,[150]

air trapped in the header that escapes through seal plugs,[144,148] weakened ICD header bonds,[147] adapter problems,[151] and incomplete contact between the lead pin and header (Fig. 10.102).[149] Most reports are limited to a one or a few cases, which presented intraoperatively or perioperatively. Any oversensing or abrupt impedance rose that occurs in the first 30 days after a new implant should be considered a connection problem, providing lead dislodgement is excluded. Although fractures or insulation failures rarely occur in the first 6 months after lead implant, they may occur early after pulse generator change, especially if a chronic lead is damaged during the procedure. In a recent study, most connection problems that were misdiagnosed as fractures presented after the perioperative period; and 46% presented more than 6 months after the last surgical

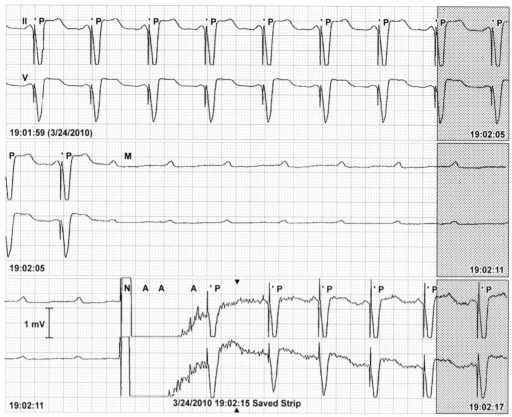

Fig. 10.99 Asystole and shock hours post-implant. Left panel: surface telemetry. Right panel: device interrogation showing from top to bottom the atrial EGM, ventricular EGM, and markers. This intracardiac tracing is diagnostic of air in the header. If minor damage to the header seal plug prevents complete closure after the torque wrench is removed, body fluid may enter into the header via the defect, forming an accessory sensing pathway that competes with normal sensing (Guidant Corporation. Preventing and detecting oversensing due to damaged, torn or missing seal plugs. Guidant Product Update Number 35, November 2003). While sensing is typically not disrupted, if there is air in the header, as the air escapes through the damaged seal plug it displaces fluid, transiently alters the impedance, and leads to nonphysiologic noise signals that can be sensed by the ICD. This form of oversensing subsides after the entrapped air has escaped from the header, and is limited to hours to 1–2 days following implant. One treatment option is to program the device to DOO with therapies off and observe for 24–48 hours. (From Friedman PA, Rott MA, Wokhlu A, Asirvatham SJ, Hayes DL, eds. A Case-Based Approach to Pacemakers, ICDs, and Cardiac Resynchronization, Vol. 2, Advanced Questions for Examination Review and Clinical Practice. Minneapolis, MN: Mayo Foundation for Medical Education and Research Cardiotext Publishing, 2011: 44–51.)

procedure.[141] Thus, connection problems are an important cause of late impedance rises.

Figure 10.103 shows a stepwise algorithm for discriminating lead fractures from connection problems and normally functioning leads using both noise oversensing and impedance. In addition to time course mentioned above, three criteria related to impedance trends discriminate fractures from connection problems (Fig. 10.104):

1 Very high impedance $\geq 10,000\,\Omega$ indicates an open or nearly open circuit and is specific for fracture. However, most programmers do not display a numerical value for impedance >2000–3000, so the actual value must be read by the manufacturer from a save-to-disk file.

2 A long period of return to baseline impedance after an abrupt rise occurs only in connection problems. It might occur if stress transiently alters a mostly ade-

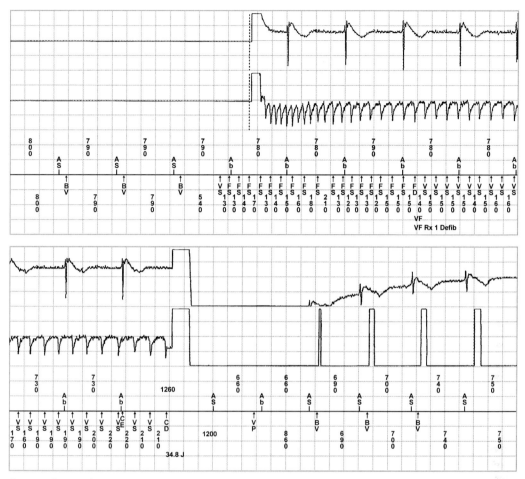

Fig. 10.99 (*Continued*)

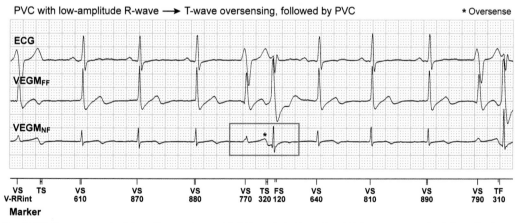

Fig. 10.100 T-wave oversensing followed by correctly sensed PVC. Shown is the T wave (asterisk) that was oversensed as indicated by the Marker Channel, resulting in a short interval between the T wave and the PVC (120 ms). Pacing impedance was normal. Such combinations of physiologic oversensing and normal physiologic sensing are the most common cause of very short interval.

A   Fracture EGM

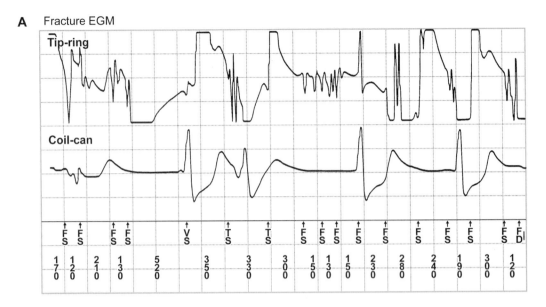

B   Connection Problem EGM

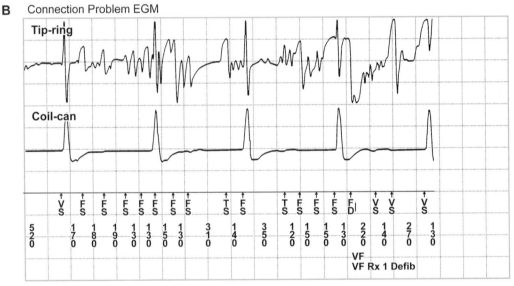

Fig. 10.101 (A and B) Electrograms from save-to-disk files. Each shows pace-sense (VTip-VRing) and high-voltage (RVCoil-Can) EGMs with ventricular marker channel. Noise is limited to the pace-sense EGM. Noise signals have high-frequency and highly variable amplitude; they occur intermittently, separated by periods of isoelectric baseline. Noise characteristics do not distinguish fractures from connection problems. FD, fibrillation detection; VS, TS, and FS, ventricular intervals in the "sinus," tachycardia, and fibrillation rate zones. (From Swerdlow CD, Sachanandani H, Gunderson BD, Ousdigian KT, Hjelle M, Ellenbogen KA. Preventing overdiagnosis of implantable cardioverter-defibrillator lead fractures using device diagnostics. J Am Coll Cardiol 2011; 57:2330–9, by permission.)

quate connection with incomplete insertion of the pin. This finding is useful when the first impedance rise occurs late after surgery or an early rise is insufficient to trigger an impedance alert; but it does not help at the first impedance rise.

3 Fractures may result in oversensing without abnormal impedance, but connection problems do not if measurements are repeated over time. The noise may originate from breaks of a few filars of the multifilar cable conductor to the ring electrode while the remain-

Before Revision

After Revision

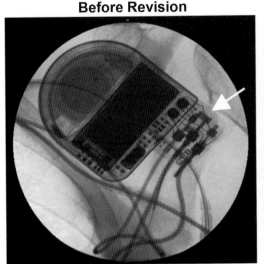
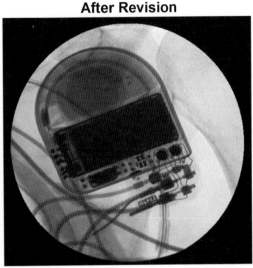

Fig. 10.102 Intraoperative fluoroscopic images corresponding to the data presented in Fig. 10.101. The ICD has been removed from the pocket to enhance image quality. Before revision, the lead connector pin was not advanced completely into the header (arrow). The proximal connection between the ring electrode and the header was intermittent, accounting for the high impedance and oversensing illustrated in Fig. 10.101. After revision, the ventricular electrode is advanced completely into the header. (From Swerdlow CD, GIllberg JG, Olson WH. Sensing and detection. In: Ellenbogen KA, Kay GN, Lau C, Wilkoff BL, eds. Cardiac Pacing and Defibrillation: A Clinical Approach, 3rd edn. Philadelphia, PA: Saunders Company, 2007: 75–160, by permission of Swerdlow, Gillberg, and Olson.)

ing filars conduct sufficiently to prevent an impedance increase at the measured resolution.

Radiography reliably diagnoses incomplete contact between the lead pin and header (Fig. 10.102) if the X-ray beam is perpendicular to the plane of the header. Intraoperative radiography may be diagnostic when preoperative images are inconclusive.

Discriminating fractures from functioning leads with high impedance Gradual, stable impedance rises without oversensing occur in normally functioning leads, presumably due to changes at the electrode–myocardial interface. Because normally functioning leads are not replaced, no report provides confirmation of criteria to discriminate such impedance rises from fractures and connection problems by return product analysis of explanted leads. Kallinen et al.[152] reported three patients with normally functioning leads who had gradual impedance increases. These leads were replaced because of concern that they might be fractured.

In one study, gradual increases in impedance or abrupt increases to stable high value occurred in 43% of apparently normally functioning leads, but only 3% of confirmed connection problems and 0% of confirmed fractures (Fig. 10.104).[141] However, the authors

could not exclude connection problems from normally functioning leads unless the connection problem was corrected surgically or the lead was replaced due to a misdiagnosis of fracture. About half of high-impedance functioning leads had impedance trends indistinguishable from connection problems with a maximum impedance <2500 Ω. Nevertheless, clinically, these leads do not require prompt replacement. In contrast, all impedance increases in fractures or connection problems were abrupt, and the subsequent impedance trend typically showed marked variability.

Approach to the patient with a suspected pace-sense lead fracture

Table 10.10 and Fig. 10.103 summarize our approach to the patient with a suspected pace-sense lead fracture. Outside the perioperative period, noise oversensing with normal impedance trend indicates a fracture. The key differential diagnosis is between noise and other causes of rapid oversensing. This finding typically requires lead replacement.

If noise oversensing and abrupt impedance rise occur, the algorithm in Fig. 10.103 assists in differentiating fractures from connection problems. Connection

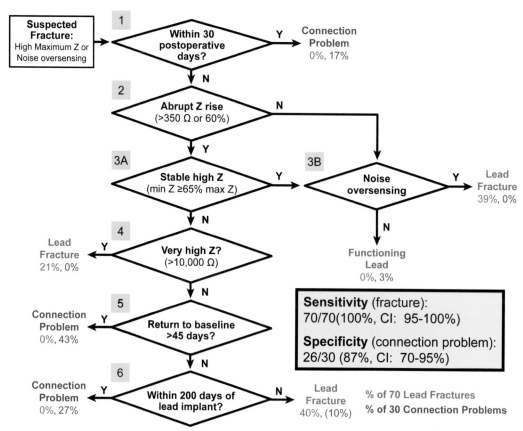

Fig. 10.103 Clinical algorithm for discrimination of pace-sense lead fractures from connection problems and functioning leads with impedance rises. Numbers in gray boxes denote algorithm steps. Percentages at each step indicate algorithm's classification for 70 fractures (maroon text) and 30 connection problems (blue text). Values in parentheses denote incorrect classification. (Reprinted with permission from Swerdlow CD, Sachanandani H, Gunderson BD, Ousdigian KT, Hjelle M, Ellenbogen KA. Preventing overdiagnosis of implantable cardioverter-defibrillator lead fractures using device diagnostics. J Am Coll Cardiol 2011; 57:2330–9.)

problems due to incomplete pin insertion of true-bipolar leads with a tight set screw may be corrected by programming integrated-bipolar sensing if that option is available because the tip connector makes an adequate connection. However, we are not aware of published follow-up data using this approach. Correspondingly, in true-bipolar leads, oversensing due to a fracture of the conductor to the ring electrode may be corrected temporarily by programming integrated-bipolar sensing. This is not recommended as a long-term solution because other elements of the lead are at higher risk for subsequent failure.

If operative intervention is required, the ICD should be inspected for incomplete insertion of the lead pin into the header, loose setscrews, and other header problems[147] *before* disconnecting the lead. Intraoperative

radiography should be performed if the diagnosis is in question. The best images are obtained by removing the generator from the pocket and orienting it perpendicular to the X-ray beam without disconnecting the leads.

For leads that present with an isolated impedance rise, limited data support intensified follow-up without operative intervention if the rise is gradual. If the rise is abrupt we recommend operative intervention if the algorithm in Fig. 10.103 indicates a fracture. If the algorithm indicates a connection problem and maximum impedance is less than 2500 Ω, we cannot make an evidence-based recommendation. About half of high-impedance functioning leads have impedance trends indistinguishable from connection problems.[141] We do not know if these represent connection problems that do not cause oversensing or changes at the electrode–

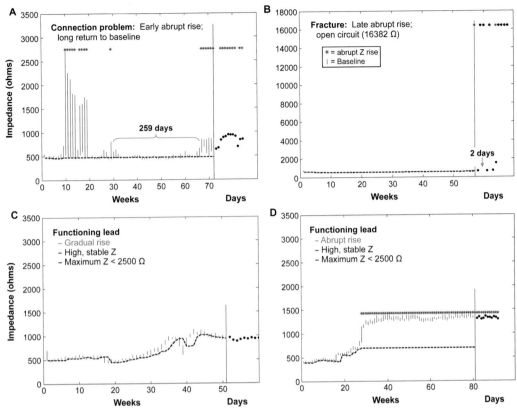

Fig. 10.104 Impedance trends for individual patients classified correctly by algorithm. To the left of the longest vertical line, data are displayed as vertical lines connecting weekly maximum and minimum values. To right, black points indicate daily values. Dotted green line denotes baseline impedance calculated for weekly values. Red stars denote impedance measurements that fulfill criteria for an abrupt rise. (A) Connection problem with first abrupt rise occurring 10 weeks post-implantation with long return to baseline (259 days). (B) Fracture with abrupt impedance rise to open circuit. Longest return to baseline is 2 days. (C) Gradual impedance rise in functioning lead. (D) Abrupt rise to high, stable impedance in functioning lead. (Reprinted with permission from Swerdlow CD, Sachanandani H, Gunderson BD, Ousdigian KT, Hjelle M, Ellenbogen KA. Preventing overdiagnosis of implantable cardioverter-defibrillator lead fractures using device diagnostics. J Am Coll Cardiol 2011; 57:2330–9.)

myocardial interface. Before deciding on conservative management, a chest X-ray should be inspected and the lead should be evaluated for pacing threshold, R-wave amplitude, oversensing induced by physical maneuvers or pacing, and high-voltage impedance.

In suspected fractures, clinical urgency is dictated by the presence of oversensing, which is the source of inappropriate shocks. Detection of VF should be disabled immediately in any patient with noise oversensing. The time course for evaluating high impedance without oversensing is less critical.

Other ICD lead failures

High-voltage conductor failures These fractures usually present either as asymptomatic abnormalities of imped-

ance or as unsuccessful cardioversion or defibrillation shocks. High voltage conductors may fail either by fracture or insulation failure. High-voltage fractures represent a minority of fractures in multilumen leads. Of fractured Sprint Fidelis leads confirmed by return product analysis fractures, 6% only had high-voltage fractures and 8% had both high-voltage and pace-sense fractures. Limited data indicate that either high-voltage impedance >100 Ω or an increase in impedance by 100% over baseline are diagnostic of a high-voltage fracture.[104] Noisy electrograms on the high-voltage leads may confirm the diagnosis, but the sensitivity of abnormal high-voltage electrograms is unknown. To date, there are no criteria for distinguishing high-voltage fractures from high-voltage connection problems.

Table 10.10 Diagnostic approach to suspected pace-sense lead fracture.

EGM Noise	Abrupt Z ↑	Diagnosis	What to do?
+	0	Lead problem	Replace lead
+	+	Lead or connection problem	Surgery: confirm connection problem noninvasively or intra-operatively; algorithm helpful. Otherwise replace lead.
0	+	Lead or connection problem; Normally functioning lead	Diagnose connection problem or normally functioning lead non-invasively. If not confirmed, evaluate intra-operatively.

Lead-can abrasions in the pocket can cause insulation failure, leading to a short-circuit during shock delivery (Fig. 10.88). Because they are often not detected by low-voltage impedance measurements, we recommend delivering a high-voltage shock at all generator replacements unless contraindicated.

Outer insulation failures Recently, failures of silicone outer insulation have been reported in St. Jude Riata® 8-Fr high-voltage leads. They present either as "outside-in" insulation failure from external abrasion in the pocket or unusually as "inside-out" insulation failure, usually at the level of the tricuspid valve.[153] Most of the inside-out failures were diagnosed by fluoroscopy, presenting a characteristic image in which the inner cables protrude outside the outer insulation (Fig. 10.105). Case reports indicate that exteriorized conductor failures may present with noise oversensing and that this

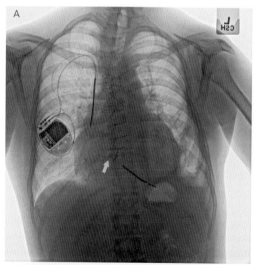

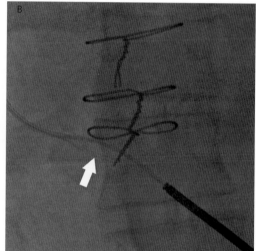

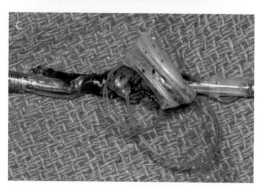

Fig. 10.105 Exteriorized conductor insulation failure of St. Jude Riata™ lead. (A) shows a PA chest X-ray, with arrow indicating region of exteriorized conductor near the tricuspid valve. (B) is a close-up image of the region indicated by the arrow. (C) shows the lead following extraction. The individual conductors are independently insulated with PTFE and had emerged from the body of the lead.

oversensing can be detected by the Medtronic Lead Integrity Algorithm.[53] Reductions in both high-voltage and pacing impedance have been reported with some Riata insulation failures, but currently data are insufficient to determine if the mechanism and location of insulation failure influences the presentation. A potential concern is high-voltage insulation failure due to lead-can abrasion, resulting in failure to defibrillate.

Lead failure diagnostics

Early diagnosis of ICD lead failure has been studied intensively since Medtronic discontinued sale of the Sprint Fidelis™ ICD lead in 2007. Present Medtronic ICDs include to algorithms to reduce inappropriate shocks if lead fractures occur.

Lead Integrity Alert™

This feature is triggered either by abnormally high impedance relative to the patient's baseline impedance or rapid oversensing that is unlikely to represent a physiologic event. Impedance is measured once daily, but oversensing is measured continuously.[53] Once an alert is triggered, Lead Integrity Alert™ (LIA) sounds an audible tone immediately and every 4 hours thereafter. Thus, the LIA alert sounds whenever the oversensing trigger is met or when daily impedance is measured. Medtronic ICDs sound the same audible tone once daily for various other alerts, but a tone that sounds every 4 hours represents an urgent alert for lead fracture. LIA alerts also reprogram the number of intervals to detect VF (NID) from the value programmed at the physician's discretion (nominally 18/24) to 30/40. This reduces inappropriate shocks caused by transient, fracture-induced oversensing.[53] A LIA alert also stores electrograms for any interval shorter than 200 ms, providing a diagnostic to determine the cause of rapid oversensing based on electrogram characteristics.[140] In newer ICDs with wireless telemetry, alerts initiate immediate internet notifications if this feature is enabled.

LIA has a specificity of approximately 70–80% for lead fractures and 80–90% for either lead fractures or connection problems.[53,154] In a prospective study of Sprint Fidelis lead fractures, LIA was associated with a 46% relative reduction in inappropriate shocks compared to conventional impedance monitoring (LIA: 38% vs. control: 70% P <0.001). Because the interval between LIA alert and inappropriate shock may be short, LIA's value depends on timely response by both patient and physician: 27% of shocked LIA patients have ≥3 days of warning.[154] Prompt response may further reduce inappropriate shocks. Once a patient presents with an alert, detection of VF should be disabled to prevent inappropriate shocks during evaluation

to determine the cause of the alert.[155] Approximately 20% of alerts are caused by events that do not require surgical revision, including previously discussed causes of rapid oversensing and impedance increases which can be managed conservatively. Thus, appropriate testing must be performed before operative intervention, including inspection of electrograms and radiographs and a thorough evaluation of lead diagnostics and function.

Lead Noise Algorithm™

This algorithm identifies lead noise by rapid signals on the pace-sense channel that correspond temporally with isoelectric periods on the high-voltage electrogram. It withholds VF therapy if it determines that noise is present (Fig. 10.106).[156] Unpublished preliminary data suggest that the nominal 45-s timeout period is too short and the algorithm (nominally "on") should be implemented without a timeout feature. It was introduced in Medtronic's Protecta™ family of ICDs.

Troubleshooting cardiac resynchronization devices

In heart failure patients with ventricular dyssynchrony, cardiac resynchronization therapy delivered via pacemakers (CRT-P) or ICDs (CRT-D) improves exercise tolerance, reduces heart failure hospitalizations, and decreases mortality.[157,158] The two widely spaced ventricular leads in resynchronization ICDs and the requirement for continuous biventricular pacing introduce novel intra-device interactions between resynchronization pacing and sensing. However, the most common problem in CRT is failure of heart failure symptoms to respond resynchronization pacing.[159]

Failure to respond to resynchronization pacing

This may be caused by patient-related factors, system-related factors, or an interaction of the patient and system (Table 10.11). In the context of this troubleshooting chapter, failure to respond refers to objective measures of LV performance after noncardiac factors (e.g. anemia, hypothyroidism, and depression) have been excluded. We assume that the patient is a good candidate for CRT and that the LV lead was positioned initially in location capable of providing effective CRT. Clinical, ECG, and echocardiographic criteria for patient selection are addressed in Chapter 3: Indication for Pacemakers, ICDs, and CRT (see Congestive heart failure section), optimizing LV lead position in Chapter 2: Hemodynamics, and optimizing pacing parameters for hemodynamic response in Chapter 8: Programming (see Cardiac resynchronization devices section).

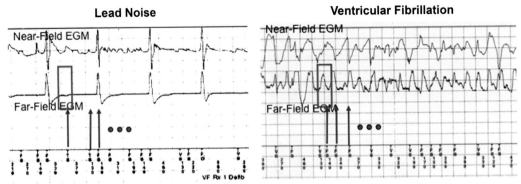

Fig. 10.106 ICD feature to discriminate pace-sense conductor failure of true bipolar ICD leads from ventricular fibrillation using far-field EGM (Medtronic Protecta ICDs). In pace-sense conductor failures, the far-field EGM has long isoelectric segments, which are not present in true VF. Stored EGM tracings during lead noise oversensing (left) and spontaneous VF (right) are shown; top tracings are the near-field (RVtip-RVring) EGM; middle tracings are the far-field EGM (RV coil-can); and the sensing markers are the lower tracing. Oversensing is identified by analyzing the peak–peak amplitudes of the far-field EGM in a 200-ms window centered at each of 12 sense markers (sensing derived from near-field EGM), as shown by the red arrows and boxes. Oversensing is identified when there are at least two far-field EGM analysis windows with isoelectric (<1 mV) amplitudes *and* at least one analysis window with peak–peak amplitude at least six times greater than the average of the two smallest amplitudes. Lead noise oversensing would have been properly discriminated from VF in these two examples. (Reproduced with permission from Swerdlow CD, Gillberg, JM, Khairy P. Sensing and detection. In: Ellengogen KA, Kay GN, Lau C, Wilkoff BL, eds. Clinical Cardiac Pacing, Defibrillation, and Resynchronization Therapy. 4th edn. Philadelphia, PA: Saunders Company, 2011: 56–126.)

Fig. 10.107 and Table 10.11 summarize our approach to troubleshooting nonresponse. Response to CRT requires effective resynchronization of at least 90% of R-R intervals. Optimal results have been associated with resynchronization of ≥92%[160] and 98%[161] of R-R intervals. The clinical goal should be biventricular pacing at or near 100%. The most common patient-related cause of nonresponse addressed by trouble-shooting is resynchronization of <90–95% of R-R intervals.

Resynchronization <90–95% of R-R intervals

Resynchronization of <90–95% of R-R intervals is caused by ventricular sensing, either related to or unrelated to conduction of the atrial rhythm.

Ventricular sensing of conducted sinus or atrial-paced rhythm Common issues resulting in ventricular sensing of conducted beats relate to programming the AV delay too long, upper rate limit behavior, functional atrial undersensing caused by trapping P waves in the PVARP, and unanticipated change to a nontracking mode.

AV delay: The AV delay may be set too long either in baseline rhythm or during exercise, resulting in intrinsic conduction of fusion of paced and conducted beats.[159] As reviewed in Chapter 2: Hemodynamics of Cardiac Pacing, optimal AV delay maximizes LV diasto-

lic filling time without causing diastolic mitral insufficiency or permitting intrinsic AV conduction. However, the optimal method of exercise-related shortening of the AV delay may differ from that of typical rate-adaptive pacing in which the goal is to mimic physiologic PR shortening due to vagal withdrawal and increased sympathetic tone. Failure to shorten the AV delay sufficiently with exercise will result in intrinsic AV conduction. Excessive programmed AV delays in baseline rhythm often are related to changes in medication (often by another physician), such as reduction in β-blocker dose.

Upper rate limit behavior: CRT patients who have normal sinus nodes and AV conduction exhibit different upper rate limit behavior than patients who require bradycardia pacing.[162] The specific response depends on the timing of sinus P waves in relation to the PVARP. In pacemaker patients with AV block, the sensed A (AS) – paced V (VP) interval prolongs when the upper rate limit is reached, resulting in pacemaker Wenckebach providing the PVARP is sufficiently short that the sinus cycle length exceeds the total atrial refractory period (TARP). However, in CRT patients with intact AV conduction, the Wenckebach response is pre-empted by native AV conduction. This typically occurs if the programmed upper rate limit is too slow. In CRT patients with normal AV conduction, a slow upper rate limit

Table 10.11 Approach to nonresponders to cardiac resynchronization.

Problem	Mechanism	Solution
Resynchronization is not delivered (pacing <95%)*		
Sensing errors		
Atrial undersense	Loss of P synchronous pacing and conduction of intrinsic ventricular complexes	Increase atrial sensitivity or reposition atrial lead. If function, shorten PVARP, increase upper tracking limit, turn off PMT algorithm
Atrial events in PVARP ("pseudo-undersensing")	Loss of P synchronous pacing and conduction of intrinsic ventricular complexes	Shorten PVARP, disable PMT and PVC response, increase upper tracking limit, consider interventricular refractory period
Atrial oversensing	Far-field R waves cause inappropriate mode switch and loss of atrial tracking	Reduce atrial sensitivey; increase PVAB; reposition lead
Ventricular oversensing	Ventricular pacing is inhibited	Reduce ventricular sensitivity; adjust ventricular refractory periods
Algorithmic inhibition of ventricular pacing	Algorithms such as rate smoothing prevent tracking abrupt increases in atrial rate	Turn algorithms off. Shorten left ventricular protection period (limits upper LV pacing rate)
Spontaneous ventricular beats		
PVCs		Alter pacing rate; determine cause of PVCs, consider additional β-blockers, amiodarone or ablation
AV conduction in sinus rhythm	Conduction of intrinsic ventricular complexes	Shorten AV delay
AV conduction in AF	Conduction of intrinsic ventricular complexes	Maintain sinus rhythm, pharmacologic rate control, pacing algorithms to cause ventricular fusion, AV junction ablation
Resynchronization is not delivered (pacing >95%, but no LV capture)*		Discussed in more detail in Chapter 2: Hemodyanmics
LV capture with slow exit from LV pacing site	Due to slow conduction of tissue around LV lead, most of ventricle activated from RV	Confirm capture by pacing LV lead alone; positive QRS complex in lead III, negative in I, and RBBB morphology in V1 indicate LV capture; If capture present, adjust V-V timing to pre-excite LV
Nonoptimal vector	Capture may be present from some LV vectors and not others; anodal capture may be present	Recheck threshold using alternate vectors
Insufficient output	LV threshold may be elevated	Increase output, or reposition LV lead
Resynchronization is delivered >95% with capture*		
Confirm patient is nonresponder	Multiple end-points have been used to define non-responders, details in text	Six-minute walk or oxygen consumption treadmill; assess ejection fraction; formal QOL assessment
Nonoptimal programming	Program parameters may not optimize intraventricular, interventricular, or atrioventricular electrical or mechanical function	Optimize V-V and AV timing with echo guidance (see Chapter 2: Hemodynamics) If frequent atrial pacing (as opposed to sensing) is disrupting left AV mechanical synchronicy, use VDD mode, consider if fusion pacing algorithms provide adequate resynchronization
Nonoptimal lead position	Insuffficient RV–LV separation to allow resynchronization	Reposition lead, particularly if in anterior vein, or small RV–LV separation radiographically and small V-V interval during intrinsic rhythm
Absence of dyssynchrony		Program to minimize ventricular pacing; CRT may not help

AV, atrioventricular; CRT, cardiac resynchronization therapy; LV, left ventricular; PMT, pacemaker-mediated tachycardia; PVAB, post-ventricular atrial blanking; PVARP, post-ventricular atrial refractory period; PVC, premature ventricular complex; RBBB, right bundle branch block; RV, right ventricular.

*In general. the closer to achieving 100% effective biventricular pacing the better, realizing that 100% effective biventricular pacing may not be possible. While older literature suggests >90% resynchronized beats is acceptable, it is probably reasonable to aim for ≥95% resynchronization.

Assessing CRT Delivery

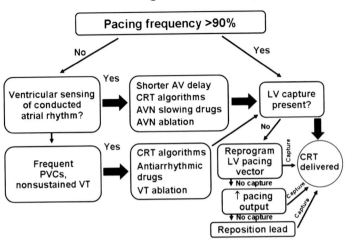

Fig. 10.107 Systematic approach to insuring delivery of cardiac resynchronization therapy. AVN, AV node; CRT, cardiac resynchronization therapy; PVC, premature ventricular complex; VTns, non-sustained VT. (From Friedman PA, Swerdlow CD, Hayes DL. Troubleshooting. In: Hayes DL, Friedman PA, eds. Cardiac Pacing and Defibrillation: A Clinical Approach, 2nd edn. West Sussex, UK: Wiley-Blackwell, 2008: 401–516, by permission of Friedman, Swerdlow, and Hayes.)

does not prevent rapid ventricular rates during sinus tachycardia. The upper rate limit should be programmed faster than the maximum sinus rate to ensure CRT during sinus tachycardia (Fig. 10.108).

If the PVARP is long, atrial tracking is lost when the P–P interval decreases below the TARP. In patients with AV block, this results in 2:1 upper rate limit behavior. However, in CRT patients with intact AV conduction, the conducted ventricular beat (VS) will initiate a new PVARP so that successive sinus P waves time in the PVARP. This is referred to as functional atrial undersensing. In CRT, the programmed sensed A_S-V delay is shorter than the intrinsic PR interval so that once AV conduction occurs at rates faster than the upper rate limit, CRT will not resume until the sinus cycle length slows to a value greater than the intrinsic PR interval + PVARP, sometimes referred to as the intrinsic TARP.[152]

Functional atrial undersensing at sinus rates below the upper rate limit due to PVARP: In CRT patients with intact AV conduction, single desynchronizing events may initiate a repetitive cycle in which sinus P waves slower than the upper rate limit are trapped in the PVARP of the preceding conducted QRS so long as the sinus cycle length is less than the intrinsic TARP (Figs 10.109 and 10.110).

This response is facilitated by first-degree AV block. When the P-wave times in the PVARP at sinus rates slower than the upper rate limit, the goals of troubleshooting are to identify the both the initiating and perpetuating events. In patients with first-degree AV block, any event that results in loss of AV synchrony by inhibiting ventricular pacing for a single beat may permit

intrinsic AV conduction. The long PR interval and resultant short RP interval causes the next sinus P wave to time in the PVARP, resulting in perpetuation of intrinsic AV conduction (Table 10.11). Multiple types of triggering events may result in the initial conducted beat. For example, atrial undersensing results in loss of atrial tracking and AV conduction of the undersensed P wave. PVARP extension after PVCs[163] traps the sinus P wave in the PVARP. R-wave double-counting (usually during PVCs) results in initiation of the PVARP at second component of double-counted R wave, effectively prolonging the PVARP.

Solutions include shortening the PVARP, deactivating the algorithm that extends the PVARP extension after PVCs, and specific algorithms that shorten the PVARP if a consistent pattern of atrial-refractory (AR)–ventricular sensed (VS) events is identified. Shortening the PVARP increases the likelihood that the next sinus P wave will be followed by a tracked, resynchronized complex after the AV interval times out. One solution to the problem of R-wave double-counting is the interventricular refractory period (IVRP) after sensed ventricular events. Ventricular sensed events during IVRP do not reset the PVARP.

Unanticipated change to a nontracking pacing mode: This is another mechanism that permits intrinsic AV conduction. The most common cause is atrial oversensing (usually of far-field R waves) resulting in reversion to the DDI mode (Fig. 10.111). Other causes include reversion to VVI mode when the elective replacement voltage is tripped or noise reversion to a nontracking mode, such as inappropriate mode switch.

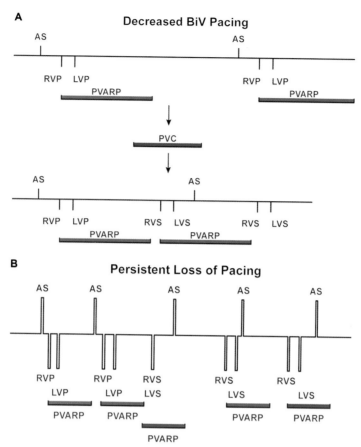

Fig. 10.108 Loss of resynchronization due to functional undersensing in the atrium, with los of tracking. A single premature ventricular complex (PVC) may result not only in inhibition of one resynchronized paced beat but in continuous promotion of intrinsic conduction and continued suppression of biventricular pacing. This results from functional undersensing in the atrium as illustrated in the left panel. With most devices, following a PVC, the post-ventricular atrial refractory period (PVARP) is extended. Either retrograde conduction from the PVC or the next sinus beat may fall in this extended PVARP and will not be tracked. Atrial pacing may then occur, but since the atrium is refractory, it will not capture, and if antegrade conduction through the AV node is present, then the sinus beats falling in the PVARP will conduct to the ventricle in the right panel, and this, in turn, will result in persistent loss of biventricular pacing and continued antegrade conduction of sinus rhythm. (From Friedman PA, Rott MA, Wokhlu A, Asirvatham SJ, Hayes DL, eds. A Case-Based Approach to Pacemakers, ICDs, and Cardiac Resynchronization, Vol. 2, Advanced Questions for Examination Review and Clinical Practice. Minnesota, MN: Mayo Foundation for Medical Education and Research Cardiotext Publishing, 2011: 113–20.)

Ventricular sensing issues unrelated to conducted atrial rhythm: PVCs inhibit ventricular pacing, and frequent PVCs reduce the fraction of resynchronized ventricular beats. Boston Scientific ICDs incorporate a programmable LV refractory period, which initiates a "LV Protection Period" during which pacing will not occur after a sensed or paced LV events. This is designed to prevent pacing in the LV vulnerable period, but it may inhibit CRT if PVCs are late-coupled, especially at high sinus rates. If the LV lead is position proximal near AV grove, this P-wave oversensing may inhibit CRT. This feature should be disabled if it interferes with CRT.

Ventricular sensing of conducted AF Conducted AF represents a particular problem for CRT[164–171] because atrial sensing cannot be used to time the next ventricular resynchronization pulse (Fig. 10.112). In CRT patients with AF, the goal of ventricular rate control is to prevent all intrinsic AV conduction. In patients with paroxysmal AF this requires high doses of β-blockers and potentially other AV nodal blocking drugs. In patients with permanent AF, AV junction ablation should be performed if pharmacologic therapy does not result in suppression of almost all AV conduction with pacing at the lower rate limit. AV junction ablation

Persistent Loss of Pacing

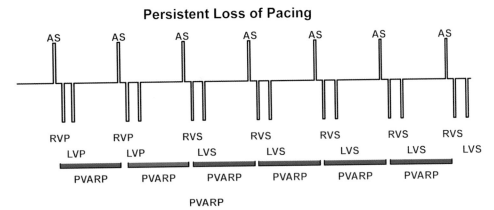

Fig. 10.109 Role of high atrial rates in preventing resynchronization. Higher atrial rates, frequent premature atrial and ventricular beats, and the presence of antegrade delayed AV conduction (a long PR interval) all may prevent biventricular stimulation, thus lowering the total "dose" of resynchronization The key interval to keep in mind when troubleshooting insufficient biventricular pacing is that the total atrial refractory period (TARP) is the sum of the sensed AV interval and the PVARP. By preventing rapid rates in the atrium (beta-blockers), PVCs and PACs (antiarrhythmic drugs, ablation), and shortening the PVARP when possible (atrial tracking, recovery, turning off PVC PVARP extension) the frequency of biventricular pacing is increased. Conversely, algorithms to terminate pacemaker-mediated tachycardia (PMT) may interrupt CRT delivery by promoting intrinsic rhythms. In the diagram, note that after the second "AS" event ventricular pacing ("RVP" and "LVP" is replaced with ventricular sensing ("RVS" and "LVS") since the third "AS" falls in the PVARP, and is therefore not tracked. (From Friedman PA, Rott MA, Wokhlu A, Asirvatham SJ, Hayes DL, eds. A Case-Based Approach to Pacemakers, ICDs, and Cardiac Resynchronization, Vol. 2, Advanced Questions for Examination Review and Clinical Practice. Minnesota, MN: Mayo Foundation for Medical Education and Research Cardiotext Publishing, 2011: 113–20.)

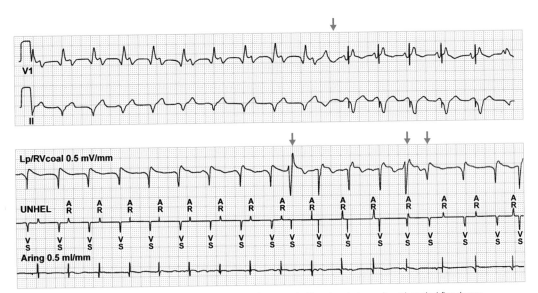

Fig. 10.110 Loss of CRT due to pseudo-atrial undersensing. Top: telemetry strip. Note sinus tachyacardia with marked first-degree atrioventricular (AV) block (P-R interval, 400 ms) and loss of atrial synchronous biventricular pacing on left. Atrial synchronous biventricular pacing is restored after premature ventricular contraction (arrow) on right. Bottom: tracking in same patient. The sinus rate exceeds the programmed upper rate limit, displacing P waves into the post-ventricular atrial refractory period (PVARP, marked as AR). Spontaneous AV conduction occurs in the form of a preempted Wencklebach upper-rate response. The first PVC (first arrow) resets the PVARP and restores atrial tracking. The second PVC (second arrow) occurs coincident with a sinus event, which falls into the post-ventricular atrial blanking period. The third PVC (third arrow) resets the PVARP and reinitiates pseudo-atrial undersensing. Atrial tracking is restored when the sinus rate slows slightly at the end of the strip. (Reproduced with permission from Swerdlow CD, Gillberg, JM, Khairy P. Sensing and detection. In: Ellengogen KA, Kay GN, Lau C, Wilkoff BL, eds. Clinical Cardiac Pacing, Defibrillation, and Resynchronization Therapy. 4th edn. Philadelphia, PA: Saunders Company, 2011, 56–126.)

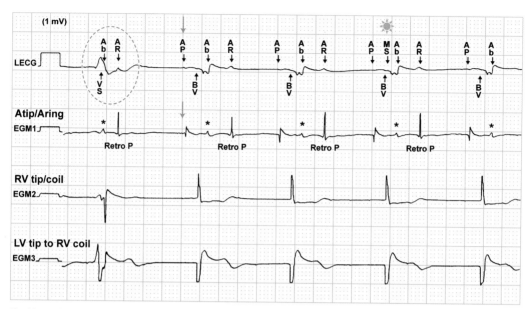

Fig. 10.111 Tracing recorded during a routine follow-up visit. From top to bottom: leadless ECG (recorded between an SVC coil and the pulse generator can), the near-field atrial signal (recorded between the atrial tip and atrial ring electrode), right ventricular EGM (RV tip to RV coil), and far-field left ventricular EGM (LV tip to RV coil). The first complex (circled) is a PVC. Note that the morphology on a leadless ECG (recorded between SVC coil and can to simulate surface ECG) is different from the subsequent complexes (which are paced, with marker "BV"), and that the first QRS is a sensed event ("VS" marker indicating a ventricular sensed event) without an antecedent atrial event. Additionally, there is far-field R-wave oversensing of the QRS complex itself on the atrial channel (Atip/ring) during the blanking period as indicated by the "Ab" marker (first atrial marker in circled complex). This results because the atrial lead is in the appendage, and records the signal generated by the ventricle (marked with an asterisk on the atrial channel). The second atrial marker is an atrial refractory sensed event ("AR" marker), and results from appropriate sensing of the retrograde P wave on the atrial channel (labeled "Retro P" on the Atip/ring). It is refractory because it occurs soon after the QRS, during the postventricular atrial refractory period (PVARP). The QRS itself is seen as a small deflection (asterisk) on the Atip/ring channel that lines up with the "Ab" marker. In the next complex (down arrow), the AP (atrial paced impulse) does not capture. Note the absence of an atrial deflection on the leadless ECG (top arrow) and stimulus artifact without capture on the Atip/ring channel (lower arrow). Following the atrial pacing artifact a biventricular paced event (BV) is oversensed on the atrial channel ("Ab" marker that aligns with small deflection on Atip/ring [asterisk]). Because atrial pacing did not result in capture, ventricular pacing leads to a retrograde P wave ("AR"). Following the third biventricular paced event (starburst/* symbol) the "MS" marker indicates an inappropriate mode switch event. In summary, atrial noncapture and far-field R-wave oversensing are both present. Markers indicate atrial pacing, far-field R-wave oversensing of ventricular depolarization, and then sensing of the actual retrograde P wave. The multiple atrial events lead to inappropriate mode switch. The problem was corrected by decreasing atrial sensitivity (eliminating far-field R-wave oversensing) and adjusting atrial outputs (eliminating noncapture). No surgery was required. (From Friedman PA, Rott MA, Wokhlu A, Asirvatham SJ, Hayes DL, eds. A Case-Based Approach to Pacemakers, ICDs, and Cardiac Resynchronization, Vol. 2, Advanced Questions for Examination Review and Clinical Practice. Minnesota, MN: Mayo Foundation for Medical Education and Research Cardiotext Publishing, 2011: 40–3.)

has been reported to improve response to CRT in patients with permanent AF.[167,168]

Some CRT devices have programmable triggered pacing modes that deliver resynchronization pacing if a ventricular sensed event occurs.[172] For example, the Medtronic Ventricular Sense Response™ feature triggers pacing in one or both ventricles after each RV-sensed event in order to achieve partial resynchronization. However, data supporting the value of the fusion pacing

that results from these features are limited.[172] Inspection of the ECG may permit identification of ineffective fusion pacing.[100]

Boston Scientific ICDs include a ventricular-rate regularization feature based on weighted average of conducted R-R intervals during mode switching. The goal is to ensure continuous ventricular pacing, even if pacing faster than the lower rate limit is required (Fig. 10.113). Concealed conduction into the AV node from

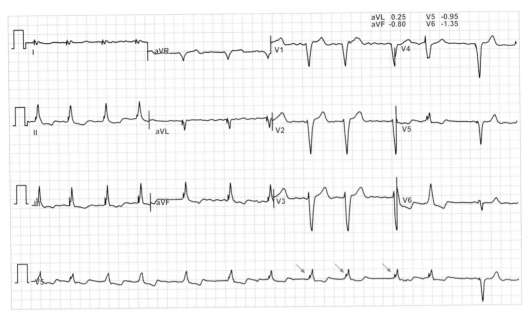

Fig. 10.112 Surface ECG from a patient with a CRT device. Arrows point to pacing artifacts. Note that most QRS complexes are not resynchronized. (From Friedman PA, Rott MA, Wokhlu A, Asirvatham SJ, Hayes DL, eds. A Case-Based Approach to Pacemakers, ICDs, and Cardiac Resynchronization, Vol. 2, Advanced Questions for Examination Review and Clinical Practice. Minnesota, MN: Mayo Foundation for Medical Education and Research Cardiotext Publishing, 2011: 136–55.)

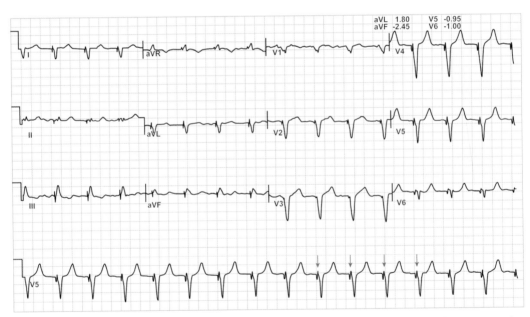

Fig. 10.113 ECG from the same patient as shown in Fig. 10.112 but with VRR (ventricular rate regularization algorithm) now programmed on. Note that stable biventricular pacing with constant rates and degree of resynchronization is present. A tradeoff with such programming, however, is that the average daily heart rate will typically now be higher, which in turn may give rise to symptoms of ischemia or ventricular dysfunction in some cases. (From Friedman PA, Rott MA, Wokhlu A, Asirvatham SJ, Hayes DL, eds. A Case-Based Approach to Pacemakers, ICDs, and Cardiac Resynchronization, Vol. 2, Advanced Questions for Examination Review and Clinical Practice. Minnesota, MN: Mayo Foundation for Medical Education and Research Cardiotext Publishing, 2011: 135–55.)

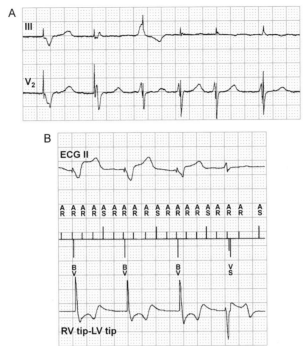

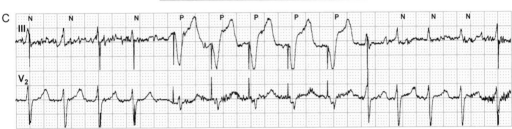

Fig. 10.114 Algorithms designed to maintain a high percent of cardiac resynchronization pacing during atrial fibrillation may be confused with inappropriate pacing. (A) Hospital telemetry shows ventricular pacing occurring after the QRS onset due to the Medtronic Ventricular Sense Response™ algorithm, which introduces a triggered biventricular pacing pulse after each RV-sensed event. (B) Surface ECG lead II, event markers and the RV tip to LV tip electrogram are displayed during atrial fibrillation. The first three complexes represent biventricular pacing ("BV"). The last complex represents a conducted complex that was sensed ("VS"). The split marker associated with the "VS" indicates that a triggered pace pulse resulted. (C) Hospital telemetry shows pacing during rapidly conducted atrial fibrillation due to an algorithm designed to maximize cardiac resynchronization pacing. This pacing, with the patient at rest, is distinct from rapid, rate-responsive pacing that is triggered by a sensor. (.) (From Friedman PA, Swerdlow CD, Hayes DL. Troubleshooting. In: Hayes DL, Friedman PA, eds. Cardiac Pacing and Defibrillation: A Clinical Approach, 2nd edn. West Sussex, UK: Wiley-Blackwell, 2008: 401–516, by permission of Friedman, Swerdlow, and Hayes.)

the paced beats may slow AV nodal conduction, thereby limiting the pacing-induced increase in ventricular rate. These and other algorithms designed to maximize cardiac resynchronization therapy may result in pacing after QRS onset on surface ECGs and pacing at "unexpected" times (Figs 10.114 and 10.115). Awareness of these algorithms prevents unnecessary intervention.)

Resynchronization ≥90–95% of RR intervals

If ≥90–95% of R-R intervals receive CRT, either pacing does not result in LV capture or LV capture does not produce resynchronization.

Loss of LV capture: This can usually be identified from the surface 12-lead ECG and confirmed by lead

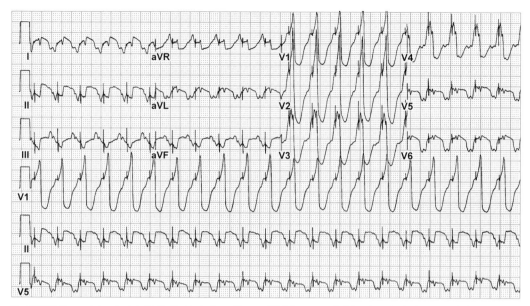

Fig. 10.115 Unexpected pacing into VT. The Ventricular Sense Response™ delivers a ventricular pacing stimulus into a ventricular event at the time of RV sensing. It is intended to provide fusion pacing to partially resynchronize contraction during rapidly conducted AF. This 12-lead ECG shows this feature delivering pulses into VT slower than the VT detection interval.

threshold testing. Threshold rise may be caused by local tissue effects, microdislodgement, or radiographically identifiable lead dislodgement. Present CRT systems permit independent programming of RV and LV outputs, facilitating determination of the RV and LV threshold. However, anodal capture may confound interpretation of LV pacing. Pacing leads are designed to capture at the cathode (negative terminal). Anodal capture occurs when the stimulus captures at the RV anode either in isolation or in conjunction with the RV or the LV cathode.[101] If anodal RV capture is mistaken for LV capture, the pacing output may be programmed to a subthreshold value in the LV, resulting in loss of resynchronization (Figs 10.116 and 10.117). Anodal capture is more common if the RV anode is a ring electrode (true bipolar pacing), which has a small surface area (high current density) that may be in direct contact with endocardium, than if the RV anode is a defibrillation coil (integrated-bipolar pacing), which has a large surface area (low current density). Most modern ICD systems offer anodes for LV pacing other than the RV ring, which should be used only when no alternatives are available.

LV capture does not produce resynchronization: LV capture will not produce resynchronization if no dyssynchrony is present or the lead is in a suboptimal location (e.g.,

anterior interventricular vein). If the LV lead is located in a region of scar, LV pacing may propagate only after marked stimulus latency or, in the end case, no propagate at all due to exit block. If the LV stimulation has marked latency, the bulk of ventricular myocardium may be activated by the wavefront initiated by the RV lead. Failure of resynchronization due to stimulus latency may be mitigated by reprogramming V-V timing to earlier pacing in the left ventricle than right the ventricle. In patients with marked right atrial–left atrial conduction delays, right atrial pacing may interfere with left-sided, mechanical AV synchrony if the programmed AV delay to short. Interatrial conduction delays may increases at higher paced rates. In patients with right-atrial pacing and marked interatrial conduction delays, echocardiographic evaluation of the mitral inflow pattern should be used to optimize the programmed AV interval.

Troubleshooting other problems in CRT systems

Phrenic nerve stimulation

The left phrenic nerve courses adjacent to the left ventricular free wall. An epicardial pacing lead in a coronary sinus tributary in juxtaposition to the phrenic nerve may stimulate it at the pacing rate, which is clinically intolerable. Phrenic stimulation may become

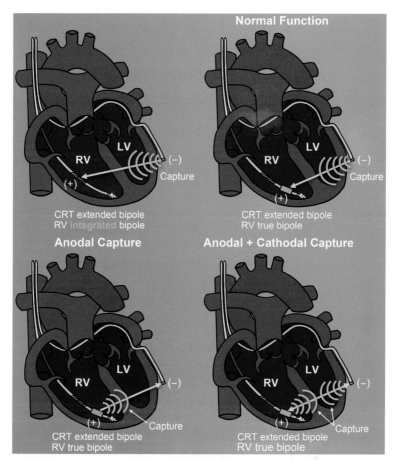

Fig. 10.116 Possible modes of anodal capture during biventricular pacing. In all examples, an extended bipole paces between LV and RV leads. The top left panel demonstrates biventricular pacing using an integratedbipolar RV lead, in which the common anode is the distal defibrillation coil. As the RV coil has a large surface area and thus a low current density, anodal capture is rare. The remaining panels depict biventricular pacing between a LV electrode and a true-bipolar RV lead, in which the common anode is the RV ring electrode. The top right panel depicts normal function, with capture only at the LV tip during LV-only pacing. The bottom left panel depicts capture only at the anode. This occurs if the anodal RV-ring threshold is lower than the LV threshold and the pacing output is between the RV anodal threshold and LV cathodal thresholds. The bottom right panel depicts anodal and cathodal capture. This may confound the determination of LV pacing threshold. (Reproduced with permission from Friedman PA, Swerdlow CD, Hayes DL. Troubleshooting. In: Hayes DL, Friedman PA, eds. Cardiac Pacing and Defibrillation: A Clinical Approach, 2nd edn. West Sussex, UK: Wiley-Blackwell, 2008: 401–516.)

apparent only after implantation due to alteration of the electode–phrenic nerve relationship with postural changes or minor lead migration. Decreasing the pacing output, reprogramming unipolar to bipolar LV pacing or changing the LV pacing vector (electronic repositioning) may eliminate phrenic stimulation non-invasively.[173] If sufficient difference between the phrenic and LV capture thresholds cannot be achieved with any of these maneuvers, the LV lead should be repositioned. Episodic phrenic stimulation may relate to transient increases in the pacing amplitude during measurement of pacing impedance. Disabling automatic measurement of pacing impedance may eliminate symptoms.

CRT proarrhythmia

On a population basis, CRT has no consistent effect on the incidence of VT/VF, with minimal effect in most studies. However, in occasional patients site-specific changes in pacing site may result in marked proarrhythmia (Fig. 10.118).[88,174–177] Proarrhythmia should be considered if there is a marked increase in VT/VF shortly after implant.

Ventricular sensing problems

CRT does not cause novel ventricular oversensing problems, but some previously described problems

A

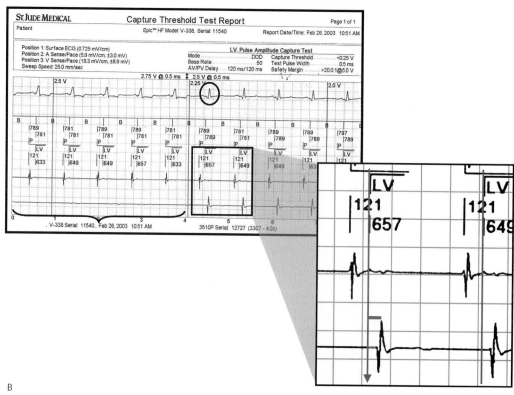

B

True LV loss of capture

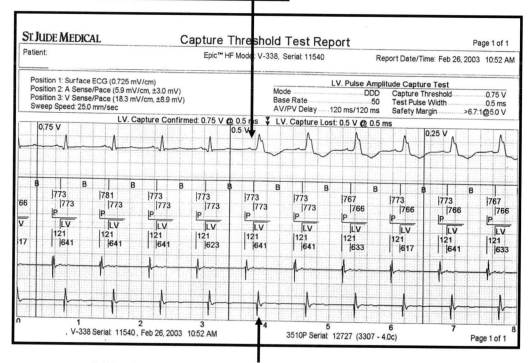

Minimal change in V sense pace

Fig. 10.117 Anodal capture during testing of LV capture threshold. LV pacing occurs between a LV cathode and a RV ring anode. (A) Upper left panel, from top to bottom: surface ECG, electrogram markers and intervals, atrial electrogram and ventricular near-field electrogram. At left, pacing output is 2.5 V and anodal capture is present, with capture occurring at both the LV electrode and the RV ring. No electrograms are visible on the LV channel due to the simultaneous RV and LV capture. With a decrement in pacing output to 2.25 V, the QRS morphology changes on the ECG (circled complex); and electrograms appear on the ventricular channel, representing local RV depolarization. Inset at lower right shows that the time between the pacing stimulus and the RV electrogram represents the interventricular conduction time during LV pacing. (B) With further decrement in LV pacing output from 0.75 to 0.5 V, true loss of LV capture occurs, with widening of the surface ECG due to left bundle branch block. The local RV depolarizations are similar during LV pacing (in A) and intrinsic AV conduction (in B). (Reproduced with permission from Blackwell Publishing.)

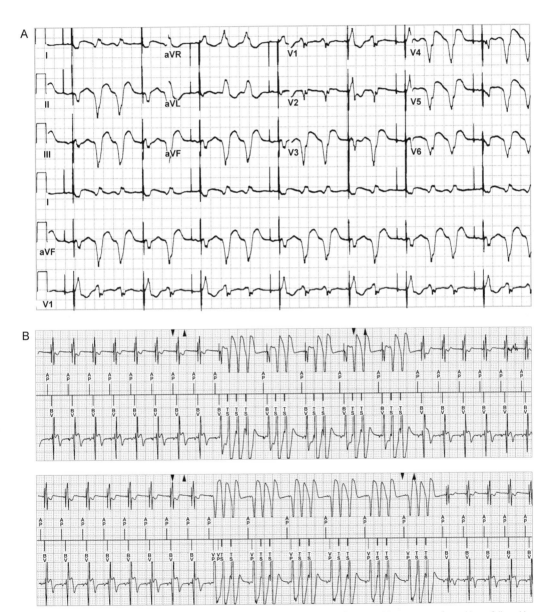

Fig. 10.118 Proarrhythmia from cardiac resynchronization pacing. (A) Twelve-lead ECG shows repetitive sequence of paced beats followed by PVC or PVC pair. (B) Real-time intracardiac EGMs during change of pacing site shows far-field EGM in upper panel and true-bipolar EGM in lower panel of each recording. Top recording shows that proarrhythmia occurs during biventricular pacing, but not LV pacing. Lower panel shows that it occurs during RV only pacing. Programming the RV output subthreshold corrected proarrhythmia.

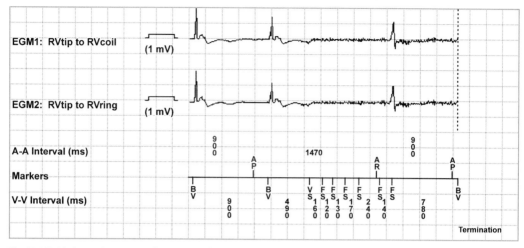

Fig. 10.119 Diaphragmatic myopotential oversensing after CRT upgrade. This patient with an integrated-bipolar lead developed oversensing after upgrade of a dual-chamber to cardiac resynchronization ICD. Stored EGMs show identical integrated-bipolar signals in top and middle position channels with marker channel. In the dual-chamber ICD, autoadjusting sensitivity after sensed R waves began at an initial value of 3 mV. After upgrade, all ventricular events are paced. Maximum post-pacing ventricular sensitivity resulted in oversensing of previously unsensed myopotentials.

occur most commonly in CRT devices. For example, R-wave double-counting is a common problem if RV capture is lost. The device counts both the paced ventricular event and the sensed response after the wavefront stimulated in the LV has propagated slowly to the RV sensing electrode (Fig. 10.63). Similarly, diaphragmatic myopotential oversensing may first be identified after "upgrade" of an ICD to a CRT-D in a patient with intact AV conduction. In the ICD configuration, the initial value of automatic adjustment of sensitivity depended on the amplitude of the sensed R wave. In the CRT-D configuration, the initial value begins at the highly sensitive post-pacing value (Fig. 10.119).

References

1 Love CJ, Hayes DL. Evaluation of pacemaker malfunction. In: Ellenbogen KA, Kay GN, Wilkoff BL, eds. Clinical Cardiac Pacing. Philadelphia: WB Saunders Co., 1995: 656–83.

2 Hauser RG, Hayes DL, Kallinen LM, *et al.* Clinical experience with pacemaker pulse generators and transvenous leads: an 8-year prospective multicenter study. Heart Rhythm 2007; 4:154–60.

3 O'Hara GE, Kristensson B-E, Lundstrom R Jr, Kempen K, Soucy B, Lynn MS. on behalf of the worldwide Kappa 700 Investigators. First clinical experience with a new pacemaker with ventricular Capture Management™ feature (abstract). Pacing Clin Electrophysiol 1998; 21:892.

4 Lee MT, Baker R. Circadian rate variation in rate-adaptive pacing systems. Pacing Clin Electrophysiol 1990; 13: 1797–801.

5 van Mechelen R, Ruiter J, de Boer H, Hagemeijer F. Pacemaker electrocardiography of rate smoothing during DDD pacing. Pacing Clin Electrophysiol 1985; 8:684–90.

6 Benditt DG, Sutton R, Gammage MD, *et al.* Clinical experience with Thera DR rate-drop response pacing algorithm in carotid sinus syndrome and vasovagal syncope. The International Rate-Drop Investigators Group. Pacing Clin Electrophysiol 1997; 20:832–9.

7 Levine PA, Sanders R, Markowitz HT. Pacemaker diagnostics: measured data, event marker, electrogram, and event counter telemetry. In: Ellenbogen KA, Kay GN, Wilkoff BL, eds. Clinical Cardiac Pacing. Philadelphia: WB Saunders Co., 1995: 639–55.

8 Levine PA. The complementary role of electrogram, event marker and measured data telemetry in the assessment of pacing system function. J Electrophysiol 1987; 1:404–16.

9 Kruse I, Markowitz T, Ryden L. Timing markers showing pacemaker behavior to aid in the follow-up of a physiological pacemaker. Pacing Clin Electrophysiol 1983; 6:801–5.

10 Irnich W. Pacemaker-related patient mortality (editorial). Pacing Clin Electrophysiol 1999; 22:1279–83.

11 Hauser R, Hayes D, Parsonnet V, *et al.* Feasibility and initial results of an internet-based North American pacemaker and ICD pulse generator and lead registry (abstract). Pacing Clin Electrophysiol 2000; 23:597.

12 Altamura G, Bianconi L, Lo Bianco F, *et al.* Transthoracic DC shock may represent a serious hazard in pacemaker dependent patients. Pacing Clin Electrophysiol 1995; 18:194–8.

13 Bianconi L, Boccadamo R, Toscano S, *et al.* Effects of oral propafenone therapy on chronic myocardial pacing threshold. Pacing Clin Electrophysiol 1992; 15:148–54.

14 Dohrmann ML, Goldschlager N. Metabolic and pharmacologic effects on myocardial stimulation threshold in patients with cardiac pacemakers. In: Barold SS, ed. Modern Cardiac Pacing. Mount Kisco, NY: Futura Publishing Co., 1985: 161–70.

15 Carnes CA, Mehdirad AA, Nelson SD. Drug and defibrillator interactions. Pharmacotherapy 1998; 18:516–25.

16 Nielsen AP, Griffin JC, Herre JM, et al. Effect of amiodarone on acute and chronic pacing thresholds (abstract). Pacing Clin Electrophysiol 1984; 7:462.

17 Schlesinger Z, Rosenberg T, Stryjer D, Gilboa Y. Exit block in myxedema, treated effectively by thyroid hormone therapy. Pacing Clin Electrophysiol 1980; 3:737–9.

18 Lee D, Greenspan K, Edmands RE, Fisch C. The effect of electrolyte alteration on stimulus requirement of cardiac pacemakers (abstract). Circulation 1968; 38 (Suppl.): VI–124.

19 O'Reilly MV, Murnaghan DP, Williams MB. Transvenous pacemaker failure induced by hyperkalemia. JAMA 1974; 228:336–7.

20 Sowton E, Barr I. Physiological changes in threshold. Ann NY Acad Sci 1969; 167:679–85.

21 Hellestrand KJ, Burnett PJ, Milne JR, Bexton RS, Nathan AW, Camm AJ. Effect of the antiarrhythmic agent flecainide acetate on acute and chronic pacing thresholds. Pacing Clin Electrophysiol 1983; 6:892–9.

22 Preston TA, Judge RD. Alteration of pacemaker threshold by drug and physiological factors. Ann NY Acad Sci 1969; 167:686–92.

23 Barold SS, Leonelli F, Herweg B. Hyperkalemia during cardiac pacing. Pacing Clin Electrophysiol 2007; 30:1–3.

24 Tworek DA, Nazari J, Ezri M, Bauman JL. Interference by antiarrhythmic agents with function of electrical cardiac devices. Clin Pharm 1992; 11:48–56.

25 Antonelli D, Freedberg NA, Rosenfeld T. Acute loss of capture due to flecainide acetate. Pacing Clin Electrophysiol 2001; 24:1170.

26 Hughes JC Jr, Tyers GF, Torman HA. Effects of acid-base imbalance on myocardial pacing thresholds. J Thorac Cardiovasc Surg 1975; 69:743–6.

27 Wilkoff BL, Hess M, Young J, Abraham WT. Differences in tachyarrhythmia detection and implantable cardioverter defibrillator therapy by primary or secondary prevention indication in cardiac resynchronization therapy patients. J Cardiovasc Electrophysiol 2004; 15:1002–9

28 Becker R, Ruf-Richter J, Senges-Becker JC, et al. Patient alert in implantable cardioverter defibrillators: Toy or tool? J Am Coll Cardiol 2004; 44:95–8.

29 Bansch D, Brunn J, Castrucci M, et al. Syncope in patients with an implantable cardioverter-defibrillator: Incidence, prediction and implications for driving restrictions. J Am Coll Cardiol 1998; 31:608–15.

30 Schreieck J, Zrenner B, Kolb C, Ndrepepa G, Schmitt C. Inappropriate shock delivery due to ventricular double detection with a biventricular pacing implantable cardioverter defibrillator. Pacing Clin Electrophysiol 2001; 24:1154–7.

31 Swerdlow CD, Russo AM, DeGroot PJ. The dilemma of icd implant testing. Pacing Clin Electrophysiol 2007; 30:675–700.

32 Brady PA, Friedman PA, Trusty JM, Grice S, Hammill SC, Stanton MS. High failure rate for an epicardial implantable cardioverter-defibrillator lead: Implications for long-term follow-up of patients with an implantable cardioverter-defibrillator. J Am Coll Cardiol 1998; 31:616–22.

33 Kron J, Herre J, Renfroe EG, et al. Lead- and device-related complications in the antiarrhythmics versus implantable defibrillators trial. Am Heart J 2001; 141:92–8.

34 Kowey PR, Marinchak RA, Rials SJ. Things that go bang in the night. N Engl J Med 1992; 327:1884.

35 Michael KA, Peterson BJ, Yue AM, et al. Use of an intracardiac electrogram eliminates the need for a surface ecg during implantable cardioverter-defibrillator follow-up. Pacing Clin Electrophysiol 2007; 30:1432–7.

36 Requena-Carrion J, Vaisanen J, Alonso-Atienza F, Garcia-Alberola A, Ramos-Lopez FJ, Rojo-Alvarez JL. Sensitivity and spatial resolution of transvenous leads in implantable cardioverter defibrillator. IEEE Trans Biomed Eng 2009; 56:2773–81.

37 Marchlinski FE, Callans DJ, Gottlieb CD, Schwartzman D, Preminger M. Benefits and lessons learned from stored electrogram information in implantable defibrillators. J Cardiovasc Electrophysiol. 1995; 6:832–51.

38 Glikson M, Swerdlow C, Daoud EG, et al. Optimal combination of discriminators for differentiating ventricular from supraventricular tachycardia by dual-chambers defibrillators. J Cardiovasc Electrophysiol 2005; 16:1–8.

39 Eberhardt F, Schuchert A, Schmitz D, Zerm T, Mitzenheim S, Wiegand U. Incidence and significance of far-field r wave sensing in a vdd-implantable cardioverter defibrillator. Pacing Clin Electrophysiol 2007; 30:395–403.

40 Sticherling C, Zabel M, Spencker S, et al. Comparison of a novel, single-lead atrial sensing system with a dual-chamber implantable cardioverter-defibrillator system in patients without antibradycardia pacing indications: results of a randomized study. Circ Arrhythm Electrophysiol 2011; 4:56–63.

41 Gunderson B, Patel A, Bounds C. Automatic identification of implantable cardioverter-defibrillator lead problems using intracardiac electrograms. Comp Cardiol 2002; 29:121–4.

42 Swerdlow C, Shivkumar K. Implantable cardioverter defibrillators: clinical aspects. In: Zipes DP, Jalife J, eds. Cardiac Electrophysiology: From Cell to Bedside. Philadephia: W.B. Saunders; 2004: 980–93.

43 Garcia-Moran E, Mont L, Brugada J. Inappropriate tachycardia detection by a biventricular implantable cardioverter defibrillator. Pacing Clin Electrophysiol 2002; 25:123–4.

44 Lloyd M, Hayes D, Friedman P. Troubleshooting. Cardiac Pacing and Defibrillation: A Clinical Approach. Armonk, NY: Futura; 2000: 347–452.

45 Callans DJ, Hook BG, Kleiman RB, Mitra RL, Flores BT, Marchlinski FE. Unique sensing errors in third-generation implantable cardioverter-defibrillators. J Am Coll Cardiol 1993; 22:1135–40.

46 Pinski SL. 2:1 tracking of sinus rhythm in a patient with a dual-chamber implantable cardioverter defibrillator:

What is the mechanism? J Cardiovasc Electrophysiol 2001; 12:503–4.

47 Ellenbogen KA, Gunderson BD, Patel AS, Ousdigian K, Abeyratne A, Swerdlow C. Lead intergrity alert performance for non-sprint fidelis® icd lead fractures. Heart Rhythm 2009; 6:S248.

48 Weretka S, Michaelsen J, Becker R, et al. Ventricular oversensing: a study of 101 patients implanted with dual chamber defibrillators and two different lead systems. Pacing Clin Electrophysiol 2003; 26:65–70.

49 Powell B, Asirvatham S, Perschbacher DL, et al. Noise, artifact, and oversensing related inappropriate ICD shock evaluation: ALTITUDE NOISE Study. Pacing Clin Elecophysiol 2012; 35:863–9.

50 Cao J, Shrivastav M, Koehler J, Swerdlow CD, Gillberg JM. Automatic identification of T-wave oversensing by patterns of alternating amplitude and frequency content in implantable cardiverter defibrillator electrograms (abstract). Heart Rhythm 2008; 5:S194.

51 Cao J, Gillberg J, Swerdlow C. A fully automatic algorithm to prevent inappropriate detection of ventricular tachycardia or fibrillation due to T-wave oversensing in implantable cardioverter-defibrillators. Heart Rhythm J 2012; 9:522–30.

52 Hsu SS, Mohib S, Schroeder A, Deger FT. T wave oversensing in implantable cardioverter defibrillators. J Interv Card Electrophysiol 2004; 11:67–72.

53 Swerdlow CD, Gunderson BD, Ousdigian KT, et al. Downloadable algorithm to reduce inappropriate shocks caused by fractures of implantable cardioverter-defibrillator leads. Circulation 2008; 118:2122–9.

54 Michaud J, Horduna I, Dubuc M, Khairy P. ICD-unresponsive ventricular arrhythmias. Heart Rhythm 2009; 6:1827–9.

55 Cao J, Gillberg J, Swerdlow C. A fully automatic, implantable cardioverter-defibrillator algorithm to prevent inappropriate detection of ventricular tachycardia or fibrillation due to T-wave oversensing in spontaneous rhythm. Heart Rhythm 2012; 9:522–30.

56 Gunderson B, Swerdlow C, Wilcox J, Hayman J, Ousdigian K, Ellenbogen K. Causes of ventricular oversensing in implantable cardioverter-defibrillators: Implications for diagnosis of lead fracture. Heart Rhythm 2010; 7:626–33.

57 Seegers J, Zabel M, Luthje L, Vollmann D. Ventricular oversensing due to manufacturer-related differences in implantable cardioverter-defibrillator signal processing and sensing lead properties. Europace 2010; 12:1460–6.

58 Sweeney MO, Ellison KE, Shea JB, Newell JB. Provoked and spontaneous high-frequency, low-amplitude, respirophasic noise transients in patients with implantable cardioverter defibrillators. J Cardiovasc Electrophysiol 2001; 12: 402–10.

59 Friedman P, McClelland R, Bamlet W, et al. Dual-chamber versus single chamber detection enhancements for implantable defibrillator rhythm diagnsois: the detect supraventricular tachycardia study. Circulation 2006; 113:2871–9.

60 Powell B, Cha Y, Jones P, et al. Diagnostic value of the ICD atrial lead in accurate discrimination of supraventricular

from ventricular arrhythmias. Heart Rhythm 2011 (Abstract)

61 Bourke T, Vaseghi M, Michowitz Y, et al. Neuraxial modulation for refractory ventricular arrhythmias: Value of thoracic epidural anesthesia and surgical left cardiac sympathetic denervation. Circulation 2010; 121:2255–62.

62 Stein KM, Euler DE, Mehra R, et al. Do atrial tachyarrhythmias beget ventricular tachyarrhythmias in defibrillator recipients? J Am Coll Cardiol 2002; 40:335–40.

63 Glikson M, Swerdlow CD, Gurevitz OT, et al. Optimal combination of discriminators for differentiating ventricular from supraventricular tachycardia by dual-chamber defibrillators. J Cardiovasc Electrophysiol 2005; 16:732–9.

64 Przibille O, Himmrich E, Nebeling R, Dorn N, Andreas K. New algorithm for discrimination of VT from SVT in patients with single chamber ICD. Heart Rhythm 2008; 5(Suppl):291.

65 Atienza L, Almendral J, Arenal Á, et al. Utilidad diagnóstica de los electrogramas almacenados por el desfibrilador automático implantable. Rev Esp Cardiol 2008; 8(Suppl A):76A–85A.

66 Swerdlow CD, Chen PS, Kass RM, Allard JR, Peter CT. Discrimination of ventricular tachycardia from sinus tachycardia and atrial fibrillation in a tiered-therapy cardioverter-defibrillator. J Am Coll Cardiol 1994; 23:1342–55.

67 Kuhlkamp V, Mewis C, Suchalla R, Bosch RF, Doernberger V, Seipel L. Rate dependence of r-r stability during atrial fibrillation and ventricular tachyarrhythmias. Circulation 1998; 98:I–713.

68 Garcia-Alberola A, Yli-Mayry S, Block M, et al. Rr interval variability in irregular monomorphic ventricular tachycardia and atrial fibrillation. Circulation 1996; 93: 295–300.

69 Swerdlow CD, Ahern T, Chen PS, et al. Underdetection of ventricular tachycardia by algorithms to enhance specificity in a tiered-therapy cardioverter-defibrillator. J Am Coll Cardiol 1994; 24:416–24.

70 Wathen MS, Volosin KJ, Sweeney MO, et al. Ventricular antitachycardia pacing by implantable cardioverter defibrillators reduces shocks for inappropriately detected supraventricular tachycardia. Heart Rhythm 2004 (abstract);1.

71 Knight BP, Zivin A, Souza J, et al. A technique for the rapid diagnosis of atrial tachycardia in the electrophysiology laboratory. J Am Coll Cardiol 1999; 33:775–81.

72 Wilkoff BL, Ousdigian KT, Sterns LD, Wang ZJ, Wilson RD, Morgan JM. A comparison of empiric to physician-tailored programming of implantable cardioverter-defibrillators: results from the prospective randomized multicenter empiric trial. J Am Coll Cardiol 2006; 48:330–9.

73 Wilkoff BL, Williamson BD, Stern RS, et al. Strategic programming of detection and therapy parameters in implantable cardioverter-defibrillators reduces shocks in primary prevention patients: results from the prepare (primary prevention parameters evaluation) study. J Am Coll Cardiol 2008; 52:541–50.

74 Klein GJ, Gillberg JM, Tang A, *et al.* Improving svt discrimination in single-chamber ICDs: a new electrogram morphology-based algorithm. J Cardiovasc Electrophysiol 2006; 17:1310–9.

75 Wilkoff BL, Kuhlkamp V, Volosin K, *et al.* Critical analysis of dual-chamber implantable cardioverter-defibrillator arrhythmia detection: results and technical considerations. Circulation 2001; 103:381–6.

76 Daubert JP, Zareba W, Cannom DS, *et al.* Inappropriate implantable cardioverter-defibrillator shocks in MADIT II: frequency, mechanisms, predictors, and survival impact. J Am Coll Cardiol 2008; 51:1357–65.

77 Kuhlkamp V, Dornberger V, Mewis C, Suchalla R, Bosch RF, Seipel L. Clinical experience with the new detection algorithms for atrial fibrillation of a defibrillator with dual chamber sensing and pacing. J Cardiovasc Electrophysiol 1999; 10:905–15.

78 Swerdlow CD. Supraventricular tachycardia-ventricular tachycardia discrimination algorithms in implantable cardioverter defibrillators: state-of-the-art review. J Cardiovasc Electrophysiol 2001; 12:606–12.

79 Sweeney MO, Ruetz LL, Belk P, Mullen TJ, Johnson JW, Sheldon T. Bradycardia pacing-induced short-long-short sequences at the onset of ventricular tachyarrhythmias: a possible mechanism of proarrhythmia? J Am Coll Cardiol 2007; 50:614–22.

80 Martinez-Sanchez J, Garcia-Alberola A, Sanchez-Munoz JJ, Penafiel-Verdu P, Giner-Caro JA, Valdes-Chavarri M. ICD proarrhythmia as a consequence of an interaction with an algorithm to prevent atrial arrhythmias. Pacing Clin Electrophysiol 2009; 32:1096–8.

81 Cron TA, Schaer B, Osswald S. Implantable cardioverter defibrillator proarrhythmia due to an interaction with "noncompetitive atrial pacing": an algorithm to prevent atrial arrhythmias. Pacing Clin Electrophysiol 2002; 25:1656–9.

82 Gronefeld GC, Israel CW, Padmanabhan V, Koehler J, Cuijpers A, Hohnloser SH. Ventricular rate stabilization for the prevention of pause dependent ventricular tachyarrhythmias: results from a prospective study in 309 ICD recipients. Pacing Clin Electrophysiol 2002; 25:1708–14.

83 Himmrich E, Przibille O, Zellerhoff C, *et al.* Proarrhythmic effect of pacemaker stimulation in patients with implanted cardioverter-defibrillators. Circulation 2003; 108:192–7.

84 Gasparini M, Menozzi C, Proclemer A, Landolina M, Iacopino S, Carboni A, Lombardo E, Regoli F, Biffi M, Burrone V, Denaro A, Boriani G. A simplified biventricular defibrillator with fixed long detection intervals reduces implantable cardioverter defibrillator (ICD) interventions and heart failure hospitalizations in patients with non-ischaemic cardiomyopathy implanted for primary prevention: the relevant [role of long detection window programming in patients with left ventricular dysfunction, non-ischemic etiology in primary prevention treated with a biventricular icd] study. Eur Heart J 2009; 30:2758–67.

85 Bourke JP, Turkington D, Thomas G, McComb JM, Tynan M. Florid psychopathology in patients receiving shocks from implanted cardioverter-defibrillators. Heart 1997; 78:581–3.

86 Hegel MT, Griegel LE, Black C, Goulden L, Ozahowski T. Anxiety and depression in patients receiving implanted cardioverter-defibrillators: a longitudinal investigation. Int J Psychiatry Med 1997; 27:57–69.

87 Kantharia BK, Patel JA, Nagra BS, Ledley GS. Electrical storm of monomorphic ventricular tachycardia after a cardiac-resynchronization-therapy-defibrillator upgrade. Europace 2006; 8:625–8.

88 Credner SC, Klingenheben T, Mauss O, Sticherling C, Hohnloser SH. Electrical storm in patients with transvenous implantable cardioverter-defibrillators: Incidence, management and prognostic implications. J Am Coll Cardiol 1998; 32:1909–15.

89 Fagundes A, LP DEM, Russo M, Xavier E. Pharmacological treatment of electrical storm in cathecolaminergic polymorphic ventricular tachycardia. Pacing Clin Electrophysiol 2010; 33:e27–31.

90 Nademanee K, Taylor R, Bailey WE, Rieders DE, Kosar EM. Treating electrical storm : Sympathetic blockade versus advanced cardiac life support-guided therapy. Circulation 2000; 102:742–7.

91 Srivatsa UN, Ebrahimi R, El-Bialy A, Wachsner RY. Electrical storm: case series and review of management. J Cardiovasc Pharmacol Ther 2003; 8:237–46.

92 Jao YT, Chen Y, Lee WH, Tai FT. Thyroid storm and ventricular tachycardia. South Med J 2004; 97:604–7.

93 Zipes DP, Camm AJ, Borggrefe M, *et al.* Acc/aha/esc 2006 guidelines for management of patients with ventricular arrhythmias and the prevention of sudden cardiac death: a report of the American College of Cardiology/American Heart Association Task Force and the European Society of Cardiology Committee for Practice Guidelines (writing committee to develop guidelines for management of patients with ventricular arrhythmias and the prevention of sudden cardiac death): Developed in collaboration with the European Heart Rhythm Association and the Heart Rhythm Society. Circulation 2006; 114:e385–484.

94 Arya A, Bode K, Piorkowski C, *et al.* Catheter ablation of electrical storm due to monomorphic ventricular tachycardia in patients with nonischemic cardiomyopathy: acute results and its effect on long-term survival. Pacing Clin Electrophysiol 2010; 33:1504–9.

95 Bansch D, Oyang F, Antz M, *et al.* Successful catheter ablation of electrical storm after myocardial infarction. Circulation 2003; 108:3011–6.

96 Shukla HH, Flaker GC, Jayam V, Roberts D. High defibrillation thresholds in transvenous biphasic implantable defibrillators: Clinical predictors and prognostic implications. Pacing Clin Electrophysiol 2003; 26:44–8.

97 Boriani G, Biffi M, Frabetti L, Maraschi M, Branzi A. High defibrillation threshold at cardioverter defibrillator implantation under amiodarone treatment: Favorable effects of d, l-sotalol. Heart Lung 2000; 29:412–6.

98 Hohnloser SH, Dorian P, Roberts R, *et al.* Effect of amiodarone and sotalol on ventricular defibrillation threshold: the Optimal Pharmacological Therapy in Cardioverter

Defibrillator patients (OPTIC) trial. Circulation 2006; 114:104–9.

99 Block M, Breithardt G. Optimizing defibrillation through improved waveforms. Pacing Clin Electrophysiol 1995; 18:536–8.

100 Kamath GS, Cotiga D, Koneru JN, et al. The utility of 12-lead holter monitoring in patients with permanent atrial fibrillation for the identification of nonresponders after cardiac resynchronization therapy. J Am Coll Cardiol 2009; 53:1050–5.

101 Dendy KF, Powell BD, Cha YM, et al. Anodal stimulation: an underrecognized cause of nonresponders to cardiac resynchronization therapy. Indian Pacing Electrophysiol J 2011; 11:64–72.

102 Swerdlow CD Russo AM, Degroot PJ. The dilemma of ICD implant testing. Pacing Clini Electrophysiol 2007; 30:675–700.

103 Daoud EG, Kalbfleisch SJ, Hummel JD, et al. Implantation techniques and chronic lead parameters of biventricular pacing dual-chamber defibrillators. J Cardiovasc Electrophysiol 2002; 13:964–70.

104 Gunderson B, Ellenbogen K, Sachanandani H, Wohl B, Kendall K, Swerdlow C. Lower impedance threshold provides earlier warning for high voltage lead fractures. Heart Rhythm (abstract). 2011.

105 Hauser RG, Hayes DL, Epstein AE, et al. Multicenter experience with failed and recalled implantable cardioverter-defibrillator pulse generators. Heart Rhythm 2006; 3:640–4.

106 Swerdlow CD, Cannom DS. ICD product reliability: lessons from electrical overstress failures. Pacing Clin Electrophysiol 2001; 24:1043–5.

107 Kolb C, Deisenhofer I, Weyerbrock S, et al. Incidence of antitachycardia therapy suspension due to magnet reversion in implantable cardioverter defibrillators. Pacing Clin Electrophysiol 2004; 27:221–3.

108 Rasmussen MJ, Friedman PA, Hammill SC, Rea RF. Unintentional deactivation of implantable cardioverter-defibrillators in health care settings. Mayo Clin Proc 2002; 77:855–9.

109 Bansch D, Steffgen F, Gronefeld G, et al. The 1 + 1 trial: A prospective trial of a dual- versus a single-chamber implantable defibrillator in patients with slow ventricular tachycardias. Circulation 2004; 110:1022–9.

110 Bansch D, Castrucci M, Bocker D, Breithardt G, Block M. Ventricular tachycardias above the initially programmed tachycardia detection interval in patients with implantable cardioverter-defibrillators: Incidence, prediction and significance. J Am Coll Cardiol 2000; 36:557–65.

111 Goldschlager N, Epstein A, Friedman P, Gang E, Krol R, Olshansky B. Environmental and drug effects on patients with pacemakers and implantable cardioverter/defibrillators: a practical guide to patient treatment. Arch Intern Med 2001; 161:649–55.

112 Brode SE, Schwartzman D, Callans DJ, Gottlieb CD, Marchlinski FE. ICD-antiarrhythmic drug and ICD-pacemaker interactions. J Cardiovasc Electrophysiol 1997; 8:830–42.

113 Monahan KM, Hadjis T, Hallett N, Casavant D, Josephson ME. Relation of induced to spontaneous ventricular tachycardia from analysis of stored far-field implantable defibrillator electrograms. Am J Cardiol 1999; 83: 349–53.

114 Brugada J, Mont L, Figueiredo M, Valentino M, Matas M, Navarro-Lopez F. Enhanced detection criteria in implantable defibrillators. J Cardiovasc Electrophysiol 1998; 9:261–8.

115 Weber M, Bocker D, Bansch D, et al. Efficacy and safety of the initial use of stability and onset criteria in implantable cardioverter defibrillators. J Cardiovasc Electrophysiol 1999; 10:145–53.

116 Klein G, Manolis A, Viskin S, et al. Clinical performance of Wavelet™ morphology discrimination algorithm in a worldwide single chamber ICD population. Circulation 2003; 110:III-345 (abstract).

117 Corbisiero R, Lee MA, Nabert DR, et al. Performance of a new single-chamber ICD algorithm: discrimination of supraventricular and ventricular tachycardia based on vector timing and correlation. Europace 2006; 8: 1057–61.

118 Lee MA, Corbisiero R, Nabert DR, et al. Clinical results of an advanced svt detection enhancement algorithm. Pacing Clin Electrophysiol 2005; 28:1032–40.

119 Gold MR, Theuns DA, Knight BP, et al. Head-to-head comparison of arrhythmia discrimination performance of subcutaneous and transvenous icd arrhythmia detection algorithms: the start study. J Cardiovasc Electrophysiol 2012; 23:359–66.

120 Gillberg JM. Medtronic Gem DR Data Base. Minneapolis, MN: 2000.

121 Gold MR, Shorofsky SR, Thompson JA, et al. Advanced rhythm discrimination for implantable cardioverter defibrillators using electrogram vector timing and correlation. J Cardiovasc Electrophysiol 2002; 13:1092–97.

122 Cohen AI, Wish MH, Fletcher RD, et al. The use and interaction of permanent pacemakers and the automatic implantable cardioverter defibrillator. Pacing Clin Electrophysiol 1988; 11:704–11.

123 Geiger MJ, O'Neill P, Sharma A, et al. Interactions between transvenous nonthoracotomy cardioverter defibrillator systems and permanent transvenous endocardial pacemakers. Pacing Clin Electrophysiol 1997; 20:624–30.

124 Glikson M, Trusty JM, Grice SK, Hayes DL, Hammill SC, Stanton MS. A stepwise testing protocol for modern implantable cardioverter-defibrillator systems to prevent pacemaker-implantable cardioverter-defibrillator interactions. Am J Cardiol 1999; 83:360–6.

125 Wathen MS, Sweeney MO, DeGroot PJ, et al. Shock reduction using antitachycardia pacing for spontaneous rapid ventricular tachycardia in patients with coronary artery disease. Circulation 2001; 104:796–801.

126 Glikson M, Beeman AL, Luria DM, Hayes DL, Friedman PA. Impaired detection of ventricular tachyarrhythmias by a rate-smoothing algorithm in dual-chamber implantable defibrillators: Intradevice interactions. J Cardiovasc Electrophysiol 2002; 13:312–8.

127 Cooper JM, Sauer WH, Verdino RJ. Absent ventricular tachycardia detection in a biventricular implantable cardioverter-defibrillator due to intradevice interaction with a rate smoothing pacing algorithm. Heart Rhythm 2004; 1:728–31.

128 Shivkumar K, Feliciano Z, Boyle NG, Wiener I. Intradevice interaction in a dual chamber implantable cardioverter defibrillator preventing ventricular tachyarrhythmia detection. J Cardiovasc Electrophysiol 2000; 11:1285–8.

129 Wietholt D, Kuehlkamp V, Meisel E, et al. Prevention of sustained ventricular tachyarrhythmias in patients with implantable cardioverter-defibrillators-the prevent study. J Interv Card Electrophysiol 2003; 9:383–9.

130 Shalaby AA. Delayed detection of ventricular tachycardia in a dual chamber rate adaptive pacing implantable cardioverter defibrillator: a case of intradevice interaction. Pacing Clin Electrophysiol 2004; 27:1164–6.

131 Dekker LR, Schrama TA, Steinmetz FH, Tukkie R. Undersensing of vf in a patient with optimal r wave sensing during sinus rhythm. Pacing Clin Electrophysiol 2004; 27:833–4.

132 Ellenbogen KA, Wood MA, Kapadia K, Lu B, Valenta H. Short-term reproducibility over time of right ventricular pulse pressure as a potential hemodynamic sensor for ventricular tachyarrhythmias. Pacing Clin Electrophysiol 1992; 15:971–4.

133 Leitch J, Klein G, Yee R, et al. Feasibility of an implantable arrhythmia monitor. Pacing Clin Electrophysiol 1992; 15:2232–5.

134 Swerdlow CD. Implantation of cardioverter defibrillators without induction of ventricular fibrillation. Circulation 2001; 103:2159–64.

135 Ruetz L, Koehler JL, Jackson TE, Belk P. Sinus rhythm R-wave amplitude does not predict undersensing of ventricular fibrillation by implantable cardioverter-defibrillators. Circ Arrhythm Electrophysiol 2009; 120: S650.

136 Hauser RG, Kallinen LM, Almquist AK, Gornick CC, Katsiyiannis WT. Early failure of a small-diameter high-voltage implantable cardioverter-defibrillator lead. Heart Rhythm 2007; 4:892–6.

137 Kallinen L, Hauser RG, Lee KW, et al. Failure of impedance monitoring to prevent adverse clinical events caused by fracture of a recalled high-voltage implantable cardioverter-defibrillator lead. Heart Rhythm 2008; 5: 755–9.

138 Krahn AD, Champagne J, Healey JS, et al. Outcome of the fidelis implantable cardioverter-defibrillator lead advisory: a report from the canadian heart rhythm society device advisory committee. Heart Rhythm 2008; 5: 639–42.

139 Kallinen LM, Hauser RG, Lee KW, et al. Failure of impedance monitoring to prevent adverse clinical events caused by fracture of a recalled high-voltage implantable cardioverter-defibrillator lead. Heart Rhythm 2008; 5: 775–9.

140 Gunderson B, Swerdlow C, Wilcox J, Hayman J, Ousdigian K, Ellenborgen KA. Causes of ventricular oversensing in implantable cardioverter defibrillators: implications for diagnosis of lead fracture. Heart Rhythm 2010; 7:626–33.

141 Swerdlow CD, Sachanandani H, Gunderson BD, Ousdigian KT, Hjelle M, Ellenbogen KA. Preventing overdiagnosis of implantable cardioverter-defibrillator lead fractures using device diagnostics. J Am Coll Cardiol 2011; 57:2330–9.

142 Swerdlow CD, Ellenbogen KA. The changing presentation of implantable cardioverter-defibrillator lead fractures. Heart Rhythm 2009; 6:478–9.

143 Chung EH, Casavant D, John RM. Analysis of pacing/defibrillator lead failure using device diagnostics and pacing maneuvers. Pacing Clin Electrophysiol 2009; 32:547–9.

144 Cheung JW, Iwai S, Lerman BB, Mittal S. Shock-induced ventricular oversensing due to seal plug damage: a potential mechanism of inappropriate device therapies in implantable cardioverter-defibrillators. Heart Rhythm 2005; 2:1371–5.

145 Schuchert A, Kuck KH, Bleifeld W. Stability of pacing threshold, impedance, and R wave amplitude at rest and during exercise. Pacing Clin Electrophysiol 1990; 13: 1602–8.

146 Shandling AH, Florio J, Castellanet MJ, et al. Physical determinants of the endocardial p wave. Pacing Clin Electrophysiol 1990; 13:1585–9.

147 Germano JJ, Darge A, Maisel WH. Weakened implantable cardioverter-defibrillator header bond: abnormality not limited to subpectoral implants. Heart Rhythm 2010; 7:701–4.

148 Lee BP, Wood MA, Ellenbogen KA. Oversensing in a newly implanted dual-chamber implantable cardioverter-defibrillator: What is the mechanism? Heart Rhythm 2005; 2:782–3.

149 Pickett RA 3rd, Saavedra P, Ali MF, Darbar D, Rottman JN. Implantable cardioverter-defibrillator malfunction due to mechanical failure of the header connection. J Cardiovasc Electrophysiol 2004; 15:1095–9.

150 Kowalski M, Ellenbogen KA, Wood MA, Friedman PL. Implantable cardiac defibrillator lead failure or myopotential oversensing? An approach to the diagnosis of noise on lead electrograms. Europace 2008; 10:914–7.

151 Haddad L, Padula LE, Moreau M, Schoenfeld MH. Troubleshooting implantable cardioverter defibrillator system malfunctions: the role of impedance measurements. Pacing Clin Electrophysiol 1994; 17:1456–61.

152 Kallinen LM, Hauser RG, Tang C, et al. Lead integrity alert algorithm decreases inappropriate shocks in patients who have sprint fidelis pace-sense conductor fractures. Heart Rhythm 2010; 7:1048–55.

153 Erkapic D, Duray GZ, Bauernfeind T, De Rosa S, Hohnloser SH. Insulation defects of thin high-voltage ICD leads: an underestimated problem? J Cardiovasc Electrophysiol 2011; 22:1018–22.

154 Swerdlow CD, Gunderson BD, Ousdigian KT, Abeyratne A, Sachanandani H, Ellenbogen KA. Downloadable software algorithm reduces inappropriate shocks caused by

implantable cardioverter-defibrillator lead fractures: a prospective study. Circulation 2010; 122:1449–55.

155 Hauser RG. Monitoring an imperfect lead. Pacing Clin Electrophysiol 2009; 32:541–2.

156 Gunderson BD, Gillberg JM, Wood MA, Vijayaraman P, Shepard RK, Ellenbogen KA. Development and testing of an algorithm to detect implantable cardioverter-defibrillator lead failure. Heart Rhythm 2006; 3:155–62.

157 Bristow MR, Saxon LA, Boehmer J, et al.; Comparison of Medical Therapy Pacing and Defibrillation in Heart Failure Investigators. Cardiac-resynchronization therapy with or without an implantable defibrillator in advanced chronic heart failure. N Engl J Med 2004; 350:2140–50.

158 Young JB, Abraham WT, Smith AL, et al.;Multicenter InSync ICDRCETI. Combined cardiac resynchronization and implantable cardioversion defibrillation in advanced chronic heart failure: the MIRACLE ICD trial. [see comment]. JAMA 2003; 289:2685–94.

159 Barold SS, Herweg B, Curtis AB. The defibrillation safety margin of patients receiving ICDs: a matter of definition. Pacing Clin Electrophysiol 2005; 28:881–2.

160 Koplan BA, Kaplan AJ, Weiner S, Jones PW, Seth M, Christman SA. Heart failure decompensation and all-cause mortality in relation to percent biventricular pacing in patients with heart failure: is a goal of 100% biventricular pacing necessary? J Am Coll Cardiol 2009; 53: 355–60.

161 Hayes DL, Boehmer JP, Day JD, et al. Cardiac resynchronization therapy and the relationship of percent biventricular pacing to symptoms and survival. Heart Rhythm 2011; 8:1469–75.

162 Wang P, Kramer A, Estes NA 3rd, Hayes DL. Timing cycles for biventricular pacing. Pacing Clin Electrophysiol 2002; 25:62–75.

163 Richardson K, Cook K, Wang PJ, Al-Ahmad A. Loss of biventricular pacing: What is the cause? Heart Rhythm 2005; 2:110–1.

164 Bartunek J, Vanderheyden M. Cardiac dyssynchrony in congestive heart failure and atrial fibrillation: integrating regularization and resynchronization. J Am Coll Cardiol 2008; 52:1247–9.

165 Boriani G, Gasparini M, Landolina M, et al. Incidence and clinical relevance of uncontrolled ventricular rate during atrial fibrillation in heart failure patients treated with cardiac resynchronization therapy. Eur J Heart Fail 2011; 13:868–76.

166 Borleffs CJ, Ypenburg C, van Bommel RJ, et al. Clinical importance of new-onset atrial fibrillation after cardiac resynchronization therapy. Heart Rhythm 2009; 6: 305–10.

167 Bradley DJ, Shen WK. Atrioventricular junction ablation combined with either right ventricular pacing or cardiac resynchronization therapy for atrial fibrillation: the need for large-scale randomized trials. Heart Rhythm 2007; 4:224–32.

168 Brignole M, Botto G, Mont L, et al. Cardiac resynchronization therapy in patients undergoing atrioventricular junction ablation for permanent atrial fibrillation: a randomized trial. Eur Heart J 2011; 32:2420–9.

169 Dong K, Shen WK, Powell BD, et al. Atrioventricular nodal ablation predicts survival benefit in patients with atrial fibrillation receiving cardiac resynchronization therapy. Heart Rhythm 2010; 7:1240–5.

170 Ferreira AM, Adragao P, Cavaco DM, et al. Benefit of cardiac resynchronization therapy in atrial fibrillation patients vs. patients in sinus rhythm: the role of atrioventricular junction ablation. Europace 2008; 10:809–15.

171 Gasparini M, Regoli F, Galimberti P, Ceriotti C, Cappelleri A. Cardiac resynchronization therapy in heart failure patients with atrial fibrillation. Europace 2009; 11(Suppl 5):v82–6.

172 Aktas MK, Jeevanantham V, Sherazi S, et al. Effect of biventricular pacing during a ventricular sensed event. Am J Cardiol 2009; 103:1741–5.

173 Gurevitz O, Nof E, Carasso S, et al. Programmable multiple pacing configurations help to overcome high left ventricular pacing thresholds and avoid phrenic nerve stimulation. Pacing Clin Electrophysiol 2005; 28:1255–9.

174 Medina-Ravell VA, Lankipalli RS, Yan GX, et al. Effect of epicardial or biventricular pacing to prolong QT interval and increase transmural dispersion of repolarization: does resynchronization therapy pose a risk for patients predisposed to long QT or torsade de pointes? Circulation 2003; 107:740–6.

175 Albert CM. Cardiac resynchronization therapy and proarrhythmia: weathering the storm. J Cardiovasc Electrophysiol 2008; 19:716–9.

176 Germano JJ, Reynolds M, Essebag V, Josephson ME. Frequency and causes of implantable cardioverter-defibrillator therapies: Is device therapy proarrhythmic? Am J Cardiol 2006; 97:1255–61.

177 Mykytsey A, Maheshwari P, Dhar G, et al. Ventricular tachycardia induced by biventricular pacing in patient with severe ischemic cardiomyopathy. J Cardiovasc Electrophysiol 2005; 16:655–8.

11 Radiography of Implantable Devices

David L. Hayes, Paul A. Friedman, Samuel J. Asirvatham
Mayo Clinic, Rochester, MN, USA

Introduction 554
Pulse generators 554
  Other types of pulse generators 556
Leads 558
  Pacemaker leads 560
    Intracardiac position 563
  Transvenous atrial leads 564
  Transvenous ventricular leads 567
  Epicardial leads 572

ICD leads 572
  Epicardial ICD leads 572
  Transvenous ICD leads 572
Coronary venous leads 577
Miscellaneous considerations 583
Conclusions 585
References 588

Cardiac Pacing, Defibrillation and Resynchronization: A Clinical Approach, Third Edition.
David L. Hayes, Samuel J. Asirvatham, and Paul A. Friedman.
© 2013 Mayo Foundation for Medical Education and Research. Published 2013 by John Wiley & Sons, Ltd.

Introduction

The chest X-ray remains an important tool in the pre-operative and postoperative evaluation of a pacemaker, implantable cardioverter-defibrillator (ICD) or cardiac resynchronization therapy (CRT) system. Additionally, the chest radiograph is essential when assessing the integrity of a pacing or ICD system. Both a poster-oanterior (PA) and a lateral view should be obtained. A systematic approach should be employed, evaluating various anatomic and device components in an orderly fashion.[1-3]

Preoperatively, the presence of clips, wires, prosthetic valves, and other hardware can provide clues to prior cardiac or thoracic surgery, which may be important when planning the operative procedure. After implantation of the pacing, ICD or CRT system, both PA and lateral radiographs should be obtained to confirm correct lead position(s) (Fig. 11.1) and to note potential surgical complications such as pneumothorax, pleural effusion, and pericardial effusion. (In addition, an oblique film may at times be helpful to determine more precisely the location of a coronary venous lead.) A chest radiograph should be performed as part of most device troubleshooting assessments. Table 11.1 provides a systematic approach to assessment of the chest radiograph of the patient with a device. Comparison with any previous radiographs is frequently useful. As part of the "total" care of the patient, inspection of the entire radiograph should be carried out, including: bony structures, aorta, cardiac silhouette, trachea, diaphragm, and lung fields.

Pulse generators

Most pulse generators are placed in a prepectoral location, inferior to the clavicle and medial to the axilla. At one time, many implants in children as well as many early ICDs were placed in an abdominal position, either below or anterior to the rectus muscle. If the pulse generator is located in an abdominal position, radiographic evaluation requires an AP radiograph of the abdomen as well as a PA and lateral chest radiograph.

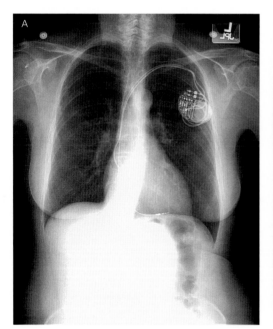
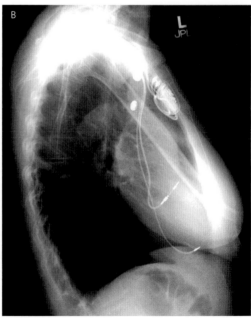

Fig. 11.1 Posteroanterior (A) and lateral (B) chest radiographs of a dual-chamber pacing system. The pulse generator is located in a left prepectoral position. The position of both atrial and ventricular leads is acceptable. The "J" on the atrial lead is adequate, and is best seen in the lateral view. The ventricular lead is not positioned in a true apical position but is well seated with adequate slack. In a true apical position, it would be seen closer to the sternum in the lateral view. (Reproduced with permission from Hayes DL. Radiography of implantable arrhythmia management devices. In: Kusumoto F, Goldschlager N, eds. Cardiac Pacing for the Clinician. New York: Springer Science + Business Media, 2007.)

Table 11.1 Systematic approach to radiographic assessment of pacemakers and ICDs.

Systematic approach	Clinical considerations
Determine pulse generator site	Any suggestion that there has been a significant shift from intended position, e.g., displaced generator, could be associated with lead dislodgment or Twiddler's
Determine pulse generator manufacturer, polarity, and model if possible	Radiographic identifiers allow determination of manufacturer – helpful if the patient comes without ID card
Inspect the connector block	Polarity of pulse generator should be determined and compared with polarity of leads

Is connector pin(s) completely through connector block? Loose connection could explain intermittent or complete failure to output or intermittent failure to capture |
Consider venous route utilized	Especially important if a pacemaker system revision is being considered, i.e., can the same venous route be accessed and how many leads are already placed in a single vein
Determine lead polarity	Does lead polarity match pulse generator polarity or has some type of adaptor been used to allow the system hardware combination?
Determine lead position	Determine where the lead was positioned, i.e., for the ventricular lead, is it in the apex, outflow tract, septal position, coronary sinus?; for the atrial lead, is it atrial appendage, lateral wall, septal position, coronary sinus?
Does lead position appear radiographically acceptable?	Inadequate lead position may explain failure to capture and/or sense. Compare current X-ray to previous X-ray if possible. Is ventricular lead redundancy or "slack" adequate; is atrial "J" adequate?
Inspect entire length of lead for integrity, i.e., fracture, compression, crimp, etc.	Intermittent or complete failure to capture/sense and/or output could be secondary to lead conductor coil fracture or loss of insulation integrity. Attempt to follow each lead along its course assessing the conductor coil. Also inspect for any "crimping" of the lead as it passes under the clavicle
Any other chest X-ray abnormality that is potentially related	For a recent implant, be certain there is no pneumothorax or hemopneumothorax. For the ICD patient with a change in defibrillation thresholds, whether acute or chronic, remember that a pneumothorax can be responsible for alterations in DFT
If no abnormality is appreciated radiographically but there is a clinical abnormality – reassess the chest X-ray in a problem-oriented fashion	As an example, if the patient has intermittent failure to output, the differential diagnosis would include a problem with the connector pin, i.e., loose setscrew, or conductor coil fracture. Go back once again and inspect these elements of the pacing system

In some patients a subpectoral position may be used in lieu of the more common prepectoral location but these positions are difficult to differentiate radiographically.

The retromammary position was once advocated for a better cosmetic result. However, given the size of contemporary devices, this surgical approach is rarely necessary and long term is more difficult because of the more involved operative techniques required (Fig. 11.2). True axillary position has also been used in an effort to obtain a better cosmetic result, but due to the somewhat more complex implant technique as well as potential discomfort of the pulse generator in this position, use of this location is uncommon.

The pulse generator manufacturer and model can usually be identified from the chest radiograph. At one time, unique shape, size, and internal circuitry pattern were sufficient to identify a manufacturer and model.

Although this no longer holds true, all current devices have a radiopaque code identifying the manufacturer and model of the device or some alpha-numeric code by which the company's technical services group can identify the "family" of devices (Fig. 11.3, Table 11.2). After identification of the manufacturer, the technical support division of that manufacturer can identify the device and should be able to provide additional information obtained at the time of implant and kept on file with the pulse generator registration (leads utilized, configurations, thresholds, etc.). The relationship of redundant, coiled lead(s) to the generator in the pocket should be noted. It may be difficult to determine which lead is connected to the pulse generator and which lead is abandoned.

The polarity of the pulse generator should be determined. This can be ascertained by the number and type of connector pins, i.e., unipolar or coaxial bipolar.

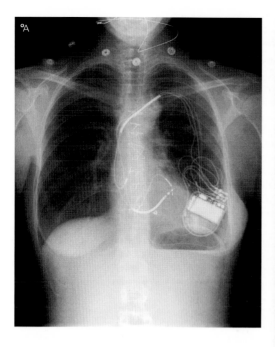
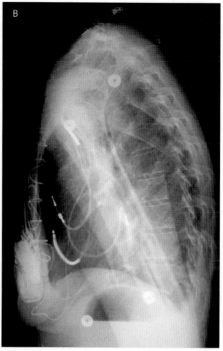

Fig. 11.2 (A) Posteroanterior and (B) lateral chest radiographs of a cardiac resynchronization therapy device (CRT-D), system with the pulse generator located in a retromammary position. Note that the right ventricular coil is in a low outflow/high septal position. The preferred view for distinguishing outflow tract and coronary sinus (CS) positions is the lateral view. In the lateral film, the right ventricular coil is just behind the sternum, whereas the CS leads wraps posteriorly in the CS, closer to the spine. (Reproduced with permission from Hayes DL. Radiography of implantable arrhythmia management devices. In: Kusumoto F, Goldschlager N, eds. Cardiac Pacing for the Clinician. New York: Springer Science + Business Media, 2007.)

(Recognition of a bifurcated bipolar lead is also possible, although there are a declining number of these leads that remain in service; Fig. 11.4.) Most contemporary pacemakers have independently programmable polarity, so the presence of bipolar leads does not necessarily imply that the device is functioning in a bipolar configuration.

Migration of a pulse generator is less common with the smaller devices used today. However, comparison of previous and current radiographs for pulse generator position is useful. The clinical concern about pulse generator migration is that tension may be placed on the lead, possibly causing dislodgment or fracture. It is not possible to determine from a radiograph whether the patient is a "twiddler," but a twisted appearance of the lead suggests Twiddler's syndrome, be it secondary to true patient manipulation of the pulse generator (Fig. 11.5)[4] or, more commonly, rotation of the pulse generator within an oversized pocket, also referred to as Reel syndrome (Fig. 11.6).[5,6]

Inspection of the generator connector block should be performed. The lead connector pin should be advanced beyond the setscrew(s) in the connector block, and the screws should be in direct contact with the pin. One cause of intermittent pacing failure, failure to output and/or failure to capture, is a loose connection between the setscrews and the connector pin (Fig. 11.7).

Other types of pulse generators

Although some implantable devices may not be readily identifiable, patient history, review of records, and assessment of available identification cards will usually reveal the type of device that has been implanted.

Implantable loop recorders are implanted with increasing frequency and appear as a small device usually in the pectoral region without an associated lead (Fig. 11.8).

Investigational devices may be more difficult to identify but most patients involved in an investigational protocol are often able to provide specific details. Figure

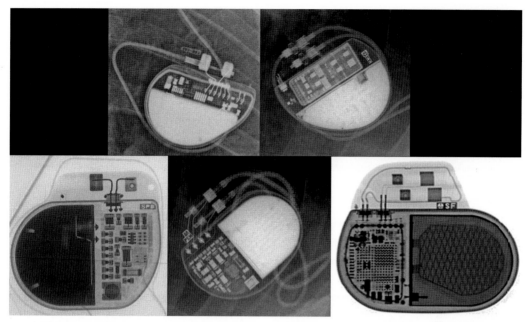

Fig. 11.3 Examples of radiographic identification of the pacemaker by radiographic codes embedded in the device. Upper left, Boston Scientific; upper right, St. Jude Medical; lower left, Sorin Medical; lower middle, Medtronic; lower right, Biotronik.

Table 11.2 Radiographic identifiers by manufacturer.

Manufacturer	
Biotronik	ICDs/CRT identified with a three-part code: year of manufacture, Biotronik logo, and a two-letter code unique to each device family; pacemakers identified with a two-part code: Biotronik logo and a two-letter code unique to each device family
Boston Scientific (Guidant)	Letters "BOS" to identify the manufacturer followed by a three-digit number which identifies which model software application is needed to communicate with the pulse generator; three-digit number does not correlate with a device model number. Note that older devices will have the designation "GDT" for devices manufactured by Guidant Corp.
Medtronic	Historically used a Medtronic-identifier symbol (Medtronic "M") followed by a unique alphanumeric identifier for each device "model." With current generation devices the radiographic identifier signifies a broader grouping or family of Medtronic devices. With the "group" identifier, technical services can provide a list of the specific models in that grouping.
St. Jude Medical	Each device has an alphanumeric series that corresponds to a specific model and can be identified from the technical manuals or by calling technical services
Sorin/ELA	ELA devices: the letters "ELA" appear and may have an additional model code. Sorin Group/Sorin Biomedica: Current devices consist of a three letter code beginning with "S" followed by both a group and a model letter. Previous Sorin Biomedica devices may have five letters

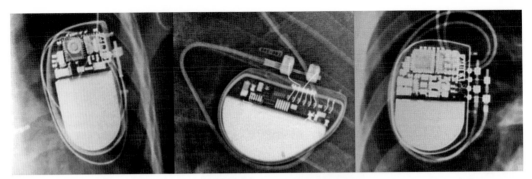

Fig. 11.4 Examples of three pulse generator polarity configurations, as described in the text. Left panel, unipolar polarity; middle panel, bipolar single-chamber pacemaker; right panel, dual-chamber bipolar configuration. (Modified with permission from Hayes DL. Radiography of implantable arrhythmia management devices. In: Kusumoto F, Goldschlager N, eds. Cardiac Pacing for the Clinician. New York: Springer Science + Business Media, 2007.)

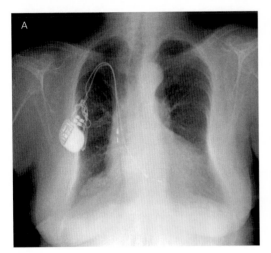
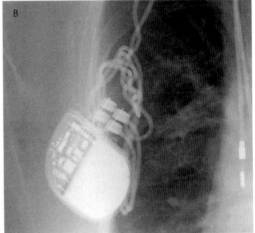

Fig. 11.5 (A) PA chest radiograph and (B) close-up in a patient with marked twisting of both leads resulting in lead retraction. This appearance is consistent with twiddler's syndrome.

11.9 demonstrates an ICD as well as an investigational device used for cardiac contractility modulation.

Always inspect the radiographic films for noncardiac hardware. Figure 11.10 demonstrates a patient with a pacemaker and a spinal stimulator.

Leads

Lead assessment is a critical component of the radiographic assessment of a pacing and/or ICD system. Standard radiographic techniques may not clearly demonstrate lead components. At one time, higher radiographic penetration and/or coning of the radiographic field was suggested to achieve better visualization of leads. However, if the radiograph has been stored digitally it may be possible to manipulate the images to better delineate the leads. Figure 11.11 demonstrates a PA chest radiograph before and after the contrast has been altered. Unfortunately, lead-insulating materials are not visualized radiographically, and loss of insulation integrity breech is a cause of lead failure that is not uncommon. Occasionally it is possible to see what appears to be a lack of continuity of the lead surface, which may correlate with a breech in the insulation (Fig. 11.12).

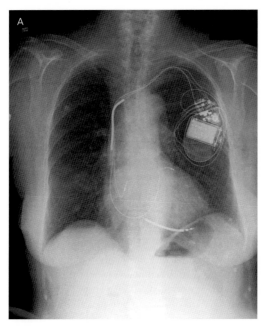
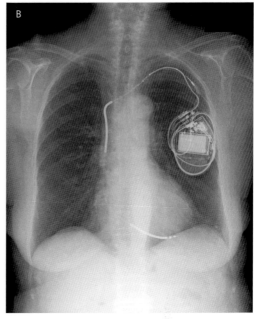

Fig. 11.6 (A) Posteroanterior radiograph from a patient following CRT-D implant. (B) Subsequent X-ray from the same patient the atrial lead and coronary sinus lead are completely retracted from the cardiac silhouette and looped or "reeled" around the pulse generator. This is a classic appearance of "Reel syndrome."

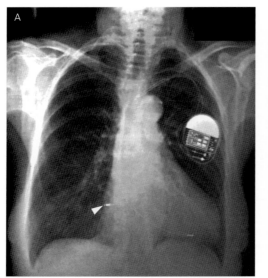
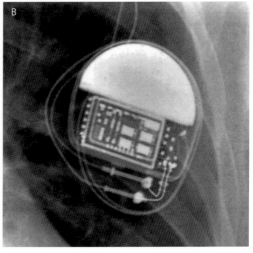

Fig. 11.7 (A) Posteroanterior radiograph and (B) close-up view from a patient with intermittent failure to pace. Comparison of the upper and lower pins reveals that the lower of the two unipolar leads is not completely advanced. This difference is more evident on the close-up view. By convention, the lower of the two leads in the connector block is the ventricular lead, so that this patient must have had intermittent or permanent ventricular failure to output. An unrelated observation, noted by the arrowhead, is shallow positioning of the atrial lead, i.e., the "J" is much wider than 90°. (From Hayes DL. Pacemaker radiography. In: Furman S, Hayes DL, Holmes DR Jr, eds. A Practice of Cardiac Pacing, 3rd edn. Mount Kisco, NY: Futura Publishing, 1993: 361–400, by permission of Mayo Foundation for Medical Education and Research.)

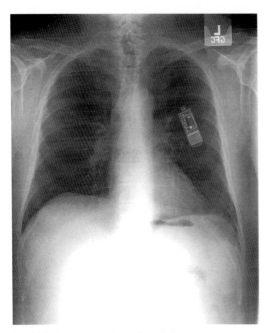

Fig. 11.8 Posteroanterior chest radiograph demonstrating an implantable loop recorder.

The number, types, location, and radiographic integrity of all leads should be determined after studying the PA and lateral radiographs. Unlike pulse generators, leads do not have characteristic radiopaque markers to aid in their identification; however, information regarding the type and functional status of various leads can be obtained by their radiographic appearance.

It is not uncommon for a patient to have a cardiac rhythm device implanted and have a variety of functional and abandoned leads, both epicardial, transvenous, and/or coronary venous. If additional procedures are required and lead extraction is required, it may be necessary to determine the type, position, and integrity of all leads.

Pacemaker leads

The vast majority of contemporary pacing leads are placed transvenously, although patients may still have epicardial (myocardial) pacing wires placed after certain types of cardiac surgical repair or due to congenital cardiac anomalies. Intravascular insertion of transvenous leads is usually through either the right or left axillary, subclavian, or cephalic veins. The internal

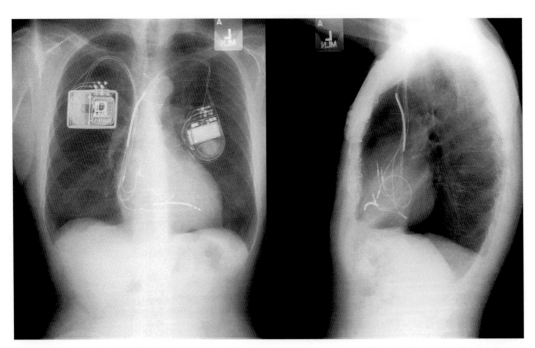

Fig. 11.9 Posteroanterior chest radiograph from a patient with a CRT-D device (pulse generator in left pectoral region) as well as a pulse generator on the right side. The right-sided pulse generator is an investigational device for the purpose of cardiac contractility modulation.

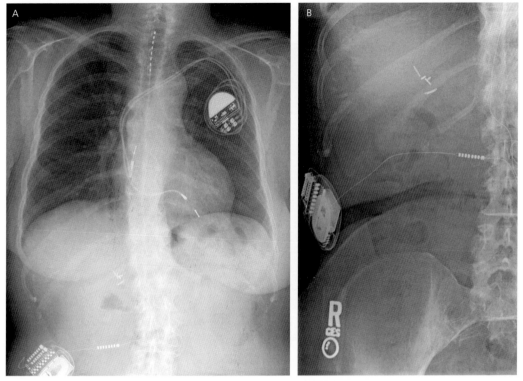

Fig. 11.10 (A) Posteroanterior chest radiograph and (B) abdominal film. A dual-chamber pacemaker is present in the left prepectoral position. In addition, on the PA film, a lead and the superior portion of another pulse generator can be seen in the lower right portion of the film. On the abdominal X-ray (B) the other pulse generator, a spinal cord stimulator and associated lead, can be more easily visualized.

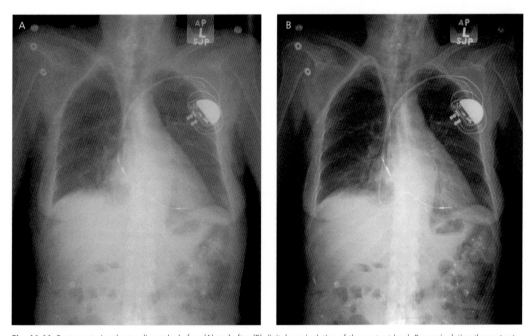

Fig. 11.11 Posteroanterior chest radiographs before (A) and after (B) digital manipulation of the contrast level. By manipulating the contrast the pacemaker leads can be more easily seen in (B).

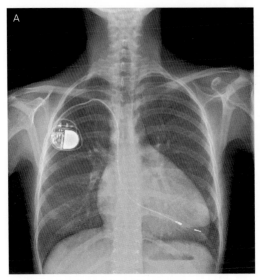

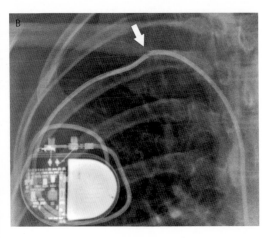

Fig. 11.12 (A) Posteroanterior chest radiograph and (B) close-up of a portion of the posteroanterior film demonstrating a disruption of the outer portion of the lead, presumably the insulation, with the appearance that the conductor coil is intact (arrowhead). In this patient, chronic pacing thresholds were considered acceptable and unchanged.

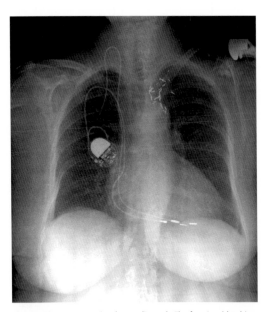

Fig. 11.13 Posteroanterior chest radiograph. The functional lead is placed in the subclavian vein; a portion of a much older transected second lead remains that was inserted through the right jugular vein. (Reproduced with permission from Hayes DL. Radiography of implantable arrhythmia management devices. In: Kusumoto F, Goldschlager N, eds. Cardiac Pacing for the Clinician. New York: Springer Science + Business Media, 2007.)

or external jugular veins have been used in the past, but should not be considered a good alternative for lead placement at this time (Fig. 11.13). Jugular vein insertion sites are usually easily identified by the lead coursing over or under the clavicle.

Clues as to the insertion site may be obtained from the chest radiograph by a change in the directional contour of the lead (Fig. 11.14). A more medial insertion site suggests a subclavian approach; a more lateral site suggests a cephalic or axillary approach.

A femoral approach may occasionally be needed if access via the superior veins is not an option. An X-ray of the pelvis and abdomen is necessary to assess adequately the course and integrity of the lead (Fig. 11.15).

The radiopaque conductor coil should be inspected in its entirety. There should be no discontinuity of the coil (Fig. 11.16); any kinking or sharp angulation may represent lead fracture. Special attention should be paid to the area between the first rib and the clavicle, as this is a frequent site of lead fracture (subclavian crush syndrome) (Fig. 11.17).[7]

Indentations caused by ligatures compressing the insulating material of a lead (Fig. 11.18) do not usually have any clinical significance. Such indentations do not imply the presence of lead damage, although it is possible to affect lead integrity with excessively tight ligatures placed around the sleeve.

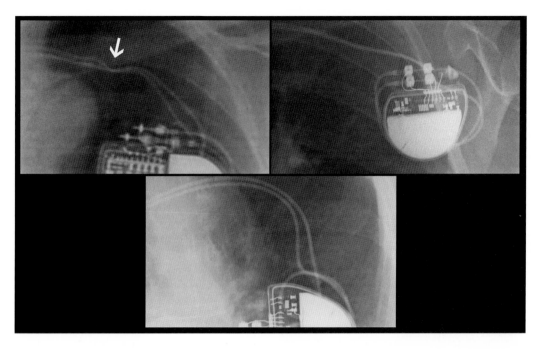

Fig. 11.14 Radiographs demonstrating different venous routes for permanent lead placement. Upper left, subclavian vein placement. Note compression of the lead as it passes between the first rib and the clavicle (arrow); upper right, axillary vein placement; bottom, cephalic vein placement.

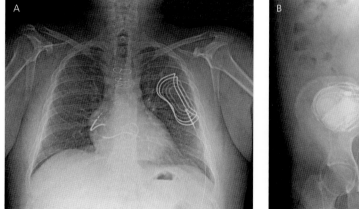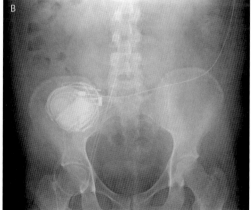

Fig. 11.15 (A) Posteroanterior chest radiograph and (B) abdominal film from a patient with the lead implanted via the femoral vein. The course of the defibrillation leads is through the inferior vena cava to the right atrium and right ventricular position. Also seen is an extravascular subcutaneous patch over the left heart, necessary to create a shocking vector encompassing the left ventricle.

It is generally difficult to make a radiographic determination regarding the diameter or "French" size of the implanted leads. Traditionally leads have been "stylet-driven." Newer leads are "lumenless" and of significantly smaller size.[8] Such leads may be more difficult to detect and follow on the radiograph (Fig. 11.19).

Intracardiac position

In order to appreciate abnormal lead position, a detailed description of the normal radiographic appearance is necessary.

Leads should have a modest amount of redundancy present. Undue tension on leads may result in poor

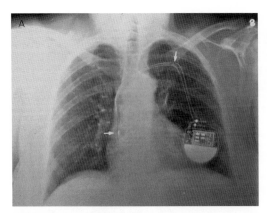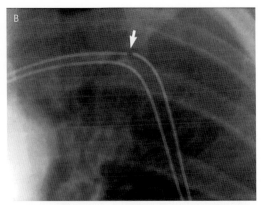

Fig. 11.16 (A) Posteroanterior chest radiograph demonstrating complete separation of the conductor coil of the ventricular lead as it passes below the clavicle (upper arrow). (The lower arrow notes a suboptimally positioned atrial lead which is too shallow.). (B) In the close-up view, the arrow again notes the separation of the conductor coil. (Reproduced with permission from Hayes DL. Radiography of implantable arrhythmia management devices. In: Kusumoto F, Goldschlager N, eds. Cardiac Pacing for the Clinician. New York: Springer Science + Business Media, 2007.)

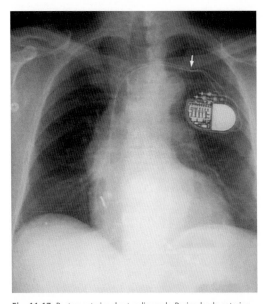

Fig. 11.17 Posteroanterior chest radiograph. Pacing leads entering via the subclavian vein. Note indentation (arrow) of the lead as it passes under the clavicle, signifying compression of the lead. (Reproduced with permission from Hayes DL. Radiography of implantable arrhythmia management devices. In: Kusumoto F, Goldschlager N, eds. Cardiac Pacing for the Clinician. New York: Springer Science + Business Media, 2007.)

pacing thresholds or frank dislodgment from the endocardial surface. In Fig. 11.20 both atrial and ventricular leads are positioned in such a way that they are too shallow. The atrial lead is most likely in the right atrial appendage. The atrial lead is not optimally positioned

and is best appreciated on the lateral view. The angle of the "J" is significantly greater than 90°. The ventricular lead is also much too shallow, and this can be appreciated in both views.

Generous lead redundancy is preferred in pediatric patients in an attempt to accommodate subsequent growth and minimize the number of lead revisions that will be required during a lifetime of pacing therapy (Fig. 11.21).

Unipolar leads have a single electrode (cathode) at the tip, whereas bipolar leads will have two electrodes separated by a variable interelectrode space (Fig. 11.22).

The type of lead fixation can often be determined by the chest radiograph (Fig. 11.23). Active fixation leads have a radiopaque screw, which is usually visible radiographically. The tines of a passive fixation lead cannot be visualized, so the absence of a "screw" would suggest a passive fixation mechanism.

Transvenous atrial leads

Atrial leads may have a preformed "J" shape, or the lead may be straight but positioned in the atrium in such a way that a "J" is formed. Preformed "J" leads are now used less frequently than standard leads for atrial application. Use of a preformed "J" may limit options to place the lead in alternative atrial positions.

Atrial leads have historically been most commonly positioned in the atrial appendage unless the atrial appendage had been surgically amputated. Regardless of whether a preformed "J" or a straight lead is implanted in the atrium, if implantation is in the right atrial appendage, the J portion of the lead is slightly medial on the PA projection and anterior on the lateral

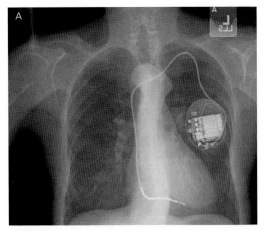

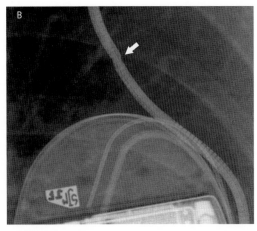

Fig. 11.18 (A) Posteroanterior and (B) close-up radiographic views of an indentation of the insulation material caused by excessive tightening of the ligature around the sleeve (see arrow). (Reproduced with permission from Hayes DL. Radiography of implantable arrhythmia management devices. In: Kusumoto F, Goldschlager N, eds. Cardiac Pacing for the Clinician. New York: Springer Science + Business Media, 2007.)

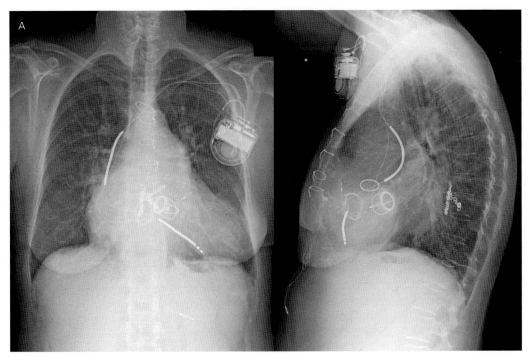

Fig. 11.19 (A) Posteroanterior and (B) lateral chest radiographs demonstrating a ventricular "lumenless" lead. The small diameter of the lead, 4 Fr, makes it somewhat more difficult to see on the radiograph.

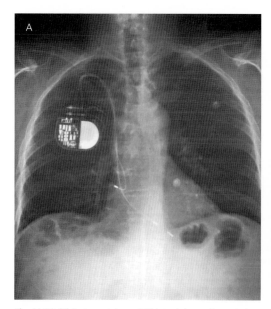

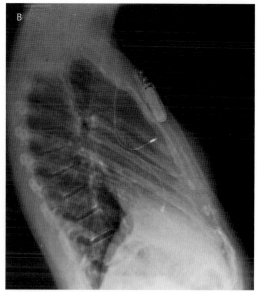

Fig. 11.20 (A) Posteroanterior and (B) lateral chest radiographs in a patient with suboptimal position of both leads. The ventricular lead position is also inadequate, i.e., too little slack has been left on the lead.

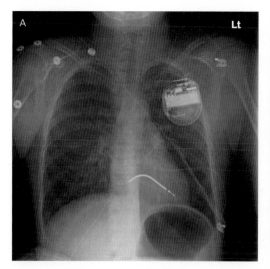

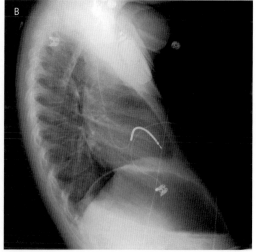

Fig. 11.21 (A) Posteroanterior and (B) lateral chest X-ray from a pediatric patient with a newly implanted pacemaker. Excessive redundancy has been left on the ventricular lead in an effort to allow for future growth.

projection. Optimally, the limits of the "J" should be no greater than approximately 80° apart. Redundancy proximal to the J within the atrium or superior vena cava should not be seen.

There is growing interest and enthusiasm for positioning the atrial lead in a septal position to avoid or minimize the intra-atrial conduction delay that may occur when the lead is positioned in the appendage (Fig. 11.24). Any portion of the free wall may also be targeted (Fig. 11.25), as long as there is mechanical stability and satisfactory thresholds can be obtained. Unlike the appendage, the remainder of the atrium is

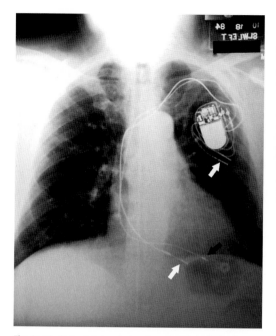

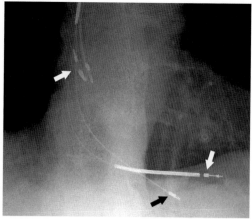

Fig. 11.23 Close-up portions of posteroanterior chest radiograph demonstrating four active fixation leads. One atrial lead is clearly bipolar (upper white arrow) and because of the projection of the other atrial lead it is difficult to determine the polarity of this lead with certainty. One ventricular lead is bipolar (lower white arrow) and the other unipolar (black arrow).

Fig. 11.22 Posteroanterior chest radiograph of a single-chamber pacing system. There is evidence of an abandoned bipolar lead in the vicinity of the pulse generator. There are two ventricular leads: one bipolar (white arrows) and one unipolar (black arrow). The bipolar lead is abandoned so the unipolar lead must be connected to this bipolar single-chamber pulse generator. This was accomplished by placing an indifferent electrode in the connector block where the (+) portion of an inline bifurcated bipolar lead would have been connected. Upon close inspection of the connector block one can discern that there is a visible difference between the pins in the (−) or lower and (+) or upper portions of the connector block.

not trabeculated, and active fixation leads are usually required to obtain mechanical stability.

Pacing for the reduction or prevention of atrial fibrillation remains somewhat controversial. However, techniques that have been used include positioning the lead in the atrial septum or the use of two atrial leads.[9–11] In Fig. 11.26, one lead is positioned in the right atrial appendage and the other lead on the posterior septum near the coronary sinus os. Pacing the atrium via the coronary sinus has also been advocated, but has never been widely performed. A large posterior curve suggests placement in the coronary sinus, although it could also suggest placement across a patent foramen ovale or atrial septal defect into the left atrium.

Special note should be made of the appearance of a type of atrial lead used many years ago, which main-

tained the "J" shape by incorporating a retention wire into the lead (Fig. 11.27).[12] This lead design had the potential for the retention wire to fracture and protrude through the insulation, resulting in cardiac and/ or vascular laceration, or to migrate into extracardiac locations. Despite their age, there are still a small number of these leads in service and they require ongoing digital fluoroscopic surveillance because the retention wire itself may be difficult to visualize on a standard radiograph, even with significant protrusion or migration of the wire.

Transvenous ventricular leads

Transvenous ventricular leads are traditionally placed in the right ventricular apex. Radiographically, the lead should have a gentle contour with the tip of the lead pointing downward in the PA view and located between the left border of the vertebral column and the cardiac apex. The position of the heart, vertical or relatively more horizontal, largely determines the position of the lead in relation to the cardiac apex and varies among patients. The lateral view is necessary to distinguish an apical position in which the lead tip is anterior and caudally directed, is directed posteriorly in the right ventricle, or is on the posterior surface of the heart, i.e., within the coronary sinus. The ventricular lead should have a gentle curve along the lateral wall of the right atrium and cross the tricuspid valve to the ventricular

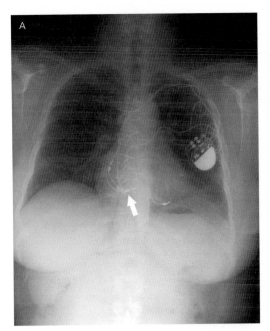
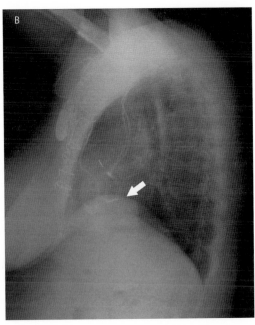

Fig. 11.24 (A) Posteroanterior and (B) lateral chest radiographs of a dual-chamber pacing system. This patient had long intra-atrial conduction time and in an attempt to normalize atrial activation the atrial lead was placed on the intra-atrial septum. Note that in the posteroanterior radiograph the atrial lead is not on the free wall and is located close to the tricuspid annulus. On the lateral radiograph the lead is seen to be posterior. This is the typical radiographic appearance of an atrial lead positioned on the low atrial septum just posterior to the coronary sinus. (Reproduced with permission from Hayes DL. Radiography of implantable arrhythmia management devices. In: Kusumoto F, Goldschlager N, eds. Cardiac Pacing for the Clinician. New York: Springer Science + Business Media, 2007.)

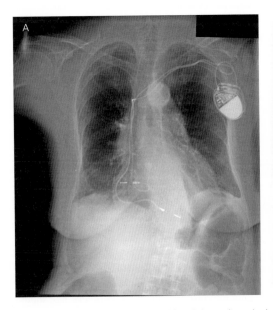
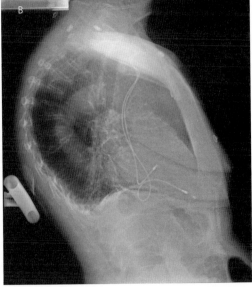

Fig. 11.25 (A) Posteroanterior (PA) and (B) lateral chest radiographs demonstrate an atrial position other than the atrial appendage. The lead is positioned laterally.

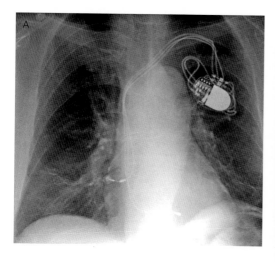

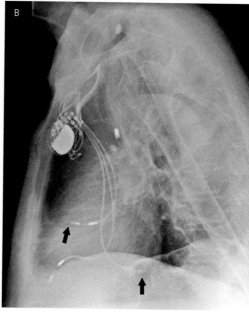

Fig. 11.26 (A) Posteroanterior and (B) lateral chest radiographs of a dual-site atrial pacing system. Leads are positioned in the pacing system. Leads are positioned in the right atrium (upper black arrow), posterior atrial septum (lower black arrow), and right ventricular apex.

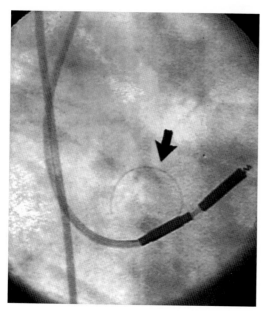

Fig. 11.27 Digital fluoroscopy of Accufix™ 330–801 active fixation atrial lead. The arrow denotes fractured and protruding retention wire. (Reproduced with permission.)

apex (Fig. 11.1). It may be preferable to place the lead on the right ventricular septum or outflow tract (Fig. 11.28).

There is growing interest in placement of the leads in a nonapical position, given the potential for adverse hemodynamics from an apically placed lead. Although the data are inconclusive regarding the long-term hemodynamic advantages of a nonapical position and the potential superiority of one nonapical position over another, i.e., low septal, mid-septal, or His bundle vicinity, there is enough experience with nonapical positioning to state that it is feasible and safe.[13–15]

A nonapical position may also be chosen for specific pacing applications. The radiographs in Fig. 11.9 contain multiple leads in multiple right ventricular positions. The patient has a right ventricular apical lead that is part of an original ICD system. The leads connected to the device located in the right pre-pectoral region are part of a cardiac contractility modulation device placed as part of a clinical investigation. The leads are positioned in the posterior septum and the anterior septum. Figure 11.29 demonstrates a patient with the ventricular lead position in the right

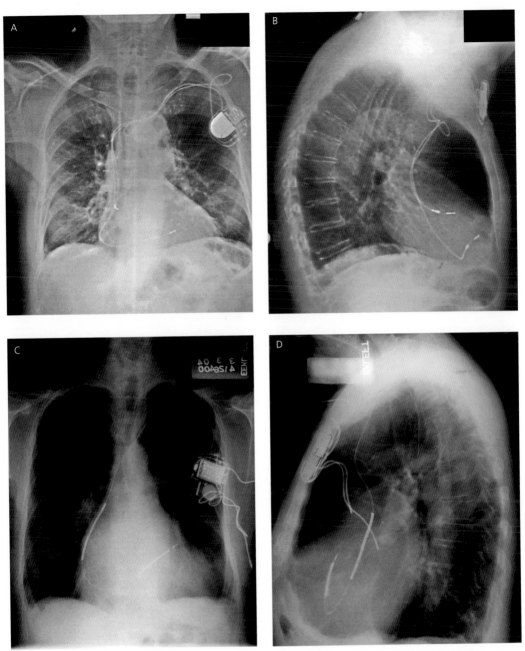

Fig. 11.28 (A) Posteroanterior and (B) lateral chest radiographs in a patient with the ventricular lead positioned in the very low right ventricular outflow tract. The lateral view is necessary for absolute determination of the position of this lead. (C) Posteroanterior and (D) lateral chest radiographs in a patient with the ventricular lead positioned in the septum. (A and B, Reproduced with permission from Hayes DL. Radiography of implantable arrhythmia management devices. In: Kusumoto F, Goldschlager N, eds. Cardiac Pacing for the Clinician. New York: Springer Science + Business Media, 2007.)

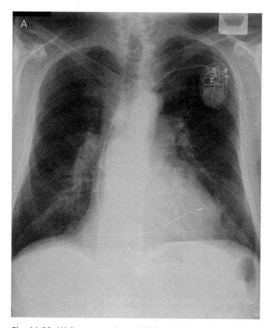
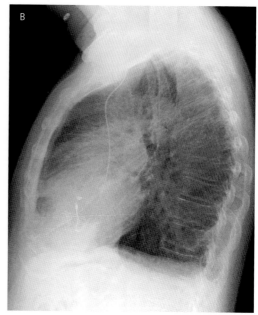

Fig. 11.29 (A) Posteroanterior and (B) lateral chest radiograph of a patient with a pulse generator and a single lead positioned in the right ventricular outflow.

ventricular outflow tract for the purpose of hemodynamic monitoring. Because of the potential benefit of avoiding the adverse consequences of right ventricular apical lead positioning, lead placement in the right ventricular outflow tract or septal positions continue to gain popularity. Figure 11.30 represents a combination of epicardial leads that are being actively used and abandoned transvenous new leads in a patient with a congenital anatomic abnormality.

A left ventricular endocardial position has historically been considered undesirable and was likely not intentionally placed within the left ventricle (Fig. 11.31).[16] Although there is a growing experience with left ventricular endocardial pacing for purposes of resynchronization,[17,18] this technique has not yet gained popularity because of concern related to the thromboembolic potential of having a lead permanently positioned in the systemic circulation. However, leads intended for right-sided placement may reach the left ventricular cavity through perforation of the ventricular septum, the lead having inadvertently crossed a patent foramen ovale, atrial septal defect, or ventricular septal defect during transvenous placement, and in the pericardial space as a result of perforation. The preferred view identifying a lead as terminating in the left ventricle is the lateral projection, in which the lead will be excessively posterior (toward the spine) (Fig. 11.32). If there is early recognition that a lead has inadvertently been placed in the left atrium or left ventricle, the lead should be withdrawn and repositioned in the right side of the heart.

Lead dislodgment may occur and may result in failure to capture and/or sense. Dislodgment may be obvious, i.e., macrodislodgment. Such dislodgment can be anywhere other than its original position, i.e., the pulmonary artery, coronary sinus, ventricular cavity, or superior or inferior vena cava. Dislodgment may not be identifiable radiographically. This has been labeled "microdislodgment" but, in the absence of X-ray documentation, there is no evidence of its presence. It is, therefore, a presumptive diagnosis. A "macrodislodged" atrial lead is shown in Fig. 11.33 and a "macrodislodged" ventricular lead is shown in Fig. 11.34.

It is often helpful to compare serial chest X-rays to confirm a lead dislodgment. In Fig. 11.35, PA chest X-rays from two consecutive days demonstrate a change in coronary venous lead position.

Single-lead VDD systems are not commonly used, but can be identified by an additional bipolar sensing electrode in the atrialized portion of the lead, which may or may not have contact with the endocardial surface (Fig. 11.36).

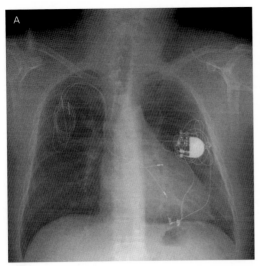

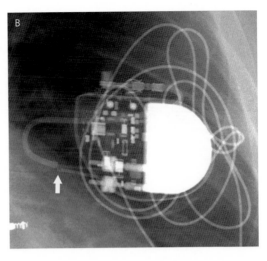

Fig. 11.30 (A) Posteroanterior (PA) chest radiograph of endocardial and epicardial pacing leads in a patient with D-transposition of the great vessel is status post Mustard procedure. From the right infraclavicular region the endocardial leads enter the heart through the superior vena cava, then into the atrium. The leads course anterior to the baffle connecting the pulmonary veins into the right ventricle. The atrial lead is in an atypical left atrial location anterior to the baffle. The ventricular lead enters the morphologic left ventricle proximal to its apex. The epicardial system is seen in the left chest with screw-in leads placed posteriorly and inferiorly into the ventricle. An atrial lead has not been placed. (B) A close-up from the PA radiograph notes the presence of a "Y" connector which connects two ventricular epicardial leads to this single chamber ventricular pacemaker. On this close-up there is a defect in the lead adaptor just as it exits the connector block (arrow).

Epicardial leads

Epicardial pacing leads are used in patients with specific congenital cardiac abnormalities, some pediatric patients, and in patients with right atrioventricular valve prostheses (Fig. 11.37). The lead(s) are tunneled to the pulse generator either in the pectoral or abdominal area. Historically, epicardial leads have had a higher incidence of lead failure, and a transvenous approach is generally preferred if possible (Fig. 11.38).

When epicardial leads are present and the pulse generator is located in an abdominal position, it should be remembered that this position seems to increase the likelihood of lead fracture. Although longevity of epicardial leads has yet to be equal to transvenous pacing leads,[19] contemporary epicardial lead function has improved.[20]

ICD leads
Epicardial ICD leads

Currently used infrequently (Fig. 11.39), such systems usually have easily recognizable patches positioned over the heart, as well as epicardial or transvenous pacing leads for sensing and pacing purposes. Depending on the manufacturer, the actual defibrillation coils may or may not be easily visualized. One manufacturer's epicardial patches feature a radiopaque marker around the periphery of the patch; this is not active, and a fracture of this marker does not reflect on the integrity of the patch. The actual coils of these patches are radiolucent and not visible on the radiograph. A frequent site of fracture in all epicardial patches is at the patch–lead junction, and this area should be carefully inspected.

Transvenous ICD leads

ICD leads most commonly have an active fixation mechanism, but may be passive, and like pacing leads should have a gentle redundancy. Leads may have a single high-voltage coil in the right ventricle, or may have an additional coil in the superior vena cava area (Figs 11.40 and 11.41).[21,22] Rarely, an additional subclavian lead, subcutaneous patch, or array[23] may be used in order to obtain satisfactory defibrillation thresholds (Fig. 11.42). As with pacing leads, the insertion into the connector block and the connection with the setscrews should be noted. All leads and patches should be

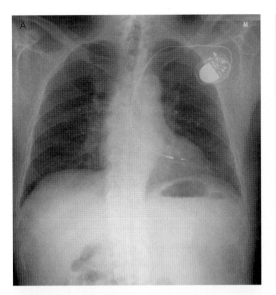
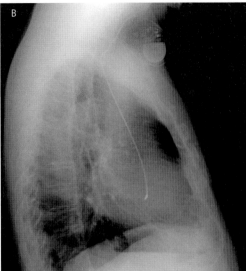

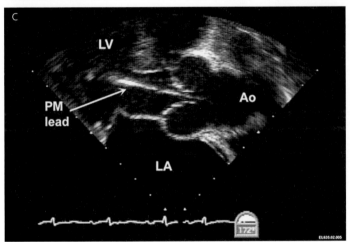

Fig. 11.31 (A) Posteroanterior and (B) lateral chest radiographs demonstrating a ventricular lead that courses over the spine, is relatively straight, and is positioned in an unusually high position when viewed on the posteroanterior film (A). On the lateral film (B), the lead is seen to course posteriorly, which is consistent with a left ventricular position. On a still frame from the two-dimensional echocardiogram (C), the lead is seen crossing the aortic valve and residing in the left ventricle. The lead had been placed inadvertently via the subclavian artery. (Reproduced with permission from Hayes DL. Radiography of implantable arrhythmia management devices. In: Kusumoto F, Goldschlager N, eds. Cardiac Pacing for the Clinician. New York: Springer Science + Business Media, 2007.)

inspected for obvious fracture, and for unusual bending or kinking. Subcutaneous patches and arrays are usually placed inferior and posterior to the axilla, and lateral and/or customized oblique views may be required to obtain satisfactory visualization of a patch.

At any given point in time there are usually one or more ICD leads that are on "advisory" because of poor performance or structural problems that develop. Occasionally, such structural problems are identifiable radiographically. A current example is one in which the conductor cable may become externalized, i.e., erode through the insulation (Fig. 11.43).[24] It is important to be aware of any radiographic appearance that may help identify a defective lead.

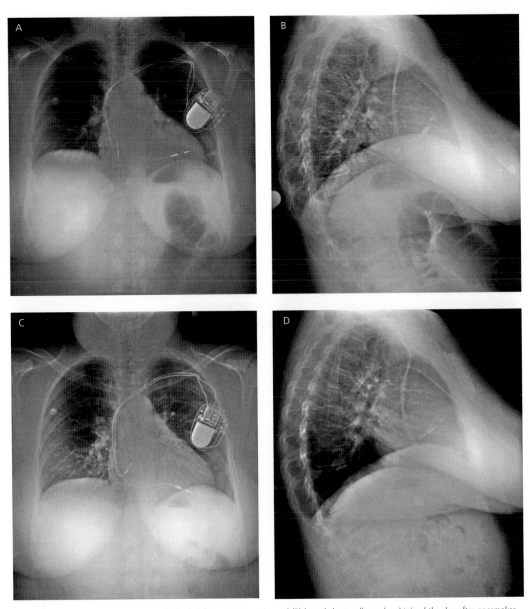

Fig. 11.32 Unusual course of the ventricular lead. (A) In posteroanterior and (B) lateral chest radiographs obtained the day after pacemaker implantation, the lead has a "high take-off," as it begins to cross to the left from the atrial position. This lead had been passed across an unknown patent foramen ovale and positioned in the left ventricle. (C) Posteroanterior and (D) lateral chest radiographs obtained the day after the lead had been withdrawn and repositioned in the right ventricular apex. (A,C, From Hayes DL. Complications; and Lloyd MA, Hayes DL. Pacemaker and ICD radiography. In: Hayes DL, Lloyd MA, Friedman PA, eds. Cardiac Pacing and Defibrillation: a Clinical Approach. Armonk, NY: Futura Publishing, 2000: 453–84, 485–517, by permission of Mayo Foundation for Medical Education and Research.)

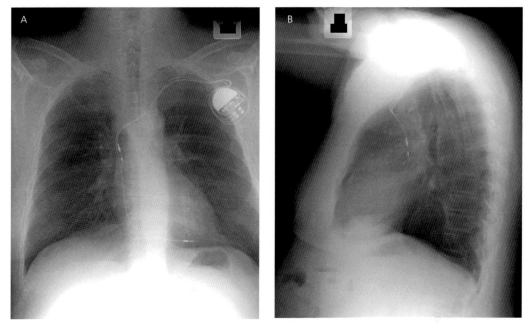

Fig. 11.33 (A) Posteroanterior and (B) lateral chest radiograph demonstrating a grossly dislodged (macrodislodgment) atrial lead.

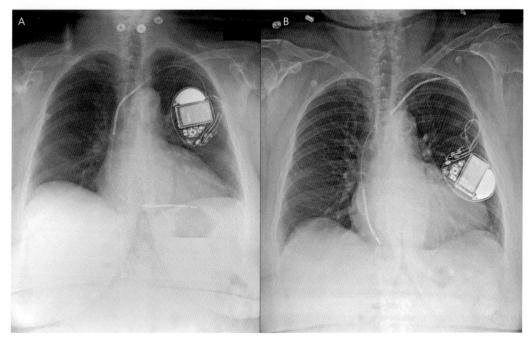

Fig. 11.34 (A) Posteroanterior chest radiograph taken after the implantation of a single-chamber ICD with a dual-coil lead. (B) A subsequent posteroanterior chest radiograph demonstrate macrodislodgement of the ventricular lead.

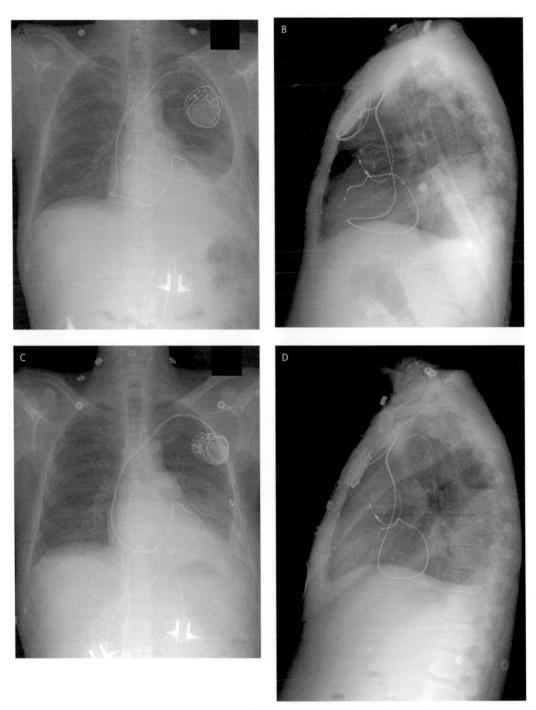

Fig. 11.35 (A) Posteroanterior (PA) and (B) lateral chest radiograph taken the day after CRT device implantation. The coronary sinus lead appears to be adequately positioned. (C) PA and (D) lateral chest radiograph taken the day after CRT device implantation. The coronary sinus lead has definitely moved, with radiographic evidence of a less distal position on the second set of radiographs. Note the absence of a right ventricular lead – all ventricular pacing is from the left ventricle in this system. (Reproduced with permission from Hayes DL. Radiography of implantable arrhythmia management devices. In: Kusumoto F, Goldschlager N, eds. Cardiac Pacing for the Clinician. New York: Springer Science + Business Media, 2007.)

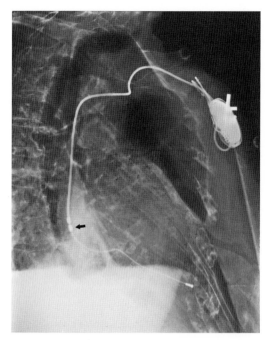

Fig. 11.36 Oblique chest radiograph of a VDD pacing system. Sensing electrodes are located on the "atrialized" portion of the lead (arrow) and the ventricular lead functions in a unipolar pacing configuration. (Reproduced with permission from Furman SF, Hayes DL, Holmes DR Jr. A Practice of Cardiac Pacing. Mt Kisco, NY. Futura Publishing Company, Inc., 1986.)

Coronary venous leads

Coronary sinus lead placement was used many years ago, but lost favor because of the high rate of lead dislodgment. However, with the advent of CRT, placing a permanent lead in the coronary venous system has become commonplace. Atrial pacing can also be achieved via the coronary venous system, but this is not commonly performed for permanent pacing.

Radiographic evaluation of a CRT system requires the caregiver assessing the radiograph to have a familiarity with coronary venous anatomy and lead placement. The placement of the left ventricular lead will vary due to variations in coronary sinus anatomy. There has been some enthusiasm for radiographic evaluation of the coronary venous system with computed tomography (CT) venography prior to attempt CRT implant.[25,26] This technique may provide additional preimplant information regarding variations in coronary venous anatomy, potential target veins, etc. (Fig. 11.44).

The ventricle or atrium can be paced from the coronary sinus, depending on where the lead is positioned. The atrium is more likely paced when leads are positioned in the coronary sinus itself; the ventricle is paced with very distal placement, or in any of the ventricular tributaries, as usually used for CRT. Figures 11.45, 11.46 and 11.47 demonstrate coronary

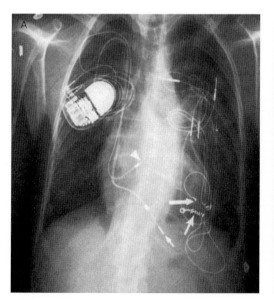
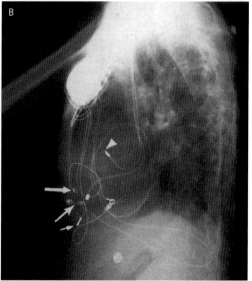

Fig. 11.37 (A) Posteroanterior and (B) lateral chest radiographs demonstrating several types of pacing leads, as described in the text. The arrowhead indicates active fixation of the atrial endocardial lead; large arrow, an abandoned stab-in epicardial lead; medium arrow, an abandoned screw-in epicardial lead; and small arrow, a passive fixation transvenous lead. (Reproduced with permission from Hayes DL. Radiography of implantable arrhythmia management devices. In: Kusumoto F, Goldschlager N, eds. Cardiac Pacing for the Clinician. New York: Springer Science + Business Media, 2007.)

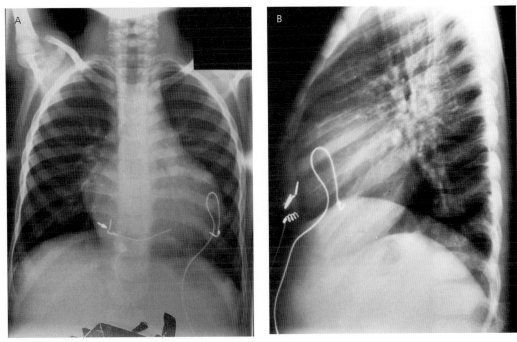

Fig. 11.38 (A) Posteroanterior and (B) lateral chest X-ray from a patient with three epicardial pacing leads. There are two "stab-in" leads, one of which is fractured (arrow). There is also a single screw-in ventricular epicardial lead. (Reproduced with permission from Furman SF, Hayes DL, Holmes DR Jr. A Practice of Cardiac Pacing. Mt Kisco, NY. Futura Publishing Company, Inc., 1986.)

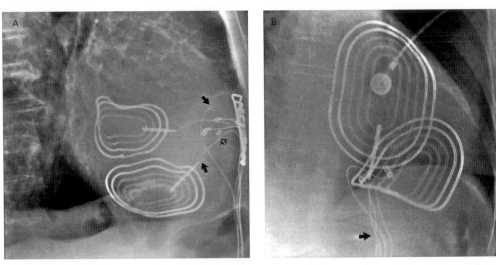

Fig. 11.39 (A) Lateral (LAT) chest radiograph (B) posteroanterior (PA) radiographs that demonstrate fracture of the epicardial patch (arrows). Note the posterior positioning of the patches in the lateral view consistent with idea location on the posterior and posterolateral left ventricle. (Reproduced with permission from Brady PA, Friedman PA, Trusty JM, Grice S, Hammill SC, Stanton MS. High failure rate for an epicardial implantable cardioverter-defibrillator lead: implications for long-term follow-up of patients with an implantable cardioverter-defibrillator. J Am Coll Cardiol 1998; 31:616–22.)

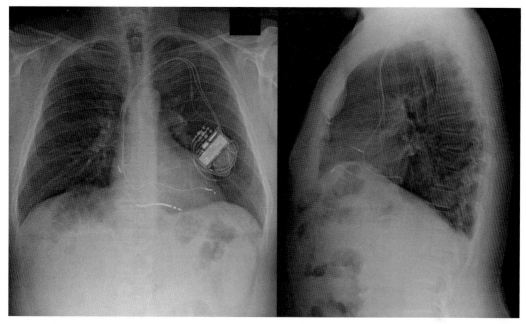

Fig. 11.40 (A) Posteroanterior and (B) lateral chest radiographs of an implantable cardioverter-defibrillator (ICD) system. The ICD is connected to a single-coil ventricular lead.

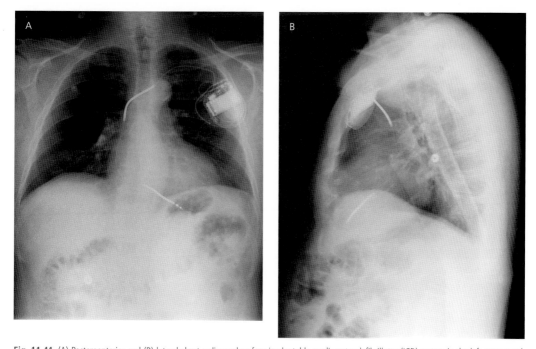

Fig. 11.41 (A) Posteroanterior and (B) lateral chest radiographs of an implantable cardioverter-defibrillator (ICD) system in the left prepectoral position. The ICD is connected to a dual-coil ventricular lead.

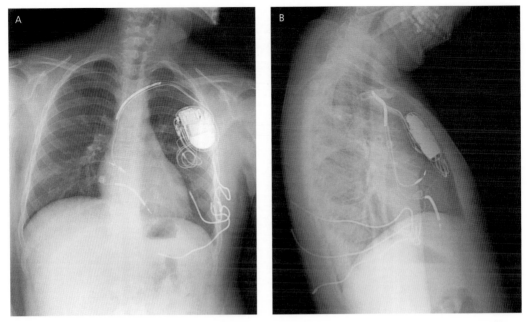

Fig. 11.42 (A) Posteroanterior and (B) lateral chest radiographs from a patient with an implantable cardioverter-defibrillator. Unacceptable defibrillation thresholds necessitated placement of a subcutaneous array.

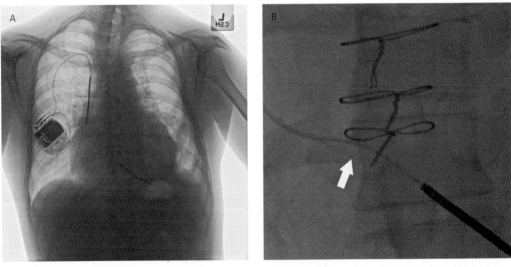

Fig. 11.43 (A) Posteroanterior chest radiograph from a patient with a St. Jude Medical Riata lead. Close inspection reveals cables that have been externalized from the lead as a result of an inside-out erosion of the insulation. (B) This is more apparent on a close-up of the specific area.

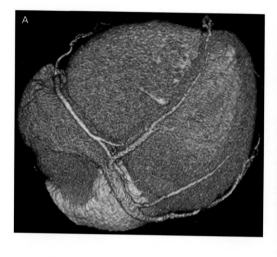

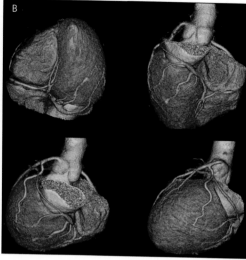

Fig. 11.44 (A) Computed tomography (CT) venography larger image of a single view and (B) a composite of images demonstrating coronary venous system by CT angiography.

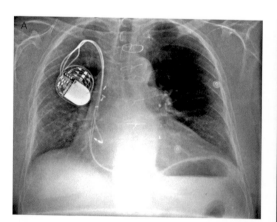

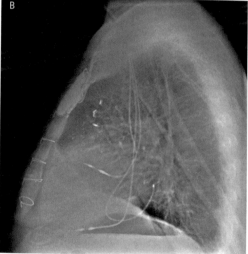

Fig. 11.45 (A) Posteroanterior and (B) lateral chest radiographs from a patient with right atrial, right ventricular, and coronary sinus leads. In the posteroanterior view the coronary sinus lead is noted to be leftward and closer to the lateral wall, where as on the lateral view the coronary sinus lead is seen to be the most posterior of the three leads. This is consistent with posterolateral cardiac venous positioning of this lead. The large distance between the left and right ventricular lead electrodes is desirable for cardiac resynchronization. (Reproduced with permission from Hayes DL. Radiography of implantable arrhythmia management devices. In: Kusumoto F, Goldschlager N, eds. Cardiac Pacing for the Clinician. New York: Springer Science + Business Media, 2007.)

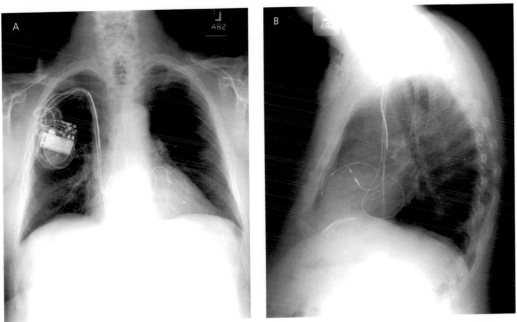

Fig. 11.46 (A) Posteroanterior and (B) lateral chest radiographs from a patient with right atrial, right ventricular (RV), and coronary sinus leads. The coronary sinus lead is positioned in a lateral branch of the anterior interventricular cardiac vein. (Reproduced with permission from Hayes DL. Radiography of implantable arrhythmia management devices. In: Kusumoto F, Goldschlager N, eds. Cardiac Pacing for the Clinician. New York: Springer Science + Business Media, 2007.)

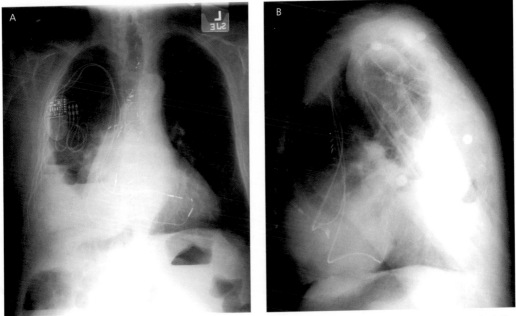

Fig. 11.47 (A) Posteroanterior and (B) lateral chest radiographs from a patient with right atrial, right ventricular, and coronary sinus leads. The coronary sinus lead has been placed on the posterolateral ventricular wall via the middle cardiac vein and then subselection into a lateral tributary of this vein. (Reproduced with permission from Hayes DL. Radiography of implantable arrhythmia management devices. In: Kusumoto F, Goldschlager N, eds. Cardiac Pacing for the Clinician. New York: Springer Science + Business Media, 2007.)

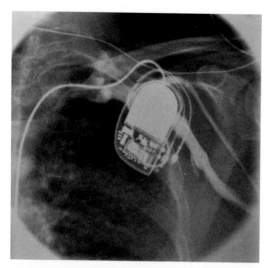

Fig. 11.48 Contrast material injection prior to pacemaker system revision demonstrates that the contrast material essentially stops, indicating extensive, if not total, obstruction of the subclavian vein. (Reproduced with permission from Furman SF, Hayes DL, Holmes DR Jr. A Practice of Cardiac Pacing. Mt Kisco, NY. Futura Publishing Company, Inc., 1986.)

sinus lead placement in the lateral anterior interventricular, and middle cardiac veins, respectively.

If assessing dislodgement of a coronary sinus lead, the lateral chest X-ray is paramount, as differentiation of a right ventricular outflow tract from coronary sinus site is difficult if not impossible on the PA image alone.

Miscellaneous considerations

Occasionally, it may be difficult to locate the subclavian vein, or the patency of the cephalic, axillary, or subclavian vein may be in question. Contrast material injected into a peripheral intravenous line in the ipsilateral upper extremity will define the venous anatomy as it flows into the central circulation, determining patency and guiding access (Fig. 11.48).[27] There is also evidence that using contrast-guided venous puncture on a routine basis will minimize the incidence of pneumothorax.[28]

There is also some interest and experience reported with contrast venograms performed with carbon dioxide, especially for those patients with allergy to standard contrast media.[29,30] We do not have any experience with this technique to date.

Management of the patient with a prosthetic tricuspid valve that requires permanent pacing requires special consideration. A single ventricular pacing lead can be placed across a bioprosthetic valve, but there is no way to predict if the lead will interfere with valve function or minimize the functional longevity of the bioprosthetic valve. Placement of the ventricular lead with echocardiographic guidance, as well as fluoroscopy, has been suggested in an effort to minimize trauma to the bioprosthetic valve. The goal of echocardiographic guidance would be to preferentially place the lead so that it was in a commissure of the bioprosthetic valve. Our experience with this approach is limited, but we have found that it is difficult, even with echocardiographic guidance, to be certain that the lead is within a commissure. Use of small French size leads that may be more "mobile" and preferentially settle in a commissure may be optimal (Fig. 11.19).[31]

A standard ventricular transvenous pacing lead cannot be placed across a mechanical prosthetic tricuspid valve. Several approaches have been used in this circumstance. If the need for permanent pacing is anticipated at the time of tricuspid valve replacement, some have advocated placing the transvenous lead outside the sewing ring of the tricuspid valve. The concern with this approach is the difficulties that would be encountered if the lead would need to be extracted at some future date or if the lead failed and another lead was necessary. Alternatively, transmural or transmyocardial ventricular pacing lead placement can be considered.[32] In this approach, a cardiac surgeon places an active fixation lead through the free wall of the right ventricle and the lead is actively fixated to the endocardial surface. A purse-string suture is placed around the lead where it passes through the right ventricular lead. Our limited but long-term success with this technique has been excellent (Fig. 11.49).[32]

Another option in the patient who has undergone tricuspid valve replacement or surgery, in whom it is desirable to avoid placing a lead across the tricuspid valve, or in the patient in whom ventricular access is limited because of congenital anomalies, would be to pace the ventricle via the coronary veins. (Fig. 11.50).[33]

The most common cardiovascular congenital anomaly encountered by the implanting physician is persistent left superior vena cava, in which the leads are placed through the left vena cava, into the coronary sinus and then into the right atrium.[34] The ventricular lead will usually need to be looped in order to direct it across the tricuspid valve into the right ventricle (Fig. 11.51). The diagnosis can be suspected by the finding of an enlarged coronary sinus at echocardiography, or by contrast injection into an ipsilateral intravenous line in the left upper extremity.

Congenital cardiovascular anomalies may require novel implantation techniques and may result in

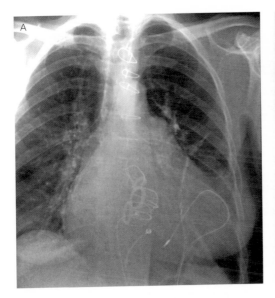

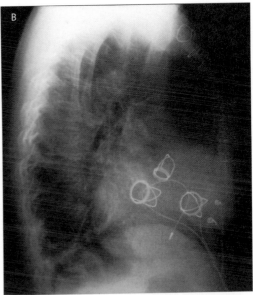

Fig. 11.49 (A) Posteroanterior and (B) lateral chest radiographs of a patient with prosthetic mitral and tricuspid valves. A ventricular lead passes through the free wall. (Reproduced with permission from Furman SF, Hayes DL, Holmes DR Jr. A Practice of Cardiac Pacing, 3rd edn. Mt Kisco, NY Futura Publishing Company, Inc., 1993.)

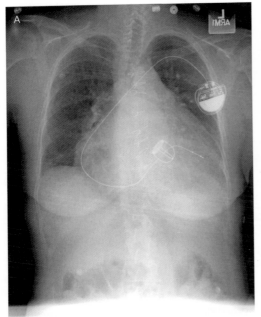

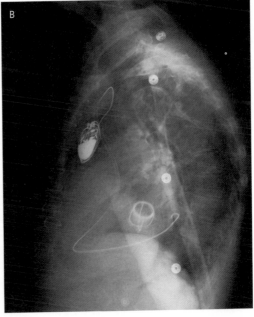

Fig. 11.50 (A) Posteroanterior and (B) lateral chest radiographs of a patient with prosthetic aortic, mitral, and tricuspid valves. A permanent pacemaker was needed for atrioventricular block. The ventricular pacing lead was placed via the coronary sinus into a lateral vein position.

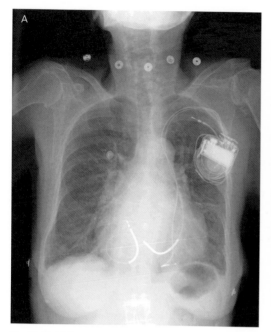
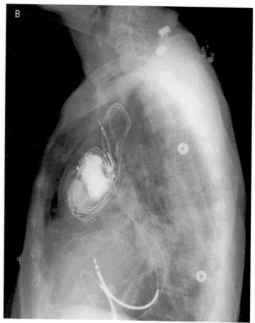

Fig. 11.51 (A) Posteroanterior and (B) lateral chest radiographs of a DDD pacing system in a patient with a persistent left superior vena cava. The atrial lead courses through the left superior vena cava and the coronary sinus and into the right atrium. The ventricular lead follows the same path, but is then looped into the right ventricle. (From Hayes DL. Implantation techniques. In: Hayes DL, Lloyd MA, Friedman PA, eds. Cardiac Pacing and Defibrillation: a Clinical Approach. Armonk, NY: Futura Publishing, 2000: 159–200. Used with permission of Mayo Foundation for Medical Education and Research.)

unusual lead placement. Knowledge of the native and corrected anatomy is essential when planning a procedure and when interpreting the chest radiograph; consultation with the congenital cardiologist or cardiovascular surgeon may be helpful (Figs 11.52 and 11.53).

As new technologies emerge there may be specific radiographic identifiers that a clinician interpreting the chest radiograph of the device patient should be aware. A recent example is a magnetic resonance imaging (MRI) conditionally safe pacemaker.[35] The pacemaker has a special radiographic identifier (Fig. 11.54) and the lead has a radiopaque helix (Fig. 11.55). Both of these can also be seen in the close-up of a patient chest radiograph in Fig. 11.56.

In some situations the chest radiograph may not provide the necessary diagnostic information and other imaging techniques may be needed. An echocardiogram may be helpful for confirmation of a lead position (Fig. 11.31C). CT may also be diagnostic in some situations when chest radiograph is not (Fig. 11.57).[36,37]

Conclusions

The chest radiograph provides important information about pacing, ICD, and CRT systems. As systems become more complex and specialized, and as indications for these devices expand, the importance of recognizing the normal and abnormal radiographic appearance of these systems is essential. A systematic evaluation of the anatomy and system components is necessary preoperatively, postoperatively, and during troubleshooting. When approaching a patient with suspected or known system malfunction, following the systematic radiographic evaluation in Table 11.1 can provide important clues to and/or the actual diagnosis. If a systematic radiographic approach is followed and no abnormalities are appreciated, the radiograph should be reassessed in a focused approach. For example, if the patient had presented with intermittent and/or consistent failure to output, both lead fracture and loose connector pin would be part of the differential diagnosis. The chest radiograph should then be

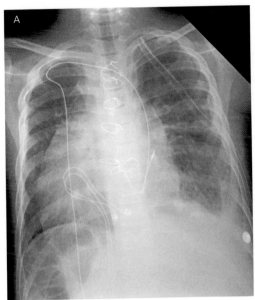
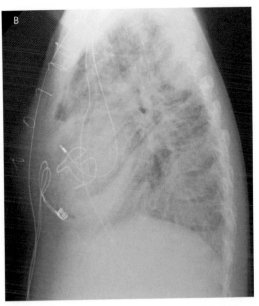

Fig. 11.52 (A) Posteroanterior and (B) lateral chest radiographs from a child with a univentricular heart after a septation procedure and implantation of a dual-chamber pacemaker. The ventricular lead has been placed in an epicardial position, and the atrial lead is transvenously positioned. (From Lloyd MA, Hayes DL. Pacemaker and ICD radiography. In: Hayes DL, Lloyd MA, Friedman PA, eds. Cardiac Pacing and Defibrillation: a Clinical Approach. Armonk, NY: Futura Publishing, 2000: 485–517, by permission of Mayo Foundation for Medical Education and Research.)

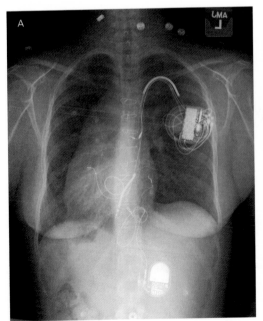
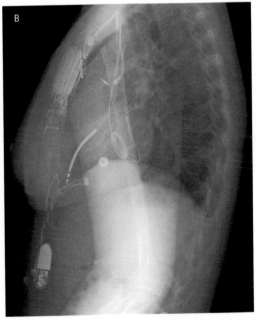

Fig. 11.53 (A) Posteroanterior and (B) lateral chest radiographs of a patient with dextrocardia, total situs inversus with congenitally corrected transposition of the great vessels. Due to progressive dysfunction of the systemic ventricle, a cardiac resynchronization device was placed. The coronary sinus lead is positioned in a right ventricular vein fairly basally in a lateral branch. With congenitally corrected transposition of the great arteries the RV is posterior and explains why the lead looks as if it is still in the coronary sinus when the lateral radiograph is examined. The ICD lead is in the morphologic left ventricular apex with the left ventricle being more anterior than the right. The atrial lead is most likely located in the region of the anterior intra-atrial septum.

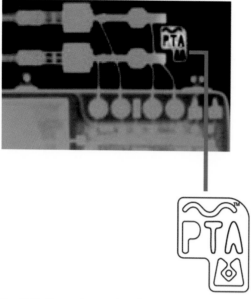

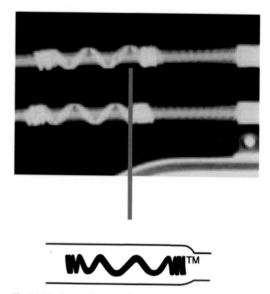

Fig. 11.54 Close-up from a radiographic image of the "header" of a pacemaker that is designated as being MRI conditionally safe. The "curved" symbol over the letter designation of the device (PTA) signifies that the pulse generator is an magnetic resonance imaging (MRI) conditionally safe device. (Image courtesy of Medtronic, Inc.)

Fig. 11.55 Close-up from a radiographic image of the proximal portion of a pacing lead that is designated as being MRI conditionally safe. The coils on the leads signify that pacing leads are MRI conditionally safe. (Image courtesy of Medtronic, Inc.)

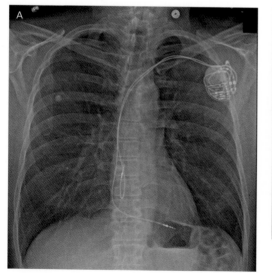

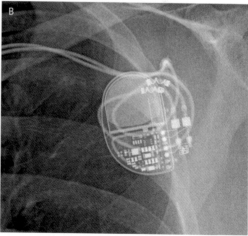

Fig. 11.56 (A) Posteroanterior chest radiograph and (B) close-up view from the PA film of a MRI conditionally safe pacing system. Note that on close inspection both of the details explained in Figures 11.54 and 11.55 can be seen.

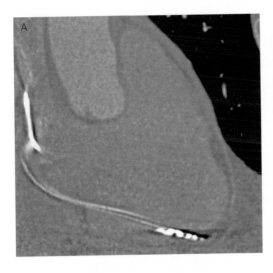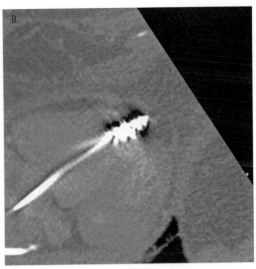

Fig. 11.57 (A) Lateral and (B) close-up slices from cardiac computed tomography (CT) scan demonstrating perforation of an active fixation lead.

reinspected with specific attention to the lead in question and the connector block.

Following this approach will allow the clinician to gain the most information possible from the radiograph.

References

1 Hayes DL. Radiography of implantable arrhythmia management devices. In: Kusumoto F, Goldschlager N, eds. Cardiac Pacing for the Clinician. New York: Springer Science + Business Media, 2007.

2 Burney K, Burchard F, Papouchado M, Wilde P. Cardiac pacing systems and implantable cardiac defibrillators (ICDs): a radiological perspective of equipment, anatomy and complications. Clin Radiol 2004; 59:1145.

3 Lanzman RS, Winter J, Blondin D, et al. Where does it lead? Imaging features of cardiovascular implantable electronic devices on chest radiograph and CT. Korean J Radiol 2011; 12:611–9.

4 Nicholson WJ, Tuohy KA, Tilkemeier P. Twiddler's syndrome. N Engl J Med 2003; 348:1726–7.

5 Cooper JM, Mountantonakis S, Robinson MR. Removing the Twiddling stigma: spontaneous lead retraction without patient manipulation. Europace 2010; 12:1347–8.

6 Wollmann CG. Reel syndrome: the ratchet mechanism. Minerva Cardioangiol 2011; 59:197–202.

7 Altun A, Erdogan O. Pacemaker lead failure suggestive of crush injury. Cardiol Rev 2003; 11:256.

8 Gammage MD, Lieberman RA, Yee R, et al. for the Worldwide SelectSecure Clinical Investigators. Multi-center clinical experience with a lumenless, catheter-delivered, bipolar,

permanent pacemaker lead: implant safety and electrical performance. Pacing Clin Electrophysiol 2006; 29:858–65.

9 Saksena S, Prakash A, Ziegler P et al. DAPPAF Investigators. Improved suppression of recurrent atrial fibrillation with dual-site right atrial pacing and antiarrhythmic drug therapy. J Am Coll Cardiol 2002; 40:1140–50.

10 Bailin SJ. Atrial lead implantation in the Bachmann bundle. Heart Rhythm 2005; 2:784–6.

11 Padeletti L, Michelucci A, Pieragnoli P, Colella A, Musilli N. Atrial septal pacing: a new approach to prevent atrial fibrillation. Pacing Clin Electrophysiol 2004; 27:850–4.

12 Lloyd MA, Hayes DL, Holmes DR Jr. Atrial "J" pacing lead retention wire fracture: radiographic assessment, incidence of fracture and clinical management. Pacing Clin Electrophysiol 1995; 18:958–64.

13 Mond HG, Vlay SC. Pacing the right ventricular septum: time to abandon apical pacing. Pacing Clin Electrophysiol 2010; 33:1293–7.

14 Vlay SC. Right ventricular outflow tract pacing: practical and beneficial: a 9-year experience of 460 consecutive implants. Pacing Clin Electrophysiol 2006; 29:1055–62.

15 Cantu F, De Filippo P, Cardano P, De Luca A, Gavazzi A. Validation of criteria for selective His bundle and para-Hisian permanent pacing. Pacing Clin Electrophysiol 2006; 29:1326–33.

16 Paravolidakis KE, Hamodraka ES, Kolettis TM, Psychari SN, Apostolou TS. Management of inadvertent left ventricular permanent pacing. J Interv Card Electrophysiol 2004; 10:237–40.

17 Bordachar P, Derval N, Ploux S, et al. Left ventricular endocardial stimulation for severe heart failure. J Am Coll Cardiol 2010; 56:747–53.

18 Spragg DD, Dong J, Fetics BJ, *et al.* Optimal left ventricular endocardial pacing sites for cardiac resynchronization therapy in patients with ischemic cardiomyopathy. J Am Coll Cardiol 2010; 56:774–81.

19 Sachweh JS, Vazquez-Jimenez JF, Schondube FA, *et al.* Twenty years experience with pediatric pacing: epicardial and transvenous stimulation. Eur J Cardiothorac Surg 2000; 17:455–61.

20 Thomson JD, Blackburn ME, Van Doorn C, Nicholls A, Watterson KG. Pacing activity, patient and lead survival over 20 years of permanent epicardial pacing in children. Ann Thorac Surg 2004; 77:1366–70.

21 Manolis AS, Chiladakis J, Maounis TN, Vassilikos V, Cokkinos DV. Two-coil versus single-coil transvenous cardioverter defibrillator systems: comparative data. Pacing Clin Electrophysiol 2000; 23:1999–2002.

22 Rinaldi CA, Simon RD, Geelen P, *et al.* A randomized prospective study of single coil versus dual coil defibrillation in patients with ventricular arrhythmias undergoing implantable cardioverter defibrillator therapy. Pacing Clin Electrophysiol 2002; 26:1684–90.

23 Verma A, Kaplan AJ, Sarak B, *et al.* Incidence of very high defibrillation thresholds (DFT) and efficacy of subcutaneous (SQ) array insertion during implantable cardioverter defibrillator (ICD) implantation. J Interv Card Electrophysiol 2010; 29:127–33.

24 Duray GZ, Israel CW, Schmitt J, Hohnloser SH. Implantable cardioverter-defibrillator lead disintegration at the level of the tricuspid valve. Heart Rhythm 2008; 5:1224–5.

25 Shepard RK, Ellenbogen KA. Challenges and solutions for difficult implantations of CRT devices: the role of new technology and techniques. J Cardiovasc Electrophysiol 2007; Suppl 1:S21–5.

26 Van de Veire NR, Schuijf JD, De Sutter J, *et al.* Non-invasive visualization of the cardiac venous system in coronary artery disease patients using 64-slice computed tomography. J Am Coll Cardiol 2006; 48:1832–8.

27 Lickfett L, Bitzen A, Arepally A, *et al.* Incidence of venous obstruction following insertion of an implantable cardio-verter defibrillator: a study of systematic contrast venography on patients presenting for their first elective ICD generator replacement. Europace 2004; 6:25–31.

28 Chan NY, Liem LB, Mok NS, Wong W. Clinical experience of contrast venography guided axillary vein puncture in biventricular pacing R1. Int J Cardiol 2003; 92:55–8.

29 Winters SL, Curwin JH, Sussman JS, *et al.* Utility and safety of axillo-subclavian venous imaging with carbon dioxide (CO) prior to chronic lead system revisions. Pacing Clin Electrophysiol 2010; 33:790–4.

30 Heye S, Maleux G, Marchal GJ. Upper-extremity venography: CO2 versus iodinated contrast material. Radiology 2006; 241:291–7.

31 Antonelli D, Freedberg NA. Endocardial ventricular pacing through a bioprosthetic tricuspid valve. Pacing Clin Electrophysiol 2007; 30:271–2.

32 Hayes DL, Vlietstra RE, Puga FJ, Shub C. A novel approach to atrial endocardial pacing. Pacing Clin Electrophysiol 1989; 12:125–30.

33 Lord SW, Clark SC. Pacing the left ventricle through the coronary sinus in a patient with a prosthetic tricuspid valve replacement. Heart 2003; 89:1442–4.

34 Ratliff HL, Yousufuddin M, Lieving WR, *et al.* Persistent left superior vena cava: case reports and clinical implications. Int J Cardiol 2006; 113:242–6.

35 Wilkoff BL, Bello D, Taborsky M, *et al.* EnRhythm MRI SureScan Pacing System Study Investigators. Magnetic resonance imaging in patients with a pacemaker system designed for the magnetic resonance environment. Heart Rhythm 2011; 8:65–73.

36 Hirschl DA, Jain VR, Spindola-Franco H, Gross JN, Haramati LB. Prevalence and characterization of asymptomatic pacemaker and ICD lead perforation on CT. Pacing Clin Electrophysiol 2007; 30:28–32.

37 Henrikson CA, Leng CT, Yuh DD, Brinker JA. Computed tomography to assess possible cardiac lead perforation. Pacing Clin Electrophysiol 2006; 29:509–11.

12 Electromagnetic Interference: Sources, Recognition, and Management

David L. Hayes, Paul A. Friedman, Samuel J. Asirvatham

Mayo Clinic, Rochester, MN, USA

Pacemaker responses to noise 593
Asynchronous pacing 593
Mode resetting (power-on reset, or electrical reset) 597
Environmental electromagnetic interference 598
Hospital environment 598
Electrocautery 598
Defibrillation 601
Catheter ablation 601
Magnetic resonance imaging 602
Extracorporeal shock wave lithotripsy 604
Transcutaneous electrical nerve stimulation 604
Electromyograms and nerve conduction studies 605
Dental equipment 605

Electroconvulsive therapy 605
Diathermy 606
Impedance plethysmography 606
Capsule endoscopy 606
New technologies 606
Industrial environment 607
Nonindustrial and home environments 608
Microwave ovens 608
Home induction ovens 609
Metal detectors 609
Electronic article surveillance equipment 609
Cellular phones 610
Therapeutic radiation 610
Clinical advice 611
References 611

Cardiac Pacing, Defibrillation and Resynchronization: A Clinical Approach, Third Edition.
David L. Hayes, Samuel J. Asirvatham, and Paul A. Friedman.

Potential sources of electromagnetic interference (EMI), often a concern for patients with cardiac devices, are often misdirected because of myth or hype by the media. It is important for the caregiver to know not only what sources of interference are of potential concern to patients with devices, but also how external interference actually affects pacemakers, implantable cardioverter-defibrillators (ICDs) and cardiac resynchronization therapy (CRT) systems. Interference refers to an inappropriate device response to electromagnetic signals resulting in absent, modified, or inappropriate detection or therapy.

Implantable devices are subject to interference from many sources. Most sources of EMI are nonbiologic but, in addition, biologic sources of interference, such as myopotentials, may cause pacemakers and defibrillators to malfunction. In general, contemporary devices are effectively shielded against commonly encountered EMI. There has always been some concern about EMI that patients may encounter in the nonhospital environment, but because of improvements in pulse generator shielding and design, EMI in the nonhospital environment is now of less concern, with the exception of some military and industrial environments. The principal sources of interference that affect pacemakers and defibrillators are in the hospital environment.

The portions of the electromagnetic spectrum that may affect implantable devices are radio waves, with frequencies between 0 and 109 Hz, including alternating current electricity supplies (50 or 60 Hz) and electrocautery, and microwaves, with frequencies between 10^9 and 10^{11} Hz[1] (Fig. 12.1). Higher frequency portions of the spectrum, including infrared, visible light, ultraviolet, X-rays, and gamma rays, do not usually interfere with implanted devices because their wavelength is much shorter. However, therapeutic radiation can damage pulse generator circuitry directly.

EMI enters the device by conduction through body tissues if the patient is in direct contact with the source, or by radiation if the patient is in an electromagnetic field in which implanted device leads acts as an antenna or the telemetry antenna picks up the signal. Implantable devices have been protected from interference by shielding of the pacemaker circuitry, filtering of the incoming signal, and reduction of the distance between the electrodes to minimize the "antenna" size, thus maximizing nearby (myocardial) signals while minimizing far-field signals. Similarly, ICD systems utilizing true bipolar sensing (tip to ring) are less susceptible to EMI than those incorporating integrated sensing (tip to distal coil) right ventricular leads due to the smaller "antenna" with the tip to ring lead. The contemporary pulse generator is protected from most sources of interference because the circuitry is shielded inside a stainless steel or titanium case. In addition, body tissues provide some protection by reflection or absorption of external radiation.

Bipolar leads sense less conducted and radiated interference because the distance between anode and cathode is smaller than that for unipolar leads. Bipolar sensing configuration largely eliminates myopotential inhibition in pacemakers. Nonetheless, contemporary pacemakers with unipolar sensing configuration are not commonly affected by myopotential inhibition. In general, although older studies have shown that there is considerably less sensing of external electrical fields and less effect from electrocautery during surgery with bipolar sensing, most patients do well clinically with unipolar sensing configuration as well.

Defibrillators incorporate variable signal amplification to permit detection of fine ventricular fibrillation (VF) electrograms while avoiding sensing of T waves, so that myopotential interference may on occasion occur. Because amplification increases with time and is

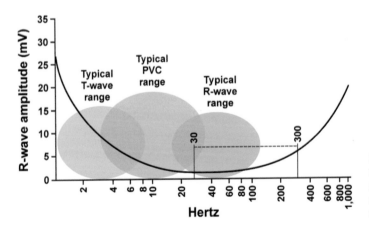

Fig. 12.1 Electromagnetic frequency spectrum of intracardiac events. PVC, premature ventricular contraction. Potential sources of external interference often fall within the 30–300 Hz range.

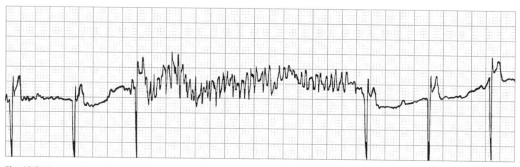

Fig. 12.2 Electrocardiographic tracing from a patient with a pacemaker programmed to the VVI mode. Isometric maneuvers performed at a ventricular sensitivity of 1.4 mV result in myopotentials and pacemaker inhibition.

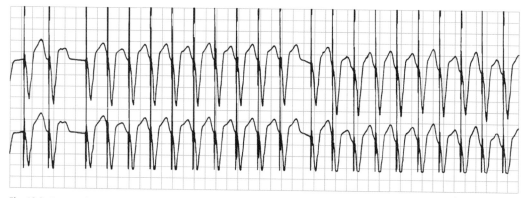

Fig. 12.3 Electrocardiographic recording taken at rest from a patient with a pacemaker programmed to the DDDR mode. During exposure to equipment emitting a radiofrequency signal close to that of the pacemaker, the external signal was sensed on the atrial sensing circuit of the pacemaker, resulting in tracking and a paced ventricular rate at the programmed upper rate limit.

augmented following paced beats, oversensing is most likely to occur at slow heart rates, particularly while pacing.

Sensed interference is filtered by narrow band-pass filters to exclude noncardiac signals. However, signals in the 5–100 Hz range are not filtered because they overlap the cardiac signal range. These signals can result in abnormal pacemaker and ICD behavior if they are interpreted as intrinsic cardiac activity.

The possible responses to external interference include the following:

• Inappropriate inhibition of pacemaker output (Fig. 12.2)
• Inappropriate triggering of pacemaker output (Fig. 12.3) and inappropriate tracking (if sensed on the atrial channel)
• Asynchronous pacing (Fig. 12.4)
• Reprogramming, usually to a backup mode (Fig. 12.5)

• Inappropriate initiation of "other" features, such as mode switching or rate drop response (Fig. 12.6)
• Inappropriate detection of EMI as a ventricular tachyarrhythmia resulting in ICD discharge (Fig. 12.7)
• Inappropriate detection of EMI as an atrial tachyarrhythmia (Fig. 12.8)
• Failure to sense VT/VF.

The most common responses to EMI are triggering or inhibition of pacemaker function, and false tachyarrhythmia detection in ICDs.

Pacemaker responses to noise
Asynchronous pacing

To protect the patient from inappropriate inhibition of pacemaker output, pacemakers have the capability of reverting to asynchronous pacing if exposed to sufficient interference. This change is usually activated by signals detected during a noise-sampling period within

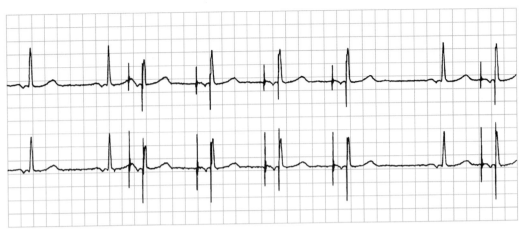

Fig. 12.4 Electrocardiographic recording taken at rest from a patient with a pacemaker programmed to the DDDR mode. During exposure to equipment emitting a radiofrequency signal close to that of the pacemaker, the external signal resulted in intermittent asynchronous (DOO) pacing.

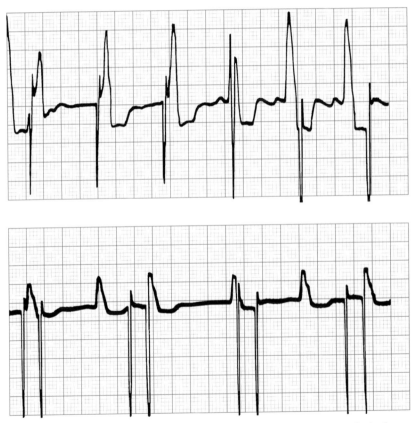

Fig. 12.5 Electromagnetic reprogramming. (A) Transtelephonic electrocardiographic tracing during magnetic application from a patient with a pacemaker programmed to the DDD pacing mode. The transmission reveals VOO pacing instead of the expected DOO response. (B) Electrocardiographic tracing obtained after reprogramming during magnetic application to the DDD mode; there is appropriate DOO pacing. A history obtained from the patient revealed that she had undergone magnetic resonance imaging of her head and not notified the caregiver that she had a pacemaker.

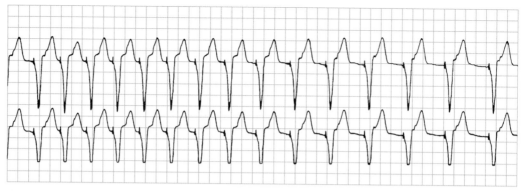

Fig. 12.6 Electrocardiographic tracing from a patient with a dual-chamber pacemaker. The electrocardiogram is obtained during exposure to a source of electromagnetic interference. The interference is sensed on the atrial sensing channel, and the pacemaker responds by rapid ventricular tracking. Criteria are met for mode switching, and the rate begins to fall back to the programmed lower rate.

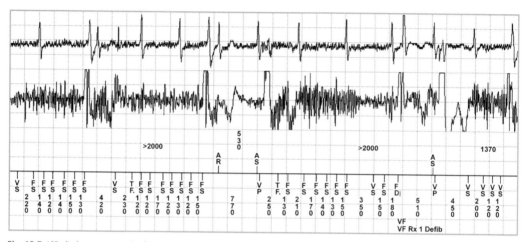

Fig. 12.7 ICD discharge as a result of EMI. (Top: atrial tip to ring EGM; middle: ventricular tip to ring EGM; bottom: marker channel.)

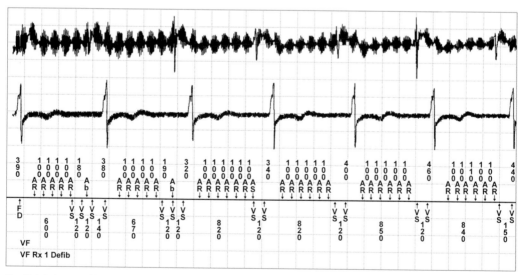

Fig. 12.8 Noise caused by electrical stimulation delivered during use of some type of chiropractic treatment equipment. The noise was sensed on both channels but more so on the atrial channel of the device. (Top: atrial tip to ring EGM; middle: ventricular tip to ring EGM; bottom: marker channel.)

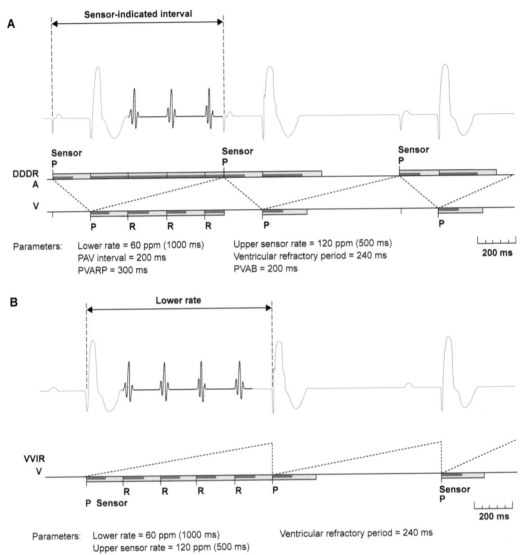

Fig. 12.9 (A) Examples of noise reversion mechanisms from one manufacturer. Noise reversion occurs in a dual-chamber pacemaker when there is continuous refractory sensing in the atrial or ventricular refractory period. During noise reversion a pacemaker in a non-rate-adaptive mode, pacing will occur at the programmed lower rate. If the pacemaker is programmed to most rate-response modes, pacing will occur at the sensor-indicated rate. (B) Although there will be some variation among manufacturers, in the VVIR mode the pacemaker will most likely pace at the programmed lower rate during noise reversion. P, paced atrial or ventricular event; R, intrinsic ventricular event; PVAB, post-ventricular atrial blanking; PVARP, post-ventricular atrial refractory period. (Reproduced with permission from Medtronic Adapta technical manual, pp. 3–28.)

the pacemaker timing cycle (Fig. 12.9). The NSP (noise-sampling period or resettable refractory period) occurs immediately after the ventricular refractory period (VRP), which follows a ventricular sensed or paced event. During the VRP the ventricular sensing channel does not react to any signals and in particular prevents oversensing of the afterpotential of the ventricular

pacing artifact or the evoked QRS and T waves. The VRP usually lasts between 200 and 400 ms, and events occurring during this period have no effect on pacemaker timing. The NSP lasts between 50 and 200 ms. If an event is sensed during this period, it is interpreted as noise, and either the VRP or the NSP is restarted. In addition, in a dual-chamber mode, the post-ventricular

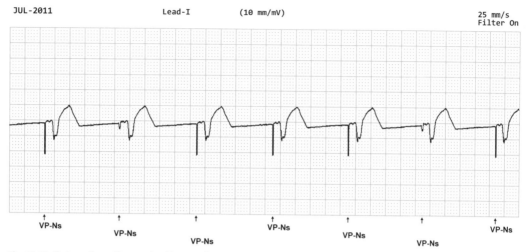

JUL-2011   Lead-I   (10 mm/mV)   25 mm/s
                                                                                              Filter On

↑ VP-Ns   ↑   ↑   ↑ VP-Ns   ↑   ↑   ↑ VP-Ns
        VP-Ns   VP-Ns
                      VP-Ns   VP-Ns

Fig. 12.10 Electrocardiographic example with ventricular pacing (VP) with noise sensing (NS). In this example from a Boston Scientific pacemaker, a paced event initiates a 50-ms fixed noise rejection period. If there is continued noise detected a 60-ms retriggerable noise rejection interval is initiated.

atrial refractory period and the upper rate interval, but not the lower rate interval, are restarted. If a further noise event is detected in the NSP, the VRP or NSP again is restarted and the pacemaker does not recognize cardiac signals. Repetitive noise events eventually cause the lower rate interval to time out, and a pacing pulse is delivered. Continuous noise thus results in asynchronous pacing at the lower rate limit.

In some pacemakers, rather than timing out the lower rate interval, repetitive detection of noise in the NSP causes temporary switching to a specific "noise reversion mode," which is usually an asynchronous mode (VOO or DOO). In some pacemakers with programmable polarity, the pacing output is unipolar in the noise reversion mode, even if the device is programmed to bipolar pacing configuration.

In other devices there is technically not a noise reversion mode but designated operation during "noise detection." For example, Fig. 12.10 depicts operation for a device in which sensing an intrinsic depolarization begins a 60-ms noise rejection interval which is retriggered in the presence of noise. Intrinsic events will not be detected during noise rejection, so that asynchronous operation results during ongoing noise sensing.

Whether noise causes inhibition or asynchronous pacing depends on the duration and field strength, and frequency of the signal. As the field strength increases, there is a greater tendency towards asynchronous pacing. At low field strengths the noise may be sensed only intermittently and thus may not be detected in the NSP, but rather in the "alert" period between the NSP

and the next pacing pulse, leading to inhibition. At higher field strengths, the noise is more likely to be sensed continuously, with sensing during the NSP resulting in asynchronous pacing. Pacemaker models vary considerably in their susceptibility to noise.

Because VT/VF can be a high-frequency low-amplitude signal, ICDs necessarily interpret some noise episodes as VF. ICDs either have no noise reversion mode or very short noise sampling windows, providing imperfect protection from exogenous interference. If the noise is sufficiently sustained, VT/VF is detected and therapies delivered. Nonetheless, due to the filtering and insulation utilized by ICDs, the real-world percentage of shocks caused by EMI is under 3%.[2]

Mode resetting (power-on reset, or electrical reset)

Transient EMI of sufficient strength can reprogram the pacing mode, as opposed to temporarily modifying function. This is most commonly caused by external defibrillation or electrocautery, and occasionally by exposure to magnetic resonance imaging (MRI) magnets, and, in contrast to noise reversion, pacing inhibition, or inappropriate shock, does not resolve when the EMI is discontinued. Following powerful EMI the device usually reverts to the "backup mode" or "reset mode," which in pacemakers is often the same as the pacemaker elective replacement indicator or "battery depletion" mode (Fig. 12.5). Confusion can arise when the "backup mode" and the default settings at battery depletion are the same. Reversion to these parameters indicates that either the pacemaker has been affected by interference or has truly reached battery depletion. In both cases, careful attention to the programmer telemetry, when available, is helpful. If the telemetered battery impedance remains low and the battery voltage is normal, the pacemaker battery is not exhausted and interference is the likely cause of the parameter change. If the etiology of revision to the "backup" mode remains unclear, reprogramming to the preset pacing mode but with maximum output and an increased rate will usually quickly result in reversion to battery depletion settings if the pacemaker battery is truly near end of life.

The backup or reset mode is usually VVI, and if the pulse generator has programmable polarity, the backup polarity is usually unipolar. Some pacemakers may reset to the VOO mode if subjected to interference, potentially resulting in competition with the intrinsic rhythm.

In some ICDs an electrical reset will result in an alert to indicate that the device has been reset and may require reprogramming. Some devices may have both a full "reset," i.e., programmed parameters are reset to default values, and a partial reset which may not affect programmed parameters. If a device reverts to default values, such values provide basic device functionality and are considered safe for the majority of patients. Reset varies among manufacturers and the technical manual and/or manufacturer's technical service group should be contacted if there is any question about device behavior with electrical reset. In ICDs, a power-on reset will usually cause the device to revert to a backup pacing mode (such as VVI at 60 ppm) and "shock only" therapies with maximum energy shocks for heart rates greater than predefined detection rates, typically >140–170 ppm. This occurs because only factory preset parameters stored in nonvolatile memory are available following the power-on reset. However, terminology may be confusing. The term "Power on Reset" (POR) is used by several manufacturers to indicate a form of device reset that may occur when the voltage drops extremely low. When the device experiences a POR, backup defibrillation therapy is not available.

Exposure to low temperatures before implantation may result in mode resetting. The cold temperatures cause an increase in the internal battery resistance, and the subsequent decrease in the battery voltage causes the end-of-life indicator or reset mode to be activated. Because this effect occurs frequently during shipment in cold climates, all pacemakers should be routinely interrogated before implantation and reprogrammed if necessary (Fig. 12.11). If an ICD interrogation before surgical implantation indicates that an electrical reset has occurred, it is best to contact the manufacturer before implanting the pulse generator.

Environmental electromagnetic interference

Electric and magnetic signals are emitted by industrial, hospital medical, and domestic sources. Each of these environments is discussed individually.

Hospital environment

The hospital is the most common environment with sources of potential EMI that can cause significant interference with implantable cardiac devices (Table 12.1).

Electrocautery Electrocautery continues to be one of the most common potential sources of EMI for patients with implanted devices. Electrocautery involves the use of radiofrequency current to cut or coagulate tissues. It is usually applied in a unipolar fashion between the cauterizing instrument (the cathode) and the indifferent plate (the anode) attached at a distance to the patient's skin. Bipolar cautery equipment is also available. The frequency is usually between 300 and 500 kHz (at frequencies of <200 kHz muscle and nerve stimulation may occur). Cutting diathermy uses a modulated signal, so that bursts of energy are applied, whereas coagulation diathermy uses an unmodulated signal to heat the tissue. Radiofrequency ablation of cardiac tissue for the treatment of arrhythmias is delivered most commonly via intracardiac unipolar electrodes at a frequency around 500 kHz, although some newer systems also use bipolar delivery between intracardiac electrodes, for a shallower lesion.

The electrocautery current a pacemaker or ICD receives is related to the distance and orientation of the cautery electrodes relative to the pacemaker and lead. High current is generated if the cautery cathode is close to the pacemaker, or if the cautery electrode and return patch surround the pacemaker.

Electrocautery can result in multiple clinical responses from an implanted pulse generator (Table 12.2). The electrocautery signal may induce currents in the pacing lead and cause local heating at the electrode–tissue interface, leading to myocardial damage with a subsequent increase in the pacing and/or sensing threshold. Threshold alteration is usually transient.

To prevent inappropriate pacemaker inhibition during cautery, a magnet may be applied over the pacemaker to convert it to an asynchronous mode. Although this maneuver may be successful, it may open some pacemakers to reprogramming by the electrocautery signal and is therefore controversial.

Pacemakers with rate-responsive functions may exhibit inappropriate responses during surgery due to

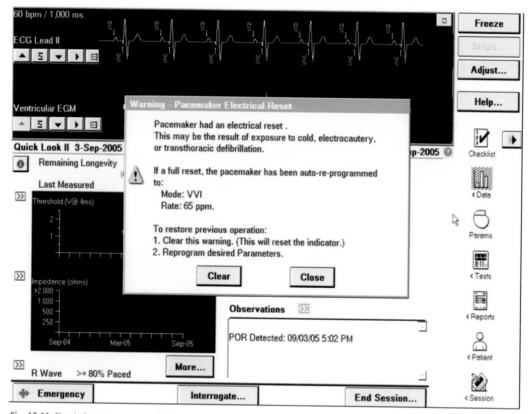

Fig. 12.11 Electrical reset programmer alert.

Table 12.1 Sources of electromagnetic interference in the hospital.

- Electrocautery
- Cardioversion-defibrillation
- Magnetic resonance imaging
- Lithotripsy
- Radiofrequency ablation
- Electroshock therapy
- Electroconvulsive therapy
- Diathermy

Table 12.2 Potential effects of electrocautery.

- Reprogramming
- Permanent damage to the pulse generator
- Pacemaker inhibition
- Reversion to a fallback or noise reversion mode, or electrical reset
- Thermal damage at the lead–myocardial interface

vibration caused by other intraoperative equipment or by the surgical procedure. The electrocautery signal may overwhelm the impedance measuring circuit of a minute ventilation rate-responsive pacemaker leading to pacing at the upper rate limit.

In ICDs, electrocautery signals may be misidentified as cardiac activity, resulting in inappropriate delivery of antitachycardia pacing or defibrillation or in failure to detect VF. For these reasons, the ICD patient should be placed on a monitor and therapies turned "off" prior to the surgical procedure. Personnel capable of recognizing tachyarrhythmias and responding to the rhythm abnormalities with external defibrillation should be available throughout the time that therapies are turned off.

If the ICD patient is pacemaker-dependent, it is important to know the ICD response to magnet application. Magnet response varies between manufacturers and sometimes between models of the same manufacturer (Table 12.3). Most commonly, but certainly not universally, magnet applications in ICDs disables tachyarrhythmia detection without altering pacing function. In this situation, it is best to use a programmer to

Table 12.3 ICD magnet response.

Medtronic	Pacing mode, pacing rate and interval as programmed. VF, FT and VFT detection is suspended. Patient Alert audible tones will occur if applicable and enabled
Boston Scientific	If "ENABLE MAGNET USE" is "on" (nominal), device will emit beeping synchronous tones on the R wave. If after 30 s the beeping does not change to a continuous tone, the magnet must be taped over the device to temporarily inhibit therapy. If beeping changes to a continuous tone after 30 s, tachy mode has gone to "off" and magnet can be removed. To turn device back to Monitor and Therapy, magnet should be placed back over the device for 30 s until R-wave synchronous tones are heard. Magnet application does not affect pacing mode/rate. If "ENABLE MAGNET USE" is programmed "off" (nominally "on"), then a magnet will *not* inhibit therapy. No tones will be emitted and a programmer will be needed to turn device off
SJM	Two programmable options for magnet response: NORMAL (Nominal) or IGNORE. In "NORMAL" response – when magnet is placed over the ICD it blinds detection and delivery of therapy. Bradycardia pacing is not affected by a magnet placed over the device and must be reprogrammed if asynchronous pacing is needed. If "IGNORE" is programmed the blinding is null and void
Sorin/ELA	When magnet is applied it disables tachy therapy and arrhythmia detection. Brady function is to pace in the programmed mode at the magnet rate (corresponding to battery voltage); pacing outputs are set to maximum; rate hysteresis and AV extension are set to zero; AV delay is set to the programmed AV delay at rest
Biotronik	When a magnet is applied, tachyarrhythmia therapy and detection will be suspended and rate-response is suspended

confirm device function before dismissing the patient from monitored care. The caregiver also needs to know whether the ICD has a programmable asynchronous mode (Table 12.4). Management of the pacing function of an ICD is particularly important at the time of surgery in order to avoid electrocautery-induced inhibition in the pacemaker-dependent patient. Many ICDs have a specific electrocautery protection mode design to be programmed on during surgery. In this mode, pacing is asynchronous and tachyarrhythmia detection is disabled.

Patients with implanted devices who are to undergo surgery in which electrocautery may be used should be assessed preoperatively. Table 12.5 summarizes perioperative pacemaker and ICD care. Preoperatively, it is most important to record and/or print the programmed settings and to determine whether the patient is pacemaker-dependent.

In the operating room, during patient preparation, the indifferent electrocautery plate is placed at a distance from the pulse generator, usually on the thigh, and good contact is ensured. The effect of electrocautery may be difficult to assess, because it generates large artifact on the surface electrocardiographic (ECG) monitor. Because pulse oximetry and arterial blood pressure monitoring are not perturbed by electrocautery, these are monitored to insure a stable cardiac rhythm and blood pressure.

Electrocautery should be used with caution in the vicinity of the pulse generator and leads. The cathode should be kept as far from the pulse generator as possible, and the lowest possible amplitude should be used.

Table 12.4 ICD asynchronous mode availability.

- *St. Jude:* All ICDs have asynchronous mode but are ONLY programmable when the ICD THERAPY/FUNCTIONS are turned "OFF"
- *Medtronic:*
  - Gem series – no (with exception of GEM III AT which can be programmed to DOO/VOO [no Patient Alert])
  - Marquis, EnTrust, Virtuoso and Concerto – yes
    - Once asynchronous for 6 hours an "urgent" alert tone occurs and will occur every 6 hours until therapies on
- *Boston Scientific:* "off electrocautery" option turns therapies off and mode to asynchronous in the following models:
  - Prizm II – 1860, 1861
  - Vitality EL-DS – T125, T127, T135
  - Vitality II EL-DS – T165, T167, T175, T177
- *ELA/Sorin:* No asynchronous mode
- *Biotronik:* No asynchronous mode

During electrocautery, device function and cardiac rhythm should be carefully assessed. The most likely response is transient inhibition or asynchronous pacing during electrocautery, which should not cause a significant hemodynamic problem. Secure connection with good skin contact with the grounding pad is essential; disconnection of the pad may result in the implanted cardiac device serving as the anode for cautery, resulting in injury at the myocardial lead interface. Use of two dispersive pads protects against this risk.

Postoperatively, it is critical that the pulse generator be interrogated and, if a reset has occurred, the preoperative settings are restored. Rechecking thresholds fol-

Table 12.5 Perioperative management of pacemakers and ICDs.

Preoperatively
- Identify pacemaker and determine "reset" mode
- Check pacemaker programming, telemetry, thresholds, battery status
- Deactivate rate response or Vario
- Record pacemaker information

Intraoperatively
- Position electrocautery-indifferent plate away from pacemaker so that pacemaker is not between electrocautery electrodes
- Monitor pulse oximetry and/or arterial blood pressure (electrocardiogram is obscured by artifact)
- Have programmer readily available
- Use bipolar cautery when possible
- Do not use cautery near pacemaker/defibrillator
- Use cautery in short bursts
- Reprogram if reset mode is hemodynamically unstable
- Rarely consider use of VVT mode if necessary

Postoperatively
- Check pacemaker programming, telemetry, thresholds
- Reprogram if necessary

lowing exposure to electrocautery and comparison with preoperative values is reasonable but not an absolute requirement. If problems are encountered during interrogation of the pacemaker or reprogramming to the original settings, the manufacturer should be consulted to determine whether a malfunction has occurred.

Defibrillation External transthoracic defibrillation delivers a large amount of electrical energy in the vicinity of a cardiac device and can potentially damage the pulse generator and injure cardiac tissue in contact with the lead. Cardiac devices are protected from external defibrillation damage by special circuitry incorporating a Zener diode that electronically regulates the voltage entering the pacemaker circuit and prevents high currents from being conducted by the lead to the myocardium. However, extremely high energies may overwhelm this protection, causing pacemaker damage or cardiac injury. Internal defibrillation (during cardiac surgery or via a separate ICD) via epicardial or subcutaneous patches or via intracardiac defibrillation electrodes delivers less energy, but at close proximity to the device and may also interfere with pacemaker function. Bipolar pacemakers are less susceptible than unipolar pacemakers to interference from defibrillation.

As with electrocautery, defibrillation may result in reprogramming to the backup or reset mode, a transient increase in pacing or sensing threshold, or damage to pacemaker circuitry.

The degree of damage may be related to the distance of the defibrillation paddles from the pulse generator. The paddles should be placed as far as possible from the generator; when possible, an anterior–posterior configuration is preferred (Fig. 12.12). However, in the anterior–anterior configuration, the paddles should be a minimum of 10 cm away from the pulse generator if possible. After defibrillation, the pulse generator should be interrogated and the programmed settings compared with those before defibrillation or cardioversion. A transient rise in threshold should be managed by increasing the energy output if necessary (Fig. 12.13). Rarely, prolonged, severe threshold increases occur that necessitate lead replacement. In patients with ICDs, shock delivery via the ICD typically results in successful cardioversion and eliminates the need for external shock delivery and potential interactions. Cardioversion of atrial arrhythmias is performed with biphasic, QRS-synchronized shocks to prevent ventricular proarrhythmia; atrial defibrillation thresholds are typically 7–10 J, so that starting with a 15-J shock is reasonable in practice.[2,3] Recommendations for management of patients undergoing cardioversion and defibrillation are summarized in Table 12.6.

Catheter ablation Catheter ablation of intracardiac tissues to control arrhythmias was first performed with direct current shock. This technique had a higher tendency to affect pacemakers than did external defibrillation, and patients frequently experienced problems, including reversion to the backup or reset mode, pacemaker circuit failure, and transient increases in pacing and sensing thresholds. Direct current catheter ablation is not used because of the superiority of radiofrequency ablation, and it is avoided in patients with permanent pacemakers.

Catheter ablation most commonly uses radiofrequency current, which is similar to coagulation electrocautery, i.e., unmodulated radiofrequency current delivered at 400–500 kHz. Effects similar to those of surgical electrocautery have been reported, including inappropriate inhibition, asynchronous pacing, and resetting to backup mode.

For most commonly targeted arrhythmias, the ablation catheter is remote from the pacing or defibrillation electrode. Infrequently, for some atrial or ventricular tachycardias, ablation energy must be delivered near implanted leads. In bipolar systems, significant myocardial injury at the site of the pacemaker electrode or pulse generator damage is rare. During the procedure, pacing is typically programmed to a backup mode (e.g. VVI 40), and in ICDs therapies are turned off. The concern is not radiofrequency energy interfering with the ICD but rather that the ICD appropriately detects

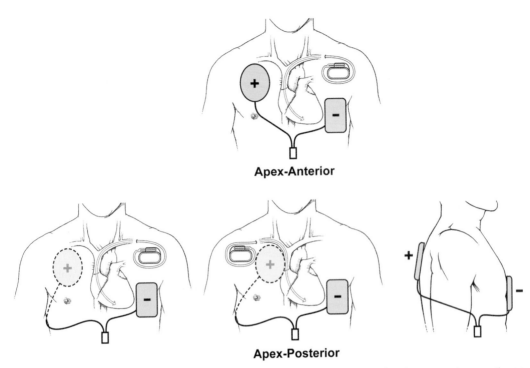

Apex-Anterior

Apex-Posterior

Fig. 12.12 For elective cardioversion, the paddles should ideally be kept at least 10–15 cm away from the pulse generator. In our practice, we use anterior–posterior paddle placement, but anterior–anterior paddle placement can also be used.

VT and delivers ATP or shocks, which may interfere with entrainment or other electrophysiology maneuvers performed as part of the ablation procedure. It is good practice to check parameters, sensing, and pacing thresholds following ablation. In the case of VT ablation, modification of the arrhythmia substrate may also necessitate parameter changes (e.g., setting a slower VT zone if slow VT is inducible post-ablation).

When atrioventricular (AV) nodal ablation is performed, some operators prefer to place the permanent pacemaker before AV nodal ablation. Performing the procedure in this sequence obviates temporary pacemaker placement.

Before radiofrequency ablation is performed, however, it is essential to interrogate the pulse generator, record its programmed settings, and measure thresholds. Rate-adaptive sensing should be programmed off. A programmer should be available during the procedure. After the procedure, the device should be checked and reprogrammed if necessary. In our experience, pacing system damage or threshold changes are extremely rare in this setting.

Magnetic resonance imaging During MRI, three types of electromagnetic fields are present that may interact with implanted cardiac devices: a static magnetic field (which may exert mechanical force and/or activate the reed switch); a rapidly changing magnetic field; and a radiofrequency field (the latter two of which may lead to heating, electrical reset, and pacing inhibition or triggering). When a pacemaker or ICD is near an MRI scanner with the electromagnet "on," the reed switch may close, resulting in asynchronous pacing. Although there may be competition with the underlying cardiac rhythm, asynchronous pacing rarely causes a clinical problem.

Reported interactions and/or atypical function with implantable devices in MRI scanners include asynchronous pacing induced by the magnet, pacing inhibition and/or rapid pacing, reprogramming, and death due to induction of a ventricular tachyarrhythmia.[4,5] There have been concerns about heating of the conductor coil with tissue damage at the electrode–myocardial interface, although in practice this seems rare.[5] Pacemaker circuitry damage by MRI scanning is very unlikely.

A number of observational studies have reported that MRI scanning can be performed safely in carefully selected patients with pacemakers and ICDs, undergoing specific imaging sequences.[6–11] There has been significant variation in study design and in patient

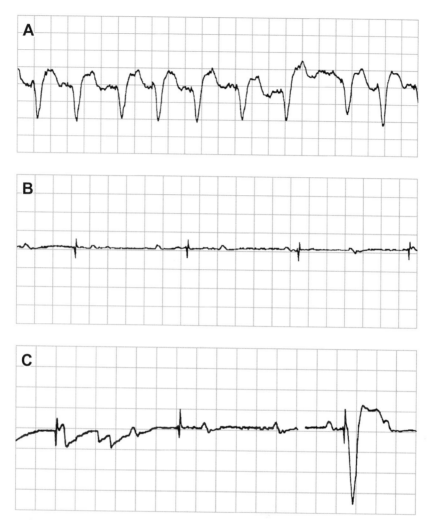

Fig. 12.13 External transthoracic defibrillation. (A) Electrocardiographic recording from a patient with a DDD pacemaker. The underlying rhythm is atrial fibrillation, and the ventricular pacing channel is irregularly tracking the atrial fibrillation, with a resulting rate of approximately 100 ppm. (B) Electrocardiographic recording immediately after elective cardioversion demonstrates ventricular asystole with ventricular pacing artifacts and failure to capture. (Device programmed to VVI in tracings B & C.) (C) A subsequent tracing demonstrates intermittent ventricular capture. (From Hayes DL, Wang PJ, eds. Cardiac Pacemakers and Implantable Defibrillators: A Multi-Volume Workbook, Vol 4. ICDs and Pacemakers. Armonk, NY: Futura Publishing Co., 2000: 37, by permission of the publisher.)

Table 12.6 Cardioversion-defibrillation in the patient with a pacemaker or ICD.

- Ideally, place paddles in the anterior-posterior position
- Try to keep paddles at least 4 in from the pulse generator
- Have the appropriate programmer available
- Interrogate the device after the procedure
- If an implantable defibrillator is in place, use it to deliver the cardioversion shock

inclusion and exclusion criteria among the published studies. Variations have included the type of device included (i.e., pacemaker only vs. pacemaker and ICD), pacemaker dependency status, body region imaged, i.e., nonthoracic vs. thoracic, MRI tesla strength and specific absorption rate (SAR).[12]

In one study of 115 extrathoracic MRI examinations using a 1.5-tesla magnet,[10] there were no significant differences between pre- and immediate- and long-term post-imaging sensing amplitudes, pacing thresholds, or lead impedances. Tests were carried out in patients in the study by Nazarian *et al.*,[11] thoracic and non-thoracic MRI examinations were performed and diagnostic questions were answered in 100% of non-thoracic and 93% of thoracic studies, i.e., artifact generated by the pulse generator can did not usually interfere with adequate image acquisition. Pacemaker-dependent and nonpacemaker-dependent patients performed with an acceptable risk–benefit ratio.

In short, the interactions between implanted cardiac rhythm devices and MRI scanners are complex, and may be influenced by imaging factors (magnet strength, imaging sequence), device factors (device type, lead type, polarity, sensitivity, and other parameter settings), and patient factors (pacemaker dependency, susceptibility to arrhythmias).

While routine MRI scanning of all patients with implanted rhythm devices cannot be recommended, MRI scanning of patients with pacemakers and defibrillators can be safely performed in selected individuals with advanced preparation. Guidelines to safely perform MRI in patients with implantable devices have been published by individual centers and professional societies.[13–15] Of paramount importance, the patient needs to be fully informed of the potential risk, which must be weighed against the potential clinical benefit of the MRI, and the medical center should have a clinical protocol and experienced personnel and equipment in place.

Given the increasing use of MRI scanning, manufacturers are responding to the need for MRI compatible devices. In 2010 the US Food and Drug Administration (FDA) approved the first pacing system that can safely undergo MRI under specified conditions. FDA approval followed publication of results of a prospective, controlled trial of 464 implanted patients randomized to an MRI or control group. Of the 258 patients randomized to undergo MRI (a 1.5-T MRI scan between 9 and 12 weeks post-implant), no MRI-related complications occurred during or after the scan. Specifically, there were no sustained ventricular arrhythmias, pacemaker inhibition or output failures, electrical resets, or other malfunctions.[16,17]

It is important to note that MRI compatibility requires specific design changes in the entire system, i.e., pulse generator and leads. If a patient with a pre-existing non-MRI conditional pacing system undergoes pulse generator replacement, MRI would remain contraindicated unless the original pacing lead(s) were removed and MRI-compatible leads used with the MRI-compatible pulse generator. Even an abandoned pacing lead that is not labeled as MRI-compatible has potential to adversely interact with the MRI as outlined above.

To date there has not been approval of an MRI safe ICD system.

Extracorporeal shock wave lithotripsy Extracorporeal shock wave lithotripsy (ESWL) is a noninvasive treatment for nephrolithiasis, cholelithiasis, and pancreatic duct stones that delivers multiple, focused hydraulic shocks, generated by an underwater spark gap, to a patient lying in a water bath. The shock is focused on the stones, and because the shock wave can produce ventricular extrasystoles, it is synchronized to the R wave.

ESWL is safe to use with implanted pacemakers, provided that the shock is given synchronously with the ECG and that dual-chamber pacemakers have safety pacing enabled. In the pacemaker-dependent patient, it is recommended that a dual-chamber pacemaker be programmed to the VVI, VOO, or DOO pacing mode to avoid ventricular inhibition. Programming of a DDD pulse generator to the VVI, VOO, or DOO mode also avoids rare instances of irregularities of pacing rate, supraventricular arrhythmias that can be tracked or induced, and triggering of the ventricular output by electromechanical interference.[18]

ESWL has not been reported to cause any damage to the pacemaker. Historically, an older activity-sensing pacemaker utilizing a piezoelectric crystal placed at the focal point of the ESWL could be damaged by shattering of the crystal.

Although data are limited, ESWL appears to be generally well tolerated by patients with ICDs. During ESWL magnet is applied to disable tachyarrhythmia therapies (or a surgery mode is enabled), the patient is continuously monitored, and a programmer and resuscitation cart are immediately available.[18] If bradycardia develops, lithotripsy is terminated immediately; atrial ectopy or controlled atrial fibrillation do not mandate cessation of therapy. If the therapeutic target is within 5 cm of the device, special care is taken.

Transcutaneous electrical nerve stimulation Transcutaneous electrical nerve stimulation (TENS) is a commonly used method for the relief of acute and chronic pain from musculoskeletal and neurologic problems. A TENS unit consists of several electrodes placed on the skin and connected to a pulse generator that applies pulses of between 1 and 200 V and 0 and 60 mA at a frequency of 20–110 Hz. The output and frequency of the unit can be adjusted by the patient to provide maximum relief of pain.

The repetition frequency of the TENS output is similar to the normal range of heart rates, so it would be expected that TENS pulses might cause pacemaker inhibition. The literature is limited and mixed results regarding the potential for device interference.[19–22]

TENS can probably be used safely in most patients with bipolar pacemakers. However, it is reasonable to take special precautions in the pacemaker-dependent patient and monitor the response during initial TENS application. If TENS results in interference in patients with unipolar pacemakers, the testing can be repeated after reprogramming the sensitivity to a less sensitive value.

TENS units are best avoided in ICD patients. The TENS unit may create EMI that could be misinterpreted as a tachyarrhythmia, leading to inappropriate device discharge. If the indication for TENS use is compelling, testing for potential interaction should be strongly considered.

Electromyograms and nerve conduction studies There have been concerns regarding the potential for clinically significant interference from electromyograms or nerve conduction studies, but the available literature is very limited.[23] As with exposure to any medical procedure with potential EMI, if the patient is pacemaker-dependent and/or has an ICD, it would be reasonable to monitor an initial study, where experts would be available who would recognize EMI if present.

Dental equipment Dental ultrasound scalers may cause inhibition or asynchronous pacing in older pacemakers, but are probably not a significant concern with contemporary devices. Dental drilling can cause enough vibration to increase the pacing rate of older activity-sensing pacemakers.

Electroconvulsive therapy Electroconvulsive therapy (ECT) is generally safe with respect to implantable device function, as only a minimal amount of electricity reaches the heart because of the high impedance of intervening body tissues and bipolar energy delivery. We routinely place ICD patients on continuous monitoring and turn tachyarrhythmia detection "off" until after ECT therapy is completed. ECG monitoring during the procedure and interrogation of the pacemaker after the procedure are advisable. In pacemakers programmed to a unipolar sensing configuration, seizure activity may generate sufficient myopotentials to result in inhibition or ventricular tracking.

The equipment used may also generate an electrical field capable of causing 60-cycle interference (Fig. 12.14).

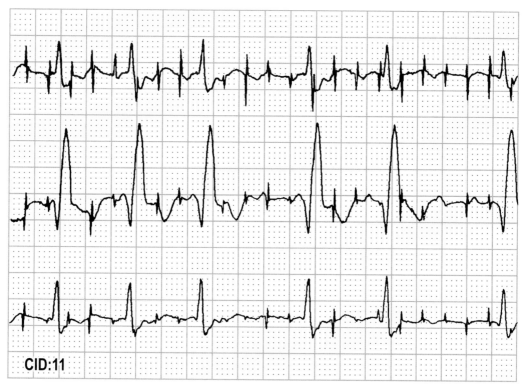

Fig. 12.14 Electrocardiographic tracing obtained after electroconvulsive therapy from a patient with a DDD pacemaker. The patient was hemodynamically stable at the time of electrocardiography. The artifacts were generated by the electroconvulsive therapy equipment, not by the pacemaker. When the power source for the equipment was turned off, the artifacts were no longer present.

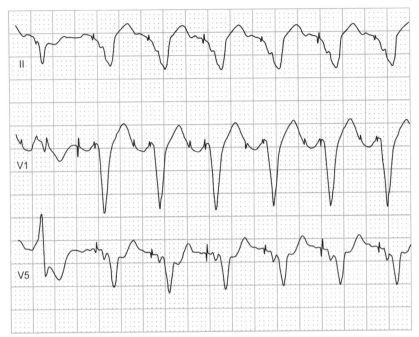

Fig. 12.15 Rate-adaptive pacemakers that utilize a minute ventilation sensor have been shown to interact with some electrocardiogram (ECG) monitors capable of documenting respiratory rate. In this example, upon connection to the monitor a paced tachycardia at a rate of 117 ppm occurs. This tachycardia stopped when the ECG leads were removed.

Diathermy Diathermy can be used to refer to several therapies. Surgical diathermy is also known as electrosurgery or electrocautery and is discussed above. Diathermy also commonly refers to use of energy to generate deep tissue heat used in physical medicine and rehabilitation. Ultrasonic diathermy heats tissues with ultrasound and electric diathermy utilizes high-frequency alternating magnetic or electric fields. Diathermy can be a source of interference, and because of its high frequency should be avoided near the pulse generator implantation site. It has the potential to inhibit the pulse generator or damage the pulse generator circuitry by excessive heating (Fig. 12.15). Diathermy may also lead to inappropriate ICD shocks due to oversensing.

Impedance plethysmography Some patient monitoring systems can cause interference with minute ventilation sensing pacemakers.[24] Specifically, interference can occur with a monitor in which impedance plethysmography is used to document the patient's respiratory rate and to detect ECG lead disconnection. Because a minute ventilation sensor also functions by detecting a change in intrathoracic impedance, the current injected

by the monitor may result in inappropriate sensor-driven pacing.

As soon as the patient is disconnected from the monitor, the heart rate returns to the programmed lower pacing rate. It is important that physicians working with such patients in the operating suite and intensive care unit be familiar with this circumstance (Fig. 12.15).

Capsule endoscopy Capsule endoscopy has gained increasing use for evaluation of the small intestine and concerns were raised whether this procedure would cause interference with implantable cardiac devices. Pacemaker noise reversion has been reported[25] and ICD oversensing during *in vitro* testing has been reported.[26]

From a multicenter retrospective analysis it appears that capsule endoscopy has a low likelihood of resulting in any significant clinical interference with implanted devices.[27]

New technologies Any new medical technologies that generate an electromagnetic field or deliver ionizing radiation, irrespective of whether they are cardiovascular in nature, should be assessed to determine whether

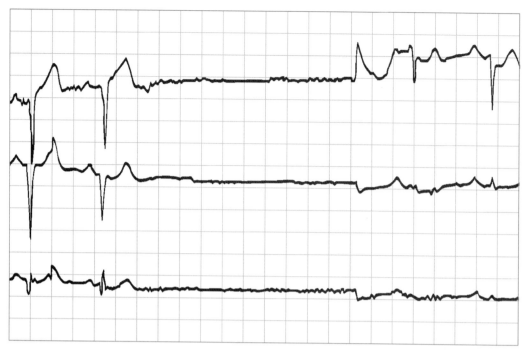

Fig. 12.16 Tracing from an ambulatory monitor from a man with intermittent high-grade AV block. He worked in an industrial environment working with very powerful induction heaters. He would become intermittently symptomatic in various portions of the work area. Ambulatory monitoring correlated intermittent pacemaker inhibition with symptoms. It was difficult to be certain if the tracings represented true inhibition or artifact. However, each episode correlated with symptoms in the patient's diary.

they generate clinically significant interference with implanted pacemakers and defibrillators.

Industrial environment

Conventional wisdom has been to advise patients to avoid arc welding and close contact with combustion engines. This advice needs to be re-examined as pacemakers become more resistant to external interference. However, as previously discussed, pacemakers using a unipolar sensing configuration remain more susceptible to EMI than pacemakers in a bipolar sensing configuration. For patients whose livelihood involves equipment with potential for EMI, a pulse generator with committed bipolar sensing configuration should be implanted.

Industrial environments with significant potential for clinically significant EMI with implantable devices include industrial-strength welding, i.e., welding equipment exceeding 500 A, use of degaussing equipment, and induction ovens. If a patient works in one of these environments or potentially some other even more obscure environment that suggests significant potential for EMI, the work environment should be carefully evaluated. If the patient is pacemaker-dependent, consideration should be given to assessment of the work environment by someone with expertise in EMI assessment. If the patient is not pacemaker-dependent, assessment may be achieved by ambulatory monitoring during exposure to the environment or by use of patient-triggered event records stored within the pacemaker (Fig. 12.16).

From a practical standpoint, most patients who claim to do arc welding use low-amperage equipment for hobby welding. If the patient uses welding equipment in the 100–150 A range, significant EMI is unlikely to occur. However, before giving the patient permission to return to this activity, the pacemaker clinician must consider the type of hardware implanted and the patient's dependency status.

Testing methods have been designed to allow exposure of the patient with a pacemaker or ICD to progressively stronger fields of EMI but this testing is not practical for the individual patient.

If the risk of clinically significant EMI is felt to be low, a simple approach can be suggested to the device patient. For example, if the patient wants to use low amperage welding equipment, have the patient stand very close to a family member or friend, as that person turns on and operates the equipment. If the patient has no ill effects, the patient can try operating the equipment while the other individual is standing very close to them and ready to take control of the welding equipment. If no ill effects are noted, the patient could continue with the equipment for a short period of observation by the other individual to assure all concerned that no problems occur. In general, patients with ICDs are advised not to use arc welders without testing the environment first to avoid inappropriate shocks. When welding must be preformed, patients are advised to limit welding current to 130 amperes, to work only in dry areas with gloves and shoes, to keep welding cables close together and far from the ICD as possible, and to keep the welding arc at least 2 feet away from the implanted device.

Nonindustrial and home environments

Many potential sources of EMI in the nonindustrial and home environments are capable of inhibition of the pacemaker (Table 12.7). However, it would be unusual for most of these sources to cause EMI of clinical significance with the exception of those listed under "special consideration."

Although few household sources cause clinically significant EMI resulting in pacemaker malfunction, the potential for interference from cellular phones and electronic article surveillance equipment has been of intense interest because of possible public health issues. Before these are discussed in detail, several other potential sources, some of historical importance only, merit discussion.

Microwave ovens One of the most common questions still asked by implantable device recipients is whether they can use a microwave oven. In many areas, signs are still in place warning the patient with an implanted device not to use a microwave oven. The original warnings were posted because ineffective microwave shielding and less effective shielding of early pacemakers created the potential for device interference. Microwave ovens are no longer considered a significant source of

Table 12.7 Potential sources of electromagnetic interference (modified from Medtronic, Inc, with permission).

No known risk*	Minimal risk†	Special consideration‡
Battery charger for household batteries	Cordless headphones, i.e. TV/Stereo	Ignition system components of car/motorcycle
Casino slot machine	Cordless telephone – from antenna and charging base	Electric fence
CD/DVD/VHS player or recorder	Electric cart, i.e., grocery or golf	Electric pet containment fence
Dishwasher	Hand-held electric kitchen appliances, e.g. electric mixer or knife	Transformer box
Electric blanket	Electric shaver – corded	Metal detector – search head (beach comber)
Electric guitar	Electric toothbrush charging base	Induction cooktop stove
Garage door opener	Hairdryer – hand-held	Electric body fat scale
Heating pad	Home wireless electronics from antenna	Abdominal stimulator
Hot tub	Magnetic therapy products	Magnetic mattress pad or pillow
Ionized air filter	Radio-controlled items – from antenna	
Iron	Sewing maching/serger – from motor	
Kitchen appliances – not hand-held, e.g., refrigerator, stove, toaster	Speakers	
Massage chair/pad	Treadmill – motorized	
Medical alert necklace	Vacuum cleaner – motorized	
Microwave oven		
Radio (excluding HAM radio)		
Remote control (CD, DVD player, TV)		
Salon hair dryer		
Shaver – battery powered		
Tanning bed		
TV		

*Being used as intended and in normal working condition – there is no known risk.
†Maintain approximately 15 cm between the item and the implanted cardiac device.
‡Maintain at least the recommended distance between the item and the implanted cardiac device.

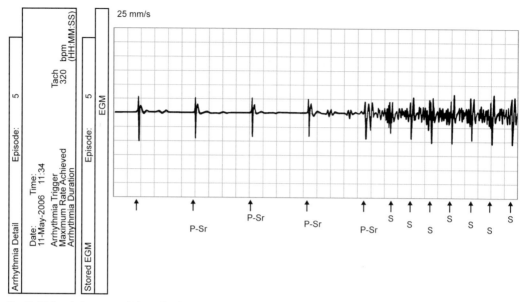

25 mm/s

Arrhythmia Detail
Episode: 5
Date: 11-May-2006   Time: 11:34
Arrhythmia Trigger
Maximum Rate Achieved
Arrhythmia Duration
Tach 320 bpm (HH:MM:SS)

Stored EGM
Episode: 5
EGM

P-Sr   P-Sr   P-Sr   P-Sr   S   S   S   S   S   S   S

Fig. 12.17 Stored electrogram which correlated with exposure to electronic article surveillance (EAS) equipment in a large retail store. The electrongram begins with a paced rhythm followed by noise generated by the EAS equipment which is sense (S) and inhibits the pacemaker resulting in asystole. (From Gimbel JR, Cox JW Jr. Electronic article surveillance systems and interactions with implantable cardiac devices: risk of adverse interactions in public and commercial spaces. Mayo Clin Proc 2007; 82:318–22. Copyrighted and used with permission of Mayo Foundation for Medical Education and Research.)

interference, partly because they have effective shielding and interlocking circuitry that prevents them from being switched on while the door is open; moreover, significant advances have been made in shielding cardiac device circuitry.

Home induction ovens Induction cooktops have the potential to cause device interference. Investigations to date have established that patients at risk are those in whom the pulse generator is unipolar and implanted on the left side. It is most likely to occur in such patients if they are standing as close as possible to the cooktop and if the pan or pot is not concentrically lined up with the induction coil.[28–30]

Metal detectors This equipment is frequently mentioned as a potential problem for patients with implantable devices, and warning signs are often seen at airport security stations. Asynchronous pacing might occur for one or two beats without ill effect to the patient.[31] The major reason to warn patients about metal detectors is that the implanted device may "set off" the detector. Patients are advised to travel with an identification card indicating the type of implanted cardiac device, and to request a manual search at the airport. Walking through

the detectors at an easy pace is well tolerated; but patients should be advised not to lean on them.

Electronic article surveillance equipment Antitheft devices (electronic article surveillance equipment) in many department stores and libraries consist of a tag or marker that is sensed by an electromagnetic field as the person walks through or by a "gate" (Fig. 12.17). Most systems consist of a "deactivator" that a cashier can use to remove or deactivate the tag after purchase of an item. This allows the customer to purchase an item and leave the store without activating an alarm. These electronic antitheft devices consist of multiple technologic systems that generate electromagnetic fields in various ranges, including the radiofrequency range of 2–10 mHz, electromagnetic fields in the 50–100 kHz range, pulsed systems at various frequencies, and electromagnetic fields in the microwave range. Some systems continue to pose potential concern for the device patient.[32] Reported abnormalities including reprogramming to backup mode or noise reversion, inhibition, and oversensing.

It is reasonable to advise patients with an implantable device to pass through any obvious electronic article surveillance equipment and avoid leaning on or

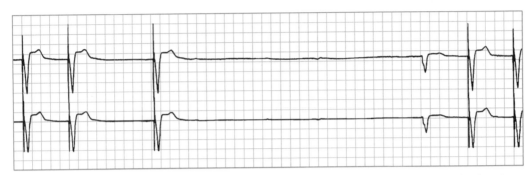

Fig. 12.18 Electrocardiographic tracing obtained during exposure to a cellular telephone from a patient with a VVIR pacemaker. The tracing reveals profound pacemaker inhibition. The patient became nearly syncopal, at which point the phone was removed. The phone used for testing is not commercially available.

standing near the electronic article surveillance equipment: "Don't linger, don't lean."

Cellular phones Although there has been a great deal of interest in cellular phones and the potential for pacemaker or ICD interference (Fig. 12.18), no significant clinical interference is seen with available phones and with normal use.[33]

Based on older investigations, the greatest chance of interference by cellular phones occurred when the phone was directly over the device. Although this position is possible if the activated phone were carried in a pocket directly over the pacemaker, it is certainly not a "normal" phone use position and could be consciously avoided. As stated earlier, minimal interference occurred at the ear position. Most adverse effects are eliminated if the phone is kept 8–10 cm from the implanted device.

Even though specific changes in pacemaker design, such as feed-through filters, have significantly reduced rates of interference, new phone technologies could result in the potential for pacemaker interference, thus requiring further testing.

Therapeutic radiation Therapeutic radiation does not technically result in EMI. However, as an external source of potential damage to an implantable pulse generator, it is incorporated in this chapter. The dose of radiation used in diagnostic X-ray procedures, including coronary angiography, barium enemas, and cerebral angiography, for example, does not significantly affect pulse generator function either immediately or cumulatively. However, computed tomography (CT) has been demonstrated to occasionally cause oversensing in implantable devices both *in vivo*[34] and *in vitro*.[35] The risk of a clinically significant adverse event from CT scanning is very low and this imaging

technique need not be restricted in patients with implantable cardiac devices.

Therapeutic radiation can cause failure in contemporary pacemakers that incorporate complementary metal oxide semiconductor (CMOS) integrated circuit technology.[36] ICDs have also been shown to fail when exposed to radiation.[37] Radiation therapy may also result in inappropriate ICD discharge.

Radiation therapy can also result in ICD "reset." The mechanism is believed to be a secondary neutron cloud that can interfere with the "memory cell" of the device and cause reset of the device. Some ICDs will result in a "patient alert" that therapies have been programmed "off." As long as the "reset" is recognized, the device can be reprogrammed to pre-existing parameters and remain in service.[38] Although it is important to be aware of this possibility and check the device as needed when the patient is undergoing therapy, the incidence of device reset is relatively low.[39]

The amount of therapeutic radiation that can cause a device failure is unpredictable and may involve changes in sensitivity, amplitude, or pulse width; loss of telemetry; failure of output; or runaway rates. If dysfunction occurs, device replacement is required. Although some changes may resolve in hours to days, the long-term reliability of the pacemaker is suspect, and it should be replaced. It should be emphasized that radiation therapy to any part of the body away from the site of the pulse generator should not cause a problem with the generator, but it should be shielded to avoid scatter.

Centers that perform therapeutic radiation should have a protocol for patients with pacemakers or defibrillators. Before radiation begins, the device should be identified and evaluated. The most common clinical situation is development of malignant disease of the

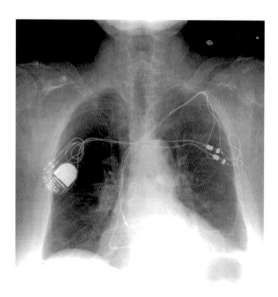

Fig. 12.19 Chest radiograph from a female patient whose pacemaker was initially implanted in the left prepectoral area. A carcinoma of the left breast was diagnosed necessitating mastectomy and subsequent radiation therapy. Prior to radiation the pacemaker was moved to the contralateral chest. This was accomplished by connecting "extenders" to the pacing leads and then tunneling subcutaneously to the right prepectoral region, where a new pacemaker pocket was formed and the pacemaker connected to the extenders and reimplanted.

breast on the ipsilateral side in a patient with a permanent pacemaker. The pacemaker must be moved out of the field of radiation, because shielding the pacemaker would result in suboptimal radiation therapy. The pacemaker can be explanted and a new system implanted on the contralateral side. Alternatively, it may be possible to explant the pacemaker, tunnel the existing long-term pacing lead through the subcutaneous tissues to the contralateral side, and form a new pacemaker pocket on the contralateral side. The pacemaker is reattached to the now-tunneled lead and reimplanted (Fig. 12.19). However, this is performed infrequently because of concerns related to erosion of leads in a subcutaneous position, and diminished long-term lead reliability.

Clinical advice
Nearly all patients can be reassured that EMI will not affect their pacemaker, ICD or CRT device during the course of daily life. Patients in specialized industrial environments should be assessed individually. Improvements in pulse generator resistance to EMI should con-

tinue to minimize clinical concerns. However, the potential for EMI should never be taken lightly and appropriate screening and monitoring should be carried out to avoid adverse clinical outcomes. In addition, despite improvements in pulse generator susceptibility to EMI, emerging technologic advances result in new challenges for the patient with an implanted arrhythmia-control device. Newer wireless technologies or any technology with electromagnetic potential must be assessed for potential interference with implantable pulse generators.

References
1 Irnich W, Steen-Mueller MK. Pacemaker sensitivity to 50 Hz noise voltages. Europace 2011; 13:1319–26.
2 Saxon LA, Hayes DL, Gilliam FR, *et al.* Long-term outcome after ICD and CRT implantation and influence of remote device follow-up: the ALTITUDE survival study. Circulation 2010; 122:2359–67.
3 Newman DM, Dorian P, Paquette M, *et al.* Worldwide Jewel AF AF-Only Investigators. Effect of an implantable cardioverter defibrillator with atrial detection and shock therapies on patient-perceived, health-related quality of life. Am Heart J 2003; 145:841–6.
4 Strach K, Naehle CP, Mühlsteffen A, *et al.* Low-field magnetic resonance imaging: increased safety for pacemaker patients? Europace 2010; 12:952–60.
5 Irnich W. Risks to pacemaker patients undergoing magnetic resonance imaging examinations. Europace 2010; 12:918–20.
6 Naehle CP, Kreuz J, Strach K, *et al.* Safety, feasibility, and diagnostic value of cardiac magnetic resonance imaging in patients with cardiac pacemakers and implantable cardioverters/defibrillators at 1.5 T. Am Heart J 2011; 161: 1096–105.
7 Buendía F, Cano Ó, Sánchez-Gómez JM, *et al.* Cardiac magnetic resonance imaging at 1.5 T in patients with cardiac rhythm devices. Europace 2011; 13:533–8.
8 Mollerus M, Albin G, Lipinski M, Lucca J. Magnetic resonance imaging of pacemakers and implantable cardioverter-defibrillators without specific absorption rate restrictions. Europace 2010; 12:947–51.
9 Boilson B, Acker NG, Payne NE, *et al.* Safety of MRI scanning in patients with permanent pacemakers: are all devices equal? J Interv Card Electrophysiol 2012; 33:59–67.
10 Sommer T, Naehle CP, Yang A, *et al.* Strategy for safe performance of extrathoracic magnetic resonance imaging at 1.5 tesla in the presence of cardiac pace-makers in non-pacemaker-dependent patients: a prospective study with 115 examinations. Circulation 2006; 114:1285–92.
11 Nazarian S, Roguin A, Zviman MM, *et al.* Clinical utility and safety of a protocol for noncardiac and cardiac magnetic resonance imaging of patients with permanent pacemakers and implantable-cardioverter defibrillators at 1.5 tesla. Circulation 2006; 114:1277–84.
12 Gimbel JR. Magnetic resonance imaging of implantable cardiac rhythm devices at 3.0 tesla. Pacing Clin Electrophysiol 2008; 31:795–801.

13 Nazarian S, Halperin HR. How to perform magnetic resonance imaging on patients with implantable cardiac arrhythmia devices. Heart Rhythm 2009; 6:138–43.

14 Levine GN, Gomes AS, Arai AE, et al. Safety of magnetic resonance imaging in patients with cardiovascular devices: an American Heart Association scientific statement from the Committee on Diagnostic and Interventional Cardiac Catheterization, Council on Clinical Cardiology, and the Council on Cardiovascular Radiology and Intervention: endorsed by the American College of Cardiology Foundation, the North American Society for Cardiac Imaging, and the Society for Cardiovascular Magnetic Resonance. Circulation 2007; 116:2878–91.

15 Roguin A, Schwitter J, Vahlhaus C, et al. ESC position paper: magnetic resonance imaging in individuals with pacemakers or implantable cardioverter defibrillator systems. Europace 2008; 10:336–46.

16 Forleo GB, Santini L, Della Rocca DG, et al. Safety and efficacy of a new magnetic resonance imaging-compatible pacing system: early results of a prospective comparison with conventional dual-chamber implant outcomes. Heart Rhythm 2010; 7:750–4.

17 Wilkoff BL, Bello D, Taborsky M, et al. EnRhythm MRI SureScan Pacing System Study Investigators. Magnetic resonance imaging in patients with a pacemaker system designed for the magnetic resonance environment. Heart Rhythm 2011; 8:65–73.

18 Platonov MA, Gillis AM, Kavanagh KM. Pacemakers, implantable cardioverter-defibrillators, and extracorporeal shockwave lithotripsy: evidence-based guidelines for the modern era. J Endourol 2008; 22:243–7.

19 Pyatt JR, Trenbath D, Chester M, Connelly DT. The simultaneous use of a biventricular implantable cardioverter defibrillator (ICD) and transcutaneous electrical nerve stimulation (TENS) unit: implications for device interaction. Europace 2003; 5:91–9.

20 Digby GC, Daubney ME, Baggs J, et al. Physiotherapy and cardiac rhythm devices: a review of the current scope of practice. Europace 2009; 11:850–9.

21 Pyatt JR, Trenbath D, Chester M, Connelly DT. The simultaneous use of a biventricular implantable cardioverter defibrillator (ICD) and transcutaneous electrical nerve stimulation (TENS) unit: implications for device interaction. Europace 2003; 5:91–3.

22 Carlson T, Andréll P, Ekre O, et al. Interference of transcutaneous electrical nerve stimulation with permanent ventricular stimulation: a new clinical problem? Europace 2009; 11:364–9.

23 Schoeck AP, Mellion ML, Gilchrist JM, Christian FV. Safety of nerve conduction studies in patients with implanted cardiac devices. Muscle Nerve 2007; 35:521–4.

24 Southorn PA, Kamath GS, Vasdev GM, Hayes DL. Monitoring equipment induced tachycardia in patients with minute ventilation rate-responsive pacemakers. Br J Anaesth 2000; 84:508–9.

25 Bandorski D, Keuchel M, Brück M, Hoeltgen R, Wieczorek M, Jakobs R. Capsule endoscopy in patients with cardiac pacemakers, implantable cardioverter defibrillators, and left heart devices: a review of the current literature. Diagn Ther Endosc 2011; 2011:376053.

26 Dubner S, Dubner Y, Rubio H, Goldin E. Electromagnetic interference from wireless video-capsule endoscopy on implantable cardioverter-defibrillators. Pacing Clin Electrophysiol 2007; 30:472–5.

27 Bandorski D, Lotterer E, Hartmann D, et al. Capsule endoscopy in patients with cardiac pacemakers and implantable cardioverter-defibrillators: a retrospective multicenter investigation. J Gastrointest Liver Dis 2011; 20:33–7.

28 Irnich W, Bernstein AD. Do induction cooktops interfere with cardiac pacemakers? Europace 2006; 8:377–84.

29 Hirose M, Hida M, Sato E, Kokubo K, Nie M, Kobayashi H. Electromagnetic interference of implantable unipolar cardiac pacemakers by an induction oven. Pacing Clin Electrophysiol 2005; 28:540–8.

30 Binggeli C, Rickli H, Ammann P, et al. Induction ovens and electromagnetic interference: what is the risk for patients with implantable cardioverter defibrillators? J Cardiovasc Electrophysiol 2005; 16:399–401.

31 Kolb C, Schmieder S, Lehmann G, et al. Do airport metal detectors interfere with implantable pacemakers or cardioverter-defibrillators? J Am Coll Cardiol 2003; 41:2054–9.

32 Gimbel JR, Cox JW Jr. Electronic article surveillance systems and interactions with implantable cardiac devices: risk of adverse interactions in public and commercial spaces. Mayo Clin Proc 2007; 82:318–22.

33 Tandogan I, Ozin B, Bozbas H, et al. Effects of mobile telephones on the function of implantable cardioverter defibrillators. Ann Noninvasive Electrocardiol 2005; 10:409–13.

34 Yamaji S, Imai S, Saito F, Yagi H, Kushiro T, Uchiyama T. Does high-power computed tomography scanning equipment affect the operation of pacemakers? Circ J 2006; 70:190–7.

35 McCollough CH, Zhang J, Primak AN, Clement WJ, Buysman JR. Effects of CT irradiation on implantable cardiac rhythm management devices. Radiology 2007; 243:766–74.

36 Hurkmans CW, Scheepers E, Springorum BG, Uiterwaal H. Influence of radiotherapy on the latest generation of pacemakers. Radiother Oncol 2005; 76:93–8.

37 Hurkmans CW, Scheepers E, Springorum BG, Uiterwaal H. Influence of radiotherapy on the latest generation of implantable cardioverter-defibrillators. Int J Radiat Oncol Biol Phys 2005; 63:282–9.

38 Thomas D, Becker R, Katus HA, Schoels W, Karle CA. Radiation therapy-induced electrical reset of an implantable cardioverter defibrillator device located outside the irradiation field. J Electrocardiol 2004; 37:73–4.

39 Kapa S, Fong L, Blackwell CR, Herman MG, Schomberg PJ, Hayes DL. Effects of scatter radiation on ICD and CRT function. Pacing Clin Electrophysiol 2008; 31:727–32.

13 Follow-up

David L. Hayes[1], Niloufar Tabatabaei[2], Michael Glikson[3], Samuel J. Asirvatham[1], Paul A. Friedman[1]

[1]Mayo Clinic, Rochester, MN, USA

[2]Olmsted Medical Center, Rochester, MN, USA

[3]Davidai Arrhythmia Center, Sheba Medical Center and Tel Aviv University, Tel Hashomer, Israel

Requirements for a device follow-up clinic 614
Space 614
Personnel 614
Equipment 615
Pacemaker follow-up 616
Trans-telephonic monitoring 616
Equipment 616
Trans-telephonic monitoring sequence 617
Internet-based remote monitoring 618
Pacemaker clinic follow-up visit 618
Retrieval of previous data and records 620
Discussion and interview 620
Assessment of stored data 621
Programming sequence 622
Rate-adaptive parameter programming 622
Radiographic assessment 624
Data storage 626
ICD follow-up 626
Assessment of the patient's clinical status 626
Pulse generator assessment 626

Capacitor status 628
Assessing lead function 630
Defibrillation efficacy assessment 631
Medications 632
Strategies to minimize shocks 634
CRT follow-up specifics 634
Remote patient monitoring 634
Practical considerations of remote monitoring 640
Patients' concerns during follow-up 640
Medical advisories and recalls 640
Lifestyle and personal concerns 644
Psychologic issues encountered following device implantation 645
Withdrawal of device support 646
Conclusions 646
References 646

Cardiac Pacing, Defibrillation and Resynchronization: A Clinical Approach, Third Edition.
David L. Hayes, Samuel J. Asirvatham, and Paul A. Friedman.
© 2013 Mayo Foundation for Medical Education and Research. Published 2013 by John Wiley & Sons, Ltd.

The complexity of device follow-up for pacemakers, implantable cardioverter-defibrillators (ICDs) and cardiac resynchronization therapy (CRT) systems has paralleled the increasing sophistication of the devices. Follow-up therefore requires a dedicated staff with a thorough understanding of implantable devices. Traditionally, the purpose of device follow-up has been to ensure appropriate device function. Implanted devices continue to acquire an increasing amount of data, both physiologic and device-related, to permit assessing health status, with the goal of notifying caregivers before clinical decompensation occurs to permit clinical intervention.

Follow-up of permanent pacemakers can be accomplished in more than one way: periodic visits to a pacemaker clinic; less frequent clinic visits in combination with trans-telephonic monitoring (TTM); and/or surveillance via web-based downloads. Follow-up of ICDs and CRTs can likewise be accomplished in more than one way: periodic visits to an ICD clinic or significantly less frequent visits in combination with remote access monitoring. In addition to routine checks, patients on a remote-monitoring network are able to transmit data if they are symptomatic which can limit travel time, clinic visits, and costs. Remote access monitoring represents the most significant advance in device follow-up in decades and is now widely embraced in the USA and Europe and gaining popularity in other parts of the world. Implanted devices may also incorporate external sensors such as a weight scale or blood pressure monitor. Physiologic information is wirelessly transmitted to a hub, from which it can be processed and sent to clinicians.

TTM for pacemakers may eventually be completely supplanted by web-based remote monitoring given the significantly greater amount of clinical decision-making information that can be gained. However, given the current penetration of TTM in the USA, this technology will probably continue to be in use to some degree for a number of years.

TTM can be performed by the implanting center or by a commercial monitoring firm. Follow-up solely by TTM is suboptimal, because some patients undergoing pacemaker implantation may not be seen again until battery depletion indicators appear. Periodic clinic visits allow thorough evaluation and, if necessary, alteration of output settings, rate-adaptive settings, and other parameters. Few patients would obtain maximum efficiency of their pacemaker if it remained at nominal or initially programmed values for the life of the pulse generator.

Remote access monitoring requires implantation of a compatible device. With inductive systems the patient holds a wand over the device to activate remote monitoring; the patient's unit is typically connected to a phone line or to the cellular phone network to transfer data via the internet to a privacy-protected website. "Wandless" systems incorporate a radiofrequency transmitter that is positioned so as to be in regular patient proximity, e.g., on a night stand. The implanted device is automatically wirelessly interrogated on a scheduled basis. Depending on specified preferences, caregivers are provided device information through fax, telephone, and/or internet. Furthermore, physicians have access to the website to follow routinely scheduled patient transmissions as well as patient-initiated transmissions. Various levels of alerts are generated by the system if a malfunction is detected, e.g., a high impedance suggesting lead failure or ICD therapies being turned "off."

Requirements for a device follow-up clinic

Requirements for a device follow-up clinic are detailed in a consensus statement developed jointly by Heart Rhythm Society (HRS) and the European Heart Rhythm Association (EHRA).[1] The text that follows, although largely consistent with the HRS/EHRA consensus statement, is based on the design of our long-standing device follow-up clinic.

Space

Because of the specialized equipment necessary for pacemaker ICD and CRT assessment and follow-up, dedicated space is desirable. There must be adequate space for:
- Patient assessment, programming, and storage of all necessary programmers (Fig. 13.1)
- Electrocardiographic monitoring
- Space for informal exercise both for assessment of rate response and determination of appropriate rate-adaptive parameters and 6-minute hall walk tests that may be used for follow-up of CRT patients
- Teaching tools, e.g., written educational information, DVDs, DVD recorder and screen, heart models (Fig. 13.2)
- Trans-telephonic receiving station or stations (the number of stations required is proportional to the overall volume of calls received) (Figs 13.3 and 13.4)
- Remote access internet stations to receive and review patient transmissions (Fig. 13.5)
- Record storage (even though most storage may be accomplished by computerized databases, in many centers some room is required for "paper storage")
- Resuscitative equipment.

Personnel

Personnel requirements in the pacemaker clinic include the following:

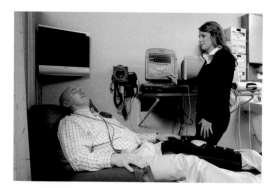

Fig. 13.1 Outpatient area for device programming. The chair reclines to a semisupine position. The programmers surround the area for easy access to any one of them.

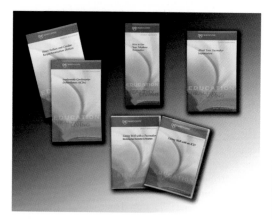

Fig. 13.2 Various teaching materials available in the outpatient area: we have an educational DVD about pacemakers and another about implantable cardioverter-defibrillators (ICDs). The patients see the DVD at the time of the device implant and are sent home with one for future reference. Also pictured are brochures that educate the patient about the basics of pacemakers, ICDs and cardiac resynchronization therapy devices.

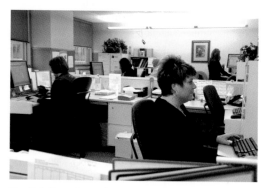

Fig. 13.3 The patient is also sent home with a folder that includes educational brochures and a cover note reiterating post-implant restrictions, future transmission dates and important phone numbers related to device follow-up.

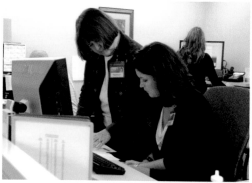

Fig. 13.4 Work area for nurses performing device follow-up, including trans-telephonic monitoring. With digital storage of electrocardiographic tracings, reliance on the electronic medical record and availability of technical manuals on-line, the computer terminal and phone are the major requirements.

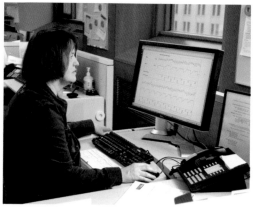

Fig. 13.5 Mayo Clinic, Rochester, has a large device follow-up area. Depicted here is the area where trans-telephonic and remote monitoring is performed with stations for up to eight registered nurses.

• Allied professionals with expertise in pacemaker and ICD programming and follow-up (among them may be registered nurses, specially trained technicians, certified technologists [in some countries], physician assistants, and nurse practitioners)
• Secretarial support may be desirable if patient correspondence, appointments, billing, etc., is not automated by the device follow-up system and/or managed by other areas of the institution.

Equipment

Equipment requirements include the following:
• Electrocardiographic (ECG) monitoring (this could be and is most commonly accomplished by the

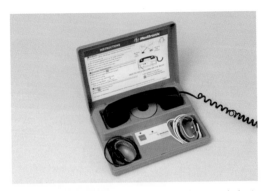

Fig. 13.6 Typical equipment used by the patient for trans-telephonic monitoring. In addition to the telephone, the patient requires a transmitter and electrodes. Various types of electrodes can be used. During electrocardiographic transmission, the patient is instructed to transmit for approximately 30 s. However, if the transmission needs to be interrupted for any reason, an alarm can be sent from the receiving center. If the patient hears the alarm, he or she is instructed to stop the transmission attempt and pick up the phone.

programmers. However, because independent monitoring is helpful in some situations, multichannel ECG monitoring should ideally be available.) Full 12-lead electrocardiography remains useful for assessment of CRT devices
• Programmers for all devices followed (Fig. 13.1)
• Reclining chair or examining table for patient evaluation (Fig. 13.1)
• Resuscitative equipment including external cardioversion defibrillation
• Trans-telephonic receiving station or stations
• Computer access to remote monitoring websites (Fig. 13.5).

Pacemaker follow-up

Trans-telephonic monitoring

TTM has been part of pacemaker follow-up for over 40 years (Fig. 13.6). For many years, this follow-up method was used primarily in the USA and never gained significant popularity in other countries. Although still used widely in the USA, this technique is increasingly being replaced by web-based remote access.

TTM is an effective method to monitor pacemaker battery status and to demonstrate normal or abnormal function. Admittedly, trans-telephonic assessment of atrial events is much more difficult than assessment of ventricular events. In large part the reason is simply the small amplitude of the atrial signal, whether paced or intrinsic. The pacemaker artifact may overwhelm the atrial event, whereas the usually larger ventricular event

is not commonly overshadowed by the ventricular pacing artifact.

Obtaining TTM tracings of good quality can be an issue. Patients with pacemakers are often elderly, and without excellent initial teaching and possibly coaching during the TTM calls, they may have difficulty handling the trans-telephonic equipment. We request that a family member or friend be present during the initial teaching session. It is often reassuring to the patients to know that someone else has the information necessary to complete the transmission should they forget a portion of the instructions. Transmission difficulties may be compounded if the patient has a significant hearing deficit. Incorrect use of the trans-telephonic transmitter and improper magnet placement may impair the quality of the transmission (Fig. 13.7).

Some types of telephones may be suboptimal for TTM. For example, with cordless phones the quality of transmission at times is decreased and there is sometimes a greater chance of being disconnected. Speaker phones and phones with altered volume controls may also present problems. Any source of electromagnetic interference close to the site of the patient's transtelephonic transmission may induce significant artifacts (Fig. 13.8). Cell phones have also been problematic but technology is being further developed to allow for cell phone transmission.

The frequency of TTM differs among centers. At this time, reimbursement for TTM generally is not allowed for more frequent follow-up than that specified by the Centers for Medicare and Medicaid Services (CMS) guidelines.

Equipment

To perform TTM, the patient must have access to the necessary TTM equipment. Typical transmitting equipment is shown in Fig. 13.6. Transmission requires contact with the patient's skin, i.e., most commonly electrodes on the wrists or the chest. After calling the pacemaker clinic or commercial follow-up center the patient places the telephone over the transmitting equipment. In the pacemaker clinic a receiving center is used to obtain the ECG tracings the patient transmits (Fig. 13.3).

Multiple varieties of electronic medical records as a repository for implantable device data exist including institution-designed, institution-specific systems; and commercial systems. The most commonly used commercial system is the Medtronic Paceart® System (www.paceart.com). The Paceart® System will organize and archive relevant patient, device, programmer, transtelephonic, and remote management system information for follow-up of arrhythmia patients with implanted cardiac devices. Paceart® supports a common workflow by managing information for all leading manufacturers'

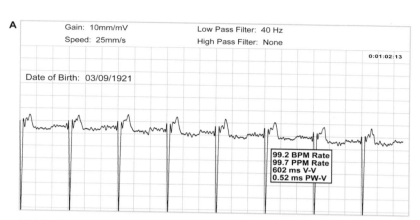

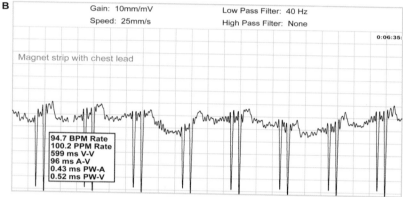

Fig. 13.7 (A) Upper tracing obtained during magnet application in a patient with a pacemaker programmed to a dual-chamber mode. Only the ventricular pacing artifact is seen. This tracing was obtained with the patient using "wrist bands" (bracelets) for the transmission. (B) Lower tracing obtained from the same patient but using a chest lead, i.e., removing the wrist band from the wrist and establishing contact between the electrode of the wrist band and the chest. Even though there is significant artifact present, both the atrial and ventricular pacing artifacts can now be seen.

devices and serves as the link to electronic health record systems.

Paceart® standardizes patient and device information. The report format is consistent across all manufacturers' devices (Fig. 13.9). It provides active device and lead information, current programming, data/telemetry information, and trending device performance. The system also provides functionality for creating physician correspondence and scheduling patient follow-ups for both in-clinic and remote systems. The system will also assist in charge and billing management and provide documentation of in-clinic and remote patient management activities.

Trans-telephonic monitoring sequence

Compared to web-based remote monitoring, the information that can be obtained trans-telephonically is limited. The order in which the information is collected may vary. The following sequence is used by our clinic.

- Brief discussion with the patient to determine general well-being and elucidate any problems the patient believes may be related to the pacemaker
- Nonmagnet "free-running" tracing (duration ≈ 30 s)*
- Magnet tracing (duration ≈ 30 s)*
- Patient informed of pacemaker status; date of next TTM transmission or clinic visit scheduled
- TTM data stored.

If the nonmagnet tracing displays intrinsic rhythm, the underlying rhythm should be noted and compared with previous transmissions. If there is intermittent pacing or pacing in only one chamber of a dual-chamber device, sensing of intrinsic activity can be assessed.

---

* The recommendation for 30 s of captured information originates from very old regulations from CMS and remains the only legislated recommendation of record.

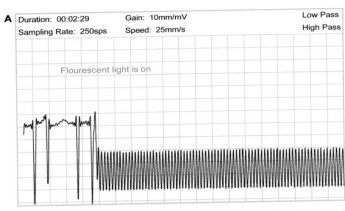

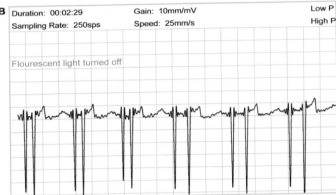

Fig. 13.8 (A) Upper tracing obtained during transtelephonic monitoring. Significant artifact is present making interpretation of the tracing impossible. When the patient was queried, it was noted that a fluorescent light next to the transmission equipment was turned "on." (B) The bottom tracing was obtained after the fluorescent light was turned "off"; artifact is no longer present.

The magnet tracing should be used to assess:
- Capture verification in all chambers paced
- Magnet rate
- Pulse width.

Magnet response varies not only from manufacturer to manufacturer, but also among models from one manufacturer (Fig. 13.10). Specific magnet response for many different devices is difficult to commit to memory. Therefore, it is helpful to have the specific magnet response recorded on the patient's records. The healthcare professional taking the transmission should be familiar with the elective replacement indicators (ERI) for the specific pacemaker (Table 13.1). Measurements from the patient's previous transmission should be available for comparison.

Other specific information can sometimes be obtained from specific pacemakers. The proprietary Threshold Margin Test (TMT) provides some information on pacing threshold at the onset of magnet application (Fig. 13.11). The first three pacemaker artifacts occur at a rate of 100 bpm. As part of the TMT, the pulse duration of the third pacemaker stimulus is 75% of the programmed pulse duration. Failure to capture with the reduced pulse duration provides some information about threshold and pacing margin of safety.

Internet-based remote monitoring

Pacemaker surveillance with internet-based remote monitoring is increasingly used with current generation pacemakers. Internet-based remote monitoring is used almost routinely in some centers for high-voltage devices. Internet-based follow-up is described below for both pacemakers and high-voltage devices.

Pacemaker clinic follow-up visit

The detail required during the pacemaker clinic visit depends on the follow-up technique or techniques used. If the pacemaker is not capable of internet-based remote monitoring, our practice is to follow the schedule and guidelines in Table 13.2 or at any time that the patient has a concern that may be device-related. At the time of each device clinic visit, the following steps are completed for the pacemaker patient:

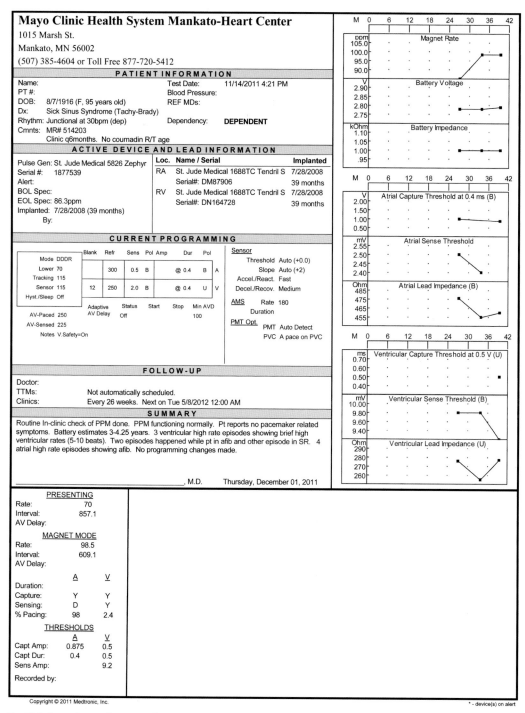

Fig. 13.9 Paceart® report format providing active device and lead information, current programming, data/telemetry information, and trending device performance.

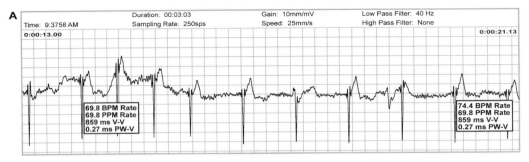

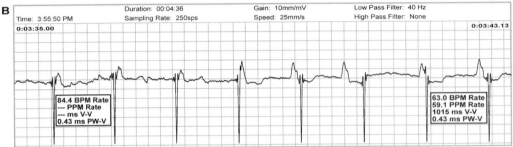

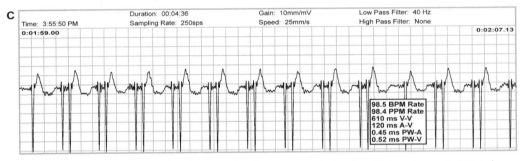

Fig. 13.10 Composite of magnet responses from three pacemakers. Magnet response, top to bottom: (A) Pacemaker goes to 100 bpm for three beats (Threshold Margin Test) followed by asynchronous pacing at programmed lower rate. (B) Asynchronous pacing at programmed lower rate. (C) Asynchronous pacing at 98 ppm.

- Retrieval of previous data and follow-up records for comparison
- Discussion with the patient about concerns and interim events
- Device interrogation
- Assessment of stored data from prior encounters (TTM/remote/in-clinic)
- Programming sequence
- Assessment of rate-adaptive parameters as needed
- Radiographic assessment if there are clinical concerns that might be addressed by a radiographic evaluation
- Update of medical record.

Retrieval of previous data and records
At the onset of the device clinic visit the patient's prior records should be available. These should include information from the patient's previous clinic visits

and most recent trans-telephonic or web-based transmissions.

Discussion and interview
The patient should be interviewed in an attempt to elucidate any clinical problems that could be pacemaker-related (Table 13.3). It is important to have some knowledge of the most commonly noted pacemaker problems. These are discussed in detail in Chapter 10: Troubleshooting.

At our institution, the pacemaker clinic does not serve as the primary healthcare or cardiac care provider and the extent of the physical examination is limited to whatever may help detect suspected problems. For example, if no clinical problem is suspected, the examination is limited to inspection of the pacemaker site.

Table 13.1 Magnet response and ERI for permanent pacemakers.

	Magnet application*
Biotronik	With "Asynchronous" magnet option*: pacing; In dual-chamber devices, the AV delay reverts to 100 ms; magnet rate dependent on battery status as follows: 90 ppm = beginning of life 80 ppm = ERI
Boston Scientific	Asynchronous pacing; In dual-chamber devices, the AV delay reverts to 100 ms; magnet rate dependent on battery status as follows: • 100 ppm = beginning of life • 90 ppm = for some devices prior to reaching ERI @ 85 ppm • 85 ppm = ERI
Medtronic	Asynchronous pacing; For dual chamber modes, PAV delay reverts to programmed value following three TMT beats with 100 ms PAV. Following three 100 ppm TMT beats all modes pace at: • 85 ppm = beginning of life • 65 ppm = when recommended replacement time (RRT/ERI) is reached or a full electrical reset has occurred • Magnet Modes are: DOO in modes with dual chamber pacing including AAI<=>DDD and AAIR<=>DDDR modes, VOO in the VDD mode and VOO/AOO in single chamber modes. • TMT reduces programmed amplitude(s) by 20% on third beat of 100 ppm TMT pacing. • Trans-telephonic Monitor: ON delays TMT 5 s and paces unipolar with magnet applied
Sorin Medical	Asynchronous pacing; In dual-chamber devices, the AV delay reverts to original programmed sensed AV interval but with magnet removal the next six cycles will have a 95-ms AV Delay to show capture at the programmed output. The final two cycles of the eight following magnet removal will again be at the rest (max.) AV Delay; magnet rate dependent on battery status as follows: • 96 ppm = beginning of life • 80 ppm = ERI • 70 ppm = when battery status results in change to VVI mode
St. Jude Medical	Asynchronous pacing; In dual-chamber devices, the AV delay reverts to 120 ms; the rate decreases in steps and final rate reveals battery status: • 100 ppm = beginning of life (earlier devices 98.6 ppm. Even older generation devices go to programmed rate with magnet) • 85 ppm = ERI; earlier devices ≤86.3 ppm. If Ventricular AutoCapture is programmed on; the device temporarily suspends beat to beat AutoCapture, increases ventricle to high output mode for duration of magnet application and initiates threshold search when magnet removed

AV, atrioventricular; ERI, elective replacement indicators; TBT, Threshold Margin Test.

*Three programmable magnet response options: Auto, Asynchronous and Synchronous; although default is Auto, asynchronous most commonly used. Synchronous mode is used for "patient-triggered monitoring." Auto mode is 90 ppm for 10 beats then reverts to programmed base rate.

At other centers the device clinic may serve as the primary healthcare provider and visits may include a complete physical examination at periodic visits.

Assessment of stored data

In some pacemakers, initial interrogation results in a printout of stored data. In other pacemakers, these data must be specifically requested. It may be necessary to obtain stored data before programming because a permanent change in programming may "clear" stored data in some devices.

Contemporary pacemakers may have the capability of storing a great deal of data. Although the storage capabilities increase with each successive pacemaker generation, at the time of manuscript preparation, select devices have the ability to store up to 1 megabyte of data.

The data can provide invaluable assistance in achieving optimal programming and in diagnosing intermittent symptoms. Although stored data has improved with each new generation of devices there are potential limitations of stored diagnostic function. Limitations include low sensitivity and specificity for some events such as device determination of a pathologic atrial tachyarrhythmia. Stored intracardiac electrograms (EGMs) are a critical component in confirmation of stored diagnostic data and follow-up of stored events.

Categories of stored information include:
- Event counters (Fig. 13.12)
- Rate histograms (Fig. 13.13)
- Electrograms (Fig. 13.14)
- Measured values (Fig. 13.15)
- Special diagnostic features (Fig. 13.16).

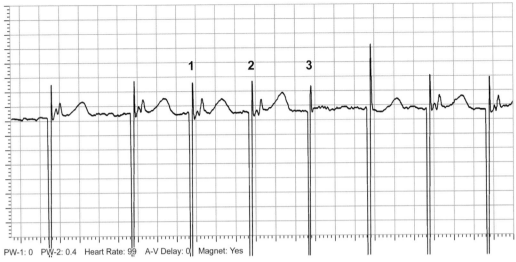

PW-1: 0   PW-2: 0.4   Heart Rate: 99   A-V Delay: 0   Magnet: Yes

Fig. 13.11 Tracing from trans-telephonic monitoring demonstrating a threshold margin test (TMT). There is failure to capture on the third artifact at 100 bpm. During the TMT the pulse width on the third artifact is decreased by 25%. Failure to capture by that artifact would demonstrate capture threshold to be very close to the programmed output.

Table 13.2 Mayo Clinic Guidelines for routine follow-up of pacemaker and ICD patients.

- Routine follow-up every 4 months for both pacemaker and ICD patients
- ICD patients should have one in-clinic visit annually (with DFT testing if necessary)
- New implants: in-clinic check 3 months from implant, then routine 4 months checks
- Pack changes: begin routine 4 month checks from pack change date
- Pacemakers using TTM:
  - Begin monthly checks when battery ≤6 months
  - When pacemaker is nearing 5 years of age, check for last estimated battery longevity. If not available, schedule in-clinic follow-up. Document estimated remaining longevity in pacemaker database*
- Status post AV node ablation (may or may not be a new implant):
  - Monthly clinic checks at 1, 2, and 3 months following AV node ablation to decrease lower rate limit of the device by 10 bpm each month from 90 to 80 bpm at 1 month, 80 to 70 bpm at 2 months, from 70 to 60 bpm at 3 months
- Annual DFT testing required if: DFT > 14 J or as directed by physician
  - Considerations for DFT testing: abdominal device, cold can, epicardial system, separate PM and ICD, SQ lead, separate defib and pace/sense leads, coaxial leads, medication change that could impact DFT

*There are specific exceptions as a result of devices that historically need battery check more frequently.

Programming sequence

A specific sequence should be adopted and followed for interrogation and programming. Our pacemaker clinic staff has adopted the in-clinic sequence detailed in Table 13.4.

It is not important that this specific sequence be followed but it is crucial that all steps be completed in some orderly manner to avoid omission of any necessary steps.

Rate-adaptive parameter programming

As discussed in Chapter 9: Rate-Adaptive Pacing, the patient's rate requirements may change over time. For example, in the chronotropically incompetent patient in whom rate response is restored, the newly found rate response may allow the patient to begin an exercise program and improve conditioning. With subsequent improvement in conditioning, a change in rate-adaptive parameters may be desired, such as higher paced rates and a faster increment in heart rate.

Conversely, if symptomatic coronary artery disease were to develop in a patient with a rate-adaptive pacemaker, it may be desirable to make the rate-adaptive parameters less sensitive to avoid rate-related angina while the coronary artery disease is being evaluated and treated.

We routinely assess exercise informally at the first clinic visit, i.e., at approximately 3 months post-implant in most patients. On subsequent visits the rate response

Table 13.3 Common symptoms and possible pacemaker related causes.

Symptoms	Considerations
Palpitations	Rapid paced ventricular rates Tracking of sinus tachycardia or supraventricular arrhythmia Pacemaker-mediated tachycardia Atrial failure to capture with retrograde conduction and tracking of the premature atrial contraction Intrinsic (nonpacemaker-related) tachyarrhythmia or extra systoles
Weakness, fatigue, malaise	Pacemaker syndrome Failure to capture Inappropriately programmed rate-adaptive parameters Disease process unrelated to the permanent pacemaker
Dyspnea	Pacemaker syndrome Underlying cardiac or pulmonary disease
Hiccups	Phrenic nerve stimulation
Muscle stimulation	Current leakage in unipolar configuration Loss of insulation integrity of the pacing lead
Presyncope, syncope	Pacemaker syndrome Failure to capture Oversensing with inhibition Vasodepression
Cough	Pacemaker syndrome
Chest pain	Pacemaker syndrome

Source: Modified from Goldschlager N, Ludmer P, Creamer C. Follow-up of the paced outpatient. In: Ellenbogen KA, Kay GN, Wilkoff BL, eds. Clinical Cardiac Pacing. Philadelphia: WB Saunders Co., 1995: 780–808, by permission of WB Saunders Co.

would be reassessed if stored rate histograms suggest that the patient is achieving a less than optimal rate distribution. If the rate histogram suggests suboptimal rate response the rate-adaptive parameters are reprogrammed and informal exercise assessment performed.

The patient is also questioned about normal and desired activity levels. This is especially important the first time rate-adaptive parameters are initiated. However, because activity levels change – increase with better conditioning and improvement in well-being or decrease because of associated medical problems – it is wise to enquire about any change in activity before assessing and possibly altering rate-adaptive parameters.

Some CRT devices provide an activity log, i.e., objective evidence of the patient's activity level. This is especially important in patients with heart failure, because decreasing activity levels may presage the onset of clinical congestive heart failure (Fig. 13.17).

Informal exercise, when needed, can be accomplished in multiple ways depending on available equipment and monitoring. If telemetry is available then the patient should be connected to a wireless monitor and asked to walk at a pace that feels "casual" for a minimum of 2 min. Rates are assessed via telemetry throughout the walk. If the paced rate achieved is felt to be inappropriately low or high for the patient, rate-adaptive parameters can be adjusted and the walk repeated. If the rate response during the "casual" walk seems appropriate for the patient and if the patient is capable of and describes more vigorous exercise as part of his or her daily activities, the process can be repeated with the patient maintaining what they perceive as a "brisk" or "vigorous" cadence. Paced rates are again assessed during this period. For any exercise assessment, formal or informal, the "onset" of the rate change as well as the rate response post-exercise should be assessed. The onset and offset of the rate-adaptive sensor is

Date of Visit: **08-Aug-2007 14:43:36**
9987 Software Version 1.5
Copyright © Medtronic, Inc. 2002

Device: **EnRhythm P1501DR**
Serial Number: **PNP427615H**

Quick Look Report   **Page 4**

Pacing	(% of Time Since 11-Jul-2006)
AS-VS	34.4 %
AS-VP	<0.1 %
AP-VS	65.1 %
AP-VP	0.5 %
MVP	On

OBSERVATIONS (0)

• No observations based on current interrogation.

Fig. 13.12 Telemetered data classifying cardiac events as paced or sensed for both atrial and ventricular channels.

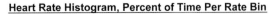

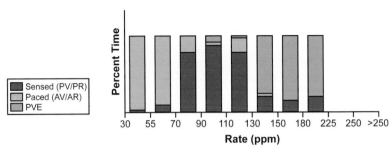

Heart Rate Histogram, Percent of Time Per Rate Bin

Event Counts

Rate (ppm)	PV	PR	AV	AR	PVE
30 - 54	6	0	166	0	0
55 - 69	148,791	29	1,196,237	361	0
70 - 89	522,321	369	129,762	351	1,285
90 - 109	131,652	2,128	5,853	155	12,536
110 - 129	6,096	238	1,518	17	187
130 - 149	0	35	4	1	127
150 - 179	0	8	0	0	45
180 - 224	0	1	0	0	4
225 - 249	0	0	0	0	0
> 250	0	0	0	0	0
Total:	**808,866**	**2,808**	**1,333,540**	**885**	**14,184**

Total Event Count: 2,160,283

Fig. 13.13 Telemetered data displaying rate histogram, i.e., distribution of heart rates since the counters were previously cleared. (Courtesy and copyrighted by St. Jude Medical.)

programmable and can be adjusted if the onset or offset appears too brisk or too slow. For a typical pacemaker patient in his or her sixties or older, with a brisk walk a heart rate of up to 100–110 is expected, and the upper rate is often set to 120. For younger patients, higher upper rate limits are usually programmed. A brisk walk typically uses 50–70% of the expected peak heart rate (calculated as 220 – age).

If wireless telemetry is not available the patient can be connected to the trans-telephonic receiver by wrist electrodes to allow single-lead ECG monitoring and the cable disconnected from the receiver, bracelets left in place, and the patient asked to hold the end of the cable. The patient is then asked to perform the type of walk(s) described above. At the end of the walk, the cable is immediately plugged in, and with the receiving mode at "standby," the ECG can be obtained at once and heart rate recorded that should be near the peak heart rate achieved. If telemetry is available, it is the preferred method of monitoring the patient during exercise. Alternatively, the rate histogram can be assessed for the focused period of informal exercise.

For the patient who exercises vigorously, formal exercise may be important. If formal (treadmill) exercise is

performed and the rate-adaptive pacemaker being optimized has an activity sensor, the patient should avoid holding on to the treadmill. Holding the treadmill railing may blunt the sensor response and lead to inappropriate programming (Chapter 8: Programming, see Rate programmability section; and Chapter 9: Rate-Adaptive Pacing).

Radiographic assessment

Radiographic assessment of the pacemaker or ICD may provide critical information. This is discussed in detail in Chapter 11: Radiography of Implantable Devices. We do not routinely obtain a chest radiograph for every visit to the device clinic. For the patient with any implanted device, a chest X-ray is obtained in the event a clinical problem occurs and it is felt that an X-ray may be valuable in the evaluation and management of the patient or before any invasive procedure, such as replacement of the pulse generator. Exceptions include specific leads that have failure modes that are detected radiographically, such as the Riata lead in which a conductor may become exteriorized from the main lead body.[2,3]

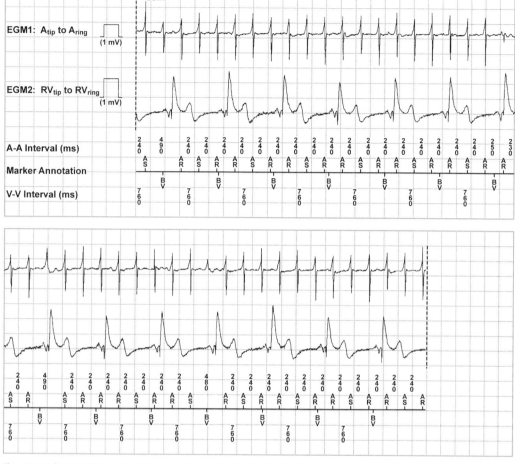

Fig. 13.14 Telemetered intracardiac electrograms from a patient with a biventricular pacemaker programmed to the DDDR mode. The atrial electrogram documents an atrial tachyarrhythmia. Biventricular pacing occurs at a regular rate consistent with mode-switching.

Device: **EnRhythm P1501DR**
Serial Number: **PNP429726H**

Date of Visit: **26-Aug-2011 13:56:05**
9987 Software Version 7.2
Copyright © Medtronic, Inc. 2010

Battery and Lead Measurements Report   **Page 1**

Last interrogation: 26-Aug-2011 13:56:05

Battery Voltage

(ERI=2.81 V on 14-Jun-2011)
26-Aug-2011 02:15:00
Voltage   2.81 V   ERI

Sensing Integrity Counter

(if >300 counts, check for sensing issues)
Since 25-May-2011 14:38:01
Short V-V Intervals   0

Atrial Lead Position Check

No measurement since reset

Lead Impedance

26-Aug-2011 02:16:45
A. Pacing   352 ohms
RV Pacing   456 ohms

Sensing

26-Aug-2011 02:20:14
P-Wave Amplitude   2.4 mV
R-Wave Amplitude   6.4 mV

Fig. 13.15 Telemetered data of battery voltage, battery impedance, lead impedance, intrinsic amplitude measurement, and sensing integrity counter from a dual-chamber ICD.

Pacemaker Model: **Medtronic.Kappa KDR933**
Serial Number: **PKU722860**

07/12/11 12:55:17 PM
Medronic.Kappa 900 Software 7.0
Copyright © Medtronic, Inc. 2001

Initial Interrogation Report	**Page 6**

Arrhythmia Summary: 03/09/11 to 07/12/11

VHR Episodes   3
AHR Episodes   237 (<0.1 hrs/day - <0.1%)
Episode Trigger   Mode Switch

Type	Date/Time	Duration hh:mm:ss	Rates (bpm): Max A	Max V	Avg V	Sensor	EGM
VHR							
Longest...	04/01/11 4:56 PM	:01	95	180	180	95	No
	05/01/11 3:12 PM	:01	108	180	180	95	Yes
Last	07/06/11 1:43 PM	:01	109	180	180	85	Yes
AHR							
First	03/11/11 7:26 AM	:10	165	102	84	81	No
Fastest	05/17/11 2:30 AM	:18	178	83	70	70	No
Longest	07/03/11 4:09 PM	:30	166	183	128	96	No
	07/10/11 4:50 AM	:19	165	120	95	78	Yes
Last	07/12/11 12:13 PM	:12	165	102	95	84	Yes

Fig. 13.16 Telemetered data of diagnostic information about atrial and ventricular events that meet criteria for "high rate."

Data storage

It is critical that the programmed data and battery and lead measurements be stored in some manner for future reference. A computerized database is preferable but if a relatively small number of patients are being followed, paper storage may be a manageable but inferior solution.

Although our data storage is entirely electronic, printouts of measured data and initial and final programmed parameters can be kept in a permanent record to allow comparison with subsequent device evaluations. This method may work well for centers with smaller volumes of patients. For large numbers of patients, paper storage becomes cumbersome.

If patient data are computerized, several additional functions may be available for data management, including the following:
• Keeping track of follow-up schedules
• Automatic reminders of patients delinquent in follow-up
• Ability to query for outcome data or to assess performance of specific leads or pulse generators
• Billing functions.

ICD follow-up

Follow-up of patients with ICDs is in many respects similar to that of patients with pacemakers. Indeed, with the progressive integration of pacemaker and ICD technology, assessing the "pacemaker" function of the ICD has become a standard part of ICD evaluation. The effectiveness and convenience of device follow-up has been significantly enhanced by the advent of remote access monitoring. Due to the increasing use of remote monitoring, and in-person clinic visit dedicated to device assessment may occur only once per year, with remote assessment at 3–4 month intervals, and for clinical events or automated alerts. The goals of ICD follow-up include assessment of patient health status, confirmation of system integrity and function, and ensuring optimal device-specific programming to minimize shocks. The approach to ICD follow-up is summarized in Table 13.5.

Assessment of the patient's clinical status

The vast majority of patients with an ICD have significant structural heart disease (Fig. 13.18), most commonly a dilated or ischemic cardiomyopathy.[4] An in-clinic evaluation provides an opportunity for review of medical status and medical regimen and for providing or arranging for additional medical evaluation as needed. Knowledge of the patient's medical status may also guide management of arrhythmias (e.g., whether to add a β-blocking agent or reprogram an ICD to manage atrial fibrillation with rapid ventricular response, provide anticoagulation to prevent stroke in patients with detected atrial fibrillation). Assessment of clinical status is aided by the use of device-based physiologic data (Fig. 13.19).

Pulse generator assessment

An important purpose of ICD generator assessment is to ensure that an adequate charge remains in the battery. Battery depletion is the single most common indication for device replacement.[5] ICDs use lithium

Table 13.4 Guidelines for routine pacemaker interrogation and programmed parameters.

1	Turn on programmer and attach ECG cables
2	Place programmer head/wand over device
3	Initiate interrogation if programmer has not already done so
4	Print initial printout of programmed parameters
5	Check battery voltage and estimated remaining longevity
6	Assess data for any mode switch episodes, atrial or ventricular high rate episodes, electrograms, % pacing, histograms, etc.
7	Obtain real-time rhythm strip
8	Check underlying rhythm @VVI 30 bpm for pacemaker dependency. Obtain rhythm strip
9	Perform sensing tests to measure P and/or R waves*
10	Obtain/record impedance values
11	Perform threshold test for all chambers paced

12	Check current programming to make sure the outputs are programmed at least 2X the threshold voltage or 3X the pulse width. Also check the programmed sensitivity is at least half the measured P or R wave. Make programming changes if necessary
	• Pacemaker nominals:
	  • Atrial – 2.0 V at 0.4 ms and 0.5 mV
	  • RV – 2.5 V at 0.3 ms and 2.5 mV
	  • LV – 1.0–1.5 V above threshold

13	Troubleshoot any problems When troubleshooting elevated LV thresholds, remember the option of programming the various configurations and assessing the threshold in each one. Steps to take: • Check the LV lead model to see if unipolar or bipolar. If unipolar, remember that bipolar configurations will not work • Check in the ICD system notes to see if patient had stimulation in any of these configurations so you would not want to select them • Program each configuration on the permanent programming screen • Go to the threshold testing screen, and check the LV threshold • Record the configuration and the threshold • Select and program another configuration, then check threshold again and record • Select the lowest threshold
14	Clear counters if required by the specific device
15	If St. Jude Medical pacemaker, demonstrate and discuss patient alert tones with patient. Document if patient unable to hear auditory alert tones
16	Print final printout of programmed parameters and measured data
17	Double-check changes with another nurse
18	Remove ECG patches and turn off programmer
19	Discuss plan for next follow-up with patient
20	Release patient
21	Clean programmer head/wand and/or ECG cables
22	Enter results in Pacemaker Database "Follow-up" note. Remember to add "Physician Reviewer"
23	Enter "Programming" note in Pacemaker Database if any programming changes
24	Add/update battery longevity information to "Reminder notes"
25	Dictate in Mayo electronic record and complete charge slip as appropriate
26	Schedule patient for next appointment if patient has routine Mayo follow-up
27	File printouts in patient's folder

*Reminder: R-wave should not be a PVC but an intrinsic beat.

silver vanadium oxide chemistry, in which the unloaded voltage provides a reasonable estimate of remaining battery life. Battery voltages gradually decline from beginning of life (BOL), to middle of life (MOL), to appearance of the elective replacement indicator (ERI), and to end of life (EOL). As battery voltage may temporarily decline after a high-voltage charge, rechecking the unloaded voltage 24 h later may show return to normal. Figure 13.20 depicts battery status determinations by manufacturers.

Once a battery is depleted to the ERI voltage, the time remaining until device malfunction varies, depending on the model, the degree of antibradycardia pacing, and the number of shocks delivered. Typically, plans are made for elective pulse generator replacement within no more than 3 months of ERI status, and often sooner.

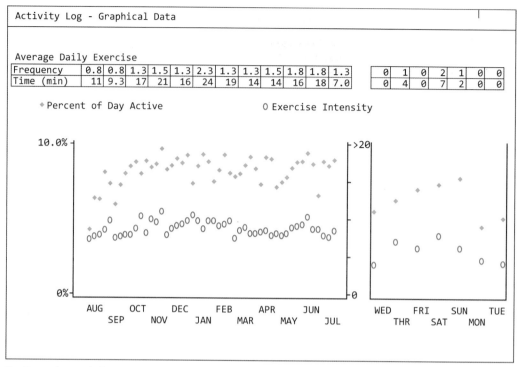

Fig. 13.17 Telemetered information depicting the patient's activity. The "solid" dots reflect the "% of day the patient was active" and the "open circles" represent the instensity of the exercise. The graph to the left depicts the trend over the prior year and the graph to the right depicts the activity trend over the prior week.

To be certain that the ERI voltage is detected, most devices will generate an audible tone or vibratory stimulus to alert the patient when ERI is reached, and an internet-based alert is sent to the clinic when remote monitoring is performed. Patients are instructed to contact the clinic following any device alert although patients at times have difficulty hearing the alerts.[6]

In contrast to the ERI voltage, which is measured in the unloaded state, the EOL voltage is the minimum loaded voltage, recorded while the battery is maximally stressed. This usually occurs during capacitor charge. If interrogation shows that the voltage has declined to EOL at any time, this signifies that during a capacitor charge or other heavy current drain, the battery voltage dipped below acceptable levels. A device should be replaced before EOL is reached, and replaced immediately if an EOL voltage is seen, as subsequent function may be unreliable.

Capacitor status

Defibrillators require the use of capacitors to accumulate and store charge before shock delivery, because a battery is unable to deliver the high level of voltage and current needed over the shock interval. Implantable devices use electrolytic capacitors, as these have a high energy density which allows a small size. However, electrolytic capacitors develop relatively large leakage currents over time, which can be reduced by recharging ("reforming") the capacitors. With early ICDs, patients had to be seen in the clinic every few months for capacitor reforming. Generally, failure to reform capacitors with sufficient frequency can result in significant delays for the first shock during therapy delivery; subsequent therapies in the same episode are not affected, because the capacitor is reformed after the first charge. Due to this, current ICDs perform automatic capacitor formations periodically, with frequency that varies by manufacturer. Excessively frequent capacitor formation does not harm the device or its functionality, although battery depletion may be accelerated.

For the clinician, the most pertinent capacitor information is the charge time, which is actually a measure of both battery and capacitor function; it is provided on device interrogation (Fig. 13.20). Some manufacturers have used charge time to indicate pulse generator EOL. Although acceptable charge time can vary from

Table 13.5 Routine follow-up evaluation of implantable cardioverter-defibrillators

Assessment of patient clinical status
- Interval history (myocardial infarction, new heart failure, syncope)
- Changes in medications, particularly antiarrhythmic drugs
- Device-based logs of physical activity and physiology

Pulse generator assessment
- Remaining battery life
- Capacitor formation and charge time
- Advisories/recalls (in many devices checked via manufacturer web page by entering specific device serial number)
- Presence of any alerts

Lead status
- Real-time telemetry with maneuvers
- Evidence of lead failure on stored electrograms
- Radiographic assessment (if there is a sign of abnormality)
- Electrogram amplitude, threshold, and impedance trends
- Parameter alerts (impedance)
- Rapid oversensed events

Patient-specific programming and therapy
- RV pacing minimized for non-CRT devices (ideally <10%, consider intervention if >40%)
- For patients with CRT devices, assessment of response
- Defibrillation efficacy:
  - Identify patients at risk for failed shocks
  - Device–device interactions (for patients with more than one implanted device)
  - Specific situations suggesting additional testing
  - Medication effects

Strategies to minimize shocks
- Sufficiently long detection in patients with nonsustained episodes
- Use of antitachycardia pacing
- Absence of T-wave oversensing on ventricular lead and far-field R-wave oversensing on atrial lead
- Appropriate use of detection enhancements

CRT, cardiac resynchronization therapy; RV, right ventricular.

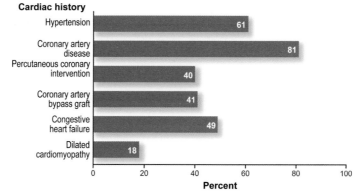

Fig. 13.18 Typical distribution of heart disease in ICD recipients. (Adapted from Wilkoff BL, Auricchio A, Brugada J, *et al*.; Heart Rhythm Society; European Heart Rhythm Association; American College of Cardiology; American Heart Association; European Society of Cardiology; Heart Failure Association of ESC; Heart Failure Society of America. HRS/EHRA expert consensus on the monitoring of cardiovascular implantable electronic devices (CIEDs): description of techniques, indications, personnel, frequency and ethical considerations. Heart Rhythm 2008; 5:907–25.)

A
Cardiac Compass®

OptiVol fluid index is an accumulation of the difference between the daily and reference impedance.

The OptiVol feature is an additional source of information for patient management and does not replace assessments that are part of standard clinical practice. Note: The OptiVol threshold and observations are not available from the Medtronic CareLink Network.

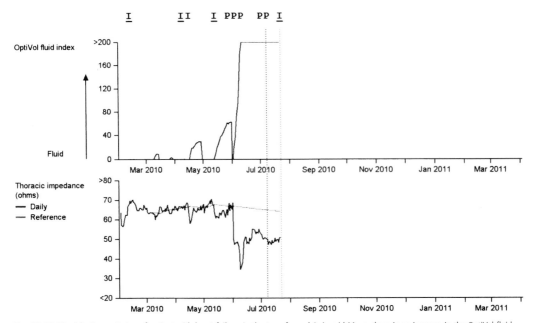

Fig. 13.19 Physiologic monitoring of patient with heart failure. In the top of panel A, in mid Mayo, there is an increase in the OptiVol fluid index (an index based on the change in impedance from a moving average), and the bottom shows a simultaneous drop in the thoracic impedance. A drop in impedance suggests increase lung fluid. At that time, the decision was made to implant a left ventricular assist device (LVAD) due to worsening heart failure; with medical therapy the impedance returns to baseline. In early June, following implant, the impedance again drops, consistent with early postoperative pulmonary edema. Impedance may also have dropped from lower impedance cause by the metal of the LVAD itself, and RV-LV function mismatch. (B) The Cardiac Compass report, which allows assessment of atrial arrhythmia burden, ventricular rate, detected tachyarrhythmia events, and physical activity to help determine causes of a changes in a patients condition. The average ventricular rate during AT/AF and during the day and night increased following LVAD implant because the pacing lower rate limit was reprogrammed to 90 bpm immediately postoperatively, and then decreased to 80 bpm about a month and a half later. The surgical team requested the increase in lower rate limit function, as it appeared to benefit LVAD function. The patient activity hours per day suddenly decreased from 1 h/day to 0 h/day due to the hospitalization and recovery period following LVAD implant. (Adapted from Erkapic, D, Duray GZ, Bauernfeind T, De Rosa S, Hohnloser SH. Insulation defects of thin high-voltage ICD leads: an underestimated problem? J Cardiovasc Electrophysiol 2011; 22:1018–22.)

device to device, a full capacitor charge generally does not exceed approximately 10 s. When it is longer than that, check with the manufacturer if it is not shortened by a capacitor formation (charge–discharge cycle).

Assessing lead function

Leads are considered the weakest link in an ICD system. ICDs record serial measurements of lead impedance and generate plots showing impedance trends. As in pacemakers, elevated impedance suggests a conductor discontinuity, whereas low impedance suggests an insulation defect or short within the lead.[7] Normal pacing impedance is a function of lead design, but for any lead (except for adapted lead combinations) impedance <200 Ω indicates an insulation defect and impedance >2000 Ω indicates conductor failure. A loose setscrew or faulty adapter can also cause abnormally high impedances.[8] Normal shocking lead impedance ranges 25–100 Ω for transvenous systems. Values outside this range suggest a conductor defect (high impedance) or insulation breach or short circuit (low impedance).

In ICDs, lead fracture may also present with characteristic nonphysiologic short intervals (<150 ms) caused by make-break electrical contact noise. Their presence

B
Cardiac Compass®

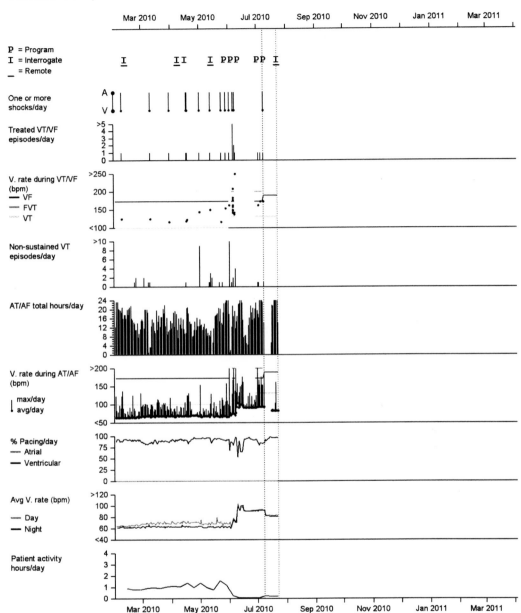

Fig. 13.19 (*Continued*)

in stored episode recordings, short interval counters, or during proactive maneuvers indicates lead failure. A detailed discussion on the approach to patients with rapid oversensing, impedance abnormalities, and suspected lead or connector abnormalities is discussed in Chapter 10: Troubleshooting, see Troubleshooting ICD lead failure section.

Defibrillation efficacy assessment

In contrast to pacing thresholds, which are easily assessed in the office environment, defibrillation testing requires intensive monitoring because of the necessity or likelihood of arrhythmia induction and shock delivery. Given the reliability of current ICD systems, the practice of routine pre-dismissal and annual follow-up

A

Last interrogation: 27-Jan-2012 15:53:40

Battery Voltage

(RRT=2.63V)
27-Jan-2012
Voltage   3.08 V

Last Capacitor Formation

13-Oct-2011
Charge Time   9.2 sec
Energy   0.0 - 35 J

Last Charge

13-Oct-2011
Charge Time   9.2 sec
Energy   0.0 - 35 J

Sensing Integrity Counter

(if >300 counts, check for sensing issues)
Since 07-Feb-2011
Short V-V Intervals   0

Atrial Lead Position Check

No measurement since reset.

Lead Impedance

A. Pacing		589 ohms	27-Jan-2012
RV Pacing		646 ohms	27-Jan-2012
LV Pacing	(LVtip to LVring)	646 ohms	27-Jan-2012
RV Defib		52 ohms	27-Jan-2012
SVC Defib		62 ohms	27-Jan-2012

Sensing

| P-Wave Amplitude | 3.4 mV | 27-Jan-2012 |
| R-Wave Amplitude | 19.8 mV | 27-Jan-2012 |

Last High Voltage Therapy

14-Jul-2010
Measured Impedance   45 ohms
Delivered Energy   14 J
Waveform   Biphasic
Pathway   B>AX

Fig. 13.20 Device status interrogation. (A) Screen shot from the Carelink® network of reporting status on a defibrillator. The battery voltage is 3.08, and recommended replacement time (RRT) is at a voltage of 2.63. Date shown is date of the last voltage check. Below is shown date, charge time, and energy charge level of the last capacitor formation (internal charge/discharge), and below that the last charge, which in this case is the same. Lead diagnostic information follows. (B) Boston Scientific battery status indicator. A gauge indicates the amount of charge available to graphically indicate relative amount of battery used, and longevity. Details regarding devices statistics used to calculate longevity (frequency pacing), remaining charge, and power consumption also provided. Capacitor information is also shown on this screen.

defibrillation threshold (DFT) testing has been abandoned by most electrophysiologists. Follow-up DFT testing is now reserved for specific clinical situations such as in the setting of marginal implant DFTs, or following the addition of antiarrhythmic drugs (although even then, the greater concern is adequate VT detection due to drug-induced VT slowing, as defibrillation is only modestly affected by antiarrhythmic drugs; Table 13.6).[9]

Medications

The interactions between medications and defibrillators require special mention in follow-up, because medications may be modified by other caregivers without full appreciation of the interaction with ICDs.

In general, the medications demonstrated to promote longevity in cardiovascular patients – β-blockers, angiotensin converting enzyme inhibitors or angiotensin receptor antagonists, antihyperlipidemic agents, statins, and aspirin – have no significant interaction with defibrillators and should be used as indicated. However, membrane-active antiarrhythmic drugs can affect pacing function, defibrillation function, and the rate and regularity of intrinsic arrhythmias. The effects of medications on defibrillator function are summarized in Table 13.7.

Use of antiarrhythmic drugs can affect pacing thresholds, so that thresholds should be rechecked when membrane-active drugs, particularly class IC agents, are prescribed. Class IC agents have use depend-

B

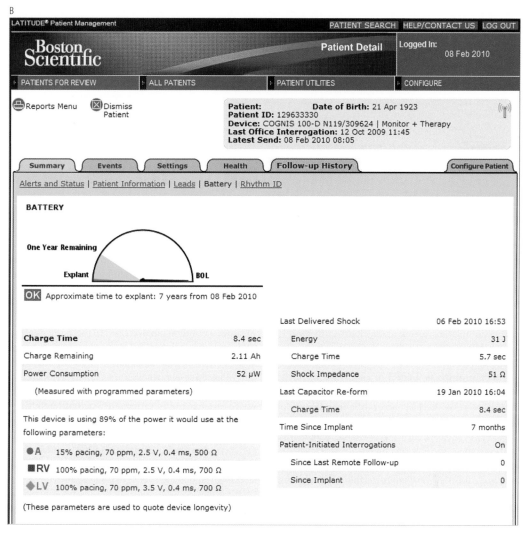

LATITUDE® Patient Management

Boston Scientific

Patient Detail

Logged In: 08 Feb 2010

PATIENT SEARCH HELP/CONTACT US LOG OUT

PATIENTS FOR REVIEW | ALL PATIENTS | PATIENT UTILITIES | CONFIGURE

Reports Menu   Dismiss Patient

Patient: **Date of Birth:** 21 Apr 1923
Patient ID: 129633330
Device: COGNIS 100-D N119/309624 | Monitor + Therapy
Last Office Interrogation: 12 Oct 2009 11:45
Latest Send: 08 Feb 2010 08:05

Summary | Events | Settings | Health | Follow-up History | Configure Patient

Alerts and Status | Patient Information | Leads | Battery | Rhythm ID

BATTERY

One Year Remaining

Explant   BOL

OK Approximate time to explant: 7 years from 08 Feb 2010

Charge Time	8.4 sec	Last Delivered Shock	06 Feb 2010 16:53
Charge Remaining	2.11 Ah	Energy	31 J
Power Consumption	52 µW	Charge Time	5.7 sec
(Measured with programmed parameters)		Shock Impedance	51 Ω
		Last Capacitor Re-form	19 Jan 2010 16:04
		Charge Time	8.4 sec
		Time Since Implant	7 months
		Patient-Initiated Interrogations	On
		Since Last Remote Follow-up	0
		Since Implant	0

This device is using 89% of the power it would use at the following parameters:

● A   15% pacing, 70 ppm, 2.5 V, 0.4 ms, 500 Ω

■ RV 100% pacing, 70 ppm, 2.5 V, 0.4 ms, 700 Ω

◆ LV 100% pacing, 70 ppm, 3.5 V, 0.4 ms, 700 Ω

(These parameters are used to quote device longevity)

Fig. 13.20 (*Continued*)

Table 13.6 Clinical circumstances suggesting the need for defibrillator evaluation and consideration of arrhythmia induction.

Clinical situation	Considerations
Recurrent shocks, therapies	Lead failure; inappropriate therapies for atrial arrhythmias; recurrent or refractory ventricular arrhythmias
New antiarrhythmic drugs (affect defibrillation threshold, ventricular tachycardia rate, or both)	Antiarrhythmic drugs can alter ventricular tachycardia rate, requiring reprogramming; can also affect defibrillation threshold
Significant change in clinical status: myocardial infarction, deteriorating cardiac function	Can affect sensing (if infarction involves tissue near sensing lead); require new medications; rarely, affect defibrillation threshold
Reprogramming to a lower sensitivity (e.g., for T-wave oversensing)	Might result in underdetection of ventricular fibrillation
Other events: pneumonectomy, patch crinkle, etc.	Can affect defibrillation threshold

Table 13.7 Interactions of antiarrhythmic medications (membrane active drugs) and implantable cardioverter-defibrillators (ICDs).

ICD function	Potential medication effect
Sensing	Diminished slew rate could affect detection (rare)
Detection	Ventricular tachycardia rate slowed below detection cut-off rate
	QRS widening can affect morphology detection enhancement criteria
	Variability in R-R intervals during VT may lead to stability detection enhancement error
Pacing	Increase pacing threshold
	Increase threshold at rapid pacing rates, affecting antitachycardia pacing (use dependency, particularly class IC agents)
	Induce bradycardia or atrioventricular block necessitating antibradycardia pacing
Defibrillation	Proarrhythmia with increased shock frequency
	Increase or decrease defibrillation threshold

ency, so that their effects are amplified at higher heart rates; thus, antitachycardia pacing (ATP) may be more affected than standard antibradycardia pacing. Defibrillators permit independent programming of ATP outputs, which should generally be set for values greater than those of the standard pacing therapies to ensure capture. A fuller discussion of the effects of medication on pacing function is found in Chapter 1: Pacing and Defibrillation.

The most important effect of antiarrhythmic drugs in patients with ICDs is the slowing of ventricular tachyarrhythmias. Ventricular tachycardia may slow below the cut-off rate and remain undetected; a useful rule of thumb is to increase the detection cycle length when initiating these medications by 30–50 ms. Drugs may also increase or decrease the defibrillation threshold, adversely affecting fibrillation termination, although clinically important elevation of defibrillation thresholds is uncommon with current biphasic systems.[10] Due to these effects, initiation of antiarrhythmic drug therapy is followed by ICD parameter assessment, with reprogramming and testing commonly performed in our practice. The effects of medication on defibrillation function are discussed in greater detail in Chapter 1: Pacing and Defibrillation.

Strategies to minimize shocks

A number of programming strategies exist to reduce the likelihood of defibrillator shock, thus to improve the tolerance of device therapy. These include use of sufficiently long detection times in patients with non-sustained arrhythmias to minimize the risk that these trigger detection or therapy; liberal use of ATP to terminate arrhythmias; programming sensing functions to prevent T-wave oversensing on the ventricular lead and far-field R-wave oversensing on the atrial lead; and appropriate use of detection enhancement to minimize the risk of inappropriate detections.[11] Screening

patients for use of these strategies at follow-up minimizes the risk of shock. These strategies are summarized in Chapter 8: Programming, see Optimizing programming section, and Tables 8.6 and 8.7.

CRT follow-up specifics

All aspects of follow-up described to this point apply to CRT evaluation during follow-up. In addition to the basics of pacing and defibrillator follow-up the clinician must also assess whether the patient is responding appropriately to CRT. The definition of response has varied among studies to include 6-minute walk time, New York Heart Association (NYHA) class, and left ventricular (LV) volumes. Outside of a clinical trial, patients' described symptoms (NYHA class), and 6-minute walk distance are practical and useful for assessing response. Response to CRT requires that a sufficient number of R-R intervals are resynchronized (as close to 100% as possible), meaning that the LV pacing frequency is sufficiently high, that LV capture occurs, and that the complexes are not fused (which may limit the degree of resynchronization and response).[12]

A detailed discussion on the approach to CRT non-response is found in Chapter 10: Troubleshooting, see Troubleshooting cardiac resynchronization devices section, and is summarized in Table 13.8.

Remote patient monitoring

TTM shows real-time pacing function (capture, non-capture) and battery status, is limited in its ability to detect intermittent malfunctions, and is primarily useful for assessing battery status.[13] Internet-based remote monitoring transmits all of the stored information available with an in-office visit, including battery voltage, capacitor charge time, impedance trends and captures threshold trends, stored episode data, real-time electrograms, rapid over-sensing counts, and detailed parameter settings. Automatic thresholds for

Table 13.8 Approach to CRT nonresponders.

Problem	Mechanism	Solution
Resynchronization is not delivered (pacing <95%)*		
Sensing errors		
Atrial undersense	Loss of P-synchronous pacing and conduction of intrinsic ventricular complexes	Increase atrial sensitivity or reposition atrial lead. If function, shorten PVARP, increase upper tracking limit, turn off PMT algorithm
Atrial events in PVARP ("pseudo-undersensing")	Loss of P-synchronous pacing and conduction of intrinsic ventricular complexes	Shorten PVARP, disable PMT and PVC response, increase upper tracking limit, consider interventricular refractory period
Atrial oversensing	Far-field R waves cause inappropriate mode switch and loss of atrial tracking	Reduce atrial sensitivey; increase PVAB; reposition lead
Ventricular oversensing	Ventricular pacing is inhibited	Reduce ventricular sensitivity; adjust ventricular refractory periods
Algorithmic inhibition of ventricular pacing	Algorithms such as rate smoothing prevent tracking abrupt increases in atrial rate	Turn algorithms off. Shorten left ventricular protection period (limits upper LV pacing rate)
Spontaneous ventricular beats		
PVCs		Alter pacing rate; determine cause of PVCs, consider additional β-blockers, amiodarone or ablation
AV conduction in sinus rhythm	Conduction of intrinsic ventricular complexes	Shorten AV delay
AV conduction in AF	Conduction of intrinsic ventricular complexes	Maintain sinus rhythm, pharmacologic rate control, pacing algorithms to cause ventricular fusion, AV junction ablation
Resynchronization is not delivered (pacing >95%, but no LV capture)*		Discussed in more detail in Chapter 2: Hemodyanmics
LV capture with slow exit from LV pacing site	Due to slow conduction of tissue around LV lead, most of ventricle activated from RV	Confirm capture by pacing LV lead alone; positive QRS complex in lead III, negative in I, and RBBB morphology in V1 indicate LV capture; If capture present, adjust V-V timing to pre-excite LV
Nonoptimal vector	Capture may be present from some LV vectors and not others; anodal capture may be present	Recheck threshold using alternate vectors
Insufficient output	LV threshold may be elevated	Increase output, or reposition LV lead
Resynchronization is delivered >95% with capture*		
Confirm patient is nonresponder	Multiple end-points have been used to define non-responders, details in text	Six-minute walk or oxygen consumption treadmill; assess ejection fraction; formal QOL assessment
Nonoptimal programming	Program parameters may not optimize intraventricular, interventricular, or atrioventricular electrical or mechanical function	Optimize V-V and AV timing with echo guidance (see Chapter 2: Hemodynamics) If frequent atrial pacing (as opposed to sensing) is disrupting left AV mechanical synchronicy, use VDD mode, consider if fusion pacing algorithms provide adequate resynchronization
Nonoptimal lead position	Insuffficient RV–LV separation to allow resynchonization	Reposition lead, particularly if in anterior vein, or small RV–LV separation radiographically and small V-V interval during intrinsic rhythm
Absence of dyssynchrony		Program to minimize ventricular pacing; CRT may not help

AV, atrioventricular; CRT, cardiac resynchronization therapy; LV, left ventricular; PMT, pacemaker-mediated tachycardia; PVAB, post-ventricular atrial blanking; PVARP, post-ventricular atrial refractory period; PVC, premature ventricular contraction; RBBB, right bundle branch block; RV, right ventricular.

*In general. the closer to achieving 100% effective biventricular pacing the better, realizing that 100% effective biventricular pacing may not be possible. While older literature suggests >90% resynchronized beats is acceptable, it is probably reasonable to aim for ≥95% resynchronization.

Alert Conditions	Enable-Urgency Tone / Monitor	Threshold
AT/AF Daily Burden Settings	Off / Off	6 hr
Avg. V. Rate During AT/AF Settings	Off / Off	6 hr at 100 bpm
Number of Shocks Delivered in an Episode	Off / Off	
All Therapies in a Zone Exhausted	Off / Off	
RV Lead Integrity	On-High / On	
A. Pacing Lead Impedance Out of Range	On-High / On	<200 or >3000 ohms
RV Pacing Lead Impedance Out of Range	On-High / On	<200 or >1000 ohms
LV Pacing Lead Impedance Out of Range	On-High / On	<200 or >3000 ohms
RV Defibrillation Lead Impedance Out of Range	On-High / On	<20 or >100 ohms
SVC Defib Lead Impedance Out of Range	On-High / On	<20 or >100 ohms
Low Battery Voltage RRT	On-High / On	2.63 V(RRT)
Excessive Charge Time EOS	On-High / On	
VF Detection OFF, 3+ VF or 3+ FVT Rx Off.	On-High / On	

Fig. 13.21 Remote monitoring alerts. This screen shot from a CareLink® session indicates alerts that can be set with programmable threshold to notify the patient of a device a medical or device condition that may warrant attention. Alerts can be based on atrial arrhythmia (AT/AF) burden, ventricular rates during atrial arrhythmias, therapy delivery, or finding that suggest hardware issues (lead impedance, battery status, capacitor charge time). In additional to patient audible notification, internet-based alerts can be sent to caregivers.

abnormal values can be established to enable internet-based caregiver alerts and device-based audible or vibratory patient alerts in the event of abnormal values (Fig. 13.21). Abnormalities may indicate device malfunction (e.g., lead impedance), or clinical events (e.g., development of atrial fibrillation, incipient pulmonary edema). Studies including large numbers of patients have demonstrated that remote monitoring shortens the time to detection and treatment of actionable events, and is associated with shortened cardiovascular hospitalization and decreased mortality (Fig. 13.22).[14] Internet-based remote monitoring saves patients clinic visits, and increases healthcare efficiency by requiring less provider care for routine follow-up, and focusing attention on potential problems.

Remote monitoring may be completely automated or, in the case of inductive systems, may require patient intervention. Automated systems utilize radiofrequency transmitters integrated into the implanted device to transmit to a hub, which then communicates to secure data servers via a cellular or land line connection (Fig. 13.23). The hub may be a transceiver kept within the home (typically on a night stand) or a portable unit that can receive implanted device data independent of patient action. In inductive systems, the patient holds a wand over his or her device to active a telemetry session, which is then transmitted via a phone connection to a secure internet site. Inductive systems primarily allow remote monitoring interface of legacy systems, i.e., devices available prior to the development of remote-monitoring systems with devices designed with wireless radiofrequency link. For wireless telemetry, the patient's radiofrequency monitor can typically be within 10 ft of the implanted device for transmissions to occur,

whereas inductive telemetry requires a wand to be placed over the device within a range of a few inches. Irrespective of the mechanism used, data are transmitted to a protected website that can be accessed by healthcare providers, and other sites (with limited data) available to the patients themselves.

Expert consensus documents for follow-up using remote access monitoring have been established by professional societies.[1,15] The Mayo Clinic follow-up schedule for patients on a remote-monitoring system (which at this time includes contemporary high-voltage, ICD and CRT-D, devices and select pacemakers) is as follows:

• Nightly/as per system: lead, battery, and other alerts check with automatic transmission with radiofrequency devices
• Third month: clinic visit
• Third month through failure: every 4 months remote access monitoring with yearly in-clinic visit.

More frequent follow-up may be required early after implantation and as the device approaches elective replacement indicators. Other factors accounting for increased frequency of follow-up include patient-initiated transmissions secondary to symptoms, system alerts, or therapy delivery. Some systems incorporate two levels of alerts: low urgency (or yellow) for less time-critical warnings such as elective battery replacement indicators and atrial lead malfunction, and high-urgency (red) alerts for ventricular lead malfunction and other critical warnings. For the clinician, adjustable alert preferences include notification frequency and mode (fax, phone, page, and/or web-based). The Latitude™ and CareLink™ systems allow patients to log in to a patient-specific website to see their alerts and

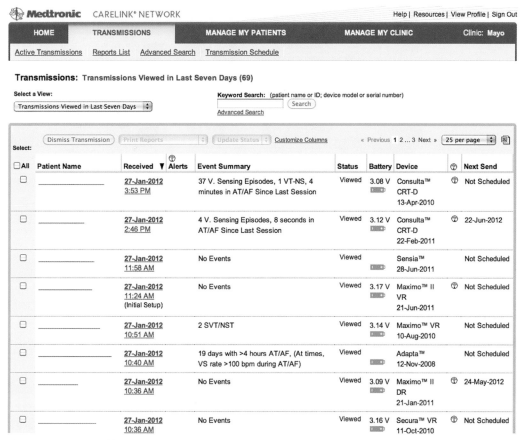

Fig. 13.22 Intenet remote follow up clinic report. All remote internet-based systems generate summaries of active patients, or patients with recent transmissions or alerts, highlighting pertinent clinical information. This example is from the CareLink® network showing recent transmissions, and summarizing date received, clinical events, battery status, device type, and next scheduled transmission.

battery status. Table 13.9 summarizes the functionality of remote monitoring systems, and Table 13.10 the web addresses for caregivers. Because remote programming is not available at this time, a clinic visit is required for parameter changes. Remote programming is technically possible but the limitations in making this available are regulatory in nature.

The role of remote monitoring to insure appropriate device function is well established and data from a remote-monitoring registry have demonstrated improved survival for those patients that are networked, i.e., followed by remote monitoring (Fig. 13.24).[14] Its role in monitoring disease states is promising and rapidly emerging. Two disease states have received significant attention: congestive heart failure (CHF) and atrial fibrillation (AF).

Congestive heart failure: The role of various physiologic parameters in predicting heart failure is the subject of continued investigation. A decline in activity levels (recorded by the accelerometer present in all ICDs) and increase in body weight may be signs of developing heart failure.[16] In one study decreased heart rate variability (a measure of the variability of R-R intervals associated with changes in autonomic tone) was shown to precede hospitalization by 16 days and automated detection had a 70% sensitivity for detection of cardiovascular hospitalizations, with 2.4 false positives per patient-year follow-up.[17] Measurement of intrathoracic impedance-based estimates of pulmonary congestion has been used as an early predictor of CHF (Fig. 13.19). However, overall the specificity and sensitivity of detecting a change in pulmonary congestion has been low and has been not demonstrated in a randomized clinical trial.[18] Therefore, the clinical utility of intrathoracic impedance monitoring remains uncertain. Clinical studies of devices implanted into the central circulation to monitor pulmonary artery pressure have

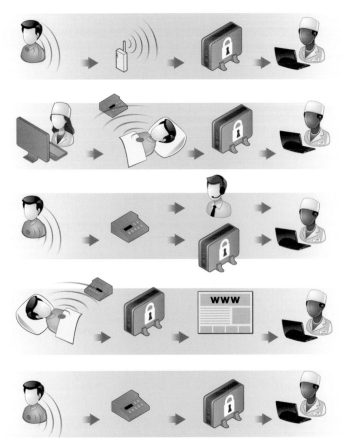

Fig. 13.23 Cartoons depicting variations in currently available remote systems. All require communication from the implanted device to a hub, which then send the information to a secure server via the internet. Systems differ in whether they provide access to the internet via a landline or dedicated cellular connection, and if a cellular connection is used, whether there is a fee to the patient for its use or not.

also shown promise in heart failure management, although their role in clinical practice is not yet defined.[19–21] Some systems also permit tracking of "external" data such as blood pressure and weight by means of wireless communication with blood pressure cuffs and scales, and patient symptoms by means of patient-completed surveys. Remote monitoring systems that incorporate a scale and blood pressure cuff have demonstrated survival benefit using these systems compared with usual care, and shortened hospitalization compared with nurse telephone support.[22,23]

Atrial fibrillation: Implanted devices that incorporate an atrial lead can effectively determine the occurrence of atrial tachycarrhythmias. Established evidence-based clinical guidelines indicate patients with atrial fibrillation and risk factors from thromboembolism (most commonly congestive heart failure, hypertension, age

75 or more, diabetes or previous stroke or transient ischemic attack) benefit from anticoagulation. However, these data are all based on atrial fibrillation diagnosed with surface electrocardiography. Recent prospective randomized trials have demonstrated an associated between device-detected atrial tachyarrhythmias and subsequent thromboembolism.[24,25] In the ASSERT study, 2580 patients aged 65 or older with hypertension, no known history of atrial fibrillation, and a standard indication for a pacemaker or defibrillator were monitored for subclinical atrial tachyarrhythmias, defined as an atrial tachycardia with atrial rate >190 bpm lasting at least 6 minutes. Subclinical atrial tachyarrhythmias were present in 10% of patients within 3 months, and significantly increased the risk of stroke (hazard ration 2.5; $P = 0.008$) (Fig. 13.25). Interventional studies to determine the effect of treating these short, subclinical arrhythmias have not been performed, optimal man-

Table 13.9 Summary of remote monitoring system characteristics.

	Biotronik Home Mooitoring™	Medtronic Ca relink™	Boston Scientific Latitude™	Sorin SMARTVIEW™	St Jude Merlin. net™
Wireless communication with implanted device	Radiofrequency	Radiofrequency	Radiofrequency	Radiofrequency	Radiofrequency
Data transmission	GSM network	Analogue phoneline and GSM network	Analogue phonetine	Analogue or GSM	Analogue or GSM
Transmitter	Mobile or stationary (GSM)	Stationary	Stationary	Stationary	Stationary
Frequency of transmissions	Scheduled FU; daily FU; alert events	Scheduled FU; alert events: on patient demand	Scheduled FU; alert events	Scheduled FU; alert events	Scheduled FU; alert events
Remote follow-up	Yes	Yes	Yes	Yes	Yes
RM	Yes	Yes	Yes	Yes	Yes
Physician notification	SMS, email, fax	SMS, email	Fax, phone	Fax, email SMS	Fax, email SMS
Feedback to patient via transmitter	LED indicating normal status or call to clinic	Confirmation for successes interrogation and transmission	Automatic text and audio messages	LED indicating HM status	LED indicating call to clinic, automated phone calls
IEGM (real-time at remote follow up)	30 s (monthly periodic EGMs)	10 s	10 s	7 s	30 s
IEGM (arrhythmic episodes)	All memorized episodes	All memorized episodes	All memorized episodes	All memorized episodes	All memorized episodes
FDA and CE Mark system approval	Yes	Yes	Yes	No	Yes
Special features	Automatic RV and LV thresholds. Send phone calls to pts	Automatic RA, RV, and LV (Consulta and Protecta XT) pacing thresholds	Optional wireless weight scales and BP cuffs	Patient initiated transmissions	Alerts fully configurable online
	Comprehensive heart failure monitor, intrathroracic impedance measurement (CE-Mark only)	Optivol® lung fluid status alert	Configurable data transmission to associated caregivers	SMARTVIEW HF featuring PhD clinical status	Send phone calls to parts. CoRVUE fluid status alert
	Configurable red and yellow alerts	Configurable red and yellow alerts	Configurable red and yellow alerts	PDF export of patient reports	Automatic RA. RV, a nd LV pacing thresholds (next generation of ICDs)
	Alerts fully configurable online. Patient callback	ILR RM	Electronic health record data export capability	Access for heart failure specialists and general cardiologist	
	Electronic health record export compatibility	PDF export of patient reports			
	Devices available for RM	Any already implanted devices available for RM			

RA, right atrial; RV, right ventricular; LV, left ventricular; IEGM, intracardiac electrogram; BP, blood pressure; GSM, global system for mobile communications.

Modified from Burri and Senouf.[6]

Source: Adapted from Dubner S, Auricchio A, Steinberg JS, et al.; Document reviewers:, Israel C, Padeletti L, Brignole M. ISHNE/EHRA expert consensus on remote monitoring of cardiovascular implantable electronic devices (CIEDs). Europace 2012; 14:278–93.

agement is not yet determined, so that a risk factor based strategy is our preferred approach at present.[26]

Practical considerations of remote monitoring

In the early years of remote monitoring there were a number of concerns expressed by caregivers. There was a perception that patients, accustomed to a face to face visit, would not accept the electronic transfer and assessment of data. To the contrary, patient satisfaction is higher with remote monitoring. The technology gives them greater reassurance because they realize there is not only greater capacity for data transmission but problems with their device, or alerts, will reach their caregiver even faster with remote monitoring.

There was also a concern that the amount of data available through remote monitoring would overwhelm the device clinic personnel. Although some debate persists on this subject, systems and processes in

place to prioritize alerts and levels of alerts generally makes data assessment reasonably straightforward to manage.

Another fear of clinicians was one of litigation. Caregivers were afraid that data would be transmitted and not acted upon before the patient suffered an adverse consequence. A specific example would be the patient with paroxysmal atrial fibrillation who suffered a cerebrovascular event before the remote monitoring transmission was assessed and therapy offered to the patient. This concern has not materialized. To our knowledge, no legal precedent has been set. In fact, based on randomized trial data,[27,28] clinical problems are recognized and responded to faster through remote monitoring than they are when patients are followed in a conventional office-based manner.

Patients' concerns during follow-up

It is impossible to predict all concerns that might be raised by the patient with an implantable cardiac device. However, several specific issues are invariably raised, and they should be included in the information, whether written or oral, provided to the patient.

Medical advisories and recalls

Despite their overall high level of reliability, over the years there have been periodic safety alerts and "recalls"

Table 13.10 Remote monitoring websites for caregivers.

LATITUDE	www.latituderemote.bostonscientific.com
CARELINK	www.medtroniccarelink.com
MERLIN	www.merlin.net
HomeMonitoring	www.biotronik-homemonitoring.com
SMARTVIEW	www.sorin-smartview.us

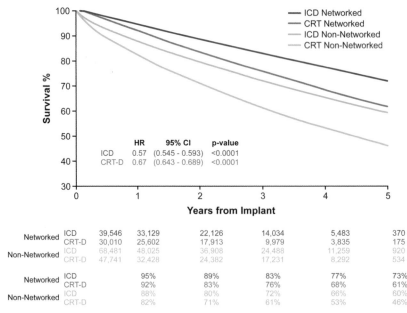

Fig. 13.24 Survival of CRT and ICD patients followed by the Latitude remote monitoring network vs. clinic only (non-networked) in a non-randomized study of over 185,000 patients. Patients selected for remote monitoring by their physicians had a 50% lower mortality than those undergoing in-office only evaluations. (From Saxon LA, Hayes DL, Gilliam FR, et al. Long-term outcome after ICD and CRT implantation and influence of remote device follow-up: the ALTITUDE survival study. Circulation 2010; 122:2359–67.)

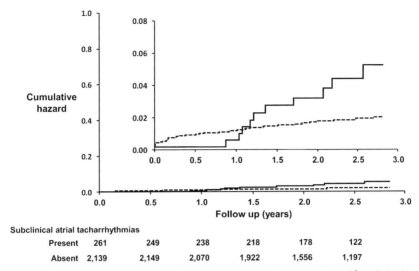

Subclinical atrial tacharrhythmias					
Present	261	249	238	218	178	122
Absent	2,139	2,149	2,070	1,922	1,556	1,197

Fig. 13.25 Risk of thromboembolism following subclinical episode of atrial tachyarrhythmias. The ASSERT study[5] enrolled 2580 patients and found that the occurrence of device detected atrial tachyarrhythmias (defined as an atrial rate above 190 bpm for more than 6 minutes) more than doubled the risk of stroke or thromboembolism.

of implantable devices and leads affecting thousands of patients. In more recent years the number of device-related alerts and advisories has increased dramatically, probably due to increased awareness, greater enforcement of reporting policy, lay press coverage, and increased device complexity.[29,30]

Dealing with medical advisories and recalls from the manufacturer or the Food and Drug Administration (FDA) and reporting device failures are responsibilities of the physician or the institution, or both, providing follow-up care.[31,32]

The FDA categorizes recalls into three classes:
• Class I: Situations in which there is a reasonable probability that the use of, or exposure to, a violative product will cause serious adverse health consequences or death
• Class II: Situations in which the use of, or exposure to, a violative product may cause temporary or medically reversible adverse health consequences or in which the probability of serious adverse health consequences is remote
• Class III: Situations in which the use of, or exposure to, a specific product is not likely to cause adverse health consequences.

Safety advisories or safety alerts are sometimes issued and are, in general, less significant than class III recalls.

When informed of a recall or advisory, the physician or institution involved in follow-up of the patient with a pacemaker or ICD is responsible for making certain that the patient is aware of the potential problem and

that appropriate steps are taken. Necessary action depends on the type of problem identified. Action may range from pulse generator or lead replacement to lead extraction, intensified follow-up, or patient notification only. Patient notification and advice should be documented in the medical record. For patients on remote monitoring, the system being used may allow some additional methods of notifying the patient of an alert.

Device clinic personnel should be available to discuss the alert or advisory with the patient after notification. They should also be knowledgeable about the specific problem and be able to explain the problem in a way the patient can understand.[33]

Under prior legislation (Safe Medical Devices Act of 1990 [Public Law 101–629] and the Medical Device Amendments of 1992), hospitals, ambulatory surgical facilities, nursing homes, and outpatient treatment facilities that are not physicians' offices must report to the FDA or the manufacturer any death, serious illness, or serious injury caused or contributed to by a medical device. Such incidents should be reported within 10 working days of the event. Patient deaths must be reported to the FDA, and serious illness and injury must be reported only to the manufacturer. (If the manufacturer is unknown, the report should be made to the FDA.)

Advisories almost always result in patient concern and often impaired quality of life. Depending on the advisory it may also result in more intensive follow-up or a surgical procedure to replace or remove affected

Table 13.11 Definition of device malfunction.

Device malfunction	Failure of a device to meet its performance specifications or otherwise perform as intended. Performance specifications include all claims made in the labeling for the device. The intended performance of a device refers to the intended use for which the device is labeled or marketed [FDA Regulations 803.3(n)]. Whenever possible, device malfunction should be confirmed by laboratory analysis
Device malfunction with compromised therapy	A device (pulse generator or lead) that has malfunctioned in a manner that compromises pacing or defibrillation therapy (including complete loss or partial degradation). Some examples include: sudden loss of battery voltage, accelerated current drain such that low battery voltage is not detected before loss of therapy and sudden malfunction resulting in nondelivery of defibrillation therapy
Induced malfunction	A malfunction caused by external factors (e.g., therapeutic radiation, excessive physical damage, etc.) including, but not limited to, hazards that are listed in product labeling. Damage to a pulse generator caused by a lead malfunction is considered to be a lead rather than a pulse generator malfunction
Malfunction without compromised therapy	A device that has malfunctioned in a manner that does not compromise pacing or defibrillation therapy. Some examples include: error affecting diagnostic functions, telemetry function, data storage; malfunction of a component that causes battery to lose power prematurely, but in a time frame that is detectable during normal follow-up before normal function is lost, and mechanical problems with connector header that do not affect therapy
Normal battery depletion	1. A device is returned with no associated complaint and the device has reached its elective replacement indicator(s) with implant time that meets or exceeds the nominal (50th percentile) predicted longevity at default (labeled) settings
	2. A device is returned and the device has reached its elective replacement indicator(s) with implant time exceeding 75% of the expected longevity using the longevity calculation tool available at the time of production introduction, calculated using the device's actual settings

Source: Carlson MD, Wilkoff B, Maisel WH, *et al.*; American College of Cardiology Foundation; American Heart Association; International Coalition of Pacing and Electrophysiology Organizations. Recommendations from the Heart Rhythm Society Task Force on Device Performance Policies and Guidelines. Heart Rhythm 2006; 3:1250–73.

hardware.[34,35] Advisories involve significant cost and burden on the healthcare system and operative morbidity and mortality for patients.[36,37] Device replacement has a higher morbidity than new implantation and for some "recall" events likely exceeds the potential morbidity of the device malfunction that necessitated the advisory.

A device malfunction is said to occur when it fails to meet its performance specification, or otherwise fails to perform as intended. Device malfunction may compromise or degrade therapy, or may only impact ancillary features such as diagnostics (see Table 13.11 for definitions of device malfunction). The approach to "recall" management depends on the mechanism of malfunction and its predictability, the impact should malfunction occur, patient factors (e.g., pacemaker dependency), and the risk of surgical interventions to correct the malfunction (e.g., device replacement). Professional societies have prepared guidelines to assist caregivers through the difficult landscape of managing device alerts and recalls.[38,39] The documents emphasize early detection of hardware malfunction, clear and timely communication to minimize patient confusion, and avoidance of unnecessary interventions to minimize surgical complications.

The recommendations emphasize the need to balance the risk caused by defective hardware with the risk associated with intervention, and the need to balance the need for patient monitoring with the need to minimize his or her level of anxiety. The following guidelines are suggested for patient management.

Suggested methods of increasing patient safety while minimizing inconvenience and anxiety include the following:
• Increased follow-up frequency for devices that are not replaced
• Maximal use of automatic alerts and home monitoring systems for early detection of malfunctions in patients with advisory hardware
• Efficient, quick, and responsible communication between manufacturers, physicians, and patients so that relevant information will reach patients through their caregivers rather than via mass media.

Recommended measures to decrease unnecessary device replacements include the following:
• Careful individual risk assessment, taking into account not only the probability of intrinsic device failure, but also potential consequences of failure related to current device indication in the individual

patient. For example, a pacemaker-dependent ICD patient with recurrent life-threatening arrhythmia is at much higher risk in the event of device failure than a patient implanted for primary prevention of sudden death. The concept of current device indication (as opposed to original indication for implantation) is important, as the clinical condition may have changed since implantation with newly developed arrhythmias or pacemaker dependence.

• The risks of the replacement operation and time to elective replacement of the device must also be considered for the individual patient.[34,35] Overall, a risk of malfunction below 1/1000 is considered low when considering replacement in a patient who is not at particularly high risk should the device malfunction.

• In some specific situations, consideration of alternative noninvasive measures of management, such as reprogramming or more frequent monitoring, may be applicable.

Given the small risk of device malfunctions in most circumstances, the physician must allay patient anxiety and confusion and objectively balance the risk of operation with continued observation. Table 13.12 sum-marizes the HRS guidelines for decisions on device recalls and notifications.

The Medtronic Fidelis lead advisory involved more than 100,000 leads worldwide.[40] These leads tend to present with conductor fracture with frequent episodes of inappropriate shocks. The magnitude and severity of this phenomenon encouraged the development by the manufacturer of a special device algorithms (Lead Integrity Alert[R], [LIA] that was designed to identify lead fracture at its earliest stages, alert the patient and the follow-up center and automatically reprogram the device to reduce the risk of inappropriate shocks.[41] In the earlier models these algorithms were downloaded to all devices of patients with Fidelis leads. Currently they are included and automatically turned on in all new Medtronic ICD models.

Our policy of follow-up for patients with Fidelis leads takes advantage of contemporary advances in technologies such as extensive use of remote monitoring, LIA algorithms, and patient alerts, and applies the principles for management of device recalls as depicted in the US and European guidelines for management of device recalls.

Table 13.12 Guidelines for decisions on device recalls and notifications.

Consider device/lead replacement if:	• The mechanism of malfunction is known and is potentially recurrent • The risk of malfunction is likely to lead to patient death or serious harm, and • The risk of replacement is less than or at least not substantially greater than the risk of device malfunction
Consider device/lead replacement in:	• Patients who are pacemaker-dependent • Patients with an ICD for secondary prevention of sudden death, and • Patients with an ICD for primary prevention of sudden death who have received appropriate device therapy for a ventricular arrhythmia
Consider device replacement if the predicted end of life (EOL) is approaching	
Consider conservative management with periodic noninvasive device monitoring when the rate of device malfunction is very low in:	• Patients who are not pacemaker-dependent and • Patients with an ICD for primary prevention of sudden cardiac death who have not required device therapy for a ventricular arrhythmia
Provide routine follow-up for patients with a device malfunction that has been mitigated or corrected by reprogramming the software	
Consider conservative management with periodic noninvasive device monitoring in patients where operative intervention risk is high or in patients who have other significant competing morbidities even when the risk of device malfunctions or patient harm is substantial	

Source: Carlson MD, Wilkoff B, Maisel WH, *et al.*; American College of Cardiology Foundation; American Heart Association; International Coalition of Pacing and Electrophysiology Organizations. Recommendations from the Heart Rhythm Society Task Force on Device Performance Policies and Guidelines. Heart Rhythm 2006; 3:1250–73.

The Riata and Riata ST leads are the most recent ICD leads on "advisory" as of the writing of this text.[2,3] The lead cables may become exteriorized with an inside-out abrasion mechanism. The lead may continue to function normally with the exteriorized ETFE-coated cables. However, the natural history of the exteriorized cables is unknown at this time and best management not yet determined. In addition, some of the electrical failures of this lead are probably due to "lead on can" abrasions and whether or not this particular family of leads has a higher incidence of "lead on can" abrasions and failure is not yet known.

Lifestyle and personal concerns

Return to driving has traditionally been less of an issue with pacemakers than with ICDs. Both the HRS and the EHRS have established guidelines for return to driving after pacemaker implantation.[42,43] These are summarized in Table 13.13. Regulations for return to driving differ from state to state.

Although regulations vary among various countries and even states within the USA, general principles have been adopted by both US and European expert panels. Patients with ICDs are generally prohibited from any commercial driving. Patients who have received an ICD for primary prevention may drive within a relatively short period of time. At our institution we ask pacemaker and CRT patients and ICD patients implanted for primary prevention to avoid driving for 10 days and explain this need as a medicolegal or liability issue. For patients with high-voltage devices for secondary prevention and primary prevention patients who subsequently receive an appropriate therapy for ventricular tachycardia or fibrillation, especially with syncope, are restricted from driving for 6 months. Furthermore, patients may have contraindications to driving without any tachycardia because of unstable medical issues, and driving privilege will need to be assessed on an individual basis.[42]

Another driving-related issue that arises not infrequently is whether a seat belt interferes with the device. The seat belt may be over the implant site for the driver with a left pectoral implant or a passenger with a right-sided implant. Seat belts are not an issue unless they result in irritation at the implant site in the early weeks after implantation. If irritation is a concern, the patient can place some padding over the pulse generator or around the seat belt in the area of pulse generator contact. This should not be an excuse not to wear a seat belt and would not be considered a justifiable reason for not wearing a seat belt if cited by the authorities.

Limitation of physical activities after device implantation must be addressed. We recommend that ipsilateral arm movement be limited to 90° abduction for 3–4 weeks. Admittedly, this may be overcautious and impossible for some patients, especially pediatric

Table 13.13 Guidelines for driving after pacemaker implantation.

	Restriction for private driving	Restriction for professional driving
EHRA driving recommendations		
ICD implantation for secondary prevention	3 months	Permanent
ICD implantation for primary prevention	4 weeks	Permanent
After appropriate ICD therapy	3 months	Permanent
After inappropriate ICD therapy	Until measures to prevent inappropriate therapy are taken	Permanent
After replacement of the ICD	1 week	Permanent
After replacement of the lead system	4 weeks	Permanent
Patients refusing ICD for primary prevention	No restriction	Permanent
Patients refusing ICD implantation for secondary prevention	7 months	Permanent
HRS driving recommendations		
Overview of recommendations		
Type of driving	Indication	Driving restriction
Private Primary prevention	Recovery from operation (≥1 week)	
	Secondary prevention	6 months
Commercial (covered by US Dept of Transportation guideline)	Primary prevention	Cannot be certified to drive
	Secondary prevention	Cannot be certified to drive

EHRA, European Heart Rhythm Association; HRS, Heart Rhythm Society.

patients. The lead is secured to the pectoral muscle near the venous insertion site, and it is unlikely that more vigorous arm movements would dislodge the lead. However, some guidelines should be given to the patient and this approach has been successful for most adult patients who are usually able to follow the restriction without difficulty. We frequently send patients home with a sling to be worn loosely for 5–7 days as a reminder to limit arm motion. This is especially helpful in the pediatric population.

Although we restrict arm motion on the side of the pulse generator implant, we are also careful to caution the patient not to immobilize the arm. Complete immobility could lead to reflex sympathetic dystrophy.[44]

We also recommend that patients limit lifting to no more than 10 lb with the ipsilateral arm for the first 2 weeks after implantation.

Issues of return to work and disability arise. Once again, the advice should be individualized. Patients who have jobs that do not involve heavy physical exertion can return to work shortly after the procedure. It is unusual for the patient to experience postoperative pain significant enough to require more than ibuprofen or acetaminophen and to limit the ability to perform the job. Patients who have jobs that involve heavy physical exertion in which performance depends on upper body strength, or activities that require that the arm ipsilateral to the new implant be lifted above shoulder level may need to wait longer to return to work. In these circumstances, it is justifiable to keep the patient away from work for up to 4 weeks.

Sports activities are important for many patients. Patients are told that they can return to most sports activities. For the younger pacemaker patient, most competitive sports are reasonable, with the exception of contact sports having a significant potential for injury. Specifically, football, wrestling, and boxing carry some risk. Patients should be informed of the risk and be given counseling to weigh the ratio of risk to benefit. The predominant concern with contact sports is direct trauma to the lead at or near the connector block. If the lead(s) has been implanted via the subclavian vein, it may be somewhat more susceptible to injury from any repetitive motion that has the potential of narrowing the interspace between the first rib and clavicle, e.g., weightlifting and basketball. Again, the issues should be discussed with the patient and the importance of the activity weighed against the risk.

Golf and swimming are two relatively common athletic activities for the average device patient. We suggest waiting 4 weeks after implantation before returning to golfing due to motion restrictions already described. Swimming can be resumed as soon as the incision is healed, but the recommendation is to limit some strokes for 4 weeks to stay within the abduction guidelines already discussed.

Hunting and marksmanship also seem to be relatively frequent activities for our patient population. If these activities will be continued, the device should be implanted on the side contralateral to that from which the patient shoots a rifle. We allow patients to return to these activities at any time so long as they stay within the shoulder movement guidelines outlined.

ICD recipients are ineligible for some competitive sports; however, noncompetitive athletics and physical activity are generally encouraged. Detailed guidelines regarding sporting activities for ICD recipients have been published.[45]

Concerns about resumption of sexual activity are frequent. Patients are often reluctant to ask questions about resuming sexual activity. Caregivers should be proactive in approaching the subject of sexual activity. Patients are told that they may resume sexual activity whenever they like, so long as they observe the shoulder motion guidelines.

Similar to the seat belt issue previously discussed, some women are concerned about irritation to the device site by their bra strap. Our patients are advised either not to wear a bra until the incision is well healed or nontender, or to place extra padding around the strap. Rarely is this a significant problem or concern.

Many unanticipated concerns arise. Initial education about the pacemaker or defibrillator and how it works is the best way to facilitate the patient's return to health.

Psychologic issues encountered following device implantation

Significant psychologic issues related to low-voltage devices, i.e., pacemakers and CRT-D do occur but are relatively infrequent compared with ICDs.

Many ICD patients naturally have some level of preoccupation about getting shocked and what a shock will feel like. People describe shocks in many different ways. Some say it feels like a kick to the chest, others compare it to a jolt from an electric fence, and so on. Patient surveys have revealed that on a pain scale ranging 1–10, with 1 representing "no pain" and 10 representing "worst pain imaginable," most patients rate an ICD shock as a 6.[46] Most patients also indicate that the shock is more sudden and frightening than it is painful. Although most ICD patients would agree with these analogies and ratings, at best they are a bit incomplete, and at worst, perhaps a bit misleading for many reasons. Patients may remember a shock as less painful if they know that it was delivered to stop a life-threatening arrhythmia, i.e., the shock was appropriate.[47] Some research suggests that patients may remember inappropriate shocks as more painful than appropriate shocks. Perhaps the knowledge that the ICD saved their life will make the patient more accepting of the shock experience. It may be helpful to remind the patient that a shock is a life-saving event as opposed to a negative experience.

A phantom shock may be a particularly difficult event and some patients will argue with their clinician that the device interrogation is wrong, insisting that they experienced a shock.

Phantom shocks often occur just as the patient is going to sleep but can happen during sleep or when fully alert. Phantom shocks may occur in patients who have had multiple shocks and are worried about more as well as patients who have never received a therapy.

Patients who are having difficulty adjusting to having a device, specifically an ICD, may benefit from an ICD support group. There are also blogs for patients with devices. If the blog is "unfiltered" patients should be warned that not all of the information may be correct.

Having the patient develop a "shock plan" and involving appropriate loved ones may help to decrease and/or avoid some of the psychologic issues. Steps involved include the following:

1   Patient understands what is recommended if they experience a shock. The recommendations given may differ, depending on whether or not the patient experiences symptoms at the time of shock and whether they received one shock or more than one shock. Typically, if the patient has experienced more than one shock within 24 hours they should seek medical attention. If a single shock has been delivered and the patient feels well, if the patient is on a remote monitoring system, an additional transmission and review of the data may be all that is needed.

2   Patients should be encouraged to talk to their family or friends about how they can help if the patient receives a shock. Identifying individuals to help in an emergent situation may help to reduce the patient's anxiety.

3   A shock plan would include family and/or significant others knowing what to do should an emergency arise, i.e., what hospital has the medical information, what medications the patient is taking, having a medical summary on hand if traveling and possibly requiring care at a facility that does not have the past medical history, etc.

4   Directing the patient to techniques and methods that may assist them in remaining calm and focused should a shock occur.

Withdrawal of device support
Although it is generally accepted that withdrawal of ICD therapies to avoid shocks for ventricular tachyar-

rhythmias in terminally ill patients is reasonable,[48–51] the role of withdrawing pacemaker therapy, especially in a pacemaker-dependent patient, is not as clear.[52–54] Discussions regarding withdrawal of pacemaker therapy are often sharply divided given the expected variation in personal beliefs. Nevertheless, a recent expert consensus statement supports the withdrawal of both ICD and pacemaker therapies in terminally ill patients if doing so is consistent with the patient's healthcare-related values, preferences, and goals.[55]

The consensus statement[55] outlines steps that should be taken if a patient or patient surrogate requests device deactivation. Three very important caveats should be remembered:

1   The patient, or surrogate, has the ultimate authority to decide if a device is to be deactivated.

2   If device deactivation is counter to the beliefs of the caregiver, no caregiver can be forced to perform the deactivation. However, the hospital or practice must have a process in place that would allow the deactivation to be completed by another caregiver.

3   Depending on the type of device being activated and clinical history of device usage, expectations should be set for patients and their family members as to what to expect when the device is deactivated.

Whether at implant or some other appropriate time, patients should be made aware that device therapy can be withdrawn if that should be their wish in the presence of defined circumstances.[55] All patients should be encouraged to have a "living will" with clear delineation of all of their wishes, including management of the implantable device.

Conclusions
Appropriate follow-up of an implantable device is required to ensure continuing integrity of the system and to detect failures before they become clinically manifest. This requires a thorough understanding of both device function and interpretation of the extensive telemetered data provided. However, with the incorporation of routine device self-assessment, with the ability of many pulse generators to alert patients effectively to potential problems, and with the advent or remote monitoring, device surveillance has changed dramatically in recent years. Furthermore, with continued maturation of device technology and monitoring, the focus of follow-up is evolving from detecting device malfunction to predicting disease progression before it becomes manifest in order intervene to maintain health.

References
1 Wilkoff BL, Auricchio A, Brugada J, et al. Heart Rhythm Society; European Heart Rhythm Association; American

College of Cardiology; American Heart Association; European Society of Cardiology; Heart Failure Association of ESC; Heart Failure Society of America. HRS/EHRA expert consensus on the monitoring of cardiovascular implantable electronic devices (CIEDs): description of techniques, indications, personnel, frequency and ethical considerations. Heart Rhythm 2008; 5:907–25.

2 Erkapic, D, Duray GZ, Bauernfeind T, De Rosa S, Hohnloser SH. Insulation defects of thin high-voltage ICD leads: an underestimated problem? J Cardiovasc Electrophysiol 2011; 22:1018–22.

3 Duray GZ, Israel CW, Schmitt J, Hohnloser SH. Implantable cardioverter-defibrillator lead disintegration at the level of the tricuspid valve. Heart Rhythm 2008; 5:1224–5.

4 Friedman P, McClelland RL, Bamlet WR, et al. Dual-chamber versus single chamber detection enhancements for implantable defibrillator rhythm diagnosis. The Detect Supraventricular Tachycardia Study. Circulation 2006; 113:2871–9.

5 Hauser RG, Hayes DL, Epstein AE, et al. Multicenter experience with failed and recalled implantable cardioverter defibrillator pulse generators. Heart Rhythm 2006; 3:640–44.

6 Simons EC, Feigenblum DY, Nemirovsky D, Simons GR. Alert tones are frequently inaudible among patients with implantable cardioverter-defibrillators. Pacing Clin Electrophysiol 2009; 32:1272–5.

7 Ellenbogen KA, Wood MA, Shepard RK, et al. Detection and management of an implantable cardioverter defibrillator lead failure: incidence and clinical implications. J Am Coll Cardiol 2003; 41:73–80.

8 Duru F, Luechinger R, Scharf C, Brunckhorst C. Automatic impedance monitoring and patient alert feature in implantable cardioverter defibrillators: being alert for the unexpected! J Cardiovasc Electrophysiol 2005; 16:444–8.

9 Curtis AB. Defibrillation threshold testing in implantable cardioverter-defibrillators: might less be more than enough? J Am Coll Cardiol 2008; 52:557–8.

10 Hohnloser SH, Dorian P, Roberts R, et al. Effect of amiodarone and sotalol on ventricular defibrillation threshold: The Optimal Pharmacological Therapy in Cardioverter Defibrillator Patients (OPTIC) Trial. Circulation 2006; 114:104–9.

11 Swerdlow CD, Friedman PA. Advanced ICD troubleshooting: Part I. Pacing Clin Electrophysiol 2005; 28:1322–46.

12 Hayes DL, Boehmer JP, Day JD, et al. Cardiac resynchronization therapy and the relationship of percent biventricular pacing to symptoms and survival. Heart Rhythm 2011; 8:1469–75.

13 Crossley GH, Chen J, Choucair W, et al. PREFER Study Investigators. Clinical benefits of remote versus transtelephonic monitoring of implanted pacemakers. J Am Coll Cardiol 2009; 54:2012–9.

14 Saxon LA, Hayes DL, Gilliam FR, et al. Long-term outcome after ICD and CRT implantation and influence of remote device follow-up: the ALTITUDE survival study. Circulation 2010; 122:2359–67.

15 Dubner S, Auricchio A, Steinberg JS, et al. ISHNE/EHRA expert consensus on remote monitoring of cardiovascular implantable electronic devices (CIEDs). Europace 2012; 14:278–93.

16 Sack S, Wende CM, Nägele H, et al. Potential value of automated daily screening of cardiac resynchronization therapy defibrillator diagnostics for prediction of major cardiovascular events: results from Home-CARE (Home Monitoring in Cardiac Resynchronization Therapy) study. Eur J Heart Fail 2011; 13:1019–27.

17 Adamson PB, Smith AL, Abraham WT, et al. Continuous autonomic assessment in patients with symptomatic heart failure: prognostic value of heart rate variability measured by an implanted cardiac resynchronization device. Circulation 2004; 110:2389–94.

18 van Veldhuisen DJ, Braunschweig F, Conraads V, et al. DOT-HF Investigators. Intrathoracic impedance monitoring, audible patient alerts, and outcome in patients with heart failure. Circulation 2011; 124:1719–26.

19 Ritzema J, Troughton R, Melton I, et al. Hemodynamically Guided Home Self-Therapy in Severe Heart Failure Patients (HOMEOSTASIS) Study Group. Physician-directed patient self-management of left atrial pressure in advanced chronic heart failure. Circulation 2010; 121:1086–95.

20 Ritzema J, Melton IC, Richards AM, et al. Direct left atrial pressure monitoring in ambulatory heart failure patients: initial experience with a new permanent implantable device. Circulation 2007; 116:2952–9.

21 Troughton RW, Ritzema J, Eigler NL, et al. HOMEOSTASIS Investigators. Direct left atrial pressure monitoring in severe heart failure: long-term sensor performance. J Cardiovasc Transl Res 2011; 4:3–13.

22 Cleland JG, Louis AA, Rigby AS, Janssens U, Balk AH. Noninvasive home telemonitoring for patients with heart failure at high risk of recurrent admission and death: the Trans-European Network-Home-Care Management System (TEN-HMS) study. J Am Coll Cardiol 2005; 45: 1654–64.

23 Goldberg LR, Piette JD, Walsh MN, et al. WHARF Investigators. Randomized trial of a daily electronic home monitoring system in patients with advanced heart failure: the Weight Monitoring in Heart Failure (WHARF) trial. Am Heart J 2003; 146:705–12.

24 Glotzer TV, Daoud EG, Wyse DG, et al. The relationship between daily atrial tachyarrhythmia burden from implantable device diagnostics and stroke risk: the TRENDS study. Circ Arrhythm Electrophysiol 2009; 2:474–80.

25 Healey JS, Connolly SJ, Gold MR, et al. ASSERT Investigators. Subclinical atrial fibrillation and the risk of stroke. N Engl J Med 2012; 366:120–9.

26 Lamas G. How much atrial fibrillation is too much atrial fibrillation? N Engl J Med 2012; 366:178–80.

27 Crossley GH, Boyle A, Vitense H, Chang Y, Mead RH. CONNECT Investigators. The CONNECT (Clinical Evaluation of Remote Notification to Reduce Time to Clinical Decision) trial: the value of wireless remote monitoring with automatic clinician alerts. J Am Coll Cardiol 2011; 57:1181–9.

28 Varma N, Epstein A, Irimpen A, Schweikert R, Love C. Efficacy and Safety of Automatic Remote Monitoring for

ImplantableCardioverter-Defibrillator Follow-Up. The Lumos-T Safely Reduces Routine Office Device Follow-Up (TRUST) Trial. Circulation 2010; 122:325–32.

29 Maisel WH. Pacemaker and ICD generator reliability: meta-analysis of device registries. JAMA 2006; 295: 1929–34.

30 Maisel WH, Moynahan M, Zuckerman BD, et al. Pacemaker and ICD generator malfunctions: analysis of Food and Drug Administration annual reports. JAMA 2006; 295:1901–6.

31 Shein MJ, Brinker JA. Pacing: FDA and the regulatory environment. In: Ellenbogen KA, Kay GN, Wilkoff BL, eds. Clinical Cardiac Pacing. Philadelphia: WB Saunders Co., 1995: 809–20.

32 Maisel WH, Hauser RG, Hammill SC, et al. Heart Rhythm Society Task Force on Lead Performance Policies and Guidelines; American College of Cardiology (ACC); American Heart Association (AHA). Recommendations from the Heart Rhythm Society Task Force on Lead Performance Policies and Guidelines: developed in collaboration with the American College of Cardiology (ACC) and the American Heart Association (AHA). Heart Rhythm 2009; 6:869–85.

33 Undavia M, Goldstein NE, Cohen P, et al. Impact of implantable cardioverter-defibrillator recalls on patients' anxiety, depression, and quality of life. Pacing Clin Electrophysiol 2008; 31:1411–8.

34 Poole JE, Gleva MJ, Mela T, et al. REPLACE Registry Investigators. Complication rates associated with pacemaker or implantable cardioverter-defibrillator generator replacements and upgrade procedures: results from the REPLACE registry. Circulation 2010; 122:1553–61.

35 Uslan DZ, Gleva MJ, Warren DK, et al. Cardiovascular implantable electronic device replacement infections and prevention: results from the REPLACE Registry. Pacing Clin Electrophysiol 2012; 35:81–7.

36 Gould PA, Krahn AD. Complications associated with implantable cardioverter-defibrillator replacement in response to device advisories. JAMA 2006; 295:1907–11.

37 Kapa S, Hyberger L, Rea RF, Hayes DL. Complication risk with pulse generator change: implications when reacting to a device advisory or recall. Pacing Clin Electrophysiol 2007; 30:730–3.

38 Auricchio A, Gropp M, Ludgate S, Vardas P, Brugada J, Priori SG. Writing Committee for the European Heart Rhythm Association Guidance Document on Cardiac Rhythm Management Product Performance. European Heart Rhythm Association Guidance Document on cardiac rhythm management product performance. Europace 2006; 8:313–22.

39 Carlson MD, Wilkoff B, Maisel WH, et al. American College of Cardiology Foundation; American Heart Association; International Coalition of Pacing and Electrophysiology Organizations. Recommendations from the Heart Rhythm Society Task Force on Device Performance Policies and Guidelines. Heart Rhythm 2006; 3:1250–73.

40 Hauser RG, Maisel WH, Friedman PA, et al. Longevity of Sprint Fidelis implantable cardioverter-defibrillator leads

and risk factors for failure: implications for patient management. Circulation 2011; 123:358–63.

41 Swerdlow CD, Gunderson BD, Ousdigian KT, et al. Downloadable algorithm to reduce inappropriate shocks caused by fractures of implantable cardioverter-defibrillator leads. Circulation 2008; 118:2122–9.

42 Epstein AE, Baessler CA, Curtis AB, et al. American Heart Association; Heart Rhythm Society. Addendum to "Personal and public safety issues related to arrhythmias that may affect consciousness: implications for regulation and physician recommendations. A medical/scientific statement from the American Heart Association and the North American Society of Pacing and Electrophysiology". Public safety issues in patients with implantable defibrillators. A Scientific statement from the American Heart Association and the Heart Rhythm Society. Heart Rhythm 2007; 4:386–93.

43 Vijgen J, Botto G, Camm J, et al. Consensus statement of the European Heart Rhythm Association: updated recommendations for driving by patients with implantable cardioverter defibrillators. Europace 2009; 11:1097–107.

44 Okada M, Suzuki K, Hidaka T, et al. Complex regional pain syndrome type I induced by pacemaker implantation, with a good response to steroids and neurotropin. Intern Med 2002; 41:498–501.

45 Zipes DP, Ackerman MJ, Estes NA 3rd, et al. Task Force 7 : arrhythmias. J Am Coll Cardiol 2005; 45:1354–63.

46 Ahmad M, Bloomstein L, Roelke M, Bernstein AD, Parsonnet V. Patients' attitudes toward implanted defibrillator shocks. Pacing Clin Electrophysiol 2000; 23:934–8.

47 Marcus G, Chan D, Redberg R. Recollection of pain due to inappropriate versus appropriate implantable cardioverter-defibrillator shocks. Pacing Clin Electrophysiol 2011; 34:348–53.

48 Mueller PS, Hook CC, Hayes DL. Ethical analysis of withdrawal of pacemaker or implantable cardioverter-defibrillator support at the end of life. Mayo Clin Proc 2003; 78:959–63.

49 Goldstein NE, Lampert R, Bradley E, Lynn J, Krumholz HM. Management of implantable cardioverter defibrillators in end-of-life care. Ann Intern Med 2004; 141:835–8.

50 Berger JT. The ethics of deactivating implanted cardioverter defibrillators. Ann Intern Med 2005; 142:631–4.

51 Lewis WR, Luebke DL, Johnson NJ, Harrington MD, Constantini O, Aulisio MP. Withdrawing implantable defibrillator shock therapy in terminally ill patients. Am J Med 2006; 119:892–6.

52 Mueller PS, Jenkins SM, Bramstedt KA, Hayes DL. Deactivating implanted cardiac devices in terminally ill patients: practices and attitudes. Pacing Clin Electrophysiol 2008; 31:560–8.

53 Zellner RA, Aulisio MP, Lewis WR. Should implantable cardioverter-defibrillators and permanent pacemakers in patients with terminal illness be deactivated? Deactivating permanent pacemaker in patients with terminal illness. Patient autonomy is paramount. Circ Arrhythm Electrophysiol 2009; 2:340–4.

54 Kay GN, Bittner GT. Should implantable cardioverter-defibrillators and permanent pacemakers in patients with

terminal illness be deactivated? Deactivating implantable cardioverter-defibrillators and permanent pacemakers in patients with terminal illness: an ethical distinction. Circ Arrhythm Electrophysiol 2009; 2:336–9.

55 Lampert R, Hayes DL, Annas GJ, *et al.* American College of Cardiology; American Geriatrics Society; American Academy of Hospice and Palliative Medicine, American Heart Association; European Heart Rhythm Association; Hospice and Palliative Nurses Association. HRS Expert Consensus Statement on the Management of Cardiovascular Implantable Electronic Devices (CIEDs) in patients nearing end of life or requesting withdrawal of therapy. Heart Rhythm 2010; 7:1008–26.

Index

Page numbers in *italic* refer to figures.
Page numbers in **bold** refer to tables.
Sorting is in letter-by-letter order
ignoring spaces so that, e.g., "fat
pad" comes after "fatigue".

1:1 AV relationship, tachycardias with
489, 492–495, *497*, 516, *518*
ATP on 495
"55D" polyurethane 140
"80A" polyurethane 139–140
110 ms phenomenon *see* ventricular
safety pacing

AA (time period) 256
AAI pacing (atrial inhibited pacing)
257–259, *260*, 328
assessment of AV conduction
195–196
indications and contraindications
135
VVI pacing *vs* 56–57
AAIR pacing 259–260
electrocardiogram *288*
indications and contraindications
135, 408
AAIR Safe Pace *60*
AAT mode *see* single-chamber
triggered-mode pacing
abandoned leads 238–240
children 200
contact with electrodes 146, 431
MRI and 604
radiography *562*
see also nonfunctional leads
abbreviations, timing cycle **256**
abdomen, device implantation 30,
574
ablation 601–602
atrioventricular node 112, 399,
537–539, 602
electromagnetic interference from
598, 601–602
for lead extraction 215
septal, heart block from 107
for tachyarrhythmias 106–107
VT storm 511
ablation catheters, lead extraction 215

aborted sudden death
arrhythmogenic right ventricular
dysplasia 121
long QT syndrome 119
acceleration times, sensors *see* reaction
time
accelerometers 410–411
dual-sensor rate-adaptive pacing
416–418
see also SonR sensor
Accufix™ atrial J lead
radiography 566, *569*
recalls 209
Accuity® leads *152*
action potentials 2–4, 17
active cans, cold cans *vs* 32
active fixation leads 10–11, *137*, 153
cardiac perforation 225, *588*
children 200–202
extraction 210–211
pacing thresholds 6–7, 194
radiography 564, *567*, *577*
active transport mechanisms 2
activity logs, CRT 623, *628*
activity sensors 409–411
activity thresholds 420–422, *423*
adaptors, connectors *198*, **198**
additional repolarization time 19, *21*
ADI mode 259, *260*, 328
advisories, pacemaker replacement 204,
640–644
AFib Rate Threshold (Boston Scientific)
387
afterpotentials 8–9, 15
air
in pockets 452
see also seal-plug problems
air embolism, avoidance 162
alcohol, on DFT 33
alerts
ICDs 472, 628
lead failure 533
internet-based 636
see also advisories
alignment, electrograms 377, *379*, *380*
alignment errors, electrograms 377
allergies 232
order sets and 205

alternating bundle branch block 101
alternating RR intervals 476–477, 481
Ambulatory Threshold Test (Boston
Scientific) **336**
American College of Cardiology,
indications for pacemakers and
ICDs 94
American Heart Association, indications
for pacemakers and ICDs 94
amiodarone
on DFT 33
on pacing thresholds 443
on ventricular tachycardia 492
AMIOVIRT trial 116–117
amplification *see* variable signal
amplification
amplitude
duration *vs* 4
electrograms 8, 9f
R waves *342*
see also intrinsic amplitude tests;
voltage amplitude
analyzers, pacing systems 192–193
anastomoses, ventricular veins *184*
anatomy 2
coronary sinus *177*, *302*
Andersen Trial 56–57
anesthesia 158–159
for VT storm 511
angiographic wires *see* guidewires
angiography *see* contrast venography
anodal capture 542, *543*, *544–545*
anodal shocking 20–21
anodal stimulation, resynchronization
and 316
anterior intraventricular vein *177*, *178*
lead placement *582*
anterior left ventricular pacing, ECG
300, *303*
anterior myocardial infarction 100
antiarrhythmic drugs
affecting pacing thresholds **435**,
443–444, *448*
Class IC 443, 492, 632–634
ICD problems, follow-up 632–634
ICDs and 33–34, 632–634
for VT storm 511
antibiotics 205, **207**, 238

Cardiac Pacing, Defibrillation and Resynchronization: A Clinical Approach, Third Edition.
David L. Hayes, Samuel J. Asirvatham, and Paul A. Friedman.
© 2013 Mayo Foundation for Medical Education and Research. Published 2013 by John Wiley & Sons, Ltd.

anticoagulants
    cardioversion and 228
    device implantation and 203
    for established thrombosis 234
    pocket hematomas 229
antitachycardia pacing (ATP) 34–35,
        390–393, **396**, *499*
    drugs and 634
    initiating lead noise *524*
    misclassification by ICDs 507, *508*
    optimizing therapy 395, 507
    on ventricular tachycardia 34–35, 495
    VT storm 511
antitheft devices 609–610
AOO (atrial asynchronous pacing) 257
apex
    lead placement 169
        assessment 298–299, 567–569
        right ventricular pacing 61, *65*, 66,
            110
        ECG 299–300
        minimization 331–332
arc welding 607–608
arm lifting restriction 205, 644–645
arrays, subcutaneous 175, *176*, *580*
arrhythmias
    causes of recurrence 246–252
    during lead implantation 228–229
    life-threatening, prevention 112–114,
        370, **396**, **397**
    see also specific arrhythmias
arrhythmogenic right ventricular
        dysplasia, ICDs 121–122
article surveillance equipment 609–610
artifacts, electrical 452–454, *455*
aspirin
    device implantation and 203
    pocket hematomas 229
asynchronous mode, ICDs 600
asynchronous pacing (SOOR pacing)
        260
    magnet response **621**
    noise reversion 593–597
    rate-modulated 261
    see also atrial asynchronous pacing;
        dual-chamber pacing, sequential
        asynchronous; ventricular
        asynchronous pacing
asystole
    avoidance in programming 321
    prevention 265–266
atria
    conduction system 51
    effect of pacing 56
    J leads *137*, *577*
        dislodgement 220
        placement 190–192
        radiography 564–567
        see also Accufix™ atrial J lead
    lead dislodgement 220, 441
    sensing thresholds 195
    trans-telephonic monitoring 616

atrial asynchronous pacing (AOO) 257
atrial-based timing systems 268–272
atrial blanking period 346–348, **349**, 384
    Boston Scientific ICDs 384, *386*
    see also post-ventricular atrial
        blanking periods
Atrial Capture Control (Biotronik) **336**
atrial defibrillators 393
atrial electrograms 8
    ICDs 474, *477*
        undersensing 501
atrial escape interval *see* ventriculoatrial
        interval
atrial fibrillation *497*
    AFib Rate Threshold (Boston
        Scientific ICDs) 387
    assessment of suppression 437
    atrial undersensing 504–506
    atrioventricular block and 99
    heart failure and **110**, 112
    ICD selection 150
    inappropriate rejection *500*
    late shock 394
    during lead implantation 228
    lead placement for 192
        radiography 567
    pacing mode on 57–58, *59*
    paroxysmal 492, *494–495*
    prevention algorithms 106
    programming **397**, 399, *401*
    remote monitoring 638–640
    sleep apnea 103
    thromboembolism and 638–640, *641*
    ventricular rate regulation for 78,
        295–296
    ventricular sensing, cardiac
        resynchronization devices
        537–541
    ventricular tachycardia *vs* 489
    VVIR pacing 134
atrial flutter 489, *497*
    during lead implantation 228
    mode switching and 276
atrial inhibited pacing (AAI pacing)
        257–259, *260*, 328
    assessment of AV conduction
        195–196
    indications and contraindications
        135
    VVI pacing *vs* 56–57
atrial oversensing
    CRT devices **535**, 536, **635**
    ICDs 476
atrial pacemakers
    lead dislodgement 220
    lead placement *170–171*
        radiography 564–569, *568*
        ventricular lead placement with
            190
    single-chamber, sick sinus syndrome
        103
    see also Accufix™ atrial J lead

atrial premature beats, biventricular
        pacing 286
Atrial Protection Interval (API™)
        276–278
atrial rate, ventricular rate *vs*, SVT-VT
        discriminators 383–387
atrial refractory period **325**
    pacing during 276–278
    see also post-ventricular atrial
        refractory period; total atrial
        refractory period
atrial rhythms
    cardiac transplantation 202
    native 332, *333*
    ventricular sensing problems 534–537
atrial sensing window 275
atrial septal defect 232
atrial synchronous
        (P-tracking/P-synchronous) pacing
        see VDD pacing
atrial tachyarrhythmias
    mode switching for 276
    risk of thromboembolism 638–640
atrial tachycardia
    ATP on 495
    caused by pacing 276–278
    during lead implantation 228
Atrial Tracking Recovery™ (Medtronic)
        398, *399*
atrial undersensing 286, *345*, *352*
    CRT devices **535**, **635**
    ICDs 384, 388
        atrial fibrillation 504–506
atrial upper interval (AUI) 278
atrial upper rate (AUR) 278
atrioventricular block 80
    as complication 228
    pacing for 94–101
    pacing mode selection 136
    PEA sensor 418
    programming for 471–472
    from septal ablation 107
    single-pass VDD pacing 136
        children 200
    sinus node dysfunction 136
    symptoms 99, 471
    see also first-degree heart block;
        second-degree heart block
atrioventricular conduction, failure of
        resynchronization 316
atrioventricular delay 269, *270*, **271**, 278,
        279, 283, 284, 292, **327**, 436
    cardiac resynchronization devices 534
atrioventricular dissociation 43–45
atrioventricular interval (AVI) 46,
        49–55, 257, 264–268, **325**
    assessment 435
    ECG 292–295
    extension 331–332
    programming 49, 307–316, 331–332,
        400, 424
    resynchronization (CRT) 70–71, 424

atrioventricular interval hysteresis 268,
    270, 283–284
  options **271**
atrioventricular node (AV node) 2, 3f
  ablation 112, 399, 537–539, 602
  assessment 195–196
atrioventricular search hysteresis (AVSH)
    60, **271**, 278–279, 331–332, 437
  symptoms 471
atrioventricular sequential, non-P-
    synchronous pacing with
    dual-chamber sensing (DDI
    pacing) 261–262, 292, 328
atrioventricular sequential, non-P-
    synchronous, rate-modulated
    pacing with dual-chamber sensing
    (DDIR pacing) 262
atrioventricular sequential pacing *see*
    dual-chamber pacing, sequential
    asynchronous
atrioventricular sequential, ventricular
    inhibited pacing (DVI pacing) 261
atrioventricular synchrony 43, 45–49
atrioventricular valve plane, fluoroscopy
    169
Attain Ability Straight 4396 lead 153
Attain Starfix LV lead 153
auto-capture algorithms 335
AutoCapture™ system 338–339, *340*,
    469
autosensing 341
AutoThreshold (Sorin Medical) **336**
autothresholds 322, 337, *338*, 433–435
AVI *see* atrioventricular interval
A wave, mitral valve inflow 52, *53*
axillary approach 160–164
  children 199–200
  radiography *563*
axillary vein 162
azygos vein, defibrillator coils *31*

Bachmann's bundle 2, 51
backfilling, defibrillation coils 145
backup modes (reset) 439
  electromagnetic interference and
    597–598
  ICDs, radiotherapy 610
  unexpected reversion to 470
bacteremia 207, 238
balloon catheters, coronary sinus
    venography 181–182
bandpass filters 15
basal location of leads, assessment
    298–299
baseline electrograms, ventricular
    fibrillation *vs* 520
batteries 14
  depletion 246, *248*, 432, *433*, 439, 452
    ICDs 626–627, *632–633*
  longevity 14, 204, 432, *433*
  voltages 14, 439, 627–628, *632–633*
battery impedance 14

BELIEVE trial 67
β-blockers, long QT syndrome 119–120
bifascicular block, chronic 101
bifocal pacing
  right ventricular, heart failure 67
  see also dual-site atrial pacing
bifurcated bipolar connectors **198**, 556
bilateral bundle branch block 101
binary search algorithms 26
bioprosthetic tricuspid valves **198**, 583
Biotronik
  Atrial Capture Control **336**
  atrioventricular interval hysteresis
    271
  blanking characteristics **349**
  CRT devices, ventricular sensing
    mechanism 281
  ICDs
    magnet response **600**
    R-wave double-counting 481–484
  magnet response and ERI **621**
  pulse generators, identification **557**
  remote monitoring **639**
  SMART® algorithm 390, *391*
  timing systems **273**
  Ventricular Capture Control **336**
biphasic waveforms, ICDs 22–24
bipolar electrograms 8
bipolar functions, switching to unipolar
    341, *347*
bipolar leads 11, *12*, 13, 138–139
  connectors 197–198
  fracture 248, *251*
  ICDs *367*
  interventricular offsets 153
  minimizing EMI 592
  radiography 556, 564, *567*
bipolar pacemakers, radiography *558*
bipolar sensing, ICDs 146–147
Bisping screwdriver 11
biventricular hysteresis 284
biventricular pacing (cardiac
    resynchronization therapy; CRT)
    13, 50
  activity logs 623, *628*
  atrioventricular interval timing 70–71
  defibrillation with (CRT-D) 117
    electrogram templates 377
  device-based optimization 399–400
  device circuit interruption 246
  device selection 151–153
  device troubleshooting 533–546
  ECG 296–299, 300–312
  follow-up 634, **635**
  heart failure 13, 67–70, 107–111, **111**
  lack of response 316
  leads, placement *108–109*
  pacemaker selection 134
  phrenic nerve stimulation 245
  programming of devices 395–400
  QRS vector fusion 72–75
  rate-adaptive pacing and 424–425

RV pacing avoidance 60–61
timing cycles 281–287
vector management 153
  see also offsets
blanked atrial flutter search 276
blanking periods 256, *267*, 445
  programming 346–348, **349**, *350*
  see also atrial blanking period;
    cross-chamber refractory
    periods; post-ventricular atrial
    blanking periods; ventricular
    blanking periods
B-LEFT HF trial 67
blood pressure
  pacemaker syndrome 467
  remote monitoring 638
Boston Scientific
  Ambulatory Threshold Test **336**
  atrioventricular interval hysteresis
    271
  battery status indicator *632–633*
  blanking characteristics **349**
  CRT devices, ventricular sensing
    mechanism 281
  ICDs 368
    asynchronous mode **600**
    atrial blanking period 384, *386*
    committed shocks 372
    effect of magnets 510, 515, **600**
    electrogram alignment 377, *380*
    far-field R-wave rejection 504
    LV refractory period 537
    primary prevention programming
      396
    sensitivity 364
    SVT-VT discriminators 376,
      387–388, 515–516
  magnet response and ERI **621**
  pulse generators, identification **557**
  remote monitoring **639**
  Retry mode **336**
  Rhythm ID™ 387–388, *389*, 516
  timing systems **273**
  Tracking Preference™ 398
  Vector Timing and Correlation
    morphology algorithm *380*, *389*
  Ventricular Automatic Capture **336**
bradyarrhythmias, cardiac
    transplantation 112
bradycardia 101, *102*, 103
  ICDs
    programming 393
    selection 150
  during lead implantation 228
  pacing mode selection 135–136
  proarrhythmic pacing 506, *507*
  programming 397, **398**
  sleep 101–104
  sudden, response algorithms
    280–281, 332–333, 437, *438*
bras 645
breast cancer, radiotherapy 611

Brugada syndrome 120–121
Bulldog lead extender *212*
bundle branch block
    alternating 101
    bifascicular block 101
    cardiac perforation 226
    left 66–67, *108*
        cardiac perforation 226
        heart failure 110
        V-V optimization 75–77
    right
        cardiac perforation 226
        resynchronization for 111–112
    trifascicular block 101
bundle branch system 2
bundle of His 2, *184*
    see also His–Purkinje system
burns, electrode–myocardial interface
    441
"burst plus" mode, ATP 507
"bursts", ATP 391

CABG-Patch trial 115
cable leads *11*, 145
calcification on leads 140
Canadian Trial of Physiologic Pacing 57
capacitors 22, 628–630
    energy 22, 24, 25
    shock dosage 24
capsule endoscopy 606
capture
    anodal 542, *543*, *544–545*
    failure 441–452, 541–542
        pseudo-malfunctions 452–454
    latency 303, 304
        see also stimulus latency
    thresholds 322, *324*
    see also Ventricular Autocapture™
Capture Management™ (Medtronic)
    336
carbon dioxide, contrast venography
    with 583
carbon electrodes 10
    vitreous 139
cardiac arrest
    congenital heart disease 125–126
    recurrence risk 113
cardiac contractility modulation (CCM)
    78
cardiac output, troubleshooting
    471–472
cardiac resynchronization therapy *see*
    biventricular pacing
cardiac transplantation, pacing after
    112, 202
cardio-inhibitory response, carotid sinus
    reflex 79, 104
cardiomyopathy
    fibrosis 116
    hypertrophic 78–79
        ICDs 122–125
        pacing for 107

septal myectomy 125
    sudden death 122, **125**
    ICDs 116–117, 122–125
    ischemic, ICDs 115
    from tachycardia 117
        pacing for 111
cardioversion **603**
    altered pacing thresholds 441, *447*,
        601, *602*
    during lead implantation 228
    low-energy 393
CareLink™ web-based follow-up system
    636–637, **639**, **640**
carotid sheath, jugular approach 165
carotid sinus reflex 79, 104
    hypersensitivity, pacing mode
        selection 136
catecholaminergic polymorphic
    ventricular tachycardia 121
catheter ablation *see* ablation
catheterization suites 158
    cardiac perforation treatment 227
cathodal shocks *21*
CAT trial 116
cefazolin **207**
cells (power sources) *see* batteries
cellular injury 7
cellular phones 610
cephalic approach 165, *166*
    radiography *563*
'Change Tachy Mode with Magnet'
    (Boston Scientific) 515
channelopathies, ICDs 120–121
    programming **397**
charge, capacitors 22
charge time, capacitors 628–630
chest pain **623**
chest radiography 553–589
    follow-up 624
    ICDs 473
    leads 558–583
        coronary sinus 577–583
        ICDs 572–577
    pacemaker troubleshooting 429, 431
    pulse generators 554–558
children
    device implantation 198–202
    rate programming 328
    redundancy of leads 199, *200–201*,
        564, *566*
    single-pass VDD pacing 136
chronaxie 4
chronic threshold 6
chronotropic incompetence 43
    bradycardia 103
circadian lower rates *see* sleep rates
circadian pattern, stimulation threshold
    7, 30–33
circuits (in devices) 15
    interruption 246–248
circuits (re-entrant) 34–35, 77
    see also endless-loop tachycardia

circus movement tachycardia *see*
    endless-loop tachycardia
classification, indications for pacemakers
    and ICD 94
CLEAR trial (Clinical Evaluation of
    Advanced Resynchronization trial)
    418, 424–425
clinical assessment, troubleshooting
    428–429
Clinical Evaluation of Advanced
    Resynchronization trial (CLEAR
    trial) 418, 424–425
clinics for follow-up 614–616
    visits 618–621
clopidogrel
    device implantation and 203
    pocket hematomas 229
closed-loop sensors 408
Closed Loop Stimulation 412–414
coaxial leads 11, 139
    ICDs 144–145, *521*
codes, pacemaker nomenclature 16, 320
codes (radiographic) 557
coils
    ICDs 29, 30, *31*, 145, 146–147
        subcutaneous 175, *176*
    see also electrodes
cold cans, active cans *vs 32*
cold temperatures 598
committed shocks 372–373
comorbidities *44*
COMPANION trial 117
competition, pace *vs* sense 460
    atrial 276–278
    biventricular pacing 284–285
compliance *see* noncompliance
complications 219–254
    of lead extraction 209–210
    local anesthesia 159
    pacemaker replacement 204–205
component malfunctions 439–440, 452,
    462, 469
computed tomography
    cardiac perforation 225
    oversensing 610
computerized data storage 626
Conducted AF Response™ (Medtronic)
    399
conduction system *see* anatomy;
    physiology
conductors 11, 139
    externalization 573–577, *580*, 644
    fracture *250*, *439*, 446–448
    ICDs 145
    radiography 562, *564*
    see also setscrews
congenital heart disease 125–126, 171,
    174, 198, 583–585, *586*
congenitally corrected transposition of
    great vessels, lead placement *586*
congenital third-degree AV block, pacing
    for 96–98

connectors 141, *142*, 196–198
    ICDs 147–148, 198
        failed shocks 514–515
    loose 234, *239*, *442*
    noise 486
        lead fracture *vs* 525–529, *530*
    radiography 556
    see also setscrews
conscious sedation 158–159
consecutive interval counting 368–370, 388
constant repolarization time 19
constant-voltage pulse generators 14–15
consultations, follow-up 620–621
contact curves, coronary venous leads 153
contact sports 645
CONTAK-CD trial, coronary sinus lead complications **223**
continuous biventricular pacing 151
contractility
    increasing 78
    left ventricle 51
contrast venography 162–163, 164, 165, 583
    coronary sinus cannulation 179, 181–183
Cook locking stylet *212*
coradial leads 11
Cordis type connectors *141*
coronary artery bypass graft, ICDs and 115
coronary artery disease
    ICDs 114–116
    resynchronization in 69, 70
    see also myocardial infarction
coronary sinus leads 175–189
    anatomy *177*, *302*
    atrial 192
    cannulation 176–179
    complications 223
    congenital heart disease 196
    dislodgement 220–223
    exit block 248–252, 441
    extraction 215
    from persistent left SVC 167
    radiography 169, 185, 232, *576*, 573–583
coronary venous leads 151–153
cough **623**
counters 256
cracks, lead surfaces 12, 140
crista supraventricularis, as landmark 66
critical mass theory 18
cross-chamber refractory periods 286–287, 518–519
cross-stimulation 441, *446*
crosstalk, ventricular output inhibition 265–268, 348, *350*, 454–455, *456*, *458*

crosstalk sensing window *see* ventricular triggering period
CRT *see* biventricular pacing
crush injury (to lead) 248, *252*, 431, 562, *564*
current device indication 643
current of injury 195
curved sheaths 178–181
curved stylets
    ventricular leads 167–169
    see also J curved stylets
curves, coronary venous leads *152–153*
cut-away sheaths 188
cutdowns, device implantation 160
cutting diathermy 598
cyclists 410

Dacron pouches 243
Danish Pacemaker Trial 56–57
DANPACE trial 58–60
databases, lead performance 142–144, 430–431
data storage 626
    in pacemakers 621–622
DAT mode 328
DAVID trial 57, *58*
DDD pacing (dual-chamber pacing and sensing with inhibition and tracking) 262–264
    indications and contraindications **135**
    right ventricular apex pacing 110
    sinus node dysfunction 136
    VDD pacing *vs* 292
    VVI pacing *vs* 48, 57
DDDR pacing
    indications and contraindications **135**
    programming procedure 357–360
    on timing cycles 272–276
DDI pacing (atrioventricular sequential, non-P-synchronous pacing with dual-chamber sensing) 261–262, 292, 328
DDIR pacing (atrioventricular sequential non-P-synchronous rate-modulated pacing with dual-chamber sensing) 262
DDT mode 284, *285*
deactivation 646
deceleration time *see* recovery time
DECREASE-HF trial 67
defibrillation 16–21, 393
    external 601, *602*, *603*, **603**
        altered pacing thresholds 441
    testing at implantation 25–33
        failure 29–33
        risk 28
    see also implantable cardioverter-defibrillators; shocks

defibrillation coils 29, 30, *31*, 145, 146–147
    subcutaneous 175
defibrillation theshold (DFT) 26–27
    drugs on 33
    testing 632
DEFINITE trial 117
deflectable catheters 140, *141*, 178–181
delayed longitudinal contraction (DLC), V-V optimization on 76
delivered energy, stored energy *vs* 25
delivery systems for leads 13–14
    over-the-wire 13, 151–153, 185–187
        see also guidewires
    sheaths 13, 178, 179, *180*, 188–189
deltopectoral groove 165
dental equipment, interference 605
depolarization 4, 17, 19, *21*, 415
    isoelectric 452
detection by ICDs 362, 364, 366–393
    duration 372, **398**, 507
    enhancements 373–376
    see also redetection; underdetection
device malfunctions 642–643
    see also component malfunctions
dextrocardia, lead placement *586*
DF-1 standard 12, 198
DF-4 standard 148
DFT *see* defibrillation threshold
diagnostics
    features for 439–440
    ICDs 473
        lead failure 533
    programming 350, *360*
    see also troubleshooting
dialysis, hyperkalemia 443–445
diameter, leads 140
diaphragm
    myopotentials 486–488
        lead fracture *vs* 522, *523*
        oversensing 546
    stimulation 245
        assessment 169, 187–188
diastolic function, left ventricle 70
diathermy 598, 606
    see also electrocautery
differential atrioventricular interval (AVDI) 48, 268, **325**
    see also interatrial conduction time
digital recording systems, pseudo-malfunctions 458, *464*, *465*
dilated cardiomyopathy, ICDs 116–117
dilated ventricular veins, lead placement 187
DINAMIT trial 115
discharge from hospital 205
dislodgement of leads 220–223, 441, *445*, *525*
    dual-chamber ICDs 149
    radiography 571, *575*, 583
dissection of coronary sinus 185, *186*
    risk of 179

DOO (dual-chamber sequential asynchronous pacing) 257, *258*
DOOR pacing *see* dual-chamber pacing, rate-modulated
Doppler tissue imaging, V-V optimization 75–76
Doppler velocity, mitral valve inflow 52, *53*
dosage (of shocks) 24–25
dose–response curve, defibrillation 25–26
dressings, post-implant 205
driving, post-implant 205, 644
drugs
  affecting pacing thresholds **435**, 443–444, *448*
  ICD problems 472
    follow-up 632–634
  for VT storm 511
  see also antiarrhythmic drugs
dual-chamber ICDs 149–153
  electrograms 488–489
  SVT-VT discriminators 382–390, 516–517
dual-chamber pacing
  clinical effects 57–58
  ECG 292–296
  leads *170–171*, 189–192
  magnet response 289
  mode switching 348–350
  pulse generators, radiography *558*
  rate adaptation 408
  rate-modulated *see* DDDR pacing
  rate-modulated asynchronous (DOOR) 261
  refractory and blanking periods 346–348
  sequential asynchronous (DOO) 257, *258*
  upper rate limits 328
dual-chamber pacing and sensing with inhibition and tracking (DDD pacing) 262–264
  indications and contraindications **135**
  right ventricular apex pacing 110
  sinus node dysfunction 136
  VDD pacing *vs* 292
  VVI pacing *vs* 48, 57
dual-chamber sensing *see* DDI pacing; DDIR pacing
dual-coil systems, ICDs 146–147, 148, 173
dual-sensor rate-adaptive pacing 415–418
dual-site atrial pacing, radiography 567, 569
dual-site pacing, heart failure 67
DUSISLOG study 416–418
DVI pacing (atrioventricular sequential, ventricular inhibited pacing) 261
dynamic sensing, ICDs 362–365
dyspnea **623**

dyssynchrony 67, *68*, 69, 70, 77
  heart failure 107–110
  interventricular 43, *44*

Easytrak® OTW leads *152*, 153
ecchymoses 229
echocardiography
  lead placement guidance 583
  optimizing therapy 399–400
    atrioventricular 52–55
    ventricular timing 75–77
  programming guidance 331–332
  tricuspid regurgitation 245
"80A" polyurethane 139–140
ejection fraction
  dilated cardiomyopathy 116–117
  ICD after myocardial infarction 115, 116
  ventricular tachycardia 113
elective replacement indicators (ERI) 204, **621**, 627
elective replacement voltages 14
electrical artifacts 452–454, *455*
electrical overstress failure 515
electrical reset 597–598
electrocardiography
  arrhythmogenic right ventricular dysplasia 121
  atrioventricular synchrony 47–49
  Brugada syndrome 120
  equipment 615–616
  equipment failure 463–464
  intrinsicoid deflection 7
  misinterpretation, causes 430, 435–439
  normal waveform *3f*, *17*
  paced 256, 288–316
  QRS vector fusion 72–75
  telemetry 439
electrocautery 598–601
electroconvulsive therapy 605
electrodes 6–7
  contact with abandoned leads 146, 431
  fractal coatings 6, *138*, 175
  materials 6, 10, 139
  minimizing EMI 592
  minute ventilation sensing 411
  myocardial interface 441
  resistance 6
  retained 240
  ring electrodes *12*
  see also coils; interelectrode distance
electrograms (intracardiac) 8, 15, 194–195, *359*
  ICDs 365, *367*, 377, *379*, *380*, 473–476, *477*, 488–495
  SVT *vs* VT 488–510
  truncation 377, *381*, **381**
electrolytic capacitors 628
electromagnetic interference 452–454, *480*, 485–486, 591–612
  trans-telephonic monitoring *618*

electromyography 605
electronic order sets 205
electrophysiology 2–4
  after cardiac arrest 113
  atrioventricular block 100
  tetralogy of Fallot 125
electrosurgical dissection sheath 213
Elgiloy 139
embolism *see* thromboembolism
embryological remnants, infra-Hisian 66
emergency management
  frequent ICD shocks 510
  VT storm 511
emergency programming, pacemakers 321
"ENABLE MAGNET USE" (Boston Scientific) **600**
end-diastolic volume 42
endless-loop tachycardia (ELT) 279–280, *281*, 348, *351*, *352*
  see also pacemaker-mediated tachycardia
endocarditis, valvular 207
end-systolic volume 42
energy
  capacitors 22, 24, 25
  ICD shocks 393
EOL voltage 628
epicardial leads 141, *142*
  children 198
  implantation 196
    for exit block 441–443
  radiography 572, *577*, *578*
    ICDs 572
epicardial patches 572, 573, *578*
episode summaries (text episode summaries) 500
epsilon waves *122*, **124**
erosion 229–230, *231*, 236–237
escape interval, extension *see* rate hysteresis
escape rhythms, atrioventricular block 99
Eustachian ridge, coronary sinus cannulation and 179
evoked responses, AutoCapture™ system 338
Evolution mechanical sheath 213
E wave, mitral valve inflow 52
examination (clinical), follow-up 620
excimer laser sheath 213
excitability 2
excitable gaps, re-entrant circuits 35
exercise
  assessment 419–420
  AV block 96
  AV optimization and 55
  ICD shocks 472
  physiology 42, *45*
  reprogramming for 623–624
  space in clinics 614

upper rate limits 328, *330*
  see also activity sensors
exit block 7, 248–252, 441–443
exit delay 303–304
experience, lead extraction 209
Expert Ease/Lifestyle option *358*
Extended High Rate (St. Jude) 516–517
extended PTFE jackets, defibrillation
  coils 145
external cardioversion 441, 601, *602*,
  603
external defibrillation 441, 601, *602*,
  603, **603**
external interference *see* electromagnetic
  interference
externalization, conductors 573–577,
  580, 644
external jugular access 165
extracardiac signals 245
  interference *see* electromagnetic
    interference
  oversensing from 476, *479*, *480*,
    485–488
  see also diaphragm; myopotentials
extracorporeal shock wave lithotripsy
  604
extraction of leads 205–215
  after cardiac perforation 227
  complications 209–210
  practitioners of 209
  techniques 210–215
extrasystoles *see* premature ventricular
  contractions; ventricular
  extrasystoles
extrathoracic subclavian approach *see*
  axillary approach
Ez locking device (LLD) *212*

failure of treatment, ICDs 29–33
failure to pace 454–458, 467–470
fallback operation 296, *298*, **325**
family history, long QT syndrome 119
far-field electrograms
  ICDs 474, *477*, 495
    oversensing 501–504, *505*, *539*
    VT *vs* SVT 489
far-field R waves 195, 384–387, 388, *390*,
  477
  oversensing 501–504, *505*, *539*
far-field sensing 259, 456, *460*, *461*
  ICDs 365, 388, *390*, *477*
far-field signal rejection 8, 146
fascicular ventricular tachycardia 127
fatigue **623**
fat pad, posteroseptal space *184*, 185
femoral vein
  lead extraction 214–215
  lead placement, radiography *562*, *563*
fibrosis 7, 10
  cardiomyopathy 116
  defibrillation coils 145
  lead extraction and 210, *211*
Fidelis leads *see* Sprint Fidelis leads

"55D" polyurethane 140
filling waves, mitral valve inflow 52
filtering
  electrograms 15, 593
  ICDs
    electrograms 474–476
    St. Jude Medical 478–480
  sensing 8
finger subcutaneous leads 175
firing rates, echocardiography 75
first-degree heart block *96*
  pacing for 94
fixation of leads 10
  see also active fixation leads; passive
    fixation of leads
FIX-HF trials 78
flashback intervals
  Medtronic ICDs 495, *496–497*, *498*
  slow VT *516*
flat surface coils 145
flexibility, leads 139
fluoroscopy
  headers 529
  lead insulation failures 532
  lead placement
    right atrium 191
    ventricular 169, 176, *177*, *181*, 185,
      232
    oblique views 169, 176, *177*, *181*, 185,
      232, *304*
  see also contrast venography
follow-up 613–649
  clinics 614–616
    visits 618–621
  history-taking 429
  ICDs 626–646
  pacemakers 616–618
  programming at 357–360, 622–624,
    627
follow-up data, in programmers *324*
Fontan corrections 196
Fontan procedure 202
Food and Drug Administration
  MedWatch 439–440
  recalls, classification 641
  website 431
fractal coatings, electrodes 6, *138*,
  175
fracture of leads 210, *243*, 248, *249*, *250*,
  251, 446–448
  connector noise *vs* 525–529, *530*
  high-voltage 512–514, 531
  ICDs 248, 522, 630–631
  impedance 522–525, 529, 530–531
  noise *480*, 486
  oversensing from *439*
  pace-sense leads 521–522
  polarity programming and 341–345
  radiography *562*, *578*
  see also Accufix™ atrial J lead; Sprint
    Fidelis leads
frame rates, echocardiography 75
Frank–Starling law 42

free-wall pacing
  lead sites 153, *172–173*
  radiography 567
  left ventricle 51, 71
    ECG 300
  right ventricle 64–66
frequencies, electrograms 8
functional failure to capture 452
functional leads, removal 207–208
functional undersensing 348, *352*,
  460–461
  atrial 536, *537*
fusion beats *see* QRS vector fusion

gap junctions 4
golf 645
great cardiac vein *177*
guidelines
  classification of indications for
    pacemakers and ICD 94
  on driving 644
  follow-up **622**, 636–637
  heart failure, pacing for **110**
  infections **242–243**
  lead extraction 205–209
  on product recalls 642–643
guidewires 178–181
  axillary approach technique 162, *163*
  cephalic approach technique 165
  see also over-the-wire lead delivery
    systems; stylets
guiding sheaths *see* sheaths

Haar transform *378*
headers 196–197
  fluoroscopy 529
  incompatible leads 457–458
  loose setscrews 446
  malfunctions *469*
    noise 522, *525*, *526–527*
heart block *see* atrioventricular block;
    first-degree heart block;
    second-degree heart block
heart failure
  monitoring *630–631*, 637–638
  pacing 66–70, 107–112
    biventricular 13, 67–70, 107–111,
      111
    programming for **397**
  sensor applications 418
  resynchronization (CRT) 424–425
heart rate 42, 43, *45*
  atrioventricular interval and 49
  PR interval *vs* 51
  variability, heart failure 637
  see also chronotropic incompetence;
    entries beginning rate…
Heart Rhythm Society
  guidelines for lead extraction
    205–209
  indications for pacemakers and ICD
    94
helices *see* screw-in leads

hematomas *225*
  pockets 229, *230*
hemostasis 159, 229
heparin
  device implantation and 203
  pocket hematomas 229
High Rate Timeout (Medtronic)
  516–517
high septum site, ventricular leads
  172–173
high-voltage leads, failure 512–514,
  521–533
His–Purkinje system 2, 3f
  see also bundle of His
histograms, rate response assessment
  420, *421*, *422*
history-taking
  ICD troubleshooting 472–473
  pacemaker troubleshooting 428–429
home monitoring 15
Home Monitoring™ (Biotronik) **639**
hospital environment, electromagnetic
  interference 598–607
hospital stay, device implantation
  203
hubs, web-based monitoring 636
hunting 645
HV interval 101
hyperkalemia 443–445
  drugs causing 472
hyperthyroidism, on pacing thresholds
  443
hypertrophic cardiomyopathy 78–79
  ICDs 122–125
  pacing for 106–107, 110
  septal myectomy 125
  sudden death 122, **125**
hypertrophic obstructive
  cardiomyopathy 78–79
hysteresis 292, *293*, 331, 435–436,
  462
  biventricular 284
  see also atrioventricular interval
      hysteresis; atrioventricular search
      hysteresis; rate hysteresis

iliac vein approach 166
image manipulation, radiography 558,
  561
immobilization 645
impedance 4–5, 139
  in batteries 14
  intracardiac 412–414
  leads 431–432, 440
    fracture 522–525, 529, 530–531
    ICDs 630
    measurement 194, 322
    management of increase 529,
      530–531
  transthoracic 411, *630–631*, 637
  see also source impedance
impedance plethysmography 606

implantable cardioverter-defibrillators
    (ICDs)
  atrial 393–394
  channelopathies 120–121
    programming **397**
  coils 29, 30, *31*, 145, 146–147
    subcutaneous 175, *176*
  connectors 147–148, 198
    failed shocks 514–515
  contraindications 126–127
  detection *see* detection by ICDs
  device selection 144–149
  driving and 644
  dual-chamber *see* dual-chamber ICDs
  electromagnetic interference 597,
    599–600
  follow-up 626–646
  inactivation 515
  indications 112–126
  interaction with pacemakers 517–518
  leads *see* leads, ICDs
  LV refractory period 537
  misclassification of antitachycardia
      pacing 507, *508*
  power-on reset 598
  programming *see* programming, ICDs
  psychologic issues 645–646
  radiotherapy 610–611
  redetection in 373, 507–510, 511
  resynchronization with 67, 107, **110**,
    117, 377
  sensing 146–147, 362–366
    minimizing EMI 592
  single-chamber *see* single-chamber
      ICDs
  sports and 645
  subcutaneous leads 30, 175, *176*
  timing cycles 287–288
  transcutaneous electrical nerve
      stimulation 605
  troubleshooting 472–533
  variable signal amplification 592–593
  ventricular lead placement 171–173
  voltage gradient 24–25
  waveform 21–24
  see also defibrillation
implantation of pulse generators
    158–160
  ICDs, testing 25–33
  replacement 203–205
  right-sided, ventricular lead
      placement 169
implantation suites *see* catheterization
    suites
inactivation of ICDs 515
incisions
  infection 207
  management 205
  pacemaker replacement 204
induction heaters/ovens 607, 609
inductive systems, web-based
    monitoring 636

industrial environments 607–608
infants, third-degree AV block 98
infection 235–238, *240*, *241*, **242–243**
  lead extraction for 205–207
  pockets 230–231, 232
inferior myocardial infarction 100
inflammation, transvenous pacing 7
inflow Doppler velocity, mitral valve 52,
  53
informed consent, pacemaker
    replacement 204
infra-Hisian block 66, *97*, 101
infra-Hisian embryological remnants 66
initial rate responses, sensors 411
injury
  cellular 7
  current of 195
"inline" connectors 197, **198**
inside-out insulation failures 532–533
insulation 11–12, 139–140
  defects 248, 449, *451*
    extracardiac stimulation 245
    polarity programming and
      341–345
  erosion through *see* conductors,
      externalization
  ICD leads 145–146, 532–533
  impedance and 431
  radiography 558, *562*
integrated bipolar leads, ICDs *367*
integrated sensing, ICDs 146–147
interatrial conduction time 47, *50*
  see also differential atrioventricular
      interval
interelectrode distance
  bipolar leads 138–139
  for SVT-VT discriminators 384
interference *see* electromagnetic
    interference
internal jugular approach 165, *167*
International Normalized Ratio, device
    implantation and 203, 229
internet *see* web-based monitoring
interrogation 321, 429
  at follow-up 621–622
    ICDs 632–633
  before implantation 598
  postoperative 600–601
interval-based SVT-VT discriminators
    373
interventricular dyssynchrony 43, *44*
interventricular offsets 72, 75, 153, 424
interviews, follow-up 620–621
intra-atrial conduction time 47, 51
intra-device interactions, ICDs 518–519
intraventricular dyssynchrony 67, *68*, 70
intrinsic amplitude tests *323*
intrinsic atrial rhythms *see* atrial
    rhythms, native
intrinsic deflection 7, 194
intrinsicoid deflection 7
INTRINSIC RV trial 58–60

intrinsic total atrial refractory period 286
introducer approach 160–161
    dual-chamber pacing 189–190
investigation devices, radiography 556, 558, *560*, 569–571
IS-1 standard 12, 141, 197
    wrong connections 458
IS-4 standard 12
    ICDs 198
ischemic cardiomyopathy, ICDs 115
ischemic heart disease *see* coronary artery disease; myocardial infarction
Ishikawa method, AV optimization 53, *54*
isoelectric depolarization 452
isoelectric events 458
isometric maneuvers *see* provocative maneuvers
iterative increment–decrement DFT 26

J curved stylets 191
J leads *137*
    dislodgement 220
    placement 190–192
    radiography 564–567
    retention wires 567, *569*
    see also Accufix™ atrial J lead
jugular approach 165, *167*, 562
junctional escape beats *102*

ladder diagrams *456*
laser sheaths 210, 213
lateral view, radiography 169, *556*, 567–569, *570*, 571, 583
Latitude™ web-based follow-up system 636–637, **639**, **640**
lead-can abrasion, ICD shocks and 514, 532
lead extenders 248
Lead Integrity Alert™ (Medtronic) 533, 643
lead–lead interactions 522
lead maturation 7
Lead Monitor warning *347*
Lead Noise Algorithm™ (Medtronic) 533, *534*
leads
    abandoned *see* abandoned leads
    damage 234–235, *240*
        see also conductors, fracture
    design 9–14
    diameter 140
    dual-chamber pacing *170–171*, 189–192
    ECG, position assessment 298–299
    epicardial *see* epicardial leads
    extraction 205–215
        after cardiac perforation 227
        complications 209–210

practitioners of 209
    techniques 210–215
failure 430–432
    high-voltage 512–514, 521–533
    rates 140
fracture *see* fracture of leads
ICDs 12, 144–149, *367*
    additional 147
    failure 512–514, 521–533
    follow-up 630–631
    fracture 248, 522, 630–631
    impedance 630
    radiography 572–577, *579*, *580*
impedance 431–432, 440
    fractures 522–525, 529, 530–531
    ICDs 630
    measurement 194, 322
implantation
    approaches 160–166, 562
    arrhythmias during 228–229
    biventricular pacing *108–109*
    children 198–202
    congenital heart disease 171, *174*
    dual-chamber pacing *170–171*, 189–192
    epicardial 196
    radiography 554, **555**
    ventricular *see* ventricular pacing, lead placement
    see also coronary sinus leads
incompatible headers 457–458
integrity 430–432
intracardiac siting
    on atrioventricular intervals 49–50, 51, 54
    biventricular pacing *108–109*
    dual-chamber pacing *170–171*
    heart failure 66–67
    prosthetic tricuspid valve *174*
    radiography 563–564, 567, *568*, 569–571
    speckle-track strain imaging 68, *69*
    for SVT-VT discriminators 384
    ventricular pacing 61–66, 71–78, 166, 185
noise 486
passive fixation *see* passive fixation of leads
performance data 142–144, 430–431
radiography 558–583
    see also under fluoroscopy
resistance 5–6
resynchronization 151–153
selection 136–144
shallowness *231*, 564
surgical examination 440
tricuspid regurgitation 150–151
tunneled, breast cancer 611
see also dislodgement of leads; Riata leads; subcutaneous leads
leads (ECG), pacing lead position assessment 298–299

left atrium, pacing 77
left bundle branch block 66–67, *108*
    cardiac perforation 226
    heart failure 107, 110
    V-V optimization 75–77
left ventricle
    contractility 51
    dysfunction
        ICD after myocardial infarction 115, 116
        resynchronization for 111
    free-wall pacing 51, 71
        ECG 300
    function 42
    leads 13–14, 175–189
        ECG 300, *301*
        inadvertent placement in 232
        radiography 571, *573*, *574*, *576*
    outflow tract velocity–time integral (LVOT VTI) 75
    pacing 66–70
        lack in resynchronization 316
    refractory period (Boston Scientific ICD) 537
    threshold elevation **627**
Left Ventricular Protection Period (LVPP™) *287*, 537
legislation, device safety 641
LEXiCon study 210
LIA *see* Lead Integrity Alert™ (Medtronic)
Liberator locking stylet *212*
life, batteries *see* longevity
ligatures
    lead damage *240*, 562, *565*
    lead fixation 189
    see also sutures
Linox® lead *152*
lipid absorption, leads 140
lithium, power sources 14
litigation, remote monitoring and 640
"living wills" 646
LLD Ez locking device *212*
lobes, Attain Starfix LV lead 153
local anesthesia, complications 159
locking stylets, lead transection and 211, *212*
LOLA ROSE study 67
longevity
    batteries 14, 204, 432, *433*
    epicardial leads, children 198
    ICDs 148–149
long-pin connectors *197*
long QT syndrome, ICDs 117–120
loop recorders, implantable 556, *560*
loops, coronary sinus leads 187, *188*
loose connectors 234, *239*, 442
loose setscrews 446, *479*
low-energy cardioversion 393
Low Energy Safety Study (LESS) trial 28–29
lower rate behavior, CRT devices 284

lower rate limits (LRL) 260, **325**
    sudden bradycardia response
        algorithms 332
    see also nominal lower rate
low-molecular-weight heparin
    device implantation and 203
    pocket hematomas 229
Low Rate Detect (Medtronic) *335*
low septum site, ventricular leads
    172–173
LRL (lower rate limits) 260, **325**
    sudden bradycardia response
        algorithms 332
    see also nominal lower rate
lumenless leads 140, *141*, 565
LV Protection Period *see* Left Ventricular
    Protection Period (LVPP™)

macrodislodgement 220, 441, 571,
    575
MADIT-II trial 58
    ICD after myocardial infarction
        114–115
MADIT-CRT trial 69, 111, **111**
magnet(s)
    artifacts *452, 453*
    ICD inhibition 510, 515
    resetting pacemakers 598
magnetic resonance imaging 208,
    602–604
    conditionally safe pacemakers 585,
        587
magnet rates 14, 289, 439
magnet response
    ICDs 599–600
    pacemakers 289–290, *291*, **325**, 618,
        620, **621**
magnet tracing, trans-telephonic
    monitoring 617–618
mains interference 452–454
malaise **623**
malfunctions 439–440, 452, 462, *469*,
    642–643
    headers *469*
    noise 522, *525, 526–527*
malignant vasodepressor syncope, SonR
    sensor 411
mammography, device siting and 160
Managed Ventricular Pacing™ (MVP)
    278, *465, 466*
Managed Ventricular Pacing trial 60
maneuvers *see* provocative maneuvers
mannitol 11
manufacturers, calling 429–430
margin testing, defibrillation 33
marker channels, ICDs 473–476
marksmanship 645
MAUDE database, website 431
maximum sensor rate (MSR) 272–276,
    325
maximum tracking rate (MTR)
    272–276, **325**

Mayo Clinic, follow-up guidelines **622**,
    636–637
mechanical AV optimization 52–55
mechanical dyssynchrony
    pacing in heart failure 69
    resynchronization on 77
mechanical sheaths, lead extraction 210,
    213
Medicare, Medicaid, ICD in non-
    ischemic cardiomyopathy 117
Medtronic
    Atrial Tracking Recovery™ 398, *399*
    atrioventricular interval hysteresis
        271
    Capture Management™ **336**
    Conducted AF Response™ *399*
    CRT devices, ventricular sensing
        mechanism 281
    ICDs
        accidental inactivation 515
        alerts 472
        arrhythmia detection 368–370, *370*
        asynchronous mode **600**
        committed shocks 372–373
        electrogram alignment 377
        electrograms 476
        far-field R-wave rejection 503–504
        far-field R waves and 384, *386*
        flashback intervals 495, *496–497,
            498*
        lead failure diagnostics 533
        magnet response **600**
        near-field sensing 365
        post-ventricular atrial blanking
            periods 503–504
        primary prevention programming
            396
        Sensing Integrity Count 522
        sensitivity 364
        SVT-VT discriminators 376, 388,
            515–516
        T-wave oversensing 478, 481,
            482–483
    Lead Integrity Alert™ 533, 643
    Lead Noise Algorithm™ 533, *534*
    Low Rate Detect 335
    magnet response and ERI **621**
    Paceart® System 616–617, *619*
    pulse generators, identification **557**
    "quiet-timer" blanking *349*
    "rate drop response" *282*
    remote monitoring **639**
    timing systems **273**
    see also Managed Ventricular
        Pacing™; Sprint Fidelis leads
MedWatch (FDA) 439–440
membrane active drugs **34**
    on DFT 33
memory, pacemakers 621–622
mental stress, sensors *409*
Merlin.net™ (St. Jude) **639, 640**
metal detectors 609

metal ion oxidation, leads 140
metals, electrodes 10
microaccelerometer, SonR sensor 411
microdislodgement 220, 441, 571
microprocessors 15
microwave ovens 608–609
middle cardiac vein *177, 178, 304*
    lead placement 188
    ECG 300
    radiography *582*
midlateral area, left ventricular pacing,
    heart failure 67
migration of pulse generators 229–230,
    243–244, 512, 556
milliseconds, paced beats per minute *vs*
    257
mineralization on leads 140
minute ventilation sensors 411, 606
    dual-sensor rate-adaptive pacing
        416–418
MIRACLE-ICD trial, coronary sinus
    lead complications **223**
mitral regurgitation 50, 77
    left bundle branch block 66
mitral valve
    function 46
    inflow Doppler velocity 52, *53*
mixed venous oxygen saturation,
    rate-adaptive pacing and 415
mobile phones 610
Mobitz types, second-degree heart block
    94–96
mode resetting 597–598
Mode Selection Trial (MOST Trial)
    57–58
    pacemaker syndrome 45
mode switching 276, *277, 279*, **325**,
    348–350, *353–354, 355, 356*
monoventricular pacing, heart failure
    66–67
morbidity, pacing mode on 56–61
morphology algorithms, Vector Timing
    and Correlation (Boston Scientific)
    380, 389
morphology analysis, ventricular
    electrograms 489, *492, 499,
    502–503*
morphology-based SVT-VT
    discriminators 373, **375**, 376–377,
    378, 379, 380, 388
    failure **381**, 515
mortality, pacing mode on 56–61
MP35N (alloy) 139, 145
M-PATHY study, hypertrophic
    obstructive cardiomyopathy
    78–79
multifilar leads *11*, 145
multiluminal leads 11, *521*
multipolar left ventricular leads 14
multisite pacing, codes 16
Mustard procedure, active fixation lead
    placement 202

MUSTIC-AF trial, resynchronization
    112
MUSTIC trial, coronary sinus lead
    complications **223**
myocardial infarction
    atrioventricular block 100
    ventricular tachyarrhythmia 114–116
myocardial twist 75
myocardium
    electrode interface, damage 441
    intracardiac impedance 412–414
    stimulation 2–4
myopotentials *479*, 592–593
    diaphragm 486–488
        lead fracture *vs* 522, *523*
        oversensing 546
    inhibition by 456–457, *463*
    oversensing 486–488
    pectoralis muscle
        on electrograms 377, **381**
        ICD electrograms 476
        oversensing 487–488

narrow-band electrograms, ICDs
    474–476
narrow band-pass filters 593
national registry, ICD in non-ischemic
    cardiomyopathy 117
native rhythms
    finding 432–433
    see also atrial rhythms, native
NBG code, pacemaker nomenclature
    16
near-field electrograms, ICDs 473–474,
    475, 495
near-field signals, sensing by ICDs 365
near-isoelectric events 458
negative RV-LV timing cycle *283*
nerve conduction studies 605
neuraxial modulation 511
neurocardiogenic syncope 79–80,
    104–105, *106*
    algorithms for 280–281
    Closed Loop Stimulation for 414
    pacing mode selection 136
neuromuscular diseases, AV block 100
night rates *see* sleep rates
noise 476, *480*, 486, 522–533, *534*
noise rejection 268, 597
noise reversion 15, 593–597
noise-sampling period 593–597
nomenclature
    right ventricular pacing sites 169–171
    see also codes
nominal atrial sensitivity 339
nominal lower rate 328
nominal upper rate limit 328
nominal ventricular sensitivity 339
noncommitted shocks 372–373, *374*
Non-Competitive Atrial Pacing™
    (NCAP) 276, *277*
noncompliance, β-blockers 119–120

nonfunctional leads 238–240
    removal 208–209
    see also abandoned leads
nonphysiologic AV delay *see* ventricular
    safety pacing
nontracking modes 276, 348–350
    unanticipated change to 536, *537*, *539*
North American Society of Pacing and
    Electrophysiology/BPG, codes 320
number of intervals to detect VF (NID),
    reprogramming 533
NYHA functional class, ICD after
    myocardial infarction 115

OAO mode 328
oblique views, fluoroscopy 169, 176,
    177, *181*, 185, 232, *304*
ODO mode 328
offsets, interventricular 72, 75, 153, 424
Ohm's law 4–5
One Button Detection Enhancements™
    (Boston Scientific) **376**
1:1 AV relationship
    tachycardias with 489, 492–495, *497*,
        516, *518*
    ATP on 495
"onset" enhancement, single-chamber
    detection **375**, 376, 382
open-loop sensors 408
operating rooms 158
    cardiac perforation 227
    see also catheterization suites
operative evaluation 440
operative intervention
    chest radiography before 554
    pace-sense lead fractures 530–531
    see also postoperative care;
        preoperative preparation
Optim® (insulator) 139
order sets, post-implant 205, *206*
orientation curves, coronary venous
    leads *153*
outpatient procedures, device
    implantation 203
output programming 333–339, *343*
    safety margins 337, 433
outputs
    failure *see* failure to pace
    maximum 441
overdrive pacing modes 228
oversensing
    CRT devices **535**, 536–541, **635**
    diaphragmatic myopotentials 546
    failure to pace 454, *457*
    ICDs 362, *363*, *364*, 476–488,
        592–593
        far-field electrograms 501–504,
            505, *539*
        far-field R waves 501
        lead fracture 522
        R waves 384–387, 388, *390*
        T waves 365–366, 476–481, 522, *525*

lead fracture *439*
P waves 522, *523*, *525*
    ICDs *480*, 485
    lead fracture *vs* *523*
    see also atrial oversensing
over-the-lead sheath removal 188
over-the-wire lead delivery systems 13,
    151–153
    left ventricle 185–187
    see also guidewires
OVO mode 328
oxygen saturation, mixed venous,
    rate-adaptive pacing and 415

P80A polyurethane 12
PA (time period) 256
Pac-A-Tach trial 57
Paceart® System (Medtronic) 616–617,
    619
paced beats per minute, milliseconds *vs*
    257
paced depolarization integral, sensor 415
paced events, defined 256
Pacemaker Lead Extraction with the
    Laser Sheath (PLEXES) study 210
pacemaker-mediated tachycardia
    470–471
    algorithms for **326**
    see also endless-loop tachycardia
Pacemaker Selection in the Elderly trial
    57
    lead dislodgement 220
pacemaker syndrome 44–45, *46*, *48*, 245
    AV block *vs* 80
    diagnostic criteria **123–124**
    symptoms 467
    from VVI pacing 134
pace-sense lead failure 521–531, **532**,
    533, *534*
    management 529–531
pacing 4–9
    device selection 134–136
    indications 94–97
pacing artifacts, assessment 289, *295*
Pacing in Cardiomyopathy study (PIC
    study) 78
pacing intervals, long 457
pacing modes 56–61, 257–264, **320**
    selection 134, 135–136
    sick sinus syndrome 60, 136
    see also mode switching; *specific modes*
pacing pads, during lead implantation
    228–229
pacing threshold *see* stimulation
    threshold
pain 230–232
    chronic 207
    local anesthesia complication 159
    subcuticular siting of pulse generators
        159
palpitations 470, 471, **623**
    before ICD shocks 472–473

parallel-wound leads 11
passive fixation of leads 10, *137*
  cardiac perforation 225
  radiography 564, *577*
patches, epicardial 572, *578*
patent foramen ovale *233, 574*
patient satisfaction, remote monitoring 640
patient-specific DFT 26–27
patient-specific testing, defibrillation 33
PAVE trial, resynchronization 112
PEA sensor (SonR sensor; peak endocardial acceleration sensor) 411–412, *413*, 418, 424–425
pectoralis muscle
  deep placement of pulse generators 160
  stimulation 245
  see also myopotentials
peel-away sheaths 188
perforation
  coronary sinus 185
  great vessels 227
  heart 225–227, *588*
performance data, leads 142–144, 430–431
pericardial effusions, ICD shocks and 512
pericarditis 228
persistent left SVC 167, 198, 583, *585*
personnel, follow-up clinics 614–615
phantom shocks 473, 646
phase duration, defibrillator waveforms 23–24
phones (cellular) 610
phrenic nerve stimulation 245, 542–543
physiology 2–4, 42–43, 51
PIC study (Pacing in Cardiomyopathy study) 78
piezoelectric crystals, activity sensors 409, *410*
pleural effusions, ICD shocks and 512
pneumopericardium *224*
pneumothorax 223–225
  contrast venography and 583
  ICD shocks and 512
pockets for pulse generators 159–160
  air 452
  complications 229–230
  infection 207, 230–231, 236
  manipulation 456–457
  pain 159, 230–232
polarity **326**
  bipolar lead fracture and 248, *251*
  connectors 197–198
  defibrillation 24
  pectoral muscle stimulation 245
  programming 341–346, *347*, 449, *450*
  pulse generators, radiography 556, *558*
polarization 2, 6
  sensing and 8–9

polytetrafluoroethylene *see* extended PTFE jackets
polyurethane 12, 139–140
  defects 248
porous electrodes 139
positive RV-LV timing cycle *283*
posterior left ventricular pacing
  ECG 300
  heart failure 67
posterolateral cardiac vein *177*
  lead placement *581*
posteroseptal space fat pad *184*, 185
post-market surveillance data 142–144
postoperative care 205, 600–601
post-pacing T-wave oversensing 477–478, *481*
post-shock electrogram diminution 146
post-ventricular atrial blanking periods (PVAB) 264, **326**, 348, *351*
  ICDs 501–504
post-ventricular atrial refractory period (PVARP) 261, *263*, 264, *265*, **326**
  atrial events in **535**, 536, *537*, *538*, **635**
  extension 275, 276, 280, **326**, 348, *351*, *352*, 462
  programming 348, *351*
  shortening 276–278
  tracking and 395
potassium ions 2
powered sheaths, lead extraction 210, 211–213
power-on reset 597–598
P-P intervals, tachycardias 489
preactivation, LV lead 76
Predictors of Response to CRT (PROSPECT study) 77
pre-ejection interval 44
  rate-adaptive pacing and 415
pre-excitation, left atrium 77
premature ventricular contractions (PVC)
  AAI pacing 257–259
  algorithms for 398–399
  biventricular pacing 286
  pause limitation 78
  PVARP extension for 280, 348
  shortening 399
  undersensing 458–459
  see also ventricular extrasystoles
preoperative preparation, device implantation 203
pressure changes, right ventricle, rate-adaptive pacing and 415
primary prevention of life-threatening arrhythmias 112–114
  programming for **396, 397**
  rate criteria 370
PR interval 2, *50*, *52*
  heart rate *vs 51*
  second-degree heart block 94

PR Logic, SVT-VT discriminators 376, 388, *390*, 516
proarrhythmic pacing 506, *507*
  cardiac resynchronization devices 543, *545*
  VT storm 511
product recalls *see* recalls
programmable waveforms, ICDs 149
programming 15, 319–407
  for atrioventricular block 471–472
  atrioventricular interval and 49, 307–316, 331–332, 400
  resynchronization (CRT) 424
  battery depletion and 246
  at follow-up 357–360, 622–624, **627**
  ICDs 360–394, **396, 397**
    emergencies 511
    for pace-sense lead fractures 530
    sensing 365–366
    troubleshooting 515–521
  magnet response 289
  optimizing therapy 394–395, **397, 398**
  output 333–339, *343*
    safety margins 337, 433
  pacemaker codes 16
  polarity 341–346, *347*, 449, *450*
  resynchronization devices 395–400
    VV (time period) 424–425
  sensitivity 339–341, *342*, *343–344*
  sensor function 418–423
  for sick sinus syndrome 104
  suggested parameters *361*
  for T-wave oversensing 481, *483*
  undocumented 462
  unexpected parameters 350–357
  see also reprogramming
progressive depolarization theory 19, *21*
prolapse of coronary sinus leads 187, 188
propafenone *448*
PROSPECT study (Predictors of Response to CRT) 77
prosthetic tricuspid valve
  epicardial systems and 196
  lead placement 171, *174*, 583, *584*
provocative maneuvers 456–457, *462*, *463*, *478*, *479*, 488, *593*
pseudo-fusion 316
pseudo-malfunctions 452–454, 458
  digital recording systems 458, *464*, *465*
pseudo-Wenckebach behavior 264, *265*, *266*, *273*, *274*
  biventricular pacing, avoidance 286
  exercise and *420*
  upper rate limit setting 328, *330*
psychologic issues 645–646
P-tracking/P-synchronous pacing *see* VDD pacing
pull-back technique, coronary sinus venography *183*

pulmonary artery
    pressure 637–638
    use in lead placement *170–171*
pulse amplitude *see* voltage amplitude
pulsed Doppler, frame rates 75
pulse duration **326**
    amplitude *vs* 4
    programming 333–339
pulse generators 14–15
    children 199
    connectors *142*
    EMI shielding 592
    failure 432, *433*, 439–440, 515
    ICDs, follow-up 626–628
    identification 429–430, 556
    lead compatibility 141
    migration 229–230, 243–245, 512, 556
    physical evaluation 440
    radiography 554–558
    replacement 203–205, 642–644
    sites of placement 30
        see also specific sites
    size 159
    see also implantation of pulse generators; pockets for pulse generators
pulse width *see* pulse duration
Purkinje fibers 2
PVAB *see* post-ventricular atrial blanking periods
PVARP (post-ventricular atrial refractory period) 261, *263*, 264, *265*, **326**
    atrial events in **535**, 536, *537, 538*, **635**
    extension 275, 276, 280, **326**, 348, *351, 352*, 462
    programming 348, *351*
    shortening 276–278
    tracking and 395
P waves *3f*
    dual-chamber pacing 292
    oversensing 522, *523, 525*
        ICDs *480*, 485
        lead fracture *vs 523*
        see also atrial oversensing
    programming sensitivity 339
    in refractory period *352, 353*
    tracking 274, *276*

QRS complex *3f, 17*
    as dyssynchrony marker 111
    heart failure 66, 69–70
    lead siting based on 71, 72
    mitral valve inflow waves *vs* 52, 53
    resynchronization 304–305, *309–311*
    second-degree heart block 95, *97*
    width on AV optimization 54
    see also stimulus–QRS interval
QRS vector fusion 72–75, 304–307
QT sensing pacemaker 414

quality of life
    dual-sensor rate-adaptive pacing 416
    pacing mode on 57
QuickFlex LV lead (St. Jude) 153
"quiet-timer" blanking (Medtronic) **349**

"R" (in codes) 320
radial strain, ventricular timing optimization 75
radiofrequency energy
    electromagnetic interference 598, 601
    lead extraction 213, 215
radiography *see* chest radiography; fluoroscopy
radiotherapy 208, 248, *250*, 462–463, 610–611
RAFT trial, biventricular pacing **111**
RAM, pulse generators 15
"ramps", ATP 391
rate-adaptive atrioventricular interval *see* rate-variable atrioventricular interval
rate-adaptive pacing *357*
    electromagnetic interference and 598–599
    indications 408
    programming at follow-up 622–624
    resynchronization (CRT) and 424–425
    sensing devices for 408–418, 437–439
    symptoms 471
Rate Branch™ (St. Jude) **376**, 388–390, *391*, 516
rate criteria, detection by ICDs 367–372
rate drop response programming *282, 334*
rate hysteresis **326**, 435–436
    see also hysteresis
rate-modulated pacing 259–261
    asynchronous 261
    DDIR pacing 262
rate programmability 328, *329, 330*
rate-responsive capability
    assessment 420, *421*, 422, *422*
    atrioventricular interval and 49
    for bradycardia 136
    codes 16
rate smoothing 295, *297*, **326**, 436–437
    intra-device interactions 518–519
rates of pacing
    assessment 435–439
    troubleshooting 462–464
rate-variable atrioventricular interval 268, *269*, **327**
reaction time **327**, 422, *424*
real-time electrograms, ICDs 476, *477*
recalls
    Accufix™ atrial J lead 209
    pacemaker replacement 204, 640–644

recharging, capacitors 628
reconfirmation, in ICDs 372–373, *375*
records
    trans-telephonic monitoring 616–617, *619*
    see also data storage
recovery time **327**, 422, *424*
recurrence of preimplantation symptoms, causes 246–252
redetection, in ICDs 373, 507–510, 511
redundancy of leads 563–564, *566*
    children 199, *200–201*, 564, *566*
    coronary sinus leads 187, 188
reed switches 602
Reel syndrome 556, *559*
re-entrant circuits 34–35, 77
    see also endless-loop tachycardia
re-entrant tachycardias, pacing for 106
reforming, capacitors 628
refractory period extension theory *see* progressive depolarization theory
refractory periods 17, *18*, 256, 257
    atrium **325**
        pacing during 276–278
        see also post-ventricular atrial refractory period; total atrial refractory period
    biventricular pacing 286–287
    programming 346–348
    P waves in *352, 353*
    resettable 593–597
    SSIR pacing 260
    ventricular (VRP) 257, **327**, 346
        resetting in response to noise 596–597
registered nurses (RNs) 205
registries
    lead failure 430
    lead performance 144, 430–431
    see also national registry; REPLACE registry
regularity of rhythm, VT *vs* SVT 489–492
reimplantation
    after infections 238
    leads 215
    see also replacement
remote access monitoring 15, 614, 634–640
repairability, leads 140
repetitive rapid oversensing 522
replacement
    pulse generators 203–205, 642–644
    see also reimplantation
replacement voltages, elective 14
REPLACE registry
    infection 235
    lead dislodgement 220
repolarization 19
    see also additional repolarization time

reprogramming
  bipolar to unipolar mode 341
  for electromagnetic interference 593, *594*
  for exercise 622–624
  finding thresholds 337
  number of intervals to detect VF (NID) 533
  for sudden bradycardia 471
  undocumented 462
reset modes *see* backup modes
resettable refractory periods 593–597
resistance 5–6
  impedance *vs* 5
  see also source impedance
respiratory rate, minute ventilation sensors 411
resynchronization *see* biventricular pacing
retained fragments 238–240, *243*, *244*
retained sponges *224*
retention wires, J leads 567, *569*
retrograde atrial excitation *see* ventriculoatrial conduction
retromammary siting, pulse generators 160
Retry mode (Boston Scientific) **336**
REVERSE trial, biventricular pacing **111**
rheobase 4, 335–337
RHYTHM II study 75
Rhythm ID™ (Boston Scientific) 387–388, *389*, 516
Rhythm ID Going Head to Head Trial (RIGHT) 388
Riata leads 532–533, *580*, 624, 644
right atrial appendage, lead placement 191–192
right atrium, lead placement 190–191
right bundle branch, pacing site 67
right bundle branch block
  cardiac perforation 226
  resynchronization for 110–111
right pectoral implantation, ICDs 30, *32*
right superior fascicles 66
right ventricle
  apex pacing (RVA pacing) 61, *65*, 66, 107
    ECG 299–300
    minimization 331–332
  arrhythmogenic dysplasia, ICDs 121–122
  defibrillator lead placement 171–173
  impedance-based sensor 412–414
  pacing 57–66
    bifocal 67
    ECG 299–300
    free-wall 64–66
    lead placement 166–175, *176*
    tricuspid regurgitation 245–246
  pressure changes, rate-adaptive pacing and 415
  resynchronization on function 77

right ventricular outflow tract
  lead position
    ECG 300
    radiography 571
  pacing 61, 64, *65*
  ventricular tachycardia *126*
ring electrodes *12*
Ritter method, AV optimization 53–54
RR intervals
  alternating 476–477, 481
  lead fracture 522
  rate smoothing 436–437
  reduced percentage resynchronized 534–542
  tachycardias 489
runaway pacemaker 462–463
R waves
  amplitude test *342*
  double-counting 481–485, 522, *525*, 546
  far-field 195, 384–387, 388, *390*, *477*
    oversensing 501–504, *505*, *539*
  ICDs, sensing 362–364, 384, 520
  programming sensitivity 339, *342*

SafeR™ algorithm 279
safety margins
  defibrillation 26–27, 28
  programming output 337, 433
  T-wave oversensing *482–483*
SAVE-PACe trial 58–60
SCD-HeFT trial 115, 117
screens, programmers 321, *322*, *323*, *324*
  "additional features" *361*
  data collection *358*
  lead warnings *432*
  "summary" *359*
screw-in leads 10–11, *137*
  extraction 210–211
seal-plug problems, headers 522, *525*, *526–527*
seat belts 644
secondary prevention of life-threatening arrhythmias 112
  programming for **397**
  rate criteria 370
second-degree heart block 97
  pacing for 94–96
second phase duration, defibrillation 23–24
sedation
  conscious 158–159
  for VT storm 511
Seldinger technique *see* introducer approach
SelectSecure™ lead 140, *141*
sensed events, defined 256
sensing 7–9
  bipolar *vs* unipolar leads 13
  CRT devices, errors **535**
  devices for rate-adaptive pacing 408–418, 437–439

electrograms 15
ICDs 146–147, 362–366
  minimizing EMI 592
pacemaker codes 16
thresholds 192–196, **327**, 435
  assessment 420–422, *423*
  programming **327**, 339–341, *345*
troubleshooting 534–549
ventricular fibrillation 33
see also atrial sensing window; far-field sensing; oversensing; undersensing
Sensing Integrity Count, Medtronic ICDs 522
sensitivity
  ICDs 364–365, *366*
  thresholds 362, *366*
  programming 339–341, *342*, *343–344*
Sensor and Quality of Life study 416
septal-to-posterior wall motion delay (SPWMD), V-V optimization on 76–77
septum
  ablation, heart block from 106
  cardiac enlargement 185
  lead siting, radiography 566, *568*, *569–571*
  myectomy, hypertrophic cardiomyopathy 125
  pacing 64, *65*, *172–173*
    in bifocal pacing 67
    ECG 300
  see also high septum site; low septum site
setscrews, loose 446, *479*
sexual activity 645
shallowness of leads *231*, 564
sheaths
  curved 178–181
  lead delivery 13, 178, 179, *180*
    removal 188–189
  lead extraction 210, 211–213
shock plans 646
shocks 393
  anodal 20–21
  for atrial fibrillation 394
  committed *vs* non-committed 372–373, *374*
  dosage 24–25
  efficacy assessment 631–632
    see also shocks, unsuccessful
  frequent 510–511
  inappropriate 472
  lead-can abrasion and 514, 532
  optimizing therapy 394–395, 506–510, 634
  psychologic issues 645–646
  symptoms before 472–473
  unsuccessful 511–521
    misclassification as 511–512
shooting 645
short–long–short sequences 506

short QT syndrome 121
shoulder movement 205
sick sinus syndrome (sinus node
        dysfunction) 101–103
    cardiac transplantation 202
    pacing mode and 60, 136
sildenafil, on DFT 33
silicone 12, 139, 140
silver, ICD leads 145
single-chamber atrial pacemakers, sick
        sinus syndrome 103
single-chamber ICDs 149–153
    electrograms 488, 489–495, 499
    SVT-VT discriminators 373–374,
        376–382, 515–516
single-chamber pacing, pulse generators,
        radiography 558
single-chamber rate-modulated pacing
        (SSIR pacing) 259–260
    see also AAIR pacing; VVIR pacing
single-chamber triggered-mode pacing
        (VVT mode) 259, 260, 328
    electrocardiogram 289
single-chamber ventricular pacing see
        VVI pacing; VVIR pacing
single element subcutaneous leads 175
single-lead VDD systems 262
    radiography 571, 577
single-pass VDD pacing
    atrioventricular block 136
    children 200
sinoatrial node (SA node) 2, 3f
sinus arrest 102
sinus node dysfunction see sick sinus
        syndrome
sinus rhythm, ventricular sensing
        problems 534–537
sinus tachycardia 489, 492–495, 496–497
siting
    pulse generators 159–160
    see also leads, intracardiac siting
situational syncope 105
situs inversus, lead placement 586
Situs® left ventricular lead 152–153
size
    ICDs 148–149
    pulse generators 159
slack see redundancy of leads
sleep, bradycardia 101–103
sleep rates 296, 325, 328, 330, 435
sleeves, lead fixation 188
    children 199
slew rates 8, 9f, 195
    see also tilt
slings 205, 645
"smaller diameter possible", leads 139
SMART® algorithm (Biotronik) 390,
        391
SMART-AV trial 70–71, 399–400
SMARTSense™, atrial blanking period,
        Boston Scientific ICDs 384
SMARTVIEW™ (Sorin) 639

snares, femoral lead extraction 214
sodium ions 2
SonR sensor (PEA sensor) 411–412,
        413, 418, 424–425
SOOR pacing (asynchronous pacing) see
        asynchronous pacing
Sorin Medical
    atrioventricular interval hysteresis
        271
    AutoThreshold 336
    blanking characteristics 349
    CRT devices, ventricular sensing and
        281
    ICDs, magnet response 600
    magnet response and ERI 621
    Parad algorithm 518
    pulse generators, identification 557
    remote monitoring 639
    SafeR™ algorithm 279
    timing systems 273
source impedance 9
speckle-track strain imaging
    lead siting based on 68, 69
    ventricular timing optimization
        75
spectrum, electromagnetic 592
sponges
    hemostasis 159
    retained 224
spontaneous rhythm see atrial rhythms,
        native; native rhythms
sports 645
Sprint Fidelis leads, fracture 531, 643
SSIR pacing (single-chamber
        rate-modulated pacing) 259–260
    see also AAIR pacing; VVIR pacing
stability, leads 153, 187–188
"stability" enhancement, single-chamber
        detection 375, 376, 377, 382,
        383–384, 516
staff, follow-up clinics 614–615
stairs, down vs up 410
standards
    leads 12, 141
    see also specific standards
staphylococci 235–236
Starling's law 42
"stat set" button 321
stenosis of veins 207, 237, 238
stents, lead removal 207
step-down to failure DFT 26, 27
step-up to success DFT 26
sternocleidomastoid muscle 165
steroid elution 6, 7, 137, 138
steroids, systemic 443
stiffness of leads 139
stimulation
    anodal, resynchronization and 316
    diaphragm 245
        assessment 169, 187–188
    myocardium 2–4
    pectoralis muscle 245

phrenic nerve 245, 542–543
    see also cross-stimulation
stimulation threshold 4–7
    circadian pattern 7, 30–33
    drugs and endocrine disorders 435,
        443–444, 448
    external cardioversion on 441, 447,
        601, 602
    measurement 192–194, 337–338
    pacemaker replacement 204
    variation 6–7
stimulus energy, voltages vs 4
stimulus latency 542
    see also capture, latency
stimulus–QRS interval 303–304
stimulus-T sensing pacemaker 414
St. Jude Medical
    atrioventricular interval hysteresis
        271
    blanking characteristics 349
    coronary sinus leads 152, 153
    CRT devices, ventricular sensing
        mechanism 281
    ICDs
        asynchronous mode 600
        committed shocks 372
        electrogram alignment 377, 379
        far-field R waves and 386, 504
        filtering 478–480
        magnet response 600
        monitor zones 372
        primary prevention programming
            396
        programmability 149
        reconfirmation 373
        sensitivity 364–365, 366
        SVT-VT discriminators 376,
            388–390, 391, 515–516
        T-wave oversensing 478, 481
    magnet response and ERI 621
    Merlin.net™ 639
    pulse generators, identification
        557
    remote monitoring 639
    timing systems 273
    Ventricular Autocapture™ 336
    see also Riata leads
storage of data 626
    in pacemakers 621–622
stored electrograms, ICDs 476, 477
stored energy 25
straight stylets
    atrial J leads 190–191
    ventricular leads 168, 169
strain imaging see speckle-track strain
        imaging
strength–duration curve 4
stress, sensors 409
stroke volume 42
    rate-adaptive pacing and 415
stylet-driven leads, over-the-wire leads vs
        185, 186

stylets
  J leads 190–191
  lead damage 235
  ventricular leads
    curved 167–169
    management 166
    sheath removal 188
  see also guidewires; locking stylets
subclavian approach 165
  crush injury (to lead) 431, 564
  extrathoracic see axillary approach
  pneumothorax 223
  radiography 563, 564
subclavian artery puncture 225, 232, 573
subclavian vein thrombosis 233–234
subcutaneous arrays 175, 176, 580
subcutaneous leads, ICDs 30, 175, 176
subcutaneous patches 573
subcuticular siting, pulse generators 159
subpectoral position, pulse generators, children 199
subselection
  ventricular veins 187, 188
success, lead extraction, defining 209
sudden bradycardia response algorithms 280–281, 332–333, 437, 438
"sudden-brady response" (SBR) 282
sudden death
  Brugada syndrome 120, 121
  hypertrophic cardiomyopathy 122, 125
  long QT syndrome 120
  prevention 113–114
  see also aborted sudden death
sudden unexplained death syndrome, ICDs 120–121
"summary" screens, programmers 359
superior vena cava
  defibrillator coils in 146–147, 173, 175
  persistent left 167, 198, 583, 585
support groups 646
supraventricular tachycardia 102
  ATP on 392–93
  dual-chamber ICDs 150
  electrograms, ICDs 475, 488–510
  pacing for 105–106
  ventricular tachycardia vs
    ICD electrograms 488–510
    misclassification 515–517
    redetection error 507–510
  see also SVT-VT discriminators
surface area, electrodes 10, 139
surgery
  preparation of patient 600
  see also operative evaluation; operative intervention
surveillance data, post-market 142–144
surveillance equipment 609–610
sustained-duration override features 516–517
sustained rate duration, single-chamber detection 375

sutures
  absorbable 199
  lead transection and 211
  see also ligatures
SVT-VT discriminators
  dual-chamber ICDs 382–390, 516–517
  failure 499–501
  failure of defibrillation due to 515–517
  optimizing therapy 395
  in redetection 507, 509
  single-chamber 373–374, 376–377, 515–516
  St. Jude Medical ICDs 376, 388–390, 392, 515–516
  see also morphology-based SVT-VT discriminators
S waves, right ventricular apex pacing 299–300
swimming 645
sympathetic denervation 511
symptoms
  atrioventricular block 99, 471
  causes of recurrence 246–252
syncope 623
  atrioventricular block 101
  Closed Loop Stimulation for 414
  drugs causing 472
  ICDs and 113, 473
  malignant vasodepressor syncope, SonR sensor 411
  neurocardiogenic see neurocardiogenic syncope
  pacing mode selection 136
  reflex 104–105
  tilt-table testing 79, 105
  see also sudden bradycardia response algorithms

tachyarrhythmias
  atrial
    mode switching for 276
    risk of thromboembolism 638–640
  mode switching for 276, 348–350, 353–354, 355, 356
  pacing for 105–106, 107
  ventricular
    myocardial infarction 114–116
    underdetection 515–521
tachycardia
  cardiomyopathy from 110, 117
  with 1:1 AV relationship 489, 492–495, 497, 516, 518
  ATP on 495
  re-entrant circuits 34–35
  see also endless-loop tachycardia
tachycardia-bradycardia syndrome 101, 102
tamponade 185, 227
TARP see total atrial refractory period
teaching, trans-telephonic monitoring 616

Telectronics/Medtronic connector type 141
telemetry 15, 439
  see also remote access monitoring
telescoping sheaths, lead extraction 211
temperatures, low 598
temperature-sensing rate-adaptive pacemakers 415
temporary programming 322
terminal illness, withdrawal of therapy 646
tetralogy of Fallot, ICDs 125
text episode summary 500
third-degree atrioventricular block 96–98
thoracotomy, lead extraction 215
Threshold Margin Test 337–338, 339, 618, 622
thresholds
  defibrillation 25–26
    antiarrhythmic drugs on 33
    causes of elevation 30, 512
    programmable waveforms for 149
    sensitivity 362, 366
    upper limit of vulnerability and 33
  elevation 441, 627
  measurement 337–338, 433–435
  output programming for 335–339, 343
  reduction 137
  see also capture, thresholds; sensing, thresholds; steroid elution; stimulation threshold
thrombin, topical 229
thromboembolism
  atrial fibrillation and 638–640, 641
  inadvertent LV lead placement 232, 233, 234
  pacing mode on 57
thrombolytic therapy 234
thrombosis 207, 232–234, 236
tidal volume 411
tilt
  defibrillator waveforms 22, 23–24
  see also slew rates
tilt-table testing, syncope 79, 105
timers, SVT-VT discriminators 382
timing circuits 15
timing cycles 255–318
  ECG 302–316
tip extrasystoles see ventricular extrasystoles
tones (audible), ICDs see alerts
torsades de pointes 118
tortuous veins, ventricular lead placement 169
total atrial refractory period (TARP) 264, 265, 328, 538
  intrinsic 286
tracking 274, 276, 395, 399
Tracking Preference™ (Boston Scientific) 398
traction, lead extraction 210

training, lead extraction 209
transcutaneous electrical nerve
    stimulation 518, 604–605
transection, lead extraction 211, *212*
transmembrane potential 2–4
transmural lead placement 583
transplantation *see* cardiac
    transplantation
transport mechanisms (active) 2
transposition of great vessels *174*
    congenitally corrected *586*
trans-telephonic monitoring 614,
    616–618, *619, 622*
transthoracic impedance 411, *630–631*,
    637
transvenous pacing, electrodes 6–7
trauma 248
treadmill exercise 419, 624
Trendelenburg position 161–162
trends, impedance measurements 322
tricuspid regurgitation 150–151, *243*,
    245–246, *247*
tricuspid stenosis 246
tricuspid valve
    abnormalities, epicardial systems and
        196
    see also prosthetic tricuspid valve
trifascicular block 101
triggered-mode pacing
    ECG 289, 292
    single-chamber *see* single-chamber
        triggered-mode pacing
triggering *see* DDT mode
trocars, for subcutaneous leads *176*
troponin, ICD candidacy after
    myocardial infarction 115
troubleshooting
    cardiac resynchronization devices
        533–546, **635**
    ICDs 472–533
    pacemakers 428–472, **627**
true bipolar leads, ICDs *367*
truncated waveforms, ICDs 22, *23*
truncation, electrograms (intracardiac)
    377, *381*, **381**
tunneled leads, breast cancer 611
T wave *17*
    oversensing, ICDs 365–366, 476–481,
        522, *525*
twiddler's syndrome 240–243, 556, *558*
twist, myocardial 75

UK Pacing and Cardiovascular Events
trial 57
ultrasound
    for subclavian approach 223
    see also echocardiography
underdetection, ventricular
    tachyarrhythmia 515–521
undersensing 458–466, **470**
    ICDs 362, *363, 364,* 388, 501,
        515–521
        ventricular fibrillation 519–521

    see also atrial undersensing; functional
        undersensing
undocumented programming 462
unifilar leads *11*
unipolar functions, switching from
    bipolar 341, *347*
unipolar leads *12*, 13, 137–139
    connectors 197–198
    electromagnetic interference and 592
    IS-1 standard 141
    radiography 564, *567*
units of timing 257
univentricular heart, lead placement *586*
univentricular sensing, biventricular
    pacing 284–285, *286*
upper limit of vulnerability 18–19, *20*,
    33
upper rate behavior
    atrioventricular interval 295
    CRT devices 285–286, 534–536
upper rate limits (URL) 260, 328, *330*
upper tracking rate (UPR) 275
URL (upper rate limits) 260, 328, *330*

VAA response to ATP 495
VA interval (ventriculoatrial interval)
    257, *258*
    DDD pacing 262
    extension 276–278
valvular endocarditis 207
vancomycin **207**
variable signal amplification, ICDs
    592–593
varicosity, coronary venous system 153
vasodepressor response
    carotid sinus reflex 79, 104
    see also malignant vasodepressor
        syncope
Vasovagal Pacemaker Study (VPS-1) 80
vasovagal syncope *see* neurocardiogenic
    syncope; syncope
Vaughan-Williams classification **34**
VAV response to ATP 495
VDD pacing (atrial synchronous
    (P-tracking/P-synchronous)
    pacing) 262, *263*
    atrioventricular block 136
    DDD pacing *vs* 292
    indications and contraindications
        135
    single-lead, radiography 571, *577*
    see also single-pass VDD pacing
VDDR pacing
    atrioventricular block 136
    indications and contraindications
        135
VDI mode 328
vectors
    ECG 298
        biventricular pacing 300–302
    far-field electrograms 489
    ICDs 29
    pacing 72–75, 153

Vector Timing and Correlation
    morphology algorithm (Boston
    Scientific) *380, 389*
vegetations *235*
vein of Marshall 192, *193*
veins
    defibrillation electrodes 175
    stenosis 207, *237, 238*
    tortuosity 169
venepuncture, axillary approach 162
venlafaxine, on DFT 33
venography 162–163, 164, 165, 583
    coronary sinuses 179, 181–183
venoplasty 233
venous approaches
    lead placement 160–166
    radiography 562
ventricles, electrograms 8, 194–195, 474,
    476, 489–495
ventricular asynchronous pacing (VOO)
    257
Ventricular Autocapture™ (St. Jude
    Medical) **336**
Ventricular Automatic Capture (Boston
    Scientific) **336**
ventricular avoidance pacing algorithms
    278–279, 331–332, 458
ventricular-based timing systems
    268–272
ventricular blanking periods (VRP)
    263–265, *267,* **327, 349,** 454–455
Ventricular Capture Control (Biotronik)
    336
ventricular depolarization gradient 415
ventricular extrasystoles
    during blanking periods 348
    during lead implantation 228
    resynchronization and 316
    see also premature ventricular
        contractions
ventricular fibrillation 18
    detection by ICDs 368–370
    self-terminating 507
    sensing 33
    undersensing 519–521
ventricular inhibited pacing (VVI
    pacing) 45, *47, 48,* 257, *258,* 320,
    328
    clinical effects 56–57
    indications 134, **135**
ventricular oversensing
    CRT devices **535,** 537–541, **635**
    ICDs 476–488
ventricular pacing
    avoidance algorithms 278–279,
        331–332, 458
    clinical effects 57–61
    ECG 300–303
    heart failure 13, 66–70, 107–111, **111**
    lead criteria 151–153
    lead placement 166–175, 542
        atrial lead placement with 190
        radiography 567–572

ventricular pacing (cont'd)
  lead siting 61–66, 71–78, 166, 185
  sick sinus syndrome 104
  see also biventricular pacing; right
      ventricle, pacing
ventricular pacing inhibition, CRT
    devices **535**
ventricular rate, atrial rate vs, SVT-VT
    discriminators 383–387
ventricular rate regulation (VRR) 78,
    295–296, 399, 539–541
ventricular refractory period (VRP)
    257, **327**, 346
  resetting in response to noise
      596–597
ventricular safety pacing 267, 268, **327**
Ventricular Sense Amplitude algorithm
    342
Ventricular Sense Response™ algorithm
    284, 285, 539, 542
"Ventricular Sensing Test" 343–344
ventricular septal defect 232
ventricular tachyarrhythmias
  myocardial infarction 114–116
  underdetection 515–521
ventricular tachycardia
  antitachycardia pacing on 34–35, 495
  catecholaminergic polymorphic 121
  detection by ICDs 368–370
    see also SVT-VT discriminators
  electrograms, ICDs 475
  fascicular 127
  indications for ICDs 113
  during lead implantation 228
  right ventricular outflow tract 126
  self-terminating 507
  slow 515, 516
  supraventricular tachycardia vs
    ICD electrograms 488–510
    misclassification 515–517
    redetection error 507–510
  VT storm 510–511
ventricular timing optimization (V-V
    optimization) 71–78

ventricular triggering period 265, 267,
    455, 468
ventricular veins 177, 178, 302
  anastomoses 184
  lead placement 187, 188, 582
ventriculoatrial conduction 44, 279,
    433–434
  1:1, ventricular tachycardia 517
ventriculoatrial interval (VA interval)
    257, 258
  DDD pacing 262
  extension 276–278
vibration sensors see piezoelectric
    crystals
vibrations from ICDs see alerts
virtual electrodes 19–21
vitreous carbon electrodes 139
voltage
  batteries 14, 439, 627–628, 632–633
  stimulus energy vs 4
voltage amplitude **326**
  minimization 151
  programming 333–339
voltage drop, within pulse 14–15
voltage gradient, ICDs 24–25
VOO (ventricular asynchronous pacing)
    257
VPS-1 (Vasovagal Pacemaker Study) 80
VR (time period) 256
V Rate > A Rate (Boston Scientific)
    387–388
VS-1A connectors 197
VS-1B connectors 197
VS-1 standard 141, 197
VT storm 510–511
vulnerable period 18–19, 20
VV (time period) 256
  resynchronization 304–307
  programming 424–425
VVI pacing (ventricular inhibited
    pacing) 45, 47, 48, 257, 258, 320,
    328
  clinical effects 56–57
  indications 134, **135**

VVIR pacing 134, **135**, 259–260, 261
  indications 408
VVT mode see single-chamber
    triggered-mode pacing

walking, assessment 419–420, 421,
  623–624
wandless systems, trans-telephonic
    monitoring 614
wands 15
warfarin
  device implantation and 203
  for thrombosis 234
waveform
  ECG 3f, 17
  ICDs 21–24
  programmable, ICDs 149
Wavelet, SVT-VT discriminators 376,
    378, 388
weakness **623**
wearable cardioverter-defibrillators,
    indications 113, 114
web-based monitoring 614, 634–637,
    638, **639**, **640**
websites
  product performance information
    431
  remote monitoring **640**
weight (body), remote monitoring 638
welding (arc welding) 607–608
Wenckebach block 94, 96, 534
  see also pseudo-Wenckebach behavior
wireless telemetry, web-based
    monitoring 636
wires, fracture see Accufix™ atrial J lead
withdrawal of therapy 646
work, return to 645
workplaces (industrial) 607–608
wrist bands, trans-telephonic
    monitoring 617

Zener diodes 15, 601
zone boundaries, rate detection 372,
    373